Nutrition & Diet Therapy: Evidence-Based Applications

FOURTH EDITION

Nutrition & Diet Therapy: Evidence-Based Applications

FOURTH EDITION

Carroll A. Lutz, MA, RN

Associate Professor Emerita
and Adjunct Professor
Jackson Community College
Jackson, Michigan

Karen Rutherford Przytulski, MS, RD

Clinical Dietitian
Sparrow Health System
Lansing, Michigan
and Clinical Dietitian
Heartland Home Care and Hospice
Mason, Michigan

F. A. DAVIS COMPANY / PUBLISHERS • PHILADELPHIA

F. A. Davis Company
1915 Arch Street
Philadelphia, PA 19103
www.fadavis.com

Printed in the United States of America

Last digit indicates print number: 10 9 8 7 6 5 4 3 2 1

Publisher, Nursing: Robert G. Martone
Developmental Editor: Arlene Chappelle
Art and Design Manager: Carolyn O'Brien

As new scientific information becomes available through basic and clinical research, recommended treatments and drug therapies undergo changes. The author(s) and publisher have done everything possible to make this book accurate, up to date, and in accord with accepted standards at the time of publication. The author(s), editors, and publisher are not responsible for errors or omissions or for consequences from application of the book, and make no warranty, expressed or implied, in regard to the contents of the book. Any practice described in this book should be applied by the reader in accordance with professional standards of care used in regard to the unique circumstances that may apply in each situation. The reader is advised always to check product information (package inserts) for changes and new information regarding dose and contraindications before administering any drug. Caution is especially urged when using new or infrequently ordered drugs or when admistering medications to children.

Library of Congress Cataloging-in-Publication Data

Lutz, Carroll A.
  Nutrition and diet therapy: evidence-based applications / Carroll A. Lutz, Karen Rutherford Przytulski. — ed. 4.
       p. ; cm.
  Includes bibliographical references and index.
  ISBN 0-8036-1336-9
  1. Dietetics. 2. Diet therapy. 3. Nutrition.
  [DNLM: 1. Diet Therapy. 2. Diet. 3. Nutrition. WB 400 L975n 2005]
I. Przytulski, Karen
  Rutherford. II. Title.
  RM217.L88 2005
  613.2—dc22   2005014731

DEDICATIONS

To Robert, my husband of 46 years.

Carroll A. Lutz

To Paul, my husband of 30 years.

Karen R. Przytulski

Preface

The fourth edition of *Nutrition and Diet Therapy* is designed to provide the beginning student with knowledge of the fundamentals of nutrition related to the promotion and maintenance of optimal health. Practical applications and treatment of pathologies with nutritional components are stressed. In addition, basic scientific information is introduced to enable students to begin to understand nutritional issues reported in the mass media. The sequential introduction of material continues to be a unique feature of this text. The authors resist the temptation to introduce concepts and examples of applications before the underlying basic science and vocabulary have been covered. The fourth edition has been extensively updated with new information. Of particular note is the evidence showing genetic differences in individuals' metabolism of nutrients. Such instances are woven into the relevant chapters and offer insight into the long history of contradictory reports concerning the effect of foods and nutrients on health outcomes.

This book was written to meet the educational needs of nursing students, dietetic assistants, diet technicians, and others. Support materials for the nursing student include case studies with examples of care plans and clinical analysis study questions. This edition continues to incorporate the standardized nursing terminology of NANDA, NOC, and NIC into each chapter's nursing care plans to show its usefulness in many different settings. Critical Thinking Questions follow the care plans and are designed to provoke imaginative thought and to foster discussion. Currently there exists an information explosion related to the science of nutrition. As researchers discover new and more effective treatments for nutrition-related disorders and health maintenance, the ability to think critically becomes increasingly important for professional growth and development. Students need not only to grasp the facts but also to apply the information in a clinical environment. This text has been developed to facilitate acquiring these skills.

The text can be used to teach a complete course in nutrition or as a desk reference for practitioners. The student using this book needs no previous exposure to anatomy, physiology, or medical terminology. Subjects are fully supported by diagrams, illustrations, figures, and tables. Depending upon the curriculum, chapters may be omitted or presented in a different sequence. We recognize that this text contains an immense amount of data and information. We hope this rich store of information permits instructors to adapt the text to the objectives of their courses while at the same time serving as a reference and directory for students satisfying their curiosities or completing solo or group projects whether in preclinical or in clinical courses.

The content of *Nutrition and Diet Therapy,* 4th ed. is organized into three units.

Unit One, **The Role of Nutrients in the Human Body,** covers basic information on nutrition as a science and how this information is applied through the nursing process. All the essential nutrients are covered, including definitions and descriptions of functions, effects of excesses and deficiencies, and food sources. The Dietary Reference Intakes, including the most recently released ones for electrolytes and water have been incorporated into this edition. Information on the use of food in the body and how the body maintains energy balance completes the unit.

Unit Two, **Family and Community Nutrition,** provides an overview of topics such as nutrition throughout the life cycle, food management, nutrient delivery via oral, enteral, and parenteral routes, and nutritional aspects of complementary therapy.

Unit Three, **Clinical Nutrition,** focuses on the care of clients with pathologies caused by or causing nutritional impairments. Pathological conditions include diabetes mellitus and hypoglycemia, cardiovascular disease, renal disease, gastrointestinal disease, cancer, and AIDS. Other pertinent topics include interactions among foods, nutrients, and drugs; weight control; nutrition during stress; and care of the client with a terminal illness.

Special features are used throughout the text to facilitate the teaching and learning process. All of the chapters include the following:

Boxes and Tables containing summaries, assessment tools, commonly prescribed diets, and research findings.

Illustrations that reinforce important points in the text or graph statistical data for clarity.

Study Aids Chapter Review Questions and Clinical Analysis Questions that are similar to those on the NCLEX examination. Answers to the Study Aids questions are printed in Appendix M.

Case Study with a proposed **Nursing Care Plan** Allows the student to see how the nutrition principles described in the chapter are applied in a specific clinical situation. The case studies were written to incorporate elements that are likely to recur in practice.

Clinical Applications Stimulate the interest of the

beginning student by showing how the information might be used in practice. Cover a variety of topics that emphasize application to clinical practice or current use in the health care professions.

Critical Thinking Questions Invite the student to think holistically with compassion and creativity. They can be used as a basis for class discussion.

Wellness Tips Emphasize nutrition's positive effect on maintaining or improving health.

Reference Lists Support the text with data sources and introduce the student to the scientific literature.

Additional features are used to clarify information:

Clinical Calculations Isolate and explain many of the mathematical calculations that are used in nutritional science.

Flowcharts of physiological and pathological processes Lead the student to an understanding of the relationship between nutrition and health.

Glossary Includes over 950 entries to aid in recalling and locating definitions of terms boldfaced in the text.

Appendix Serves as a ready source of information for students in class discussions or group assignments.

Accompanying the text for instructors who adopt it for their classes are:

Power Point Presentations More than 650 Power Point slides covering all the chapters of the book are a new offering for instructors who adopt the text. These presentations provide a ready source of material to select for classroom use.

Test Bank An electronic test bank contains over 1100 questions arranged by chapter. Some items have the new NCLEX formats: multiple response, ordered response, and fill-in-the-blank.

Electronic Updates As new information becomes available, updates will be posted on the F.A. Davis Web site accessible under the authors' names and this edition of Nutrition and Diet Therapy.

We believe that *Nutrition and Diet Therapy*, 4th ed. provides the clinical information necessary for a fuller understanding of the relationship between the knowledge about nutrition and diet and its clinical application. This text balances direct explanations of the underlying science with an introduction to the clinical responsibilities of the health care professional.

Acknowledgments

Writing a book, even a fourth edition, is a huge task, requiring the assistance of many people. Our colleagues contributed to this project, sometimes with information and critiques, sometimes just by being supportive. We would like to thank all the organizations and publishers that gave permission for the use of their materials. John and Judy Przytulski deserve special recognition for the many clerical tasks they completed and the new computer skills they taught us. The staff at the Jackson Community College Learning Resource Center, especially Marion VanLoo, obtained literature from distant sources through interlibrary loans. Martin Frigg, PhD, from Sight and Life supplied long distance consultation on vitamin A from Switzerland. Kent Clark, CNSD, RD, provided valuable input for Chapter 24, Nutrition During Stress. Our editorial and production staff at F.A. Davis Company, including Bob Martone, Kristin Kern, Shirley Kuhn, Carolyn O'Brien, Danielle Barsky, Frank Musick, and Steve Latrelle, shared their knowledge and expertise in all phases of our joint project. Our Developmental Editor, Arlene Chappelle, Copy Editor, Amy Peterson, and Project Manager, Donna Hibbs, served admirably, picking up the pieces dropped along our paths. To all of them go our heartfelt thanks.

Contents

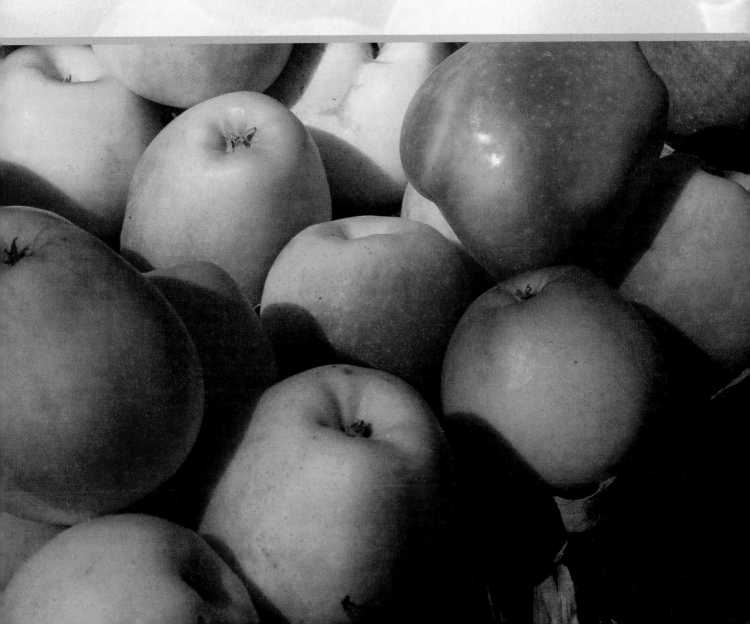

The Role of Nutrients in the Human Body

CHAPTER 1

Evolution and the Science of Nutrition

After completing this chapter, the student should be able to:

1. Discuss the relationship between the biologic evolution of the human body and present-day nutritional concerns.
2. State the three functions of nutrients.
3. Identify the six classes of nutrients.
4. Discuss the effects of malnutrition on health and provide examples.
5. Describe the relationship between nutrition and health.

Food and health have always been connected. In this chapter, we compare food habits and their effect on the health of our ancestors with those of present-day people. The chapter highlights past and present views about health and health care and discusses the effect of these views on the role of health-care professionals. It also examines the science of nutrition and introduces some basic terminology.

Evolution of the Human Body and Emergence of Health Issues

Throughout history our ancestors survived on a variety of diets. What prehistoric humans (prehistoric refers to the period in time before humans were able to write) ate in any particular geographic area depended in large part on the climate in which they lived, their hunting and gathering skills, their food-processing technology, and available foods. Clues from pictures painted on cave walls and artifacts suggest that the earliest humans were hunter-gatherers: people who ate wild game and any plants, fish, seeds, and honey they could find (Fig. 1–1). Stone tools excavated from sites suggest that the use of tools accompanied a big increase in meat consumption. Fossil remains showing jaw size and shape and tooth size, shape, and

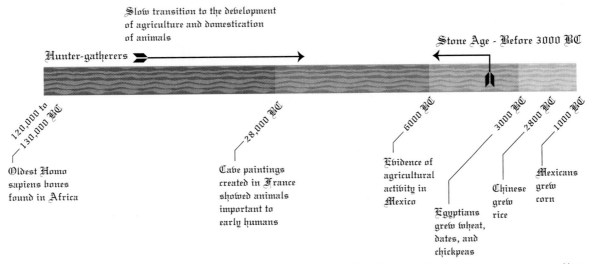

Figure 1–1 Timeline from the discovery of the oldest Homo Sapiens to 120000 BC, when Mexican farmers grew corn. Humans evolved slowly and adapted to a wide vareiety of foodstuffs.

wear patterns suggest our ancestors had large variability in their diets (Cullen, 2003).

The human body evolved the capability to subsist on a wide variety of foodstuffs of both plant and animal origin. The traditional diet of Eskimos, for example, consists of mostly fish, whereas some other groups subsist mostly on grains. Humans' ability to adapt makes it possible for them to survive for long periods on inferior diets.

Effect of Agriculture

Early Mexican farmers began to grow crops about 8000 years ago. Evidence suggests that they started growing corn about 3000 years ago. The Egyptians grew wheat, dates, and chickpeas more than 5000 years ago. Remnants of cooked bread found in a 5000-year-old man discovered a decade ago suggest the beginnings of agriculture. About 4800 years ago, the Chinese began to grow rice.

The emergence of agriculture led to population expansion. Individuals learned to work together to grow crops and began to live together in larger groups to protect their cultivated fields and harvested food stores. The formation of such communities led to the development of villages and towns. Food distribution systems for the rationing of the harvest from one growing season to the next evolved to help ensure an adequate food supply in the event of a poor harvest or natural disaster.

Agriculture, however, especially single-crop agriculture, limited the variety of foods available to a given community. Today we understand that growth deficiencies can result from a diet based on single-crop agriculture; no single food can furnish all the raw materials necessary for optimal human growth and health maintenance. Variety, moderation, and balance in the diet are all necessary for health (Wellness Tip 1–1).

  1–1 • Variety, moderation, and balance promote good health.

Adaptation to Feast and Famine

Seasonal and cyclical variations in food availability affected our ancestors. An example of a **seasonal variation** is an abundance of food during summer and fall compared with a scarcity of food late in winter. A **cyclical variation** is a recurring series of events such as a period of drought and famine followed by a period of plentiful rainfall.

Biologically, the human body adapted to such feast-or-famine conditions by developing the capacity to store energy as fat. This adaptation enabled humans to survive famine, but it did not ensure optimal nourishment. The situation is much the same today. Famine still exists in many countries in the world, and even in developed countries some population groups—notably, poor, very young, pregnant, and elderly people—suffer from malnutrition. For other population groups—those with unlimited access to food—the human body's capacity to store fat in unlimited amounts has lead to an epidemic of chronic disease related to overnutrition.

Food Safety Issues

Many people like to imagine the so-called natural man or woman who lived a healthy, happy life on unprocessed foods. Although the food our ancestors ate may have been free of pesticides and additives, it was not always safe. Meat, for example, could turn **rancid** and harbor parasites; fungal infestations could contaminate both stored grain and grain in the fields; and heavy metals (such as lead) leached out of utensils into food, often with fatal effects.

Our Ancestors' View of Health

In the past, it was commonly held that health was subject to supernatural laws. For example, the recurrent epidemics of bubonic plague that swept Europe in the Middle Ages (between 1340 and 1660 AD) were thought to result from witchcraft and the work of the devil. The discovery of bacteria in the late 1880s and the subsequent development of antibiotics in the 1940s rendered many diseases treatable.

Until recent decades, health care focused mainly on curing disease. Slowly, in part because of scientific progress, the impetus behind health-care delivery has shifted to disease prevention. The use of vaccines is one form of prevention. The consumption of certain food substances that can help prevent certain diseases and enhance recovery from disease is another.

Current Attitudes Towards Health and Health Care

Today many diseases are known to be linked to lifestyle behaviors such as smoking, lack of adequate physical activity, and poor nutritional habits. The World Health Organization (WHO) reports that nearly one-third of early death and disability stems from nutritional or dietary causes, including too little food in the poorest countries and too much food (or the wrong kind) in the richest (WHO, 2002). WHO predicts that in Canada and the United States, healthy life expectancy can increase by 6.5 years by changing negative lifestyle behaviors. Health-care providers emphasize the relationship between lifestyle and the risk of disease. Many people, at least in industrialized countries, are increasingly managing their health problems and making personal commitments to lead healthier lives.

Nutrition is, in part, a preventive science. Given sufficient resources, how and what one eats is a lifestyle choice. **Health** is defined as a state of complete physical, mental, and social well-being and not just the absence of disease or infirmity.

The ability to detect disease early using highly sophisticated technology is another major focus of the health-care system. Early disease detection not only reduces suffering and mortality but also enables people to alter the behaviors, including food habits, that affect disease progression. A new area of research called nutritional genomics identifies individuals through genetic testing who are predisposed to specific diseases. People who know what health problems they are likely to acquire may be willing to modify their diets to maximize their health. The greatest potential for benefit from dietary modification is likely to be in health maintenance, blocking or slowing the early signs of disease development (Elliott and Ong, 2002). Early identification of disease frequently results in a cost saving to individuals. Although educating and screening clients for disease is expensive for society as a whole, society has increasingly come to realize that it is less costly than treating disease. For this reason, all health-care providers should take advantage of each encounter with clients to educate them.

The Changing Role of Health-Care Professionals

Changing attitudes about health have altered the role of health-care professionals. No longer are clients totally reliant on physicians; their care is now in the hands of a multidisciplinary team.

Clients are the focus of the health-care team. It is a fact that clients who participate in their own care are more likely to achieve the set goals or objectives. Clients are more likely to change negative behaviors if they believe the benefits of therapy are worth the consequences, express or show a readiness to change, have adequate memory skills, express confidence, and are literate. When a patient is aware and accepts his or her medical con-dition, requests and accepts information, and can describe how learning is best achieved (written instructions, verbal instructions, demonstration, etc), a readiness to change becomes apparent. Family members, caregivers, or desig-nated guardians who care for clients unable to care for themselves need to be involved with the health-care team.

An institutionalized client's health-care team may include more than 15 members. The respective titles and responsibilities of the major members of the health-care team are outlined in the following sections.

Registered Nurses

Registered nurses (RNs) are responsible for clients' daily health care, including their nutritional care. RNs communi-cate with physicians and dietitians regarding clients' response to food, including intake and tolerance. They also provide nutrition education, if needed, and record infor-mation on clients' charts. Box 1–1 discusses in more detail nursing roles pertinent to nutrition.

Box 1–1 **Nursing Roles Pertinent to Nutrition**

Nurses classify their functions by role. Although we divide them here for purposes of discussion, the roles often all come into play in a single client interaction.

Care Provider

Nurses monitor clients' food intake and report and record deficits. Nurses coordinate clients' diagnostic tests and promote compensatory food and fluid intake when tests are completed. Nurses prepare clients and their surroundings for meals, prepare food served for self-feeding, and feed clients who are unable to feed themselves.

Teacher

Nurses provide information and coach clients in required skills to maximize nutritional care. To accomplish this end, the nurse needs to assess client's readiness to learn, cultural issues, motor skills, and availability of care-giver support. Nurses tailor the educational materials used to clients' reading levels. A general rule for health education is that printed materials should be written at a maximum of the eighth-grade reading level. Pilot testing material on intended audience will reveal weaknesses.

The desired outcome of health education is behav-ior, not increased knowledge. A prerequisite to making a behavior change, however, is the knowledge necessary to make the change. An objective measure to evaluate if a change in behavior has occurred is helpful. For exam-ple, body weight can be used to evaluate instruction. Multiple teaching sessions are preferable to a single lesson.

Counselor

Nurses assist clients in making decisions affecting their health. A counselor focuses on attitudes, feelings, and behaviors to encourage the client in achieving self-control. The nurse needs to ensure that clients receive a diet that they are willing to follow and that is adapted to their home situation. Studies have shown that facilita-tion skills of customizing, adapting, and including the client in decision making exert the strongest force on client satisfaction and intention to comply with dietary counseling (Trudeau and Dube, 1995). An imperfect diet that is followed is preferable to a perfectly designed one that is ignored. The role of counselor contrasts with that of teacher who helps the client to acquire new knowl-edge and skill.

Client Advocate

Nurses act to protect and support the client's rights. Nurses impart necessary information so that individuals may make informed decisions. Basic to these rights is the client's right to be informed of treatment options, risk, and expected outcomes.

Health Team Member

Modern health care requires the cooperation of many individuals of varied professions. On the team's side, communication skills, the quality of information and instructions, and a willingness to identify and address barriers influence patient compliance (White, 2002). **Compliance** is the extent to which a patient's behavior coincides with medical advice. Nutrition instruction can be provided by anyone on the health-care team, including physicians, nurses, pharmacists, and dietitians. Sometimes the nurse may have the knowledge, interest, and time to provide nutrition instruction. When the nurse is unable to teach the client, it is important to refer the client to another team member. The member of the team with the most education and training on the nutri-tional care of clients is the registered dietitian. Most clients are referred to this team member as needed. Nurses are often responsible for coordinating the care among members of the multidisciplinary team.

Licensed Practical Nurses/ Licensed Vocational Nurses

Licensed practical nurses (LPNs) and licensed vocational nurses (LVNs), supervised by RNs, feed clients, monitor food consumption, measure intake and output, and record data.

Clinical Pharmacists

Pharmacists (RPhs) prepare, preserve, and compound medicines and dispense them according to the prescriptions of physicians. They counsel clients about food-drug and drug-drug interactions and function as valuable resources for all team members.

Physicians

Physicians are responsible for the diagnosis and treatment of medical conditions. They manage medical care, order laboratory tests, prescribe medications and diet, and explain treatment plans to clients.

Registered Dietitians

Registered dietitians (RDs), together with physicians, have the responsibility to meet clients' nutritional needs. This responsibility includes interpreting the physician's diet order in terms of clients' food habits and food choices, calculating clients' nutritional requirements, evaluating clients' response to therapeutic diets, and providing nutrition education and counseling for clients. The registered dietitian is usually the team member with the most education and training in the nutritional sciences.

Dietetic Technicians

Dietetic technicians (DTs) assist dietitians by taking nutrition histories and body measurements, reviewing records, and monitoring clients' food intake.

Other Health-Care Personnel

Other health-care personnel who may be involved in client care include licensed social workers, medical technologists, nurse practitioners, and physical and occupational therapists.

Nutrition Is a Science

Stated simply, **nutrition** is the science that studies the relationship of humans to food. The discussion of nutrition in this text involves the following topics:

- The chemical content of food
- The body's use of food
- The relationship of food to health
- Selection of food
- Techniques to modify food habits
- Diet as treatment for disease
- The relationship between medications and food intake

As this list suggests, the science of nutrition encompasses ideas from many other sciences: biology, chemistry, economics, educational theory, nursing, medicine, pharmacology, physiology, psychology, and sociology. This connection with other disciplines suggests the far-reaching implications of good nutrition.

Nutrients

The science of nutrition historically has been based on the nutrients found in food. **Nutrients** are the chemical substances supplied by food that the body needs for growth, maintenance, and repair. Nutrients can be divided into six groups:

1. Carbohydrates (often abbreviated as CHO)
2. Fats (lipids)
3. Proteins
4. Minerals
5. Vitamins
6. Water

Each group is discussed in a separate chapter.

Nutrients are considered either **essential** or **nonessential,** depending on whether the body can or cannot manufacture them. When the body requires a nutrient for growth or maintenance but lacks the ability to manufacture it in amounts sufficient to meet bodily needs, this essential nutrient must be supplied by foods in the diet. Vitamin C, vitamin A, and calcium are 3 of the more than 40 essential nutrients. Nutrients not needed in the diet because the body can make them are called nonessential. For example, the amino acid alanine is a nonessential nutrient because the body can manufacture it from other raw materials.

Functions of Nutrients

All nutrients perform one or more of the following functions:

1. Serve as a source of energy or heat
2. Support the growth and maintenance of tissue
3. Aid in the regulation of basic body processes

These three life-sustaining functions collectively are part of **metabolism,** the sum of all physical and chemical changes that take place in the body. Nutrients have specific metabolic functions and interact with one another to maintain the body.

Source of Energy

Energy is defined in the physical sciences as the capacity to do work. Energy exists in a variety of forms: electric, thermal (heat), chemical, mechanical, and others.

All food enters the body as chemical energy. The body processes the chemical energy of food and converts it into other energy forms. Chemical energy is transformed into electric signals in nerves, for example, and mechanical energy in muscles.

Carbohydrates, fats, and proteins, the nutrients that supply energy, are referred to as the **energy nutrients.** The energy both in foods and in the body is measured in kilocalories, abbreviated kcal (see Glossary). Because energy cannot be seen, heard, or felt, it is one of the most difficult biological concepts to understand. For this reason, it warrants an entire chapter of its own in this book (see Chapter 6).

Growth and Maintenance of Tissues

Some nutrients provide the raw materials for building the body structures and participate in the continued growth and maintenance of necessary tissues. Water, proteins, fats, and minerals are the nutrient classes that contribute in a major way to building body structures.

Regulation of Body Processes

Some nutrients control or regulate chemical processes in the body. For example, certain minerals and proteins help regulate how water is distributed in the body. Vitamins are necessary in the series of reactions involved in generating energy. Vitamins themselves are not energy sources, but if the body lacks a particular vitamin, it will not produce energy efficiently.

Malnutrition

Ingesting too much or too little of a nutrient can interfere with health and well-being. There is a beneficial range of intake for any nutrient; an intake below or above that range is incompatible with optimal health. Thus, **malnutrition** (poor nutrition) occurs when body cells receive too much or too little of one or more nutrients. For example, a single-food diet, such as a grapefruit diet to lose weight, will result in malnutrition if followed for an extended period.

Undernutrition

Malnutrition includes **undernutrition,** the result of a deficiency of one or more nutrients. Undernutrition may be related to:

- An individual's inability to obtain safe foods that contain the essential nutrients
- An individual's failure to consume essential nutrients
- The body's inability to use the nutrients in food
- Disease conditions that increase the body's need for nutrients
- A disease process that causes nutrients to be excreted too rapidly from the body

Undernutrition occurs in many different circumstances. For example, stress from trauma, surgery, or a burn frequently produces a state of undernutrition. People exposed to such severe and prolonged stressors may be undernourished even if they consume an apparently normal diet. Prolonged physical stress causes the body to break down internal protein stores, and protein is excreted as a result.

Although undernutrition is not widespread in the United States, it does exist as a result of poverty, illness, neglect, poor dietary planning, or environmental hazards. It can occur as well in institutional settings if caregivers fail to provide adequate nourishment, monitor clients' food intake, and make sure they have help eating. Groups especially vulnerable to undernutrition are children, pregnant women, and elderly people. Malnourished children grow at a slower rate than adequately nourished ones, and they are prone to infections and more likely to have mental and developmental problems.

Overnutrition

Overnutrition, which is an excessive intake of nutrients, is another form of malnutrition. Overnutrition often results from the use of self-prescribed over-the-counter vitamin and mineral supplements. For example, when ingested in very high doses once or habitually, preformed vitamin A can cause headache, vomiting, bone abnormalities, and liver damage. Vitamin D toxicity can lead to the deposit of calcium in soft tissues and irreversible kidney and cardiovascular damage. Overnutrition is associated also with eating too much food and hence having an excessive intake of many nutrients rather than of a single one.

Phytochemicals and Zoochemicals

The philosophy that food can be health promoting beyond its traditional value as a source of nutrients is gaining acceptance among scientists and health professionals (American Dietetic Association, 1999). Knowledge of physiologically active food ingredients in plant sources (**phytochemicals**) and animal sources (**zoochemicals**) has expanded our understanding of the role of diet in health. Foods that contain phytochemicals and zoochemicals are called **functional foods.**

Substances in animal products that have been associated with reduced risk of disease have been identified. For example, fermented dairy products, such as yogurt, that contain probiotics have been shown to improve gastrointestinal health. **Probiotics** are bacteria found in food that reduce the duration of acute diarrhea in children (Wanke, 2002). The positive attributes of yogurt are most pronounced during the course of treatment with antibiotics. The prefix *phyto-* comes from the Greek word for *plant*. Phytochemicals are nonnutrient food components (food chemicals) that provide medical or health benefits, including the prevention or treatment of a disease (Table 1–1).

Table 1–1 Selected Functional Foods, Phytochemicals, and Reported Health Benefits

FUNCTIONAL FOODS	PHYTOCHEMICAL(S) IDENTIFIED	REPORTED HEALTH BENEFIT
Tomatoes, grapefruit	Lycopene	Reduce risk for prostate cancer Reduce risk for heart attack
Garlic, onions, chives	Allyl sulfides	Reduce risk for stomach and colon cancer Reduce risk for heart disease
Soy products, legumes, peanuts	Isoflavones: genistein, diadzein	Reduce risk for breast, prostate, and endometrial cancer Reduce risk for heart disease Reduce risk for osteoporosis May assist in the treatment of menopausal symptoms

(Continued on the following page)

Table **1–1**   **Selected Functional Foods, Phytochemicals, and Reported Health Benefits** *(Continued)*

FUNCTIONAL FOODS	PHYTOCHEMICAL(S) IDENTIFIED	REPORTED HEALTH BENEFIT
Whole flaxseed	Lignans, phytoestrogens	Increase laxation (increased frequency and bulk of feces) May protect against heart disease, cardiac arrhythmia, and stroke Reduce risk for hormone-sensitive cancers Favorably affects the immune system by reducing inflammation May prevent retinopathy in premature infants
Green tea	Polyphenols	Reduce risk for gastric, esophageal, and skin cancers Reduce risk for heart disease
Broccoli, cabbage, Brussels sprouts, cauliflower, kohlrabi, watercress, turnips	Sulforaphanes, indoles, isothiocyanates	May reduce risk of breast, stomach, and lung cancers May protect the retina from light-induced oxidative damage May be responsible for reversing eye damage or macular degeneration in very early stages
Fruits, vegetables, nuts, tea, wine, oregano	Flavonoids	May reduce cancer risk; acts as an **antioxidant**

Large studies that examined the dietary patterns among different cultures have revealed the first clues about fruits', vegetables', and whole grains' protective role against heart disease and cancer.

Research techniques have allowed scientists to study the functions of such plant constituents in the laboratory as well as in animals and humans. Phytochemicals seem to be able to stop a cell's conversion from healthy to cancerous at many different stages of cell division and growth. Phytochemicals also may decrease risk for chronic diseases, such as cardiovascular disease, cancer, and diabetes. It is not known whether each of the more than 400 phytochemicals produces its reported health benefits by functioning alone or in combination with others. Most experts advise eating a wide variety of fruits, whole grains, and vegetables (Fig. 1–2) and not narrowing intake to particular foods.

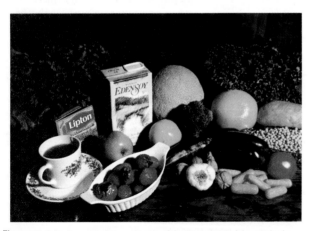

Figure **1–2** Eating a wide variety of fruits, vegetables, whole grains, tea, soy, and flaxseed is an excellent way to obtain a natural supply of phytochemicals.

Nutrition and Health

Good nutrition is essential for good health and important for physical growth and development, good body composition, and mental development. People's nutritional state can protect them from or predispose them toward chronic disease. Medical treatment for many diseases includes diet therapy. Nutrition is thus both a preventive and a therapeutic science.

Physical Growth and Development

Although heredity determines much of individual growth patterns and genetic potential, malnutrition can delay or prevent individuals from achieving that potential. Without enough calcium, phosphorus, and protein, for example, bones cannot grow properly. Children who are malnourished may never reach their genetic potential for height.

Slowed growth is one of the first clinically measurable indicators of inadequate dietary intake in children. For this reason, health-care providers measure an infant's height and weight and record them on growth charts on each visit. Examples of growth charts for the height and weight of infants and children are in Appendix D.

Body Composition

Nutrient intake can affect body composition, which in turn can affect health. The human body is composed of four main types of substances (water, fat, ash, and protein) and one minor substance (carbohydrate) (Fig. 1–3). One-half to three-quarters of the body is made up of water. A normally active woman has a body fat content between 18 and 22 percent. A normally active man has a body fat content between 15 and 19 percent. Body **ash,** which accounts for approximately 6 percent of body weight, is the body's mineral content. It includes, for example, the calcium and phosphorus that are constituents of the human skeleton.

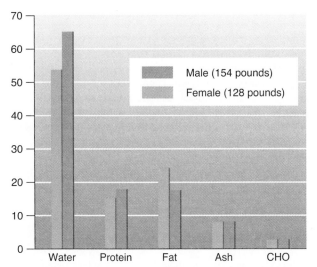

Figure **1–3** Approximate body composition of a typical 25-year-old man (154 lb) and woman (128 lb). Note that the typical woman has a higher percentage of body fat than does the typical man. The man has a higher percentage of lean body mass. The percentage of ash content is equal in both sexes. The human body has minimal carbohydrate content.

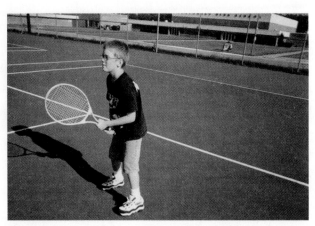

Figure **1–4** A young man developing muscle tissue while enjoying a sport.

Approximately 15 percent of the body's weight is protein; the male body contains more protein than the female body. With age, body composition typically becomes higher in fat and lower in protein. Protein is stored primarily in muscle tissue, organs, and certain body chemicals. When the body loses protein, it is losing muscle tissue, organ mass, the protein stored in body substances, or combinations thereof. Preservation of body protein is necessary for optimal health. A loss of structural body content (heart muscle, kidney, liver, or blood proteins) is undesirable and leads to illness.

A person's body fat and protein content can be modified by food intake, exercise, or both. Exercise increases body protein content by increasing muscle content (Fig. 1–4). Eating too much food (ingesting more calories than the body expends) increases the fat content of the body because fat is stored for future use.

Mental Development

Research continues on the relationship between undernutrition and brain development in the child. It has been found that undernourished babies have smaller and fewer brain cells, but the relationship between intelligence and the size and number of brain cells is not clear. There is some evidence that the mental development of infants younger than 6 months of age is particularly vulnerable to the effects of malnutrition. Some nutritional deficiencies may cause permanent impairment of the central nervous system (CNS) in young infants.

Some conditions that affect the CNS may be reversible through diet. Nutrition plays an important role, for example, in the prevention and management of some forms of dementia. **Dementia** is an impairment of intellectual function that is usually progressive and interferes with normal social and occupational activities (impairment refers to any condition that causes a person to deteriorate; **progressive** means it becomes more severe or spreads to other parts). Excessive alcohol intake or nutritional deficiencies may result in dementia. Correcting the deficiency or eliminating alcohol from the diet may improve intellectual function. Not all forms of dementia are directly related to poor nutrition.

Diet has been found to enhance mental function even short term. In one study, children who consumed less than half of the energy recommended for breakfast has significantly poorer attendance, punctuality and grades at school than children who ate more for breakfast. The poor eaters also had more behavioral problems. After getting breakfast at school, the poor eaters attendance, math grades, and behavior improved (Kleinman, et al, 2002). Another study showed that elderly people also have better memory and task performance after consumption of carbohydrates (Korol, 2002). It seems starvation impedes concentration.

Diet as Therapy

A **modified diet** is often an important component of a client's total health care. A modified diet is one that has been altered to include more or fewer nutrients, to effect a change in the texture or consistency of what is ingested, or to restrict the intake of any substance. For example, diet is an important part of the treatment for clients with a metabolic disease such as diabetes. Special dietary measures are often required to maintain the lives of patients who have chronic heart, kidney, liver, and gastrointestinal diseases. These diets must also take into consideration the effects of medications on nutrients. Adjustments in diet are also necessary in other situations, such as after highly stressful or traumatic events, including severe burns, broken bones, and surgery.

Although deficiency of a single nutrient is rare, it is seen in some clients. In such cases, adding foods to the diet that contain the missing nutrient is often sufficient to solve the problem. The last section of this book describes various diets for specific clinical situations.

SUMMARY

Nutrition is the science of food and its relation to people. The human body evolved by adapting to a wide variety of diets. Although survival is possible on an inferior diet, optimal health is not. Health is a state of complete physical, mental, and social well-being, not just the absence of disease or infirmity. Nutrition is vital to optimal health. The principles of nutrition are applied by the health-care team to promote health and treat many diseases. The science of nutrition is based on chemical constituents of foods called nutrients, which function to provide fuel, support tissue growth and maintenance, and regulate body processes. A nutrient is called essential if the body requires it and cannot manufacture it in sufficient amounts to meet bodily needs. A balanced nutrient intake is vital for physical growth and development, optimal body composition, mental development, and disease prevention.

>>> CHAPTER REVIEW

1. Women's bodies normally contain more _____ and less _____ than men's bodies.
   a. Carbohydrate, protein
   b. Fat, protein
   c. Protein, ash
   d. Water, fat

2. The human body has adapted to feast-or-famine conditions by developing the capacity to store:
   a. Fluid
   b. Carbohydrate
   c. Fat
   d. Protein

3. Which of the following is not one of the traditional groups of nutrients?
   a. Zoochemicals
   b. Vitamins
   c. Minerals
   d. Proteins

4. An example of an energy nutrient is:
   a. Water
   b. Fat
   c. Vitamins
   d. Minerals

5. Malnutrition always occurs as a result or part of:
   a. The aging process
   b. A low income
   c. Infirmity
   d. Overnutrition

✚ CLINICAL ANALYSIS

1. Mrs. A believes she can cleanse her body of toxic compounds by abstaining from all food for 10 days. You should:
   a. Tell Mrs. A she needs to drink extra fluids for this approach to succeed.
   b. Ignore Mrs. A because you think she will not listen to you.
   c. Pretend to agree with Mrs. A. because you do not want to make her angry.
   d. Explain to Mrs. A the importance of variety, balance, and moderation in the diet.

2. Mr. and Mrs. J are members of a local fitness club and have recently had their body fat content analyzed. Mr. J expresses concern because his wife's body fat content (20%) is higher than his body fat content (15%). He asks, "Why is there a difference?" An appropriate response would be:
   a. A normally active woman has a body fat content between 18 and 22 percent.
   b. A normally active woman has a body fat content between 15 and 19 percent, so his wife should exercise more.
   c. A person's body fat content is not that important.
   d. If his wife would increase her protein intake, her body fat content would decrease.

3. Billie is an 18-month-old boy who weighs 25 lb and is 32 1/2 inches long. His mother asks you to evaluate his growth. (Hint: Use the growth chart in Appendix D for boys, birth to 36 months.) You should tell her:
   a. Billie weighs too much for his height.
   b. Billie weighs too little for his height.
   c. Billie is in the 90th percentile.
   d. Billie is in the 50th percentile, or about average.

REFERENCES

American Dietetic Association: Functional foods—position of the American Dietetic Association. J Am Diet Assoc 99:1278, 1999.

American Dietetic Association: Tracking Trends. J Am Diet Assoc, Chicago, 2002, p. 2.1 supp l.

Cullen, B: Testimony from the iceman. Smithsonian February: 42, 2003.

Elliott, R and Ong, TJ: Nutritional genomics. BMJ 3245:1438, 2002.

Fernandez-Armesto, F: Near a Thousand Tables: A History of Food. Free Press, New York, 2002.

Kleinman, RE, et al: Diet, breakfast, and academic performance in children. Ann Nutr Metab 46(supp l):24, 2002.

Kaplan, RJ, et al: Cognitive performance is associated with glucose regulation in healthy elderly persons and can be enhanced with glucose and dietary carbohydrates. Am J Clin Nutr 72:825, 2000.

Korol, DL: Enhancing cognitive function across the life span. Ann N Y Acad Sci 959:167, 2002.

Lampe, JW: Health effects of vegetables and fruits: assessing mechanisms of action in human experimental studies. Am J Clin Nutr 70:4755, 1999.

Lichtenstein, PL, et al: Environmental and heritable factors in the causation of cancer: Analyses of cohorts of twins from Sweden, Denmark, and Finland. N Engl J Med 343:78, 2000.

Mukamal, KJ, et al: Tea consumption and mortality after acute myocardial infarction. Circulation 105:2476, 2002.

Panel on Macronutrients, Panel on the Definition of Dietary Fiber, Subcommittee on Upper Reference Levels of Nutrients, Subcommittee on Upper Reference Levels of Nutrients, Subcommittee on Interpretation and Uses of Dietary Reference Intakes, and the Standing Committee on the Scientific Evaluation Dietary Reference Intakes for Energy, Carbohydrate, Fiber, Fat, Fatty Acids, Cholesterol, Protein, and Amino Acids. National Academy Press, Washington, DC, 2002.

Pollitt, E, Cueto, S, and Jacoby, ER: Fasting and cognition in well- and undernourished school children: A review of three experimental studies. Am J Clin Nutr 67:779S, 1998.

Shell, ER: The Hungry Gene. Atlantic Monthly Press, New York, 2002, p 85.

Szajewska, H, Mrukowicz, JZ: Probiotics in the treatment and prevention of acute infectious diarrhea in infants and children: A systematic review of published randomized double blind, placebo-controlled trials. J Pediatr Gastrenterol Nutr 33 (suppl):517, 2001.

Teaford, MF and Ungar, PS: Diet and evolution of the earliest human ancestors. Proc Natl Acad Sci USA 97:13506, 2000.

Trudeau, E, and Dube, L: Moderators and determinants of satisfaction with diet counseling for patients consuming a therapeutic diet. J. Am Diete Assoc 95:34,1995.

U.S. Department of Agriculture and U.S. Department of Health and Human Services. Nutrition and Your Health: Dietary Guidelines for Americans, ed 5. Washington, DC, U.S. Department of Health and Human Services, 2000, Home and Garden Bulletin No. 232.

Wanke, CA: Do probiotics prevent childhood illness? BMJ 322:1318, 2001.

White, JR, et al: Clarifying the role of insulin in type 2 diabetes management. Clin Diabetes 21:1, 2003.

WHO (World Health Organization): World Health Report 2002: Reducing Risks, Promoting Healthy Life. Geneva, Switzerland, World Health Organization, 2002.

USDA: The Interactive Healthy Eating Index. www.forcevbc.com/good/food.htm

Individualizing Client Care

After completing this chapter, the student should be able to:

1. Define the terminology used in the nursing process and in nutrition assessment.
2. Describe methods of nutrition assessment.
3. Demonstrate the use of three techniques to analyze dietary status.
4. Describe the dietary exchange system and identify the exchange lists of foods.
5. Identify components of the health belief systems of large cultural groups that affect their nutrition.
6. Explain the components of various religious customs that affect individual food intake.
7. Discuss strategies to provide culturally competent nutritional care.

This chapter introduces the steps of the nursing process as they apply to nutrition, as well as the terminology and methodology used for measuring and evaluating nutritional status. Because cultural traditions influence the way people regard certain foods and the effects of those foods on health, the last section of this chapter covers culturally competent care.

The **nursing process,** a systematic method of planning, delivering, evaluating, and documenting care, is used by nurses in different cultures (Thoroddsen and Thorsteinsson, 2002). The nursing process, summarized in Box 2–1, also serves as part of the organizing framework of the licensing examinations for registered nurses and licensed practical/vocational nurses.

Fictional case studies throughout this book integrate the steps of the nursing process: **assessment** or data collection, **analysis** yielding a **nursing diagnosis, planning** for desired outcomes, **implementation** of nursing actions, and **evaluation.**

Terminology

Nurses and dietitians have defined the terminology used in the practice of their professions. Knowledge of this termi-nology will help students understand the clinical examples in the following chapters.

Standardized Nursing Languages

Computerized information systems hold great potential for collecting and analyzing data pertaining to health care. For the system to work, however, the data must be in an appropriate form. Words must have standardized meanings regardless of the health-care setting. The integrated language selected for use in this text is NANDA-NOC-NIC, described in Table 2–1. Several nursing languages have been developed throughout the world, some for specialty practices and some that integrate NANDA-NOC-NIC into the database. Institutions have expanded upon these nursing languages to incorporate other health-care providers' documentation in an electronic patient record.

NANDA, Formerly the North American Nursing Diagnosis Association

Since 1982, the **North American Nursing Diagnosis Association (NANDA)** has worked to define and clarify the client problems nurses are licensed to treat. This work is proceeding on an international level and encompasses all of nursing, not just client problems related to nutrition. The nursing diagnoses have been arranged in patterns and assigned code numbers within the patterns. The codes permit computerization of client records, comparison of client outcomes, and validation of nursing's contribution to health care.

Nursing Outcomes Classification

In 2004, the third edition of Nursing Outcomes Classification (NOC) was published. It includes nursing-sensitive outcomes with definitions, indicators, and measurement scales (Moorhead, Johnson, and Maas, 2004). The scales are being tested for validity and reliability and hold promise to measure progress toward a goal rather than determining only whether or not a goal has been achieved. Even though many disciplines contribute to health-care outcomes, nursing care is a major component to the outcomes

---

| Box 2–1 | Steps in the Nursing Process |

Assessment

Assessment, or data collection, is an organized procedure to gather facts necessary to help the client. A physical examination of the client follows the taking of his or her history. The two types of data pertinent to the nursing process are subjective data and objective data.

The **symptoms** the client recounts are **subjective data** and not verifiable by another. **Objective data** can be observed and verified by someone other than the client. These data are called **signs,** obtainable by physical examination or through laboratory tests and diagnostic studies.

Analysis

Analysis of the data involves comparing it against standards to identify problem areas. The assessment findings are shared with the client (and family or caregiver as appropriate), and the problem is defined using input from the client or his or her representative.

In many areas of health maintenance, the client's active participation is essential. Often clients must learn about their diseases and treatments. If clients do not participate in the nursing diagnostic process and their priorities are not respected, they may not cooperate with treatment plans. When the treatment plan includes diet change, the client elects to follow it or not several times a day. The analysis of the client's subjective and objective data leads to a nursing diagnosis, a statement of a client's nursing problem that the nurse is licensed to treat.

Planning

Planning the care appropriate for the client's nursing problems encompasses two parts: a desired outcome or goal and the actions necessary to achieve it. The **desired outcome** describes a successful resolution to (or a significant improvement in) the nursing problem. To facilitate later evaluation of the nursing process, desired outcomes are most useful when they are client-centered, realistic, and measurable and contain a desired deadline for completion.

Implementation

Implementation of the plan of care includes directions for the health-care providers to produce a unified effort on behalf of the client. These nursing actions or interventions should be clear and specific so that a new person assigned to care for a client can proceed without hesitation. A correct **nursing action** is one that is likely to produce the desired outcome. The reason for selection of a nursing action to produce a certain outcome is called a **rationale.** The nursing care plans in this text contain statements of rationale to demonstrate the logical connection between desired outcomes and nursing actions.

Evaluation

Evaluation is the process of comparing the client's status after the nursing implementation has been completed with the stated desired outcome. The nurse and client judge whether the problem has been resolved. If it has not, the nursing process is again set in motion, beginning with an assessment.

---

included in NOC. The outcomes and definitions are to be used as written. The selection of outcomes depends on the nurse's clinical judgment. The outcomes are not designed to be used as goals, but an individual indicator at a specified level of attainment may serve as a goal. Linkages to nursing diagnoses by NANDA are suggested.

Nursing Interventions Classification

In 2004, the fourth edition of Nursing Interventions Classification (NIC) was published, listing interventions and definitions, each followed by many nursing activities that a nurse could select to treat the client's problem (Dochterman and Bulechek, 2004). To retain the standardized language, the interventions and the definitions are used as written, but the nursing activities may be changed to fit each situation. This work carefully distinguishes the ongoing assessment activities that are part of the intervention by using the words *monitor* or *identify* to denote this use, rather than the term *assess,* which is the first step in the nursing process. Linkages to nursing diagnoses by NANDA are also suggested.

Examples of some of the nursing diagnoses, nursing outcomes, and nursing interventions pertinent to nutrition are listed in Table 2–1. Neither the outcomes (NOC) nor the

interventions (NIC) are prescriptive. Nurses are free to select any outcomes or interventions they believe to be appropriate. The selections in Table 2–1 illustrate a variety of outcomes and interventions. Some of this standardized terminology is used in the case studies and care plans in this text.

Nutritional Terms

Nutritional terminology involves specific meanings. **Nutritional status** refers to the body's condition as it relates to the intake and use of nutrients. All members of the health-care team have roles in the effective evaluation of a client's nutritional status. **Dietary status** describes what a client has been eating. Although a client's dietary status may be adequate, his or her nutritional status may nevertheless be poor. An evaluation of a client's dietary status can help to determine the reason for this poor nutritional status, or it may rule out poor diet as the source of the client's problem.

Two levels of methodology are commonly used to identify clients at nutritional risk. Box 2–2, a validated screening tool, is an example of the first level of nutritional care, screening, which is used to quickly identify persons at nutritional risk. A nutritional screening should be brief

Table 2–1   **Examples of Nursing Diagnoses, Nursing-Sensitive Outcomes, and Nursing Interventions Pertinent to Nutrition**

NURSING DIAGNOSIS (CLIENT STATES IDENTIFIED FOR IMPROVEMENT OR RETENTION)	NURSING-SENSITIVE OUTCOME (VARIABLE CLIENT OR CAREGIVER STATE, BEHAVIOR, OR PERCEPTION THAT IS RESPONSIVE TO A NURSING INTERVENTION)	NURSING INTERVENTION (NURSE BEHAVIOR OR ACTIVITY)
NANDA terminology (NANDA, International, 2003, with permission)	NOC terminology (Moorhead, Johnson and Maas, 2004, with permission)	NIC terminology (Dochterman and Bulechek, 2004, with permission)
Imbalanced nutrition: more than body requirements	Nutritional status: nutrient intake	Weight reduction assistance
Imbalanced nutrition: less than body requirements	Nutritional status: food and fluid intake	Eating disorders management
Risk for imbalanced nutrition: more than body requirements	Nutritional status: nutrient intake	Nutrition management
Excess fluid volume	Electrolyte and acid/base balance	Fluid management
Deficient fluid volume	Hydration	Hypovolemia management
Risk for deficient fluid volume	Fluid balance	Fluid/electrolyte management
Feeding self-care deficit	Self-care: eating	Self-care assistance: feeding
Impaired swallowing	Self-care: eating	Swallowing therapy

enough that the information can be gathered in a short time. The time to administer the tool presented in Box 2–2 may be extremely brief; if one factor is found to be present, the screening is stopped and the client is declared at nutritional risk and referred to a dietitian.

More comprehensive than screening, a nutritional assessment is the second level of methodology. A **nutritional assessment** is the evaluation of a client's nutritional status (nutrient stores) based on a physical examination, **anthropometric measurements,** laboratory data, and food

intake information. Many members of the health-care team are involved in a comprehensive nutritional assessment, including the physician, dietitian, nurse, social worker, and laboratory staff.

Because it requires many resources, this second level of nutritional care is usually completed only in the cases of clients at high nutritional risk. For example, a surgeon may order a comprehensive nutritional assessment before surgery to determine whether the client could tolerate a procedure better after nutritional rehabilitation.

Box 2–2   **Admission Nutrition Screening Tool**

A. Diagnosis
   If the patient has at least ONE of the following diagnoses, circle and proceed to section E to consider the patient AT NUTRITIONAL RISK and stop here.
   Anorexia nervosa/bulimia nervosa
   Malabsorption (celiac sprue, ulcerative colitis, Crohn's disease, short bowel syndrome)
   Multiple trauma (closed-head injury, penetrating trauma, multiple fractures)
   Decubitus ulcers
   Major gastrointestinal surgery within the past year
   Cachexia (temporal wasting, muscle wasting, cancer, cardiac)
   Coma
   Diabetes
   End-stage liver disease
   End-stage renal disease
   Nonhealing wounds
B. Nutrition intake history
   If the patient has at least ONE of the following symptoms, circle and proceed to section E to consider the patient AT NUTRITIONAL RISK and stop here.
   Diarrhea (>500 mL × 2 days)
   Vomiting (>5 days)
   Reduced intake (<1/2 normal intake for >5 days)
C. Ideal body weight standards
   Compare the patient's current weight for height to the ideal body weight chart. If at <80% of ideal body weight, proceed to section E to consider the patient AT NUTRITIONAL RISK and stop here.

(Continued on the following page)

Box 2-2 **Admission Nutrition Screening Tool** *(Continued)*

D. Weight history
Any recent unplanned weight loss? No _____ Yes _____ Amount (lbs or kg) _____
If yes, within the past _____ weeks or _____ months _____
Current weight (lbs or kg) _____
Usual weight (lbs or kg) _____
Height (ft, in or cm) _____

Find percentage of weight lost: $\dfrac{\text{usual wt} - \text{current wt}}{\text{Usual wt} \times 100}$ = _____ % wt loss

Compare the % wt loss with the chart values and circle appropriate value

Length of time	Significant (%)	Severe (%)
1 week	1–2	>2
2–3 weeks	2–3	>3
1 month	4–5	>5
3 months	7–8	>8
5+ months	10	>10

If the patient has experienced a significant or severe weight loss, proceed to section E and consider the patient AT NUTRITIONAL RISK.
E. Nurse assessment
Using the above criteria, what is this patient's nutritional risk? (check one)
_____ LOW NUTRITIONAL RISK
_____ AT NUTRITIONAL RISK
From Kovacevich, et al, 1997, p 22, with permission

The Nursing Process—Assessment

The first and most basic step of the nursing process is assessment. An organized and systematic search for pertinent subjective and objective data (Table 2–2) creates a sound foundation upon which to build health care.

Table 2-2 **Sample Subjective and Objective Nutritional Data**

SUBJECTIVE	OBJECTIVE
Usual diet and fluid intake	Accurate actual height and weight
Number of meals per day	Body build or frame
Last meal: time, foods, beverages, and amounts	Skin **turgor** and/or dryness
Food and nutrient supplements	Condition of teeth and gums
Appetite	Hair quantity and quality
Problems with digestion and/or elimination	Body fat measurements
Allergies or food intolerances	Complete blood count
Usual alcohol consumption	Serum albumin
Chewing and/or swallowing problems	Serum electrolytes
Use of dentures	
Usual weight and recent changes	
Likes and dislikes	

Subjective Data

Subjective data as they relate to nutrition include the client's history from an interview or questionnaire. When more detailed food intake information is required, one of the five techniques listed in Table 2–3 may be used; some of the advantages and disadvantages of each are given.

It is interesting to note that not every technological change has an immediate benefit for an individual client. Computerized programs for taking diet histories, for example, have been evaluated and judged to be adequate for epidemiological studies but not for assessment of individuals (Landig et al, 1998).

Neither reported dietary intake nor any other item of assessment data is suitable as the sole criterion of nutritional status.

Objective Data

A physical examination can include general appearance, anthropomorphic measurements, and laboratory or other diagnostic tests. Table 2–2 lists objective data relevant to a nutritional assessment.

General Appearance

Well-nourished people generally look healthy and usually have an optimistic perspective. Table 2–4 compares the appearance of a well-nourished individual with that of an individual who is less well nourished. A person need not display all of the abnormal signs listed in Table 2–4 to be regarded as malnourished.

Table 2-3 **Commonly Used Techniques to Obtain Food Intake Information**

TECHNIQUE	COMMENTS
COMPARISON WITH THE MYPYRAMID MODEL Health-care provider asks client what he or she eats and compares this reported food intake with MyPyramid Model.	Can be used to screen many clients quickly. Does not require a trained interviewer. Is not comprehensive. May overlook some clients who would benefit from nutritional care.
FOOD FREQUENCY Health-care provider requests client to fill out a question-naire asking about **usual food intake** during specified times, such as "What do you usually eat for breakfast?"	Questionnaire can be tailored to particular nutrients of interest (e.g., lactose, gluten). May assess food usage for any length of time: day, week, month, weekends versus weekdays, summer versus winter, etc. Initial client contact does not require a trained interviewer. May require special resources (e.g., computerized database) to evaluate the information collected. Provides limited information on a client's food behaviors such as meal spacing, length of usual mealtime, etc.
FOOD RECORDS Health-care provider asks client to record his or her food intake for a specified length of time (1, 3, or 7 days).	A motivated client will provide reasonably accurate information. A less highly motivated client will "forget to keep" part or all of the food record. Research shows some clients will change their food habits while keeping a food record; therefore, this technique works poorly in determining a client's dietary and/or nutritional status. This technique works well when a behavior change is desired. May require special resources (e.g., a computerized database) to evaluate the information obtained. Client needs to be available for a follow-up visit to review the evaluated food records. Analysis of results is time-consuming.
24-HOUR DIETARY RECALL Health-care provider asks client what he or she has eaten during the previous 24 hours.	Is a fairly simple technique. Interviewer should be trained not to ask leading questions. Yields limited information only about the kinds of foods and beverages consumed within the previous 24 hours. The previous 24 hours may not have been usual for the client. Frequently clients may not remember what they ate and the amounts they ate.
DIET HISTORY Health-care provider conducts an in-depth interview to obtain information about usual food intake, drug and medication usage, alcohol and tobacco use, financial ability to obtain food, special dietary needs, food allergies and intolerances, weight history, cultural and religious preferences that may influence food selection, ability to chew and swallow foods, previous dietary instructions received, client knowledge about nutrition, and elimination patterns.	Is comprehensive. Requires a trained interviewer, usually a dietitian. An analysis of the results obtained can usually be provided on the same day the information is collected. Is a good technique for high-risk clients when information is needed to evaluate the need for nutritional support. Is highly dependent on the willingness of the client to reveal information to the interviewer. Client must be a good historian. Is time-consuming.

SOURCE: Adapted from Moore, MC: Pocket Guide, Nutrition and Diet Therapy. Mosby, St. Louis, 1993, p 10, and from Mason, M, Wenberg, BG, and Welsch, PK: The Dynamics of Clinical Dietetics, John Wiley & Sons, New York, 1982, p 10.

Anthropometric Data

For clinical purposes, body size, weight, and proportions are determined by **anthropometry,** the science of measuring the body. Such measurements are used to determine growth, body composition, and nutritional status. The body's energy and protein stores also can be derived from these measurements.

The collection of anthropometric data on height and weight— **triceps skinfold,** midarm circumference, abdominal circumference, and waist and hip measurements—is described briefly in the following sections. Other measurements may also be selected.

HEIGHT AND WEIGHT. Height may be measured in inches or centimeters. Adults and older children are

(Table 2–4) **General Appearance as an Indicator of Nutritional Status**

	NORMAL	ABNORMAL
Demeanor	Alert, responsive Positive outlook	Lethargic Negative attitude
Weight	Reasonable for build	Underweight Overweight, obese
Hair	Glossy, full, firmly rooted Uniform color	Dull, sparse Easily, painlessly plucked
Eyes	Bright, clear, shiny	Pale conjunctiva Redness, dryness
Lips	Smooth	Chapped, red, swollen
Tongue	Deep red Slightly rough One longitudinal furrow	Bright red, purple Swollen or shrunken Several longitudinal furrows
Teeth	Bright, painless	Caries, painful, mottled, or missing
Gums	Pink, firm	Spongy, bleeding, receding
Skin	Clear, smooth, firm, slightly moist	Rashes, swelling Light or dark spots Dry
Nails	Pink, firm	Spoon shaped or ridged Spongy bases
Mobility	Erect posture Good muscle tone Walks without pain or difficulty	Muscle wasting Skeletal deformities Loss of balance

measured standing with head erect; infants and young children are measured lying on a firm, flat surface.

Weight may be recorded in pounds or kilograms. The agency policy regarding calibration of the scale should be followed. Each time the client is weighed, it should be on the same scale at the same time of the day, and the client should be wearing the same kind of clothing.

TRICEPS SKINFOLD. The measurement of subcutaneous tissue over the triceps muscle in the upper arm provides an estimate of the amount of body fat. The **triceps skinfold** measurement helps to differentiate between a person who is heavy because of muscle mass and one who is heavy because of excess fat.

The ability to take accurate measurements requires practice. Often research designs require the same researcher to take all measurements and record the average of two or three values at each site. Body areas other than the triceps can also be used to measure skinfolds. Although nurses usually do not make skinfold measurements, they do need to be able to answer clients' questions regarding the procedure and the information obtained from it.

MIDARM CIRCUMFERENCE. Because 50 percent of the body's protein stores are located in muscle tissue, the circumference (circumference is the outside edge of a circle) of the midarm provides information about body protein stores. The upper arm is measured between the shoulder and the elbow. Because bone mass variations, age, and gender are not considered in this measurement (Flanigan,

1997), the **midarm circumference** measurement must be interpreted as part of a complete assessment.

BODY FRAME SIZE. Elbow width has been used as an indication of frame size and is the measure used in the 1983 Metropolitan Height-Weight tables (Shils, 1999). Clinical Calculation 2–1 describes a procedure to determine body frame size without calipers.

ABDOMINAL CIRCUMFERENCE (GIRTH). The measurement of the abdomen, in inches or centimeters, is often taken at the umbilicus. **Abdominal circumference (girth)** provides information when an individual is accumulating fluid in the abdominal cavity, a condition called **ascites.** Girth is also measured to monitor growth of a fetus or of abnormal tissue within the abdomen.

WAIST AND HIP MEASUREMENTS. Within an agency, a standard procedure should be used for waist and hip measurements. With the person standing, the waist is measured at the narrowest site and the hips are measured at the greatest circumference. The tissue should not be compressed.

BODY DENSITY MEASURES. Muscle and fat tissue have different rates of metabolism. Therefore, the proportions of each in the body influence whether a person is overweight. These proportions can be determined by several techniques, including underwater weighing, dual-energy x-ray absorptiometry, and bioelectrical impedance.

Underwater weighing (hydrodensitometry) compares the person's scale weight with his or her weight underwa-

Clinical Calculation 2-1

Determining Body Frame Type

Extend your arm and bend your elbow so that your forearm is upward at a 90-degree angle. While keeping your fingers straight, turn the inside of your wrist toward your body. Place your thumb and index finger of the opposite hand on the two prominent bones of the elbow. Measure the space between thumb and index finger. Elbow width less than given in the following table designates a small frame, whereas larger measurements indicate a large frame.

HEIGHT IN 1″ HEELS	ELBOW BREADTH FOR MEDIUM FRAME
Men	
5′2″ to 5′7″	2 1/2″ to 2 7/8″
5′8″ to 6′3″	2 3/4″ to 3 1/8″
6′4″	2 7/8″ to 3 1/4″
Women	
4′10″ to 5′3″	2 1/4″ to 2 1/2″
5′4″ to 6′0″	2 3/8″ to 2 5/8″

SOURCE: Reprinted courtesy of Met Life Insurance Company, Statistical Bulletin, with permission.

ter. After correcting for lung volume, the examiner calculates the proportion of body fat. Underwater weighing provides the most accurate assessment of the amount of fat in the body. It is not easily determined, however. Even in research studies, several measurements must be taken and averaged to obtain a value that minimizes error. Because the technique is cumbersome and time consuming and requires special equipment, its main use is in research.

In **dual-energy x-ray absorptiometry (DEXA),** two x-ray beams are passed through the body. The amount of energy detected after the beams pass through the body varies with bone, fat, and muscle tissue. DEXA has been validated against underwater weighing and is another research tool (Daniels, Khoury, and Morrison, 1997). In clinical practice, DEXA is used to measure bone mineral density as an indicator of conditions marked by bone loss, such as osteopenia and osteoporosis (Chapter 8). A screening test to determine a person's level of risk for those conditions can be conducted with an **ultrasound bone densitometer** that involves no radiation exposure.

In the **bioelectrical impedance test,** electrodes on the extremities are stimulated. The greater electrolyte content and conductivity of the body's **fat-free mass** is compared with that of fat or bone. Tissues rich in water and electrolytes allow an electrical current to pass with greater ease than do denser fat and bone (Heymsfield, Nunez, and Pietrobelli, 1997). Measurements are not painful and usually are not felt at all because the frequencies used do not stimulate nerves and muscles (Jacobs, 1997).

Body composition is predicted in the bioelectrical impedance test from a measure of total body water. The client's fat-free mass is predicted, and his or her percentage of body fat is determined by comparing body weight with the predicted fat-free mass. The measurements obtained are percentage of body water, percentage of lean body mass, and percentage of body fat. These procedures were validated on healthy adults and are not necessarily applicable to ill adults (Jacobs, 1997), children (Horlick et al, 2002), or athletes (Houtkooper et al, 2001). For instance, anthropometric equations were superior to bioelectrical impedance in estimating body composition in power athletes (Huygens et al, 2002). Bioelectrical impedance tends to overestimate percentage of body fat in lean subjects and underestimate it in obese persons (Sun, et al, 2005). Because bioelectrical impedance is based on total body water, any factors disturbing water balance may alter the results. Examples are diuretic use, excessive sweating, hemodialysis, premenstrual edema, and alcohol consumption within the 24 hours before the test.

Laboratory Tests

Body fluids and excretions are analyzed by laboratory tests. These data include results from blood, urine, and stool tests. From these tests, much information can be obtained concerning what a person has eaten, what his or her body has stored, and how the body is using nutrients. Blood can be analyzed for glucose, protein, or fat content. Vitamin and mineral status can be determined directly by examining the blood or indirectly by examining enzymes related to the vitamin or mineral. Many experts doubt, however, that vitamin or mineral body stores can be accurately determined by blood samples. The uncertainty lies in whether the nutrient in the blood reflects body stores, a transport form of the nutrient, or the amount in one specific body compartment.

Good clinical judgment must be used in selecting tests and interpreting results. Reliance upon a single test or single reading is not recommended. Several studies have shown that a thorough nutritional history and physical examination is as effective in identifying malnutrition as a battery of laboratory tests (Moore, 1993).

The Nursing Process—Analysis

The health-care provider uses subjective or objective data or both to identify the level of the client's wellness regarding nutrition. The client's data are compared with standard nutritional parameters. Those in common use include height-weight tables, body mass index, waist-to-hip ratio (WHR), the Dietary Guidelines and MyPyramid from the U.S. Departments of Agriculture and Health and Human Services, the Food and Nutrition Board of the Institute of Medicine's Recommended Dietary Allowances (RDAs) and Adequate Intakes (AIs), and the ADA Exchange Lists. Making a judgment on the basis of a single parameter is not recommended.

Basic Nutritional Parameters

The data collected from the client are compared with various norms and recommendations to determine an appropriate nursing diagnosis (see Table 2–1). The parameters commonly used for comparison are included in the next section.

Height-Weight Tables

Many height-weight tables are currently in use, each based on a different underlying assumption (see Chapter 18). Table 2–5 shows the Metropolitan Life Insurance Table, which lists weights for height based on the lowest mortality (but it is not certain that the specified weights in this table are equated with maximum health). A reliable height-weight table should stipulate allowable shoe heel height and the weight of clothing. The information from height-weight tables is used to calculate a person's percentage of **healthy body weight (HBW)**. If a range of weights is given, the midpoint of the range is used. Clinical Calculation 2–2 illustrates the process.

Body Mass Index (BMI)

The **body mass index (BMI),** also called **Quetelet's Index** (Keys et al, 1972), is derived from weight and height (BMI = wt in Kg divided by (ht in meters)^2. It can also be calculated with reasonable accuracy using common American measures as shown below.

1. Multiply weight in pounds by 705.
2. Divide the result by height in inches.
3. Divide the second result by height in inches.

Table 2–5 **Metropolitan Life Insurance Company Height-Weight Table**

			MEN (INDOOR CLOTHING†)					
HEIGHT (IN SHOES*)			SMALL FRAME		MEDIUM FRAME		LARGE FRAME	
FEET	INCHES	CENTIMETERS	POUNDS	KILOGRAMS	POUNDS	KILOGRAMS	POUNDS	KILOGRAMS
5	2	157.5	128–134	58.2–60.9	131–141	59.5–64.1	138–150	62.7–68.2
5	3	160.0	130–136	59.1–61.8	133–143	60.4–65.0	140–153	63.6–69.5
5	4	162.6	132–138	60.0–62.7	135–145	61.4–65.9	142–156	64.5–70.9
5	5	165.1	134–140	60.9–63.6	137–148	62.3–67.2	144–160	65.5–72.7
5	6	167.6	136–142	61.8–64.5	139–151	63.2–68.6	146–164	66.4–74.5
5	7	170.2	138–145	62.7–65.9	142–154	64.5–70.0	149–168	67.7–76.4
5	8	172.7	140–148	63.6–67.2	145–157	65.9–71.4	152–172	69.1–78.2
5	9	175.3	142–151	64.5–68.6	148–160	67.2–72.7	155–176	70.5–80.0
5	10	177.8	144–154	65.5–70.0	151–163	68.6–74.1	158–180	71.8–81.8
5	11	180.3	146–157	66.4–71.4	154–166	70.0–75.5	161–184	73.2–83.6
6	0	182.9	149–160	67.7–72.7	157–170	71.4–77.3	164–188	74.5–85.5
6	1	185.4	152–164	69.1–74.0	160–174	72.7–79.1	168–192	76.4–87.3
6	2	188.0	155–168	70.5–76.4	164–178	74.5–80.9	172–197	78.2–89.5
6	3	190.5	158–172	71.8–78.2	167–182	75.9–82.7	176–202	80.0–91.8
6	4	193.0	162–176	73.6–80.0	171–187	77.7–85.0	181–207	82.3–94.1

			WOMEN (INDOOR CLOTHING†)					
HEIGHT (IN SHOES*)			SMALL FRAME		MEDIUM FRAME		LARGE FRAME	
FEET	INCHES	CENTIMETERS	POUNDS	KILOGRAMS	POUNDS	KILOGRAMS	POUNDS	KILOGRAMS
4	10	147.3	102–111	46.4–50.0	109–121	49.5–55.0	118–131	53.6–59.5
4	11	149.9	103–113	46.8–51.4	111–123	50.0–55.9	120–134	54.5–60.9
5	0	152.4	104–115	47.3–52.3	113–126	51.4–57.2	122–137	55.5–62.3
5	1	154.9	106–118	48.2–53.6	115–129	52.3–58.6	125–140	56.8–63.6
5	2	157.5	108–121	49.1–55.0	118–132	53.6–60.0	128–143	58.2–65.0
5	3	160.0	111–124	50.5–56.4	121–135	55.0–61.4	131–147	59.5–66.8
5	4	162.6	114–127	51.8–57.7	124–138	56.4–62.7	134–151	60.9–68.6
5	5	165.1	117–130	53.2–59.0	127–141	57.7–64.1	137–155	62.3–70.5
5	6	167.6	120–133	54.5–60.5	130–144	59.0–65.5	140–159	63.6–72.3
5	7	170.2	123–136	55.9–61.8	133–147	60.5–66.8	143–163	65.0–74.1
5	8	172.7	126–139	57.3–63.2	136–150	61.8–68.2	146–167	66.4–75.9
5	9	175.3	129–142	58.6–64.5	139–153	63.2–69.5	149–170	67.7–77.3
5	10	177.8	132–145	60.0–65.9	142–156	64.6–70.9	152–173	69.1–78.6
5	11	180.3	135–148	61.4–67.3	145–159	65.9–72.3	155–176	70.5–80.0
6	0	182.9	138–151	62.7–73.6	148–162	67.3–73.6	158–179	71.8–81.4

*Shoes with 1-inch heels.
†Allow 3 lb.
NOTE: The weights presented are those associated with the lowest mortality. They are not necessarily the weights of which people are healthiest, perform their jobs optimally, or even look their best.
SOURCE: Reprinted courtesy of Met Life Insurance Company, Statistical Bulletin, with permission.

Clinical Calculation 2–2

Percent Healthy Body Weight

The formula for calculating percent healthy body weight is:

$$\frac{\text{Client's weight}}{\text{Weight from table}} + 100 = \frac{\text{Percent healthy}}{\text{body weight}}$$

For example, according to the height-weight table (Table 2–5), a 5-ft 5-in woman with a medium frame has a range of 130 to 144 lb, including 3 lb of clothing. Assuming she is 5 ft 5 in barefoot, the table is entered at 5 ft 6 in to allow for 1-in heels. The midpoint of the range is 137 lb.

If the woman weighed 137 lb, her HBW would be 100 percent. If she weighed 159 lb, her HBW would be 116 percent, calculated as follows:

$$\frac{159\ lb}{137\ lb} \times 100 = 116\ \text{percent}$$

Someone with 90 percent HBW is considered underweight. A person at 111 to 119 percent HWB is overweight. A person at 120 percent HWB or more is obese.

BMI was designed to provide a measure of weight independent of height. Although the BMI has been used as an indicator of obesity, it fails to distinguish **adipose tissue** from muscle or water weight. Gallagher et al (1996) determined that the BMI varied with age and gender but not with ethnicity in their sample of healthy adults who did not engage in extensive physical activity or exercise training. They concluded that BMI cannot be used as a comparable measure of fatness in men and women, because women have significantly more body fat than men for equal BMIs for all age groups. Daniels, Khoury, and Morrison (1997) documented that BMI varies with gender, race, stage of maturation, and waist-to-hip ratio in 7- to 17-year-olds. Figure 2–1 shows a means to quickly estimate a BMI with only a straight edge and Table 18–1 lists BMIs for weights of 91 to 443 pounds correlated with heights of 58 to 76 inches. Nevertheless, as suggested earlier, clinical judgment is required to apply these findings to individuals. In general, the following classifications are used:

- BMI of 18 or less—Underweight
- BMI of 19 to 24—Normal
- BMI of 25 to 29—Overweight
- BMI of 30–39—Obese
- BMI of 40 or more—Morbidly Obese

Waist Measurements

Waist circumferences of more than 40 inches in men and 35 inches in women are related to increased risk of cardiovascular disease (Krauss et al, 2000), but the specific cutoff points are best documented for white populations (Zhu, et al, 2005). Similarly, waist-to-hip ratios (WHR) greater than 0.8 in women and greater than 0.95 in men indicate increased risk of problems related to obesity

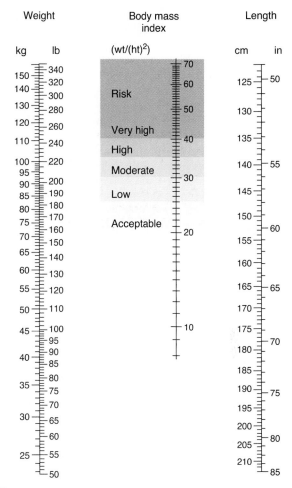

Figure **2–1** Using a straight edge to connect a person's weight with length, the point of intersection on the middle scale shows an approximate BMI. The likely level of health risk is also shown. (United States Department of Agriculture, 2000.)

(Gropper, Smith, and Groff 2005). To attain **waist-to-hip ratio (WHR),** the waist measurement is divided by the hip measurement.

The chances of developing health problems are increased when a person is overly fat. Excess body fat is correlated with cardiovascular disease, the most common form of diabetes, certain cancers, and other illnesses. Obesity and overweight in adulthood are associated with large decreases in life expectancy and increases in early mortality (Peeters et al, 2003).

Dietary Guidelines for Americans

The U.S. Departments of Agriculture and Health and Human Services have jointly published Dietary Guidelines for Americans every 5 years since 1980. This publication can be read or downloaded from the Web site at http://www.healthierus.gov/dietaryguidelines. The 2005 guidelines for health promotion can be found in Clinical Application 2–1. Additional information on the specified nutrients can be found in later chapters. A summary graphic promoting the Dietary Guidelines appears as Figure 2–2.

Clinical Application 2–1

Dietary Guidelines—Key Recommendations for the General Population

ADEQUATE NUTRIENTS WITHIN CALORIE NEEDS

- Consume a variety of nutrient-dense foods and beverages within and among the basic food groups while choosing foods that limit the intake of saturated and trans fats, cholesterol, added sugars, salt, and alcohol.
- Meet recommended intakes within energy needs by adopting a balanced eating pattern, such as the U.S. Department of Agriculture (USDA) Food Guide or the Dietary Approaches to Stop Hypertension (DASH) Eating Plan (see Chapter 20).

WEIGHT MANAGEMENT

- To maintain body weight in a healthy range, balance calories from foods and beverages with calories expended.
- To prevent gradual weight gain over time, make small decreases in food and beverage calories and increase physical activity.

PHYSICAL ACTIVITY

- Engage in regular physical activity and reduce sedentary activities to promote health, psychological well-being, and a healthy body weight.
  - To reduce the risk of chronic disease in adulthood: Engage in at least 30 minutes of moderate-intensity physical activity, above usual activity, at work or home on most days of the week.
  - For most people, greater health benefits can be obtained by engaging in physical activity of more vigorous intensity or longer duration.
  - To help manage body weight and prevent gradual, unhealthy body weight gain in adulthood: Engage in approximately 60 minutes of moderate- to vigorous-intensity activity on most days of the week while not exceeding caloric intake requirements.
  - To sustain weight loss in adulthood: Participate in at least 60 to 90 minutes of daily moderate-intensity physical activity while not exceeding caloric intake requirements. Some people may need to consult with a health-care provider before participating in this level of activity.
- Achieve physical fitness by including cardiovascular conditioning, stretching exercises for flexibility, and resistance exercises or calisthenics for muscle strength and endurance.

FOOD GROUPS TO ENCOURAGE

- Consume a sufficient amount of fruits and vegetables while staying within energy needs. Two cups of fruit and 2 1/2 cups of vegetables per day are recommended for a reference 2000-calorie intake, with higher or lower amounts depending on the calorie level.
- Choose a variety of fruits and vegetables each day. In particular, select from all five vegetable subgroups (dark green, orange, legumes, starchy vegetables, and other vegetables) several times a week.

- Consume 3 or more ounce-equivalents of whole-grain products per day, with the rest of the recommended grains coming from enriched or whole-grain products. In general, at least half of the grains should come from whole grains.
- Consume 3 cups per day of fat-free or low-fat milk or equivalent milk products.

FATS

- Consume less than 10 percent of calories from saturated fatty acids and less than 300 mg/day of cholesterol, and keep trans fatty acid consumption as low as possible.
- Keep total fat intake between 20 to 35 percent of calories, with most fats coming from sources of polyunsaturated and monounsaturated fatty acids, such as fish, nuts, and vegetable oils.
- When selecting and preparing meat, poultry, dry beans, and milk or milk products, make choices that are lean, low-fat, or fat-free.
- Limit intake of fats and oils high in saturated and/or trans fatty acids, and choose products low in such fats and oils.

CARBOHYDRATES

- Choose fiber-rich fruits, vegetables, and whole grains often.
- Choose and prepare foods and beverages with little added sugars or caloric sweeteners, such as suggested by the USDA Food Guide and the DASH Eating Plan.
- Reduce the incidence of dental caries by practicing good oral hygiene and consuming sugar- and starch-containing foods and beverages less frequently.

SODIUM AND POTASSIUM

- Consume less than 2300 mg (approximately 1 teaspoon of salt) of sodium per day.
- Choose and prepare foods with little salt. At the same time, consume potassium-rich foods, such as fruits and vegetables.

ALCOHOLIC BEVERAGES

- Those who choose to drink alcoholic beverages should do so sensibly and in moderation—defined as the consumption of up to one drink per day for women and up to two drinks per day for men.
- Alcoholic beverages should not be consumed by some individuals, including those who cannot restrict their alcohol intake, women of childbearing age who may become pregnant, pregnant and lactating women, children and adolescents, individuals taking medications that can interact with alcohol, and those with specific medical conditions.
- Alcoholic beverages should be avoided by individuals engaging in activities that require attention, skill, or coordination, such as driving or operating machinery.

(Continued on the following page)

FOOD SAFETY

- To avoid microbial foodborne illness:
  - Clean hands, food contact surfaces, and fruits and vegetables. Meat and poultry should not be washed or rinsed.
  - Separate raw, cooked, and ready-to-eat foods while shopping, preparing, or storing foods.
  - Cook foods to a safe temperature to kill microorganisms.

- Chill (refrigerate) perishable food promptly and defrost foods properly.
- Avoid raw (unpasteurized) milk or any products made from unpasteurized milk, raw or partially cooked eggs or foods containing raw eggs, raw or undercooked meat and poultry, unpasteurized juices, and raw sprouts.

Accessed 3/25/2005 at http://www.health.gov/dietaryguidelines/dga2005/recommendations.htm

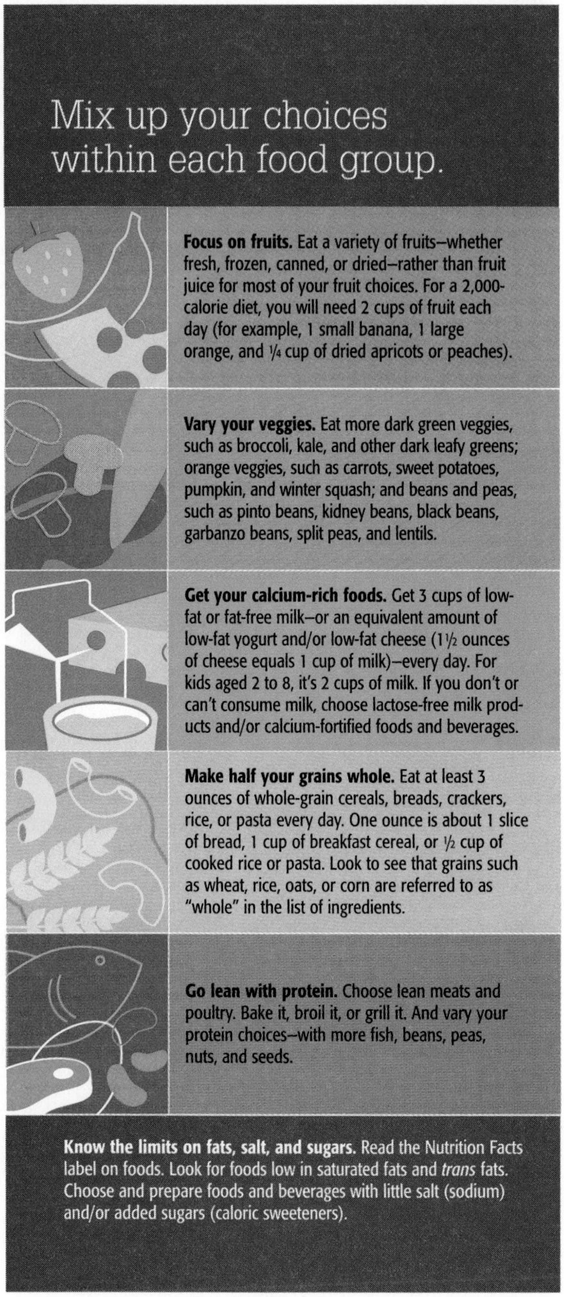

Mix up your choices within each food group.

Focus on fruits. Eat a variety of fruits—whether fresh, frozen, canned, or dried—rather than fruit juice for most of your fruit choices. For a 2,000-calorie diet, you will need 2 cups of fruit each day (for example, 1 small banana, 1 large orange, and ¼ cup of dried apricots or peaches).

Vary your veggies. Eat more dark green veggies, such as broccoli, kale, and other dark leafy greens; orange veggies, such as carrots, sweet potatoes, pumpkin, and winter squash; and beans and peas, such as pinto beans, kidney beans, black beans, garbanzo beans, split peas, and lentils.

Get your calcium-rich foods. Get 3 cups of low-fat or fat-free milk—or an equivalent amount of low-fat yogurt and/or low-fat cheese (1½ ounces of cheese equals 1 cup of milk)—every day. For kids aged 2 to 8, it's 2 cups of milk. If you don't or can't consume milk, choose lactose-free milk products and/or calcium-fortified foods and beverages.

Make half your grains whole. Eat at least 3 ounces of whole-grain cereals, breads, crackers, rice, or pasta every day. One ounce is about 1 slice of bread, 1 cup of breakfast cereal, or ½ cup of cooked rice or pasta. Look to see that grains such as wheat, rice, oats, or corn are referred to as "whole" in the list of ingredients.

Go lean with protein. Choose lean meats and poultry. Bake it, broil it, or grill it. And vary your protein choices—with more fish, beans, peas, nuts, and seeds.

Know the limits on fats, salt, and sugars. Read the Nutrition Facts label on foods. Look for foods low in saturated fats and *trans* fats. Choose and prepare foods and beverages with little salt (sodium) and/or added sugars (caloric sweeteners).

Figure 2–2 The 2005 Dietary Guidelines encourage Americans to choose foods wisely, emphasizing variety and limiting fat, salt, and sugar. More detail on the Guidelines can be accessed at http://www.healthierus.gov/dietaryguidelines.

These guidelines target the healthy general population older than 2 years of age to assist in the prevention of chronic and degenerative diseases. They do not apply to individuals who have diseases or conditions that alter normal nutritional requirements, but some of those modifications are covered in the complete document accessible from the Web site.

The guidelines are intended to be applied to several days' intake; it is inappropriate to use them to evaluate individual food items, a single meal, or one day's intake (Callaway, 1997). Wellness Tip 2–1 suggests ways to incorporate the Dietary Guidelines into a person's life.

Wellness Tip **2–1 •** Adding a healthy behavior is easier than eliminating a less healthy one. With the establishment of the healthy behavior, the unhealthy one may diminish.

- Eating 2 cups of fruits and and 2 1/2 cups of vegetables every day would provide many nutrients known to affect health for the better.
- If milk intake is low, selecting equivalent items from this food group would also improve long-term health.
- Small increases in physical activity can help to start a person on the path to recommended levels of exercise.
- Keep score. Add one additional serving of desirable food or 10 more minutes of physical activity every week or two.
- Keep at it. Instant success at anything is rare; it seems to occur only because outsiders just don't see the work that preceded the success or the restarts after failure.
- Evolutionary changes in lifestyle are more likely to be lasting than revolutionary ones
- Control portion sizes. Portion sizes and energy intake for specific food types have increased markedly since 1977, with greatest increases registered for food consumed at fast food establishments and in the home (Neilson and Popkin, 2003).

The New Food Guide Pyramid

In 2005, the U.S. Department of Agriculture created **MyPyramid,** which includes healthful diet choices balanced with appropriate activity (Fig. 2–3). Foods are grouped into categories—(1) grains; (2) vegetables; (3) fruits; (4) oils; (5) milk; (6) meat and beans—on the basis of similar nutrient content. For example, foods in the milk group are high in calcium, riboflavin, and protein. Each of the food groups supplies some but not all of the essential nutrients, thus some foods from each of the groups should be eaten daily.

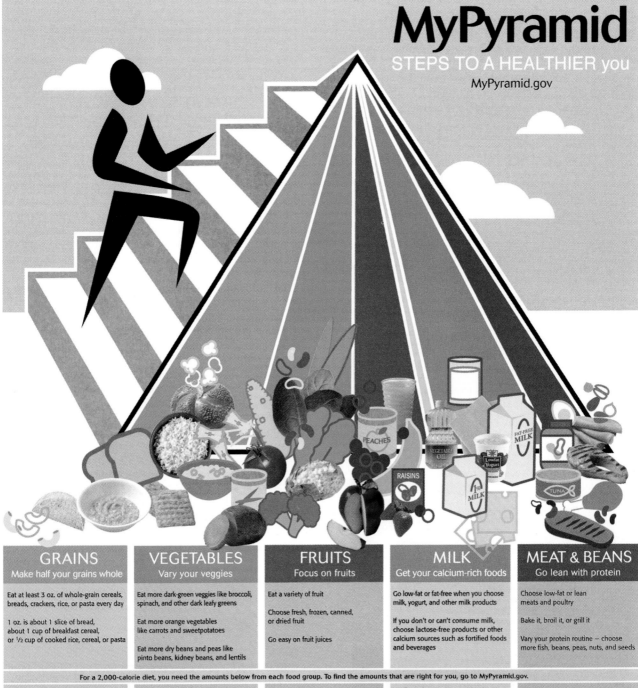

MyPyramid
STEPS TO A HEALTHIER you
MyPyramid.gov

GRAINS	VEGETABLES	FRUITS	MILK	MEAT & BEANS
Make half your grains whole	Vary your veggies	Focus on fruits	Get your calcium-rich foods	Go lean with protein
Eat at least 3 oz. of whole-grain cereals, breads, crackers, rice, or pasta every day	Eat more dark-green veggies like broccoli, spinach, and other dark leafy greens	Eat a variety of fruit	Go low-fat or fat-free when you choose milk, yogurt, and other milk products	Choose low-fat or lean meats and poultry
1 oz. is about 1 slice of bread, about 1 cup of breakfast cereal, or ½ cup of cooked rice, cereal, or pasta	Eat more orange vegetables like carrots and sweetpotatoes	Choose fresh, frozen, canned, or dried fruit	If you don't or can't consume milk, choose lactose-free products or other calcium sources such as fortified foods and beverages	Bake it, broil it, or grill it
	Eat more dry beans and peas like pinto beans, kidney beans, and lentils	Go easy on fruit juices		Vary your protein routine — choose more fish, beans, peas, nuts, and seeds

For a 2,000-calorie diet, you need the amounts below from each food group. To find the amounts that are right for you, go to MyPyramid.gov.

| Eat 6 oz. every day | Eat 2½ cups every day | Eat 2 cups every day | Get 3 cups every day; for kids aged 2 to 8, it's 2 | Eat 5½ oz. every day |

Find your balance between food and physical activity
- Be sure to stay within your daily calorie needs.
- Be physically active for at least 30 minutes most days of the week.
- About 60 minutes a day of physical activity may be needed to prevent weight gain.
- For sustaining weight loss, at least 60 to 90 minutes a day of physical activity may be required.
- Children and teenagers should be physically active for 60 minutes every day, or most days.

Know the limits on fats, sugars, and salt (sodium)
- Make most of your fat sources from fish, nuts, and vegetable oils.
- Limit solid fats like butter, margarine, shortening, and lard, as well as foods that contain these.
- Check the Nutrition Facts label to keep saturated fats, *trans* fats, and sodium low.
- Choose food and beverages low in added sugars. Added sugars contribute calories with few, if any, nutrients.

MyPyramid.gov
STEPS TO A HEALTHIER YOU

U.S. Department of Agriculture
Center for Nutrition Policy and Promotion
April 2005
CNPP-14

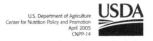

Figure 2–3 MyPyramid, designed to permit individualized assessment and tracking, is available online for consumers at *http://www.mypyramid.gov.*

The width of the colored bands in MyPyramid offers a general guide as to the proportion of the food intake that should be consumed from the indicated food group. The stepping person is a reminder to balance kilocaloric intake with suitable activity. Detailed information for professionals including

- Kilocaloric intake by age, gender, and activity level and
- Food intake patterns by kilocalorie level is available at http://www.mypyramid.gov/professionals/index.html.

All of the materials now specify amounts of the various foods in household measures rather than "servings" used in the previous edition of the Food Guide Pyramid that could be easily misinterpreted in favor of overconsumption.

Tools for Analysis of a Client's Situation

A client's reported or recorded food intake must be analyzed to reach a conclusion. The foods can be grouped according to the classifications in MyPyramid, or individual foods can be analyzed using a table of food composition or a computerized diet analysis program.

Tables of Food Composition

Food composition tables list foods and the amounts of selected nutrients for a specified volume or weight of the food. The U.S. Department of Agriculture (USDA) publishes a food composition table entitled Nutritive Values of the Edible Part of Foods (abridged in Appendix B). The database can be searched via the Internet at http://www.nal.usda.gov/fnic/cgi-bin/nut_search.pl. Tables of food composition serve as a practical reference in which to look up the nutritive content of a particular food or ingredients in a recipe. Such a process is helpful for comparing individual items but is very time consuming to use to analyze even a day's intake. Fortunately, computerized analysis is readily available.

Computerized Diet Analysis

Many computer software programs are available to compare an individual's intake with that recommended for someone of the same age and gender. Some of them include height, weight, and activity level. Even before the easy availability of computer software, some nutrient databases contained blank spaces for one or more nutrient values for a given food item, and such missing data affect the final value obtained for the nutrient. To be correct, software programs must also reflect recent changes in the Recommended Dietary Allowances (RDAs).

Computerized diet analysis programs can save time, but care must be taken when inputting data. For example, selection of "orange juice concentrate" instead of "orange juice" will skew the analysis. Even with excellent databases, the information gained from such a program needs to be interpreted. The only scientifically correct statement to be made is that the intake for a given period does or does not meet the RDA. It is inappropriate to base a judgment of nutritional or dietary status solely on a comparison to the RDA.

HEALTHY EATING INDEX. The Healthy Eating Index (HEI) is a measure of diet quality devised by the United States Department of Agriculture Center for Nutrition Policy and Promotion. It has 10 components scored with up to 10 points each for a possible perfect score of 100. The first five components are based on consumption of grains, vegetables, fruits, milk, and meat, numbers 6 through 8 are based on fat consumption (total, saturated, and cholesterol), number 9 is based on sodium, and number 10 is based on variety. A Healthy Eating Index score above 80 implies a good diet, one between 51 and 80 a diet that needs improvement, and one less than 51 a poor diet. Diets of various population groups have been analyzed with the HEI and are reported in this text. Box 2–3 shows the HEI analysis of the data given in Case Study 2–1 obtained at http://209.48.219.53/. The site is being updated.

The Nursing Process—Planning

Having assessed and analyzed a client's nutritional status, the nurse's next step is to plan a strategy that addresses any identified problems to treat or strengths to reinforce. The Nursing Outcomes Classification lists indicators which can then be used to track progress toward a particular outcome. The strategy may include referral to a dietitian.

In addition to traditional library sources, the Internet can deliver much information. To help evaluate the wealth of material available in cyberspace, Tufts University's Web site, http://www.navigator.tufts.edu, rates nutrition sites for content (accuracy, depth of information, and last update) and for usability. In evaluating literature, it is also wise to regard findings cautiously, especially those of a single study, until the study has been replicated (repeated with similar results). Often, findings related to health and nutrition are publicized in the general press before being critiqued by the scientific community. In general, good advice is to avoid extremes of dietary practices in favor of *balance, moderation,* and *variety.*

A fundamental decision in planning client care is whether to treat the client's nutritional problems within the nursing department or to refer the client to the dietary department. Many factors affect this decision. A nurse is likely to refer the client to a dietitian if the nutritional problem is severe or complex. A lack of nursing time and resources also may necessitate a referral.

The referral system has two functions. First, it ensures that the client and his or her family receive comprehensive care. Second, it arouses clients' and families' awareness of their needs for and the benefits of nutritional services.

If the nurse decides to treat the client directly, an efficient approach is to teach the client using the same nutritional tool, such as MyPyramid, that was used during the assessment. When the nurse chooses to treat the client's nutritional problems, it is crucial to prioritize the problems with the client and to select acceptable interventions. One or two changes may be easier for the client to sustain than a complete dietary overhaul. For that reason, it is important to select those interventions most likely to make a major difference in the client's health status.

The following section describes the **Recommended Dietary Allowances (RDAs)** and **Adequate Intakes (AIs)** that can also be used to establish dietary goals for individuals.

Dietary Reference Intakes

A new system of dietary reference values has replaced the old system of Recommended Dietary Allowances (RDAs).

Box 2–3

Here is the food displayed for Case Study 2–1

Select your serving sizes and specify how many servings you consumed for each. When you are done, click on **Save & Analyze** to save your food entry information and to analyze your food intake. If you want to make more than one day's food entry, click on **Return to Login** to save a day's food entry information and make another day's food entry. For a record of today's food entry, click **Print Food Record** prior to saving food entry. To return to initial values, click on the **Reset Values**. To add or remove food items, click on **Enter Foods**.

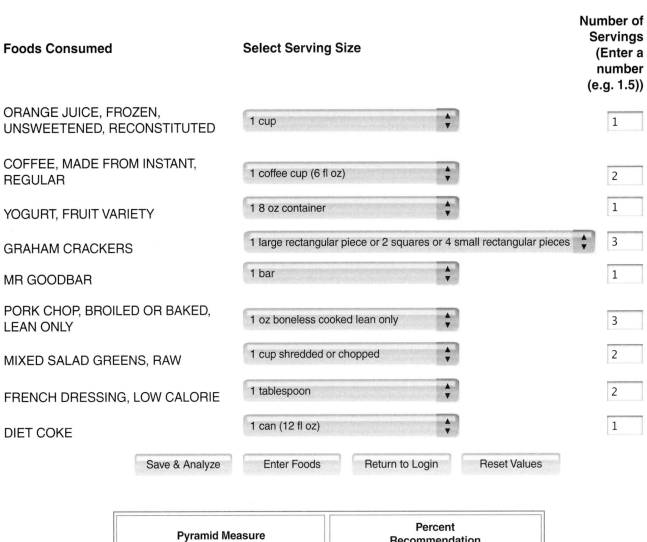

Foods Consumed	Select Serving Size	Number of Servings (Enter a number (e.g. 1.5))
ORANGE JUICE, FROZEN, UNSWEETENED, RECONSTITUTED	1 cup	1
COFFEE, MADE FROM INSTANT, REGULAR	1 coffee cup (6 fl oz)	2
YOGURT, FRUIT VARIETY	1 8 oz container	1
GRAHAM CRACKERS	1 large rectangular piece or 2 squares or 4 small rectangular pieces	3
MR GOODBAR	1 bar	1
PORK CHOP, BROILED OR BAKED, LEAN ONLY	1 oz boneless cooked lean only	3
MIXED SALAD GREENS, RAW	1 cup shredded or chopped	2
FRENCH DRESSING, LOW CALORIE	1 tablespoon	2
DIET COKE	1 can (12 fl oz)	1

Save & Analyze   Enter Foods   Return to Login   Reset Values

Pyramid Measure	Percent Recommendation
Fat	Fats, Oils and Sweets are not part of HEI
Milk	37%
Meat	54%
Vegetables	50%
Fruits	50%
Grains	20%

Back   **Nutrient Intakes**   **HEI Score**   **Calculate History**

Box 2-3   (Continued)

HEI Score For Case Study 2–1

Click directly on the [?] [?] [?] emoticon (face) for more detailed dietary information.

HEI Component	Emoticon	Score (Out of 10)	Number of Pyramid Servings Eaten	Number of Pyramid Servings Recommended
Grain	[?]	2.0	1.8	9
Vegetable	[?]	5.1	2.0	4
Fruit	[?]	5.0	1.5	3
Milk	[?]	3.7	1.1	3
Meat	[?]	5.3	1.3	2.4

HEI Component	Emoticon	Score (Out of 10)	Amount Eaten	Recommendation or Goal
Total Fat	[?]	10.0	28.9% of total calories	no more than 30%
Saturated Fat	[?]	7.7	11.1% of total calories	less than 10%
Cholesterol	[?]	10.0	79 mg	less than 300 mg
Sodium	[?]	10.0	1099 mg	less than 2400 mg
Variety	[?]	6.0	6	8

Total HEI Score: **64.8** out of a possible 100

More information about the Healthy Eating Index - To view this document you need Adobe Acrobat Reader

Here the food intake in Case Study 2–1 has been entered into an online diet analysis site. The case study student's intake is compared to the Food Guide Pyramid and is scored against the Healthy Eating Index. Source: United States Department of Agriculture, Center for Nutrition Policy and Promotion, accessed at http://147.2089.133 on February 22, 2003.

Although the term RDA remains, its meaning has been changed. Since 1993, the Food and Nutrition Board of the Institute of Medicine has worked to re-evaluate the RDAs, which originally focused on preventing deficiency diseases. Recent research findings support a role for certain nutrients in reducing the risk of chronic diseases. This information is evaluated as part of the process of establishing the new standards (National Academy of Sciences, 1997a, 1997b, 1997c). In addition to RDAs for vitamins and minerals, DRIs have been established for the macronutrients (carbohydrate, fat, and protein) and for water and electrolytes. The effort, in collaboration with Canada, has produced nutrient recommendations for North America.

Dietary Reference Intakes (DRIs) are composed of four nutrient-based reference values that can be used for assessing and planning diets. As with the old RDAs, the DRIs are intended to apply to the healthy general population.

All DRIs refer to average daily intakes for 1 or more weeks. The four components of the DRIs are the following:

- Estimated Average Requirements (EARs)
- Recommended Dietary Allowances (RDAs)
- Adequate Intakes (AIs)
- Tolerable Upper Intake Levels (ULs)

The **Estimated Average Requirement (EAR)** is the intake that meets the estimated nutrient need of 50 percent of the individuals in a life-stage and gender group. It is used to set the RDA and to assess or plan the intake of groups.

The newly defined **Recommended Dietary Allowance (RDA)** is the intake that meets the needs of 97 to 98 percent of healthy individuals in a life-stage and gender group. It is intended for use as a goal for daily intake by individuals, not for assessing the adequacy of an individual's nutrient intake. It does serve as a benchmark, however, in that if a healthy person's average intake meets or exceeds the RDA, the intake is likely to be adequate. If average intake is less than the RDA, there is risk of inadequate nutrient intake.

The RDA is expressed as a single absolute value and does not take into account a person's height or weight. One might expect nutrient need to vary with body size, but present knowledge does not permit finer distinctions.

Adequate Intake (AI) is the average observed or experimentally determined intake by a defined population or subgroup that appears to sustain a defined nutritional state, such as normal circulating nutrient values, growth, or other functional indicators of health. Information on the reduction of disease risk is incorporated into the setting of AIs.

If an EAR or RDA cannot be set because of the scarcity of information, the AI may be used as a goal for an individual's nutrient intake. AIs may also be used to set tentative goals for group intakes.

The values listed for EARs, RDAs, and AIs represent the quantities of nutrients found in typical diets in the United States and Canada. If clients take supplements for the sources of nutrients or if they follow very unusual diets (such as diets consumed by particular ethnic groups), it may be necessary for caregivers to make adjustments in planning clients' nutritional intakes.

The Tolerable Upper Intake Level (UL) is the highest average daily intake by an individual that is unlikely to pose risks of adverse health effects in 97 to 98 percent of individuals in specified life-stage and gender groups. Ordinarily the UL refers to intake from food, fortified food, water, and supplements; exceptions are noted in the listing. UL is not intended to be a recommended level of intake, because there is no established benefit for healthy individuals associated with nutrient intakes above the RDA or AI levels.

The Dietary Reference Intakes showing RDAs and AIs are given in Appendices F, H, and I. The table of ULs is Appendix G.

Desired Outcomes/Evaluation Criteria

Clearly worded outcome and evaluation statements are essential to facilitate later evaluation of a client's progress toward a goal. Table 2–6 gives several examples of statements describing desired outcomes or goals. Correctly and incorrectly formulated outcomes are shown, with a critique of the faulty ones.

The Nursing Process— Implementation

Once the nurse has developed a care plan with the client and his or her family, putting it into effect is the next step. It may take time and patience on the nurse's part to select appropriate interventions for an individual client or family.

Nursing Interventions

For clients requiring basic nutritional information, the activities listed as part of Nursing Interventions Classification (see Table 2–1) may simplify the task of implementing and documenting the nursing process. A given diet prescription may be implemented in various ways, but finding the approach a client will use faithfully is not only a challenge but also the key to success.

The concept of food exchanges is an effective system for educating and counseling clients about nutrition and meal planning.

Table 2–6 **Correctly and Incorrectly Stated Desired Outcomes**

CORRECT	INCORRECT	CRITIQUE OF INCORRECT
Client will lose 2 lb per week for the next 4 weeks.	Client will lose 20 lb in 2 weeks.	Not realistic
	Client will lose 20 lb.	No deadline
Client will consume a vegetable rich in vitamin A every other day for the next 6 weeks.	Client will increase intake of vitamin A.	Not measurable
	Teach client to consume vegetables rich in vitamin A.	Not client centered

American Dietetic and Diabetes Associations Exchange Lists

A food guide called the ADA **Exchange Lists** is published jointly by the American Dietetic Association and the American Diabetes Association. The ADA Exchange Lists are used for some clients with diabetes (Chapter 19) and also for clients who are attempting to achieve a healthier body weight (Chapter 18). Exchange lists are used to calculate a client's food intake, to educate the client about nutrition and meal planning, and to counsel the client about food choices.

The system is composed of six lists of foods grouped by nutrient composition. For example, corn is on the starch list because it is closer in composition to a slice of bread than to green beans. It is possible to approximate a client's carbohydrate, fat, protein, and kilocalorie intake with exchange lists.

There are six basic exchange lists: (1) starch; (2) fruit; (3) milk in three groups: skim, low fat, and whole; (4) vegetable; (5) meat in four groups: very lean, lean, medium fat, and high fat; and (6) fat in three groups: monounsaturated, polyunsaturated, and saturated. Table 2–7 identifies typical foods in each exchange list. In addition, some foods are considered "free" and are permitted in large amounts because they contain little energy (few kilocalories). Free foods are on a separate list. Note that some free foods have limitations on the amount to be consumed in a day or at one time. An adaptation of the exchange list appears in Appendix A.

Table 2–8 shows the amount of carbohydrate, protein, fat, and kilocalories (energy) in one exchange on each list. As you can see from the table, one exchange on the fruit list is not equal to one exchange on the starch list. To correctly use this method of meal planning, it is necessary for clients to choose the correct number of items from each appropriate list.

Understanding the meaning of the term *exchange* is important. In this context, it means a defined quantity of food within an exchange list. For example, one bread exchange is a single slice (a defined quantity). Individual

Table 2–7 Typical Foods in Each Exchange List

EXCHANGE LIST	FOOD ITEMS
Starch	Cereals, grains, pasta, dried beans, peas, lentils, starchy vegetables, bread, crackers
Meat	Beef, pork, veal, poultry, fish, wild game, cheese, eggs, tofu, peanut butter
Fruit	Fresh, frozen, or unsweetened canned fruit; dried fruit; fruit juice
Vegetable	Raw or cooked nonstarchy vegetables, vegetable juices
Milk	Milk, yogurt, evaporated milk, powdered milk
Fat	Avocado, margarine, mayonnaise, nuts, seeds, oil, salad dressing, bacon, coconut, powdered coffee whitener, cream, sour cream, whipped cream, cream cheese

food items within an exchange list are essentially equal to each other in nutrient composition and can thus be exchanged or "swapped" for each other. Portion sizes for various items have been adjusted to make each exchange approximately equal. For example, Table 2–9 shows items equal to one starch exchange.

Using the Exchange Lists

Exchange lists can be adapted for any prescribed kilocalorie, protein, fat, or carbohydrate level. A specific meal plan for the client to follow should be given with the exchange lists.

A meal plan is a food guide that shows the number of choices or exchanges the client should eat at each meal or snack. Table 2–10 illustrates two different meal plans for two different kilocalorie levels. One example is provided for distributing the various exchanges among meals. It is also possible to calculate different meal plans for the same kilocalorie level. Table 2–11 illustrates two 1200-kilocalorie meal plans.

Table 2–8 Energy Composition of the Six Exchange Lists

EXCHANGE LIST	CARBOHYDRATE (GRAMS)	PROTEIN (GRAMS)	FAT (GRAMS)	KILOCALORIES
Starch	15	3	0–1	80
Meat				
Very lean	0	7	0–1	35
Lean	0	7	3	55
Medium fat	0	7	5	75
High fat	0	7	8	100
Vegetable	5	2	0	25
Fruit	15	0	0	60
Milk				
Skim	12	8	0–3	90
2 percent	12	8	5	120
Whole	12	8	8	150
Fat (all)	0	0	5	45

SOURCE: The exchange lists are the basis of a meal planning system designed primarily for people with diabetes and others who must follow special diets. The exchange lists are based on principles of good nutrition that apply to everyone. © With permission 1995 American Diabetes Association and American Dietetic Association.

Table 2–9 **Examples of One Starch Exchange**

Puffed cereal	1 1/2 cups
Bread	1 slice
Corn, whole kernel	1/2 cup
Rice, cooked	1/3 cup

Exchange lists and meal plans give clients a selection of food choices that necessitates minimal calculation. This method can also be used to control the distribution of nutrients throughout the day. For clinical reasons, many clients need to modify meal frequency.

The Nursing Process—Evaluation

At the time of the deadline stated in the desired outcome, the nurse and the client decide whether or to what degree the objective has been met. If the progress has been unsatisfactory, they explore the reasons, such as unrealistic expectations, not enough time elapsed, or nursing actions not appropriate or not implemented.

A diet can be measured against three criteria: *balance, moderation,* and *variety.* A **balanced diet** includes sufficient foods from each of the five major food groups daily. Moderation means avoiding too much or too little of any one food or food group. A varied diet contains many different foods within each major food group.

Impact of Culture on Nutrition

Culture comprises the learned, shared, and transmitted values, beliefs, and norms of a particular group that guide thinking, decisions, and actions in patterned ways (Leininger, 1991). Although nation of origin, ethnic identity, and religious affiliation are prime examples of culture, other alliances such as colleges, corporations, professions,

Table 2–11 **Two 1200-kcal Meal Plans Using Exchanges for 1 Day**

EXCHANGES	MEAL PLAN 1	MEAL PLAN 2
Starch	5	6
Meat, lean	4	1
Meat, medium	1	3
Vegetable	2	4
Fruit	3	2
Milk, skim	2	1
Fat	4	4

political parties, and service clubs also imbue people with values and norms.

Health practices draw together people of similar habits, such as athletes or vegetarians. Thus, some aspects of culture are passed on from birth, but other aspects are voluntarily selected. All aspects of culture, including the family's food ways, ethnicity, and religion, may influence an individual's food choices. Figure 2–4 shows a multigenerational birthday party shaped in part by culture.

Even among individuals of similar cultural heritage, differences exist. Dietary preferences, for example, differ among people of Hispanic descent from such diverse places as Cuba, Puerto Rico, and Mexico (Loria et al, 1995). Just because a person belongs to a certain ethnic or religious group does not mean that he or she has adopted its traditional lifestyle and practices.

Ethnocentrism

The belief that one's own group's view of the world is superior to that of others is **ethnocentrism.** The dominant cultural group in the United States has been white descendants of northern Europeans who are middle class and Protestant. Education, work, punctuality, independence,

Table 2–10 **1500- and 1800-kcal Meal Plan Using Exchanges for 1 Day**

	1500 KCAL	1800 KCAL
Starch	7	7
Meat, lean	1	3
Meat, medium	3	3
Vegetable	4	5
Fruit	3	5
Milk, skim	2	2
Fat	6	7

DISTRIBUTION OF EXCHANGES THROUGHOUT THE DAY

	1500-KCAL MEAL PLAN			
	BREAKFAST	LUNCH	DINNER	SNACK
Starch	2	2	2	1
Meat, lean	0	1	0	0
Meat, medium	0	0	3	0
Vegetable	0	2	2	0
Fruit	1	1	1	0
Milk, skim	1	0	0	1
Fat	2	2	2	0

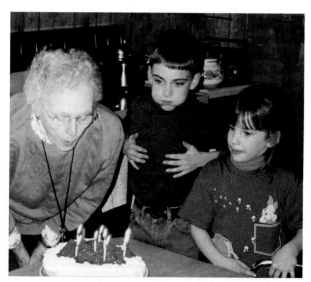

Figure 2–4 Many cultures have their own ways to observe life's milestones: births, birthdays, weddings, deaths. These children are sharing a birthday tradition with their 88-year-old great-grandmother.

and a future orientation—important values of this dominant culture—are reflected in the health-care system.

Health-care providers have tried, often unsuccessfully, to deliver this version of health care to clients without regard to the clients' cultures. Clients who failed to achieve goals that were imposed on them were labeled "noncompliant" (Wuest, 1993). Clients unable to communicate in the dominant culture's language were defined as having "altered communication" (Eliason, 1993; Levine, Ortmann, and Lunney, 1994).

The validity of a single standard of health regardless of ethnicity is questionable, because research involving health care has systematically excluded large subgroups of the population. For example, the rate of metabolism of caffeine, as well as of many other drugs, varies widely with ethnicity (Burroughs, Maxey, and Levy, 2002); thus standards of health related to caffeine intake that were set for white populations may not apply equally to other groups. Similarly, waist-to-hip ratio norms used to identify high risk for cardiovascular disease may need to be developed for specific racial groups (Zhu, 2005).

Acculturation

The process of adopting the values, attitudes, and behavior of another culture, **acculturation,** often puts people at risk in their overall health. For example, Latino women most acculturated into norms of the United States were least likely to initiate and to continue breastfeeding (Rassin et al, 1994).

Another adverse effect of acculturation is seen in the increase in diabetes in native populations. The major disease affecting widely scattered indigenous populations undergoing acculturation is type 2 diabetes mellitus, also called non–insulin-dependent diabetes mellitus (NIDDM). The incidence of the disease in Pima Indians is the highest in the world (Krosnick, 2000). In native residents of Canada and Australia, the incidence of type 2 diabetes is higher than in the general population of those regions (Daniel and Gamble, 1995; D'Alessio, 1995). The death rate from diabetes for native Hawaiians is more than three times that of the general U.S. population, and their mortality from heart disease is 44 percent higher (Mokuau, Hughes, and Tsark, 1995).

Culturally Competent Care

Knowledge of, acceptance of, and respect for other cultures are necessary to provide culturally competent care. The goal is a treatment plan that successfully blends the client's cultural beliefs with the practices of modern medicine. Clinical Application 2–2 illustrates the adaptation of diabetic teaching to Native American mythology.

Food Preferences of Ethnic Groups

Food items considered appropriate for human consumption vary widely by culture. Choices are influenced by economic and geographic constraints. The Seminole language, for instance, has no word for *vegetables,* for which the word *weeds* is substituted (Nelson, et al, 1993).

Rituals of preparation may be culturally determined, and allocation of food resources within a household may

---

Clinical Application 2–2

Using Ojibway Mythology in Diabetic Teaching

The Native American adage to walk in another's moccasins offers insight into culturally competent care. A program in Toronto capitalized upon Ojibway mythology to provide instruction on the self-care of diabetes. The program was organized at the request of Native Canadians and included day-long educational workshops. These sessions were conducted by an elder, and all participants sat in a circle. The circle confers equal status on every individual and represents harmony with nature. The beginning focus was on Nanabush, a legendary teacher of the Ojibway who symbolizes moderation and balance. Traditional narratives show him conversing with Diabetes. The moral of the story is to learn about "Diabetes," to live with him, and to control one's life through spiritual strength. Workshop activities included exercise breaks and a buffet lunch that allowed participants to choose their meals. Practitioners learned that avoiding a rigid diet prescription would enhance the individual's freedom, which was highly valued among the Ojibway (Hagey, 1984).

---

reflect the culture's values. Ethnic identity is important in determining staple foods, meal structure, and traditional holiday feasts.

In addition, certain foods may be culturally endorsed treatments for disease. Many other cultures espouse variations of the "hot/cold" systems described below under Hispanic Americans and Chinese Americans. Foods traditionally given to children when they are sick may also bring comfort to ill adults. The following brief summaries describe traditional foods of five cultural groups and suggest possible applications for adapting nutritional needs to accommodate these preferences.

African Americans

The traditional African American cuisine began from the necessity of making do with ingredients available to slaves. One-pot dinners serve to tenderize the meat and flavor the vegetables. These stews often contain pork and greens such as dandelion, turnip, and collard. Other foods often served are dried beans, sweet potatoes, rice, grits, cornbread, and specialty gravies (red-eye, sausage, or cream).

Soul food signifies a shared heritage and loving preparation, not just favorite and familiar foods. African Americans who choose this type of food should be encouraged to use beans, rice, and sweet potatoes but to cook without a lot of fat, such as by steaming. Traditional foods can be prepared to decrease fat consumption by baking, braising, broiling, or grilling instead of frying. Fat-free broths can be substituted for rich gravies.

Hispanic Americans

The dietary pattern covered below is that of Mexican Americans. Table 2–12 lists characteristic foods consumed by Puerto Rican and Cuban people as well as other ethnic groups.

Table 2–12 **Characteristic Eating Patterns of Selected Cultural Groups**

GROUP	GRAINS AND STARCHES	FRUITS	VEGETABLES	MEATS AND MEAT SUBSTITUTES	MILK AND MILK SUBSTITUTES	TO DECREASE FAT
Latino Mexican	Tortillas, corn products, potatoes, corn		Chili peppers, tomatoes, onions, beets, cabbage, pumpkins, string beans	Meat, poultry, eggs; pinto, calico, garbanzo beans	Cheese; milk seldom consumed	Encourage: • Salsa as dip or topping • Baked corn tortillas, especially stuffed with chicken to make tamales, tostados, or enchiladas • Rice with chicken or beans • Reduced-fat cheeses Discourage: • Fried tortillas • Sour cream and regular cheese as toppings • Refried beans that are cooked in lard • Deep-fried foods such as chimichangas
Puerto Rican	Plantains (starchy vegetable that looks like a large banana), Puerto Rican bread (resembles Italian bread), rice, viands (starchy vegetable whose roots and tubers are peeled, boiled, and eaten as a side dish)	Guava, canned peaches, pears, fruit cocktail	Beets, eggplant, carrots, green beans, onions	Legumes (especially red kidney beans), eggs, pork, chicken, cod, fish, pigeon, peas, garbanzo beans	Flan (custard); milk seldom consumed	
Cuban	Rice		Green peppers, onions, tomatoes	Black beans, pork, chicken, chorizo (a highly seasoned sausage)	Milk seldom used	
Italian	Pasta, yeast breads, starchy root vegetables		Green peppers, onions, tomatoes	Spiced sausages, fish, tomato-based meat sauces	Cheese; milk seldom consumed (high incidence of lactose intolerance)	Encourage: • Salad with no-fat dressing • Minestrone soup • Pasta with tomato or clam sauce • Grilled meat or seafood Discourage: • White sauces made with cream, butter, or cheese • Breaded and fried meats and vegetables • Sausages and other fatty meats such as prosciutto (spiced ham)
Southern Black American	Cornbread, biscuits, white bread, butter beans, corn, sweet potatoes, grits, rice, white potatoes, corn, yams	Melons, bananas, peaches	Kale, collards, mustard greens, okra, tomatoes, cabbage, summer squash	Catfish, pork, chicken, black-eyed peas, other dried beans and peas	Buttermilk, evaporated milk, ice cream (high incidence of lactose intolerance)	Encourage: • Baked fish and chicken • Steamed vegetables • Fresh melon • Grilled foods

	Grains/Starches	Fruits	Vegetables	Protein Foods	Milk Products	Recommendations
Asian Southern Chinese	Rice	All	Mushrooms, bean sprouts, Chinese greens, bok choy	Beef, pork, poultry, seafood	Limited except for ice cream	Encourage: • Hot and sour soup; wonton soup • Steamed (not fried) dumplings • Lightly stir-fried chicken or seafood • Steamed whole fish • Steamed vegetables and steamed rice Discourage: • Egg rolls • Crispy fried noodles • Fried rice • Deep-fried entrees • Spareribs • Tempura
Northern Chinese	Wheat, millet seed used in noodles, bread, dumplings		Chinese greens, bamboo, alfalfa sprouts, bok choy	Beef, poultry, seafood, eggs, tofu, soybeans	None (high incidence of lactose intolerance among all Chinese)	
Japanese	Rice, most other complex carbohydrates		All	Fish, beef, pork, eggs, poultry, shellfish, soybean products	None (high incidence of lactose intolerance)	
Asian Indian	Rice, wheat, millet, barley, maize, ragi (Old World cereal grain)	Mangoes, bananas	Cabbage, cauliflower, onions, chilies, tomatoes, potatoes, green leafy, okra, green beans, root vegetables	Legumes, nuts (Many vegetarians depending upon region)	Yogurt, buttermilk, milk added to coffee and tea	Encourage: • Broiled, poached, or steamed lean meats and poultry if nonvegetarian and religious practice permits • Steamed, stir fried, baked, or roasted vegetables • Olive oil, canola oil • Low-fat dairy products Discourage: • Deep fried breads and snacks • Coconut oil
European Middle Eastern	Pita bread, rice, couscous, bulgur wheat	Figs, peaches, dates	Grape leaves, tomatoes, peppers, olives, eggplant, onions, squash, fennel, okra, peas	Lamb, chicken, goat, legumes, fish, squid	Yogurt, Feta cheese	Encourage: Baked or grilled lean meats and vegetables, legumes, Fresh fruit, Yogurt dressings Discourage: Fried meats and fish, excess cheese, butter between layers of phyllo (pastry), sour cream

(Continued on the following page)

Table 2–12 **Characteristic Eating Patterns of Selected Cultural Groups** *(Continued)*

GRAINS AND GROUP	STARCHES	FRUITS	MEATS AND MEAT VEGETABLES	MILK AND MILK SUBSTITUTES	SUBSTITUTES	TO DECREASE FAT
Northern European	Dark breads, wheat breads, potatoes	All	All, especially onions, carrots, beans	Beef, pork, poultry, fish, shellfish, eggs, sausages	All cheese and milk products	Encourage: • Broiled, poached, or steamed lean meats • Wine- and tomato-based sauces • Consommé Discourage: • Creamed soups and sauces • Sausages • Whole milk and whole-milk products • Fried potatoes • Sour cream
Native American	Corn, wild oats and rice, Indian biscuits (Bannock bread)	Wild berries, choke cherries, black cherries, crab apples	Wild rhubarb, Indian celery, wild mushrooms and roots	Game, seafood, acorns, hazelnuts, pinenuts	Few used (high incidence of lactose intolerance)	Encourage: • Game with visible fat removed • Broiled, poached, or steamed meats Discourage: • Excessive fish oil • Fried food • Lard in cooking

Corn is the staple crop of Mexico. Vegetables and meat often are incorporated into a main dish and served with salsa. Foods are frequently stewed or fried in oil or lard. Fruits are popular. Sweet foods, such as yeast pastries, are common in the traditional Mexican diet, and sugar is often added to foods.

A health belief that may influence a Mexican American's food choices is the "hot-cold" system. Illness and physiological conditions are categorized as "hot" or "cold." Foods of the opposite category are eaten in an attempt to return balance to the body. Because these categories vary widely from region to region, it is best simply to ask clients what foods they would like to eat.

The traditional Mexican diet can be adapted to the recommendations of the Dietary Guidelines with some changes in preparation. Beans can be boiled, for example, instead of refried; beef can be grilled instead of fried; diet drinks can be substituted for lemonade or soda. The starches and fruits that are part of the Mexican American diet can still be used.

Native Hawaiians

Before the arrival of Westerners, native Hawaiians consumed a diet based on taro (a starch root similar to potato), sweet potatoes, breadfruit, fruit, greens, and seaweed. Fat content was approximately 10 percent of kilocalories. Foods were eaten raw or steamed.

Adopting a Western diet has been detrimental to native Hawaiians' health. Among all of the population groups in the United States, the prevalence of obesity among native Hawaiians is second only to that of the Pima Indians. Longevity is greater in Hawaii than in any other state, except among native Hawaiians, who have the shortest lifespan of the ethnic groups.

An experimental diet was introduced to native Hawaiians to determine whether short-term diet changes could alter their risk factors for cardiovascular disease. At the start, these individuals had an average BMI of 39.6. All of the food was provided in two on-site meals and take-home snacks. The evening meal included a cultural or health education session. During the 3-week experiment, the participants were encouraged to eat as much of the traditional Hawaiian foods as they wanted but limited amounts of fish and chicken. Average energy intake decreased 41 percent. Average weight loss was 17.1 pounds (7.8 kilograms). Serum cholesterol decreased 14 percent (Shintani et al, 1991).

As detailed in later chapters, total fat and cholesterol intakes are connected to an increased risk of chronic disease. Adopting a diet that resembled that of their ancestors, dramatically altered risk factors for diabetes mellitus and heart disease in these native Hawaiians. Some of the success was attributed to the stimulation of pride in their heritage.

Chinese Americans

As throughout the world, Chinese cooking is based on the availability of foodstuffs. Wheat is produced in northern China, where noodles and dumplings are a major part of the cuisine, whereas in the south that grows rice, it is the staple grain.

Cooking technique involves cutting meats into bite-sized pieces in the kitchen. Experience with diseases resulting from poor sanitation led to avoidance of cold water and raw fruits and vegetables. Fruits and vegetables are quickly cooked to retain a crisp texture.

Chinese medicine views sickness as an imbalance between yin and yang forces, a system that some compare to the parasympathetic and sympathetic nervous systems. Certain illnesses, foods, and medicines are categorized as *yin* or *yang*. *Yin*, or "cold," foods include pork, most vegetables, boiled foods, foods served cold, and white foods. *Yang*, or "hot" foods include beef, chicken, eggs, fried foods, foods served hot, and red foods. Noodles and soft rice are neutral, neither *yin* nor *yang*.

To maintain fluid intake, Chinese Americans prefer hot tea to ice water. Dairy products are rarely used. A caregiver interested in increasing a Chinese American's calcium intake would probably achieve better results advocating green leafy vegetables or tofu rather than milk. Family members may cook food at home to provide the hospitalized client with "hot" or "cold" foods. Because *yin* and *yang* cover various categories of foods, cooking methods, and colors, the perceptive nurse or dietitian can suggest items or procedures that also fit the diet prescribed by Western medicine. Clinical Application 2–3 relates such a case.

Jewish Americans

Orthodox Jews interpret dietary laws stringently. There are three key characteristics of strict kosher food preparation: (1) only designated animals may be eaten, (2) some of those animals must be ritually slaughtered and dressed,

---

Clinical Application 2–3

Bridging Yin and Yang Beliefs and the Germ Theory of Disease

A Chinese infant was experiencing repeated bouts of diarrhea. Several tests were performed, and changes were made in the child's formula to no avail. Finally a nurse made a home visit. She discovered several bottles of home-prepared formula on the windowsill, while others were in the refrigerator. The family lived in an apartment in New York without air-conditioning, and it was midsummer. When the nurse asked about the procedure used to store the formula, the mother stated that because childbirth is regarded as a cold condition and she should therefore avoid cold, her husband removed the day's bottles from the refrigerator before he left for work in the morning so they would be "warm" for the mother's condition. The nurse explained that storage at room temperature permitted bacteria to grow in the formula, which was the cause of the baby's diarrhea. Together, the mother and nurse searched for another procedure to bridge the cultural belief and the germ theory of disease. The mother decided to don a coat, hat, and gloves before opening the refrigerator to retrieve each bottle at feeding time. The nurse wisely guided the mother to a solution that left her belief system intact. The infant suffered no further episodes of diarrhea (Jackson, 1993).

Table 2–13 **Selected Religious Customs That Affect Food Intake**

RELIGION	RESTRICTED FOODS AND BEVERAGES
Buddhism	1. All meat
Catholicism	1. Meat prohibited by some denominations on holy days such as Good Friday and Ash Wednesday 2. Alcoholic beverages by some denominations
Hinduism	1. Beef, pork, and some fowl
Islam	1. All pork and pork products 2. All meat must be slaughtered according to ritual letting of blood. 3. Carnivorous animals, birds of prey, and land animals without external ears 4. Blood and blood byproducts 5. Alcohol and intoxicants
Orthodox Judaism	1. All pork and pork products 2. All fish without scales and fins 3. Dairy products should not be eaten at the same meal that contains meat and meat products. 4. All meat must be slaughtered and prepared according to Biblical ordinances. Since blood is forbidden as food, meat must be drained thoroughly. 5. Bakery products and prepared food mixtures must be prepared under acceptable kosher standards. 6. Leavened bread and cake are forbidden during Passover.
Seventh-Day Adventist	1. All pork and pork products 2. Shellfish 3. All flesh foods (some members) 4. All dairy products and eggs (some members) 5. Blood 6. Highly spiced foods 7. Meat broths 8. All alcoholic beverages 9. Coffee and tea

and (3) dairy products and meats must not be eaten at the same meal. Separate cooking and serving utensils are used for dairy meals and meat meals, although glass utensils, being nonabsorbent, can be used for either (Purnell and Paulanka, 2003). Fruits, vegetables, and starches need no special preparation and can be served with either meat or dairy meals.

When a preplanned kosher meal is unavailable, a cottage cheese fruit plate is a good choice for an orthodox Jew. The cottage cheese should be transferred to a paper plate with new disposable plastic utensils because neither the plate nor the utensils used can have ever touched meat. If bread or crackers are served, labels must indicate that they contain no meat products.

Table 2–12 lists the characteristic eating patterns of selected cultural groups with suggested means of decreasing fat intake. Table 2–13 lists selected religious customs that affect food intake.

SUMMARY

The assessment of a client's nutritional status includes subjective data (knowledge of nutrition and usual intake) and objective data (general appearance, anthropometric data, body density measures, and diagnostic tests). Nursing diagnoses are derived by comparing the client's data with nutritional standards (height-weight tables, body mass index, U.S. Dietary Guidelines, MyPyramid, and Recommended Dietary Allowances). Dietary changes may require the nurse to monitor the client's knowledge and practices as well as to provide feeding assistance.

Diet prescriptions and instructions may use the American Dietetic Association and American Diabetes Association Exchange Lists or other diets covered in Unit III of the text.

To avoid stereotyping individuals because of their ethnic or religious affiliations, the best practice is to ask clients to describe their dietary preferences. Nurses can then design nursing actions that will be meaningful to the client.

CASE STUDY 2-1

A student in a beginning nutrition course is showing a friend the textbook. "You could help me improve my diet," the friend says. "I know I am not eating right." At the time the friend was eating a chocolate bar. She described herself as 18 years old and sedentary. The student asks the friend to list what she has eaten during the past 24 hours. From the friend's list, the student gathers the following data:

Breakfast: 8 ounces of orange juice, 2 cups of black coffee

Lunch: 8 ounces of fruit yogurt and 6 square graham crackers

Midafternoon snack: Mr. Goodbar

Dinner: 3-ounce boneless pork chop, 2 cups of green salad, 2 tablespoons low-calorie French dressing, 12 ounces of diet Coke

Comparing the friend's intake to the tables for 18-year-old women available at MyPyramid, the student finds her friend's intake should be 1800 kilocalories distributed as the following:

	FRIEND'S INTAKE	MYPYRAMID
Oils	1/2 teaspoon	5 teaspoons
Milk	1 cup	3 cups
Meat and beans	3 ounces	5 ounce equivalents
Vegetables	1 cup	2 1/2 cups
Fruits	1 cup	1 1/2 cups
Grains	3 ounce equivalents	6 ounce equivalents
Discretionary kilocalorie allowance	267	195

In this situation, the student probably would not formalize a nursing care plan for the friend, but the following plan illustrates the thought process involved in developing a nursing care plan for this case.

NURSING CARE PLAN

SUBJECTIVE DATA Client expresses need for instruction in healthy diet. A 24-hour recall shows fewer than the recommended MyPyramid intake for all food groups. She consumed excessive discretionary kilocalories.

OBJECTIVE DATA Client is observed eating a chocolate bar at 3 P.M.

NURSING DIAGNOSIS NANDA: Health-Seeking Behavior (NANDA 2003, with permission) related to expressed desire to improve nutritional intake.

DESIRED OUTCOMES EVALUATION CRITERIA	NURSING ACTIONS/INTERVENTIONS	RATIONALE
NOC: Health-Seeking Behavior (Moorhead, Johnson, and Maas, 2004, with permission)	NIC: Nutrition Management (Dochterman and Bulechek, 2004, with permission.)	
Friend will keep a food record for 3 days.	Instruct friend to list everything she eats or drinks for 3 days.	Food record will gather facts about the friend's food intake to use as an instructional tool.
Friend will read the section on MyPyramid in student's textbook by this evening.	Lend friend textbook to read.	Providing literature utilizes expert opinion to reinforce student's teaching. Reading and seeing illustrations elicits active participation and employs senses other than hearing.
Friend will meet with student in 4 days to compare food record to MyPyramid and design a plan of action.	Meet with friend in 4 days to sort and analyze food record data. Provide apples at meeting to model healthy snack food.	Setting follow-up visit just after food record is completed will maintain the friend's interest. Modeling desirable behavior is a technique to encourage change.

CTQ CRITICAL THINKING QUESTIONS

1. When the student meets with the friend 4 days later, the friend says she has not been keeping the requested food diary. "I'm hopeless. I'll never be able to change," she moans. What steps might be taken to refocus her attitude?

2. You have a friend or relative who displays food intake similar to that described in Case Study 2–1. You care deeply for this person. How might you approach the subject of healthy eating if the person does not ask for assistance?

3. In what way has geography impacted ethnic eating patterns listed in Table 2–14? In what way has geography affected the typical diet in the United States?

≫ CHAPTER REVIEW

1. Which of the following statements about a nutrient analysis calculated by a computer is correct?
   a. The results obtained will not vary from one nutrient database to another.
   b. Nutrient databases using the RDA to compare and analyze results may be outdated.
   c. The results obtained are self-explanatory and need not be clarified to the client.
   d. The results are always more accurate than those obtained from manual calculations using a table of food composition.

2. Which of the following is not a part of the U.S. Dietary Guidelines?
   a. Choose a diet low in fat, saturated fat, and cholesterol.
   b. Eliminate salt and sugar from the diet.
   c. Maintain a healthy weight.
   d. Vary the foods you consume.

3. Which statement about the use of the ADA Exchange Lists is true?
   a. Two starch exchanges can be substituted for two meat exchanges.
   b. Exchange lists are used to calculate an individual's RDA.
   c. An exchange is a defined quantity of food on a particular exchange list.
   d. All 1200-kilocalorie meal plans contain six starch exchanges and only lean meat exchanges.

4. Which of the following is true of the traditional Chinese yin and yang health belief system?
   a. A cold, or yin, condition is balanced by consuming hot, or yang, foods.
   b. A hot condition is flushed with large quantities of cold water.
   c. Rice is considered magical and is consumed at every meal.
   d. Yang, or hot, foods include only foods served hot.

5. Which of the following adheres to strict kosher regulations?
   a. Avoiding cheese and cheese products.
   b. Eating only certain cuts of pork.
   c. Keeping separate utensils and dishes for meat and dairy meals.
   d. Serving lobster, clams, and shrimp only on festive occasions.

✚ CLINICAL ANALYSIS

1. Ms. G has just been diagnosed with type 2 diabetes (NIDDM). She is a Native American who has left her reservation for employment in town. Which of the following actions by the nurse shows respect for Ms. G's culture?
   a. Instructing her to increase her intake of vegetables.
   b. Telling her to lose weight and avoid alcohol and fast-food restaurants.
   c. Giving Ms. G an instruction sheet based on the ADA exchange system.
   d. Asking Ms. G how she "sees" or perceives diabetes in her life.

2. Mr. P is a 65-year-old man, recently widowed, whose physician is recommending weight loss. Mr. P has had little experience with grocery shopping or cooking. Which of the following systems for instructing Mr. P would the nurse select to offer the best chance of success?
   a. A computerized diet analysis program
   b. MyPyramid
   c. The ADA Exchange Lists
   d. The RDA/AI tables

3. Ms. E attended a community health fair where she entered her recalled intake for the previous 24 hours into a computer for analysis. On the basis of the printout she was given, she now thinks she should begin taking vitamin and mineral supplements. A friend who is a nurse correctly bases her advice on the following:
   a. A 1-day diet recall is inadequate data on which to base supplementation.
   b. A hand recalculation should be done to verify the accuracy of the computer printout.
   c. The RDAs on which computer programs are based are intended for only the 50 percent of the population who are obsessed with health.
   d. Undoubtedly, the operators of the computer at the fair had a product to sell: "Let the buyer beware."

REFERENCES

American Dietetic Association and American Diabetes Association: Exchange Lists for Meal Planning. American Dietetic Association and American Diabetes Association, Chicago and Alexandria, Va, 1995.

Burroughs, VJ, Maxey, RW, and Levy, RA: Racial and ethnic differences in response to medicines: Towards individualized pharmaceutical treatment. J Nat Med Assoc 94:1, 2002.

Callaway, CW: Dietary guidelines for Americans: An historical perspective. J Am Coll Nutr 16:510, 1997.

D'Alessio, V: Running a Band-aid service. Nursing Standards 9:22, 1995.

Daniel, M, and Gamble, D: Diabetes and Canada's aboriginal peoples: The need for primary prevention. Int J Nurs Stud 32:243, 1995.

Daniels, SR, Khoury, PR, and Morrison, JA: The utility of body mass index as a measure of body fatness in children and adolescents: Differences by race and gender. Pediatrics 99:804, 1997.

Dochterman, J, and Bulechek, G (eds): Nursing Interventions Classification (NIC), ed 4. Mosby, St. Louis, 2004.

Eliason, MJ: Ethics and transcultural nursing care. Nurs Outlook 41:225, 1993.

Flanigan, KH: Nutritional Aspects of Wound Healing. Adv Wound Care 10:48, 1997.

Gallagher, D, et al: How useful is Body Mass Index for comparison of body fatness across age, sex, and ethnic groups? Am J Epidemiol 14:143, 1996.

Gropper, SS, Smith, JL, and Groff, JL: Advanced Nutrition and Human Metabolism, ed 3. Wadsworth, Belmont, CA, 2005.

Hagey, R: The phenomenon, the explanations and the responses: Metaphors surrounding diabetes in urban Canadian Indians. Soc Sci Med 18:265, 1984.

Heymsfield, SB, Nunez, C, and Pietrobelli, A: Bioimpedance analysis: What are the next steps? Nutr Clin Pract 12:201, 1997.

Horlick, M, et al: Bioelectrical impedance analysis models for prediction of total body water and fat-free mass in healthy and HIV-infected children and adolescents. Am J Clin Nutr 76: 991, 2002.

Houtkooper, LB, et al: Body composition profiles of elite American heptathletes. J Sport Nutr Exerc Metab 11:162, 2001.

Huygens W, et al: Body composition estimations by BIA versus anthropometric equations in body builders and other power athletes J Sports Med Phys Fitness 42:45, 2002.

Jackson, LE: Understanding, eliciting and negotiating clients' multicultural health beliefs. Nurse Pract 18:30, 1993.

Jacobs, DO: Bioelectrical impedance analysis: Implications for clinical practice. Nutr Clin Pract 12:204, 1997.

Keys, A, et al: Indices of relative weight and obesity. J Chronic Dis 25:329, 1972.

Kovacevich, DS, et al: Nutrition risk classification: A reproducible and valid tool for nurses. Nutr Clin Pract 12:20, 1997.

Krauss, RM, et al: AHA Dietary Guidelines, Circulation 102:2284, 2000.

Krosnick, A: The diabetes and obesity epidemic among the Pima Indians. N J Med 97:31, 2000.

Landig, J et al: Validation and comparison of two computerized methods of obtaining a diet history. Clin Nutr 17:113, 1998.

Leininger, M: The theory of culture care diversity and universality. In Leininger, M (ed): Culture Care Diversity and Universality: A Theory of Nursing. National League for Nursing Press, New York, 1991.

Levine, MA, Ortmann, D, and Lunney, M: Nursing diagnosis in crosscultural settings. Nurs Diag 5:158, 172, 1994.

Loria, CM, et al: Macronutrient intakes among adult Hispanics: A comparison of Mexican Americans, Cuban Americans, and mainland Puerto Ricans. Am J Public Health 85:684, 1995.

Mason, M, Wenberg, BG, and Welsch, PK: The Dynamics of Clinical Dietetics. John Wiley & Sons, New York, 1982.

Metropolitan Life Insurance Company Height-Weight Table. Metropolitan Life, Warwick, RI, 1983.

Mokuau, N, Hughes, CK, and Tsark, JAU: Heart disease and associated risk factors among Hawaiians: Culturally responsive strategies. Health Soc Work 20:46, 1995.

Moore, MC: Pocket Guide, Nutrition and Diet Therapy. Mosby, St. Louis, 1993.

Moorhead, S, Johnson, M, and Maas, M (eds): Nursing Outcomes Classification (NOC), ed 3. Mosby, St. Louis, 2004.

NANDA International: NANDA Nursing Diagnoses: Definitions and Classification, 2003–2004. NANDA International, Philadelphia, 2003.

National Academy of Sciences: Dietary Reference Intakes. Nutr Rev 55:319, 1997a.

National Academy of Sciences: Origin and framework of the development of Dietary Reference Intakes. Nutr Rev 55:332, 1997b.

National Academy of Sciences: Uses of Dietary Reference Intakes. Nutr Rev 55:327, 1997c.

Nelson, M, et al: Problem of changing food habits: Reaching disadvantaged families through their own food cultures. In Karp, RJ (ed): Malnourished Children in the United States. Springer, New York, 1993.

Neilson, SJ and Popkin, BM: Patterns and trends in food portion sizes, 1997–1998. JAMA 289:450, 2003.

Purnell, LD, and Paulanka, BJ: Transcultural Health Care, ed 2. FA Davis, Philadelphia, 2003.

Peeters, A, et al: Obesity in adulthood and its consequences for life expectancy: A life table analysis. Ann Intern Med 138:24, 2003.

Rassin, DK, et al: Acculturation and the initiation of breastfeeding. J Clin Epidemiol 47:739, 1994.

Shils, ME, et al (eds): Modern Nutrition in Health and Disease, ed 9. Williams & Wilkins, Baltimore, 1999.

Shintani, TT, et al: Obesity and cardiovascular risk intervention through the ad libitum feeding of traditional Hawaiian diet. Am J Clin Nutr 53:1647S, 1991.

Sun, G, et al: Comparison of multifrequency bioelectrical impedance analysis with dual-energy X-ray absorptiometry for assessment of percentage body fat in a large, healthy population. Am J Clin Nutr 81:74, 2005.

Thoroddsen, A and Thorsteinsson, HS: Nursing diagnosis taxonomy across the Atlantic Ocean: Congruence between nurses' charting and the NANDA taxonomy. J Adv Nurs 37:372, 2002.

United States Department of Agriculture: Dietary guidelines for Americans, ed 5. Washington, DC, 2000. Accessed 6/26/2000 at http://www.usda.gov.cupp/Dietgd.pdf.

United States Department of Agriculture and Center for Nutrition Policy and Promotion: Interactive Healthy Eating Index, Washington, DC. Accessed 3/25/2005 at http://209.48.219.53.

Wuest, J: Removing the shackles: A feminist critique of noncompliance. Nurs Outlook 41:217, 1993.

Zhu, S, et al: Race-ethnicity-specific waist circumference cutoffs for identifying cardiovascular risk factors. Am J Clin Nutr 81:409, 2005.

CHAPTER 3

Carbohydrates

Learning Objectives

After completing this chapter, the student should be able to:

1. Describe the types of carbohydrates, identify food sources of each, and indicate the body's needs for them.
2. List the major functions of carbohydrates and methods by which the body stores them.
3. Discuss dietary fiber and list its functions; identify dietary food sources.
4. Describe the relationship between carbohydrates and dental health.
5. List the carbohydrate content (in grams) of each appropriate exchange list.
6. Discuss dietary recommendations relating to fiber, added sugar, and total carbohydrate intake.

Carbohydrates, fats, and proteins all meet the body's basic energy needs. Carbohydrates, however, are recommended as the major source of energy because they break down rapidly and are therefore readily available for use by the body. This chapter discusses the body's use of carbohydrates and the way carbohydrates relate to the other energy nutrients.

Green plants manufacture carbohydrates during a complex process called **photosynthesis.** In this process, carbon dioxide from the air and water from the soil are transformed into sugars and **starches.** Sunlight and the green pigment **chlorophyll** are necessary for this conversion. All the food we eat is a product of photosynthesis. If this process did not occur, the whole food chain would collapse and life would cease to exist. Figure 3–1 illustrates this amazing process.

Based on their chemical structure, carbohydrates are divided into two major groups: sugars and starches. Sugars have a simple structure, whereas starches are more complex. Therefore, sugars are often called **simple carbohydrates** and starches **complex carbohydrates.** The abbreviation for carbohydrate is CHO.

Composition of Carbohydrates

Understanding the composition of carbohydrates involves understanding three structures: molecule, element, and atom. A **molecule** is the smallest quantity into which a substance may be divided without loss of its characteristics. For example, water's formula is H_2O. If the hydrogen atoms are pulled apart from the oxygen atom, the resulting products are hydrogen and oxygen, which bear no resemblance to water. Molecules are made of elements. In the case of water, H_2O, the elements are hydrogen and oxygen. An **element** is a substance that cannot be separated into simpler parts by ordinary means. An **atom** is the smallest particle of an element that retains its physical characteristics.

Classification of Carbohydrates

Carbohydrates are composed of the elements carbon, hydrogen, and oxygen. The ratio of hydrogen to oxygen is the same as that for water, two parts of hydrogen to one

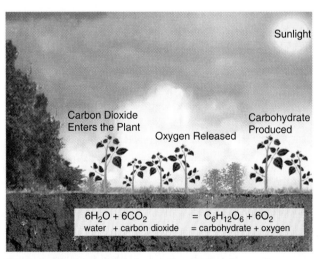

Figure **3–1** Photosynthesis is a vital process that transforms carbon dioxide and water into carbohydrates.

part of oxygen. The simplest carbohydrates have the formula $C_6H_{12}O_6$. Carbohydrates in general are frequently abbreviated CHO.

Simple carbohydrates, sugars, include monosaccharides and disaccharides (*mono* means one, *di* means two, and *saccharide* means sweet). Starches are also called polysaccharides.

Simple Carbohydrates

A **monosaccharide** contains one molecule of $C_6H_{12}O_6$. A **disaccharide** is composed of two molecules of $C_6H_{12}O_6$ joined together (minus one unit of H_2O). When the body joins two molecules of monosaccharides together, a molecule of water is released in the process. Both monosaccharides and disaccharides are classified as simple carbohydrates.

Monosaccharides

The monosaccharides are the building blocks of all other carbohydrates. The three monosaccharides of importance in human nutrition are *glucose, fructose,* and *galactose.* Note the *ose* ending in the name of each of these sugars. All monosaccharides and disaccharides end with the letters *ose.*

GLUCOSE

The monosaccharide glucose in the body is commonly called the blood sugar. It is the major form of sugar in the blood. Normal **fasting blood sugar (FBS)** is 70 to 100 milligrams per 100 milliliters of serum or plasma. Regardless of the form of sugar consumed, the body readily converts it to glucose. Glucose is present in only small amounts in some fruits and vegetables and is moderately sweet.

Another name for glucose is **dextrose.** Clients in healthcare facilities often receive intravenous feedings. **Intravenous** simply means within or into a vein. The most common intravenous feeding is D_5W, used primarily to deliver fluids to the client.

FRUCTOSE

Found in fruits and honey, fructose is commonly referred to as the honey sugar. It is the sweetest of all the monosaccharides. Relatively new on the list of food sweeteners is **high-fructose corn syrup (HFCS).** Fructose is used extensively in soft drinks, canned foods, and various other processed foods. The human body readily converts fructose to glucose after ingestion.

GALACTOSE

The monosaccharide galactose comes mainly from the breakdown of the milk sugar lactose. Yogurt and unaged cheese may contain free galactose. It is the least sweet of all the monosaccharides. The body converts galactose into glucose after ingestion.

Disaccharides

When two monosaccharides are linked together, a disaccharide is formed. The three disaccharides of importance are sucrose, lactose, and maltose.

Clinical Calculation 3–1

Converting Grams of Sugar into Teaspoons of Sugar

An added sugar intake of 60 grams doesn't mean much to average American consumers, because most Americans are not familiar with the metric system. Food labels use the metric system to list the nutritional content of a product. To enhance understanding of label reading, let's convert grams of sugar into teaspoons. One teaspoon of sugar contains 4 grams of CHO. Therefore, 60 grams of sugar is equal to 15 teaspoons.

SUCROSE

The most prevalent disaccharide, sucrose, is ordinary white table sugar made commercially from sugar beets and sugar cane. Brown, granulated, and powdered sugars are all forms of sucrose. Sucrose is also found in molasses, maple syrup, and fruits. The two monosaccharides joined together to form sucrose are glucose and fructose. The average U.S. sugar utilization per capita on the basis of food disappearance data was 120 pounds per year in 1970, and it reached 150 pounds in 1995. This is almost 1/2 pound per person per day (Howard and Wylie-Rosett, 2002). One half pound of sugar per day is approximately 60 grams. Another study showed the intake of added sugar may be as high as 82 grams or 20 1/2 teaspoons per day (Guthrie and Morton, 2000). Data gathered by researchers indicate that soft drinks and sugars added at the table are two of the top four carbohydrate sources for U.S. adults.

The Food and Nutrition Board of the National Academy of Sciences suggests a *maximum* intake of added sugar not to exceed 25% of calorie intake. Distinguished from natural sugars such as lactose found in milk and fructose found in fruits, added sugars are those incorporated into foods and beverages during production. Major sources include candy, soft drinks, fruit drinks, pastries, and other sweets. Food and Nutrition Board Institute of Medicine, Food and Nutrition Board, 2002).

LACTOSE

Because it occurs naturally only in milk, lactose is commonly referred to as the milk sugar. Lactose is the least sweet of the disaccharides. The two monosaccharides that make up lactose are glucose and galactose.

FOOD LABELS

Information on the amount of sugar in a food product can be found on the product's food label. The total amount of sugar in grams can be found on the Nutrition Facts portion of the label. The federal government regulates the use of terms such as *sugar free* and *reduced sugar* or *less sugar.* Terms such as these can be located anywhere on the food's label. Box 3–1 is a list of standards or definitions for legally defined label descriptors:

Box 3–1

TERM	STANDARD
Sugar-free	Contains less than 1/2 gram of sugars per serving
Reduced sugar or less sugar	At least 25% less sugar or sugars per serving than a standard serving size of a traditional food
No added sugar or without added sugar	No sugars added during processing or packing, including ingredients that contain sugar, such as juice or dry fruit
Low sugar	May not be used as a claim on a food label

MALTOSE

The disaccharide maltose is produced when starches are broken down by the body into simpler units. This disaccharide is present in malt, malt products, beer, some infant formulas, and sprouting seeds. Maltose consists of two units of glucose joined together.

SUGAR ALCOHOLS

Food labels use the term *sugar alcohols.* Sugar alcohols have various names, such as sugar replacers, polyols, nutritive sweeteners, and bulk sweeteners. Lactitol, maltitol, isomalt, sorbitol, xylitol, and mannitol are all sugar alcohols (also called sugar replacers) and currently are approved for use in the United States. Sugar alcohols are commonly used on a one-for-one replacement basis for sugars in recipes. For example, 1 cup of sugar would be replaced with 1 cup of isomalt in a recipe. Sugar alcohols add not only sweetness but also bulk to recipes. Sugar alcohols have the following characteristics:

- Generally do not promote tooth decay
- Commonly have a cooling effect on the tongue
- Are slowly and incompletely absorbed from the intestine into the blood
- May have a laxative effect for some people if consumed in excess

Intense sweeteners, unlike sugar replacers, do not add bulk or volume to a food product; they only add sweetness. They are 150 to 500 times as sweet as sugar and are mostly artificial/synthetic. Intense sweetener is still relatively new terminology for nonnutritive sweeteners or artificial sweeteners such as aspartame, saccharin, and sucralose. See Table 3–1.

Complex Carbohydrates (Polysaccharides)

More chemically complex carbohydrates are called **polysaccharides.** *Poly* means many, and polysaccharides are many molecules of $C_6H_{12}O_6$ joined together with many molecules of water released. Polysaccharides can be composed of various numbers of monosaccharides and disaccharides. The three types of complex carbohydrates of nutritional importance are starch, glycogen, and fiber. Table 3–2 summarizes the composition of carbohydrates.

Starch

Starch, the major source of carbohydrate in the diet, is found primarily in grains, cereals, breads, pasta, starchy vegetables, and legumes. Legumes include dried peas and beans such as black beans, pinto beans, kidney beans, navy beans, soybeans, black-eyed peas, split green or yellow peas, chick peas (garbanzo beans), and lentils. Strictly speaking, all starches yield simple sugars on digestion;

Table 3–1   Artificial Sweeteners

ARTIFICIAL SWEETENER	TRADE NAME	COMMENTS
Aspartame	Nutrasweet	Used in sweetened products such as puddings, gelatins, frozen desserts, yogurt, hot cocoa mixes, powdered soft drinks, carbonated beverages, teas, breath mints, chewing gums, some vitamins, and cold preparations. Also used as a tabletop sweetener. Reviewed by such regulatory agencies as the Centers for Disease Control (CDC) and Food and Drug Administration (FDA) and found to be safe. Should not be used by individuals with a rare genetic disease called phenylketonuria (PKU). www.aspartame.org
Saccharin	Equal	Artificial sweetener.
	Sweet N Low	Carbonated beverages, toothpaste, cold remedies, dietetic puddings, cakes, cookies.
	Sugar Twin	Saccharin was banned in Canada in 1977. The U.S. Food and Drug Administration also proposed a ban on saccharin, but Congress passed a moratorium on the ban. Although high doses of saccharin were shown to cause bladder cancer in male rats, numerous human studies have shown no association between saccharin and cancer at human levels of consumption.
Sucralose	Splenda	Only noncaloric sweetener made from sugar. Approved for use by the Food and Drug Administration (FDA).
Stevia	Stevia	Natural alternative sweetener that is classified as an herb. It is sold as a dietary supplement. Stevia has not gone through the FDA approval process as a sweetener.

Table 3–2   **Composition of Carbohydrates**

Elements	C (carbon)
	H (hydrogen)
	O (oxygen)
Molecule	$C_6H_{12}O_6$
Monosaccharide (simple)	One unit of $C_6H_{12}O_6$
Disaccharide (simple)	Two units of $C_6H_{12}O_6$ minus one unit of H_2O
Polysaccharide (complex)	Many units of $C_6H_{12}O_6$ minus many units of H_2O

starchy foods are mostly low in fat and high in carbohydrates, and some starchy foods have the advantage of containing much fiber (discussed in a later section).

Glycogen

The polysaccharide **glycogen** is commonly called the *animal starch,* because it is found in liver and muscle tissue. Although it is not a significant source of dietary carbohydrate, glycogen is crucial to the function of the human body. Glycogen is continually broken down and built up to provide immediate fuel for muscle action. Glycogen represents the body's carbohydrate stores. Liver glycogen helps sustain blood glucose levels during sleep.

The typical human body has an available store of glucose in the form of glycogen for about 1 day's energy needs. Because the body's ability to store carbohydrate in the form of glycogen is limited, an adequate intake of dietary carbohydrates is essential. When glycogen is stored, water is also stored. Each glycogen molecule attracts many molecules of water because of the way the elements are arranged. With glycogen stores completely filled, the average person weighs about 4 pounds more than when glycogen stores are empty.

DIETARY FIBER

Dietary fiber refers to foods, mostly from plants, that the human body cannot break down to digest. Fiber is eliminated from the body in the intestinal waste. Sometimes called roughage or bulk, fiber adds almost no fuel or energy value to the diet, but it does add volume. Bulk or volume fills the stomach, and most experts believe a full stomach contributes to a feeling of satisfaction after eating. When satisfied, further eating ceases.

The recommended daily adequate intake (AI) for fiber is as follows (Food and Nutrition Board, 2002):

- Men 50 years and younger: 38 grams
- Women 50 years and younger: 25 grams
- Men over 50: 30 grams
- Women over 50: 21 grams

In the United States, the average person consumes less than the recommended amount of dietary fiber and few people consume even the recommended levels. Recent research indicates the average fiber intake for U.S. adults is only 15 grams per day (USDA, 2005).

Eating too much fiber can also cause problems. Much evidence suggests that eating more than 50 grams of fiber a day can interfere with mineral absorption, which can lead to problems such as anemia and osteoporosis. The current recommendation is that a desirable fiber intake be achieved by healthy people *not* by adding fiber concentrates (such as psyllium) to the diet but by the consumption of fruits, vegetables, legumes, and whole-grain cereals, because these excellent sources of fiber also provide minerals, vitamins, and phytochemicals.

Fiber is classified as either soluble or insoluble. **Solubility** is the ability of one substance to dissolve in another. For example, oil does not dissolve in water, so oil is insoluble in water. Insoluble fiber does not dissolve in water, whereas soluble fiber does. Soluble and insoluble fiber react differently in the body and are needed for different reasons.

SOLUBLE FIBER

Sources of soluble fibers include beans, oatmeal, barley, broccoli, and citrus fruits; oat bran is a particularly good source of soluble fiber. Soluble fiber dissolves in water and thickens to form gels. The reported health benefits of soluble fibers include reduced cholesterol levels, regulated blood sugar levels, and weight loss (by helping dieters control their appetites).

INSOLUBLE FIBER

Examples of sources of insoluble fibers include the woody or structural parts of plants, such as fruit and vegetable skins, and the outer coating (bran) of wheat kernels. Insoluble fibers have been reported to promote regularity of bowel movements and reduce the risk of diverticular disease and some forms of cancer. Table 3–3 lists the food sources of each type of fiber and their reported health benefits.

Functions of Carbohydrates

Carbohydrates play the following roles in the body:

1. Provide fuel
2. Spare body protein
3. Help prevent ketosis
4. Enhance learning and memory processes

Provide Fuel

Carbohydrates, fats, and proteins provide the body's energy needs. **Energy** is the capacity to do work. To understand the concept of energy, it may be helpful to think of the human body as a machine. Just as gasoline is a car's fuel, so carbohydrates, proteins, and fats are the human machine's fuel. Without fuel, a car ceases to operate. Without fuel sources over an extended period of time, death by starvation results for the human machine. Just as you cannot efficiently substitute something other than gasoline for a car (with a gasoline engine), you cannot efficiently substitute something other than carbohydrate, protein, and fat for fuel in your body.

The brain, other nervous tissue, and the lungs use carbohydrate as a primary source of fuel. Because the brain cannot store carbohydrate, it must have an uninterrupted,

Table 3–3 **Food Sources and Reported Benefits of Fiber**

	INSOLUBLE FIBER	SOLUBLE FIBER
Solubility	Does not dissolve in water	Dissolves in water
Food Sources	Wheat bran	Oatmeal
	Corn bran	Oat bran, barley
	Vegetables	Some fruits such as apples, oranges
	Nuts	
	Fruit skins	Broccoli
	Some dry beans*	Some dry beans*
Reported Benefit	Promotes regularity	May help reduce cholesterol levels
	May help reduce risk of some forms of cancer	May assist in regulating blood sugar levels
	May reduce risk of diverticular disease	May promote weight loss by increasing **satiety**†

*Current laboratory methods to assay soluble fiber content of individual foods are imprecise. This is the subject of much research.
†Satiety is defined as the sensation of fullness after eating.

ongoing source of carbohydrate. This has many clinical applications that will be discussed throughout the book.

Spare Body Protein

When we eat an inadequate amount of carbohydrates, our bodies suffer. We must have a continuous supply of glucose for all cells to function, particularly those of the central nervous system. Remember that our glycogen stores are limited. But the body can convert protein to glucose. Therefore, the body will break down internal protein stores (muscle tissue) before fat stores if carbohydrate intake is inadequate. An adequate supply of dietary carbohydrates spares body protein stores from being partially converted into glucose and allows protein to be used for growth and repair of body tissue. This principle has important ramifications for human nutrition, which will be discussed throughout the text.

Help Prevent Ketosis

A balanced intake of energy nutrients is vital. If a person's carbohydrate intake is too low, the body will break down both stored fat and internal protein stores to meet its fuel needs. The human machine cannot optimally handle the excessive breakdown of stored body fat because it lacks the necessary equipment. As a result, partially broken-down fats accumulate in the blood in the form of ketones, and the person is said to be in a state of **ketosis.** Survival is possible on a very low carbohydrate diet, but good health is not.

Fatigue, nausea, and lack of appetite are some of the undesirable consequences of ketosis. Coma and death have occurred in severe cases. The presence of ketosis is easily determined by testing for the presence of acetone or diacetic acid in the urine. **Acetone** and **diacetic acid** are ketone bodies. A minimum of 50 to 100 grams of carbohydrate each day is usually enough to prevent ketosis.

Enhance Learning and Memory

Considerable evidence exists that blood glucose concentrations regulate neural and behavioral processes. Glucose enhances learning and memory in humans throughout the life cycle. Findings across many laboratories demonstrate that glucose consumed early in the morning facilitates specific forms of cognitive function, particularly verbal

declaration memory (intentional memory for words and narratives). Children score higher on tests when they eat breakfast. Improvements include both enhanced memory and retrieval of information from long-term memory. Glucose enhanced cognitive function in elderly test subjects who had some mild age-related memory deficits (Korol, 2002).

Consumption Patterns

Most of the world's population subsists primarily on carbohydrates. Foods rich in carbohydrates are easily grown in most climates, are low in cost, and are easily stored. Many carbohydrates do not require refrigeration or electricity, and their shelf life may stretch to years. In Asia, where rice is a dietary staple, carbohydrates provide as much as 80 percent of the fuel in the diet.

In 1909, Americans obtained about 66 percent of their total carbohydrate intake from starches such as corn, potatoes, wheat, and beans and about 33 percent from sugars such as table sugar, maple sugar, molasses, jelly, and jam. By 1980, sugars furnished more than 50 percent of the carbohydrates in the food supply. Between 1994 and 1996, Americans aged 2 years and older consumed 20 1/2 teaspoons per day of added sugar (Guthrie and Morton, 2000). The largest source of added sweeteners was regular soft drinks, which accounted for one-third of intake.

The most recent nationwide data on dietary intakes are based on the United States Department of Agriculture's (USDA) Continuing Survey of Food Intake by individuals. Findings included (USDA, 2005):

- U.S. adults averaged only one serving per day of whole grains
- 2% of adults consumed no whole grain
- Consumption of milk decreased by 16% since the late 1970s, whereas consumption of carbonated soft drinks increased by 16%
- Only 54% of individuals ate fruit on a given day

Health Benefits of Carbohydrates

The kinds of carbohydrates eaten are an important health consideration. Epidemiological data support the association between a high intake of vegetables and fruits and low risk of chronic disease (Lampe, 1999). Legumes are low in fat and are excellent sources of protein, dietary fat, micronutrients, and phytochemicals (Messina, 1999). Numerous studies have linked regular consumption of whole grains with a lower risk of certain cancers and heart disease. Many nutrition experts attribute these health benefits to both the fiber contained in whole grains and the phytochemicals.

Research has been done to study the relationship between sugar and chronic disease and other health problems. Long-term data relating sugar consumption to heart disease are unavailable. However, short-term studies show excessive sugar consumption may accelerate heart disease and worsen diabetes control (Howard and Wylie-Rosett, 2002). Sugary foods also often displace other more nutritious foods in the diet. For example, carbonated beverages are consumed instead of milk and fruit juices. Also, as with any food or beverage, too much sugar can lead to undesirable weight gain. On the other hand, sugar can be used to make nutritious foods more appealing and increase a person's desire to eat them.

Several studies have shown a relationship between carbohydrate consumption and dental caries. **Dental caries** is the gradual decay of the teeth. A dental cavity is a hole in a tooth caused by dental caries. Dental caries results from the interaction of four factors: a genetically susceptible tooth, **bacteria,** carbohydrate, and time. All four must occur simultaneously for a cavity to form, as Figure 3–2 illustrates.

Genetic Susceptibility

Genetic susceptibility is an individual's likelihood of developing a given trait as determined by heredity. We cannot control our genetic susceptibility for cavities, and bacteria are always present in our mouths and difficult to eliminate. However, we can control the length of time carbohydrate-containing foods are in our mouths and the kinds of carbohydrates we eat.

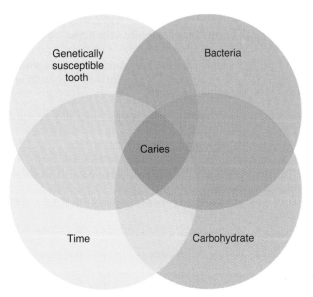

Figure **3–2** Interactions necessary for dental cavity formation.

Risk Factors for Cavity Formation

Bacteria, carbohydrate-containing foods, and the length of time that teeth are exposed to sugars influence cavity formation. Bacteria normally present in the mouth interact with dietary carbohydrates and produce acids. The acids, not the sugar, cause decay. All types of sugars can promote cavity formation, including fructose, glucose, maltose, lactose, and sucrose. A strong relationship exists between the length of time sugars are actually present in the mouth and the development of caries. For example, sticky foods such as caramels and raisins, which adhere to the tooth surface for longer periods, are more likely than other foods to lead to tooth decay in susceptible people. Sipping sweetened beverages continually throughout the day can lead to tooth decay. **Nursing-bottle syndrome** is a dental condition caused by the frequent and prolonged exposure of an infant or young child to liquids containing sugars. Milk, formula, fruit juice, and other sweetened drinks can all cause rampant dental cavities.

Typically, nursing-bottle syndrome occurs when a caretaker habitually puts a baby to bed with a bottle of milk, juice, or other sweetened liquid. During sleep, the flow of saliva decreases, which allows liquids from the nursing bottle to pool around the teeth, undiluted for extended periods. Parents need to be cautioned against this practice.

The main ways to maintain oral health include (Holt, Roberts, and Graham, 2000):

- Reduce consumption, and especially frequency of food and drink containing sugar
- Consume sugar only as part of a meal
- Snacks and drinks should be sugar-free
- Avoid frequent consumption of acidic drinks

Eating Right to Prevent Cavities

Certain foods may help counteract the effects of the acids produced by oral bacteria. Aged cheese (cheddar, Swiss, blue, Monterey jack, Brie, Gouda), as well as processed American cheese, may inhibit tooth decay. Cheese stimulates the production of saliva. Chewing fibrous foods such as apples or celery stimulates the production of generous amounts of saliva. Saliva helps clear the mouth of food and counteracts acid production. Because saliva production is increased during a meal, sugars eaten with a meal are less likely to cause decay than those eaten between meals.

Food Sources

As indicated earlier, carbohydrates fall into two general groups: sugars and starches. All starches contain fiber; however, all starches do not provide equal amounts of fiber.

Sugars

Table sugar contains 4 grams of carbohydrates per teaspoon. When determining a person's sugar consumption, we consider not only the simple sugars such as honey, jam, and jelly but also the sugars present in carbonated beverages, ice cream, sherbet, cakes, pies, cookies, and donuts. Tables of food composition may be used to approximate the actual intake a person may have from combination foods (see Appendix B). The new sugar

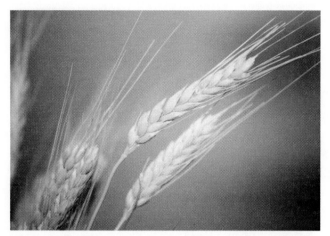

Figure **3–3** The most nutritious parts of wheat germ are the bran and endosperm, which are removed during the milling of grain.

replacers contain on average about 2 grams of carbohydrate per teaspoon.

Starches

Starches are complex carbohydrates and are important sources of fiber and other nutrients. Figure 3–3 illustrates a typical cereal grain. Its main parts are the germ, bran, and endosperm. Most of the nutrients in cereal are in the bran and germ.

Whole grains are more nutritious than refined grains. Products made from the **milling** process are said to be refined. During the milling of grain, the germ and bran from the grain kernel are removed. White flour results from the milling of wheat, white rice from the milling of rice. Oat products are not normally milled. The nutritive value of cereal depends on the amount of bran and germ retained during the milling process. For this reason, the use of whole grains should be encouraged whenever possible. Examples of whole grains include:

- Cornbread made from whole ground cornmeal
- Ground cornmeal
- Cracked wheat bread
- Oatmeal and oatmeal bread
- Pumpernickel bread
- Rye bread
- Whole-wheat bread
- Breads made from bran
- Barley
- Graham crackers

Enrichment is the process of adding nutrients that were previously present in a food but that were removed during processing or lost from storage. Nearly all white bread in the United States is enriched with certain B vitamins and iron. Other enriched products include macaroni, noodles, spaghetti, and ready-to-eat cereals. Enriched products are not nutritionally equal to their whole-grain counterparts because not all the nutrients lost during milling are replaced. For example, the fiber lost during milling is not replaced by enrichment. Anyone who prefers not to eat

whole grains should be encouraged at least to select enriched grain products.

Carbohydrate counting is a technique that those who provide health care use to teach clients about both the carbohydrate content of foods and healthful portion sizes. According to a recent study, portion sizes and energy intake have increased markedly between 1977 and 1998 for food consumed at both fast food restaurants and in the home (Nielson and Popkin, 2003). A serving is not the amount commonly eaten but a defined amount of a particular food according to nutrition experts. Because of the large number of defined portion sizes in The American Diabetic and Dietetic Associations Exchange Lists for Menu Planning and the widespread use of this meal-planning system throughout health care, this text uses Exchange Lists. One serving or exchange of milk, fruit, grain, cereal, bread, or starchy vegetable is considered 15 grams of carbohydrate. Figure 3–4 illustrates portion sizes of various food items that contain approximately 15 grams of CHO. Figure 3–5 illustrates the concept that a small bagel contains two exchanges of CHO (30 grams), whereas a large bagel contains four exchanges of CHO (60 grams). Eating too much of any of the energy nutrients can result in an unhealthful weight gain. Perhaps no other concept is more important to understanding nutrition than healthful portion sizes.

Exchange List Values

Exchange lists were introduced in Chapter 2. This section focuses on exchange lists that contain carbohydrates. A complete copy of the exchange lists is included in Appendix A. Exchanges that include carbohydrates are the starch/bread, vegetable, fruit, and milk lists.

Starch/Bread Exchange List

One American Dietetic Association/American Diabetes Association (ADA) exchange of starch contains approximately 15 grams of carbohydrate. For example, each of the food items in Figure 3–4 is equal to one starch exchange. Whole-grain products average about 2 grams of fiber per serving. Some foods are higher in fiber (Table 3–4). As a general rule, 1/2 cup of cooked cereal, grain, or pasta or 1 ounce of a bread product is one starch exchange.

Vegetable Exchange List

Raw and cooked vegetables are also good sources of carbohydrates. Vegetables contain between 2 and 3 grams of

Table 3–4 Selected Starch Exchanges

Bran cereal*	1/2 cup
Cooked cereal	1/2 cup
Ready-to-eat, unsweetened cereal	3/4 cup
Sugar-frosted cereal	1/2 cup
Beans and peas (cooked)*	1/3 cup
Corn, whole kernel	1/2 cup
Potato, baked	1 small (3 ounces)
Whole-wheat bread	1 slice (1 ounce)

General rule: 1/2 cup of cereal, grain, or pasta or 1 oz of a bread product is equal to one starch exchange.
*Higher in fiber.

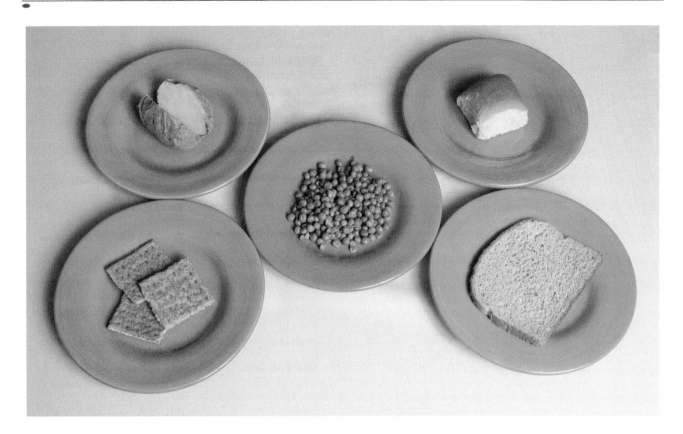

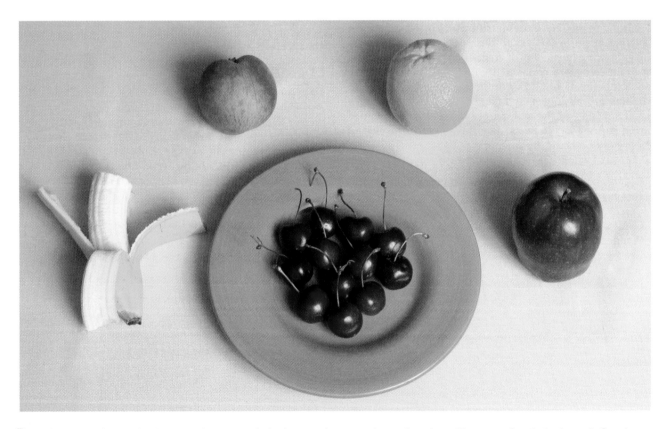

Figure 3–4 Each of these foods is equal to one carbohydrate exchange and contains about 15 grams of carbohydrate. A, Starches; B, Fruits.

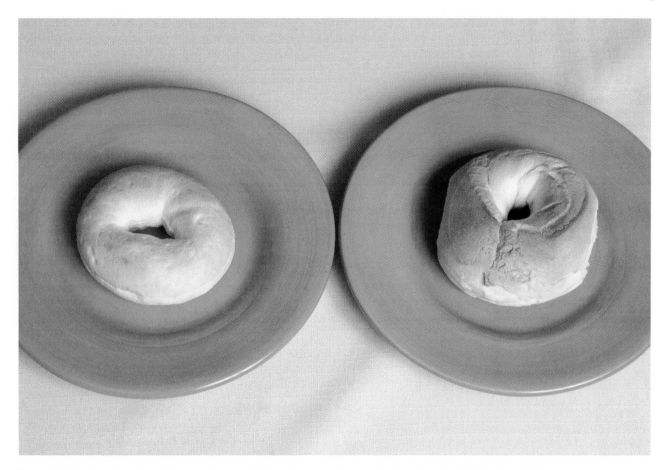

Figure 3–5 The bagel on the left is equal to two CHO exchanges, whereas the bagel on the right is four CHO exchanges.

fiber per serving. One vegetable exchange contains approximately 5 grams of carbohydrate. Table 3–5 defines one vegetable exchange. Vegetables also contribute vitamins and minerals to the diet.

Fruit Exchange List

Fruits are another source of carbohydrates. One ADA exchange of fruit contains approximately 15 grams of carbohydrate (Table 3–6). Many fruits are excellent sources of fiber and contain vitamins and minerals.

Milk Exchange List

Milk, with its lactose content, is an important source of carbohydrates. One cup of milk contains 12 grams of carbohydrates. Skim, whole, and 2 percent milk all contain approximately the same amount of carbohydrates. Eight ounces of plain low-fat yogurt (with added nonfat milk solids), 1/3 cup dry nonfat milk, 1/2 cup evaporated milk, and 1 cup of buttermilk are each equal to one exchange.

Estimating the Fiber Content of Foods

Table 3–7 lists the carbohydrate and approximate fiber content in one serving from each of the carbohydrate-containing exchange lists. Because the fiber content of starches, fruits, and vegetables is highly variable, using the exchange list to approximate a client's fiber intake provides only an estimate. For example, 1/3 cup of All-Bran cereal contains 10 grams of fiber, several more grams than the exchange list value of 2 grams would suggest.

The fiber values given in Table 3–7 may be useful to screen large numbers of clients to identify individuals with

Table 3–5 Vegetable Exchanges

1/2 cup of cooked vegetables or 1/2 cup of vegetable juice or 1 cup of raw vegetables.

Table 3–6 Selected Fruit Exchanges

Apple (raw, 2 in across)	1 apple
Banana (small)	1 banana
Blueberries*	3/4 cup
Grapefruit (medium)	1/2 grapefruit
Nectarine, small	1 nectarine
Strawberries (raw whole)*	1 1/4 cup
Prunes (dried)*	3 medium
Orange (2 1/2 in across)	1 orange
Orange juice	1/2 cup

*Contains 3 g or more of fiber.

Table 3–7 **Carbohydrate and Fiber Content of ADA Exchanges**

	CARBOHYDRATE (G)	FIBER (G)
Milk	12	0
Fruit	15	2*
Starch	15	2*
Vegetable, nonstarchy	5	2–3

*Unless identified as a food with 3 g or more of fiber per serving.

a potential fiber deficiency. If a more accurate estimate of a client's fiber intake is necessary, other techniques include using a computerized nutritional analysis or looking up individual food items in a table of food composition (Appendix C).

Dietary Recommendations

The Food and Nutrition Board of The National Academy of Sciences, Institute of Medicine issued new dietary recommendations that pertain to carbohydrates in 2002. To meet the body's daily energy and nutritional needs while minimizing risk for chronic disease, adults should get 45 to 65 percent of their kcalories from carbohydrates. The committee reasoned that because carbohydrates, fat, and protein all serve as energy sources and can substitute for one another to some extent to meet kcaloric needs, the recommended ranges for consuming energy nutrients should be useful and flexible for dietary planning, hence, the 45 to 65 percent range. The ranges for children are similar to adults in respect to carbohydrates.

Both children and adults should consume at least 130 grams of carbohydrate each day. However, this newly set RDA is based on the minimum amount of carbohydrates needed to produce enough glucose for the brain to function. The report suggests added sugars should comprise no more than 25 percent of total kcalories eaten. This suggested maximum level stems from evidence that people with diets high in added sugars have lower intakes of essential nutrients.

SUMMARY

Carbohydrates are comprised of sugars and starches. All carbohydrates are composed of $C_6H_{12}O_6$ in single units or joined together. The average American's intake of sugars is considered excessive, whereas the intake of starches is considered low. Many Americans would also benefit by increasing their fiber intake through the consumption of more starches, fruits, and vegetables. The consumption of whole-grain starches should be encouraged. Dietary carbohydrates promote tooth decay in susceptible individuals. The ADA Exchange Lists that contain carbohydrates are the starch, vegetable, fruit, and milk lists.

Adverse consequences follow inadequate carbohydrate consumption. The human body must have a continuous source of glucose for proper central nervous system function, but its glycogen stores are limited. Therefore, when there is no carbohydrate in the diet and the body uses protein or fat for a fuel source, the body in effect cannibalizes itself for glucose. Muscle and organ mass is lost in the process. A minimum of 50 to 100 grams of carbohydrate a day is usually adequate to prevent these consequences.

CASE STUDY 3-1

K.L. is a 19-year-old college student. He is interested in bodybuilding and spends much of his time on strength conditioning. He lifts weights or uses the Stairmaster (an aerobic conditioning machine) daily. He is 6 feet tall and weighs 175 lb. For the past 3 weeks, he has been drinking a powdered protein supplement (that contains no carbohydrate) instead of eating the dorm food, which he claims "isn't any good anyway." He also takes a high-stress vitamin and mineral tablet. He arrived at the clinic today with complaints of fatigue, nausea, a lack of appetite, light headedness, and memory loss. His urine tested positive for ketones.

NURSING CARE PLAN

SUBJECTIVE DATA Client has chosen not to eat any foods that contain carbohydrates for approximately 3 weeks.

OBJECTIVE DATA Urine positive for ketones

NURSING DIAGNOSIS NANDA: Imbalanced Nutrition: Less than body requirements (NANDA, 2003, with permission) for CHO, related to knowledge deficit as evidenced by verbal statements that he has not been eating CHO-containing foods and by urine positive for ketones.

DESIRED OUTCOMES EVALUATION CRITERIA	NURSING ACTIONS/INTERVENTIONS	RATIONALE
NOC: Nutritional Status Moorhead, Johnson, and Maas, 2003, with permission)	NIC: Nutrition Management (Dochterman and Bulechek, 2004, with permission)	
Client will state one reason why he needs CHO by the end of the appointment.	Encourage client to consume foods from the Food Pyramid, including milk, starches, fruits, and vegetables. Refer to the dietitian for instruction on normal nutrition and protein needs for athletes.	Explaining why carbohydrates are necessary in the diet may motivate the client to eat carbohydrates. Milk, vegetables, fruits, and starches are all good sources of CHO. The nurse may need to educate the client about dietary sources of carbohydrates.
Schedule the client for a return visit in 1 week. Client will keep a food record until next visit.	On next visit, ask client to demonstrate knowledge gained. (For example, "How many servings of starch, fruits, and vegetables do you need daily?") Test the urine for ketones at the next visit. Review the client's food record and determine if he is eating at least 50 to 100 grams of CHO each day.	The minimum recommended intake to prevent ketosis is 50 to 100 grams of CHO per day.

CTQ CRITICAL THINKING QUESTIONS

1. At the client's next visit, what would you do if the food records showed a recorded carbohydrate intake of only 30 grams for most days? What if the client said, "I don't want to eat any more because I feel better"?

2. At the next client visit, what would you do if the food records showed that the client ate only sugar to increase his carbohydrate intake because "Sugar is a quick energy food"?

CHAPTER REVIEW

1. Which of the following is a disaccharide?
   a. Glucose
   b. Lactose
   c. Fructose
   d. Galactose

2. A healthy adult needs _____ grams of fiber each day.
   a. 5 to 10
   b. 11 to 19
   c. 20 to 35
   d. More than 50

3. Twelve grams of simple carbohydrate is equal to _____ teaspoon(s) of sugar.
   a. 1
   b. 2
   c. 3
   d. 8

4. One slice of bread contains approximately _____ grams of carbohydrates.
   a. 5
   b. 8
   c. 10
   d. 15

5. Which of the following may cause diarrhea?
   a. A medication that contains sorbitol
   b. A lack of dietary fiber
   c. A lack of exercise
   d. An insufficient fluid intake

CLINICAL ANALYSIS

1. Ms. C is concerned about the dangers associated with the consumption of artificial sweeteners and wants to know if they are safe. As a health-care worker, it is appropriate for you to:
   a. Ignore Ms. C's comments because you think she is overly concerned
   b. Assure her that the government wouldn't allow a food or herbal product to be sold if it was hazardous to her health
   c. Explain to her that no food is guaranteed to be 100% safe and it is best to avoid artificial sweeteners if she is not comfortable with these products
   d. Refer her to the local health food store
2. Mr. J claims he is trying to lose weight, and his urinalysis shows that there are ketones in his urine (ketonuria). You should ask him:
   a. When he ate last
   b. How much milk, fruit, and starch he usually eats
   c. What else he usually eats
   d. All of the above
3. Mr. P complains of constipation. As his nurse, you would like to teach him to eat more insoluble fiber to help alleviate his discomfort. You should encourage the intake of:
   a. Wheat and corn bran, nuts, fruit skins, and dried beans
   b. Eggs, cheese, and chicken
   c. Milk, yogurt, and ice cream
   d. Oatmeal, barley, and broccoli

REFERENCES

American Dietetic Association: ADA's Nutrition trends survey result. J Am Diet Assoc 102:7(suppl), 2002.

American Diabetes Association, American Dietetic Association: Exchange lists for meal planning. American Dietetic Association, Alexandria, VA, 2003.

Dochterman, J, and Bulechek, G (eds): Nursing Interventions Classification (NIC), ed 4. Mosby, St. Louis, 2004.

Duyff, LD: American Dietetic Association Complete Food and Nutrition Guide, ed 2. John Wiley & Sons, Hoboken, New Jersey, 2002.

Food and Nutrition Board, National Academy of Science, Institute of Medicine: Dietary Reference Intakes for Energy, Carbohydrate, Fiber, Fat, Fatty Acids, Cholesterol, Protein, and Amino Acids. National Academy Press, Washington, 2002.

Guthrie, JF, and Morton, JF: Food sources of added sweeteners in diets of Americans. J Am Diet Assoc 100:43, 2000.

Holt, R, Roberts, G, and Scully, C: Dental damage, sequelae, and prevention. Ann N Y Acad Sci 959:167, 2002.

Howard, BV, and Wylie-Rosett, J: Sugar and cardiovascular disease: A statement for healthcare professionals from the Committee on Nutrition of the Council on Nutrition, Physical Activity, and Metabolism of the American Heart Association. Circulation 106:523, 2002.

Korol, DL: Enhancing cognitive function across the life span. Ann N Y Acad Sci 959:167, 2002.

Lampe, JW: Health effects of vegetables and fruit: Assessing mechanisms of action in human studies. Am J Clin Nutr 70:439s, 1999.

Moorhead, S, Johnson, M, and Maas, M (eds): Nursing Outcomes Classification (NOC), ed 3. Mosby, St. Louis, 2003.

Messina, MJ: Legumes and soybeans: Overview of their nutritional profiles and health effects. Am J Clin Nutr 70:439s, 1999.

NANDA International: Nursing Diagnosis Association: Definitions and Classifications, 2003–2004. NANDA International, Philadelphia, 2003.

Nielson, SJ, and Popkin, BM: Patterns and trends in food portion sizes, 1977–1998. JAMA 289:450, 2003.

Uhlman, M, and Ridder, K: Nutrition information, questionable serving sizes confuse Americans. The Salt Lake City Tribune, October 20, 2002.

USDA: Continuing survey of food intake by individuals, 1994–1996. Accessed April 2005 at www.usda.gov.

Fats

The descriptive name for fats of all kinds, lipids, is used in clients' medical records. The **lipids** include true fats and oils as well as related fat-like compounds such as **lipoids** and **sterols.** Fats and oils are present in the body and in foods. Fats are typically thought of as solids, whereas oils are regarded as liquids. For example, the body produces oil adjacent to hair. Not as readily apparent to some people is the layer of fat beneath the skin, which is solid. At room temperature, dietary fats such as lard and butter are solid, whereas corn and olive oils are liquid.

Lipids are **insoluble** in water and are greasy to the touch. When two insoluble substances are mixed together, they separate readily, such as vinegar and oil. You can shake the vinegar and oil combination repeatedly, but it will still separate after the agitation stops.

Composition of Fats

Lipids are composed of the elements carbon, hydrogen, and oxygen. These are the same three elements that make up carbohydrates, but the proportion of oxygen to carbon and hydrogen is lower in fats (the implications of which are discussed later). The basic structural unit of a true fat is one molecule of **glycerol** joined to one, two, or three fatty acid molecules. Glycerol is thus the backbone of a fat molecule.

A **fatty acid** is composed of a chain of carbon atoms with hydrogen and a few oxygen atoms attached. The fatty acid chains joined to the glycerol molecule vary in length (depending on the number of carbon atoms present) and composition. The different taste, smell, and physical appearance of each fat results from the variety of fatty acids and their physical arrangement in the fat molecules. Beef tastes, smells, and looks different from chicken mostly because of the difference in fatty acid composition. All fats contain fatty acids.

A fat can have from one to three fatty acids. As you will see, the number of fatty acids a fat contains has important implications for both diet and health.

Monoglycerides and Diglycerides

When a single fatty acid is joined to a glycerol molecule, the resulting fat is called a **monoglyceride.** When two fatty acids are joined to a glycerol molecule, the fat is called a **diglyceride.** The terms monoglyceride and diglyceride are commonly seen on food labels.

Triglycerides

When three fatty acids are joined to a glycerol molecule, a **triglyceride** is formed. Most of the fat found in our diets and in the body is in the form of triglycerides. Excess triglycerides are stored in the specialized **adipose cells** that make up **adipose tissue.** The human body has a virtually unlimited capacity to store fat. Figure 4–1 illustrates the structure of monoglycerides, diglycerides, and triglycerides.

Length of Fatty Acid Chain

Fatty acids vary in the length of their fatty acid chains. The length of each fatty acid chain is determined by the number of carbon atoms present and can vary from 2 to 24 carbons. The length of the fatty acid chain determines how the body transports the fat in the body, since fatty acid

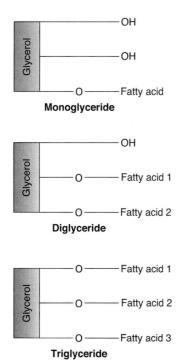

Figure **4–1** Monoglycerides, diglycerides, and triglycerides. A monoglyceride has one fatty acid attached to the glycerol molecule, a diglyceride has two fatty acids attached to the glycerol molecule, and a triglyceride has three fatty acids attached to the glycerol molecule.

chains of short length (<6 carbon atoms) and medium length (8 to 12 carbon atoms) are processed differently than longer chains. This is a fact that has implications for diet in many diseases. For example, in certain diseases of malabsorption, the client cannot tolerate foods with long-chain fatty acids. This problem is discussed in more detail in later chapters.

Degree of Saturation

The terms *saturated, unsaturated, monounsaturated,* and *polyunsaturated* have become household words. *Trans-fatty acid* is a more recent addition to this list. Consumers and clients ask sophisticated questions about fats and expect health-care professionals to define and explain the terminology. Technically, all of these terms refer to the chemical structure of fatty acids, based on the degree or nature of the hydrogen atom saturation.

The degree of saturation of a fatty acid depends on the extent to which hydrogen is joined to the carbon atoms present. A **saturated fatty acid** is filled with as many hydrogen atoms as the carbon atoms can bond with and has no double bonds between carbons. In this case, a **double bond** describes the type of chemical connection between two neighboring carbon atoms, each lacking one hydrogen atom. In an **unsaturated fatty acid,** the carbon atoms are joined together by one or more of such double bonds.

Wellness Tip **4–1** • Read food labels. Some products (those with health claims) will list the amount of saturated, monounsaturated, *trans*-fatty acids, and polyunsaturated fat in the item. Avoid saturated fat and *trans*-fatty acids.

Wherever a double bond occurs, another hydrogen atom could potentially join the chain. In other words, the fatty acid chain is lacking hydrogen atoms and is thus less saturated than a chain that is completely filled. A fatty acid with only one carbon-to-carbon double bond is **monounsaturated.** A fatty acid with more than one carbon-to-carbon bond is **polyunsaturated.** See Figure 4–2 for a structural comparison of saturated, monounsaturated, and polyunsaturated fatty acids.

In addition to the fats in the body, the fats found in foods are combinations of saturated and unsaturated fatty acids. They are designated as follows:

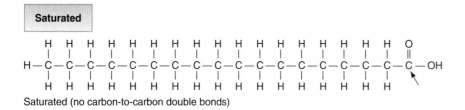

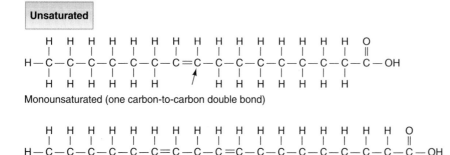

Figure **4–2** Saturated, monounsaturated, and polyunsaturated fatty acids. A saturated fatty acid has no carbon-to-carbon double bonds. A monounsaturated fatty acid has one carbon-to-carbon double bond. A polyunsaturated fatty acid has more than one carbon-to-carbon double bond.

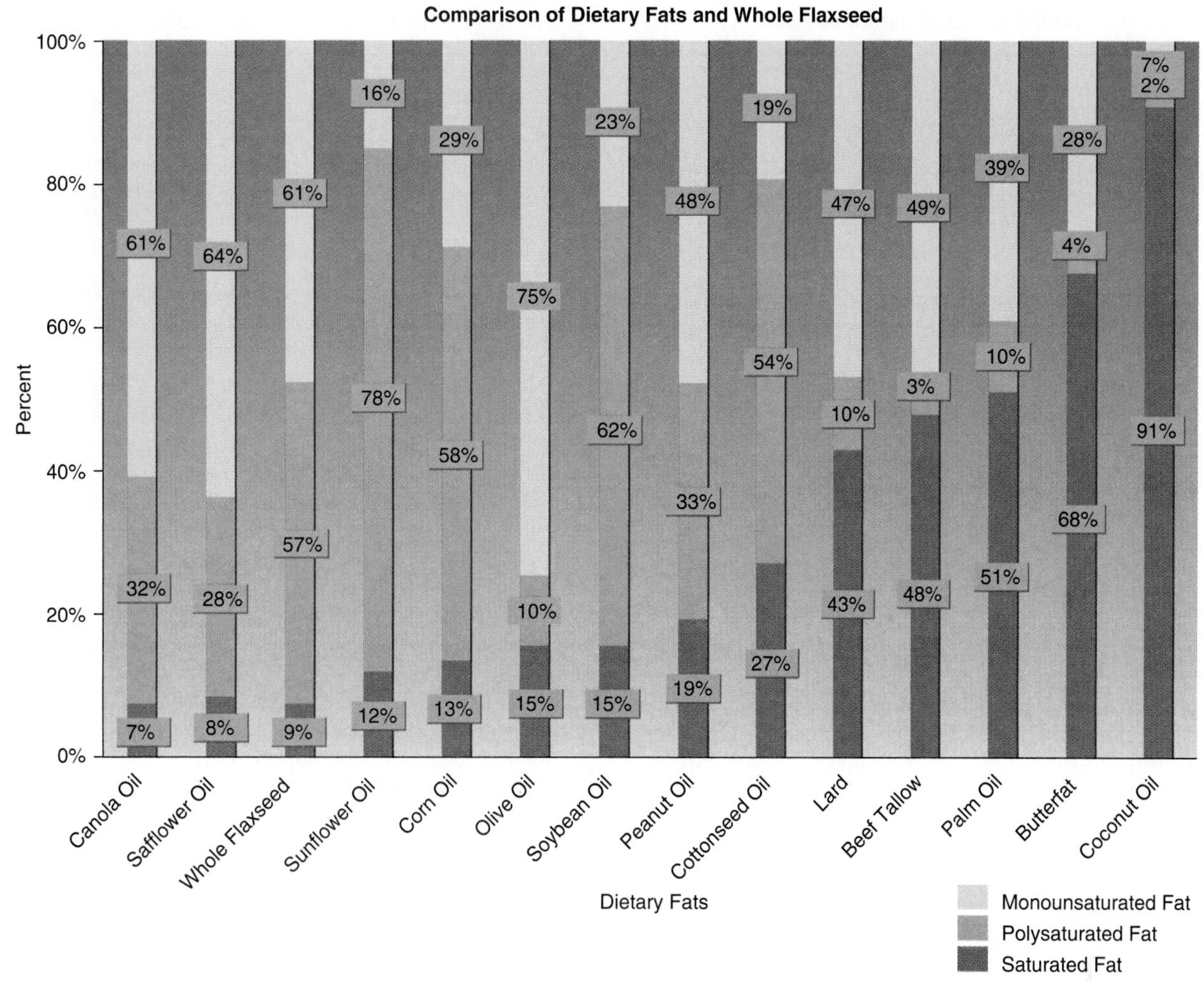

Comparison of Dietary Fats and Whole Flaxseed

Figure **4–3** Comparison of fatty acid composition of edible fats, oils, and flaxseed. The oil with the highest monounsaturated fat content is olive oil. The oil with the lowest saturated fat content is canola.

- Saturated fat: Composed mostly of saturated fatty acids
- Unsaturated fat: Composed mostly of unsaturated fatty acids
- Monounsaturated fat: Composed mostly of monounsaturated fatty acids
- Polyunsaturated fat (PUFA): Composed mostly of polyunsaturated fatty acids
- *Trans*-fatty acids: Composed of partially hydrogenated fatty acids

Figure 4–3 graphs the concept that dietary fats contain mixtures of fatty acids. See Wellness Tip 4–1.

Physical Properties and Food Sources

Saturated Fats

Saturated fats are likely to be solid at room temperature. They are usually found in animal products such as meat, poultry, and whole milk. The exceptions are tropical coconut and palm-kernel oils and cocoa butter, which are vegetable sources of saturated fat. See Tables 4–1

and 4–2 for a more complete list of foods containing saturated fat.

Saturated fats become rancid very slowly because the chemical bond between carbon and hydrogen is very stable. A rancid fat has an offensive odor and taste caused by the partial chemical breakdown of the fat's molecular structure. Consumers usually discard **rancid** foods because of the highly offensive odor. Products made with saturated fats have a longer **shelf life** (the time a product can remain in storage without deterioration) because the fat in the product is more stable. Saturated fats have been targeted for reduction in the average American's diet by health authorities because of their unhealthful effects when ingested in excess of the body's needs.

Unsaturated Fats

Unsaturated fats are likely to be liquid at room temperature and of plant origin; they tend to become rancid more quickly than saturated fats. The double carbon bonds in unsaturated fatty acids are very unstable and therefore easily broken. For this reason, many convenience products have traditionally been made with saturated fats to

Table 4–1 Food Sources of Saturated Fats

Meat products	Visible fat and marbling in beef, pork, and lamb, especially in prime-grade and ground meats, lard, suet, salt pork
Processed meats	Frankfurters Luncheon meats such as bologna, corned beef, liverwurst, pastrami, and salami Bacon and sausage
Poultry and fowl	Chicken and turkey (mostly beneath the skin), Cornish hens, duck, and goose
Whole milk and whole-milk products	Cheeses made with whole milk or cream, condensed milk, ice cream, whole-milk yogurt, all creams (sour, half-and-half, whipped)
Plant products	Coconut oil, palm-kernel oil, cocoa butter
Miscellaneous	Fully hydrogenated shortening and margarine, many cakes, pies, cookies, and mixes

lengthen their shelf life. The food industry is changing this practice; increasingly, more convenience products are made with unsaturated fats. Examples of unsaturated fats are corn, cottonseed, safflower, soybean, and sunflower oils. See Table 4–3 for a more complete list of unsaturated fats.

Hydrogenation

Commercial food processing frequently involves hydrogenation—adding hydrogen to a fat of vegetable origin (unsaturated) to either extend the fat's shelf life or make the fat harder. This process of adding hydrogen to a fat is called **hydrogenation.** If only some of the fat's double bonds are broken by the hydrogenation, the product becomes partially hydrogenated. If all of the double bonds are broken, the product becomes completely hydrogenated. Completely hydrogenated fats are highly saturated.

Table 4–2 Selected Foods High in Cholesterol and/or Saturated Fat

FOOD	AMOUNT	CHOLESTEROL (mg)	SATURATED FAT (mg)
Liver	3 oz	410	2.4
Cream puff	1	228	10.0
Baked custard	1 cup	213	7.0
Egg, hard cooked	1	215	5.0
Waffles, homemade	2	204	8.0
Coconut custard pie	1 piece	183	8.0
Cheesecake	3.25 oz	170	10.0
Shrimp, boiled	6 large	167	0.2
Eggnog, commercial	1 cup	149	11.0
Bread pudding/raisins	1 cup	142	4.5
Whole milk	1 cup	124	5.0
Ground beef, 21 percent fat	3 oz cooked	76	7.0

Table 4–3 Food Sources of Unsaturated Fats

FOODS HIGH IN MONOUNSATURATED FATTY ACIDS	FOODS HIGH IN POLYUNSATURATED FATTY ACIDS
Canola, olive, peanut oils	Corn, cottonseed, mustard seed, safflower, sesame, soybean, and sunflower seed oils
Almonds, avocados, cashews, filberts, olives, and peanuts	Halibut, herring, mackerel, salmon, sardines, fresh tuna, trout, whitefish

rated fats; that is, they have no carbon-to-carbon double bonds. For example, a completely hydrogenated corn oil is closer to lard in saturation than a partially hydrogenated corn oil. All vegetable spreads, such as corn oil margarine, have been hydrogenated to some extent. If these spreads had not been hydrogenated, they would be liquids (except for the saturated tropical oils). Clients are usually advised to avoid products that contain completely hydrogenated fats when the therapeutic goal is to decrease saturated fat intake.

A health consequence of hydrogenation is the formation of **trans-fatty acids.** Trans-fatty acids are produced by the partial hydrogenation of unsaturated vegetable oils. As illustrated in Figure 4–4, a cis configuration double bond between carbon atoms in a fatty acid has a kink or bend. A trans configuration double bond between carbon atoms in a fatty acid is straighter. During hydrogenation, many of the fatty acids are converted from the cis to the trans configuration. There is evidence that the trans configuration is detrimental to health (Dausch, 2002). If the goal is to decrease consumption of trans fatty acids, it is desirable to decrease consumption of hydrogenated foods. Foods that may be high in trans fatty acids include:

- Commercially baked goods
- Fried foods in restaurants
- Hard margarines and shortenings
- Crackers
- Biscuit and some cake mixes
- Some candy
- Animal crackers and cookies
- Frozen waffles and pancakes
- Microwave popcorn

The food industry is currently in the process of reformulating many of these products to decrease their trans-fatty acid content.

Classification

Lipids can be classified according to three criteria: whether the fat is emulsified or nonemulsified, whether the fat is visible or invisible, and whether the fat is simple or compound.

Emulsified or Nonemulsified Fats

Fats can be classified as emulsified or nonemulsified. Fat does not mix with water, because fat is less dense than

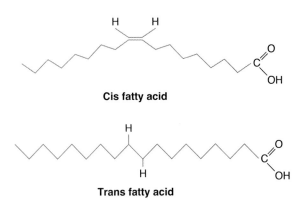

Cis fatty acid

Trans fatty acid

Figure 4–4 A *cis* fatty acid and a *trans* fatty acid. Whenever there is a change from *cis* to *trans* configuration in a fatty acid, the three-dimensional shape of the molecule is altered.

water and will rise to the surface of any water and fat mixture. An **emulsion** is a mixture in which the fat and water molecules are evenly dispersed throughout. An **emulsifier** is an agent that prevents fat from rising to the surface of any fat and water mixture. This is possible because an emulsifier has a molecule with two different kinds of ends. One end attracts one molecule of fat, and the other end attracts one molecule of water. Whole milk is an example of a food that is naturally emulsified. Egg yolk is an example of a natural emulsifier.

Visible or Invisible Fats

Dietary fat is classified as either visible fat or invisible fat according to whether it can or cannot be seen. About 40 percent of dietary fat is ingested as **visible fat.** This 40 percent includes vegetable oils, butter, margarine, lard, mayonnaise, salad dressings, bacon, and cream (USDA, usda.gov/dietaryguidelines/dga2000). People trying to decrease the fat content of their diets should try to eliminate visible fats first.

Invisible fats cannot be identified as readily. These fats are present in egg yolks, poultry, emulsified milk and milk products, the marbling in meat, and many baked goods and snacks. Invisible fat accounts for the remaining 60% of fat in the American diet. Even if clients eliminate all visible forms of fat from their diet, large amounts of invisible fat may be present. Clients should be taught to identify the invisible forms of fat. Food labels and a knowledge of food composition help teach clients the many sources of invisible fat. Exchange lists can be used to increase knowledge of food composition. See Wellness Tip 4–2.

Wellness Tip **4–2** • Serving sizes are important. A 1-tablespoon serving has three times the amount of fat of a 1-teaspoon serving.

Simple or Compound Fats

Fats are also classified as simple or compound. **Simple fats** are lipids that have only fatty acids or a hydroxyl molecule joined to glycerol. Think of the hydroxyl molecule as being just a simple chemical filler. Monoglycerides, diglycerides, and triglycerides are all simple fats.

When a protein replaces one of the fatty acid chains joined to the glycerol molecule, the result is a **compound fat.** This structure is then called a **lipoprotein.** Lipoproteins are composed of fat, protein, and fat-related components. They transport fat in the blood stream. The human body makes four types of lipoproteins: chylomicrons, very low-density lipoproteins (VLDLs), low-density lipoproteins (LDLs), and high-density lipoproteins (HDLs). As is evident by their names, the lipoproteins vary in density. The higher the protein content of the lipoprotein, the greater the density. Lipoproteins also vary in the proportional amounts of fat and protein each contains. The type and amount of lipoproteins in people's blood can protect them or predispose them to heart disease. Lipoproteins are discussed further in Chapter 20 on cardiovascular disease.

Functions of Fats

Lipids are important in the diet and serve many functions in the human body.

Fats in Food

Fats serve several functions in food. Fats in food serve as a fuel source and act as a vehicle for fat-soluble vitamins.

Fuel Source

Fats are the major dietary source of fuel. Because fats have proportionately more carbon and hydrogen and less oxygen than carbohydrates, fats have a greater potential for the release of energy. In practical terms, this means that fats are a concentrated source of fuel or kilocalories. Fats furnish more than twice as many kilocalories, gram for gram, as carbohydrates. Each gram of fat yields 9 kilocalories, so 1 teaspoon of fat, which is equivalent to 5 grams of fat, yields 45 kilocalories. Compare these numbers with those for carbohydrates, each gram of which yields only 4 kilocalories. A teaspoon of sugar contains 4 grams of carbohydrate and therefore yields only 16 kilocalories.

Vehicle for Fat-Soluble Vitamins

In foods, fats act as a vehicle for vitamins A, D, E, and K. In the body, fats assist in the absorption of these fat-soluble vitamins.

Satiety Value

Fats also contribute flavor, satiety value, and palatability to the diet. They supply texture to food, trap and intensify its flavor, and enhance its odor. **Satiety** is defined as a person's feeling of fullness and satisfaction after eating. Fat contributes to the sensation of satisfaction after consumption because it leaves the stomach more slowly than carbohydrates. Consider for a moment the different sensations felt when eating 2 cups of ice cream versus 2 cups of chopped apples. Ice cream has a high fat content, and apples have no fat. The individual may feel full after eating 2 cups of apples but complain of a bloated feeling and a lack of gratification. Satiety is feeling full and completely satisfied and the feeling that enough or too much food has been eaten.

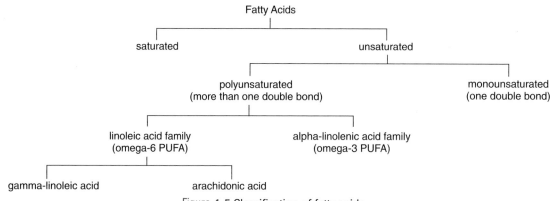

Figure **4–5** Classification of fatty acids.

Sources of Essential Fatty Acids

An **essential nutrient** is one that must be supplied by the diet because the body cannot manufacture it in sufficient amounts to prevent disease. Fat contains the essential fatty acids **linoleic, arachidonic,** and **linolenic.** Linolenic acid is subdivided into two groups, alpha and gamma. Figure 4–5 diagrams the pathways of these fatty acids.

Although the body can manufacture gamma-linoleic (γ-linolenic) acid and arachidonic acid from linoleic acid, all three of these fatty acids are now considered essential. Linoleic is called an omega-6 fatty acid. Omega is the last letter in the Greek alphabet and is used by chemists for naming fatty acid classes by their chemical structure. The six designation means that the first double bond is located six carbons down the chain (counting from the omega end).

Linoleic acid strengthens cell membranes and has a major role in the transport and metabolism of cholesterol. The omega-6 fatty acids together prolong blood-clotting time, hasten fibrolytic activity, and are involved in the development of the brain. **Prostaglandins,** compounds with extensive **hormone**-like actions, require arachidonic acid for synthesis.

Another name for alpha-linolenic fatty acid is omega-3 polyunsaturated fatty acid (PUFA). The omega-3 PUFA has a variety of biological effects that may influence the risk of cardiovascular disease and reduce the risk of incident Alzheimer disease (Morris et al, 2003). Some of this research is discussed further in Chapter 20 on cardiovascular disease.

A deficiency of linoleic acid can occur in infants and hospitalized clients under certain conditions. Linoleic acid deficiency was first observed in infants fed formulas deficient in linoleic acid; drying and flaking of the skin has been observed (Wiese, Hansen, and Adam, 1958). This deficiency was again observed in the early 1970s in hospitalized clients fed exclusively with intravenous fluids containing no fat. The symptoms included scaly skin, hair loss, and impaired wound healing. Linoleic acid deficiency is still seen occasionally with intravenous feeding.

Fats in the Body

Fat serves six major functions in the body, as described in the following sections. Fats in the body supply fuel to most tissues, function as an energy reserve, insulate the body,

support and protect vital organs, lubricate body tissues, insulate the body and nerve fibers, and form an integral part of cell membranes.

Fuel Supply

Fat serves as a fuel that supplies body tissues with needed energy.

Fuel Reserve

Fat also functions as the body's main fuel or energy reserve. Excess kilocalories consumed are stored in specialized cells called **adipose cells.** When an individual does not eat enough food to meet the energy demands of the body, the adipose cells release fat for fuel.

Organ Protection

Fatty tissue cushions and protects vital organs by providing a supportive fat pad that absorbs mechanical shocks. Examples of organs supported by fat are the eyes and kidneys.

Lubrication

Fats also lubricate body tissue. The human body manufactures oil in structures called **sebaceous glands.** Secretions from the sebaceous glands lubricate the skin to retard loss of body water to the outside environment.

Insulation

The subcutaneous layer of fat beneath the skin helps to insulate the body by protecting it from excessive heat or cold. A sheath of fatty tissue surrounding nerve fibers provides insulation to help transmit nerve impulses.

Cell Membrane Structure

Fat serves as an integral part of cell membranes and in this capacity plays a vital role in drug, nutrient, and metabolite transport and provides a barrier against water-soluble substances.

Cholesterol

Cholesterol is not a true fat but belongs to a group called **sterols.** Cholesterol is a component of many of the foods in our diet. In addition, the human body manufactures about

1000 milligrams of cholesterol a day, mainly in the liver. The liver also filters out excess cholesterol and helps to eliminate it from the body.

Functions

Cholesterol has several important functions: it is a component of bile salts that aid digestion; it is an essential component of all cell membranes; and it is found in brain and nerve tissue and in the blood. Cholesterol is necessary for the production of several hormones, including cortisone, adrenaline, estrogen, and testosterone. A **hormone** is a substance produced by the endocrine glands and secreted directly into the bloodstream. Hormones stimulate functional activity of organs and cells or stimulate secretion of other hormones to do so.

Blood Cholesterol Levels

An elevated level of cholesterol in the blood is a major risk factor for coronary artery disease. Lowering blood cholesterol levels reduces the risk of heart attacks due to coronary disease. Cholesterol levels of >200 mg per deciliter (mg/dL) are desirable. Levels between 200 and 239 mg/dL are considered borderline to high risk for coronary heart disease (CHD). A cholesterol level >240 mg/dL places the individual at a high risk for coronary artery disease (Gundy, 2001).

Food Sources

Cholesterol is present in the foods we eat. In fact, many of the products sold in supermarkets are targeted to shoppers interested in controlling their blood cholesterol levels through diet. Cholesterol occurs naturally in all animal foods and is produced only in liver tissue. When we ingest animal products, we also ingest the cholesterol the animal made. For this reason, the American Heart Association advocates the consumption of low-fat or nonfat dairy products, fish, legumes, poultry, and lean meats (Pearson, 2002). Table 4–2 lists selected foods high in cholesterol. Note that one egg supplies about 215 milligrams of cholesterol. Eggs are the major contributor of cholesterol into the average American's diet. The American Heart Association recommends that consumers limit their intake of egg yolks to no more than four per week.

The current thought among most nutrition experts is that an individual's total diet be evaluated for risk prevention. An overall healthy eating pattern that includes fruits, vegetables, and grains is important for risk reduction. No one food, even if it contains cholesterol, is unhealthy if eaten in appropriate amounts.

Fats in the American Diet

Fat available in the national food supply increased from an average of 124 grams per day per person in 1909 to 172 grams per day per person in 1985. There are approximately 5 grams of fat in a teaspoon; therefore, 124 grams converts to 25 teaspoons of fat and 172 grams to 34 1/2 teaspoons. Thus, as of 1985, Americans were eating about 9 1/2 more teaspoons of fat per day than they did in 1909. The Federal government issued the *Dietary Guidelines for Americans* in 1990. A specific recommendation was made in these guidelines to decrease fat intake to 30 percent or less of calories and 10 percent from saturated fat (USDA, 1995). As a percent of

kilocalories eaten, fat intake rose from about 34 percent in the 1930s to a high of 40 percent to 42 percent in the mid-1960s and then steadily declined to 34 percent in 1991. Although this sounds like a healthy change, it is not. Results of recent studies attribute the decreased contribution of fat to total kilocaloric intake to a higher total intake of kilocalories, not a decrease in the absolute intake of fat (Chanmugan, 2003). Many people in the developed world are eating not only too much dietary fat but also too much food.

Calculating the amount of fat as a percentage of total kilocalories is a convenient way of evaluating the level of fat in a food item. Clinical Calculation 4–1 demonstrates how to calculate the percent of kilocalories from fat in a food item. If a food item contains more than 30 percent fat, it should be balanced with other items that contain less fat, such as fruits and vegetables. What is important is the concept of balance. The main objective is to reduce overall fat intake.

Fat Intake a World-Wide Concern

Eating too much energy dense food (dietary fat) is a concern world-wide. The combination of underweight in children and overweight in adults, frequently coexisting in same family, is a new phenomenon in developing countries undergoing nutrition transition (Caballero, 2005). Changes in diet, food availability, and lifestyle are all components of nutrition transition as developing countries modernize. The obesity in adults has been linked to the availability of cheap energy-dense foods (including those from street vendors and fast-food restaurants) that facilitate the consumption of more fat. The introduction of low-cost vegetable oils from industrialized countries greatly increase the amount of fat in the average diet in countries undergoing nutrition transition. Healthier foods, including fruits and vegetables, are usually more expensive and not available to the world's poorest people. Many health experts believe messages should focus on the benefits of increasing fruit and vegetable intake, improving overall diet quality, and increasing physical activity (Doak, 2005). However, education does not address the reality that much of the world's population can not afford a quality diet and more fruits and vegetables.

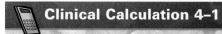

Clinical Calculation 4–1

Percent of Kilocalories From Fat

The following formula can be used to determine the percentage of kilocalories from fat in many packaged foods:

$$\frac{\text{Kilocalories from fat per serving}}{\text{*Kilocalories per serving}} \times 100 = \text{Percent kilocalories from fat}$$

Example: kilocalories from fat = 30
kilocalories per serving = 90

---

*Food labeling regulations require manufacturers to list both the number of kilocalories in a serving and the number of kilocalories from fat.

Table **4–4** **Recommended Range of Fat Intake at Selected Kilocalorie Levels**

KILOCALORIE LEVEL	TOTAL FAT (g)
1200	26–46
1500	33–58
1600	35–62
1800	40–70
2000	44–78
2200	49–85
2400	53–93
2500	55–97

Dietary Recommendations Concerning Fat

The National Academy of Science report on Dietary Reference Intakes for Macronutrients issued new guidelines pertaining to fats in 2002 ((Food and Nutrition Board, Institute of Medicine, 2002). The recommended range for adults is 20 to 35 percent of kilocalories from fat. The range for infants and young children is 25 to 40 percent of kilocalories from fat. Before this, most government health authorities and professional groups recommended that the fat content of the U.S. diet not exceed 30 percent of kilocaloric intake. The rationale for the change is that because carbohydrates, fat, and protein all serve as fuel sources and can substitute for one another to some extent to meet fuel needs, the recommended ranges for consuming these nutrients should, therefore, be useful and flexible for dietary planning (Food and Nutrition Board, Institute of Medicine, 2002). Table 4–4 lists the recommended ranges in grams of fat for various kilocalorie levels.

The report stated that saturated fat and cholesterol provide no known beneficial role in preventing chronic diseases and are not required at any level in the diet. However, the complete elimination of saturated fat and cholesterol from the diet would make it very difficult to meet other nutritional guidelines. Some monounsaturated and polyunsaturated fatty acids are required to provide the essential fatty acids. The recommended intakes for linoleic acid was set at 17 grams per day for men and 12 grams per day for women. Linoleic acid is found in both safflower and corn oil. For alpha-linolenic acid, found in milk and some vegetable oils such as soybean and flaxseed oils, the recommendations are 1.6 and 1.1 grams per day for men and women, respectively. The committee was also asked to address the subject of *trans*-fatty acids. The committee concluded that because *trans*-fatty acids are not essential and provide no known health benefits, there is no safe level for *trans*- fatty acids in the diet. People should eat as little of them as possible while consuming a nutritionally adequate diet.

Dietary Fat Intake and Health

Dietary Fat

A diet that has an appropriate balance of both fat and carbohydrate is important for optimal health. Chronic consumption of either a low-fat high-carbohydrate or a high-fat low-carbohydrate diet may result in the inadequate intake of nutrients (Food and Nutrition Board, 2002). A diet too low in fat not only lacks satiety and palatability but also may lack adequate levels of the essential fatty acids, zinc, and certain B vitamins (Food and Nutrition Board, 2002). Excessive dietary fat has been associated with an increased risk of cardiovascular disease, the development of obesity and diabetes, and an increased risk of certain cancers. Although it is difficult to predict exactly what factors will lead to a disease in a particular individual, scientists have been able to develop a list of factors closely associated with particular diseases in large population groups. These factors are called risks. Saturated fat and *trans*-fatty acids increase the risk of coronary heart disease independent of other factors. High dietary cholesterol also contributes to the development of atherosclerosis and increased coronary heart disease risk in the population, but to a lesser extent.

One of the major issues concerning kilocalorie distribution is whether eating a high-fat diet predisposes one to the development of overweight/obesity. Some experts argue that it is far from proven that eating low-fat foods automatically helps individuals keep off excess weight. The food industry has cut the amount of fat in foods, such as reduced-fat cakes, cookies, ice cream, luncheon meats, salad dressings, and other foods. Yet Americans are still getting heavier. Many experts attribute this weight gain to the substitution of sugar and refined carbohydrates for fat. A healthier choice would be to substitute vegetables and whole grains for fat. All carbohydrates are not equal in the promotion of health benefits.

Some professionals dispute the guidelines of the Food and Nutrition Board. For example, Dr. Dean Ornish in the United States uses a very low-fat diet (<10 grams of fat per day) to treat clients with heart disease (Ornish, 2004). In some Asian countries, people derive only about 10 percent of their kilocalories from fat, whereas in some Mediterranean countries, many people derive up to 44 percent of kilocalories from fat. Some nutritionally vulnerable groups are so obsessed with their fat intake that their food intake is so inadequate that they may suffer from poor nutrition. No one really knows the optimal level of dietary fat. Experts do agree that fat intake cannot be evaluated in isolation. A diet that contains all the essential nutrients and a lifestyle that balances total kilocalorie intake with sufficient activity is essential for optimal health.

Monounsaturated Fats

The health benefits of monounsaturated fatty acids have been a better-understood phenomenon. Most health educators recommend that the average American increase his or her intake of monounsaturated fats intake while decreasing his or her intake of saturated and polyunsaturated fats. There is evidence that individuals with a high intake of monounsaturated fats, a low intake of saturated fats, and a low total fat intake may have a decreased risk of coronary heart disease. Monounsaturated fats are found in canola, olive, and peanut oil. Many nutrition experts advocate the consumption of fats derived from plant sources, such as avocado, olives, nuts, peanut butter, sesame seeds,

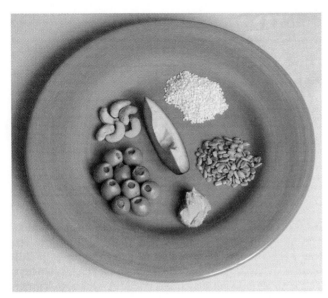

Figure **4–6** Plant sources of fats include avocado, nuts, olives, peanut butter, and some seeds.

and paste, because these foods also contribute fiber, antioxidants, and phytochemicals to the diet. Figure 4–6 illustrates plant sources of fat.

Polyunsaturated Fats

The average healthy American should not increase his or her intake of polyunsaturated fat. At very high levels of polyunsaturated fat intake, animal studies consistently show an increase in colon and mammary cancers. Observations in humans have shown that a polyunsaturated fat intake of less than 10 percent of kilocalories does not increase the population's risk of cancer.

Body Fat

Both the amount of body fat a person carries and its distribution on the body are related to health risk. Many experts feel that the ratio of body fat to total weight is more important than total weight. Healthy ranges for body fat are 15 to 19 percent for men and 18 to 22 percent for women. A high percentage of body fat has been associated with increased risk of disease, even when total body weight is normal.

The location of excess body fat is also important. Excessive fat on the lower body, specifically on the hips and thighs, seems to be less dangerous than excessive fat on the abdomen and upper body, which is associated with a much higher risk of diseases such as cancer, heart disease, and diabetes. The exchange lists in the next section can be used to assist in planning meals low in fat and teach clients about food composition.

Exchange Lists

Exchange lists can be used to learn food composition and portion control and assist in planning meals lower in fat. For example, many people do not know that sugar and fruit contain no fat and oil contains no carbohydrate. Exchange

Table **4–5** Grams of Fat in One Milk Exchange

TYPE	FAT (g)	PERCENT KILOCALORIES FROM FAT
Whole milk	8	48
2 percent (low fat)	5	38
Skim milk	Trace	<1

categories that include fat are the milk, meat, and fat lists. The amount of fat in one exchange of meat or milk varies within the list. Some foods not listed on the exchange lists are also high in fat. Many of these foods may be found in the Nutritive Values of Edible Parts of Food Tables (see Appendix B).

Milk Exchange List

The fat content of milk varies according to the type of milk—whole, 2%, 1%, or skim. Table 4–5 shows the grams of fat and percent of kilocalories from fat in one milk exchange for each kind of milk. Although whole milk and 2% milk contain saturated fat and cholesterol, the protein, carbohydrate, vitamin, and mineral content of whole, 2%, 1%, and skim milk are comparable. Skim milk contains only a trace of fat and is thus a nutritional bargain. See Wellness Tip 4–3.

 4–3 • Choose nonfat or reduced-fat dairy products, such as nonfat milk and yogurt and reduced-fat cheese.

Meat and Meat Substitute Exchange List

The meat exchange list is divided into four subgroups: one very lean meat exchange contains less than 1 gram of fat; one lean meat exchange contains 3 grams of fat; one medium-fat meat exchange contains 5 grams of fat; and one high-fat meat exchange contains 8 grams of fat. Table 4–6 lists selected food examples from each of these meat exchanges.

Many clients have misconceptions about meat. Some clients avoid all red meat because they believe it contains excessive fat. In fact, some beef and pork products are not excessively high in fat. Many consumers are not aware of the lean cuts of beef or pork. Conversely, not all fish and poultry items are lean meat exchanges. Nurses and other health educators can help clients by giving them this kind of information.

Different methods of food preparation can greatly influence the fat content of these foods (Wellness Tip 4–4). Some clients have the misconception that if they eat only lean meats, they can eat as much as they like prepared anyway they like. For example, a 3-ounce breaded fried chicken breast contains more fat than a grilled hamburger patty.

 4–4 • Bake, boil, broil, grill, or roast meat and poultry.

Meat exchanges are usually 1 ounce, but a usual portion is 3 ounces. For example, half a chicken breast is 3 ounces. Table 4–7 totals the fat content of three meat exchanges. Typically, Americans eat large amounts of meats such as

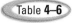

Table 4–6 **Examples of Very Lean, Lean, Medium-Fat, and High-Fat Meat Exchanges**

EACH OF THE FOLLOWING IS ONE VERY LEAN MEAT EXCHANGE AND CONTAINS LESS THAN 1 G OF FAT:

Poultry	Chicken or turkey (white meat, no skin)	1 oz
Fish	Fresh or frozen cod, flounder, haddock	1 oz
Game	Venison	1 oz
Cheese	Nonfat cottage cheese	1/4 cup
	Fat-free cheese	1 oz
Other	Egg whites	2
	Hot dogs with less than 1 g of fat	1 oz
	Egg substitute	1/4 cup

EACH OF THE FOLLOWING IS ONE LEAN MEAT EXCHANGE AND CONTAINS 3 G OF FAT:

Beef	Round, sirloin, or flank steak	1 oz
Fish	Salmon (fresh or frozen)	1 oz
Pork	Tenderloin	1 oz
Veal	Lean chop or roast	1 oz
Poultry	Chicken, dark meat, no skin	1 oz
Game	Goose, no skin	1 oz
Cheese	4.5 percent fat cottage cheese	1/4 cup
	Cheeses with less than 3 g of fat per oz	1 oz
Other	Hot dogs with less than 3 g of fat per oz	1 oz
	Processed lunch meat with less than 3 g of fat per oz	1 oz

EACH OF THE FOLLOWING IS ONE MEDIUM-FAT MEAT EXCHANGE AND CONTAINS 5 G OF FAT:

Beef	Ground beef, corned beef	1 oz
Pork	Chops	1 oz
Poultry	Chicken, dark meat, with skin	1 oz
Fish	Any fried fish product	1 oz
Cheese	Mozzarella	1 oz
Other	Egg (high in cholesterol)	1
	Tofu	1/2 cup

EACH OF THE FOLLOWING IS ONE HIGH-FAT MEAT EXCHANGE AND CONTAINS 8 G OF FAT:

Pork	Spareribs, pork sausage	1 oz
Cheese	All regular cheeses such as cheddar, Swiss, and American	1 oz
Other	Bologna	1 oz
	Knockwurst, bratwurst	1 oz
	Bacon	3 slices

Table 4–7 **Total Fat in Three Meat Exchanges**

MEAT	SUBGROUP	GRAMS OF FAT/ EXCHANGE	GRAMS OF FAT PER SERVING
Cod	Very lean	1	3
Sirloin steak	Lean	3	9
Hamburger patty, broiled*	Medium fat	5	15
Spareribs†	High fat	8	24

*About 4 oz raw
†Boneless

used on meat, poultry, seafood, or game meat products only if the product contains less than 10 grams of fat, less than 4 grams of saturated fat, and less than 95 milligrams of cholesterol per 100-gram serving (3 1/2 ounces). The legal term *lean* thus equals the ADA exchange list definition for a lean meat exchange. The term *extra lean* can be used only if the product contains less than 5 grams of fat, less than 2 grams of saturated fat, and less than 95 milligrams of cholesterol per serving and per 100 grams (3 1/2 ounces).

Clients may choose for many reasons not to eat animal products. Health-care workers should always accommodate their client's religious, ecological, and ethical beliefs and values. Appendix A details the Exchange Lists of the American Dietetic and American Diabetes Associations, which include meat substitutes in detail. Many low-fat meat substitutes are not derived from animals, including dried beans, peas, and lentils. Medium-fat vegetarian meat exchanges include soymilk, tempeh, and tofu. Peanut butter, which contains 8 grams of fat per exchange (2 tbsp), is a high-fat meat exchange.

Fat Exchange List

Each fat exchange provides 5 grams of fat. Figure 4–7 illustrates three fat exchanges. The fat list is subdivided into two groups: unsaturated fats (monounsaturated and

prime rib (from 6-ounce to 16-ounce servings). Teaching clients about meat portion sizes is usually indicated when the goal is to decrease fat intake.

Whether the meat is classified as a very lean, lean, medium-fat, or high-fat meat exchange, the grams of fat in each exchange are calculated based on the following assumptions:

- Visible fat on meat is not consumed.
- Meat is weighed after cooking.
- Meat is cooked by a low-fat method—baked, boiled, broiled, grilled, or roasted (unless otherwise indicated).

Since 1994, food-labeling regulations have become more comprehensive. Regarding the fat content labeling of meat, poultry, seafood, and game meats, two terms now have legal definitions: *lean* and *extra lean*. The term *lean* can be

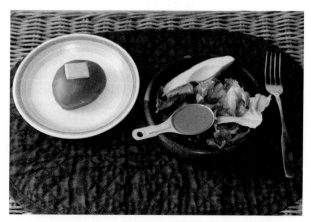

Figure 4–7 One teaspoon of margarine, one tablespoon of regular French dressing, and 1/8 of an avocado are each equal to one fat exchange and contains about 5 grams of fat.

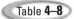 Table **4–8** **Examples of Monounsaturated, Polyunsaturated, and Saturated Fat Exchanges**

EACH OF THE FOLLOWING IS ONE FAT EXCHANGE HIGH IN MONOUNSATURATED FATTY ACIDS AND CONTAINS 5 G OF TOTAL FAT:

Olives	10 large
Canola oil	1 tsp
Peanut butter	2 tsp
Pecans	4 halves

EACH OF THE FOLLOWING IS ONE FAT EXCHANGE HIGH IN POLYUNSATURATED FATTY ACIDS AND CONTAINS 5 G OF TOTAL FAT:

Margarine, stick or tub	1 tsp
Mayo, regular	1 tsp
Corn oil	1 tsp
English walnuts	4 halves

EACH OF THE FOLLOWING IS ONE FAT EXCHANGE HIGH IN SATURATED FATTY ACIDS AND CONTAINS 5 G OF TOTAL FAT:

Bacon	1 slice (20 slices/lb)
Butter, stick	1 tsp
Cream cheese, regular	1 tbsp (1/2 oz)
Cream cheese, reduced-fat	2 tbsp (1 oz)
Sour cream, regular	2 tbsp
Sour cream, reduced-fat	3 tbsp

polyunsaturated) and saturated fats. Table 4–8 lists selected exchanges from each group.

Additional Food Sources of Fat

It is important to advise clients that snack foods, including crackers, cakes, pies, donuts, and cookies, may be high in both total fat and *trans*-fatty acids. Often, potato chips, gravies, cream sauces, soups, pizza, tacos, and spaghetti are high in fat. Microwave popcorn is higher in fat than air-popped popcorn (without added fat).

Consumers who desire low-fat foods need not avoid eating out, but they do need to make wise food choices. It is possible to eat a low-fat meal at a fast-food restaurant. However, many of the specialty fast-food hamburgers are high in fat. A small hamburger is the best burger choice. A small side salad with low-fat dressing is a better low-fat choice than French fries. Skim milk is lower in fat than either a milkshake or whole milk. A grilled chicken breast salad with a fat-free dressing is also a good choice. Consumers who desire low-fat foods need not avoid eating out, but they do need to make wise food choices. This is especially important for people who eat most of their meals in restaurants to understand.

Food labeling regulations spell out what terms may be used to describe the level of fat in a food and how they can be used. *Fat-free* on a food label means that the food contains no more than 0.5 grams of fat per serving. Synonyms for *free* include *without, no,* and *zero. Nonfat* is another synonym for *fat-free.* These terms legally can be used on a food label only if the product contains no amount of—or only trivial or "physiologically inconsequential" amounts of—fat, saturated fat, and cholesterol.

Low-fat is legally defined as a food that contains no more than 3 grams of fat in a serving. *Low saturated fat* is legally defined as a food that contains no more than 1 gram of saturated fat per serving. *Low cholesterol* is defined as a food that contains less than 20 milligrams of cholesterol per serving. Synonyms for *low* include *little, few,* and *low source of.* Additionally, serving sizes listed on food labels are standardized to make nutritional comparisons of similar products easier.

Fat Replacers

Consumers demand food products that are both low in fat and taste good. Fat helps determine texture and taste of food. For example, fat adds the smooth texture in salad dressings, the mouth feel of ice cream, the moist and tender texture of cake, and the consistency of cheese. Fat contributes to satiety. The ideal fat replacers would be able to fulfill all of these roles.

The Food and Drug Administration approved the use of fat replacers in January of 1996. A fat replacer is a nonabsorbable calorie-free fat substitute. Initially these products were approved for use in savory snack foods such as potato chips, corn chips, and crackers. The use of fat replacers such as Olestra in food has been controversial. Olestra is one example of a noncalorie fat replacer. Olestra remains inside the gastrointestinal tract after consumption and exits the body in the fecal material. It is not absorbed.

Some consumer groups object to FDA approval of a food product that may produce abdominal cramping, diarrhea, and loose stools. Any food that is not absorbed and exits the body in fecal material can produce side effects in susceptible people. The FDA studied Olestra extensively before approving its use. Several studies have shown that modest portions of salty foods made with fat replacers are no more likely to result in diarrheas, loose stools, or abdominal cramping than the consumption of snacks with conventional fats (Zorich et al, 1997; Cheskin et al, 1999).

Some fat replacers are made from ingredients commonly found in food. Some are made from chemically synthesized ingredients. They can be protein-based, carbohydrate-based, or fat-based. Each type of fat replacer has uses, advantages, and limitations.

Protein-Based

Using whey (an ingredient in milk), egg, or sometimes corn protein, protein-based fat replacers are made by special cooking and blending processes. Among the uses for protein-based fat replacers are cheese, mayonnaise, butter, salad dressings, sour cream, spreads, dairy products, ice cream, baked goods, and yogurt. Protein-based fat replacers are suitable for use in many food products and are often used with a carbohydrate-based fat replacer in frozen products and baked goods. One limitation of protein-based fat replacers is that they cannot be used in high-temperature applications.

Carbohydrate-Based

Carbohydrate-based fat replacers are made of modified food starch, gums, and grain or fruit-based fiber. They are used in dairy products, sauces, frozen desserts, salad dressings, baked goods, confections, meat products, chewing gum, dry cake, cookie mixes, and frostings. A carbohydrate-based fat reducer retains moisture and adds texture to foods. One limitation of this type of replacer is that it cannot be used for frying.

Fat-Based

A fat-based fat-replacer is made from various fats and oils, like soybean oil, and linked to another compound such as sugar (sucrose). Examples of fat-based fat replacers are Olestra and Salatrim. These products work well in savory and salty snacks, chocolate, confections, and baked products. A fat-based fat replacer can partially or fully replace fats and/or oils in all typical consumer and commercial uses. They provide the same mouth feel and flavor as fat in foods. They can be used in high-temperature cooking and frying. With some fat-based fat replacers, a few individuals may experience digestive changes similar to those people experience when eating many common foods, such as some types of fruit and high-fiber foods. The fat-soluble nutrients, vitamins A, D, E, and K, are not absorbed as readily when eaten with fat replacers.

Plant Stanols and Sterols

Foods that contain plant stanols and sterols have been shown to reduce blood cholesterol levels (USDA, 2000). Plant sterols and stanols work by blocking dietary cholesterol's entrance into the body. Foods that contain plant stanols and sterols include certain margarine spreads and salad dressings. *Benecol, Take Control,* and *Smart Balance* are brand names currently available in grocery stores (Cunningham and Marcason, 2002). *Minute Maid Premium Heart Wise* orange juice, released in November 2003, is the first orange juice to contain plant sterols.

SUMMARY

The group name for all fats is lipids. Lipids include true fats and oils and related fat-like compounds such as lipoids and sterols. Lipids are insoluble in water and greasy to the touch. Hydrogen, oxygen, and carbon are the primary elements in fats. Gram for gram, fats contain more than twice the kilocalories of carbohydrates. All fats contain fatty acids. The number of fatty acids in a fat determines whether it is a monoglyceride, diglyceride, or triglyceride. Most fats in foods and in body stores are triglycerides. The length of a fatty acid chain determines how the body transports a fat. The degree of hydrogen atom saturation or the presence or absence of carbon-to-carbon double bonds determines whether a fatty acid is saturated or unsaturated.

Fats are labeled according to the amount and type of fatty acids they contain as saturated, unsaturated, monounsaturated, or polyunsaturated. The amount of *trans*-fatty acids in a product is also listed on the food label. Fats can also be classified as emulsified or non-emulsified, visible or invisible, and simple or compound. Fats serve many important functions in our diets and our bodies.

A balanced intake of carbohydrate and fat is essential for optimal health. Chronic consumption of a low-fat high-carbohydrate or a high-fat low-carbohydrate diet may result in the inadequate intake of certain essential nutrients (Food and Nutrition Board, 2002). Excess fats in our diets are associated with cardiovascular disease, obesity and diabetes, and some types of cancer. Cholesterol is a fat-like substance that is present in animal food sources and produced by the human body. The National Academies of Science on Dietary Reference Intakes for Macronutrients did not set a tolerable upper limit for saturated fat, *trans*-fatty acids, and cholesterol (Food and Nutrition Board, 2002). Many Americans would benefit from decreasing their intake of cholesterol, *trans*-fatty acids, and saturated fat. The National Academies of Science on Dietary Reference Intakes for Macronutrients recommends that adults consume between 20 and 35 percent their of kilocalories from fat (Food and Nutrition Board, 2002). *Dietary Guidelines for Americans* recommends a saturated fat intake of less than 10 percent of kilocalories and dietary cholesterol intake of less than 300 milligrams per day. The ADA exchanges that contain fat are the milk, meat, and fat lists.

CASE STUDY 4-1

Mr. D had his cholesterol level analyzed during a routine physical examination. The nurse employed in the office of Mr. D's doctor is responsible for the following:

1. Scheduling the patient for follow-up with the physician
2. Developing a nursing care plan that addresses the patient's nursing problem to complement the medical diagnosis

Mike Rod, the nurse, scheduled the appointment. Mr. D was instructed by the nurse to write down all food he consumed for 1 day prior to the appointment. The client was advised to choose a typical day to record his food intake to provide a more accurate analysis of his usual diet. Mr. D arrived on the appropriate day and handed his food record to the nurse for review. Mike calculated the grams of fat in Mr. D's food record based on a combination of ADA exchanges and a table of food composition similar to the table in the Appendix. Mr. D's food record and Mike's calculations are as follows:

11:00 AM Restaurant	
Food	**Grams of Fat**
Salad bar:	
Assorted vegetables and lettuce	0
2 tbsp blue cheese dressing	10 (2 fats)
1 oz shredded cheese	8 (1 high-fat meat)
1 oz diced ham	3 (1 lean meat)
1/2 cup potato salad	7*
Dinner roll	0
1 tsp butter	5 (1 fat)
1 cup clam chowder	7*

7:00 PM Restaurant	
Food	**Grams of Fat**
4 oz hamburger, checked weight	20 (4 medium-fat meats)
1 oz cheese	8 (1 high-fat meat)
1 tbsp mayo	15 (3 fats)
Bun	0
6 onion rings	15*
Tossed salad	0
2 tbsp blue cheese dressing	10 (2 fats)

11:00 PM Home	
Food	**Grams of Fat**
1 cup 2% milk	5
1 orange	0
Total fat for the day	113 g of fat

*Values obtained from a table of food composition.

The physician has just seen the client, reviewed Mr. D's food record and Mike's calculations, and determined that the client's elevated cholesterol level is secondary to his dietary habits. Mr. D's cholesterol level was 225 mg/dL; he weighed 135 lb. and is 5 feet, 6 inches tall. Mr. D stated, "I cannot understand why my cholesterol is elevated. My weight is stable. I always select the salad bar for lunch, avoid sweets, and drink low-fat milk."

NURSING CARE PLAN

SUBJECTIVE DATA Admitted knowledge deficit. Food record for 1 day contained 116 grams of fat.

OBJECTIVE DATA Cholesterol level: 225 mg/dL; Height: 5 ft, 6 in; Weight: 135 lb

NURSING DIAGNOSIS NANDA: Deficient Knowledge: Diet (NANDA, 2003, with permission) more than body requirements related to admitted lack of understanding and a cholesterol level of 225 mg/dL.

DESIRED OUTCOMES EVALUATION CRITERIA	NURSING ACTIONS/INTERVENTIONS	RATIONALE
NOC: Treatment Behavior: Illness (Johnson, Maas, and Moorhead, 2003, with permission)	NIC: Nutrition Counseling (Dochterman and Bulechek, 2004, with permission)	
Client will decrease his visible fat intake.	Instruct the client on efficient means of recording.	Keeping food records will remind the client of the importance of decreasing his or her fat intake. Reviewing them with the nurse permits positive reinforcement and correction of misperceptions.
	Review food records with him at 6-week intervals.	
Client will keep a diary over the next 3 months.	Review visible dietary sources of fat with the client; concentrate on blue cheese dressing, butter, and mayonnaise. Suggest alternatives to using visible fats. Review the diet selected by the physician with the client.	It is prudent to eliminate visible fats first from an individual's diet because they are easily identifiable.
	Tell client to call the nurse if he is having trouble interpreting dietary instructions at home.	Offers the client support between visits.

C T Q CRITICAL THINKING QUESTIONS

1. Although this client is likely to respond to diet therapy, many clients do not. What would you do if after 3 months a client's food diary shows greatly reduced dietary fat but his or her cholesterol has not dropped? The physician would probably decide to prescribe medication to lower the cholesterol. How would you explain this therapy to the client?

2. What would you do if, at the following visit, the food diary shows that the client has returned to his former eating habits, thinking fat consumption no longer matters because he is taking medication?

⟫ CHAPTER REVIEW

1. Monoglycerides and diglycerides are names of lipids commonly seen:
   a. In clients' medical records
   b. On laboratory reports
   c. On food labels
   d. On clients' skin
2. Cholesterol is found:
   a. Only in saturated fats
   b. Only in foods of animal origin
   c. Mostly in eggs
   d. Only in triglycerides
3. Saturated fats are:
   a. Liquid at room temperature
   b. More likely to become rancid than other types of fats
   c. Primarily of animal origin
   d. Composed of many double carbon bonds
4. According to most health authorities, the average American would benefit by increasing his or her intake of which of the following fats while decreasing intake of other fats?
   a. Corn oil
   b. Canola oil
   c. Safflower oil
   d. Lard
5. One ounce of very lean meat contains 1 gram of fat and 35 kilocalories. What percent of kilocalories come from fat?
   a. 9
   b. 20
   c. 26
   d. 49

✚ CLINICAL ANALYSIS

1. Mrs. S, 50 years old, has a cholesterol level of 233 milligrams per deciliter. She weighs 125 pounds and is 5 feet, 5 inches tall. The dietitian has estimated her body fat content to be 35 percent. When taking a nursing history, the nurse asks Mrs. S if she eats any foods that may be related to her elevated cholesterol level. Which of the following groups of foods are most related to an elevated cholesterol level?
   a. Vegetable oils such as corn, cottonseed, and soybean
   b. Fruits and vegetables
   c. Starches such as bread, potatoes, rice, and pasta
   d. Animal fats such as butter, meats, lard, and bacon
2. Mr. B buys as many low-fat foods as possible. He eats fat-free muffins for breakfast, eats low-fat brownies or cookies for lunch each day, uses only fat-free ice cream, and buys fat-free salad dressings. He eats very little meat and chooses fat-free dairy products. He wonders why he hasn't lost more weight. The best advice is to encourage him to:
   a. Consider the amount of soda and sugar he consumes
   b. Eat even less meat
   c. Consume fewer dairy products
   d. Quit trying to lose weight
3. When Mrs. L describes her regular intake of foods, you observe that her diet is especially low in monounsaturated fats. Which of the following oils would you recommend be used in place of corn oil to increase her intake of monounsaturated fats?
   a. Sunflower seed
   b. Soybean
   c. Olive
   d. Cottonseed

REFERENCES

Agricultural Research Service Dietary Guidelines Committee: Dietary Guidelines for Americans 2000. www.ars.usda.gov/dgac.

American Dietetic and Diabetic Associations: Exchange Lists for Meal Planning. American Dietetic Association, Chicago, 2003.

Blumberg, JB: Should you be eating more fat and fewer carbohydrates? Tufts University Health and Nutrition Letter V.16; No. 12:1; February 1999.

Caballero, B: A nutrition paradox-underweight and obesity in developing countries. N Engl J Med, 352:1514, 2005.

Chanmugan, P, et al: Did fat intake in the United States really decline between 1989–1991 and 1994–1996? J Am Diet Assoc 103:867, 2003.

Cheskin, LJ, et al: Gastrointestinal symptoms following consumption of olestra or regular triglyceride potato chips. JAMA 279:150, 1998.

Cunningham, E, and Marason, W: Should my client's diet contain plant sterol/sterol esters to lower cholesterol? J Am Diet Assoc 102:81, 2002.

Dausch, J: Trans-fatty acids: A regulatory update. J Am Diet Assoc 102:18, 2002.

Doak, CM, et al: The dual burden household and the nutrition transition paradox. Int J of Obesity Res 29:129, 2005.

Dochterman, J, and Bulechek, GM: Nursing Interventions Classification (NIC), ed 4. Mosby, Philadelphia, 2004.

Ellias, SL, and Innis, SM: Bakery foods are the major source of trans-fatty acids among pregnant women with diets providing 30 percent energy from fat. J Am Diet Assoc 102:46, 2003.

Etherton-Kris, PM, and Nicolosi, RJ: Trans fatty acids and coronary heart disease risk. International Life Sciences Institute, Washington, 1995.

Food and Nutrition Board, Institute of Medicine: Dietary Reference Intakes for Energy, Carbohydrate, Fiber, Fat, Fatty Acids, Cholesterol, Protein, and Amino Acids. Washington: National Academies Press, 2002.

Freeland-Graves, J, and Nitzke, S: Position of the American Dietetic Association: Total diet approach to communicating food and nutrition information. J Am Diet Assoc 102:100, 2002.

Gundy, SM, et al: National Cholesterol Education Program (NCEP): Third Report of the NCEP Expert Panel on Detection, Evaluation, and Treatment in Adults (Adult Treatment Panel III), Full Report. National Institutes of Health, National Heart, Lung, and Blood Institute, Washington, Pub No. 01-3670, 2001.

International Food Information Council (IFIC) and The Food and Drug Administration (FDA): The Benefits of Balance: Managing Fat in Your Diet. International Food Information Council and Food and Drug Administration, Washington, 1998.

Kendler, BS: Recent nutritional approaches to the prevention and therapy of cardiovascular disease. Prog Cardiovasc Nurs 12:3, 1997.

Lichtenstein, AH: Trans fatty acids and hydrogenated fat: What do we know? Nutr Today 30:102–107, 1995.

Lichtenstein, AH, et al: Dietary fat consumption and health. Nutr Rev 56:53, 1998.

Moorehead, S, Johnson, M, and Maas, M: Nursing Outcomes Classification (NOC), ed 3. Mosby, Philadelphia, 2004.

Morris, MC: Consumption of fish and n-3 fatty acids and risk of incident Alzheimer disease. Arcg Neryil 60:940, 2003.

NANDA International: Nursing Diagnoses: Definitions and Classification, 2003–2004. NANDA International, Philadelphia, 2003.

National Institutes of Health, National Heart, Lung, and Blood Institute: Clinical Guidelines on the Identification and Treatment of Overweight and Obesity in adults. U.S. Department of Health and Human Services, Bethesda, 1998.

National Institutes of Health: NCEP issues major new cholesterol guidelines. May 15, 2001. www.nhlbi.nihi.gov/new.

Ornish, D: Ornish's Program for Reversing Heart Disease. Ballantine Publishing Group, New York, 2004.

Pearson, TA, et al: AHA Guidelines for Primary Prevention of Cardiovascular Disease and Stroke: 2002 Update. Consensus Panel Guide to Comprehensive Risk Reduction for Adult Patients Without Coronary or Other Vascular Diseases. Circulation 106:388, 2002.

Tucker, KL, et al: The combination of high fruit and vegetable and low saturated fat intakes is more protective against mortality in aging men than is either alone: Baltimore longitudinal study of aging. J Nutr 135:556, 2005.

U.S. Department of Agriculture (USDA) and U.S. Department of Health and Human Services. Dietary guidelines for Americans, ed 4. USDA Home and Garden Bulletin No. 52. Washington, 1995.

USDA Center for Nutrition Policy and Health Promotion: Nutrition Insights: The role of nuts in a healthy diet. www.usda.gov.cnpp.

USDA: Continuing survey of food intake by individuals, 1994–1996. www.usda.gov/bbnrc/foodsurvey.

USDA: The food guide pyramid. www.usda:gov8001/py.

USDA: www.usda.gov/dietaryguidelines/dga2000.

U.S. Department of Health and Human Services: The Surgeon General's Report on Nutrition and Health. Washington, DHHS Publication No. (PHS) 88-55 210, 1988.

World Health Organization: Years of healthy life can be increases 5–10 years. www.who.int/mediacentre/releases/pr84/en/print.html.

Wiese, HF, Hansen, AE, and Adam, DJD: Essential fatty acids in infant nutrition. J Nutr 58:345, 1958.

Willett, WC: Diet, nutrition, and the prevention of cancer. In Shils, ME (ed): Modern Nutrition in Health and Disease, ed 9. Williams & Wilkins, Baltimore, 1999.

Zorich, NL, et al: Randomized double blind, placebo-controlled, consumer rechallenge test of Oolean salted snacks. Regul Toxicol Pharmacol 26:200, 1997.

CHAPTER 5

Protein

Learning Objectives

After completing this chapter, the student should be able to:

1. Discuss the functions of protein for humans in health and in illness.
2. Explain the difference between complete and incomplete proteins and give examples of food sources of each.
3. Define anabolism and catabolism and list possible anabolic and catabolic conditions.
4. List the grams of protein in each exchange list containing significant amounts of protein.
5. Design a daily meal plan with adequate protein intake for a healthy adult.
6. Prepare an outline of topics to discuss with a client consuming a vegan diet.

The importance of protein in nutrition and health was first emphasized by an ancient Greek who called this nutrient *proteos,* meaning primary or taking first place. Protein is essential for body growth and maintenance. If kilocaloric intake is inadequate to support fuel requirements, dietary protein may be used for energy rather than for tissue growth and maintenance. As is true of carbohydrates and fats, protein eaten in excess can contribute to body fat stores.

Proteins are the building blocks of the body's tissues and organs. Almost half the dry weight of the body's cells is protein. It is second only to water in amounts present in the body. A description of some of the tissues composed of protein appears in Box 5–1.

Box 5–1 | Examples of Protein in the Human Body

Most of the cells of the body require periodic maintenance or replacement. Even bone tissue undergoes change in the healthy adult. However, the body cannot effectively repair tooth enamel that is destroyed by decay, hence the need for dental restoration or fillings.

Scar Tissue

The healing of the simplest wound requires proteins. Many blood clotting factors, such as the protein prothrombin, form a blood clot. The fibrin threads that form the mesh to hold the scar tissue in place are composed of protein. Low serum protein levels have been significantly associated with prolonged healing (Agrawal et al, 2003).

Hair Growth

Hair cells are dead. Hence, haircuts do not hurt. The new growth of hair does require protein building blocks, how-

ever. One sign of malnutrition is hair that can be easily and painlessly plucked.

Blood Albumin

Albumin is a transport protein that carries nutrients or elements to where they are needed. In addition to transporting substances to all the cells of the body, albumin also has functions relating to water balance (see Chapter 9) and plays a significant role in medication absorption and metabolism (see Chapter 17).

Hemoglobin

Another transport protein, **hemoglobin,** is the oxygen-carrying part of the red blood cell. The **globin** part of this molecule is a simple protein.

Small wonder, then, that people need a steady intake of protein for normal maintenance of the body. When the person is growing or has diseased or injured tissue to repair, the need for protein is even greater.

In parts of Africa, a staple of the diet is cassava root, which contains varying amounts of cyanide. If the roots are not adequately processed and the diet also is low in sulfur-containing amino acids (methionine and cysteine) that the body can use to detoxify the cyanide, a paralytic disease of the legs called **konzo** can result. It affects tens of thousands of women and children in sub-Sahara Africa (Boivin, 1997), primarily in remote areas (Bonmarin, Nunga, and Perea, 2002; Diasolua Ngudi, Kuo, and Lambein, 2002).

Although the paralysis is permanent, a rehabilitation clinic in Mozambique assists victims in maximizing the use of their legs. Kits have been developed to test the amount of cyanide in the roots and flour made from cassava roots as well as in a person's urine to monitor status.

Cassava, a hardy, drought-resistant plant that thrives in poor soil, produces cyanide as a defense mechanism. Varieties of the plant are also grown in Central and South America and the South Pacific. Different cultures have designed various means to decrease the cyanide in the plant before consuming the product. In Africa, the main methods involve drying the roots.

Composition of Proteins

To understand the functions of protein in the body, it is necessary first to comprehend their basic structure: their chemical elements and how those elements are arranged.

Proteins are composed of carbon, hydrogen, oxygen, and nitrogen. Sometimes phosphorus, sulfur, iron, and iodine form part of the protein molecule, but nitrogen is the element that distinguishes proteins from carbohydrates and fats. These elements are arranged in building blocks called amino acids.

The importance of a balanced diet along with correct food processing techniques is illustrated by the occurrence of an irreversible paralytic disease called **konzo** that is detailed in Box 5–2. This devastating condition results from consumption of a diet deficient in sulphur-based amino acids along with a food that contains cyanide because of inadequate processing.

Amino Acids

The amino acids are linked by **peptide bonds** in an exact order to make a particular protein. A chain of two or more amino acids joined together by peptide bonds is called a **polypeptide.** A single protein may consist of a polypeptide comprising from 50 to thousands of amino acids. Scientists have estimated that the body contains up to 50,000 different proteins, of which only about 1000 have been identified. Thus, an enormous variety of combinations is possible.

To visualize these combinations, examine Figure 5–1, a schematic representation of the beef insulin molecule. It might also help to think of the elements as the letters of the

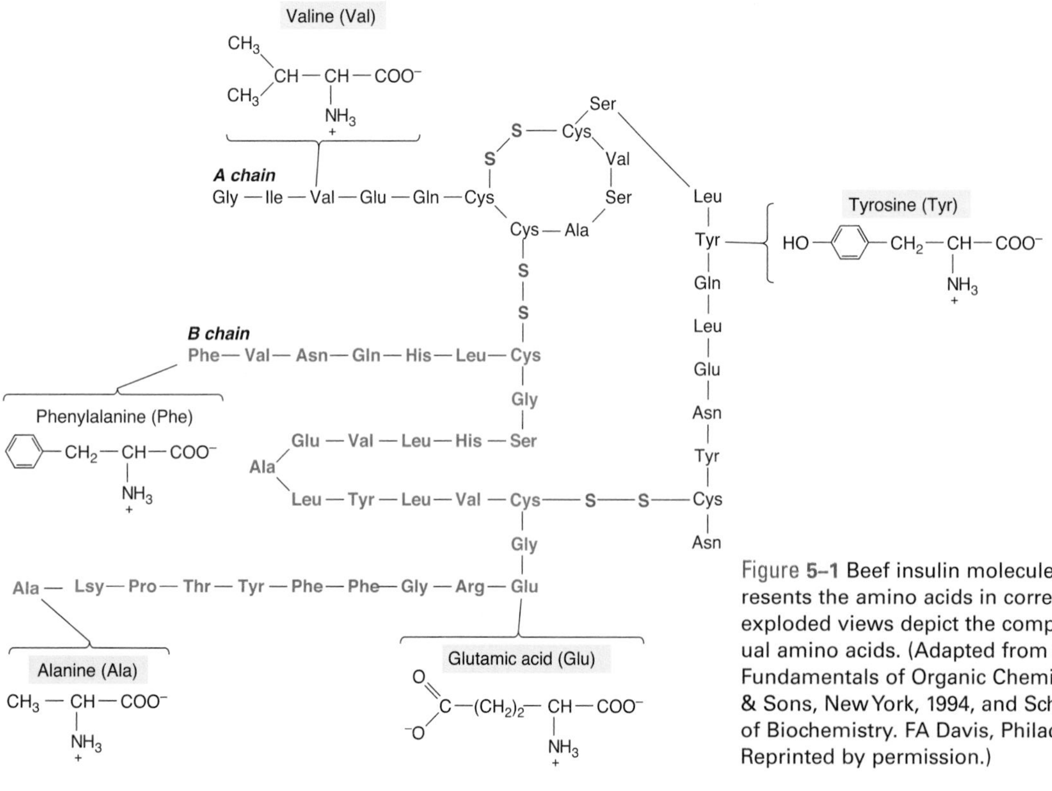

Figure **5–1** Beef insulin molecule. The central core represents the amino acids in correct sequence. The six exploded views depict the composition of the individual amino acids. (Adapted from Solomons, TWG: Fundamentals of Organic Chemistry, ed 4. John Wiley & Sons, New York, 1994, and Schumm, DE: Essentials of Biochemistry. FA Davis, Philadelphia, 1988. Reprinted by permission.)

Table 5–1 Comparison of Language and Anatomy

COMPONENT OF LANGUAGE	COMPONENT OF ANATOMY
Letters	Elements such as carbon, hydrogen, oxygen, nitrogen, sometimes sulfur
Word	Amino acid
Sentence	Protein
Paragraph	Cell
Chapter	Tissue
Book	Organ
Books on a given subject	System
Library	Human body

alphabet and amino acids as words. There are countless ways to make words (amino acids) from the 26 letters (the elements). Words put into a certain order make up sentences that have a specific and unique meaning. In this comparison, a sentence is a protein. Each protein has a specific and unique sequence of amino acids. To complete the analogy of language to anatomy, see Table 5–1.

Animal proteins that we eat are disassembled in the digestive process into component amino acids. They are then reassembled to form human proteins (see Chapter 10). Precision is necessary to manufacture proteins. A slight error in the construction of a protein, such as occurs in sickle cell disease, can have severe consequences (see Clinical Application 5–1).

Twenty-three amino acids have been identified as important to the body's metabolism. These amino acids are classified as essential, conditionally (or acquired) essential, or nonessential.

Essential Amino Acids

As is true of other nutrients, an amino acid is classified as essential if the body is unable to make it in sufficient amounts to meet metabolic needs. All **essential amino acids** must be available in the body simultaneously and in sufficient quantity for the synthesis of body proteins (Fig. 5–2). These amino acids may come from recently ingested food or from the body's own cells as they age and are broken down and replaced. Approximately 340 g of amino acids enter the free pool each day, but only about 90 g are derived from the diet (Matthews, 1999).

A person's physiologic state influences the need for essential amino acids. Thus, for infants and young children, 30 percent of protein should be constituted

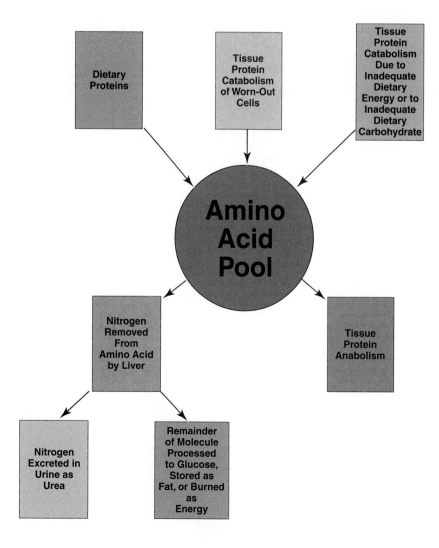

Figure **5–2** Anabolism/catabolism of protein. The body obtains amino acids from dietary protein and the catabolism of body tissue, enzymes, and secretions. The body uses amino acids to build new tissue or for immediate or future energy use. Every meal or snack does not have to contain every essential amino acid to permit anabolism. To maximize health, all essential amino acids should be supplied in adequate amounts by diet daily or at least every 2 to 3 days.

Sickle Cell Disease

Hemoglobin (Hgb) consists of 146 amino acids combined in a specific order. In the hemoglobin of a person with sickle cell disease, one amino acid, glutamic acid, has been replaced by valine at one specific location on the protein chain. In sickle cell disease the body has 99.3 percent of the amino acids in the correct sequence in the red blood cell, but early death results from the 0.7 percent error.

Sickle cell disease, an **autosomal recessive** disease, is most common among black people but also occurs in Mediterranean people. It affects one of every 375 black babies born in the United States (United States Department of Health and Human Services, 2003). About 120,000 babies with sickle cell disease are born annually (1000 in the United States). Fewer than 2 percent live to the age of 5 years (Steinberg, 1999), but in the United States, mean survival ages are 42 years for males and 48 years for females (Platt, Brambilla, and Rosse, 1994).

In sickle cell disease the red blood cells (RBCs) have a lifespan of 10 to 12 days compared with the normal 120 days, leading to chronic anemia. Additionally, the RBCs become rigid and crescent-shaped. These abnormal cells tend to clump together and block small blood vessels in many different organs, leading to strokes, acute chest syndrome (a life-threatening, pneumonia-like illness), and pain crises (see Figure 5–3).

The only cure is a bone marrow transplant from a matched sibling donor (Gaziev and Lucarelli, 2003) until alternative sources of stem cells such as cord blood become widely available (Hughes, 2000). Gene therapy is promising, but progress has been slow (Vichinsky, 2002). Comprehensive care includes red cell exchange transfusion (Lawson et al, 1999), antibiotic treatment, pneumococcal vaccination, and newborn screening programs, which in

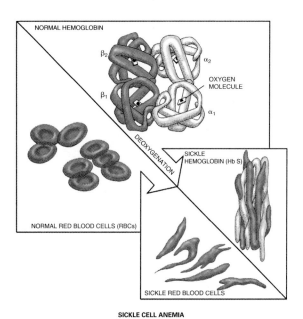

Figure **5–3** Normal red blood cells (RBCs) and hemoglobin (Hgb) compared with those in sickle cell anemia. (Reprinted from Venes, D [ed]: Taber's Cyclopedic Medical Dictionary, ed 19. FA Davis, Philadelphia, 2001, p 106, with permission.)

1999 were operative in all states except Utah, Montana, and the Dakotas (Ashley-Koch, Yang, and Olney, 2000). Pilot studies using nitric oxide to dilate blood vessels or its precursor, L-arginine as an oral supplement, show promise for managing vaso-occlusive crisis (Morris et al, 2000; Vichinsky, 2002). Techniques to diagnose the disease in a fetus in the first 3 months of pregnancy are available.

---

of essential amino acids. That figure drops to 20 percent in later childhood and to 11 percent in adulthood (Matthews, 1999).

Special preparations that the body converts to six of the essential amino acids are available but not for lysine, histidine, and **threonine.** For this reason, some authorities list only those three amino acids as totally indispensable (Gropper, Smith, and Groff, 2005).

Conditionally (Acquired) Essential Amino Acids

Other amino acids are conditionally essential or can become essential, depending on the biochemical needs of the body and the health of its organs. For example, cysteine and tyrosine become indispensable in immaturity, in metabolic disorders, and during severe stress. In PKU (see Clinical Applications 5–3), tyrosine becomes essential because normally it is produced from phenylalanine by the same enzyme that is lacking in PKU clients (Gropper, Smith, and Groff, 2005).

Nonessential Amino Acids

Nonessential amino acids are those that the body ordinarily can build in sufficient quantities to meet its needs. Often they are derived from other amino acids. Nonessential amino acids are necessary for good health, but under normal conditions adults do not have to obtain them from food. Table 5–2 lists the amino acids that have been classified as essential, conditionally and/or acquired essential, and nonessential.

Functions in the Body

Protein serves six major functions in the body:

- Provision of structure
- Growth and maintenance of tissue
- Regulation of body processes
- Development of immunity
- Circulation of blood and nutrients
- Backup source of energy

Table 5–3 lists examples of each function.

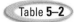

Table 5–2 Essential, Conditionally and/or Acquired Essential, and Nonessential Amino Acids

ESSENTIAL	CONDITIONALLY AND/OR ACQUIRED ESSENTIAL	NONESSENTIAL
Histidine	Arginine	Alanine
Isoleucine	Carnitine[1]	Asparagine
Leucine	Citrulline[2]	Aspartic acid
Lysine	Cysteine[3,7]	Glutamic acid
Methionine[7]	Glutamine[4]	Glycine
Phenylalanine	Serine[5]	Proline
Threonine	Taurine[6]	
Tryptophan	Tyrosine	
Valine		

[1]In newborns, can enhance the use of fat as an energy source; can be made from lysine and methionine in adults.
[2]Not used in protein synthesis, but critical in the urea cycle.
[3]Also called cystine.
[4]In major trauma or surgery, sepsis, bone marrow transplantation, intense chemotherapy, and radiotherapy (Tapiero et al, 2002); used by intestinal cells as primary source of energy (Gropper, Smith, and Groff, 2005).
[5]In some kidney diseases.
[6]Not used in protein synthesis, but essential in retinal functioning, especially in young children.
[7]Sulfur-containing amino acids.

Provision of Structure

Proteins provide much of the mass of the body. Contractile proteins, actin and myosin, are found in muscles. Fibrous proteins, such as collagen, elastin, and keratin, are found in blood vessels, bone, cartilage, hair, nails, tendons, skin, and teeth.

Maintenance and Growth

Because protein is a part of every cell (half the dry weight), adults as well as growing children require adequate protein intake. As cells of the body wear out, they must be replaced.

Anabolism Versus Catabolism

Two processes of building up or breaking down of body tissues are anabolism and catabolism. **Anabolism** is the building up of tissues as occurs in growth or healing.

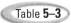

Table 5–3 Functions of Protein in the Body, With Examples

FUNCTION	EXAMPLE
Provision of structure	Muscle mass
Maintenance and growth	Hair growth
Regulation of body processes	Glucagon (actions opposite those of insulin)
Immunity	Antibodies against measles
Energy source	If adequate carbohydrate and fat are lacking
Contribution to blood volume and blood pressure	Albumin draws fluid back into capillaries from interstitial (between the cells) spaces

Catabolism is the breaking down of tissues into simpler substances that the body can reuse or eliminate.

Both processes occur simultaneously in the body. For example, tissue proteins are constantly being broken down into amino acids, which are then reused for building new tissue and repairing old tissue. Anabolism and catabolism, however, are not always in balance; at times, one process may dominate the other.

Nitrogen Balance

Foods or artificial feedings containing protein are the body's only external sources of nitrogen. Nitrogen is excreted in the urine, feces, and sweat and is sometimes lost through bleeding or vomiting. A person is in nitrogen equilibrium or nitrogen balance when the amount of nitrogen eaten is equal to the amount excreted (Clinical Calculation 5–1). A healthy adult at a stable body weight is usually in nitrogen equilibrium. Under certain circumstances, however, nitrogen balance may be either positive or negative.

POSITIVE NITROGEN BALANCE. When a person consumes more nitrogen than he or she excretes, the condition is called positive **nitrogen balance.** In other words, the body is building more tissue than it is breaking down. This state is desirable during periods of growth such as infancy, childhood, adolescence, and pregnancy.

NEGATIVE NITROGEN BALANCE. When a person consumes less nitrogen than he or she excretes, the condition is termed negative nitrogen balance. Such a person is receiving insufficient protein, and the body is breaking down more tissue than it is building. Situations marked by negative nitrogen balance include undernutrition, illness, and trauma.

Although skipping food for one day may create a temporary negative nitrogen balance, noticeable physical signs are not likely to occur. A prolonged negative nitrogen balance, however, can adversely affect children's growth rate and diminish a person's capacity to resist infections.

Disruption of body integrity by surgery, burns, or fractures causes an acute protein loss. People who are well nourished before the disruption are better prepared to weather the resulting catabolism. Poorly nourished people

Clinical Calculation 5–1

Nitrogen Balance Studies

To calculate an individual's nitrogen balance, the amount of nitrogen in the foods he or she consumes is compared with the amount of nitrogen excreted in the urine. Other potential losses are estimated. Protein is approximately 16 percent nitrogen, so to calculate the nitrogen content in the foods, the amount of protein consumed (in grams) is multiplied by 0.16. Thus, a person who ingests 50 g of protein has a nitrogen intake of 8 g. To be in nitrogen equilibrium, he or she would therefore be expected to excrete or lose 8 g of nitrogen.

are at increased risk for weight loss, anemia, and infection. Even healthy people subjected to strict bed rest for 2 weeks had protein synthesis decreased by 14 percent and skeletal muscle protein synthesis by almost 50 percent. The latter loss did not occur in subjects given a moderate exercise regimen (Ferrando, Paddon-Jones, and Wolfe, 2002).

Some individuals may be undernourished even when their total food intake is sufficient. Public health studies from Asia and Latin America describe economic and cultural factors within households that produce a relative deprivation of women and children. Women and girls in some parts of India may receive sufficient kilocalories in staple foods but not enough animal protein, fruits, and vegetables.

In some African societies, women don't eat because it is believed to interfere with fertility. In Nepal, some adolescent and adult women deprive themselves in order to follow cultural "hot-cold" food rules for reproductive-aged women, avoiding nutrient-rich fruits and vegetables (Messer, 1997). In the United States, the unwise and constant dieting practiced by some women and girls determined to achieve the cultural ideal of a slim body deprives them of nutrients necessary for good health.

Severe undernutrition results in specific clinical pictures. Starvation in poor countries may be due to famine, but the term is also used to describe clients who receive inadequate food, sometimes for days, because of treatments or diagnostic tests. The alert nurse intervenes as client advocate or coordinator of care in such cases to rearrange meal schedules or obtain food supplements.

Clients in institutions are also susceptible to **protein–energy malnutrition (PEM)** or **protein–calorie malnutrition (PCM)** when they are unable to feed themselves. In the developed world, PEM most often accompanies a disease process. Surveys of hospitalized children in this country found PEM in 20 to 40 percent of them (Baker, 1997). **Lean body mass,** chiefly skeletal and visceral muscle, is the critical element that is lost in PEM. Additional information on lean body mass appears in Chapters 18 and 24.

Individuals with wasting diseases may suffer from PCM. Two types of PCM are marasmus and kwashiorkor. **Marasmus** occurs when the victim consumes too few kilocalories and insufficient protein. The person appears to be wasting away. Marasmus is often seen in children in developing countries, but it also occurs in debilitating diseases such as cancer or AIDS.

Kwashiorkor classically occurs in a child shortly after weaning from breast milk. The child receives more kilocalories than one with marasmus but not enough protein to support growth. Clinically, he or she may look chubby, especially in the abdominal area, but the cause of this swelling is fluid retention, not fat (Fig. 5–4). Kwashiorkor is **endemic** in areas where the staple diet has a low protein to energy ratio. It seems to disrupt the slowing of metabolism that would normally be expected in response to inadequate diet (Lunn, Morley, and Neale, 1998).

Clinical Application 5–2 presents a firsthand account of the desperate situation of people in a developing country. Although rare, kwashiorkor also occurs in industrialized nations, not because of lack of food but because of parental ignorance about nutrition (Lunn, Morley, and Neale, 1998).

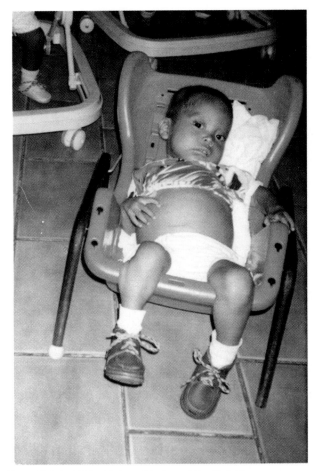

Figure **5–4** A child with kwashiorkor at the Nutrition Rehabilitation Center in San Carlos, Bolivia.

Regulation of Body Processes

Protein contributes to the regulation of body processes. Hormones and enzymes are prime examples. Table 5–4 lists these regulators and gives examples of each. Nucleoproteins, also containing protein, are essential to normal body functioning.

Hormones

Hormones are chemicals secreted by various organs to regulate body processes. Hormones are secreted directly into the bloodstream rather than into a duct or an organ. **Insulin** and **glucagon** are two important protein hormones that help control glucose metabolism. Growth hormone regulates cell division and protein synthesis to produce growth. Parathyroid hormone increases the withdrawal of calcium from the bones to maintain serum calcium levels, whereas calcitonin inhibits the release of calcium from the bones.

Enzymes

The body makes specialized proteins called **enzymes.** Enzymes are crucial to many body processes, such as digestion. The breakdown of foods in the stomach and small intestine involves enzymes, which act as **catalysts**

Letters from Valle de Sacta, Bolivia

By Constance O'Connor BSN, RN

Your letter arrived January 17th, the first mail since a week before Christmas. Mail here is an event … no TV, no newspapers. Shortwave BBC is about it for input. Much of what I do is aimed at keeping us healthy, such as ironing all line-dried clothes to get rid of any tiny insects or larvae. All fruits and vegetables are washed in chlorine bleach solution before use. We have gotten so used to the taste we may have to put a bottle on the table like a condiment when we get back home. Water we consume is either bottled or boiled for 20 minutes.

The people here are very poor, most living out in the bush, clearing land to grow bananas, pineapples, oranges, lemons, and coca. They usually construct a two-story hut on stilts so they can get out of the water with the rains. There are half-walls, if any, no screens, no toilets, rarely a well. It is a hard life. Few people survive past 55 and many children die at birth or in the first year.

Statistics are hard to obtain, as reporting even of births and deaths is minimal. A WHO report for 1963 to 1973 estimated there were 9.5 million children aged 0 to 5 years in Latin America affected by protein-energy malnutrition. A study done in our area in 1998 found 38.9% of children under 5 years of age suffering from chronic malnutrition, and 0.6% with acute malnutrition.

One acute case we saw, an 18-month-old boy, was so jaundiced and had such swelling in his lower extremities, we thought he had a kidney or liver problem. We did get care for him and learned the doctors here call that edema "the edema of hunger." These parents were motivated to get treatment as their first child died at 18 months with the same symptoms.

We took a 3-year-old girl to an ophthalmologist because she had a whitish membrane over one eye and could not see well. She was known to be anemic, but the eye doctor said her main problem was kwashiorkor. Sadly, the family refused placement in a hospital, a center for disnutrition, or even the orphanage run by our nuns. We thought this was unusual until we visited a center for disnutrition about 50 miles from us. Of the 54 children, all under three years old, 21 had kwashiorkor.

Today I am taking a 3-year-old child to a malnutrition center about a 3-hour drive from us, hoping that it is not too late to save her life. The parents refused care for her up to this point though our pueblo elders, neighbors, and other family members pleaded with them. She has protein-energy malnutrition with kwashiorkor syndrome.

We personally pay for the children we send to these centers. Obviously, if the parents had money their children would not be starving. Most poor parents just accept that the children will die. They will dress them in their nicest clothes, hold them almost constantly during this dying process, and bury them soon after death. No funeral, no coffin.

Malnutrition is a factor in many of the measles, pneumonia, shigellosis, staphylococcal disease, and of course, tuberculosis cases Jim and I care for here. On our first Christmas here we were in the middle of a yellow fever outbreak. I have had to cope with children dying from malnutrition, dehydration, infections that did not get treated in time. I think I will always see their faces.

I hope to see you in March when I'm home begging for medicines and supplies. Many thanks for your letters.

(chemicals that influence the speed at which a chemical reaction takes place but do not actually enter into the reaction). All of the examples of enzymes listed in Table 5–4 are detailed in Chapter 10. Without the aid of enzymes, many of the processes in the body would proceed too slowly to be effective.

Table 5–4   **Examples of Regulators of Body Processes**

REGULATOR	EXAMPLES
Hormones	Calcitonin
	Growth hormone (Somatotropin)
	Insulin and glucagon
	Parathyroid hormone
Enzymes	Lactase
	Lipase
	Peptidase
	Sucrase

An enzyme provides a place (its surface) for two substances to meet and react with each other. If it were not for enzymes, these two substances would be less likely to encounter one another, and basic body functioning would be impossible.

The lack of a specific enzyme can have devastating effects on health and even on life itself. Such a condition is addressed in Clinical Application 5–3.

Nucleoproteins

Nucleoproteins are regulatory complexes that include proteins. These complexes are located in the cell nucleus where they direct the maintenance and reproduction of the cell. **Deoxyribonucleic acid (DNA)** and **ribonucleic acid (RNA)** are nucleoproteins that control the protein synthesis in the cell. A **gene** is a part of the DNA that carries the code to direct the synthesis of a single protein. The kinds of proteins the cell makes vary with the nature of the cell, whether an intestinal or skin cell or an ovum or sperm cell.

Phenylketonuria (PKU)

PKU is the most common of all amino acid pathologies (de Freitas et al, 1999). About 1 in 60 whites, mostly of Northern European ancestry, is a carrier for this autosomal recessive disorder, which occurs once in 15,000 live births annually in the United States. Clients with **phenylketonuria** are unable to convert the essential amino acid **phenylalanine** to tyrosine because the enzyme phenylalanine hydroxylase is lacking or defective.

Phenylalanine occurs in all protein foods, including milk. Affected infants are immediately at risk of accumulating high blood levels of phenylalanine with consequent mental retardation.

In the United States, screening tests, using a few drops of blood from the infant's heel, are mandated by all states. The test is highly accurate when performed 24 hours after birth through the seventh day of life (March of Dimes, 2003). With mothers and infants discharged from the maternity unit within 24 hours, efforts must be made to ensure proper timing of the screening test. The American Academy of Pediatrics recommends that infants tested when they are less than 24 hours old be rescreened at 1 to 2 weeks of age (March of Dimes, 2003).

Ideally, treatment to establish metabolic control should begin in the first 7 to 10 days of life, and metabolic control should be maintained throughout the client's lifespan, requiring regular blood tests, recording of food intake, and a highly restrictive diet (National Institutes of Health, 2000). Until the 1980s, restrictions were relaxed as the client grew, so new concerns have arisen that women who cease treatment for PKU may harm their unborn children. The diet for these women is stricter than for nonpregnant adults because phenylalanine crosses the placenta such that the fetus is exposed to higher phenylalanine concentrations than the mother (Cleary and Walter, 2001). Most defects arise in the first trimester, including microcephaly, mental deficiency, and congenital heart disease (National Institutes of Health, 2000). Because most of these infants have not inherited PKU but instead were injured by their mothers' high blood levels of phenylalanine, even the rigorous standard treatment for PKU cannot help them (March of Dimes, 2003). Careful history-taking may tease out the fact that a woman was on a special diet as a small child and thus may need to have phenylalanine levels tested and to resume the diet before attempting pregnancy. An alert nurse could identify this situation before significant damage is done.

The artificial sweetener **aspartame** (Equal, NutraSweet), which is composed of aspartic acid and phenylalanine, bears a warning label regarding PKU. Clients with PKU and their families may have to be reminded regularly of the importance of dietary compliance.

Research is proceeding into nondietary treatments such as gene therapy, discovery of enzymes to degrade phenylalanine (National Institutes of Health, 2000), and supplementation with amino acids that compete with phenylalanine for transport across the blood-brain barrier (Cleary and Walter, 2001).

Immunity

A specific protein called an **antibody** is produced in the body in response to the presence of a foreign substance or a substance that the body senses to be foreign. Antibodies provide **immunity** to certain diseases and other toxic conditions. A specific antibody is created for each foreign substance.

If a person is exposed to a certain kind of disease-producing organism, the body designs an antibody that neutralizes the harmful effects of only that particular species or strain of organism. For some diseases, once the body has produced many copies of a given antibody, it can respond quickly to another attack, making the individual immune to that disease. All antibodies belong to a group of blood proteins called **immunoglobulins.**

Circulation

The main protein in the blood is albumin. It helps to maintain blood volume by drawing fluid back into the veins from body tissues. Thus it plays a major role in maintaining blood pressure. In addition, some proteins aid in maintaining the acid base balance of the body. This buffering action is described in Chapter 9.

Some proteins serve as transport vehicles for nutrients or drugs, such as the proteins that attach to fats to become lipoproteins. Drugs bind with albumin in the bloodstream. The term *protein-bound* refers to the portion of a dose of a drug that is inactive because it is attached to albumin. This process has implications that are elaborated in Chapter 17.

Energy Source

Glucose is the most efficiently used source of energy, but fat and protein can be adapted as backup sources. Most other body systems use fat for energy more readily than the nervous system does. When the body has insufficient glucose available for nervous system energy needs (as in a carbohydrate dietary deficit of longer than 12 hours), the body will utilize body protein tissue to meet the energy needs of the brain and spinal cord. Thus, adequate carbohydrate intake is necessary to (1) spare protein for its unique contribution to tissue building and (2) avoid the undesirable consequences—ketosis and muscle loss—of obtaining energy from the less efficient sources—fat and protein. Long term, the potential exists for excessive protein intake to overtax the kidneys because of their role in removing the nitrogen from amino acids to convert them to energy sources (see Chapter 10). The amount of energy obtained from a gram of protein is the same as the amount obtained from a gram of carbohydrate: 4 kilocalories.

Loss of about 30 percent of body protein is likely to be fatal. Contributing to the outcome are reduced muscle strength for breathing, impaired immune function, and decreased organ function (Matthews, 1999).

Classification of Food Protein

Few foods contain only protein. The white of an egg comes close, deriving 80 percent of its kilocalories from protein. Most foods embody various combinations of protein, fat, and carbohydrates. Some foods, however, are better sources of protein than others.

Protein foods are classified by the number and kinds of amino acids they contain. **Complete proteins** are foods that supply all nine essential amino acids in sufficient quantity to maintain tissue and support growth. **Incomplete proteins** lack one or more of the essential amino acids.

Scoring systems have been devised to rate the quality of proteins on the basis of their amino acid composition. The reference foods often used are eggs and cow's milk. It is difficult to compare foods in this way because certain factors intervene between the test situation and the family table. Some plants, for example, contain substances that inhibit digestion of protein. These inhibitors can be destroyed by heat processing but heating can also damage amino acids (Matthews, 1999).

Complete Protein

With few exceptions, single foods containing complete protein come from animal sources such as meat, poultry, fish, eggs, and cheese. Although gelatin is an animal product, it is an incomplete protein because it lacks the essential amino acid tryptophan.

Meat and milk products are both good sources of complete protein. An adult requiring 2000 kilocalories per day who follows MyPyramid would consume the equivalent of 5 1/2 ounces from the meat group and three cups of milk daily. MyPyramid categorizes cheese with milk, whereas the exchange-group system places it with meat.

Each exchange of meat contains 7 grams of protein regardless of the amount of fat. All beef is not high in fat, just as all fish and poultry are not low in fat. Figure 5–5 shows a 3-ounce portion of beef tenderloin equal to three lean meat exchanges providing 21 grams of protein. Table 5–5 com-

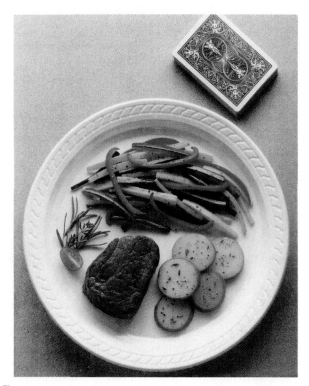

Figure **5–5** The 3-oz beef tenderloin pictured equals three lean meat exchanges. A standard deck of playing cards is shown for size comparison. (From the National Live Stock and Meat Board, 444 North Michigan Ave, Chicago, IL 60611, with permission.)

pares selected meat, fish, and poultry products. It is evident that all except the sausages offer significant protein but vary in the percent of kilocalories from fat due to the source of the item and the method of preparation. The sausages contain approximately half the protein of the other meats and twice the percentage of kilocalories from fat.

Each milk exchange furnishes 8 grams of protein. Examples of one milk exchange are 1 cup of milk, buttermilk, or yogurt; 1/2 cup of canned evaporated milk; or 1/3 cup of dry skim milk. All of these milk products offer equal protein nutrition, but all are not nutritionally equivalent because their fat content varies.

Table **5–5** **Comparison of Meat Products**

FOOD ITEM	WEIGHT OR MEASURE	METHOD OF PREPARATION	KILOCALORIES	PROTEIN GRAMS	FAT GRAMS	PERCENT OF KILOCALORIES FROM FAT
Beef chuck, lean only	3 oz	Braised	213	26	11	46
Beef round, lean only	3 oz	Braised	178	27	7	35
Pork chop, loin, lean only	3 oz	Fried	197	27	9	41
Ham, lean only	3 oz	Roasted	133	21	5	34
Salmon, red	3 oz	Baked or broiled	184	23	9	44
Ocean perch	3 oz	Baked or broiled	103	20	2	17
Chicken, light meat only	3 oz	Fried	163	28	5	28
Turkey, light meat	3 oz	Roasted	133	25	3	20
Bologna	3 oz		270	11	24	80
Salami	3 oz		215	12	17	71

Table 5-6   Grams of Protein per Exchange

EXCHANGE	GRAMS OF PROTEIN
Milk	8
Meat	7
Starch/Bread	3
Vegetable	2

Incomplete Protein

Plant foods that contain protein lack sufficient amounts of one or more of the essential amino acids. Thus, the protein of plants is called incomplete. But the term *incomplete* does not mean these foods are undesirable or should be avoided. Plant proteins are valuable because they supplement the animal proteins in the diet. In addition, different types of plant foods can be combined to provide all the essential amino acids. Grains, vegetables, legumes, nuts, and seeds are sources of incomplete protein.

The vegetable and starch/bread exchanges are sources of incomplete protein. Some vegetables such as corn, peas, and dried beans are closer in energy content to a slice of bread than to most vegetables. For this reason they appear on the Starch/Bread Exchange List. A vegetable exchange contains 2 grams of protein. One vegetable exchange would be 1/2 cup of asparagus or 1/2 cup of chopped broccoli. One starch/bread exchange, containing 3 grams of protein, would be 1/2 cup of corn, one small potato, 1/2 cup of winter squash, one slice of bread, 1/2 bagel or 1/2 English muffin, or three square graham crackers.

It is important to note the size of the item; specialty bagels and muffins may be much larger than the referenced item on the exchange list. The protein content of the four exchange lists is summarized in Table 5-6.

Limiting Amino Acids and Complementation

Plants are classified as incomplete protein sources because they lack one or more essential amino acids. This undersupplied amino acid is called the **limiting amino acid.** In cereal grains, the limiting amino acid is **lysine;** in legumes, it is **methionine.**

Based on animal studies, the principle of **complementation** was promulgated. It stated that plant foods should be combined to provide all the essential amino acids in a given meal. There are two major flaws in projecting the results of these animal studies to humans. Animals have greater protein needs than humans. Also, the experimental animal diets were completely lacking in the amino acid being studied, a situation not likely to occur in humans with the selection of whole foods (Johnston, 1999).

Adult humans can derive adequate nutrition when they consume a balanced assortment of plant protein throughout the day. As shown in Figure 5-2, supplying the amino acid pool is a dynamic process. Young children did show less effective use of protein if the complementary protein was fed at intervals greater than 6 hours, but this is an unusually long time between meals or snacks for young children (Johnston, 1999).

Vegetable Sources of Protein

For vegetarians or other individuals who limit their intake of animal foods, **legumes** are an important protein source. Legumes are plants having roots containing **nitrogen-fixing bacteria** that lock nitrogen into the plant's structure, thus increasing its nitrogen content. Legumes contain two to three times as much nitrogen as most other vegetables.

Commonly consumed legumes are peas, beans, lentils, and peanuts. Not all peas and beans are legumes. Figure 5-6 compares the protein content of peas, beans, and nuts. Examples of one exchange of legumes are 1/2 cup of peas, 1/3 cup of kidney beans, or 1/4 cup of baked beans. On the exchange lists, these legumes are classified as starch/bread. Because many legumes are not only low in fat but also high in fiber, they are valued by health-conscious people.

Nuts appear on the fat exchange list. One tablespoon of cashews or 20 small peanuts is one exchange. Peanut butter appears on two exchange lists: high-fat meat and monounsaturated fat (see Appendix A).

Textured vegetable protein products made from soybeans, peanuts, and cottonseed can enhance the vegetarian diet. The protein is spun into fibers and flavored, colored, and shaped for use as a meat substitute. In their natural form, plant proteins are less digestible than animal proteins, but well-processed soybean isolates are as digestible as egg protein (Johnston, 1999).

Vegetarianism Can Be a Healthy Lifestyle

The American Dietetic Association and Dietitians of Canada have stated that appropriately planned vegetarian diets are healthful, nutritionally adequate, and provide benefits in the prevention and treatment of certain diseases (2003). There are many degrees of vegetarianism, depending on the beliefs of the individual or family. Some people eat animal products such as milk and eggs but not animal flesh. Others eat only plant foods. Some eat only fruits. The more restrictive the diet, the more care required in monitoring intake for adequacy of protein and other nutrients.

Embracing a healthful vegetarian lifestyle encompasses more than just eliminating foods derived from animals. It is necessary to find substitutes for the nutrient-dense animal products. Many traditional regional or ethnic dishes combine a grain with a legume; the two incomplete proteins eaten together complement each other and provide adequate protein. Some favorite combinations such as a peanut butter sandwich or baked beans with brown bread are grain-and-legume combinations. The Mexican burrito, a thin cornmeal bread filled with beans, is another example. Clinical Application 5-4 distinguishes various vegetarian diets.

Health-conscious vegetarians must read labels carefully. Eliminating meat does not automatically decrease a person's fat intake, especially when prepared meals are used. Vegetable oils and cheeses used in sauces to enhance flavor increase the number of kilocalories from fat.

Vegetarian diets can be healthful as long as foods are selected and prepared appropriately. Pregnant women, infants, children, and elderly people who are vegetarians need special assessment and instruction in the use of fortified foods and supplements to ensure adequate nutrition.

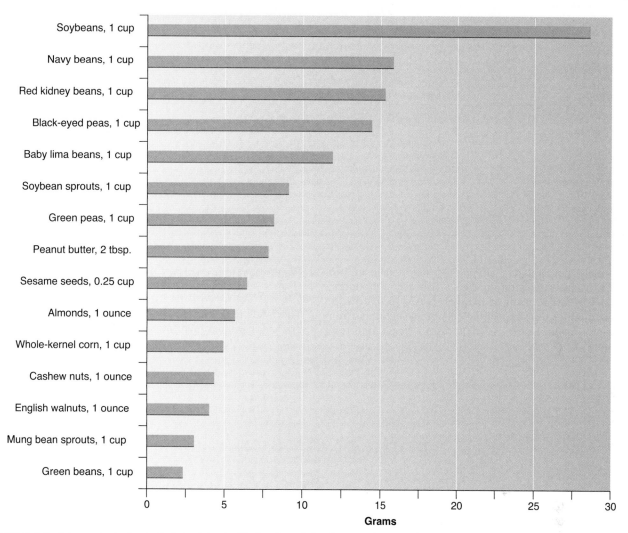

Figure 5–6 Protein content of selected plant foods. Notice that all foods named peas or beans are not legumes. Green beans offer just 2 g of protein, whereas navy beans contain 16 g.

Clinical Application 5–4

Vegetarian Diets

Vegetarians practice different degrees of strictness. From most liberal to most restrictive, the vegetarian diets are ovolactovegetarian, lactovegetarian, ovovegetarian, and strict vegetarian or vegan. The prefixes *ovo-* and *lacto-* mean eggs and milk. So an ovovegetarian will consume eggs, a lactovegetarian milk, and an ovolactovegetarian both. A vegan eats no animal products. Persons following macrobiotic diets consume unrefined/unprocessed grains, small amounts of fruits, vegetables, and legumes, and sometimes milk products. A fruitarian consumes only raw fruits, nuts, seeds, and berries.

Foods Permitted in the Various Vegetarian Diets

	MEAT, FISH, POULTRY	DAIRY PRODUCTS	EGGS
Ovolactovegetarian	No	Yes	Yes
Lactovegetarian	No	Yes	No
Ovovegetarian	No	No	Yes
Strict Vegetarian (vegan)	No	No	No

Adequate assessment of the client's physiological state, knowledge, and values will enable the nurse to provide appropriate nutritional care for vegetarian clients, including referral to registered dietitians as necessary.

(Continued on the following page)

Nutrients Vegetarians May Need to Obtain From Supplements or Designated Food Sources

NUTRIENT	SITUATION TO CONSIDER SUPPLEMENTATION
Vitamin B$_{12}$	Individuals consuming few or no animal products
Vitamin D	Individuals consuming few or no animal products; Vitamin D$_2$ may be preferred source (see Chapter 7)
Calcium	Individuals not consuming dairy products
Omega-3 Fatty Acids (American Dietetic Association: Manual of Clinical Dietetics, 2000)	Individuals consuming few or no animal products Recommended servings: 1–2 daily; 2 for pregnant or lactating women Source of 1 serving: 1 tsp flaxseed oil or 3 tbsp walnuts, or 4 tsp canola or soybean oil, or 6 oz tofu

Usually hospital or care facility dietitians can provide a balanced vegetarian diet. When a nurse encounters a vegetarian client, it is much better to inform the dietitian rather than expect the client to select items from a general menu. Figure 5–7 illustrates a vegetarian food pyramid.

Recommended Dietary Allowances

The adult RDA for protein is 56 grams for men and 46 grams for women (Institute of Medicine, 2002). Pregnancy and lactation increase the need for protein to 71 grams.

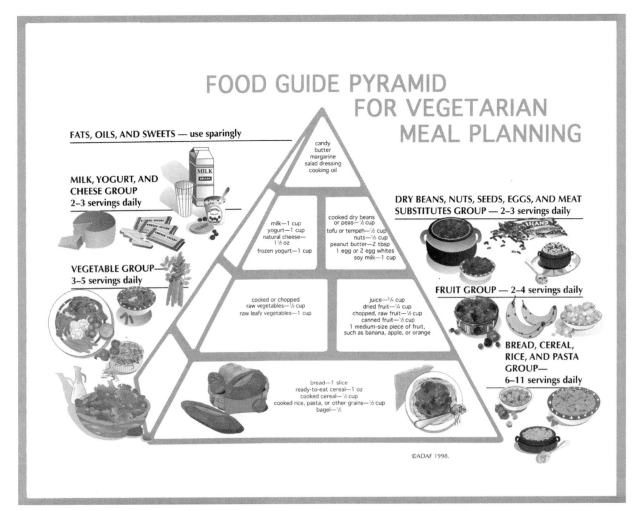

Figure **5–7** An adaptation of the food guide pyramid for vegetarians. (From the National Center for Nutrition and Dietetics, American Dietetic Association, 1998, with permission.)

Table 5–7 **Comparative Sources of 10 Grams of Protein With Kilocalories and Costs**

FOOD	PORTION	KILOCALORIES	COST/AMOUNT	COST/PORTION
Peanut butter	2 tbsp	190	$3.99/28 oz	$0.11
Tuna, canned in water	1 oz	45	$0.79/6 oz	$0.13
Large eggs, poached	1.7	126	$0.99/doz	$0.14
1% milk	1 1/4 cups	128	$1.99/gal	$0.16
Cottage cheese, 2% low fat	1/3 cup	68	$1.59/lb	$0.27
American cheese	1.7 oz	175	$5.19/2 lb	$0.28
Boneless sirloin steak	1.1 oz	66	$5.99/lb	$0.41
Bean soup, condensed, prepared with water	1 1/4 cups	215	$1.09/11.5 oz	$0.47
Bologna	2.9 oz	261	$2.99/lb	$0.54
Cracked wheat bread	5 slices	325	$2.49/24 oz	$0.57

Overeating protein foods can adversely affect a person's health. Intake of protein greater than two or three times the RDA over time may cause bone loss due to increased urinary calcium excretion. Intake of animal protein has been directly related to kidney stones, so individuals predisposed to kidney disease should limit protein intake to the RDA. High-protein diets taken by clients with diabetes mellitus may interfere with glucose control (Eisenstein et al, 2002). In clients with both hypertension and diabetes mellitus, high dietary protein intake is associated with increased microalbuminuria (Wrone et al, 2003).

Choosing Protein Foods Wisely

Producing meat is expensive. For every 5 pounds of vegetable or fish protein fed to livestock, only 1 pound of meat protein is produced. In the United States, the consumption of animal protein between 1910 and 1991 nearly doubled. Now, meat, fish, and poultry contribute 42 percent of the protein intake, dairy products 20 percent, and grains 18 percent (Smit et al, 1999).

Nurses can help clients who have limited funds and those who wish to decrease their meat intake. Table 5–7 lists equivalent sources of 10 grams of protein. The regular prices of nationally advertised brands were used, except for bread, cottage cheese, eggs, milk, and steak. Peanut butter provided 10 grams of protein for 11 cents. Water-packed tuna has the most protein per kilocalorie of the foods listed and was the least expensive complete protein food. The most expensive source in the list is cracked wheat bread. The nurse could make similar calculations for clients' favorite foods or frequently purchased foods to assist them to choose wisely. Substituting store brands or buying on sale likely would lessen the cost for peanut butter, tuna, American cheese, bean soup, bologna, and cracked wheat bread. Wellness Tip 5–1 lists other general principles nurses can teach clients.

  5–1 • Note portion size to avoid overconsumption of protein. Occasionally measure amounts that are served.
- Share restaurant entrees with another person or take a portion home to consume for another meal.
- Replace less-liked items with others in the same category: substitute yogurt or cheese for milk; substitute eggs or legume-grain casseroles for meat or fish.
- Try to incorporate meatless meals or ethnic dishes into your eating pattern regularly.

SUMMARY

Protein is necessary for provision of body structure, tissue maintenance and growth, the regulation of body processes, the development of immunity, the circulation of blood and nutrients, and as a backup source of energy. Protein provides 4 kilocalories per gram. The element that distinguishes protein from carbohydrates and fats is nitrogen. The body combines carbon, hydrogen, oxygen, and nitrogen in certain ways to form amino acids, which then become the building blocks of various proteins.

Complete protein foods contain all essential amino acids in amounts sufficient to support growth. Complete protein foods usually come from animal sources, especially the meat and milk groups.

Incomplete protein foods are grains, vegetables, legumes, nuts, and seeds. A person who eats a grain product and a legume at the same meal, however, is likely to receive all essential amino acids at that meal. Overall daily balance in intake of protein foods is more important than individual meals for most healthy adults.

A normal healthy adult male should consume 56 grams of protein daily, a woman 46 grams. A simple method of estimating protein intake uses the exchange list system. Milk exchanges provide about 8 grams of protein, meat exchanges 7 grams, bread/starch exchanges 3 grams, and vegetable exchanges 2 grams.

CASE STUDY 5-1

Mrs. F is a 72-year-old widow who eats independently in her family homestead. Her usual meals are tea and toast for breakfast, canned fruit and a muffin for lunch, and frozen potpie or canned hash for dinner. She complains that she has been having trouble chewing and has not been eating as much food as she usually does. She does not like milk.

NURSING CARE PLAN

SUBJECTIVE DATA   Food deficit as evidenced by usual food intake information

Has trouble chewing
Does not like milk

OBJECTIVE DATA   Height: 5 ft 4 in

Weight: 106 lb
Elbow width: 2 1/4 inches

NURSING DIAGNOSIS   NANDA: Imbalanced nutrition: less than body requirements (NANDA, 2003, with permission) for protein and kilocalories, related to difficulty chewing, as evidenced by stated usual intake of 28 to 32 g of protein per day and body weight 7 percent under minimum for height and frame

DESIRED OUTCOMES EVALUATION CRITERIA	NURSING ACTIONS/ INTERVENTIONS	RATIONALE
NOC: Nutritional Status: Nutrient Intake (Moorhead, Johnson, and Maas, 2004, with permission)	NIC: Nutritional Counseling (Dochterman and Bulechek, 2004, with permission)	
Client will gain 1 lb per week during the next 2 weeks.	Encourage easily chewed sources of complete protein: cheese, eggs, ground meat, and fish.	Complete protein foods contain all essential amino acids necessary for tissue building.
Client will increase her total protein intake by 14 to 18 g per day.	Create a model meal plan with Mrs. F using the Exchange Group system to count grams of protein.	Mrs. F requires 46 g of protein. The meal plan she described in her history contains only 28 to 32 g depending on dinner selection.
Client will call for dental appointment within next 2 weeks.	Explore sources of financial assistance for dental care if necessary.	Better fitting dentures would permit Mrs. F a wider variety of foods.

C T Q   CRITICAL THINKING QUESTIONS

1. What other food groups are lacking in Mrs. F's usual diet? Would you have given any of them a higher priority than protein? Why or why not?
2. Speculate on the reasons Mrs. F has developed her present meal pattern. What additions could you make to the care plan to improve her nutritional intake?

3. When following up after 2 weeks, the nurse finds that Mrs. F has gained one-half pound instead of 2 as set in the desired outcome. She has increased her intake of eggs and cheese as instructed but says she feels full before finishing her meal. What additional information should the nurse obtain? What modifications to the nursing care plan might she and Mrs. F institute?

⟫⟫ CHAPTER REVIEW

1. For which of the following functions of protein can other nutrients be substituted?
   a. Energy source
   b. Immunity
   c. Maintenance and growth
   d. Regulation of body processes
2. Which of the following foods is a complete protein?
   a. Baked beans
   b. Broccoli
   c. Beef kabobs
   d. Bread sticks
3. If a person has difficulty purchasing meat to serve every day, which of the following foods should the nurse suggest as offering the best source of protein?
   a. Bran muffins with raisins
   b. Red beans and rice
   c. Green bean, onion, and mushroom casserole
   d. Sweet potatoes and cornbread

4. How much protein would a person receive from a glass of milk?
   a. 7 grams
   b. 8 grams
   c. 14 grams
   d. 21 grams

5. Which of the following people would the nurse treat as being in a catabolic state?
   a. Adolescent boy who is into bodybuilding
   b. Lactating mother
   c. Pregnant woman in the second trimester
   d. Surgical client, first day after a stomach resection

 ## CLINICAL ANALYSIS

Mr. P, a 65-year-old man, widowed for 6 months, has been referred to your home health agency for assistance in managing his nutritional intake. He has lost 10 pounds over the past 6 months. A physical examination within the past month revealed no disease processes requiring treatment.

1. In assessing Mr. P, which of the following data would the nurse gather first?
   a. List of current medications the client takes.
   b. Blood protein levels analyzed during the recent physical examination.
   c. A description of the procedure Mr. P uses to weigh himself.
   d. Dietary recall of Mr. P's food and fluid intake.

2. Which of the following plans would be most appropriate to increase Mr. P's protein consumption immediately?
   a. Refer client to nutrition education program.
   b. Have Mr. P apply for home-delivered meals.
   c. Recommend that Mr. P supplement his meals with one of the milk-based liquid breakfast products.
   d. Suggest to Mr. P that he sign up for cooking lessons at the local high school or community college.

3. Which of the following outcomes would indicate achievement of the nutritional objective for Mr. P?
   a. A gain in weight of 2 pounds in 2 weeks.
   b. An invitation to the nurse to join him for a dinner he has learned to cook.
   c. A report by Mr. P that he is eating better.
   d. A visual inspection of Mr. P's refrigerator revealing fresh meat and milk products in abundance.

REFERENCES

Agrawal, S, et al: Nutritional and vitamin status of non-healing wounds in patients attending a tertiary hospital in India. J Dermatol 30:98, 2003.

American Dietetic Association and Dietitians of Canada: Manual of Clinical Dietetics, ed 6. American Dietetic Association, Chicago, 2000.

American Dietetic Association and Dietitians of Canada: Position on vegetarian diets. J Am Diet Assoc 103:748, 2003.

Ashley-Koch, A, Yang, Q, and Olney, RS: Sickle hemoglobin (Hb S) allele and sickle cell disease: A HuGE review. Am J Epidemiol 151:839, 2000.

Baker, SS: Protein-energy malnutrition in the hospitalized pediatric patient. In Walker, WA, and Watkins, JB (eds): Nutrition in Pediatrics. BC Decker, Hamilton, Ontario, 1997.

Boivin, MJ: An ecological paradigm for a health behavior analysis of "konzo," a paralytic disease of Zaire from toxic cassava. Soc Sci Med 45:1853, 1997.

Bonmarin, I, Nunga, M, and Perea, WA: Konzo outbreak, in the south-west of the Democratic Republic of Congo, 1996. J Trop Pediatr 48:234, 2002.

Cleary, M, and Walter, JH: Assessment of adult phenylketonuria. Ann Clin Biochem 38:450, 2001.

de Freitas, O, et al: New approaches to the treatment of phenylketonuria. Nutr Rev 57:65, 1999.

Diasolua Ngudi, D, Kuo, YH, and Lambein F: Food safety and amino acid balance in processed cassava "Cossettes." J Agric Food Chem 50:3042, 2002.

Dochterman, J, and Bulechek, G (eds): Nursing Interventions Classification (NIC), ed 4. Mosby, St. Louis, 2004.

Eisenstein, J, et al: High-protein weight-loss diets: Are they safe and do they work? A review of the experimental and epidemiologic data. Nutr Rev 60:189, 2002.

Ferrando, AA, Paddon-Jones, D, and Wolfe, RR: Alterations in protein metabolism during space flight and inactivity. Nutrition 18:837, 2002.

Gaziev, J, and Lucarelli, G: Stem cell transplantation for hemoglobinopathies. Curr Opin Pediatr 15:24, 2003.

Gropper, SS, Smith, JL, and Groff, JL: Advanced Nutrition and Human Metabolism, ed 4. Wadsworth, Belmont, CA, 2005.

Hughes, VC: Cord blood transplantation: Hallmarks of the 20th century. Lab Med 31:672, 2000.

Institute of Medicine of the National Academy of Sciences: Dietary Reference Intakes: macronutrients. Accessed November 5, 2003 at http:// www.iom.edu/file.asp?id=7300.

Johnston, PK: Nutritional implications of vegetarian diets. In Shils, ME, et al (eds): Modern Nutrition in Health and Disease, ed 9. Lippincott Williams & Wilkins, Philadelphia, 1999.

Lawson, SE, et al: Red cell exchange in sickle cell disease. Clin Lab Haematol 21:99, 1999.

Lunn, PG, Morley, CJ, and Neale, G: A case of kwashiorkor in the UK. Clin Nutr 17:131, 1998.

March of Dimes: PKU. 2003. Accessed August 6, 2003 at http:// www.modimes.org.

Matthews, DE: Proteins and amino acids. In Shils, ME, et al (eds): Modern Nutrition in Health and Disease, ed 9. Lippincott Williams & Wilkins, Philadelphia, 1999.

Messer, E: Intra-household allocation of food and health care: Current findings and understandings—introduction. Soc Sci Med 44:1675, 1997.

Moorhead, S, Johnson, M, and Maas, M (eds): Nursing Outcomes Classification (NOC), ed 3. Mosby, St. Louis, 2004.

Morris, CR, et al: Arginine therapy: A novel strategy to induce nitric oxide production in sickle cell disease. Br J Haematol 111:498, 2000.

NANDA International: Nursing Diagnoses: Definitions and Classification 2003–2004. NANDA International, Philadelphia, 2003.

National Institutes of Health: NIH Consensus Statement: Phenylketonuria (PKU) Screening and Management, 2000. Accessed June 3, 2003 at http://consensus.nih.gov/cons/113/113_statement.pdf.

Platt, OS, Brambilla, DJ, and Rosse, WF: Mortality in sickle cell disease: Life expectancy and risk factors for early death. N Engl J Med 330:1639, 1994.

Schumm, DE: Essentials of Biochemistry. FA Davis, Philadelphia, 1988.

Smit, E, et al: Estimates of animal and plant protein intake in US adults: Results from the Third National Health and Nutrition Examination Survey, 1988–1991. J Am Diet Assoc 99:813, 1999.

Solomons, TWG: Fundamentals of Organic Chemistry, ed. 4. John Wiley & Sons, New York, 1994.

Steinberg, MH: Management of sickle cell disease. N Engl J Med 340:1021, 1999.

Tapiero, H, et al: Glutamine and glutamate. Biomed Pharmacother 56:446, 2002.

United States Department of Health and Human Services: Better access to quality outpatient care for sickle cell disease could reduce patients' heavy reliance on expensive ER care. Res Activities 273:11, 2003.

Venes, D (ed): Tabor's Cyclopedic Medical Dictionary, ed 19. FA Davis, Philadelphia, 2001.

Vichinsky, E: New therapies in sickle cell disease. Lancet 360:629, 2002.

Wrone, EM, et al: Association of dietary protein intake and microalbuminuria in health adults: Third National Health and Nutrition Examination Survey. Am J Kidney Dis 41:580, 2003.

Energy Balance

After completing this chapter, the student should be able to:

1. Describe energy homeostasis.
2. List two reasons the body needs energy.
3. Describe how energy is measured both in foods and in the human body.
4. Discuss the effect of body composition on energy output.
5. Name the energy nutrient that has the highest kilocalorie density and identify two substances usually found in foods with a low kilocalorie density.

A complete understanding of the human body's energy balance system eludes experts. In approximately 40 percent of the U.S. population, the human body regulates energy intake and expenditure automatically to maintain an **energy balance.** This balance occurs even when the amount of energy needed varies and food intake is erratic. The body can also compensate during food restriction or starvation by conserving energy. Maintenance of a reduced or elevated body weight is associated with compensatory changes in energy expenditure, which oppose the maintenance of a body weight that is different from the usual body weight (Leibert, 1995). The energy balance system in about 60 percent of the U.S. population has a malfunction. This is evident by the limited ability of the medical community to successfully treat energy imbalances in clients. Most experts agree that the human body's energy balance system is the most complex of all the biological systems.

This chapter focuses on energy balance (Chapter 18 on weight control focuses on energy imbalance), and in particular on the effect of energy intake and energy expenditure on energy balance. Topics include energy measurements, factors that can influence the body's need for energy, energy consumption patterns, the kilocaloric content and nutrient density of foods, energy allowances, and current recommendations concerning energy consumption.

A basic understanding of what is known about the energy balance system in the human body is a necessary foundation for understanding energy imbalance.

Homeostasis

The human body seeks **homeostasis**—that is, equilibrium or balance. Homeostasis, in terms of energy balance, occurs when the number of kilocalories eaten equals the number used to produce energy. An individual who maintains a stable body weight is usually in energy balance.

Energy Intake

The typical adult eats 500,000 to 850,000 kilocalories per year. Eating an excess of only 1 percent or 15 extra kilocalories per day would result in a weight gain of 1.5 pounds per year—the kilocalories in 1/3 teaspoonful of butter or a quarter of a small apple. Individuals at a stable, healthy weight give little thought to the amount of food that they eat each day, yet their body weight remains constant.

Eating appears to be a voluntary act influenced by the external environment, but it is regulated internally as well. The internal regulation of energy balance involves the gastrointestinal tract, the endocrine system, the brain, and body fat stores. Physiologic regulation is evidenced by the constancy of body weight in adults and the fact that after weight gain or loss this constant body weight is reestablished. Over the long term, food energy intake is regulated to balance energy expenditure.

Energy Expenditure

Energy expenditure, which varies daily, is measured by the number of kilocalories an individual uses to meet the body's demand for fuel. A person uses many more kilocalories to run a marathon than to sleep all day. Physical activity expends energy.

Adaptive Thermogenesis

Energy expenditure frequently adapts to large increases or large decreases in food intake of several days' duration by means of a process called **adaptive thermogenesis.** Adaptive thermogenesis is one example of how the human body evolved to cope with feast-or-famine conditions. Energy expenditure decreases during food restriction or starvation. Kilocalories are burned more efficiently. Adaptive thermogenesis causes an individual who is trying to lose weight either to lose at a slower rate or to stop losing weight. It makes weight loss difficult for many people but not impossible. Overeating for several days will cause an increase in energy expenditure. Energy expenditure has been found to be higher than predicted during the refeeding of previously starved patients, especially within the first week (Hoffer, 1999). Researchers do not yet understand why some people are unable to maintain energy balance. However, for about 40 percent of the population, the human body maintains energy balance.

Measurement of Energy

Both the energy (fuel) foods contain and the amount of energy the body uses can be measured. The methods used to measure energy are fairly universal.

Units of Measure

The energy content of food is measured in kilocalories, often abbreviated as kcalories or kcal. A **kilocalorie** is the amount of heat required to raise 1 kilogram of water 1°C. Kilocalories are what the media and people who are not health-care professionals incorrectly call "calories." In chemistry, a **calorie** is the amount of heat required to raise 1 gram of water 1°C. One kilocalorie contains 1000 times as much energy as one calorie. This is important for students to understand if they are dually enrolled in both a nutrition and chemistry class. *Kilocalorie* is the term used throughout this text. Using kcalories for nutritional measurement eliminates the large numbers that use of the chemical term would necessitate.

The **joule** is another unit increasingly used to measure energy; you may encounter this term as you read scientific journals. One **kilojoule** is the amount of energy required to move a mass of 1 kilogram with an acceleration of 1 meter per second. The kilojoule is equal to 0.239 kilocalorie; a kilocalorie equals 4.184 kilojoules. With the ease of access to international research via the Internet, an understanding of the term joule is necessary to interpret research.

Energy Nutrient Values

The energy nutrients are carbohydrates, fat, and protein. Alcohol (ethanol) also yields energy. A food's kilocalorie value is determined by its content of protein, fat, carbohydrates, and alcohol. To review:

- 1 gram of carbohydrate equals 4 kilocalories (or 17 kilojoules)
- 1 gram of protein equals 4 kilocalories (or 17 kilojoules)
- 1 gram of fat equals 9 kilocalories (or 37.6 kilojoules)
- 1 gram of alcohol equals 7 kilocalories (or 29.3 kilojoules).

Water, fiber, vitamins, and minerals do not provide kilocalories. Clinical Calculation 6–1 demonstrates how to determine the energy content of a food item.

Clinical Calculation 6–1

Calculating the Energy Content of a Food Item

If you know the carbohydrate, fat, and protein content of a food item, you can readily calculate the food item's kilocalorie content. Two examples are shown below. One starch exchange contains 3 g of protein and 15 g of carbohydrate. Adding the protein and carbohydrate content in the starch exchange together equals 18.

	Carbohydrate (g)	Protein (g)	Fat (g)	Total (g)
One starch exchange	15	+ 3	+ 0	= 18

There are 4 kcal in 1 g each of carbohydrate and protein so all you need to do to obtain the kilocalorie content of the starch exchange is to multiply 4 by 18. Thus, there are 72 kcal in one starch exchange.

One fat exchange contains 5 g of fat.

	Carbohydrate (g)	Protein (g)	Fat (g)	Total (g)
One fat exchange	0	+ 0	+ 5	= 5

There are 9 kcal in a gram of fat. To obtain the kilocaloric content of one fat exchange, multiply 5 by 9. Thus, one fat exchange contains 45 kcal.

Determination of Energy Values

Foods

The energy content of individual foods is measured by a device called a **bomb calorimeter,** illustrated in Figure 6–1. A bomb calorimeter is an insulated container that has a chamber in which food is burned. The amount of heat (kilocalories) produced by the burning of the food is determined by the change in the temperature of a measured amount of water that surrounds the chamber. All energy in food is in the form of chemical energy. In a bomb calorimeter, the chemical energy stored in the food sample is transformed into heat energy. The following equation may facilitate understanding of this concept:

$$\text{Protein} + \text{oxygen} = \text{heat energy} + \text{water} + \text{carbon dioxide}$$

(Carbohydrate or fat may be substituted for protein in the equation.)

Human Body

A process similar to the combustion of food in the bomb calorimeter occurs in the body. The amount of energy the human body uses can be measured directly or indirectly. Direct measurement of energy used by the human body requires expensive equipment that is used only in scientific research. Energy is measured directly by placing a person in an insulated heat-sensitive chamber and measuring the heat emitted by the body. Indirect measurement of energy is discussed in Clinical Application 6–1.

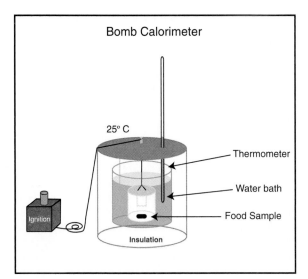

Figure **6–1** Illustration of a bomb calorimeter. The food sample is ignited and burned. The heat produced is absorbed by the known volume of water in the surrounding section. Change in temperature provides a measure of the heat produced.

Components of Energy Expenditure

The human body requires energy to meet its resting energy expenditure needs and its physical activity requirements. Physical activity includes the energy needed for voluntary activities, which are consciously controlled, such as running, walking, and swimming, and involuntary activities. Energy is also expended to digest, absorb, transport, and utilize nutrients.

Resting Energy Expenditure

Resting energy expenditure represents the energy expended or used by a person at rest. Resting energy

Clinical Application 6–1

Measurement of REE by Indirect Calorimetry

There are two techniques to indirectly measure resting energy expenditure. One method measures the amount of carbon dioxide exhaled and the amount of oxygen inspired for a given period of time. From this data, the number of kilocalories expended can be calculated. The device used to compute the intake of oxygen and output of carbon dioxide is called a respirator or metabolic machine. The health-care worker is most likely to observe this procedure in the intensive care unit of an acute care hospital. The second less-expensive method to measure REE is relatively new and measures only the amount of oxygen consumed. Using this data, the machine calculates the client's REE. The manufacturer of this machine claims it will be useful for determining the REE for routine nutritional assessment services and for clients on weight-management programs (www.korr.com).

expenditure (REE) requires more total kilocalories than physical activity in most people. Another term still in use in some scientific literature is basal metabolic rate (BMR). The major difference between resting energy and basal metabolic rate is that basal metabolic rate is always measured beginning at least 12 hours after the last meal and under certain conditions, such as controlled temperature and humidity.

Clinical Application 6–1 discusses the measurement of REE in clients. The term REE is generally associated with the use of a respirometer or a device that measures oxygen consumption. In practice, BMR and REE differ by less than 12 percent in healthy well-nourished clients, and the terms are used interchangeably.

The kilocalories necessary to support the following contribute to resting energy expenditure:

1. Contraction of the heart
2. Maintenance of body temperature
3. Repair of the internal organs
4. Maintenance of cellular processes
5. Muscle and nerve coordination
6. Respiration (breathing)

REE accounts for approximately 66 percent of most people's total energy requirements. Body composition influences resting energy expenditure. Individuals of similar age, sex, height, and weight with a higher percentage of muscle (lean body mass) have a higher REE than those with less muscle. It takes more energy, or kilocalories, to support lean body mass (protein) than to support body fat. Muscle tissue requires more kilocalories than does fat tissue, even when muscle tissue is resting. Therefore, the higher a person's body protein content, the more kilocalories he or she can eat and still maintain a stable body weight.

In clinical practice, estimating a person's resting energy expenditure is commonly done by using the Harris-Benedict equation found in Table 6–1. A different equation is used for men and women. These equations take into account age, sex, and weight but ignore differences in body composition, climate, and genetic variability (discussed in the following sections). Although these equations are not completely accurate for all individuals, they can serve as a guide for menu planning and the initial calculation of tube and intravenous feedings. The ultimate test of how kilocalories eaten work in the body is to monitor body weight and kilocaloric intake over time—one reason nurses

Table **6–1** **Harris-Benedict Equation to Calculate REE**

To convert weight in pounds to kilograms (kg): 1 kg = 2.2 pounds; divide body weight in pounds by 2.2
To convert height in inches to centimeters (cm): 1 inch = 2.54 cm; multiple height in inches by 2.54
- REE for men: 66.6 + (13.7 × wt in kg) + (5 × height in cm) – (6.7 × age in years)
- REE for women: 655.1 + (6 × wt in kg) + (1.8 × height in cm) – (4.7 × age in years).

monitor clients' body weight and food intake and dietitians calculate clients' kcaloric intake.

Age

Resting energy expenditure varies with lean body mass, which varies with age. The highest rates of energy expenditure per pound of body weight occur during infancy and childhood. In adults, REE declines about 2 percent per decade because of a decline in lean body mass. The result is a reduced need for kilocalories. Individuals can slow the decline in lean body mass somewhat by increasing their exercise. An individual who fails either to decrease kilocaloric intake to compensate for this reduced need or to increase physical activity may experience a slow weight gain (see Wellness Tip 6–1).

 6–1 • To compensate for a decrease in resting energy expenditure as you grow older, increase exercise and decrease food intake.

Sex

Differences in body composition between men and women occur as early as the first few months of life. The differences are relatively small until the child reaches age 10. During adolescence, body composition changes radically. Men develop proportionately greater muscle mass than women, who deposit fat as they mature. Consequently, REE differs by as much as 10 percent between men and women.

Growth

Human growth is most pronounced during the growth spurts that take place before birth and during infancy and puberty. Kilocalories required per kilogram of body weight are highest during these growth spurts, because the kilocaloric cost of anabolism is greater than the kilocaloric cost of catabolism.

Body Size

People with large bodies require proportionately more energy than smaller ones. A tall individual uses more energy because he or she has a greater skin surface through which heat is lost than does a shorter person. A shorter person also has less muscle tissue or lean body mass than a taller person. Most health care professionals are surprised at the large volume of food needed to maintain a tall male's body weight (>6′0″) and how small a volume of food is needed to maintain weight in a short female (<5′0″). In proportion to total body weight, the infant has a large surface area, loses more heat through the skin, and therefore has a proportionately high REE.

Genetics

REE is strongly influenced by individual genetic patterns. Each person, it seems, is programmed with a need to burn a certain number of kilocalories to maintain energy balance. This fact becomes apparent to health-care workers when counseling two very similar clients. Both clients may be of the same sex, of equal weight, perform similar types of physical activity, and have about the same body fat content. Yet each client may need to eat a different number of kilocalories to maintain a stable body weight. Many individuals have little control over the number of kilocalories required to meet the needs of REE.

Climate

Climate affects REE because kilocalories are needed to maintain body temperature. This fact pertains to extreme differences in external temperatures, whether cold or hot. In the United States and Canada, most people do not need to eat more kilocalories during colder months because most living environments range from 68°F to 77°F. Outside, people usually protect themselves from extreme cold and shivering, which causes an increase in REE, by wearing warm clothes.

Clients with fevers also need extra kilocalories. Clinical Application 6–2 discusses this need.

Thermic Effect of Food

After a meal, the heat produced by the body is called the **thermic effect of food** (TEF). An older term for this energy cost is specific dynamic action (SDA). Energy is needed to chew, swallow, digest, absorb, and transport nutrients. **Metabolism** increases after eating. As metabolism increases, more kilocalories are used.

The consumption of protein and carbohydrates results in a larger thermic effect than the consumption of fat. Fat is metabolized efficiently, with only 4 percent wastage, compared to 25 percent wastage when carbohydrate is converted to fat (Frary and Johnson, 2004). If an individual eats as many kilocalories from carbohydrate or protein as from fat, he or she will store fewer of the nonfat kilocalories as body fat.

Kilocalories do count, however, regardless of the source. Consumers need to read food labels carefully. Sometimes a regular version of a food may actually contain fewer kcalories than the fat-free or reduced-fat version. For example, a regular fig cookie contains 50 kcalories, and one fat-free version contains 70 kcalories. One-half cup of regular ice cream contains 180 calories, and the same amount of one kind of reduced-fat ice cream contains 190 kcalories. Sometimes consumers are under the illusion that because the food they are eating is low-fat, they can eat unrestricted amounts and maintain body weight (see Wellness Tip 6–2).

Clinical Application 6–2

Fever

Heat acts as a catalyst in most chemical reactions. A **catalyst** is a substance that speeds up a chemical reaction. Fever increases resting energy expenditure by about 7 percent for every 1°F increase in body temperature. Frequently, an individual with a fever is too ill to eat. Fruit juices with added glucose polymers or a nutritional supplement will give the client needed energy.

6–2 • Choose sensible portion sizes: Fat-free and reduced-fat foods may not be low in kcalories.

• Kcalories count regardless of the source (fat, protein, or CHO).

Physical Activity

For most of the U.S. population, the second component of total energy expenditure is physical activity (see Wellness Tip 6–3). Some very active individuals may need more kilocalories as a result of physical activity than as a result of REE (Fig. 6–2). Professional athletes may burn a large number of kilocalories as a result of training and engaging in competition. Table 6–2 describes a second method to estimate energy needs that includes those needed for both REE and activity. This method of calculating kilocalories expended to perform physical activity provides only an estimate. As Table 6–3 shows, the intensity and duration of any physical activity enormously influences kilocalorie expenditure. For example, a 180 pound male who trains by weight lifting will expend almost 600 kilocalories in a one-hour training session. The most accurate method to determine a client's kilocalorie requirement is to monitor both food intake and body weight over time. The energy cost of physical activity is frequently referred to as the **thermic effect of exercise (TEE).**

 6–3 • Be active.

Physical activity can greatly influence energy requirements (Table 6–3). For example, a 154-pound man of normal weight may require only 2002 kilocalories on a very sedentary day and as many as 2772 kilocalories on a very active day. A 128-pound woman of normal body weight may require only 1664 kilocalories on a very sedentary day and as many as 2304 kilocalories on a very active day.

Thermic Effect of Exercise

Energy expended during exercise is only a portion of the total energy cost of physical activity. Exercise may also affect both REE and the TEF. Some clients' REE increases for up to 48 hours after exercise. Although the exact reason for this increase in REE is not known, the most plausible explanation is that the glycogen stores need to be refilled. Because exercise depletes glycogen stores, there is an energy cost to refill these stores during the postexercise period.

Adaptive Response to Exercise

An individual with well-developed muscles performs more efficiently—uses fewer kilocalories to perform a given amount of physical work—than an individual with less well-developed muscles. As exercise is repeated, the body learns how to get the job done with the least effort (the body's adaptive response to exercise). If an individual has a weight loss due to increased exercise, he or she will eventually use fewer kilocalories to do a specific activity. This is the reason body builders need to continually increase the amount of weight lifted to achieve maximum results. Lighter people require fewer kilocalories for

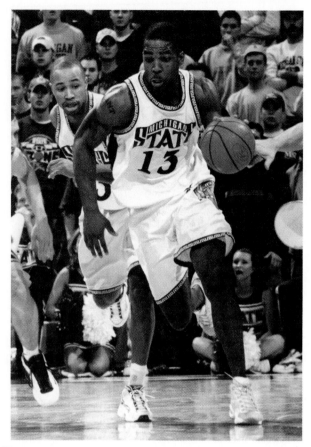

Figure **6–2** A trained athlete may burn more kcalories as a result of physical activity than as a result of resting energy expenditure. (Courtesy of Kevin Fowler, Sports Information, Michigan State University)

a given amount of exercise than heavier people do; it takes fewer kilocalories to move a smaller mass than a larger one.

Although heavier people burn more kilocalories than lighter people when they exercise because they move more weight, a heavy body is a disincentive for movement and physical activity. Heavier people tend to do fewer of those energy demanding activities (Swinburn, 2004). This has been attributed to mechanical problems associated with increased body weight. These include arthritis,

Table **6–2** Energy Needs Based on Weight and Activity

	Energy Needs in Kilocalories per Pound of Body Weight		
	SEDENTARY*	**MODERATELY ACTIVE†**	**ACTIVE‡**
Overweight	9–11	13	16
Normal weight	13	16	18
Underweight	13	18	18–23

*Patients with severely limited mobility; †Active students, sales clerks, many farm workers; ‡Full-time athletes, unskilled laborers, Army recruits.

Table 6–3 Kcalories Expended in 30 Minutes at Various Activities by 140- and 180-Pound Individuals

ACTIVITY	KCALORIES EXPENDED BY A 140-POUND PERSON	KCALORIES EXPENDED BY A 180-POUND PERSON
Sitting quietly	39	51
Walking	228	291
Running	396	510
Jogging	324	417
Cycling	192	246
Gardening	177	225
Golf (pull/carry clubs)	162	210
Golf (power cart)	75	96
Swimming (crawl, moderate pace)	270	348
Social dancing	192	246
Weight training	228	294

arthralgia (pain in a joint), low back pain, chest and wall diaphragm restriction, incontinence, obstructive sleep apnea, and cellulites (Swinburn, 2004).

Exercise and Appetite

Many exercise researchers think that exercise decreases appetite. **Appetite** is defined as a strong desire for food (or by extension for a pleasant sensation) based on previous experience that causes one to seek food for the purpose of tasting and enjoying. After exercise, a person's appetite may be less—that is, he or she may be satisfied with less food. Some types of exercise release a chemical in the brain called **beta-endorphin.** Beta-endorphin has an effect similar to that of natural morphine; it produces a state of relaxation. In effect, exercise can be a safe substitute for overeating in individuals who eat to decrease stress and tension.

Aerobic Exercise

Aerobic exercise is any activity during which the energy metabolism needed is supported by the amount of increase in oxygen inspired. Aerobic exercises increase physical fitness and involve large muscle groups. Vigorous workouts that last at least 30 minutes, such as fast walking, cycling, swimming, skating, rope jumping, aerobic dancing, hiking, jogging, and rowing, require an increase in the amount of oxygen inspired. Any exercise that raises your pulse to **target heart rate** is an aerobic activity. To determine your target heart rate, see Clinical Application 6–3.

Aerobic exercise provides many health benefits, including:

- Decreased risk of cardiovascular disease
- Improved blood sugar control for people with diabetes
- Decreased risk of obesity
- Reversal or prevention of varicose veins
- Decreased risk of osteoporosis

Clinical Application 6–3

Determining a Theoretical Target Heart Rate

The theoretical target heart rate is the rate you need to reach to achieve maximal aerobic effect. Determine your theoretical* target heart rate as follows:

1. Subtract your age from the number 220.
2. Multiply this number first by 65 percent and then by 80 percent. The two numbers should represent the range of heart beats per minute that you should try to maintain during aerobic exercise. Example of an 18-year-old woman:

$$220 - 18 = 202$$
$$202 \times 0.65 = 131$$
$$202 \times 0.80 = 161$$

This individual should exercise sufficiently to reach a heart rate of between 131 and 161 beats per minute.

*To monitor your heart rate during exercise, count the number of times your heart beats for 6 seconds and multiply by 10.

- Improvement in the quality of sleep
- Improved hypertension control

Anaerobic Exercise

Exercise during which energy needed is provided without an increase in the use of inspired oxygen is **anaerobic exercise.** Short bursts of vigorous activity, such as resistance or muscle strength training (weight lifting, for example), are forms of anaerobic exercise. Anaerobic exercise allows for muscle toning, the building of muscular strength and endurance, and the building of bone mass. This kind of training provides added strength and toughness, which help to reduce injury during aerobic exercise, prevents lower back problems, and allows for a more muscular appearance.

Diet and Activity

A healthy lifestyle depends on much more than diet alone. Physical activity makes a vital contribution to health, function, and performance. The greatest benefit derived from physical activity is gained when a person moves from sedentary to moderate levels of activity. The combination of a balanced diet and regular physical activity has a stronger effect on energy balance than either strategy alone (Jakicic, 2002).

Every adult should engage in 60 minutes or more of moderate-intensity physical activity on most, preferably all, days of the week—that is, a total of 60 minutes per day of brisk walking, stair climbing, calisthenics, heavy gardening, or dancing. The activity need not be continuous but may be broken up into short sessions. For example, six brisk 10-minute walks would meet the minimum requirement. A person performing these activities for 60 minutes expends 400 total kilocalories. The President's Council on Physical Fitness and Activity has published an Activity Pyramid (Fig. 6–3). Some health benefits can be achieved

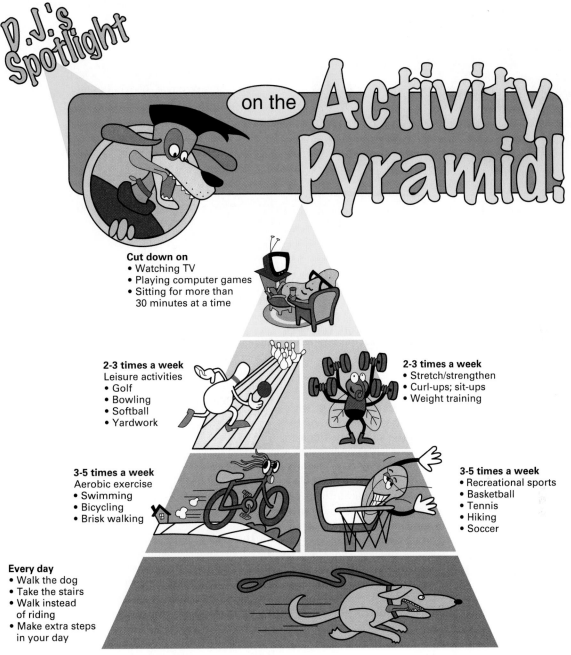

Cut down on
- Watching TV
- Playing computer games
- Sitting for more than 30 minutes at a time

2-3 times a week
Leisure activities
- Golf
- Bowling
- Softball
- Yardwork

2-3 times a week
- Stretch/strengthen
- Curl-ups; sit-ups
- Weight training

3-5 times a week
Aerobic exercise
- Swimming
- Bicycling
- Brisk walking

3-5 times a week
- Recreational sports
- Basketball
- Tennis
- Hiking
- Soccer

Every day
- Walk the dog
- Take the stairs
- Walk instead of riding
- Make extra steps in your day

Figure **6-3** The President's Council Activity Pyramid for Children. Children should have some activity every day, vigorous activity two to three times a week, and minimal sedentary activity such as watching television and playing computer games.

with a minimum of 30 minutes of moderate intensity physical activity on most days of the week; however, this is insufficient to maintain energy balance in most people.

Energy Intake

The average daily reported energy intakes for men were between 1821 and 2840 kilocalories per day. The average daily reported intakes for women were between 1381 and 1901 kilocalories per day. The average reported intakes for women are of special concern because of the difficulty in incorporating all nutrients at recommended levels in a diet

so low in kilocalories. The need for the average woman to increase energy output or physical activity is well documented.

Information from the Nationwide Food Consumption Survey has been used to compare energy intakes in 1965 with those in 1977. These data suggest that energy intake declined for both sexes by approximately 10 percent during those 10 to 20 years (National Research Council, 1989). The percentage of overweight men and women has been increasing despite the decrease in energy intake. Many experts attribute increased obesity to decreased

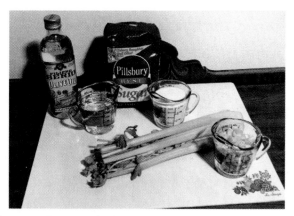

Figure **6-4** One cup of celery contains 17 kcalories, 1 cup of sugar contains 770 calories, and 1 cup of oil contains 1925 kcalories. Celery is the least kcalorically dense of the foods pictured, and oil is the most dense. Sugar is between celery and oil in kcaloric density.

energy expenditure. America is becoming an increasingly sedentary society. The current recommendation is that the typical person increase physical activity rather than decrease kilocalorie intake below the recommended energy allowance to achieve energy balance.

Kilocaloric Density of Foods

Some foods are more kilocalorically dense than other foods. Density is the quantity per unit volume of a substance. **Kilocaloric density** refers to the kilocalories contained in a given volume of a food. Foods with a high water and fiber content tend to have a lower kilocaloric density. Fruits and vegetables such as lettuce, watermelon, and celery are high in water content and low in kilocalories. A given volume of grapes has fewer kilocalories than an equal one of raisins because grapes contain more water than raisins.

Fats or foods high in fat have the highest kilocaloric density (Fig. 6–4). Whole-milk products, high-fat meat exchanges, fat exchanges, and foods made with these ingredients all contain appreciable amounts of fat. Box 6–1 lists several tips for decreasing the kilocaloric density of a diet.

Nutrient Density of Foods

Kilocaloric content alone should not be the criterion to decide whether to include a food in one's diet. The **nutrient density** of a food—the concentration of nutrients in a food compared with the food's kilocaloric content—is also an important consideration. If a food is high in kilocalories and low in nutrients, the nutrient density of the food is low. **Empty kilocalories** means that the food contains kilocalories and almost no nutrients; table sugar is an example of such a food. If a food is low in kilocalories and high in nutrients, the nutrient density of the food is high.

Cantaloupe is an example of a food with a high nutrient density—it is low in kilocalories and high in vitamin C and contains a moderate amount of vitamin A. Skim milk and whole milk are similar in nutrient content; both types of milk contain about the same amounts of protein, calcium, and riboflavin. Eight ounces of skim milk provides about 90

Box 6-1 **Tips for Decreasing the Kilocaloric Density of a Diet**

- Use low-fat or nonfat dairy products including skim milk, cheese, and yogurt.
- Brown meats by broiling or cooking in nonstick pans with little or no fat. Avoid fried foods.
- Chill soups, stews, sauces, and broths. Lift off and discard hardened fat.
- Trim all visible fat from meat before cooking.
- Use water-packed, canned foods such as fruits and tuna.
- Use fresh fruits and vegetables often. Try to eat at least 2 1/2 cups of these foods each day.
- Use low-kilocalorie salad dressings.
- When you eat out, do not look at the menu. Instead, have an idea of what you would like to eat before you arrive at the restaurant. Explain to the waitress or waiter what you would like to eat.
- Eat smaller portion sizes of all foods but particularly sandwiches (Roll et al, 2004).

kilocalories compared with 150 kilocalories in 8 ounces of whole milk. Skim milk thus has a higher nutrient density than whole milk.

In 2002, the federal government issued the Dietary Intake Reference (DRIs) Values for Energy for Active Individuals. See Table 6–4. Note that the values for pregnant and lactating women are increased. For example, a 19 year old female in her third trimester needs about 450 more kilocalories beyond her nonpregant value. A 19 year old lactating women nursing a 6 to 12 mo infant needs 400 kilocalories beyond her nonlactating value.

Dietary Recommendations

All the major national health organizations recommend that individuals maintain a healthy body weight. The American Heart Association recommends maintaining a healthy body weight to decrease the risk of heart and circulatory diseases. The American Cancer Society cites numerous studies suggesting that lower kilocaloric intake may lower an individual's risk of cancer. Most individuals would benefit by monitoring their weight and increasing their energy expenditure or decreasing their energy intake as necessary to maintain a healthy body weight.

The Food and Nutrition Board of the National Academy of Sciences (NAS) revised their guidelines on energy nutrient distribution in 2002. Box 6–2 compares the 1996 guidelines to the 2002 guidelines. Their rationale is that carbohydrate and fat are both energy sources and can substitute for one another to some extent.

Box 6-2 **National Academy of Sciences Guidelines**

	1996	2002
Kcal from CHO	50% or more	45% to 65%
Kcal from fat	30% or less	20% to 35%
Kcal from protein	10% to 35%	10% to 35%

Table 6–4   **Dietary Reference Intake Values for Energy for Active Individuals: Food and Nutrition Board, Institute of Medicine, National Academies**

| LIFESTYLE GROUP | CRITERION | Active PAL EER (kcal/day) | |
		MALE	FEMALE
Infants	Energy expenditure + energy deposition		
0–6 mo	Energy expenditure + energy deposition	570	520 (3 mo)
7–12 mo	Energy expenditure + energy deposition	743	676 (9 mo)
Children			
1–2 yr	Energy expenditure + energy deposition	1046	992 (24 mo)
3–8 yr	Energy expenditure + energy deposition	1742	1642 (6 yr)
9–13 yr	Energy expenditure + energy deposition	2279	2071 (11 yr)
14–18 yr	Energy expenditure + energy deposition	3152	2368 (16 yr)
Adults			
>18 yr	Energy expenditure	3067*	2403* (19 yr)
Pregnant women			
14–18 yr	Adolescent female EER + change in TEE + pregnancy energy deposition		
First Trimester			2368 (16 yr)
Second Trimester			2708 (16 yr)
Third Trimester			2820 (yr)
19–50 yr	Adult female EER + change in TEE + pregnancy energy deposition		
First Trimester			2403 (19 yr)
Second Trimester			2743 (19 yr)
Third Trimester			2855 (yr)
Lactating Women	Adolescent female EER + milk energy output – weight loss		
14–18 yr			
First 6 mo			2698 (16 yr)
Second 6 mo			2768 (16 yr)
19–50 yr	Adult female EER + milk energy output – weight loss		
First 6 mo			2733 (19 yr)
Second 6 mo			2803 (19 yr)

SOURCE: Copied with permission from Krause's Food, Nutrition, and Diet Therapy, ed 11. Elsevier, Philadelphia, 2004.
Data compiled from Institutes of Medicine of The National Academies Press.
For healthy active Americans and Canadians at the reference height and weight.
PAL, physically active level; EER, estimated energy requirement; TEE, total energy expenditure.
*Subtract 10 kcal/day for men and 7 kcal/day for women for each year above 19.

SUMMARY

Energy balance exists when energy intake equals energy output. A person whose body weight remains stable is usually in energy balance. In about 40 percent of the U.S. population, the capability of regulating energy intake and expenditure to accommodate daily variations is normal. When an individual is not in energy balance, he or she is gaining or losing body weight.

The human body needs energy for resting energy expenditure and voluntary physical activity. The Harris-Benedict equation is commonly used in clinical practice to provide an initial estimate a client's REE. Kilocalories needed for physical activity must be added to REE to estimate total kilocaloric need. However, the most accurate method to determine kilocalorie need is to monitor both food intake and body weight over time.

Foods high in water and fiber (fruits and vegetables) are low in kilocaloric density. Foods high in fat (fatty meats, oils, spreads, salad dressings, and food made with these ingredients) are high in kilocaloric density. Foods that are low in kilocalories and contain substantial amounts of one or more nutrients are high in nutrient density. Individuals should try to consume nutritionally dense foods. The recommended range of energy nutrient intake is 45 to 65 percent for carbohydrate, 20 to 35 percent for fat, and 10 to 35 percent for protein.

The current recommendation is that individuals who gain weight while consuming their energy RDA should increase their activity to maintain energy balance. Most Americans are eating too much of one, two, or three of the energy nutrients to maintain energy balance.

CASE STUDY 6-1

The Fairview Nursing Home holds a weekly client care conference. All of the facility's residents have their nursing care plans reviewed on a rotating basis, with each client's nursing care plan being reviewed once every 3 months. All members of the health-care team are often present at the conference. Team members may include the administrator, the physician, the director of nursing, the staff nurse, the nursing assistant, the activities director, the social worker, the dietitian, and the client or a family member representing the client.

Mr. G has been experiencing a slow weight gain. His weight history follows:

1/89	175 lb
3/89	177 lb
7/89	178 lb
9/89	180 lb
12/89	181 lb

Mr. G is 5 ft 8 in tall and 79 years old. He is alert, feeds himself, and has normal bowel and bladder function. Mr. G walks to the dining room three times a day. His favorite activity is watching television. He has good dentition and is on a regular diet. According to the appetite records kept by the nurse's aide, Mr. G's intake is good to excellent. He accepts all of the major food groups. He admits to overeating at social activities, especially those sponsored by the facility in the evenings. Mr. G is concerned with his slow weight gain but claims he does not know what to do. To address the slow weight gain problem, the health-care team and Mr. G developed the following nursing care plan.

NURSING CARE PLAN

SUBJECTIVE DATA Client expressed concern about his slow weight gain.

OBJECTIVE DATA Height is 5 ft, 8 in. Weights and percent healthy body weight:

1/89   175 lb   103 percent healthy body weight
12/89   181 lb   106 percent healthy body weight

NURSING DIAGNOSIS NANDA: Imbalanced nutrition: More than body requirements (NANDA, 2003, with permission) related to sedentary activity level and eating in response to external cues.

DESIRED OUTCOMES EVALUATION CRITERIA	NURSING ACTIONS/INTERVENTIONS	RATIONALE
NOC: Nutritional Status: (Moorhead, Johnson, and Maas, 2003, with permission)	NIC: Nutritional Counseling (Dochterman and Bulechek, 2004, with permission)	
Client will select fresh fruits for desserts at 75 percent of all social activities.	Provide encouragement to the client to select fresh fruit at all social activities. Congratulate the client when he is able to refrain from eating rich desserts. Remind the Dietary Department to serve fresh fruit at social functions.	Replacing kilocalorically dense cakes, pies, and cookies with fresh fruit will promote weight maintenance.
Client will keep a food diary and exercise log for 1 day per week for the next 3 months.	Review the client's food record with him each week. Note all empty kilocalories consumed. Discuss the client's food selections and exercise log with him. Document results.	Self-monitoring of food intake and exercise will help the client focus on controlling his behaviors. Nurse's review of food records with the client while pointing out kilocalorically dense foods will educate the client about his negative behaviors.
Client will participate in the exercise program provided by the activities director at least seven times per week for the next 3 months.	Encourage the client to attend the exercise program or to walk 20 minutes before each meal. Document the activity.	Exercise burns kilocalories and increases body protein content. A high body protein content is associated with increased energy expenditure.

C T Q CRITICAL THINKING QUESTIONS

1. What would you do at the next client care conference if Mr. G changed his mind about weight control and said, "All I have left in life is food. I don't want to lose weight"?

2. What would you do at the next client care conference if Mr. G had done everything asked but only managed to maintain his weight at 181 pounds?

⟫ CHAPTER REVIEW

1. The components of energy expenditure are:
   a. Mental activity and physical activity
   b. Thermic effect of exercise and thermic effect of foods
   c. Resting energy expenditure, physical activity, and to a lesser extent the thermic effect of foods
   d. Thermic effect of foods, physical activity, and thermic effect of exercise

2. Energy homeostasis exists when:
   a. Kilocalories from food intake equal kilocalories used for energy expenditure
   b. Kilocalories used for physical activity equal kilocalories used for energy expenditure
   c. An individual is gaining weight
   d. Kilocalories from food intake equal kilocalories used for resting energy expenditure

3. A kilocalorie is used to measure both:
   a. Weight and percentage body fat
   b. Height and weight
   c. The units of energy used in the body and contained in foods
   d. Leanness and body-fat content

4. Kilocalories required per kilogram of body weight are highest during:
   a. Starvation
   b. Growth
   c. Weight loss
   d. Old age

5. Which of the following foods is the most kilocalorically dense?
   a. 1 cup of sugar
   b. 1 cup of celery
   c. 1 cup of skim milk
   d. 1 cup of margarine

✚ CLINICAL ANALYSIS

1. Monitoring a resident's weight is a government requirement in long-term care facilities. The goal is to prevent a slow weight loss, which, over time, can have health consequences. Mr. I, resident of Sunnybrook Nursing Home, has been experiencing an undesirable slow weight loss. His weight history is as follows:

   Feb   180 pounds
   June   175 pounds
   Oct   170 pounds

   As Mr. I's nurse, you should first:
   a. Encourage Mr. I to eat only twice a day
   b. Call the doctor
   c. Wait for the next client care conference to act on this problem
   d. Monitor Mr. I's food intake and physical activity

2. A teacher noticed that many students in her fifth grade class were overweight. As a school project, the class kept food records for 3 days. A computer software program analyzed the records. Many students were eating less than their recommended dietary allowance for kilocalories but gaining weight nonetheless (a common problem among our nation's young). The teacher asked the class by a show of hands what they did after school and on weekends. Many of the same children who were overweight raised their hands when asked if they played mostly video games and watched television when not in school. The teacher shared this information with the school nurse and asked her to speak to the class. The school nurse correctly decided that:
   a. The teacher is overly concerned, because the percent of overweight students approximates the percent of overweight adults in the community.
   b. The computer program must be in error.
   c. All the students need to increase their total intake, including foods from the major food groups.
   d. Many students would benefit from an increase in physical activity.

3. A client appears to be totally concerned with the kilocaloric density of foods and not at all concerned with the nutrient density of foods. You need to encourage the consumption of both types of foods. Which of the following behaviors do you need to discourage?
   a. The substitution of skim milk for 2% milk
   b. The avoidance of all meat, fish, and poultry
   c. The inclusion of dark green and yellow fruits and vegetables in the diet
   d. The inclusion of whole grains in the diet

REFERENCES

Dochterman, JC, and Bulechek, GM: Nursing Interventions Classification (NIC), ed 4. Mosby, Philadelphia, 2004.

Food and Nutrition Board, Institute of Medicine: Dietary reference intakes for energy, carbohydrate, fiber, fatty acids, cholesterol, protein, and amino acids. National Academies Press, Washington, 2002.

Frary, CD, and Johnson, RK: Energy. In Mahon, K, and Escott-Stump, S (eds): Krause's Nutrition and Diet Therapy, ed 11. Elsevier, Philadelphia, 2004.

Groff, JL, and Gropper, SS: Advanced Nutrition and Human Metabolism, ed 3. Wadsworth, St. Paul, 1999.

Guthrie, HA: Introductory Nutrition, ed 7. Times Mirror/Mosby College Publishing, St. Louis, 1989.

Hoffer, LJ: Metabolic consequences of starvation. In Shils, ME (ed): Modern Nutrition in Health and Disease, ed 9. Williams & Wilkins, Baltimore, 1999.

Jakicic, M, et al: Relationship of physical activity to eating behaviors and weight loss in women. Med Sci Sports Exerc 34:1653, 2002.

Krause, LK, and Escott-Stump, S (eds): Krause's Food, Nutrition, & Diet Therapy, ed 11. Elsevier, Philadelphia, 2004.

Krahn, DD, et al: Changes in resting energy expenditure and body composition in anorexia nervosa during refeeding. J Am Diet Assoc 93:4, 1993.

Leibel, RL, Rosenbaum, M, Hirsch, J: Changes in energy expenditure resulting from altered body weight. N Engl J Med 332:621, 1995

Maffeis, C, et al: Meal-induced thermogenesis and obesity: Is a fat meal a risk factor for fat gain in children? J Clin Endocrinol Metab 1:214, 2001.

Moorhead, S, Johnson, M, Maas, M: Nursing Outcomes Classification (NOC), ed 3. Mosby, Philadelphia, 2004.

NANDA International: Nursing Diagnoses: Definitions and Classification, 2003–2004. NANDA International, Philadelphia, 2003.

National Research Council: Diet and Health: Implications for Reducing Chronic Disease Risk. Report of the Committee on Diet and Health, Food and Nutrition Board, Commission on Life Sciences. National Academy Press, Washington, 1989, p. 110.

Pi-Sunyer, EX (ed): Clinical Guidelines on the Identification, Evaluation, Treatment of Overweight and Obesity in Adults. National Heart, Lung, and Blood Institute, Obesity Education Initiative. U.S. Department of Health and Human Services, Bethesda, 1998.

Roll, BJ, et al: Increasing the portion size of a sandwich increases energy intake. J Am Dietet Assoc 104:367, 2004.

Swinburn, B: The runaway weight gain train: too many accelerators, not enough brakes. BMJ 329:736, 2004.

Subcommittee on the 10th Edition of the RDAs. Food and Nutrition Board. Commission of Life Sciences. National Research Council: Recommended Dietary Allowances. National Academy Press, Washington, 1989, pp. 24–38.

Treuth, MS, et al: Metabolic adaptation to a high-fat and high-carbohydrate diets in children and adolescents. Am J Clin Nutr 77:479, 2003.

Vitamins

The importance of vitamins was first recognized by the effects of their absence. Some deficiency diseases have been known for centuries, but it was not until the twentieth century that vitamins were isolated in the laboratory. This chapter considers the importance of vitamins in the body and in the diet, the general functions of vitamins, the classification of vitamins, and the use of vitamin supplements. Information is given on metabolism, functions, sources, dietary reference intakes, deficiencies, toxicities, and factors affecting stability.

The Nature of Vitamins

Vitamins are organic substances needed by the body in small amounts for normal metabolism, growth, and maintenance. Organic substances are derived from living matter and contain carbon. Vitamins are not sources of energy, and they do not become part of the structure of the body. Vitamins act as regulators or adjusters of metabolic processes and as **coenzymes** (substances that activate enzymes) in enzymatic systems.

Specific Functions

Vitamin functions are specific; the bodily processes do not permit substitutes. Thus, vitamins are similar to keys in a lock. All the notches in a key have to fit the lock or the key will not turn. Overall, one vitamin cannot perform the func-tions of another. If a person does not consume enough vitamin C, for instance, taking vitamin D will not correct the deficiency. Vitamin D is the wrong key for that lock.

Classification

A major distinguishing characteristic of vitamins is their solubility in either fat or water. This physical property is used to classify vitamins and is also significant for storage and processing of foods that contain vitamins and for the utilization of the vitamins in the body. Vitamins A, E, D, and K are fat-soluble. The eight B-complex vitamins and vita-min C are water-soluble. See Table 7-1 for a list of the 13 tra-ditionally recognized vitamins. Choline, not a vitamin by strict definition but recently added to the DRI list, appears last.

Dietary Reference Intakes

The amounts of vitamins recommended in the United States to meet the needs of almost all healthy individuals are listed by age and physiological status (Appendix F). Complete reports are accessible at http://www.nap.edu and a summary table at http://www.iom.edu/file.asp?id= 7296. Within this chapter, examples are given for healthy adults, not pregnant or lactating women. Recommended amounts vary in other countries.

Vitamins A, D, and E historically have been measured in International Units, a dosage amount that still appears on some labels. The RDAs and AIs, however, are listed in the metric system: **micrograms** and milligrams. There are no generic units that can be converted directly to the metric system. The amount designated by a unit is specific for each vitamin. The formulae to convert **International Units** to the metric system are given in Clinical Calculation 7-1.

Fat-Soluble Vitamins

More or less of the vitamin may be retained in the food, depending on the methods of processing and storing. Compared with water-soluble vitamins, the fat-soluble vitamins A, D, E, and K are more stable and more resistant to the effects of oxidation, heat, light, and **pH**. Exposure to

Table 7–1	Classification of Vitamins
FAT SOLUBLE	**WATER SOLUBLE**
Vitamin A	
Vitamin D	Thiamin
Vitamin E	Riboflavin
Vitamin K	Niacin
	Vitamin B_6
	Folic Acid
	Vitamin B_{12}
	Biotin
	Pantothenic acid
	Vitamin C

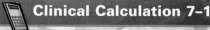

Clinical Calculation 7–1

The Elusive International Unit

Formerly, fat-soluble vitamins were measured in International Units (IU), as defined by the International Conference for Unification of Formulae. *A unit of vitamin A is not an equal measure of vitamin D or of vitamin E.* Because the old system is familiar to many people and still appears in laws, on labels, and in research reports, the formulas to convert International Units to metric measures are given below. The results may be approximate because the amounts in natural foods may vary and activation rate of provitamin A will differ in individuals.

VITAMIN A

Animal Foods: 3.3 IU = 1 microgram of **Retinol Activity Equivalents (RAE)** (formerly RE, Retinol Equivalents)
Plant Foods: 10 IU = 12 micrograms of beta-carotene or 24 micrograms of other provitamin A carotenoids*
Supplements: 10 IU of provitamin A = 1 microgram Retinol Activity Equivalents

VITAMIN D

40 IU = 1 microgram of cholecalciferol

VITAMIN E

Natural form: 1.4 IU = 1 milligram of alpha-tocopherol†
Synthetic form: 1 IU = 1 milligram of alpha-tocopherol†

---

*Includes alpha-carotene and beta-crytoxanthin in some food tables. A vitamin A calculator is available at http://www.nutrisurvey.de/vac/vac.htm.
†Averages. Conversion factors vary for different compounds of the vitamin. See http://books.nap.edu/books/0309069351/html/192.html/#pagetop Accessed April 10, 2005.

---

the sun and other kinds of dehydration, however, can adversely affect the fat-soluble vitamins.

Fat-soluble vitamins are absorbed from the intestine in the same way as fats, and like fats, they can be stored in the body, giving the potential for health problems due to excessive intake. Toxicity from vitamins A and D can be fatal.

Vitamin A

Vitamin A comes in two forms: preformed vitamin A, **retinol,** and **provitamin A,** found in **beta-carotene** and other **carotenoids,** 50 of which have some provitamin A activity. A **preformed vitamin** is already in a complete state in ingested foods whereas a **provitamin** requires conversion in the body to be in a complete state. Provitamin A is converted to retinol in the intestine. The term *precursor* is often used interchangeably with the term *provitamin*. A **precursor** is a substance from which another substance is derived.

Absorption, Metabolism, and Excretion

Of preformed vitamin A, 70 to 90 percent is absorbed if consumed with at least 10 grams of fat, but less than 5 percent of carotene is absorbed from raw vegetables (Gropper, Smith, and Groff, 2005). Vitamin A is transported bound to a retinol-binding protein. This complex is too large for the kidney to filter, so it is retained in the body. Consequently, poor protein status interferes with the transportation and usage of vitamin A. About 40 percent of vitamin A metabolites are excreted via the bile in feces and about 60 percent in urine (Gropper, Smith, and Groff, 2005).

Up to a year's supply of vitamin A is stored in the body, 90 percent of it in the liver. Excessive carotene is stored in adipose tissue, giving fat a yellowish tint, but it is apparently harmless for most people. (See the following section on Vitamin A toxicity and Clinical Application 23-5 for information on exceptional situations.)

Functions of Vitamin A

Several crucial body functions depend on vitamin A, or retinol. It is necessary for vision, for healthy epithelial tissue, for proper bone growth, and for energy regulation.

CHEMICAL NECESSARY FOR VISION. The eye is like a camera. It has a dark layer to keep out excess light, a lens

to focus light, and a light-sensitive layer at the back of the eye, called the **retina.** In the retina, light rays are changed into electrical impulses that travel along the **optic nerve** to the back of the brain. The vitamin A metabolite retinol is part of the molecules of a chemical in the retina that is responsible for this conversion. The body can synthesize this chemical, called **rhodopsin,** or visual purple, only if it has a supply of vitamin A.

When the eye is functioning in dim light, rhodopsin is broken down into a protein, called **opsin,** and vitamin A. In darkness or during sleep, opsin and vitamin A are reunited to become rhodopsin. Figure 7-1 diagrams this reaction. The body can keep reusing the vitamin A, but some of it is depleted during each visual cycle. It is for this reason that a dietary deficiency produces **night blindness** or impaired dim-light vision. Clinical Application 7-1 relates a practical method used to conserve a person's rhodopsin for night vision. The rhodopsin system in the rod cells of the retina is more sensitive to vitamin A deficiency than is the iodopsin system in the cone cells used for color vision (McLaren and Frigg, 2001).

HEALTH OF EPITHELIAL TISSUE. Epithelial tissue covers the body and lines the organs and passageways that open to the outside of the body. Skin is epithelial tissue, as are the surface of the eye and the lining of the gastroin-

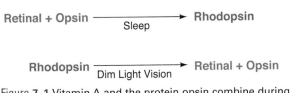

Figure 7–1 Vitamin A and the protein opsin combine during sleep to form rhodopsin. When we need to see in dim light, the rhodopsin breaks down into vitamin A and opsin.

testinal tract. Epithelial tissue has a protective function, often producing mucus to wash out foreign materials. Vitamin A in the form of retinoic acid helps to keep epithelial tissue healthy by aiding the differentiation of specialty cells. This function, control of gene expression, has led some scientists to believe that vitamin A may play a role in cancer prevention. See Clinical Application 7-2 for more information on vitamin A and cancer.

NORMAL BONE GROWTH. Animal studies have shown that retinoic acid, a metabolite of vitamin A, suppresses osteoblast (anabolism of bone) activity and stimulates osteoclast (catabolism of bone) formation while antagonizing vitamin D's maintenance of serum calcium levels. In humans, long-term intake of large amounts of vitamin A has led to bone abnormalities (Feskanich et al, 2002), and high serum retinol levels have been associated with fracture risk in men (Michaelsson et al, 2003).

ENERGY REGULATION. Vitamin A has a role in heat production and the management of energy balance. Retinoic acid regulates the synthesis of an enzyme in brown adipose tissue that controls cellular production of energy as heat (McLaren and Frigg, 2001). The reason Arctic animals store large amounts of vitamin A may be related to these functions (see Hypervitaminosis A in the section on Vitamin A Toxicity). Researchers are investigating retinoids as physiological regulators of energy homeostasis and of adipose tissue development and function in laboratory animals and its implications for obesity control (Kumar, Sunvold, and Scarpace, 1999; Ribot et al, 2001).

Vitamin A Deficiency

Even though vitamin A is stored in the body, deficiencies can occur. In some parts of the world, vitamin A deficiency is widespread. Cases are common in India, south and east Asia, Africa, and Latin America, affecting an estimated 140 million preschool children and 7.2 million pregnant women

Clinical Application 7–1

Red Light Conserves Rhodopsin

Red light breaks down rhodopsin more slowly than do other wavelengths of light. For this reason, aviators spend time in a red-lit room before flying at night. In the presence of red light, a build-up of rhodopsin occurs in the rods of the retina. Vision in dim light is thus enhanced. Red light is used on navigational instruments and in some automobiles for the same reason.

Clinical Application 7–2

Vitamin A and Cancer

Fifty percent of fatal cancers begin with abnormal differentiation of epithelial cells. Vitamin A plays a hormone-like role in normal cell differentiation throughout the body (McLaren and Frigg, 2001). It also functions as an antioxidant to neutralize **free radicals.** These highly reactive atoms or molecules can damage DNA, with resultant abnormal cell growth.

(Sommer and Davidson, 2002). In addition, many countries do not have enough data to analyze the extent of the problem (McLaren and Frigg, 2001). Vitamin A deficiency is second only to protein-calorie malnutrition as a nutritional problem affecting young people.

Vitamin A deficiency in the United States is most often due to disease. For example, clients with long-lasting infectious disease, fat absorption problems, or liver disease are at risk of vitamin A deficiency. Vision loss attributed to hypovitaminosis A due to malabsorption following ileal-jejunal bypass for morbid obesity 20 years earlier was treated successfully with vitamin A supplementation (Purvin, 1999). Xerophthalmia and ophthalmic signs of increased intracranial pressure appeared within 8 years in a 27-year-old woman after a biliopancreatic bypass for obesity. Both symptoms were relieved by vitamin A therapy (Panozzo, Babighian, and Bonora, 1998).

SIGNS AND SYMPTOMS. Lack of vitamin A as retinol causes night blindness. In this condition, the resynthesis of rhodopsin is too slow to allow quick adaptation to dim light. Because vitamin A is related to normal bone growth and development, a deficiency causes cessation of bone growth that can lead to brain and spinal cord injury. A deficiency also can cause fetal malformations (Ross, 1999).

All epithelial tissue suffers because of vitamin A deficiency with consequent lack of retinoic acid. One pathologic change is the replacement of mucus-secreting cells by keratin-producing ones in many epithelial tissues (McLaren and Frigg, 2001). The person so affected may have sinus trouble, a sore throat, and abscesses in the ears, mouth, and salivary glands. The most serious effect is the thickening of the epithelial tissue covering the eye. **Xerophthalmia,** an abnormal thickening and drying of the outer surface of the eye, is a leading cause of blindness in some developing countries. Figure 7-2 shows a characteristic lesion. Xerophthalmia occurs almost exclusively in children between 6 months and 6 years of age, usually affecting both eyes but not necessarily to the same degree (McLaren and Frigg, 2001). An estimated 3 million children are clinically affected, causing approximately 500,000 to lose their sight every year, about 70 percent of whom die within 1 year. Xerophthalmia is the only vitamin deficiency disease to have reached epidemic proportions and to persist at those levels today (Sight and Life, 2003).

TREATMENT AND PREVENTION. Active corneal xerophthalmia is a medical emergency demanding high-dose vitamin A. High doses are also recommended for

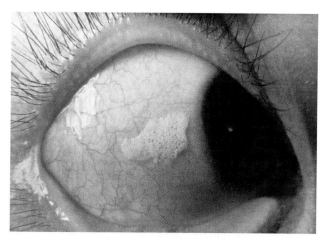

Figure **7–2** Bitot spot, a triangular shiny gray spot on the conjunctiva seen in vitamin A deficiency. (McLaren and Frigg, 2001. Reproduced with permission of Sight and Life.)

infants and young children with xerophthalmia, severe malnutrition, or measles (Ross, 2002). Vitamin A supplementation to children hospitalized with measles reduced the risk of death about 60 percent overall and 90 percent in infants. In Japan, children with measles or respiratory syncytial virus infection given vitamin A had symptoms of shorter duration than children not supplemented, even in the absence of malnutrition (Kawasaki et al, 1999). Precisely how vitamin A is involved in the immune response is unclear, but cell-mediated immunity is impaired in vitamin A deficiency (McLaren and Frigg, 2001).

Improved vitamin A status may be attributable to general economic and social development rather than to vitamin A interventions. Assessment of the local conditions and consideration of cultural preferences are key to sustainable programs. For instance, sometimes usual dietary intake might be adequate if intestinal parasites did not impair absorption, and other times carotene sources might be readily available but not favored because the traditional dietary staple is a starch (McLaren and Frigg, 2001).

Prevention of vitamin A deficiency involves multiple strategies: breast feeding, vitamin A supplementation, fortification of foods, and diet diversification, often in combination. Because breast milk contains preformed vitamin A, the World Health Organization recommends exclusive breast feeding for 4 to 6 months and breast feeding continuing up to 2 years of age, with complementary foods added at about 6 months of age. The WHO also recommends vitamin A supplementation in conjunction with immunization clinics. Other schedules vary with the location and demonstrated need.

During World War I in Denmark, substitution of margarine for butter produced an epidemic of xerophthalmia. Since then, margarine has frequently been fortified with vitamin A. Other foods selected for fortification include sugar in Central America, grain products, tea, dairy foods, oils, and formula foods. In some countries, more than 20 food items have been fortified with vitamin A, suggesting there is a potential for excessive intake (McLaren and Frigg, 2001).

Another approach to prevention of vitamin A deficiency is dietary diversification. Education of the populace regarding available but underutilized and perhaps unrecognized sources of vitamin A is one strategy. Extending the storage life of foods through preservation methods is a second. Introduction of new plants to home gardens is a third relatively simple intervention using existing local resources. All of these methods require local knowledge and time to stimulate behavioral change. More complex means of diet diversification include developing plants that are richer in vitamin A and changing the country's economic structure to make food sources of vitamin A more affordable (McLaren and Frigg, 2001).

A global humanitarian effort to eliminate vitamin A deficiency by DSM Nutritionals provides free vitamin A capsules as well as free educational materials (wall posters, books, videos, Power Point slides) in English, French, German, Spanish, and other languages. Sight and Life is based at P.O. Box 2116, CH 4002 Basel, Switzerland or can be accessed via the Web site at http://www.sightandlife.org.

Dietary Reference Intakes

The RDA for vitamin A is 700 micrograms of Retinol Activity Equivalents (RAE) for women and 900 micrograms for men. (See Clinical Calculation 7-1.) The UL for both genders is 3000 micrograms RAE per day.

Food Sources and Interfering Factors

Preformed vitamin A (retinol) is found in animal foods such as liver, kidney, egg yolk, and fortified milk products. Retinol is also obtained from provitamin A carotenoids present in fruits and vegetables. Carotenoids provide 26 percent of men's vitamin A activity and 34 percent of women's activity (National Academy of Sciences, 2000). The best-utilized sources are ripe colored fruits and cooked yellow tubers, followed by dark green leafy vegetables. The provitamin-to-retinol conversion ratios have been altered to reflect new data on the body's ability to metabolize provitamin A to retinol. **Carotene,** a yellow pigment found mostly in fruits and vegetables, can be readily seen in foods such as carrots, sweet potatoes, squash, apricots, and cantaloupe. Although not as noticeable because chlorophyll masks the yellow color, carotene is also present in dark leafy green vegetables, including spinach, collards, broccoli, and cabbage.

Vitamin A is fairly stable to heat, but sunlight, ultraviolet light, air, and oxidation easily destroy it. Carotene content of a species of vegetable can vary with the vegetable's maturity, handling, and preparation. Carrots that come packaged in plastic bags are better protected from light and air than the bouquets secured by a rubber band. Beta-carotene is more available to the body in carrots cooked with a small amount of fat than in raw carrots, an exception to the general rule that cooking depletes vitamins, but overcooking may lead to destruction of carotene by oxidation (McLaren and Frigg, 2001). Fiber intake and excessive vitamin E consumption can decrease carotenoid absorption (Gropper, Smith, and Groff, 2005). Zinc deficiency impairs the conversion of carotene to vitamin A (McLaren and Frigg, 2001).

Vitamin A Toxicity

Whereas most other vitamin toxicities are a result of supplementation, hypervitaminosis A can be caused by foods. Fetal malformations can be caused by deficiency or excess of vitamin A. The hazard of excessive vitamin A to the fetus is explained in Chapter 11. Some experts warn of possible ill effects from consumption of a healthy diet that includes multiple supplemented foods and vitamin supplements (Denke, 2002).

CAROTENEMIA. Beta-carotene is recognized by the Food and Drug Administration as Generally Recognized as Safe (**GRAS**) as a dietary supplement and a colorant. Nevertheless carotene can be consumed to excess. The condition resulting from ingesting too much carotene is called **carotenemia.** The person's skin becomes yellow, first on the palms of the hands and the soles of the feet. The whites of the eyes do not become yellow, however, as they do in people with **jaundice** caused by liver disease. Carotenemia has occurred in infants fed too much squash and carrots. The skin returns to normal within 2 to 6 weeks after stopping the excessive intake.

Recently, the assumption that carotene is harmless has been challenged, particularly by studies in which beta-carotene supplementation was associated with increased occurrence of lung cancer (see Chapter 23). More research in this area is needed.

HYPERVITAMINOSIS A. Vitamin A toxicity is called **hypervitaminosis A.** Symptoms of vitamin A toxicity are similar to those of a brain tumor causing increased intracranial pressure. Clients may complain of headaches and blurred vision and display signs of increased pressure within the skull. Other symptoms include pain in the bones and joints, dry skin, and poor appetite. Some clients have developed symptoms after consuming beef liver once or twice a week. A case of idiopathic intracranial hypertension was attributed to consumption of 2 to 3 pounds of raw baby carrots per week for 16 months (Donahue, 2000).

Self-prescribed vitamin A supplements also have produced liver disease. For one such client, the liver signs and symptoms did not appear until 24,700 International Units daily for 17 years and 270,000 IU daily for 1 year had been ingested (Miksad et al, 2002). Another client died after consuming 25,000 International Units (IU) daily for 6 years (Kowalski et al, 1994).

One hazard of excessive vitamin A intake is unique to the Arctic. Polar bear liver has made both men and dogs sick. It contains 354,545 micrograms of retinol equivalents (RE) per 3-ounce serving—394 times the RDA for men. Other Arctic game poses similar hazards.

Vitamin D

Recently, vitamin D, which promotes bone growth, has come to be regarded as a hormone rather than a vitamin because of the way it works. Vitamin D receptors have been found in tissues not usually associated with bone metabolism such as those of the heart, muscle, pancreas, brain, and skin, as well as in tissues of the blood forming and immune systems (Gropper, Smith, and Groff, 2005).

Absorption, Metabolism, and Excretion

Two forms of vitamin D are metabolically active. Vitamin D_2, **ergocalciferol,** is formed when ergosterol (provitamin) in plants is irradiated by sunlight. Vitamin D_3, **cholecalciferol,** is formed when 7-dehydrocholesterol (another provitamin) in the skin of animals or humans is irradiated by ultraviolet light or sunlight.

Both forms are absorbed into the blood. About 50 percent of dietary vitamin D is absorbed, most rapidly in the duodenum but the greatest amount in the distal small intestine (Gropper, Smith, and Groff, 2005). Like other fat-soluble vitamins, it is transported in the blood bound to protein. The liver alters the vitamin to **calcidiol,** an inactive form of vitamin D. By enzyme action, the kidney converts the calcidiol to **calcitriol,** the active form of vitamin D. Figure 7-3 diagrams the path of these processes.

Functions of Vitamin D

Vitamin D promotes normal bone mineralization in three ways. First, vitamin D stimulates DNA to produce transport proteins, which bind calcium and phosphorus, thus increasing intestinal absorption of these minerals. Second, once these minerals have been absorbed into the blood, vitamin D stimulates bone cells to use them to build and maintain bone tissue. Third, vitamin D stimulates the kidneys to return calcium to the bloodstream rather than to excrete it in the urine.

Another control mechanism is also at work. **Parathyroid hormone** is secreted in response to a low serum calcium level. Parathyroid hormone causes the catabolism of bone to maintain a correct serum calcium level. The body's priority goal is maintenance of correct serum calcium for blood clotting, nerve function, and muscle contraction. Without this mechanism to sustain vital functions, a person would not live long enough to develop rickets, the bone disease of vitamin D deficiency.

Vitamin D Deficiency

Lack of sunshine or vitamin D, chronic liver or kidney disease, and rare genetic disorders cause vitamin D deficiency. Low levels of vitamin D and decreased bone mass have been found in some vegan populations in northern geographic areas (American Dietetic Association, 2003). Of particular concern are children whose bones are still growing.

RICKETS. Vitamin D deficiency in children is called **rickets.** In 1921, an estimated 75 percent of infants in New York City were afflicted, and in 1933 nationwide, there were 339 deaths (Backstrand, 2002). Although nutritional rickets is a preventable disease, cases are still being reported. Four cases were reported in New York, all in children under 24 months who were breast fed without formula supplements (Pugliese et al, 1998), and two cases were reported in Philadelphia in children 14 and 15 months old breast fed without supplements by mothers who eliminated dairy products from their own diets (Herman and Bulthuis, 1999). Additional cases of rickets in dark-skinned children being breast fed but not receiving vitamin D supplements were reported in New England (Fitzpatrick et al, 2000), north

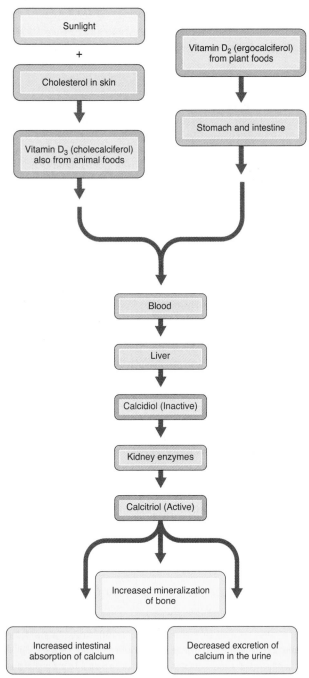

Figure **7–3** Vitamin D, whether from food or synthesis in the skin, is metabolized by the liver and the kidneys to its active form.

Texas (Shah et al, 2000), North Carolina (Kreiter et al, 2000), and Georgia (Centers for Disease Control, 2001). At greatest risk in the United States are dark-skinned children in northern, smoggy cities and breast-fed infants not exposed to sunlight. To prevent such deficiency diseases or to diagnose them early, health-care providers should pay special attention to assessing the client's whole situation and not just concentrate on the immediate reason for the visit.

In Great Britain, evidence of subnormal serum levels of vitamin D without evidence of rickets was documented among Asian 2-year-old (Lawson and Thomas, 1999) and preschool children (Davies et al, 1999). In both studies, the lowest levels were predicted or found during the winter, when exposure to sunshine and perhaps outdoor play are less common. Also in Great Britain, six cases of rickets were documented in Asian children who were breast fed without vitamin D supplementation, four of whom had mothers who wore concealing clothing as practicing Muslims and three of whom had well-educated graduate students for parents (Mughal et al, 1999). Even in summer in the United Arab Emirates, 82 percent of breast-feeding infants and 61 percent of their mothers had hypovitaminosis D (Dawodu et al, 2003).

Both vitamin D and sufficient calcium are needed for bone growth, however. Analysis of 43 children with nutritional rickets in Connecticut found that 86 percent were of African American, Hispanic, or Middle Eastern descent, 93 percent had been breast fed, and despite the fact that only 15 percent had received vitamin D supplements, low serum vitamin D levels were discovered in just 22 percent of the children. Of those with food histories available, 86 percent were weaned to diets with minimal dairy products, illustrating the importance of sufficient nutrients provided by milk products as well as vitamin D in preventing rickets (DeLucia, Mitnick, and Carpenter, 2003).

OSTEOMALACIA. Vitamin D deficiency in adults is called **osteomalacia.** This deficiency disease occurs most often in women who have insufficient calcium intake and little sunlight exposure and frequently among those who are pregnant or lactating. Women who immigrate to Europe and North America from Asia and the Middle East are particularly at risk (McLaren, 1999).

Environmental factors involved in osteomalacia are similar to those described for rickets. People whose skin is not exposed much to sunlight are at increased risk: cloistered nuns, office workers, residents of smoggy areas, and institutionalized elderly people. Low serum vitamin D levels were found in **free-living** elderly Europeans (van der Wielen et al, 1995), in vegans in Finland in winter (Outila et al, 2000), in veiled premenopausal Turkish women (Guzel et al, 2001), and in toddlers living in an area of air pollution in Delhi, India (Agarwal et al, 2001). A study of adults admitted to a medical service in a New England hospital determined that 22 percent had severe hypovitaminosis D and 34 percent had moderate deficiency (Thomas et al, 1998). Independent predictors of hypovitaminosis D in the Thomas research were inadequate vitamin D intake, winter season, and being housebound. Careful attention to a client's lifestyle and circumstances during assessment may uncover potential problems.

Because of the complex processes involved in vitamin D metabolism, liver or kidney disease can lead to bone deterioration. Chronic kidney failure has caused osteomalacia due to the inability of the kidneys to convert vitamin D to its active form. Dialysis unit protocols frequently call for pharmaceutical vitamin D supplementation.

SIGNS AND SYMPTOMS. Children with rickets have soft, fragile bones. Classic deformities occur, such as bowlegs, knock knees, and misshapen skulls. **Tetany** in infants may be due to low levels of blood calcium. One such 4-month-old child was admitted in seizures and respiratory arrest (Lamb, 1999).

Adults with osteomalacia also have increasing softness of the bones, causing deformities due to loss of calcium. The bones most commonly affected are those of the spine, pelvis, and lower extremities.

Dietary Reference Intakes

Vitamin D is measured in micrograms of cholecalciferol. Adequate Intake for vitamin D is 5 micrograms for everyone through age 50, 10 micrograms from age 51 through 70, and 15 micrograms after age 70. Intestinal absorption of vitamin D decreases with age, as does the capacity of the skin to synthesize cholecalciferol. The Tolerable Upper Intake Level (UL) is 50 micrograms for adults and children older than 1 year and 25 micrograms for infants.

Sources of Vitamin D

Two sources of vitamin D are readily available to most people. Vitamin D is synthesized by the body, and it is added to most dairy products in the United States.

SUNLIGHT. A major source of vitamin D is the body itself. Vitamin D is manufactured in the skin. Children with low dietary intakes may escape rickets if their exposure to sunlight is adequate.

Light-skinned adults can obtain the necessary 5 micrograms of cholecalciferol by exposing their hands, arms, and face to sunlight for 15 minutes twice a week, depending on latitude and season. Sunscreens with a sun protection factor of 8 or greater will block the ultraviolet rays that produce vitamin D. It is not possible to overdose on vitamin D from sunshine.

FOOD. If a person is not exposed to sunshine, food sources of vitamin D become increasingly important. Few natural foods contain enough vitamin D to provide the recommended intakes. The major food source of vitamin D in the United States is fortified milk. Milk is the ideal food to link with vitamin D because it also contains calcium and phosphorus, which are necessary for bone anabolism. See Clinical Application 7–3 on the **fortification** of foods.

SUPPLEMENTS. Historically, the means to obtain vitamin D was cod liver oil. One teaspoonful contains 226 percent of children's Adequate Intake. Although it is a natural product, cod liver oil is a supplement, not a food. The form that many vegans will accept is vitamin D_2 because it is of plant origin (American Dietetic Association, 2003).

Stability and Interfering Factors

Vitamin D is stable to heat and not easily oxidized. Little special handling of foods is necessary but a high-fiber diet interferes with the absorption of vitamin D. Abnormalities of absorption such as diarrhea, fat malabsorption, and biliary obstruction also may lead to vitamin D deficiency.

Vitamin D Toxicity

Because vitamin D is stored in the body, it is possible to ingest too much. Vitamin D from supplements or even foods can be hazardous to health.

Clinical Application 7–3

Fortification of Foods: Use and Misuse

Fortification is the addition of nutrients to foods in amounts greater than normally present to prevent deficiencies. Many cereals are fortified with vitamins and minerals not normally found in grains. Fluid milk must be fortified with vitamin D in the United States, but there are no mandates for other dairy products.

Occasionally, intentions are better than practices. Between 1985 and 1991, 56 cases of hypervitaminosis D were identified in Massachusetts. Two individuals died as a result, and nine were discharged from the hospital with residual effects. Although state law required an upper limit of 500 IU (12.5 micrograms) of vitamin D per quart, the implicated dairy's milk exceeded this by 70 to 600 times (Blank et al, 1995).

Even without considering errors in processing, experts are concerned that voluntary fortification of multiple foods by the producers could lead to excessive intakes (American Dietetic Association, 2001; Backstrand, 2002).

MOST TOXIC OF VITAMINS. Dietary intake of vitamin D is more likely to cause toxicity than any other vitamin. Daily doses of 250 micrograms over several months has produced toxicity in adults (Gropper, Smith, and Groff, 2005). Infants face increased risk from multiple fortified foods. Cases have been reported involving not dietary intake but errors of prescribing or dispensing supplemental vitamin D (Muhlendahl and Nawracala, 1999).

SIGNS AND SYMPTOMS. Clinical manifestations of hypervitaminosis D include loss of appetite, nausea, vomiting, polyuria, muscular weakness, and constipation. The more serious consequences of vitamin D overdose result from calcium deposits in the heart, kidney, and brain.

Vitamin E

The third fat-soluble vitamin is vitamin E. Much less is known about vitamin E than about vitamins A and D. Observational studies have linked it to prevention of cardiovascular disease and of cancer, but intervention studies of specific supplements have not supported the finding (Morris and Carson, 2003). A possible explanation is that whole foods contain many phytochemicals that act in concert to reduce risk of disease (Liu, 2003). More information on relevant research and interpretation of research findings is provided in Chapters 20 and 23.

Absorption, Metabolism, and Excretion

About 45 percent of vitamin E from ordinary foods is absorbed along with fat (Meydani and Hayes, 2003). The primary site of absorption is the jejunum and of excretion is via bile in the feces. Most vitamin E is stored in adipose tissue. Maximum transfer of vitamin E across the placenta occurs just before term delivery. The significance of this phenomenon will become clearer in the sections on vitamin E deficiency below and on premature infants in Chapter 12.

Functions of Vitamin E

The major function of vitamin E is as an **antioxidant.** The process by which a substance combines with oxygen is called **oxidation.** Several substances can be destroyed by oxidation, including vitamin E, vitamin A, and vitamin C. Some molecules become very unstable when they are oxidized. Their accelerated movements can damage nearby molecules. Vitamin E accepts oxygen instead of allowing other molecules to become unstable. In this role, vitamin E protects vitamin A and unsaturated fatty acids from oxidation. Vitamin E in lung cell membranes provides an important barrier against air pollution. It also protects the stability of the polyunsaturated fatty acids in the red blood cell membranes from oxidation in the lungs.

Oxidation is suspected of contributing to cataract formation and macular degeneration of the retina, although early research produced inconsistent findings. Clinical Application 7-4 describes some of the results of investigations into antioxidants and eye disease.

Other neurodegenerative diseases associated with oxidative stress, such as Alzheimer's disease, Parkinson's disease, amyotrophic lateral sclerosis (Lou Gehrig's disease), tardive dyskinesia, Huntington's chorea, and multiple sclerosis, are the subjects of ongoing research (Butterfield et al, 2002). Studies of vitamin E and Alzheimer's disease showed a lowered risk (Englehart et al, 2002) and no effect (Luchsinger et al, 2003). High intake of vitamin E from foods, not supplements, was associated with reduced risk of Parkinson's disease (Zhang, 2002).

The role of vitamin E in immunity is under investigation. Supplementation with 200 IU per day significantly improved immune response in healthy elderly persons (Meydani and Hayes, 2003).

Deficiency of Vitamin E

In animals, vitamin E deficiency produces sterility. In several species of animals, a deficiency of vitamin E suppresses the immune system, whereas supplementation stimulates it.

In humans, degenerative neurological problems and hemolytic anemia occur (Gropper, Smith, and Groff, 2005). Severe vitamin E deficiency has profound effects on the central nervous system (Benomar et al, 1999). Even with adequate vitamin E intake, defects in the alpha-tocopherol transfer protein gene have produced ataxia and mental symptoms (Hoshino et al, 1999; Schuelke et al, 1999). In cases of chronic fat malabsorption, muscle weakness and forms of **muscular dystrophy** are seen. Premature infants with inadequate reserves of vitamin E develop anemia. Without sufficient vitamin E, the membranes of the red blood cells break down easily when exposed to oxygen or an oxidizing agent.

Dietary Reference Intakes

The RDA for vitamin E considers only **alpha-tocopherol,** the predominant form of vitamin E in tissues and supplements. Previous adjustments for other forms of the vitamin have been eliminated (Gropper, Smith, and Groff, 2005). The RDA is 15 milligrams for persons 14 years of age and older. The UL is 800 milligrams for 14- to 18-year-olds and 1000 milligrams for other adults. The need for vitamin E

Antioxidants and Zinc in Eye Disease

In the Western world, age-related macular degeneration (AMD) is the most common cause of blindness among whites. The center of the retina, or macula, deteriorates so that the person loses the ability to read, drive a car, or perform fine tasks but still retains some peripheral vision. The cause is unknown, but risk factors include ultraviolet light and smoking. No cure has been discovered.

The Age-Related Eye Disease Study Research Group reported a 27 percent reduction in the risk of advanced AMD in persons receiving high-dose vitamins C, E, beta-carotene, and zinc over an average of 6.3 years of follow-up and recommended this protocol to ophthalmologists for clients meeting certain criteria (2001b). Two other carotenoids, lutein and zeaxanthin, have been investigated in relation to macular degeneration. Observational studies linked high intakes of lutein- and zeaxanthin-rich foods such as spinach, broccoli, and eggs with a 40 percent reduction in risk of AMD (Moeller, Jacques, and Blumberg, 2000). In another retinal disease, retinitis pigmentosa, short-term vision improvements, more pronounced in blue-eyed subjects, were attributed to lutein supplementation (Dagnelie, Zorge, and McDonald, 2000).

In the United States, the most common surgery performed on people over the age of 65 is to treat cataracts. A cataract is the clouding of the lens of the eye. Predisposing factors, in addition to age, are ultraviolet radiation, diabetes, smoking, and alcohol consumption.

The Age-Related Eye Disease Study Research Group reported that high doses of vitamins C, E, and beta-carotene had no apparent effect on cataract development or progression in relatively well-nourished older adults in an 11-center study over 6.3 years (2001a). A later study reported a 57 percent reduction in risk of cataract in women older than 60 years who consumed 362 milligrams of vitamin C per day and a 60 percent reduction in risk in women who used vitamin C supplements for 10 years or more (Taylor et al, 2002). In a 2-year study, lutein supplements were shown to improve visual function in persons with cataracts (Olmedilla et al, 2003). Many researchers conclude by recommending five servings of fruits and vegetables daily. They also note that health-conscious individuals who take vitamin supplements often consume nutrient-dense diets.

increases as the intake of polyunsaturated fatty acids (PUFA) increases. The recommended ratio of vitamin E/PUFA is 0.4 milligrams of d-a-alpha-tocopherol per gram of PUFA (Meydani and Hayes, 2003).

Food Sources, Stability, and Interfering Factors

The best natural source of vitamin E is vegetable oil, and the vegetable oils highest in alpha-tocopherol are the ones high in monounsaturated fatty acids, such as olive and canola oils. In contrast, corn and soybean oils have a greater proportion of gamma-tocopherol, the less well-retained form of vitamin E (Traber, 1999) that no longer is counted as contributing to vitamin E intake (Gropper, Smith, and Groff, 2005). Other sources are whole grains (especially fortified ready-to-eat cereals), wheat germ, nuts, and leafy vegetables.

Vitamin E is fairly stable on exposure to heat and acid. Normal cooking temperatures do not destroy it, but frying does. Vitamin E is unstable to light, alkalis, and oxygen. Persons who limit fat in their diets are likely limiting their vitamin E intake also.

Vitamin E Toxicity

Very large supplemental doses of more than 600 milligrams of alpha-tocopherol daily (40 times the RDA) for a year or longer may cause excessive bleeding, impaired wound healing, and depression. Clinical Application 7-5 describes a client with vitamin E toxicity.

Vitamin K

Nurses should understand the functions of vitamin K, because it is frequently prescribed as a medication. Vitamin K also impacts the effectiveness of a commonly prescribed anticoagulant. Therefore, nurses may have to give instructions regarding food intake to clients who are taking warfarin (see Chapter 17).

Clinical Application 7–5

Vitamin E Toxicity

A client was admitted to the hospital for **narcolepsy,** a disorder characterized by recurrent, uncontrollable, brief periods of sleep from which the individual is easily awakened. This client would fall asleep while driving his car.

Narcolepsy can be a sign of uremia, hypoglycemia, diabetes, hypothyroidism, increased intracranial pressure, tumor of the brainstem or hypothalamus, or absence epilepsy. If all of these causes are ruled out, the medical diagnosis is either classical or independent narcolepsy.

During her assessment, the dietitian discovered only one unusual nutritional practice. A clerk in a health foods store had recommended vitamin E. The patient had begun and continued this self-prescribed supplement.

The dietitian's investigation of vitamin E's adverse effects led her to suggest to the physician that the narcolepsy could be caused by excessive vitamin E. The client discontinued the vitamin E, and the narcolepsy disappeared.

In this case, a thorough nutritional assessment and an inquiring attitude saved the client much discomfort (and his insurance company many dollars) by eliminating the need for extensive diagnostic tests. Often, clients do not regard dietary supplements as medications. The nurse should always ask specifically about what vitamin and mineral preparations the client is taking and in what doses.

Absorption, Metabolism, and Excretion

Two forms of vitamin K can meet the body's needs. Vitamin K_1, or **phylloquinone,** is the one found in plant foods. Vitamin K_2, or **menaquinone,** is synthesized by intestinal bacteria. A synthetic, water-soluble pharmaceutical form of vitamin K_1, **phytonadione,** can be administered orally or by injection. Because of the risk of anaphylaxis, intravenous use should be limited to clients with serious hemorrhage due to vitamin K deficiency (Fiore et al, 2001).

Phylloquinone is absorbed primarily in the jejunum and menaquinone in the distal small intestine and the colon but absorption and utilization of menaquinone has not been satisfactorily documented. Vitamin K is found in large amounts in the liver with lesser amounts in the heart and other tissues. Turnover of vitamin K in the body occurs every 2.5 hours. Unused vitamin K is excreted in urine and feces via the bile (Gropper, Smith, and Groff, 2005).

Functions of Vitamin K

The role of vitamin K in blood clotting has been known and used clinically for a long time. More recently, a protein has been identified in bone that depends on vitamin K. Vitamin K participates with vitamin D in synthesizing this bone protein, which helps to regulate serum calcium levels. In addition, vitamin K-dependent proteins have been found in brain, heart, kidney, liver, lung, and spleen although the mode of action remains to be discovered (Gropper, Smith, and Groff, 2005).

BLOOD CLOTTING. At least 13 different proteins plus the mineral calcium are involved in blood clotting. Vitamin K is necessary for the liver to make factors II (**prothrombin**), VII, IX, and X. Three additional coagulation proteins are vitamin K-dependent. These factors and proteins are key links in the chain of events producing a blood clot.

BONE METABOLISM. Vitamin K influences bone metabolism by facilitating the synthesis of **osteocalcin,** a hormonally regulated calcium-binding protein made almost exclusively by the bone-building cells called **osteoblasts** (Collins and Gernacy, 1998; Xiao et al, 1997; Kanai et al, 1997). Subclinical vitamin K deficiency may be linked to decreased bone mineral density and increased fracture rates but the evidence is not conclusive (Gropper, Smith, and Groff, 2005).

Deficiency of Vitamin K

The intestinal tract of the newborn infant is sterile. For this reason, the baby is unable to produce vitamin K until the intestine is colonized with bacteria from the infant's environment, usually within 24 hours. To prevent bleeding problems, a dose of vitamin K is usually given to the infant immediately after birth. In developing countries, vitamin K deficiency in the breast-fed newborn is a major cause of infant **morbidity** and **mortality** (Olson, 1999).

Deficiencies have been associated with disease and with drug therapy. Fat absorption problems may hinder vitamin K absorption, resulting in prolonged blood clotting time. Antibiotics kill the normal bacteria in the intestine along with the organisms that are causing the infection being treated. Coagulation abnormalities attributed to decreased intestinal flora were seen in children, leading to the recommendation for prophylactic vitamin K administration for severely ill clients, those on prolonged courses of antibiotics, and persons taking inadequate diets (Bhat and Deshmukh, 2003).

Vitamin K may be useful for maintaining a positive balance of bone metabolism. One month of vitamin K supplementation in female athletes who showed low estrogen levels at baseline produced a 15 to 20 percent increase of bone formation markers and a 20 to 25 percent decrease of bone resorption markers (Craciun et al, 1998). The lack of vitamin K has also been linked to poor bone health. In hemodialysis clients, suboptimal plasma vitamin K levels were associated with increased risk of bone fracture (Kohlmeier et al, 1997).

The clinical decision-making path is not always clear. Priorities have to be set after weighing therapeutic and adverse effects of drugs. For example, vitamin K antagonist drugs are given after heart surgery to prevent clotting problems. In one set of these clients, 1 year of oral vitamin K antagonist therapy showed significantly lower osteocalcin (the calcium-binding protein made by the bone-building cells) levels than clients who were not receiving anticoagulants, although changes in bone mineral density were not detected in this period of time (Lafforgue et al, 1997).

Individuals at risk of vitamin K deficiency include newborn infants and adults who avoid green leafy vegetables or are undergoing long-term antibiotic therapy and clients with malabsorption syndromes. Careful assessment of dietary factors in these clients is warranted.

Dietary Reference Intakes

The AIs for adults 19 years of age and older for vitamin K are 90 micrograms for women and 120 micrograms for men. A UL is not determinable. The typical U.S. diet supplies 300 to 500 micrograms.

Sources of Vitamin K

The body is capable of manufacturing some vitamin K. Many common foods also contain adequate amounts.

INTESTINAL SYNTHESIS. The amount of bacterially produced vitamin K that is absorbed and utilized varies from one individual to another. Nevertheless, it is clear that bacterial synthesis alone will not meet the needs of healthy individuals (Gropper, Smith, and Groff, 2005).

FOOD SOURCES. Green leafy vegetables and vegetables of the cabbage family are the best sources of vitamin K. Examples of commonly used vegetables highest in vitamin K include broccoli, Brussels sprouts, cabbage, collards, salad greens, and spinach. This information is pertinent to obtaining the desired effectiveness of a common anticoagulant drug, warfarin (see Chapter 17).

Stability and Interfering Factors

Vitamin K resists heat but is unstable in the presence of oxygen, light, alkalis, and strong acids. Overconsumption of some vitamins can trigger a deficiency of others. In this case, megadoses of vitamins A and E have interfered with vitamin K. The anticoagulant **warfarin** interferes with the liver's use of vitamin K—the desired effect of the medication.

Vitamin K Toxicity

The naturally occurring forms of vitamins K_1 and K_2 have not been associated with adverse effects but caution is warranted, particularly if high doses are taken. Phytonadione, the pharmaceutical preparation of vitamin K_1, causes fewer adverse effects than earlier, stronger formulations but intravenous administration is not recommended except in rare cases. As always, special care must be taken when administering any medication, including vitamin K, to infants.

Table 7-2 summarizes the information on the fat-soluble vitamins. Table 7-3 summarizes the stability of vitamins to environmental conditions. See Clinical Application 7-6 for a description of two conditions that mimic deficiencies of fat-soluble vitamins.

Water-Soluble Vitamins

Vitamins that dissolve in water are vitamin C, or **ascorbic acid,** and the B vitamins. The B vitamins include **thiamin, riboflavin, niacin,** vitamin B_6, **folic acid,** vitamin B_{12}, **pantothenic acid,** and **biotin.** Another substance, **choline,** has sometimes been classified as a B vitamin and sometimes not a B vitamin. It has recently been given DRIs and is included toward the end of this chapter.

Cooking easily destroys water-soluble vitamins. For example, one-third to one-half of the vitamin content is lost in the cooking water of boiled vegetables. In addition, keeping foods hot longer than 2 hours results in a more than 10 percent loss of folate and vitamins C and B_6 (Fletcher and Fairfield, 2002).

Vitamin C

Most animals manufacture vitamin C in their livers. Humans, along with other primates, guinea pigs, some birds, and fruit-eating bats, cannot synthesize vitamin C.

Absorption, Metabolism, and Excretion

Vitamin C is absorbed from the small intestine. The adrenal and pituitary glands have the highest concentrations of vitamin C, but the greatest total amount is found in the liver.

Clinical Application 7–6

Conditions Mimicking Deficiencies of Fat-Soluble Vitamins

PROTEIN DEFICIENCY

Water and fat do not mix. To circulate fats in the water-based blood, the liver attaches fat-soluble vitamins to protein carriers. Sometimes a protein deficiency hinders the use of the fat-soluble vitamins.

ZINC DEFICIENCY

Vitamin A is carried from storage in the liver to the tissues by a zinc-containing protein. For this reason, zinc deficiency can mimic vitamin A deficiency.

Table 7–2 **Fat-Soluble Vitamins**

VITAMIN	ADULT RDA/AI AND FOOD PORTION CONTAINING IT	FUNCTIONS	DEFICIENCY DISEASE	SIGNS AND SYMPTOMS OF DEFICIENCY	BEST SOURCES
A	700 to 900 μg 5 or 6 medium raw baby carrots 5 to 15 μg	Dim light vision Differentiation of epithelial cells Normal bone growth	Night blindness Xerophthalmia	Night blindness Sore throat, sinus trouble, ear and mouth abscesses Dry and thick outer covering of eye Blindness	*Preformed:* liver, kidney, egg yolk, fortified milk *Provitamin:* carrots, sweet potatoes, squash, apricots, cantaloupe, spinach, collards, broccoli, cabbage
D	5 to 15 μg 2 to 6 cups fortified milk	Increases intestinal absorption of calcium Stimulates bone production Decreases urinary excretion of calcium	Rickets Osteomalacia	Bowlegs, knock-knees, misshapen skull Tetany in infants Soft fragile bones, especially of spine, pelvis, lower extremities	Sunlight on skin Fortified milk Cod liver oil
E	15 mg 3 tbsp safflower oil	Antioxidant Protects polyunsaturated fatty acids in red blood cell membranes from oxidation in lungs	No specific term	Animals: sterility, suppression of immune system Humans: Muscle weakness; forms of muscular dystrophy Anemia in premature infants	Vegetable oils Whole grains, wheat germ
K	90 to 120 μg 10 raw broccoli flowerets	Used in manufacture of several clotting factors, including prothrombin Assists vitamin D to synthesize a regulatory bone protein	No specific term	Prolonged clotting time	Green leafy vegetables Synthesis in intestine

As the amount of vitamin C consumed increases, the proportion of the vitamin that is absorbed decreases. In a study of healthy volunteers, 100 percent of a 200-milligram dose was absorbed. Seventy percent of a 500-milligram dose was absorbed, but 70 percent of the absorbed dose was excreted in the urine. Of the 1250-milligram dose, only 50 percent was absorbed, and nearly all of it was excreted in the urine (Levine et al, 1996).

Functions of Vitamin C

Vitamin C has diverse functions in the body. It contributes to wound, burn, and fracture healing, serves as an antioxidant, and assists in the synthesis of neurotransmitters and steroid hormones. It enhances the absorption of iron and converts folic acid, a B vitamin, to an active form.

COLLAGEN SYNTHESIS. Vitamin C is necessary in the formation of **collagen,** the strong fibrous protein in connective tissue. Bone, skin, blood vessels, soft dental structures, and scar tissue all contain collagen. Without vitamin C, collagen molecules are inadequately cross-linked, resulting in weak tissue.

ANTIOXIDANT. Vitamin C is a powerful antioxidant. By preventing the uptake of oxygen by other molecules, it deters the destruction of tissue by unstable molecules. Vitamin C is more sensitive to oxidation than either vitamin E or vitamin A and will be oxidized before they are. Thus it is called the *antioxidants' antioxidant.*

Table 7–3 **Factors Affecting Stability of Vitamins**

VITAMIN	OXYGEN	HEAT	LIGHT	ACIDS	ALKALIES
			STABLE TO		
Fat soluble					
A	No	Yes	No	No	*
D	Yes	Yes	Yes	*	*
E	No	Yes	No	Yes	No
K	No	Yes	No	No	No
Water soluble					
C	No	No	No	Yes	Yes
Thiamin	No	No	No	Yes/No†	No
Riboflavin	Yes	Yes	No	Yes	No
Niacin	Yes	Yes	Yes	Yes	Yes
B₆	*	Yes	No	Yes	No
Folic acid	No	No	No	No	Yes
B₁₂	No	Yes	No	No	No

*Data unavailable.
†Destroyed by tannic and caffeic acid; protected by ascorbic and citric acid.

ADRENAL GLAND FUNCTION. High concentrations of vitamin C are found in the **adrenal glands.** These are the organs that secrete adrenalin, the "fight or flight" hormone, in times of stress. Vitamin C aids in the release of adrenalin from the adrenal glands. Emotional and physical stress increases the body's need for vitamin C by three to four times.

IRON ABSORPTION. Vitamin C facilitates iron absorption. It acts with hydrochloric acid to keep iron in the more absorbable **ferrous** form. Four ounces of orange juice nearly quadruples the iron a person absorbs from plant foods he or she eats with it.

FOLIC ACID CONVERSION. Vitamin C converts folic acid to an active form. For this reason, deficiency of vitamin C can lead to **anemia** due to inefficient use of iron and folic acid.

Deficiency of Vitamin C

Until the 17th century, sailors on long voyages often died of **scurvy** due to lack of vitamin C. The disease develops within 3 months after vitamin C is eliminated from the diet. Signs and symptoms of scurvy usually appear when the total body pool is less than 300 milligrams (Gropper, Smith, and Groff, 2005). Although not great enough to produce scurvy, up to 16 percent of American adults may be vitamin C deficient, as determined by plasma concentrations less than 11 micromols per liter (Johnston and Bowling, 2002).

SIGNS AND SYMPTOMS. Early signs of scurvy are tender, sore gums that bleed easily and small skin hemorrhages due to weakened blood vessels. The late manifestations of scurvy relate to the breakdown of collagen. Wound healing is delayed; even healed scars may separate. The ends of long bones soften and become malformed and painful, and fractures appear. The teeth loosen in their sockets and fall out. Hemorrhages occur about the joints, stomach, and heart. Untreated scurvy often progresses to sudden death, probably from internal bleeding.

Diagnosis can be made based on history and physical examination, confirmed by serum ascorbic acid findings. Relief of symptoms upon administration of ascorbic acid is diagnostic as well as curative (Bingham, Kimura, and Imundo, 2003).

TREATMENT. Moderate doses of vitamin C will cure scurvy. A daily dose of 300 milligrams replenishes the body tissues in 5 days.

RISK FACTORS AND CONTEMPORARY CASES. Low blood levels of vitamin C are more common in men than women and in people of lower socioeconomic status. The highest prevalence (20 percent) is reported in poor elderly men, who frequently live alone and consume a diet devoid of fresh fruits and vegetables (Jacob, 1999). People who avoid acidic foods and clients receiving dialysis for kidney failure are also at increased risk of vitamin C deficiency. Case reports still appear in medical journals describing scurvy in developed countries:

- An elderly, alcoholic woman diagnosed in an emergency room—Utah (Stephen and Utecht, 2001)
- A 54-year-old rural Appalachian man who twice developed scurvy by subsisting on cooked foods—Virginia (Levin and Greer, 2000)
- A 49-year-old man with a spinal cord injury, limited transportation, and alcohol abuse—Florida (Harrow et al, 2003)
- A 43-year-old man who eliminated fruits and vegetables from his diet—Massachusetts (Pangan and Robinson, 2001)
- A 16-year-old boy who ate no fruits or vegetables after a bout of diarrhea 7 months earlier—New York (Bingham, Kimura, and Imundo, 2003)
- A 9-year-old boy with a restricted eating pattern—Australia (Akikusa, Garrick, and Nash, 2003)
- A 9-year-old developmentally delayed girl with extremely limited food preferences—Canada (Weinstein, Babyn, and Zlotkin, 2001)
- A 5-year-old boy who refused fruits, vegetables, juices, and chewable vitamin tablets for 5 months—Tennessee (Tamura et al, 2000)

Six of those clients presented with musculoskeletal complaints, and five of them underwent extensive testing before the diagnosis was made. Nutritional assessment entered late in the diagnostic process. In the case of the 5-year-old, the authors suggested that underlying psychiatric disorders in the client or the family merited assessment. Expanding the nursing assessment to include the social situation might uncover persons at increased risk of vitamin C deficiency.

Dietary Reference Intakes

The RDA of vitamin C for adults 19 years of age and older is 75 milligrams for women and 90 milligrams for men. Individuals who smoke require an additional 35 milligrams, and those exposed to second-hand smoke are urged to regularly obtain the RDA amount. A daily intake of 200 milligrams completely saturates the tissues and will prevent deficiency for more than a month if intake is stopped (Levine et al, 1999). After major surgery or extensive burns, a client may need up to 1000 milligrams of vitamin C per day. The UL of vitamin C is 2000 milligrams for adults 19 years of age and older.

Food Sources of Vitamin C

Citrus fruits are excellent sources of vitamin C. Other good sources include papaya, cantaloupe, broccoli, Brussels sprouts, green peppers, strawberries, white potatoes, cabbage, chard, kale, turnip greens, asparagus, berries, pineapple, and guavas. Three foods high in vitamins A and C are shown in Figure 7-4.

Stability and Preservation

Air, light, heat, and alkalis destroy vitamin C. Cooking reduces vitamin C content in a food by 20 to 40 percent (Bingham, Kimura, and Imundo, 2003). Orange juice from frozen concentrate contains more vitamin C than ready-to-

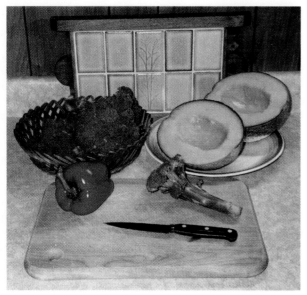

Figure **7-4** Broccoli, cantaloupe, and red pepper are excellent sources of vitamins A and C.

drink juices. The frozen concentrates have 86 milligrams per cup when prepared and 39 to 46 milligrams per cup after 4 weeks of storage. In contrast, ready-to-drink juices have 27 to 65 milligrams per cup on opening and 0 to 25 milligrams at expiration 4 weeks later (Johnston and Bowling, 2002).

Easily implemented food preparation procedures can minimize loss of vitamin C. Store orange juice in an opaque container that holds no more than an amount that can be consumed in a short time. Buy ready-to-drink orange juice 3 to 4 weeks before expiration and use within 1 week (Johnson and Bowling, 2002). Cook vegetables as quickly as possible; crisp-cooked is better than limp-cooked for retaining the vitamin C content. Boiling the cooking water for 1 minute before adding the food eliminates the dissolved oxygen that would otherwise oxidize the vitamin C. Controlling the **pH** is also important. In years past, many food establishments routinely added baking soda to vegetables to enhance their color, but the alkali also destroyed the vitamin C. Fortunately, this practice is now illegal.

Interfering Factor

Smokers deplete vitamin C stores faster than nonsmokers do. Plasma vitamin C concentrations increased significantly in smokers given a supplement of 500 milligrams of vitamin C daily for 4 weeks (Aghdassi, Royall, and Allard, 1999). Unfortunately, many smokers do not consume even the RDA. Children exposed to second-hand smoke, even at low levels, had significantly lower plasma ascorbate levels then unexposed children (Preston et al, 2003).

Vitamin C Toxicity

Megadoses in amounts of 1000 to 2000 milligrams per day have produced nausea, abdominal cramps, and diarrhea. Because vitamin C increases the amount of iron absorbed, persons with diseases characterized by iron overload should avoid megadoses of ascorbic acid. Individuals prone to kidney stones are sometimes advised not to take megadoses of vitamin C because it is metabolized to oxalate, and kidney stones are often composed of calcium oxalate. By a different mechanism competing with uric acid for reabsorption by the kidney, megadoses of vitamin C theoretically could increase the risk of urate stones (Gropper, Smith, and Groff, 2005).

Excessive vitamin C causes false readings in two common laboratory tests. Some urine glucose tests will read falsely positive. Stool guaiac for occult blood will read falsely negative.

An occasionally reported consequence of taking megadoses of vitamin C and then abruptly discontinuing them is **rebound scurvy.** The body cannot adjust quickly enough and continues to absorb a meager proportion of the now smaller dose (DePaola, Faine, and Palmer, 1999). A similar condition was reported in newborns whose mothers took supplemental vitamin C during pregnancy (Cochran, 1965). Even without megadose supplements, however, plasma vitamin C levels fall to deficiency levels within 1 to 3 weeks of removal of vitamin-rich fruits and vegetables from the diet (Johnston, 1999).

B-Complex Vitamins

The B-complex group encompasses eight vitamins: thiamin, riboflavin, niacin, vitamin B_6, folic acid, vitamin B_{12}, pantothenic acid, and biotin. They all function as coenzymes. A **coenzyme** joins with an enzyme to activate it. If a person lacks the coenzyme, the effect is the same as lacking the enzyme itself.

The fact that many of the actions of the B-complex vitamins are interrelated gives rise to a theory that combinations of low vitamin intakes may have a greater impact on health than the sum of their individual effects. In 1992 to 1993, an epidemic of peripheral neuropathy in Cuba was attributed to deficiencies of thiamin, folate, vitamin B_{12}, and sulfur-containing amino acids. Increased risk was found among those who smoked, missed meals, drank alcohol, lost weight, or consumed excessive sugar (Roman, 1994). A follow-up study of Havanan men 2 years after the epidemic reported deficiencies in all the B vitamins except B_6 (Arnaud et al, 2001). Some diseases, including beriberi and pellagra, are associated with deficiencies of a single B vitamin.

Thiamin

Beriberi is the deficiency disease due to a lack of **thiamin,** a vitamin originally named B_1. The neurological symptoms of beriberi were recognized in China in 2600 BC, but it was not until 1937 that lack of thiamin was identified as the cause. The enrichment of food products has almost eliminated this disease, but it is still seen in alcoholics and artificially nourished persons in the West and in persons in developing countries where enrichment may not be a standard practice.

ABSORPTION, METABOLISM, AND EXCRETION. The human body contains about 30 milligrams of thiamin, about one-half of it located in the skeletal muscles, but the liver, heart, kidneys, and brain also have relatively high concentrations (Gropper, Smith, and Groff, 2005). Thiamin is absorbed in the small intestine, primarily in the jejunum. The need for thiamin increases proportionately with carbohydrate intake. Excess thiamin is mainly excreted in the urine.

FUNCTIONS OF THIAMIN. Thiamin serves as a coenzyme in carbohydrate metabolism and may play a role in nerve conduction besides its contribution to energy metabolism (Tanphaichitr, 1999). It is involved in the production of energy from glucose and helps oxidize glucose to form a compound that stores energy. Thiamin is required to convert the essential amino acid **tryptophan** to niacin, another B vitamin.

DEFICIENCY. People at increased risk of thiamin deficiency include breast-fed infants of thiamin-deficient mothers, people whose carbohydrate intake is chiefly milled rice, and chronic alcoholics (Tanphaichitr, 1999). In the Orient, beriberi causes sudden death in young migrant workers who subsist on rice (McLaren, 1999). Individuals whose thiamin status is marginal may become deficient with an increased need for energy during strenuous activity, pregnancy, a growth spurt, or fever. Cases have been reported of cardiovascular disease (wet beriberi) 20 years after a gastrojejunostomy (Astudillo et al, 2003) and of peripheral neuropathy (dry beriberi) 2 months to 39 years after gastrectomies (Koike et al, 2001).

Despite what is known about the functions of thiamin on a cellular level, that knowledge does not explain all the manifestations of the deficiency disease (Gropper, Smith, and Groff, 2005). Initially, symptoms of beriberi such as anorexia, indigestion, and constipation occur because the digestive process is disrupted by impaired glucose metabolism. Without a continual supply of glucose for the central nervous system (CNS), apathy, fatigue, and muscle weakness set in. The **myelin sheaths** covering peripheral nerves eventually degenerate, resulting in paralysis and muscle atrophy. If the thiamin deficiency continues, cardiac failure and death result. In infantile beriberi, death may occur within a few hours if no thiamin is administered (Tanphaichitr, 1999).

Wernicke-Korsakoff syndrome is a neurological disorder caused by thiamin deficiency. Clients with **Wernicke's encephalopathy** display many motor and sensory deficits often involving eye muscles, balance, and memory. Clients with **Korsakoff's psychosis** have short-term memory deficits. Wernicke's encephalopathy is most likely to be seen in alcoholic clients who receive carbohydrates without adequate thiamin replacement (McLaren, 1999). Thirty-two cases of Wernicke's encephalopathy were reported in Australia over a period of 33 months before 1991, when mandatory thiamin enrichment of bread-making flour began (Wood and Currie, 1995). In other cases, extraordinary losses of thiamin have occurred through vomiting (Ohkoshi, Ishii, and Shoji, 1994) or dialysis (Jagadha et al, 1987).

Artificial feeding with intravenous glucose without thiamin supplementation for more than a week produced cases of Wernicke's encephalopathy and lactic acidosis. One malnourished woman in the United Kingdom received a glucose-containing intravenous solution without the thiamin that had been suggested by the referring physician

(Bamber, 1998). In the United States, six cases have been publicized by the Centers for Disease Control. Some clients demonstrated signs of Wernicke's encephalopathy, whereas others developed acidosis from the accumulation of lactate due to the incomplete metabolism of glucose. Three clients died from lactic acidosis due to a shortage of multivitamins for total parenteral nutrition in 1989 (Centers for Disease Control, 1989), but although a similar shortage in 1996 produced three cases, it did not result in fatalities (Centers for Disease Control, 1997). The severe deficiencies developed in 7 to 34 days, highlighting the need to regard vitamin additives to intravenous solutions as essential, not just optional, therapy.

An additional use has been proposed: to minimize the cognitive side effects following electroconvulsive therapy (ECT). Three elderly patients being treated for depression were reported to have benefited from thiamin, suggesting deficiency of the vitamin may contribute to the confusion that follows ECT (Linton et al, 2002.)

DIETARY REFERENCE INTAKES. The RDAs for thiamin are 1.2 milligrams for adult males and 1.1 milligrams for adult females. The need for thiamin increases as kilocaloric consumption increases. An athlete consuming 4000 kilocalories needs twice as much as an office worker consuming 1800 kilocalories. Fasting does not decrease the need for thiamin, however, because the need is proportional to energy expenditure, not simply food intake. An UL is not determinable.

FOOD SOURCES. Pork, wheat germ, yeast, black beans, black-eyed peas, sunflower seeds, and fortified cereals are the best sources. Many other commonly consumed foods contain lesser amounts. A person who chooses enriched grains and eats a balanced diet should have no problems with lack of thiamin.

STABILITY AND INTERFERING FACTORS. Air and heat destroy thiamin. The destruction is especially pronounced in the presence of alkalis. For this reason, adding baking soda to green vegetables to retain their color or to dried beans to soften them inactivates the thiamin in the vegetables. An enzyme in raw fish, **thiaminase,** destroys up to 50 percent of thiamin but cooking inactivates the enzyme. Tannic and caffeic acids found in coffee, tea, blueberries, black currants, Brussels sprouts, and red cabbage are also thiamin **antagonists,** but their actions may be prevented by vitamin C and citric acid (Gropper, Smith, and Groff, 2005).

TOXICITY. Thiamin is rapidly excreted from the body by the kidneys. Thus, no evidence of toxicity after oral administration of thiamin has been reported (Tanphaichitr, 1999). Excessive thiamin by injection, however, has been associated with adverse effects, including convulsions, cardiac arrhythmias, and anaphylactic shock (Gropper, Smith, and Groff, 2005).

Riboflavin

Riboflavin was encountered late in the 19th century when laboratory workers observed a yellow-green fluorescent pigment that formed crystals. The complex, originally named vitamin B_2, also contained niacin and vitamin B_6. Not until 1933 was riboflavin isolated and its identity as a vitamin established.

ABSORPTION, METABOLISM, AND EXCRETION. Absorption of riboflavin occurs in the small intestine. Although the greatest concentrations of riboflavin are found in the liver, kidneys, and heart, only small amounts are stored in the liver and kidneys, so daily needs must be met in the diet. The kidneys excrete excess riboflavin so that even an intake of 1.7 milligrams of riboflavin imparts a bright orangish-yellow color to the urine. Excretion is enhanced by diabetes mellitus, stress, and trauma (Gropper, Smith, and Groff, 2005).

FUNCTIONS. Riboflavin is a coenzyme in the metabolism of protein and of other vitamins. Thyroid and adrenal hormones control the conversion of riboflavin to its active coenzymes, which are involved in many oxidative enzyme systems.

DEFICIENCY. Riboflavin deficiency often occurs with thiamin and niacin deficiencies. A person who avoids all dairy products, however, may be deficient in riboflavin alone, a condition called **ariboflavinosis.** Signs of this deficiency include lesions on the lips and in the oral cavity, seborrheic dermatitis, and normocytic anemia. Other individuals at risk are those with congenital heart disease, some cancers, excessive alcohol intake, and women taking oral contraceptives (Gropper, Smith, and Groff, 2005).

DIETARY REFERENCE INTAKES. The RDAs for riboflavin are 1.3 milligrams for adult males and 1.1 milligrams for adult females. ULs are not determinable.

Riboflavin needs increase as protein needs increase. Clients undergoing major healing processes, such as those with extensive burns, require more riboflavin than the average person.

FOOD SOURCES. Milk and dairy products contribute the most riboflavin to the diet. Other good sources include eggs, organ meats, legumes, and fortified cereals.

STABILITY. Riboflavin is relatively stable to heat but is sensitive to ultraviolet light. Thus, cardboard milk cartons or opaque plastic bottles would be more protective of the vitamin than clear glass bottles.

A proposed use for riboflavin is the inactivation of pathogens in blood products. Studies have shown that riboflavin when exposed to light can inactivate bacteria and viruses, including intracellular HIV-1, in plasma, platelets, and red blood cells (Corbin, 2002; Goodrich, 2000). Research is continuing, because riboflavin is likely to be safe for this use.

INTERFERING FACTORS. Iron, zinc, copper, and manganese have been shown to inhibit riboflavin absorption. Drinking alcohol impairs digestion and absorption of riboflavin (Gropper, Smith, and Groff, 2005).

TOXICITY. Large oral doses have not yielded reports of toxicity, however the potential for adverse effects still exists. High doses have been used in clinical trials as migraine prophylaxis without adverse effects (Gropper, Smith, and Groff, 2005).

Niacin

Niacin, once called vitamin B_3 and "anti-black tongue factor in dogs", includes nicotinic acid and nicotinamide (Gropper, Smith, and Groff, 2005). Lack of niacin causes a specific disease, pellagra.

ABSORPTION, METABOLISM, AND EXCRETION. Not all nutrients present in a food are available to the body. Niacin is found in corn but in a bound form that cannot be absorbed. Treating the corn with lye, as is done in some Latin American cultures, frees the niacin for the body's use.

Not all of the body's niacin has to come from preformed niacin in food. The liver can convert the amino acid tryptophan to niacin, however protein synthesis is given a higher priority than niacin formation (Cervantes-Laurean, McElvaney, and Moss, 1999). This is the only known vitamin with an amino acid for a provitamin.

FUNCTIONS OF NIACIN. Requisite for over 200 enzymes, niacin is a coenzyme required for energy metabolism. Niacin also participates in the synthesis of fatty acids.

DEFICIENCY. Pellagra is the deficiency disease caused by the lack of niacin. It is endemic in India and parts of China and Africa (Cervantes-Laurean, McElvaney, and Moss, 1999) and was so in the early twentieth century in the rural southern United States, where poverty and consumption of corn were risk factors. Between 1907 and 1912, an estimated 25,000 cases of pellagra were identified in the southeast, of which approximately 40 percent were fatal (Backstrand, 2002).

To have a deficiency, a person must have a diet lacking in both niacin and tryptophan. Adults can obtain up to 67 percent of their niacin from complete protein foods. In developed countries, alcoholism, homelessness, malabsorption disorders, gastrointestinal diseases, psychiatric disorders, and diseases causing cachexia and anorexia are risk factors (Kertesz, 2001; Ozturk et al, 2001).

Pellagra has serious effects and is fatal if untreated. The "three Ds" are its major symptoms: dermatitis, diarrhea, and dementia; however, the full triad of symptoms occurs in just 22 percent of clients, and seldom do all of them appear in children (Ozturk et al, 2001). The dermatitis is a red rash on the face, neck, hands, and feet. The rash is bilaterally symmetrical; on the hands and arms it sometimes resembles gloves. A recent case involved a 48-year-old man with alcoholism and a rash on his hands, forearms, and neck that had been present for 2 years. Treatment with nicotinamide cured his rash in 2 weeks (Isaac, 1998).

DIETARY REFERENCE INTAKES. Niacin allowances are related to energy intake and are measured in **niacin equivalents (NEs).** One milligram of niacin equivalent is the same as 1 milligram of preformed niacin or 60 milligrams of tryptophan. The RDAs for niacin are 16 milligrams NE for adult males and 14 milligrams NE for adult females. The UL is 35 milligrams obtained from supplements or fortified foods. Although food composition tables report only preformed niacin, the average American diet contains approximately 900 milligrams of tryptophan equal to 15 milligrams NE (Gropper, Smith, and Groff, 2005).

FOOD SOURCES. Preformed niacin occurs in significant amounts in meat, fish, poultry, and grain products that are enriched or fortified. Coffee also contains niacin and prevents pellagra in cultures with low protein and high coffee intakes. The process of roasting coffee beans increases the niacin content by 30 times as nicotinic acid is formed from an alkaloid in the beans (Cervantes-Laurean, McElvaney, and Moss, 1999).

STABILITY. Niacin is a water-soluble vitamin. Small amounts are lost in cooking water. Niacin is stable to heat, light, air, acid, and alkalis. It is the most environmentally stable vitamin.

TOXICITY. Pharmacological doses of niacin cause flushing. Even reformulation of breakfast cereal to 100 percent of the RDA of vitamins, including niacin, has caused flushing and a rash in a person who consumed six cupfuls for breakfast (Morse, Morse, and Patterson, 1999). The large doses prescribed to lower blood lipid levels over the long term can cause liver damage. A case of niacin toxicity from food is reported in Clinical Application 7-7. It explains how food poisoning outbreaks are investigated and what the nurse's responsibilities are when assisting with the inquiry.

Vitamin B₆

Vitamin B_6 serves in many roles, but no deficiency disease is associated with its lack. The name for the pharmaceutical preparation of vitamin B_6 is **pyridoxine.**

ABSORPTION, METABOLISM, AND EXCRETION. Vitamin B_6 is absorbed in the small intestine, mainly in the jejunum. It is found throughout the body, but 80 to 90 percent of it is in muscle tissue (Leklem, 1999). Most excess is excreted in the urine with very little eliminated via the feces.

FUNCTIONS. Vitamin B_6 is a coenzyme in the synthesis and catabolism of amino acids. It is involved in the metabolism of more than 100 enzymes. Vitamin B_6 functions as a coenzyme in the conversion of tryptophan into niacin. It helps to manufacture antibodies. The synthesis of the hormone epinephrine and the neurotransmitters **dopamine** and **serotonin** all require vitamin B_6 as a coenzyme.

DEFICIENCY. A deficiency of B_6 is unlikely, because large amounts are present in the general diet. Nonetheless, factors such as drug interactions or errors in food processing may cause a deficiency. In the past, improperly processed commercial infant formula produced vitamin B_6 deficiencies.

Clinically, a person with a vitamin B_6 deficiency may present with anemia, neurological abnormalities, or impaired immune function. Infants usually display abnormal electroencephalogram tracings or convulsions. Adults more often suffer from various mouth lesions, depression, and confusion (Leklem, 1999).

DIETARY REFERENCE INTAKES. The RDAs for vitamin B_6 are 1.3 milligrams for men and women through age 50, 1.7 milligrams for older men, and 1.5 milligrams for older women. An increase in protein metabolism increases the need for vitamin B_6. The UL is 100 milligrams for adults.

FOOD SOURCES. Vitamin B_6 is widely distributed in foods. Rich natural sources include sirloin steak, salmon, and chicken breast. Whole grain products, vegetables, some fruits (bananas), and nuts are excellent sources (Gropper, Smith, and Groff, 2005). Topping the list of rich sources, however, are fortified beverages and cereals (Nutrition Data, 2003).

STABILITY. As with other water-soluble vitamins, vitamin B_6 is preserved when vegetables are cooked as quickly as possible. Vitamin B_6 is relatively stable to heat and acids but very sensitive to light and easily destroyed by alkalis.

TOXICITY. Pyridoxine toxicity has resulted from taking 2 to 6 grams per day for 2 to 40 months. These megadoses, 1100 to 3500 times the older males' RDA, were self-prescribed. Excessive amounts appear to cause degeneration of dorsal root ganglia in the spinal cord, loss of myelination, and degeneration of sensory fibers in peripheral nerves (Gropper, Smith, and Groff, 2005). Signs and symptoms include sensory loss and numbness of the hands and feet, resulting in clumsiness and severe **ataxia.** Cessation of the drug has permitted the return of some, but not all, functions. Even 200 milligrams per day has produced sensory neuropathy (Feinman and Lieber, 1999).

Folic Acid

Total body folate (the salt of folic acid) levels are estimated to range from 11 to 28 milligrams, about half of which is stored in the liver (Gropper, Smith, and Groff, 2005). **Folic acid** is involved in protein synthesis, including that of DNA, and in the maturation of red blood cells. In the latter function, it is closely involved with vitamin B_{12}.

Clinical Application 7–7

Niacin Toxicity

In late 1980, almost half the clients in a small nursing home in Illinois became ill after breakfast. Their faces became flushed or they developed a rash 15 to 30 minutes after the meal. As in suspected food poisoning outbreaks, the foods consumed were compared. Which food was eaten by all those who became ill but by none of those who did not become ill? In this case, it was cornmeal mush.

Careful observation and documentation are important in food poisoning cases. The sequence of signs and symptoms may steer the investigators in the right direction. Often the signs and symptoms have disappeared by the time the physician arrives. In this nursing home, the signs and symptoms lasted only an average of 50 minutes.

If food poisoning is suspected, health authorities take samples of the food to examine in the laboratory. None of the leftover food should be discarded before health authorities arrive. The Food and Drug Administration tested the cornmeal from the nursing home's kitchen. It contained more than 1000 milligrams of niacin per pound. The recommended amount for cornmeal is 16 to 24 milligrams per pound.

Often a food poisoning epidemic has run its course by the time the source of the outbreak is known. In this case, the offending food was identified but the method of contamination never was positively determined.

ABSORPTION, METABOLISM, AND EXCRETION.
Approximately 50 percent of the folic acid in food, where it is usually bound to amino acids, is absorbed (Gropper, Smith, and Groff, 2005). The enzyme needed to separate the folic acid from the amino acids is **folate conjugase.** It is found in salivary, gastric, pancreatic, and jejunal secretions. The unbound folate is absorbed throughout the small intestine, most efficiently in the jejunum, and transported to the liver. In the liver, some of the folate is processed for storage in the tissues and the liver, which holds about half the body's supply. Some folate is secreted into bile. When the gallbladder releases bile into the duodenum, the folate may again be split off and absorbed. This recycling process is important in allowing folate stores to be adequate for 2 to 4 months, compared with 1 to 4 weeks for thiamin stores. Excretion of folic acid occurs via bile and urine.

FUNCTIONS. Folic acid is necessary for the formation of DNA. Thus, folate participates in the reproduction of every cell. Folic acid is active in cell renewal, and adequate amounts are particularly necessary for rapidly growing cells, including those in the gastrointestinal tract, blood, and fetal tissue.

DEFICIENCY. Folic acid deficiency is probably the most common vitamin deficiency due to inadequate food intake. Only one fresh fruit or fresh vegetable daily is considered sufficient to eliminate this deficiency (Herbert, 1999). At risk are poorly nourished children and poverty-stricken people. Pregnant women, infants, and young children are also at risk, because increased folic acid is needed during periods of rapid growth. An estimated one-third of the world's pregnant women are affected by folate deficiency (Herbert, 1999). The link between folic acid and neural tube defects in the developing fetus is explained in Chapter 11. Causes of folic acid deficiency include inadequate intake, inadequate absorption, inadequate use, increased requirement, increased destruction, and increased excretion. In clients with chronic alcoholism, the fact that all six causes may coexist explains why about 80 percent of these individuals are folate deficient. A deficiency may also occur in conditions causing increased metabolic rates, such as infections and hyperthyroidism, and those characterized by increased cell turnover, such as severe burns and cancer (Herbert, 1999).

Folic acid deficiency results in impaired cell division and protein synthesis, including the faulty synthesis of red blood cells. Concentrations in the red blood cells are diminished after about 4 months of low folate intake, and after about 5 months, **megaloblastic anemia** occurs (Gropper, Smith, and Groff, 2005). In addition to laboratory blood changes, signs and symptoms include a red, smooth, and swollen tongue, heartburn, diarrhea, fainting, and fatigue. Although clients with folate deficiency do not develop the nerve damage seen in vitamin B_{12} deficiencies, they do manifest neurologic symptoms that include irritability, forgetfulness, and hostile and paranoid behavior. These symptoms improve markedly 24 hours after beginning treatment with folic acid (Herbert, 1999).

One positive result of folate deficiency occurs in tropical countries, where it protects against malaria. The lack of folic acid stops the spread of the parasite by preventing its DNA from replicating (Herbert, 1999).

DIETARY REFERENCE INTAKES. Folic acid RDAs and AIs are given in Dietary Folate Equivalents (DFEs).
One DFE equals

- 1 microgram of food folate
- 0.6 microgram of folate from fortified food or as a supplement consumed with food
- 0.5 microgram of a supplement taken on an empty stomach

The RDA for folic acid is 400 micrograms for adults. Women capable of becoming pregnant should consume 400 micrograms of folic acid from fortified foods or supplements in addition to food folate. Pregnant women have an RDA of 600 micrograms. UL for synthetic folic acid obtained from supplements and/or fortified foods is 1000 micrograms for adults.

FOOD SOURCES. Green, leafy vegetables such as spinach, asparagus, Brussels sprouts, and broccoli provide folic acid. Other vegetables and fruits containing appreciable folic acid are lima and kidney beans and oranges and strawberries. From the meat group, liver is a good source of folic acid. Because folate was recently added to the U.S. fortification protocol for grains to reduce the occurrence of neural tube defects, grain products are now major sources of folic acid.

STABILITY. Folic acid is stable in the presence of alkalis, but it is easily oxidized by light and acids. Some forms are easily destroyed by heat, so that cooking losses may be as high as 50 to 95 percent. To minimize losses, cook vegetables as quickly as possible.

INTERFERING FACTORS. Zinc deficiency and chronic alcohol intake can impair conjugase activity and diminish absorption of folic acid. Conjugase inhibitors in certain foods prevent the digestion of polyglutamate forms of folate and thus prevent its absorption. Some of the foods containing these conjugase inhibitors are legumes, lentils, cabbage, and oranges (Gropper, Smith, and Groff, 2005).

Methotrexate, an anticancer drug, is a folic acid antagonist. Its purpose is to interfere with DNA in cancer cells, but it simultaneously affects normal cells. A more commonly used drug, aspirin, displaces folic acid from its carrier protein; the displaced folic acid is then excreted.

TOXICITY. Folic acid toxicity is rare. Dose levels of over-the-counter vitamins have been limited to 400 micrograms to make it inconvenient to overdose. The limitation is not to prevent toxicity from folic acid but to avoid masking signs of pernicious anemia. The current opinion of the scientific community, however, is that intake of folate and folic acid up to 5000 micrograms per day would have no adverse effects and that a more sophisticated blood test can be used to diagnose pernicious anemia (Workshop, 1999).

Recommended doses in healthy humans have not been reported to be toxic, but very large doses in laboratory animals have produced renal toxicity and convulsions. The interaction of folic acid with antiepileptic drugs is elaborated upon in Chapter 17.

Vitamin B_{12}

Vitamin B_{12} is an essential coenzyme in the synthesis of DNA, RNA, and myelin and is necessary for normal red blood cell formation. Vitamin B_{12} is stored to a greater extent than the other B vitamins, but diverse causes can precipitate vitamin B_{12} deficiency, leading to serious consequences and a specific disease condition.

ABSORPTION, METABOLISM, AND EXCRETION. Efficient absorption of vitamin B_{12} requires an explicit protein-binding factor called **intrinsic factor,** secreted by the gastric mucosal cells in the stomach. Vitamin B_{12}, also called **extrinsic factor,** combines with intrinsic factor in the proximal small intestine. In this way, intrinsic factor protects vitamin B_{12} from digestive enzymes and intestinal bacteria until the complex reaches the ileum, where the vitamin is absorbed. About 1 percent of large pharmacological doses of vitamin B_{12} circumvents this process and is absorbed by passive diffusion in the intestine (Weir and Scott, 1999).

Vitamin B_{12} is not freely absorbed. The amount absorbed depends on the body's storage levels and the amount ingested. At low levels of intake, a large amount of the vitamin is absorbed and vice versa. In addition, in healthy persons, the vitamin can be recycled from bile and intestinal secretions (Gropper, Smith, and Groff, 2005). Vitamin B_{12} has a long half-life, so that a person's stores last from 3 to 5 years. The principal storage site is the liver, which contains 50 percent of the body's supply.

FUNCTIONS. Vitamin B_{12} is required in a series of reactions that precede the use of folic acid in DNA replication. In fact, without vitamin B_{12}, folic acid is unable to assist in the manufacture of red blood cells. Vitamin B_{12} is also essential for the synthesis and maintenance of myelin, the fatty insulation that permits speedy transmission of impulses along the nerves. Perhaps because of the vital role of vitamin B_{12} in DNA replication, a deficiency has been linked to early recurrent abortion (Reznikoff-Etievant et al, 2002).

DEFICIENCY. Persons may be at increased risk of vitamin B_{12} deficiency because of stomach pathology, intestinal disease, or diet. When a person lacks intrinsic factor, the result is a condition called **pernicious anemia.** The prevalence of the disease increases with age and is attributed to antibodies against gastric parietal cells and intrinsic factor. Pernicious anemia can also occur after the surgical removal of the stomach or a large portion of the stomach. In those cases, vitamin B_{12} is not absorbed because intrinsic factor is missing. Causation by a different mechanism can occur as well. Gastric acid facilitates separation of vitamin B_{12} from the foods containing it. Thus, vitamin B_{12} deficiency can be caused by atrophic gastritis and by prolonged use of medications that block gastric acid (Oh and Brown, 2003).

People with **Crohn's disease** involving the ileum and those whose ileum has been removed do not absorb vitamin B_{12} efficiently. Other intestinal causes of deficiency include conditions causing bacterial overgrowth and parasites.

Vitamin B_{12} deficiency can be caused by a diet devoid of animal products. People particularly at risk are the elderly who choose tea and toast for meals, persons with alcoholism who eat poorly, and strict vegetarians. A 33-year old-man who had been a strict vegetarian for many years without taking vitamin supplements became irreversibly blind as a result of severe bilateral optic neuropathy. The condition was attributed to deficiencies of vitamin B_{12} and thiamin (Milea, Cassoux, and LeHoang, 2000).

Traditional treatment of pernicious anemia involves periodic intramuscular injections of vitamin B_{12}. The pharmaceutical names for vitamin B_{12} are **cyanocobalamin** and **hydroxocobalamin.** Recent evidence suggests oral medication in large amounts may be effective for some clients (Andres et al, 2001; Nyholm et al, 2003; Oh and Brown, 2003), but data are inadequate to support oral treatment in clients with severe neurologic involvement (Lane and Rojas-Fernandez, 2002). Cyanocobalamin can also be given intranasally.

Symptoms of vitamin B_{12} deficiency are, in usual order of appearance, numbness and tingling in the hands and feet, red blood cell changes, moodiness, confusion, depression, **delusions,** and overt **psychosis.** Eventually, irreparable nerve damage occurs and, finally, death. One study reported 28 percent of clients with neuropsychiatric disorders caused by vitamin B_{12} deficiency displayed no red blood cell pathology, suggesting cobalamin deficiency should be ruled out in clients with unexplained neuropsychiatric disorders (Lindenbaum et al, 1988). A case of acute dementia in a 52-year-old client caused by vitamin B_{12} deficiency without other symptoms led the researchers to recommend screening psychiatric clients for vitamin B_{12} and folic acid regardless of age or previous health (Lerner and Kanevsky, 2002).

Diagnosing vitamin B_{12} deficiency by examining red blood cells is difficult if the person consumes ample folic acid. The folic acid enables the body to continue manufacturing red blood cells in the correct size and number, but the neurological deterioration of pernicious anemia continues unabated. The potential for masking pernicious anemia with folic acid intake led to some concern about fortification of foods with folic acid. One study indicated that food fortification has not caused a major increase in masking of vitamin B_{12} deficiency (Mills et al, 2003). Other blood tests, such as serum methylmalonic acid and homocysteine, are more effective than serum vitamin B_{12} in diagnosing vitamin B_{12} deficiency (Oh and Brown, 2003).

DIETARY REFERENCE INTAKES. The adult RDA for vitamin B_{12} is 2.4 micrograms. One ounce of beef liver contains 13 times this amount. Because 10 to 30 percent of older people may not absorb vitamin B_{12} from food effectively, the RDA for men and women older than 50 specifies that fortified foods or a vitamin supplement be used as the source for vitamin B_{12}. An UL is not determinable.

FOOD SOURCES. Vitamin B_{12} is synonymous with animal products that have derived their cobalamins from microorganisms. Healthy young adults who regularly consume meat, milk, cheese, or eggs are not at risk of vitamin B_{12} deficiency. Some plant foods may contain vitamin B_{12} from bacterial contamination or, in the case of legumes, from the nitrogen-fixing bacteria on their roots. For strict vegetarians, nutritional yeast and vitamin B_{12}-fortified products (soymilk or tofu) are more appropriate food sources than reliance on bacterial contamination. Undependable sources due to variable vitamin content or inactive vitamin B_{12} analogs are sea vegetables, unfortified yeast, beer, and other fermented foods (American Dietetic Association, 2000). Products that list vitamin B_{12} rather than cobalamin may include nonbioavailable sources (Centers for Disease Control, 2003).

STABILITY AND INTERFERING FACTORS. Vitamin B_{12} is stable to heat. However, light, acids, and alkalies inactivate it. Megadoses of vitamin C interfere with vitamin B_{12} absorption and utilization. The body's use of vitamin B_{12} is also impaired by a deficiency of vitamin B_6 and by gastritis.

TOXICITY. No toxicity from vitamin B_{12} has been recorded. Neither has benefit from excessive intake been noted in nondeficient individuals (Gropper, Smith, and Groff, 2005).

Recently Emphasized Vitamins

Two B vitamins are so widely distributed in foods that only special circumstances have produced deficiencies. Long-term **total parenteral nutrition (TPN)** is one such situation. That therapy is detailed in Chapter 15.

PANTOTHENIC ACID. The vitamin **pantothenic acid** plays a role in the metabolism of carbohydrates, fats, and proteins and in the synthesis of the neurotransmitter **acetylcholine** No cases of deficiency of pantothenic acid have been documented in people who eat a variety of foods, but deficiencies have occurred in prisoner-of-war camps and have been produced experimentally (Plesofsky-Vig, 1999). The AI is 5 milligrams for adults, and an UL is not determinable. The average U.S. diet supplies 7 milligrams. People with alcoholism, diabetes mellitus, and inflammatory bowel diseases may have an increased need for pantothenic acid (Gropper, Smith, and Groff, 2005). Rich food sources include liver, egg yolk, legumes, whole grain cereals, potatoes, and broccoli. Bacteria in the colon are able to synthesize pantothenic acid (Said, 1999).

BIOTIN. Closely related to folic acid and vitamin B_{12}, **biotin** is a coenzyme in **gluconeogenesis** fatty acid metabolism, and amino acid catabolism (Pacheco-Alvarez, Solorzano-Vargas, and Del Rio, 2002). Small amounts are stored in the muscle, liver, and brain (Gropper, Smith, and Groff, 2005). Biotin is required to form **purines** which are essential components of DNA and RNA. Oral biotin, even in pharmacological doses, is completely absorbed (Zempleni and Mock, 1999). Food sources include liver, egg yolk, legumes, nuts, tomatoes, and cereals. Deficiencies have been seen in children displaying the chief sign of skin rash and also may occur in clients fed intravenously who also receive antibiotics. Antibiotics kill the bacteria in the large intestine that synthesize biotin. Besides the rash, symptoms include alopecia, muscle pain, paresthesia, depression, and hallucinations (Gropper, Smith, and Groff, 2005). Other clients who have developed biotin deficiency are children with an inborn error of biotinidase metabolism, persons with alcoholism or gastrointestinal diseases, and those on long-term anticonvulsant therapy or receiving long-term hemodialysis (Mock, 1999). The AI for biotin is 30 micrograms for adults. The UL is not determinable.

Avidin a protein in raw egg white, binds with biotin. Humans given six raw egg whites per day developed dermatitis in 3 to 4 weeks. A week or two later, they displayed mental changes, muscle pain, nausea, and loss of appetite. Five days of biotin therapy cured the symptoms. Good food sources of biotin include liver, soybeans, egg yolk, cereals, legumes, and nuts (Gropper, Smith, and Groff, 2005).

Choline

The organic compound **choline** has been recognized as an essential nutrient partly because of experience with clients receiving long-term total parenteral nutrition (TPN). Choline occurs in the structure of membranes, modulates signaling within cells, and plays a vital role in brain development (Zeisel, 1999). Although not a vitamin by strict definition (Linus Pauling Institute, 2003), choline has been given an Adequate Intake under the Dietary Reference Intake system and appears in the vitamin section (Institute of Medicine, 2003). Choline is found in most animal tissues and is widely distributed in foods.

Choline facilitates movement of fat into the cells and decreases liver fat content by increasing phospholipid turnover. Deficiency of choline can result in fatty liver and hepatic cirrhosis. Choline is a precursor of the neurotransmitter acetylcholine and a particular formulation, choline alfoscerate, reportedly produced improvement in clients with Alzheimer's disease (De Jesus, 2003), a disease that is associated with decreased acetylcholine in the brain (Linus Pauling Institute, 2003).

The AI for choline is 550 milligrams for men and 425 milligrams for women. Estimated intake for adults is between 730 and 1040 milligrams per day. The UL for choline is 3500 milligrams per day for adults. Effects of excessive intake include sweating, salivation, hypotension, hepatotoxicity, and a fishy body odor. The last is due to excessive production and excretion of trimethylamine, a metabolite of choline (Linus Pauling Institute, 2003). The best food sources of choline are milk, eggs, liver, and peanuts. People at increased risk of choline deficiency include growing infants, pregnant or lactating women, strict vegetarians, people with cirrhosis of the liver or severe malabsorption syndromes, and clients receiving total parenteral nutrition (TPN). All of these individuals, especially those on limited diets or being artificially fed, may be at risk for deficiencies of other nutrients as well as choline.

Of the water-soluble vitamins, ascorbic acid is the most vulnerable to processing loss and niacin the most resistant. Table 7-4 summarizes information on vitamin C and six of the B-complex vitamins. In it and Table 7-2, although examples of food portions containing the RDA are given, it is for clarity only, not as a recommendation to use those specific foods to the exclusion of others. Table 7-5 and Figure 7-5 summarize the sources of vitamins by food groups.

Vitamins as Medicine

Some vitamins are available over the counter in many different formulations that can serve as dietary supplements. In certain cases, vitamins can be given in pharmacological amounts to counteract disease conditions.

Supplements

Vitamin supplements are not intended to be substitutes for a healthy diet. It should be clear from reading the chapter that knowledge of vitamins is not complete. New functions and relationships are being discovered every year. The new Dietary Reference Intakes are designed to consider

Table 7–4 Water-Soluble Vitamins

VITAMIN	ADULT RDA AND FOOD PORTION CONTAINING IT	FUNCTIONS	DEFICIENCY DISEASE	SIGNS AND SYMPTOMS OF DEFICIENCY	BEST SOURCES
C Ascorbic acid	75 to 90 mg 0.75 to 1 cup orange juice, prepared from frozen concentrate	Antioxidant Formation of collagen Function of adrenal glands Facilitation of iron absorption Conversion of folic acid to active form	Scurvy	Bleeding mucous membranes Poor wound healing or reopening of scars Softened ends of long bones Teeth loosen, may fall out Death due to internal hemorrhage	Orange juice, grapefruit juice, cantaloupe, strawberries Peppers, Brussels sprouts, broccoli
B_1 Thiamin	1.1 to 1.2 mg 3.6 oz pork chop, lean only	Coenzyme in CHO metabolism	Beriberi	Anorexia, indigestion, constipation Apathy, fatigue, muscle weakness Deterioration of myelin sheaths— paralysis, muscle atrophy Wernicke-Korsakoff syndrome Death due to cardiac failure	Pork Black beans, black-eyed peas Sunflower seeds Fortified cereals Wheat germ
B_2 Riboflavin	1.1 to 1.3 mg 2.4 to 2.8 cups nonfat milk	Coenzyme in protein metabolism	Aribino-flavinosis	Lesions on lips and in mouth Seborrheic dermatitis Normocytic anemia	Milk and dairy products Organ meats Fortified cereals Eggs
B_3 Niacin	14 to 16 mg niacin equivalents 3.6 oz water-packed tuna	Coenzyme in production of energy from glucose Participant in synthesis of fatty acids	Pellagra	Bilaterally symmetrical dermatitis on face, neck, hands, and feet Diarrhea Dementia	Tuna Chicken breast Enriched grains Coffee
B_6 Pyridoxine	1.3 to 1.7 mg 2.6 bananas	Coenzyme in synthesis and catabolism of amino acids	No specific term	Dermatitis Glossitis Convulsions	Sirloin steak Salmon Chicken breast Whole grains, fortified cereals
Folate Folic acid	400 μg 7.5 tbsp wheat germ	Essential to the formation of DNA Participant in formation of heme	No specific term	Red, smooth, swollen tongue Heartburn, diarrhea Fatigue, fainting Confusion, depression Macrocytic anemia	Beef liver Fortified grain products Broccoli Cooked asparagus Brussels sprouts Cooked spinach
B_{12} Cyanocobalamin	2.4 μg 3.2 oz cooked lean beef	Necessary for folic acid use in DNA replication Synthesis and maintenance of myelin	Pernicious anemia (lack of intrinsic factor, not dietary)	Sore tongue Numbness and tingling of hands and feet Macrocytic anemia Moodiness, confusion Depression Delusions, psychosis	Meat Fish Eggs Poultry Milk

the effect of vitamin intake on chronic disease occurrence, rather than simply to prevent deficiency diseases; however, the U.S. Preventive Services Task Force has stated that the evidence is insufficient to recommend for or against supplemental vitamins A, C, or E, multivitamins with folic acid, or antioxidant combinations as an intervention to prevent cardiovascular disease or cancer. Furthermore, the Task Force recommended against the use of beta-carotene to prevent cardiovascular disease and cancer (U.S. Preventive Services Task Force, 2003). More information on beta-carotene and cancer appears in Chapter 23. The single piece of advice given most frequently in the conclusions of researchers, however, is the admonition to eat five servings of fruits and vegetables every day. Figure 7-6 is a reminder that fruit eaten out of hand is the original fast food.

If a person wishes to take supplements, it is best not to exceed 150 percent of the RDA for each vitamin. This amount will prevent deficiency in young, well individuals, and toxicity is unlikely. A multivitamin preparation is preferred to a medley of single vitamins and generic preparations offer the lowest cost with no known difference in

bioavailability compared with specialty brands (Fletcher and Fairfield, 2002). Even so, people ought to consider vitamins as medications when their primary care providers ask what medications they are taking. In fact, between 24 and 51 percent of individuals reported taking various single or combinations of vitamins and minerals between 1988 and 1994, as detailed in Table 7-6.

For the first time, the RDAs specify fortified foods or supplements for certain life-stage groups. It is recommended that people over 50 years of age obtain vitamin B_{12} from fortified foods or supplements. For all women who may become pregnant, the recommendation is to consume 400 micrograms of folic acid from fortified foods or supplements in addition to food folate to reduce the risk of neural tube defects in the fetus, an abnormality included in Chapter 11.

Pharmacological Uses

Vitamins can be used to treat dietary deficiencies or to compensate for diseases causing malabsorption. They also have been given for some conditions unrelated to dietary deficiency.

Table 7–5 Good Sources of Vitamins by Food Groups

VITAMIN	SYNTHESIS/ MISCELLANEOUS	MEATS	MILK	FRUITS/VEGETABLES	GRAINS
A		Liver	Fortified	Deep yellow, dark green leafy	
D	In skin	Eggs from hens fed vitamin D Some fatty fish	Fortified		Fortified cereals
E				Vegetable oil	Wheat germ Whole grains Fortified cereals
K	In intestine			Green leafy	
C				Fresh fruit, especially citrus Vegetables	
Thiamin		Pork		Black beans Black-eyed peas	Wheat germ Fortified cereals
Riboflavin		Organ meats Eggs	Milk	Legumes	Fortified cereals
Niacin	Coffee	Meat Fish Poultry			Whole grains Fortified cereals
B_6		Beef Salmon Chicken breast		Bananas Nuts	Whole grains Wheat germ Fortified cereals
Folic acid		Liver		Dark green leafy Cabbage family Lima and kidney beans Cantaloupe Oranges	Fortified grain products Whole grains
B_{12}		Meat Eggs	Milk Cheese		
Pantothenic acid	In intestine	Liver Egg yolk		Legumes Broccoli Potatoes	Whole grain cereals
Biotin	In intestine	Liver Egg yolk		Tomatoes Legumes Nuts	Cereals

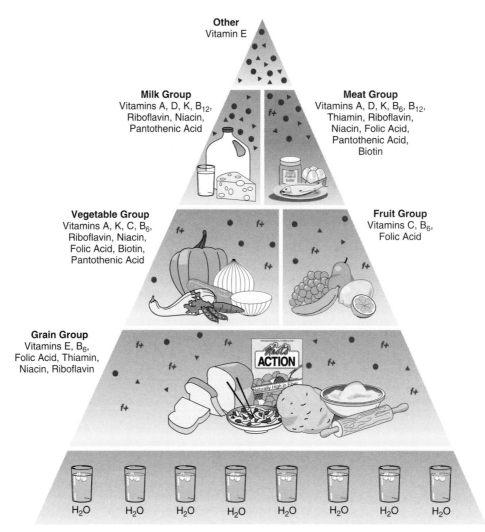

Other
Vitamin E

Milk Group
Vitamins A, D, K, B$_{12}$,
Riboflavin, Niacin,
Pantothenic Acid

Meat Group
Vitamins A, D, K, B$_6$, B$_{12}$,
Thiamin, Riboflavin,
Niacin, Folic Acid,
Pantothenic Acid,
Biotin

Vegetable Group
Vitamins A, K, C, B$_6$,
Riboflavin, Niacin,
Folic Acid, Biotin,
Pantothenic Acid

Fruit Group
Vitamins C, B$_6$,
Folic Acid

Grain Group
Vitamins E, B$_6$,
Folic Acid, Thiamin,
Niacin, Riboflavin

ACTION

H$_2$O   H$_2$O   H$_2$O   H$_2$O   H$_2$O   H$_2$O   H$_2$O   H$_2$O

Figure **7–5** This pyramid illustrates the sources of vitamins by food groups.

Treatment of Deficiencies

The obvious use of vitamins is to treat vitamin deficiencies. Vitamin C is the treatment for scurvy, vitamin D for rickets, niacin for pellagra, and vitamin B$_{12}$ for pernicious anemia. Common uses in diseases causing malabsorption are included in Unit Three on Clinical Nutrition.

Other Uses

Vitamins have been used in very large doses in attempts to prevent or to mitigate certain diseases. Results have been mixed.

MEGADOSES. A dose 10 times the RDA is called a **megadose.** Some individuals take huge doses of vitamin C in an attempt to prevent the common cold. Evidence of effectiveness has not been proven to the satisfaction of many scientists. A review of the literature, however, indicated that although vitamin C supplementation failed to reduce the incidence of colds in the normal population, it did reduce the risk of developing a cold by 50 percent in marathon runners, skiers, and soldiers on sub-arctic exercises. Similarly, beginning vitamin C supplementation at

the onset of a cold was not effective in reducing duration of symptoms, but prophylactic intake of the vitamin reduced the duration of colds by 8 percent in adults and 13 percent in children (Douglas et al 2004.) Rebound scurvy has been reported when megadoses of vitamin C were discontinued abruptly, but the evidence is scanty.

Large doses of vitamin E supplements beyond the amount that could reasonably be obtained from food are

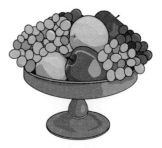

The Original Fast Food

Figure **7–6** A reminder that fruits eaten out-of-hand are the original fast foods.

Table 7–6 Vitamin/Mineral Supplement Use by Age and Sex

AGE	MALE	FEMALE
2 months to 11 years	40 percent	38 percent
12 to 19 years	24 percent	38 percent
20 to 39 years	32 percent	44 percent
40 years and over	38 percent	51 percent

SOURCE: Ervin, 2003.

the subject of investigations into neurodegenerative diseases and immunological functioning. Widespread use of such supplements awaits confirmatory research.

TREATING NONNUTRITIONAL DISORDERS. Many vitamins have uses unrelated to prevention or treatment of deficiencies. Vitamins A, E, and C, riboflavin, niacin, and pyridoxine are examples. Vitamin A derivatives are often prescribed to control acne and the wrinkles of aging. The hazards to the fetus are elaborated in Chapter 11. Clinical Application 7–8 shows vitamin C to be a food additive intended to reduce the formation of cancer-causing compounds. Riboflavin is being investigated as a preventive agent against migraine headaches (Maizels, Blumenfeld,

Clinical Application 7–8

Vitamin C and Smoked Meat

Vitamin C blocks the formation of nitrosamines from nitrates. *Nitrates* are chemicals added to smoked and cured meats to preserve them and enhance their flavor. In the small intestine, however, nitrates combine with amino acids to form nitrosamines, which have been linked to some cancers. For this reason, meat packers have begun adding vitamin C to protect against nitrosamine formation.

and Burchette, 2004; Schoenen, Jacquy, and Lenaerts, 1998). Topical application of niacin is being tested as an aid in diagnosing schizophrenia (Puri et al, 2001; Smesny et al, 2003). High doses of niacin, usually 3 to 6 grams per day, have been used to lower serum cholesterol, but doses of 2 to 4.5 grams per day have caused macular edema and vision loss until the niacin was discontinued (Callanan, Blondi, and Martin, 1998). Pyridoxine has been recommended to treat carpal tunnel syndrome (Holm and Moody, 2003) and **tardive dyskinesia,** a side effect of some psychotropic drugs (Lerner et al, 2001).

SUMMARY

Vitamins are organic substances required in minute quantities that are necessary for many bodily processes. They do not become part of the structure of the body. Some deficiency diseases have been known and treated for centuries. It was not until the twentieth century, though, that each of the known vitamins was isolated in the laboratory.

Vitamins A, D, E, and K are fat-soluble and stable to heat. Sufficient dietary fat intake and adequate fat digestion and absorption are required for the proper utilization of these vitamins. Fat-soluble vitamins, especially A and D, can be stored in excess by the body, and for that reason can be sources of toxicity. Both vitamins A and D cause clear-cut deficiency diseases: xerophthalmia and night blindness for vitamin A and rickets for vitamin D.

The water-soluble vitamins, C and the B-complex vitamins, are not stored in the body in appreciable amounts. Vitamins C, B_{12}, thiamin, and niacin have specific diseases associated with deficiency: scurvy, pernicious anemia, beriberi, and pellagra, respectively.

Because of the interdependent functions of vitamins, people without special needs are advised to rely mainly on a varied, balanced, moderate diet for vitamins (Wellness Tips 7-1). Vitamin supplements will not compensate for a poor diet. People who take vitamins should limit their intake to 150 percent of the RDA in a multivitamin product, except individuals with special needs. Two large groups of people for whom synthetic vitamins in fortified food or supplements are recommended are women who are capable of becoming pregnant (folate) and individuals older than 50 years (vitamin B_{12}).

Wellness Tip **7-1** • Eat five servings of fruits and vegetables each day. Whole foods contain nutrients and phytochemicals not found in vitamin tablets.

- Select whole-grain products rather than refined ones to maximize vitamin content.
- Follow MyPyramid. Limiting fat does not mean eliminating fat. Absorption of fat-soluble vitamins requires fat intake.
- Seek advice from the health-care provider if a whole food group is excluded from the diet.
- If using a vitamin supplement, choose a multivitamin preparation instead of individual vitamins unless the health-care provider recommends them to treat particular conditions.
- Follow the recommended dosages, not to exceed 150 percent (one and a half times) the RDA. In certain situations, vitamin supplementation has been associated with increases in infections or cancer. Bacteria and cancer cells also need these nutrients (see Chapters 12 and 23).
- When asked, be sure to include vitamin supplements on the list of medications you take.
- Treat dietary supplements as medicine. Lock them in childproof cupboards. Do not take medicines in front of children lest they imitate you.
- Do not attempt to implement the findings of every new study on vitamins that is reported.
- Take all vitamin A preparations cautiously. Seek advice from your health-care provider.

CASE STUDY 7-1

Mr. J, a 79-year-old widowed man, prides himself on caring for himself in the past year since his wife died. His typical meal pattern is:

- Breakfast—egg, toast, jam, coffee
- Lunch—cheese or lunchmeat sandwich, tea
- Dinner—canned stew or hash

Although Mr. J has a refrigerator, he avoids buying fresh fruit or vegetables. He says he has difficulty consuming produce before it spoils. He seldom goes out to eat.

For the past few months, Mr. J has noticed that his gums are tender. He stopped wearing his dentures when his gums began to bleed.

The visiting nurse confirmed the inflammation of the gums. When the nurse took Mr. J's blood pressure, she noted a red, flat rash on Mr. J's forearm.

NURSING CARE PLAN

SUBJECTIVE DATA   Sore gums
Diet lacks fresh fruits and vegetables

OBJECTIVE DATA   Inflamed gums
Erythematous **petechiae** related to blood pressure measurement

NURSING DIAGNOSIS   NANDA: Imbalanced Nutrition, less than body requirements, possible vitamin C deficiency (NANDA, 2003, with permission). Related to lack of fresh fruit and vegetables as evidenced by sore bleeding gums and petechiae after sphygmomanometer use.

DESIRED OUTCOMES EVALUATION CRITERIA	NURSING ACTIONS/INTERVENTIONS	RATIONALE
NOC: Nutritional Status: Nutrient Intake (Moorhead, Johnson, and Maas, 2004, with permission)	NIC: Nutritional Counseling (Dochterman and Bulechek, 2004, with permission)	
Will consume foods containing 90 mg of vitamin C every day within 3 days	Teach importance of daily vitamin C	Little vitamin C is stored in the body; must be consumed every day.
	Explore acceptability of good sources of vitamin C; list amounts necessary to obtain 90 mg; recommend purchasing small quantities.	Foods would be better sources than vitamin supplements because other nutrients supplied also.
	If client selects frozen vegetables, teach to boil water 1 minute before adding vegetables and to cook quickly until crisp-tender.	Heat and oxygen destroy vitamin C.

CTQ CRITICAL THINKING QUESTIONS

1. What additional assessment data would be helpful as you work with Mr. J to increase his fruit and vegetable intake?
2. Speculate on the reasons the visiting nurse is calling on Mr. J. Can you think of medical conditions that would be directly affected by lack of vitamin C?

3. Mr. J wants to keep his present meal pattern and "take a vitamin pill" to correct his nutritional deficiencies. How would you respond?

))) CHAPTER REVIEW

1. Which of the following vitamins are water-soluble?
   a. A and C
   b. A, D, E, and K
   c. B and C
   d. B, D, E, and K
2. The vitamin that is essential to the synthesis of several blood clotting factors is:
   a. Vitamin A
   b. Vitamin B_6
   c. Vitamin C
   d. Vitamin K
3. Which of the following groups of foods would be the best sources of carotene?
   a. Apricots, cantaloupe, and squash
   b. Asparagus, beets, and sweet potatoes
   c. Broccoli, lettuce, and lima beans
   d. Lemons, oranges, and strawberries
4. Deficiency of vitamin D causes:
   a. Rickets
   b. Pellagra
   c. Night blindness
   d. Beriberi
5. In general, individuals who elect to take a vitamin supplement should:
   a. Buy the most economical product
   b. Limit the amounts to 150 percent of RDA levels
   c. Obtain a physician's prescription
   d. Select the most advertised product

✚ CLINICAL ANALYSIS

1. Ms. C is bringing her 3-month-old baby girl to the well-baby clinic. Ms. C states that the baby is taking 6 ounces of a commercial baby formula every 4 hours. Ms. C has not added solid foods to the baby's diet. She was told to wait until the baby is 4 to 6 months old before adding cereal. Ms. C is giving the baby the multivitamin preparation prescribed. She also has added cod liver oil to the infant's diet. "It's only a teaspoonful," she said. Ms. C's grandmother gave Ms. C cod liver oil as a child. Ms. C credits her grandmother's care during her own childhood for her strong bones and teeth. She admires her grandmother, who at age 75 still stands straight and tall. Which of the following pieces of information should the nurse gather first to focus on the situation presented?

   a. The amount of vitamin C in the multivitamin supplement
   b. The conditions under which the vitamins are stored
   c. Ms. C's technique for measuring the vitamins
   d. The total amount of vitamin D the infant receives each day

2. Mr. S has expressed interest in improving his diet. The nurse assessed Mr. S's usual intake, noting the absence of citrus fruit. He stated the acids upset his stomach. Which of the following suggestions to maximize vitamin C content in vegetables is appropriate?
   a. Adding baking soda to the cooking water
   b. Cooking thoroughly to kill any bacteria
   c. Eating good sources raw when possible
   d. Keeping food in a mesh bag to allow air to circulate

3. Ms. M is a Seventh-Day Adventist who has elected a vegan lifestyle and who lives an indoor life. For which of the following vitamin deficiencies would she be at greatest risk without professional dietary advice?
   a. Vitamins A, C, and E
   b. Vitamins B_{12}, D, and niacin
   c. Vitamins B_6, folate, and thiamin
   d. Vitamin K, riboflavin, and biotin

REFERENCES

Agarwal, KS, et al: The impact of atmospheric pollution on vitamin D status of infants and toddlers in Delhi, India. Arch Dis Child 87:111, 2001.

Age-related Eye Disease Study Research Group: A randomized, placebo-controlled, clinical trial of high-dose supplementation with vitamins C and E and beta-carotene for age-related cataract and vision loss. Arch Ophthalmol 119:1439, 2001a.

Age-related Eye Disease Study Research Group: A randomized, placebo-controlled, clinical trial of high-dose supplementation with vitamins C and E, beta-carotene, and zinc for age-related macular degeneration and vision loss. Arch Ophthalmol 119:1417, 2001b.

Aghdassi, E, Royall, D, and Allard, JP: Oxidative stress in smokers supplemented with vitamin C. Int J Vitam Nutr Res 69:45, 1999.

Akikusa, JD, Garrick, D, and Nash, MC: Scurvy: Forgotten but not gone. J Paediatr Child Health 39:75, 2003.

American Dietetic Association: Position of the American Dietetic Association: Food fortification and dietary supplements. J Am Diet Assoc 101:115, 2001.

American Dietetic Association: Position of the American Dietetic Association and Dietitians of Canada: Vegetarian diets. J Am Diet Assoc 103:748, 2003.

American Dietetic Association: Manual of Clinical Dietetics, ed 6. American Dietetic Association, Chicago, 2000.

Andres, E et al: Oral cobalamin therapy for the treatment of patients with food-cobalamin malabsorption. Am J Med 111:126, 2001.

Arnaud, J, et al: Vitamin B intake and status in healthy Havanan men, 2 years after the Cuban neuropathy epidemic. Br J Nutr 85:741, 2001.

Astudillo, L, et al: Development of beriberi heart disease 20 years after gastrojejunostomy [letter]. Am J Med 113:157, 2003.

Backstrand, JR: The history and future of food fortification in the United States: A public health perspective. Nutr Rev 60:15, 2002.

Bamber, MG: Wernicke's encephalopathy [letter]. Lancet 352:655, 1998.

Benomar, A et al: Vitamin E deficiency ataxia associated with adenoma. J Neurol Sci 162:97, 1999.

Bhat, RV, and Deshmukh, CT: A study of Vitamin K status in children on prolonged antibiotic therapy. Indian Pediatr 40:36, 2003.

Bingham, AC, Kimura, Y, and Imundo, L: A 16-year-old boy with purpura and leg pain. J Pediatr 142:560, 2003.

Blank, S, et al: An outbreak of hypervitaminosis D associated with the overfortification of milk from a home-delivery dairy. Am J Public Health 85:656, 1995.

Butterfield, DA, et al: Vitamin E and neurodegenerative disorders associated with oxidative stress. Nutr Neurosci 5:229, 2002.

Callanan, D, Blodi, BA, and Martin, DF: Macular edema associated with nicotinic acid (niacin) [letter]. JAMA 279:1702, 1998.

Centers for Disease Control: Deaths associated with thiamine-deficient total parenteral nutrition. MMWR 38:43, 1989. Accessed July 15, 1999 at http://www.cdc.gov/epo/mmwr/preview/ mmwrhtml/00001339.htm.

Centers for Disease Control: Lactic acidosis traced to thiamine deficiency related to nationwide shortage of multivitamins for total parenteral nutrition—United States, 1997. MMWR 38:523, 1997. Accessed July 15, 1999 at http://www.cdc.gov/epo/mmwr/preview/mmwrhtml/00001339.htm.

Centers for Disease Control: Neurologic impairment in children associated with maternal dietary deficiency of cobalamin—Georgia, 2001. MMWR 52:61, 2003. Accessed December 18, 2003 at http://www.cdc.gov/mmwr/PDF/wk/mm5204.pdf

Centers for Disease Control: Severe malnutrition among young children—Georgia, January 1997—June 1999. MMWR 50:224, 2001. Accessed June 19, 2003 at http://www.cdc.gov/mmwr/preview/mmwrhtml/nn5012a3.htm.

Cervantes-Laurean, D, McElvaney, NG, and Moss, J: Niacin. In Shils, ME, et al (eds): Modern Nutrition in Health and Disease, ed 9. Lippincott Williams & Wilkins, Philadelphia, 1999.

Cochran, WA: Overnutrition in prenatal and neonatal life: A problem? Can Med Assoc J 93:893, 1965.

Collins, M, and Gernaey, A: Osteocalcin—the oldest surviving bone protein? Last updated May 1, 1998. Accessed August 5, 1999 at http://nrg.ncl.ac.uk/research/ancient-biomols/osteocalcin.html.

Corbin, F, 3rd: Pathogen inactivation of blood components: current status and introduction of an approach using riboflavin as a photosensitizer. In J Hematol 76(Suppl 2):253, 2002.

Craciun, AM, et al: Improved bone metabolism in female elite athletes after vitamin K supplementation. Int J Sports Med 19:479, 1998.

Dagnelie, G, Zorge, IS, and McDonald, TM: Lutein improves visual function in some patients with retinal degeneration: A pilot study via the Internet. Optometry 71:147, 2000.

Davies, PS, et al: Vitamin D: Seasonal and regional differences in preschool children in Great Britain. Eur J Clin Nutr 53:195, 1999.

Dawodu, et al: Hypovitaminosis D and vitamin D deficiency in exclusively breast-feeding infants and their mothers in summer: A justification for vitamin D supplementation of breast-feeding infants. J Pediatr 142:169, 2003.

Denke, MA: Dietary retinol—a double-edged sword. JAMA 287:102, 2002.

De Jesus, MMM: Cognitive improvement in mild to moderate Alzheimer's dementia after treatment with the acetylcholine precursor choline alfoscerate: A multicenter, double-blind, randomized, placebo-controlled trial. Clin Ther 25:178, 2003.

DeLucia, MC, Mitnick, ME, and Carpenter, TO: Nutritional rickets with normal circulating 25-hydroxyvitamin D: A call for reexamining the role of dietary calcium intake in North American infants. J Clin Endocrinol Metab 88:3539, 2003.

DePaola, DP, Faine, MP, and Palmer, CA: Nutrition in relation to dental medicine. In Shils, ME, et al (eds): Modern Nutrition in Health and Disease, ed 9. Lippincott Williams & Wilkins, Philadelphia, 1999.

Dochterman, J, and Bulechek, G (eds): Nursing Interventions Classification (NIC), ed 4. Mosby, St. Louis, 2004.

Donahue, SP: Recurrence of idiopathic intracranial hypertension after weight loss: The carrot craver. Am J Ophthalmol 130:850, 2000.

Douglas, RM, et al: Vitamin C for preventing and treating the common cold. [Computer software]. The Cochrane Library, Oxford, 2004 issue 4. Abstract accessed through Medline, accession no. PMID: 15495002.

Englehart, MJ, et al: Dietary intake of antioxidants and risk of Alzheimer disease. JAMA 287:3223, 2002.

Ervin, B: Leading dietary supplements used by various sex and age groups in NHANES III. National Center for Health Statistics, Centers for Disease Control and Prevention, U.S. Department of Health and Human Services, 2003. Presented at American Dietetic Association Food and Nutrition Conference and Expo, San Antonio, TX, October 26, 2003.

Feinman, L, and Lieber, CS: Nutrition and diet in alcoholism. In Shils, ME, et al (eds): Modern Nutrition in Health and Disease, ed 9. Lippincott Williams & Wilkins, Philadelphia, 1999.

Feskanich, D, et al: Vitamin A intake and hip fractures among postmenopausal women. JAMA 287:47, 2002.

Fiore, LD, et al: Anaphylactoid reactions to vitamin K. J Thromb Thrombolysis 11:175, 2001.

Fitzpatrick, S, et al: Vitamin D-deficient rickets: A multifactorial disease. Nutr Rev 58:218, 2000.

Fletcher, RH, and Fairfield, KM: Vitamins for chronic disease prevention in adults. JAMA 287:3127, 2002.

Goodrich, RP. The use of riboflavin for the inactivation of pathogens in blood products. Vox Sang 78(Suppl 2):211, 2000.

Gropper, SS, Smith, JL, and Groff, JL: Advanced Nutrition and Human Metabolism, ed 4. Wadsworth, Belmont, CA, 2005.

Guzel, R, et al: Vitamin D status and bone mineral density of veiled and unveiled Turkish women. J Womens Health Gender Based Med 10:765, 2001.

Harrow, JJ, et al: Diagnostic pitfalls: case report of scurvy in a man with spinal cord injury. J Spinal Cord Med 26:163, 2003.

Herbert, V: Folic acid. In Shils, ME, et al (eds): Modern Nutrition in Health and Disease, ed 9. Lippincott Williams & Wilkins, Philadelphia, 1999.

Herman, MJ, and Bulthuis, DB: Incidental diagnosis of nutritional rickets after clavicle fracture. Orthopedics 22:254, 1999.

Holm, G, and Moody, LE: Carpal tunnel syndrome: Current theory, treatment, and the use of B_6. J Am Acad Nurse Pract 15:18, 2003.

Hoshino, M, et al: Ataxia with isolated vitamin E deficiency: A Japanese family carrying a novel mutation in the alpha-tocopherol transfer protein gene. Ann Neurol 45:809, 1999.

Institute of Medicine of the National Academy of Sciences: Dietary Reference Intakes: Vitamins. Washington, DC. Accessed November 5, 2003 at http://www.iom.edu/file.asp?id=7296.

Isaac, S: The "gauntlet" of pellagra. Int J Dermatol 37:599, 1998.

Jacob, RA: Vitamin C. In Shils, ME, et al (eds): Modern Nutrition in Health and Disease, ed 9. Lippincott Williams & Wilkins, Philadelphia, 1999.

Jagadha, V, et al: Wernicke's encephalopathy in patients on peritoneal dialysis or hemodialysis. Ann Neurol 21:78, 1987.

Johnston, CS: Biomarkers for establishing a tolerable upper intake level for vitamin C. Nutr Rev 57:71, 1999.

Johnston, CS, and Bowling, DL: Stability of ascorbic acid in commercially available orange juices. J Am Diet Assoc 102:525, 2002.

Kanai, T, et al: Serum vitamin K level and bone mineral density in post-menopausal women. Int J Gynecol Obstet 56:25, 1997.

Kawasaki, Y, et al: The efficacy of oral vitamin A supplementation for measles and respiratory syncytial virus infection. Kansenshogaku Zasshi 73:104, 1999.

Kertesz, SG: Pellagra in 2 homeless men. Mayo Clin Proc 76:315, 2001.

Kohlmeier, M, et al: Bone health of adult hemodialysis patients is related to vitamin K status. Kidney Int 51:1218, 1997.

Koike, H, et al: Postgastrectomy polyneuropathy with thiamine deficiency. J Neurol Neurosurg Psychiatry 71:357, 2001.

Kowalski, TE, et al: Vitamin A hepatotoxicity: A cautionary note regarding 25,000 IU supplements. Am J Med 97:523, 1994.

Kreiter, SR, et al: Nutritional rickets in African American breast-fed infants. J Pediatr 137:153, 2000.

Kumar, MV, Sunvold, GD, and Scarpace, PJ: Dietary vitamin A supplementation in rats: Suppression of leptin and induction of UCP1 mRNA. J Lipid Res 40:82, 1999.

Lafforgue, P, et al: Bone mineral density in patients given oral vitamin K antagonists. Rev Rhum Engl Ed 64:249, 1997.

Lamb, E: Vitamin D deficiency presenting acutely in an infant [letter]. BMJ January 30, 1999. Accessed September 15, 1999 at http://www.bmj.com/cgi/eletters/318/7175/39.

Lane, LA, and Rojas-Fernandez, C: Treatment of vitamin B_{12} deficiency anemia: Oral versus parenteral therapy. Ann Pharmacother 36:1268, 2002.

Lawson, M, and Thomas, M: Vitamin D concentrations in Asian children aged 2 years living in England: Population survey. BMJ 318:28, 1999.

Leklem, JE: Vitamin B_6. In Shils, ME, et al (eds): Modern Nutrition in Health and Disease, ed 9. Lippincott Williams & Wilkins, Philadelphia, 1999.

Lerner, V, and Kanevsky, M: Acute dementia with delirium due to vitamin B_{12} deficiency: A case report. Int J Psychiatry Med 32: 215, 2002.

Lerner, V, et al: Vitamin B_6 in the treatment of tardive dyskinesia: A double-blind, placebo-controlled, crossover study. Am J Psychiatry 158:1511, 2001.

Levin, NA, and Greer, KE: Scurvy in an unrepentant carnivore. Cutis 66:39, 2000.

Levine, M, et al: Criteria and recommendations for vitamin C intake. JAMA 281:1415, 1999.

Levine, M, et al: Vitamin C pharmacokinetics in healthy volunteers: Evidence for a recommended dietary allowance. Proc Nat Acad Sci USA 93:3704, 1996.

Lindenbaum, J, et al: Neuropsychiatric disorders caused by cobalamin deficiency in the absence of anemia or macrocytosis. N Engl J Med 318:1720, 1988.

Linton, CR, et al: Using thiamine to reduce post-ECT confusion. Int J Geriatr Psychiatry 17:189, 2002.

Linus Pauling Institute: Choline. Accessed November 5, 2003 at http://lpi.oregonstate.edu/infocenter/othernuts/choline.

Liu, RH: Health benefits of fruit and vegetables are from additive and synergistic combinations of phytochemicals. Am J Clin Nutr 78:517S, 2003.

Luchsinger, JA, et al: Antioxidant vitamin intake and risk of Alzheimer disease. Arch Neurol 60:203, 2003.

Maizels, M, Blumenfeld, A, and Burchette, R: A combination of riboflavin, magnesium, and feverfew for migraine prophylaxis: a randomized trial. Headache 44:885, 2004.

McLaren, DS: Clinical manifestations of human vitamin and mineral disorders: A resume. In Shils, ME, et al (eds): Modern Nutrition in Health and Disease, ed 9. Lippincott Williams & Wilkins, Philadelphia, 1999.

McLaren, DS, and Frigg, M: Sight and Life Manual on Vitamin A Deficiency Disorders (VADD), ed 2. Sight and Life, Basel, Switzerland, 2001.

Meydani, M, and Hayes, KC: Vitamin E. American Society for Nutritional Sciences. Accessed October 7, 2003 at http://www.nutrition.org/nutinfo/content/vie.shtml.

Michaelsson, K: Serum retinol levels and the risk of fracture. N Engl J Med 348:287, 2003.

Miksad, R, et al: Hepatic hydrothorax associated with vitamin A toxicity. J Clin Gastroenterol 34:275, 2002.

Milea, D, Cassoux, N, and LeHoang, P: Blindness in a strict vegan [letter]. N Engl J Med 342:897, 2000.

Mills, JL, et al: Low vitamin B_{12} concentrations in patients without anemia: The effect of folic acid fortification of grain. Am J Clin Nutr 77:1474, 2003.

Mock, DM: Biotin. In Shils, ME, et al (eds): Modern Nutrition in Health and Disease, ed 9. Lippincott Williams & Wilkins, Philadelphia, 1999.

Moeller, SM, Jacques, PF, and Blumberg, JB: The potential role of dietary xanthophylis in cataract and age-related macular degeneration. J Am Coll Nutr 19:522S, 2000.

Moorhead, S, Johnson, M, and Maas, M (eds): Nursing Outcomes Classification (NOC), ed 3. Mosby, St. Louis, 2004.

Morris, CD, and Carson S: Routine vitamin supplementation to prevent cardiovascular disease: A summary of the evidence for the U.S. Preventive Services Task Force. Ann Intern Med 139:56, 2003.

Morse, JW, Morse, SJ, and Patterson, J: Niacin reaction: Common vitamin, uncommon ED diagnosis. Am J Emerg Med 17:320, 1999.

Mughal, MZ, et al: Florid rickets associated with prolonged breast feeding without vitamin D supplementation. BMJ 318:39, 1999. Accessed September 15, 1999 at http://www.bmj.com/cgi/content/full/318/7175/39.

Muhlendahl, KE, and Nawracala, J: Vitamin D intoxication. Eur J Pediatr 158:266, 1999.

NANDA International: Nursing Diagnoses: Definitions and Classification 2003–2004. NANDA International, Philadelphia, 2003.

National Academy of Sciences: Dietary Reference Intakes for Vitamin A, Vitamin K, Arsenic, Boron, Chromium, Copper, Iodine, Iron, Manganese, Molybdenum, Nickel, Silicone, Vanadium, and Zinc. National Academy Press, Washington, D.C., 2000. Nutrition Data: Fifty foods highest in vitamin B_6. Accessed November 2, 2003 at http://www.nutritiondata.com.

Nyholm, E, et al: Oral vitamin B_{12} can change our practice. Postgrad Med J 79:218, 2003.

Oh, RC, and Brown, DL: Vitamin B_{12} deficiency. Am Fam Physician 67:979, 2003.

Ohkoshi, N, Ishii, A, and Shoji, S: Wernicke's encephalopathy induced by hyperemesis gravidarum, associated with bilateral caudate lesions on computed tomography and magnetic resonance imaging. Eur Neurol 34:177, 1994.

Olmedilla, B, et al: Lutein, but not alpha-tocopherol, supplementation improves visual function in patient with age-related cataracts: A 2-y double-blind, placebo-controlled pilot study. Nutrition 19:21, 2003.

Olson, RE: Vitamin K. In Shils, ME, et al (eds): Modern Nutrition in Health and Disease, ed 9. Lippincott Williams & Wilkins, Philadelphia, 1999.

Outila, TA, et al: Dietary intake of vitamin D in premenopausal, healthy vegans was insufficient to maintain concentrations of serum 25-hydroxyvitamin D and intact parathyroid hormone within normal ranges during the winter in Finland. J Am Diet Assoc 100:434, 2000.

Ozturk, F, et al: Pellagra: A sporadic pediatric case with a full triad of symptoms. Cutis 68:31, 2001.

Pacheco-Alvarez, D, Solorzano-Vargas, RS, and Del Rio, AL: Biotin in metabolism and its relationship to human disease. Arch Med Res 33:439, 2002.

Pangan, AL, and Robinson, D: Hemarthrosis as initial presentation of scurvy. J Rheumatol 28:1923, 2001.

Panozzo, G, Babighian, S, and Bonora, A: Association of xerophthalmia, flecked retina, and pseudotumor cerebri caused by hypovitaminosis A. Am J Ophthalmol 125:708, 1998.

Plesofsky-Vig, N: Pantothenic acid. In Shils, ME, et al (eds): Modern Nutrition in Health and Disease, ed 9. Lippincott Williams & Wilkins, Philadelphia, 1999.

Preston, AM, et al: Influence of environmental tobacco smoke on vitamin C status in children. Am J Clin Nutr 77:167, 2003.

Pugliese, MT, et al: Nutritional rickets in suburbia. J Am Coll Nutr 17:637, 1998.

Puri, et al: The niacin skin flush test in schizophrenia: A replication study. Int J Clin Pract 55:368, 2001.

Purvin, V: Through a shade darkly. Surv Ophthalmol 43:335, 1999.

Reznikoff-Etievant, MF, et al: Low vitamin B_{12} level as a risk factor for very early recurrent abortion. Eur J Obstet Gynecol Reprod Biol 104:156, 2002.

Ribot, J, et al: Changes of adiposity in response to vitamin A status correlate with changes of PPAR gamma 2 expression. Obes Res 9:500, 2001.

Roman, GC: An epidemic in Cuba of optic neuropathy, sensorineural deafness, peripheral sensory neuropathy and dorsolateral myeloneuropathy. J Neurol Sci 127:11, 1994.

Ross, AC: Vitamin A and retinoids. In Shils, ME, et al (eds): Modern Nutrition in Health and Disease, ed 9. Lippincott Williams & Wilkins, Philadelphia, 1999.

Ross, DA: Recommendations for vitamin A supplementation. J Nutr 132:2902S, 2002.

Said, HM: Cellular uptake of biotin: Mechanisms and regulation. J Nutr 129(2S Suppl):490S, 1999.

Schoenen, J, Jacquy, J, and Lenaerts, M: Effectiveness of high-dose riboflavin in migraine prophylaxis. Neurology 50:466, 1998.

Schuelke, M, et al: Treatment of ataxia in isolated vitamin E deficiency caused by alpha-tocopherol transfer protein deficiency. J Pediatr 134:240, 1999.

Shah, M, et al: Nutritional rickets still afflict children in north Texas. Tex Med 96:64, 2000.

Sight and Life: Manual and Newsletters obtained from sightandlife.org on CD, September 2003.

Smesny, S, et al: Potential use of the topical niacin skin test in early psychosis—a combined approach using optical reflection spectroscopy and a descriptive rating scale. J Psychiatr Res 37:237, 2003.

Sommer, A, and Davidson, FR: Assessment and control of vitamin A deficiency: The Annecy Accords. J Nutr 132:2945S, 2002.

Stephen, R, and Utecht, T: Scurvy identified in the emergency department: A case report. J Emerg Med 21:235, 2001.

Tamura, Y, et al: Scurvy presenting as painful gait with bruising in a young boy. Arch Pediatr Adolesc Med 7:732, 2000.

Tanphaichitr, V: Thiamin. In Shils, ME, et al (eds): Modern Nutrition in Health and Disease, ed 9. Lippincott Williams & Wilkins, Philadelphia, 1999.

Taylor, A, et al: Long-term intake of vitamins and carotenoids and odds of early age-related cortical and posterior subcapsular lens opacities. Am J Clin Nutr 75:540, 2002.

Thomas, MK, et al: Hypovitaminosis D in medical patients. N Engl J Med 338:777, 1998.

Traber, MG. Vitamin E. In Shils, ME, et al (eds): Modern Nutrition in Health and Disease, ed 9. Lippincott Williams & Wilkins, Philadelphia, 1999.

U.S. Preventive Services Task Force: Vitamin Supplementation to Prevent Cancer and Cardiovascular Disease. Agency for Health-care Research and Quality, Rockville, MD, 2003. Accessed November 3, 2003 at http://www.ahrq.gov/clinic/uspstf/uspsvita.htm.

van der Wielen, RPJ, et al: Serum vitamin D concentrations among elderly people in Europe. Lancet 346:207, 1995.

Weinstein, M, Babyn, P, and Zlotkin, S: An orange a day keeps the doctor away: Scurvy in the year 2000. Pediatrics 108:E55, 2001.

Weir, DG, and Scott, JM: Vitamin B_{12} "Cobalamin." In Shils, ME, et al (eds): Modern Nutrition in Health and Disease, ed 9. Lippincott Williams & Wilkins, Philadelphia, 1999.

Wiafe, B: Food and Eyes—are they related? Sight and Life Newsletter 4:20, 1999. Manual and Newsletters obtained on CD from sightandlife.org, September 2003.

Wood, B, and Currie, J: Presentation of acute Wernicke's encephalopathy and treatment with thiamin. Metab Brain Dis 10:57, 1995.

Workshop on Folate, B_{12}, and Choline. Nutrition 15:92, 1999.

Xiao, G, et al: Ascorbic acid-dependent activation of the osteocalcin promoter in MC3T3-E1 proosteoblasts: Requirement for collagen matrix synthesis and the presence of an intact OSE2 sequence. Mol Endocrinol 11:1103, 1997. Accessed August 5, 1999 at http://endo.edoc.com/mend/v11n8/1103-abs.html

Zeisel, SH: Choline and phosphatidylcholine. In Shils, ME, et al (eds): Modern Nutrition in Health and Disease, ed 9. Lippincott Williams & Wilkins, Philadelphia, 1999.

Zempleni, J, and Mock, DM: Bioavailability of biotin given orally to humans in pharmacologic doses. Am J Clin Nutr 69:504, 1999.

Zhang, SM, et al: Intakes of vitamins E and C, carotenoids, vitamin supplements, and PD risk. Neurology 59:1161, 2002.

Minerals

After completing this chapter, the student should be able to:

1. Compare and contrast minerals and vitamins.
2. Describe one or more functions of the main nutritive minerals.
3. List at least two food sources for each mineral and identify any nonfood sources.
4. Identify individuals at increased risk for mineral deficiencies.
5. Devise strategies to increase clients' calcium or iron intakes.

In a broad sense, minerals are obtained from the earth's crust. Through the effects of the weather, rocks that contain minerals are ground into smaller particles, which then become part of the soil. Growing plants absorb the minerals from the soil. Animals eat the plants, and humans eat both the plants and the animals. In this way, minerals become part of the food chain.

Minerals in Human Nutrition

Minerals make vital contributions to the growth and maintenance of health in the body. This chapter covers the minerals important in human nutrition and the role each plays in the body. It describes some of the general functions of minerals and explains how minerals are classified in nutrition. It details the nutritional implications of the 7 major and 10 trace minerals. A note on the use of mineral supplements concludes the chapter.

Functions of Minerals

Like vitamins, minerals help to regulate bodily functions without providing energy and are essential to good health. Minerals differ from vitamins in two ways: minerals are inorganic substances, and minerals become part of the composition of the body. Minerals represent 4 percent of total body weight.

Minerals become part of the body's structure and part of the body's enzymes. For instance, calcium and phosphorus combine to give bones and teeth their hardness. Iron becomes attached to the protein globin to form hemoglobin. Iodine becomes part of the thyroid hormones.

Most minerals serve a variety of functions in the body's regulatory and metabolic processes. Sodium is essential for maintaining fluid balance. Sodium, potassium, and calcium have critical functions in nerve and muscle activity. Potassium and phosphorus play significant roles in acid-base balance. A disruption of the body's balance of any one of these minerals, albeit not necessarily caused by diet, can be life threatening.

Classification of Minerals

In nutrition, two groups of minerals exist: major and trace. **Major minerals,** also called macrominerals, are present in the body in quantities greater than 5 grams (approximately 1 teaspoonful). The body needs a daily intake of 100 milligrams (approximately 1/50 teaspoonful) or more of each of the major minerals.

Trace minerals, often called microminerals or trace elements, are present in the body in amounts of less than 5 grams. Humans need a daily intake of less than 100 milligrams of each of the trace minerals. The term *trace* does not mean unimportant. Trace minerals make vital and often unique contributions to the body's functioning.

Major Minerals

The seven major minerals include calcium, sodium, and potassium, which are familiar to many people in a dietary context. The other four major minerals are phosphorus, magnesium, sulfur, and chloride.

Calcium

The body of a 150-pound adult contains approximately 3 pounds of calcium. Ninety-nine percent of this amount is in the bones and teeth. The remaining 1 percent of the calcium circulates in the body fluids. Of this 1 percent, one-quarter to one-half is bound to plasma proteins, while the rest travels as ions, free particles that carry an electrical charge (see Chapter 9). The ionized calcium moves freely from one fluid compartment to another and serves several important functions in the body.

Functions of Calcium

Calcium, with phosphorus, forms the hard substance of bones and teeth. Ample calcium and phosphorus alone will not guarantee strong bones and teeth, however. Vitamin D is necessary for calcium absorption. Exercise, particularly weight-bearing exercise, is also essential for strong bones. Very little calcium is deposited in fully formed teeth. Consequently, if calcium is lost from the teeth, it cannot be replaced. This is the reason dental cavities or caries need restoration.

Maximum accumulation of calcium in the bones occurs during the pubertal growth spurt, during which time bone mass increases 7 to 8 percent per year. The body's peak bone mass is achieved shortly after adult height is reached. Total body bone mass remains fairly constant through the reproductive years, although various sites, such as the skull and the shaft of the femur, continue to add bone throughout life (Weaver and Heaney, 1999), but the balance is upset in the aging adult, and with age, total body bone mass decreases. Age-related bone loss is most marked in postmenopausal women but also occurs in men.

Calcium also performs several vital metabolic functions in the nervous, muscular, and cardiovascular systems.

1. Calcium assists in manufacturing **acetylcholine,** a neurotransmitter (a chemical that enhances transmission of nerve impulses).
2. Calcium acts as a catalyst in initiating and controlling muscle contraction and relaxation. At the beginning of a muscle contraction, calcium is released from its storage area inside the muscle cell. At the end of a contraction, the calcium is again gathered into its storage area.
3. Calcium is a catalyst in the clotting process: it aids in the conversion of platelets to thromboplastin and in the conversion of **fibrinogen** to **fibrin.**
4. Calcium controls the passage of substances across cell membranes by affecting membrane permeability.
5. Calcium activates certain enzymes, such as **pancreatic lipase,** and is necessary for absorption of vitamin B_{12}.

Control Mechanisms for Calcium

Although it may seem to be a permanent substance, bone is 2 to 5 percent living cells that are constantly undergoing change. Bone is the body's bank account or storage area for calcium. As much as 700 milligrams of calcium is moved in and out of the bones each day. The bone calcium pool turns over every 10 to 12 years on average, but this turnover does not occur in the teeth (Weaver and Heaney, 1999). One reason for the changes in bone composition is to maintain the adult serum calcium concentration within the normal limits of 9 to 11 milligrams per 100 milliliters of serum. Another reason for the movement of calcium in and out of the bones is to renew the bone tissue. In this process, bone cells called **osteoclasts** produce enzymes to destroy the protein matrix that holds the calcium phosphate in place. Other bone cells, called **osteoblasts** produce new matrix protein, which chemically attracts calcium and other nutrients to rebuild the bone.

Several hormones work together to accomplish these activities. Vitamin D is one of these hormones. Parathyroid hormone and calcitonin are the other two. Vitamin D is actually a hormone because it regulates tissue functions. It increases calcium absorption by the small intestine and increases calcium deposition in the bones and teeth.

Tiny glands behind the thyroid gland in the neck secrete **parathyroid hormone.** When the serum calcium level falls, the parathyroid glands secrete the hormone, which increases the withdrawal of calcium from the bone, thereby raising the serum calcium level. Additionally, parathyroid hormone increases the serum calcium level by stimulating the kidneys to return more calcium to the bloodstream instead of excreting it in the urine and by increasing the production of the active form of vitamin D, calcitriol.

To balance the action of parathyroid hormone, the thyroid gland secretes another hormone, **calcitonin,** when the serum calcium level is high. It inhibits the release of calcium from bone by the osteoclasts. Figure 8–1 illustrates the complementary actions of parathyroid hormone and calcitonin.

Other hormones affect the body's use of calcium. One prominent one is estrogen. Its exact mechanism of action in bone metabolism is unknown, but research is continuing in efforts to explain the dramatic loss of bone structure after menopause. Evidence suggests that normal women's bone resorption increases when estradiol levels are low during the menstrual cycle so that fluctuating rates of bone resorption occur from menarche to menopause (Chiu et al, 1999). One mechanism proposed for the action of estrogen on bone metabolism is that estrogen suppresses inflammatory cytokines that promote production of osteoclasts. Thus, when estrogen levels fall during menopause, the cytokines are more active, permitting greater numbers of osteoclasts to be synthesized (Sunyer et al, 1999).

Dietary Reference Intakes for Calcium

The Adequate Intake (AI) for calcium for adults aged 19 to 50 years is 1000 milligrams. For those older than 50, the amount is 1200 milligrams. The UL is 2500 milligrams. Unfortunately, the average intake for all adults is below the AI amounts. Men 19 to 50 years old have an average intake of 939 milligrams, and those over 50 years of age have an average intake of 778 milligrams. Women 19 to 50 years old consume just 665 milligrams of calcium on average, and those over 50 years of age consume 606 milligrams (U.S. Department of Agriculture, 2000).

Even with the bones as a reservoir, daily intake of calcium is important. Calcium can be obtained from animal or vegetable sources, but calcium from animal sources is more readily absorbed.

Sources of Calcium

ANIMAL SOURCES. Milk and milk products are the best animal sources of calcium, followed by sardines, clams, oysters, and salmon. In milk, calcium is combined with

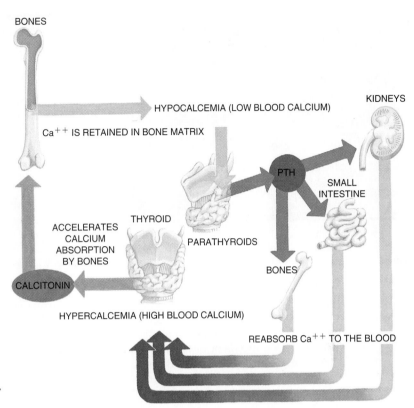

Figure **8–1** Parathyroid hormone raises serum calcium levels when they are too low. Calcitonin from the thyroid gland lowers serum calcium levels when they are too high. (Reprinted from Venes, D [ed]: Taber's Cyclopedic Medical Dictionary, ed 19. FA Davis, Philadelphia, 2001, p 304, with permission.)

lactose, which increases absorption. Even so, only 28 percent of the available calcium in milk is absorbed. Another advantageous component of milk is the protein the osteoblasts need to rebuild the bone matrix. In sum, milk is such an important source of calcium that it is virtually impossible to obtain adequate calcium without milk or dairy products. Figure 8–2 shows a child drinking milk with a "fast food" meal.

Table 8–1 lists the quantity of foods containing approximately 300 milligrams of calcium, the amount in 1 cup of milk. "Bargain" foods listed that are high in calcium but low in kilocalories include skim milk and plain yogurt. The most expensive sources of calcium, considering kilocalories, are ice cream, large-curd, creamed cottage cheese, and sherbet. Table 8–1 reveals that not all dairy products are equally beneficial as sources of calcium, but this is not a call to abandon all fat intake. Consuming some fat with calcium increases the absorption of the mineral by slowing peristalsis.

Obtaining calcium from supplements is less desirable than obtaining it from foods. Milk products supply other nutrients, such as vitamin D and lactose, which assist in calcium absorption. Milk is also a major source of riboflavin and protein. Figure 8–3 shows the percentages of the AIs or RDAs for vitamins A and D, protein, thiamin, and riboflavin an adult woman could obtain from 3 cups of skim milk. Clinical Application 8–1 describes some of the contaminants in "natural" calcium supplements.

PLANT SOURCES. Good plant sources of calcium include rhubarb, spinach, greens (turnip, beet), broccoli,

kale, tofu, and legumes. In all cases, vegetables yield more calcium when cooked. Some experts question how much the body is actually able to absorb owing to multiple interfering factors.

Another good plant source is calcium-fortified orange juice (Martini and Wood, 2002). An unusual source of

Table 8–1 Quantities of Food Containing Approximately 300 Milligrams of Calcium, Equal to One Cup of Milk, in Order of Energy Content

FOOD	AMOUNT	KILOCALORIES
Skim milk	1.0 cup	86
Grated Parmesan cheese	4.3 tbsp	99
Plain low-fat yogurt	0.7 cup	101
Swiss cheese	1.1 oz	118
2 percent milk	1.0 cup	121
Whole milk	1.0 cup	150
Cheddar cheese	1.5 oz	171
Processed American cheese	1.7 oz	180
Low-fat yogurt with fruit	0.9 cup	199
Blue cheese	2.0 oz	200
Vanilla milkshake	0.9 cup	273
Cottage cheese, 2 percent low-fat	2.0 cups	410
Hard ice cream, vanilla	1.7 cups	459
Soft ice cream	1.3 cups	479
Cottage cheese, creamed, large curd	2.25 cups	529
Sherbet	2.9 cups	786

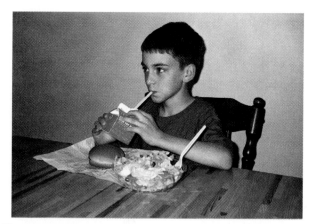

Figure **8–2** This child has a balanced meal from a fast food restaurant: a small hamburger, a salad, and milk. Growing bones and teeth need calcium from milk products.

Contents of Natural Calcium Supplements

Shells, bones and dolomite are natural sources of calcium that are used as dietary supplements. Much of the calcium found in shells and bones is in the form of calcium phosphate, one of the most difficult calcium compounds to absorb. In addition, shells and bones often contain excessive amounts of mercury and lead (Ross, Szabo, and Tebbett, 2000; Scelfo and Flegal, 2000).

Dolomite is a limestone that is rich in both calcium and magnesium. It also may contain lead, mercury, arsenic, and aluminum. Because of the possibility of contamination, it is best to obtain calcium from food sources whenever possible. When this is not possible, pharmaceutical products are preferable to natural supplements.

calcium for Navajo Americans is the ash derived from the branches and needles of the juniper tree. The ash is used to flavor various foods, such as cornmeal mush and pancakes and Navajo tea. One teaspoon of the ash supplies roughly the calcium in one glass of milk (Christensen et al, 1998). This is an example of the contribution of traditional food selection and processing to health.

Absorption and Excretion

Calcium is absorbed throughout the small intestine, especially the ileum. Growing children absorb up to 75 percent of dietary calcium, compared to 30 percent absorbed by adults (Gropper, Smith, and Groff, 2005). In general, the percentage of available calcium absorbed from vegetables is considerably less than that absorbed from milk. For example, only 5 percent of the total calcium found in spinach is absorbed. Several factors can interfere with the absorption and retention of calcium: oxalates, phytic acid,

and excessive intakes of protein, dietary fiber, and magnesium (see Table 8–2).

Some plants contain salts of oxalic acid called **oxalates** that bind with the calcium present in the vegetable to produce calcium oxalate, an insoluble substance that is excreted in the feces. The calcium content not bound to oxalates is available for absorption, however, and oxalates do not interfere with the absorption of calcium from other foods. Chard, spinach, beet leaves, rhubarb, cranberries, and gooseberries all contain oxalic acid. Unusually high intake of these foods may cause oxalic acid poisoning (see Clinical Application 8–2).

Cereals contain a substance that forms an insoluble complex with calcium. This interfering substance is **phytic acid,** the storage form of phosphorus in seeds. Foods with heavy concentrations of phytate, such as legumes, nuts, and cereals, reduce calcium absorption significantly. For other plants rich in calcium, such as broccoli and cabbage, the calcium is as easily absorbed as that in milk. The difficulty becomes the volume necessary to absorb the quantity of calcium equal to that in a glass of milk: 2.3 servings of cabbage or 4.5 servings of broccoli (Weaver and Heaney, 1999).

The overall effect of oxalic and phytic acids on calcium availability in most diets usually is not significant. People who avoid dairy products, however, need careful attention to meal planning. Ovovegetarian and vegan clients should

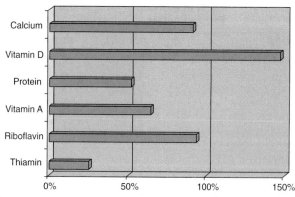

Figure **8–3** Milk supplies many nutrients in addition to calcium. Three cups of skim milk provide a woman between 25 and 50 years of age with 91 percent of her AI for calcium, 147 percent of her AI for vitamin D, 52 percent of her RDA for protein, 64 percent of her RDA for vitamin A, 93 percent of her RDA for riboflavin, and 25 percent of her RDA for thiamin. The kilocaloric cost for all of these nutrients is a miniscule 258 kilocalories.

Table **8–2** **Factors Affecting Calcium Absorption and Excretion**

INCREASE ABSORPTION	DECREASE ABSORPTION	INCREASE EXCRETION
Acidity	Alkalinity	Excessive animal protein
Estrogen	Caffeine	Excessive sodium
Lactose or sucrose	Excessive magnesium or zinc	Caffeine
Protein	Insoluble dietary fiber	
Vitamin D	Oxalic acid	
	Phytic acid	
	Vitamin D deficiency	

Oxalic Acid Poisoning

It is possible to be poisoned by ingesting too much of one or more foods that contain oxalic acid. Cranberries, gooseberries, chard, spinach, beet leaves, and rhubarb are high in oxalic acid. For example, one normal serving of rhubarb contains one-fifth the toxic dose. Rhubarb leaves contain three or four times as much as the stalks. Ingesting a fairly small amount of leaf can poison a child.

One way to minimize the chance of oxalic acid poisoning is to consume foods that contain calcium with foods high in oxalic acid. The calcium combines with the oxalate, which then passes through the intestine harmlessly. Calcium absorption will be decreased, however.

be instructed to seek calcium-fortified products, such as orange juice and calcium-set tofu, to bolster their intake of the mineral.

Adequate protein intake facilitates calcium absorption through the production of an insulin-like growth factor that promotes osteoblast bone formation, but excessive intake of protein increases urinary loss of calcium. Increasing calcium intake may offset the urinary losses (Dawson-Hughes, 2003), and the negative effects of protein are seen mainly at low calcium intakes (Heaney, 2000). In contrast, higher protein intake was favorably associated with increased bone mineral density in individuals supplemented with calcium and vitamin D (Dawson-Hughes and Harris, 2002). Moreover, when protein is accompanied by a high phosphorus intake, the calcium loss is lessened considerably. Fortunately, in the American diet, foods high in protein usually are also high in phosphorus. The possibility of influencing bone health by reducing the impact of the acid load from protein foods via generous consumption of fruits and vegetables requires further investigation (New, 2003b). See section on potassium.

Calcium absorption is hindered by excessive intake of insoluble dietary fiber. It passes through the alimentary canal undigested and speeds the contents through the intestine, thus decreasing the time available for calcium absorption.

Because calcium and other minerals use the same absorption mechanism, excessive intake can impair the absorption of calcium, especially in situations where calcium intake is low. Two such minerals are magnesium and zinc (Gropper, Smith, and Groff, 2005).

Two substances interfering with calcium retention in the body are sodium and caffeine. For every 500-milligram increase in sodium intake, an additional 10 milligrams of calcium is spilled in the urine (Krall and Dawson-Hughes, 1999), which is a small amount compared to the RDA. A direct effect of high sodium intake on bone loss at the hip has been demonstrated (Lau and Woo, 1998), but other experts state that higher urinary calcium occurs in response to salt only in a minority of individuals (Cohen and Roe, 2000).

Caffeine has a clear but small depressant effect on intestinal absorption of calcium (Heaney, 2002) as well as a stimulating effect on excretion via the urine and feces (Gropper, Smith, and Groff, 2005) that may become important when caffeinated beverages replace milk in the diet. The caffeine equal to 2 to 3 cups of coffee accelerated bone loss from the spine and total body in postmenopausal women who consumed less than 744 milligrams of calcium per day (Weaver and Heaney, 1999). Therefore, it seems probable that if a person's calcium intake is low or marginal, drinking many caffeinated beverages could make a difference in bone health.

Gastric acidity increases the solubility of calcium salts. Calcium supplements taken with a meal are better absorbed than when taken without food, possibly due to delayed emptying time of the stomach (Weaver and Heaney, 1999).

Calcium Deficiencies

Calcium deficiency in children can contribute to poor bone and tooth development. Rickets is more directly related to vitamin D deficiency than calcium deficiency except in premature infants, whose skeletons still need much added mineral. Two other conditions related to calcium balance are osteoporosis and tetany.

OSTEOPOROSIS. According to the World Health Organization, **osteopenia** is bone mineral density 1 to 2.5 standard deviations below the mean of healthy young adults, whereas **osteoporosis** is bone mineral density greater than 2.5 standard deviations below the mean. Osteoporosis permits minimal trauma to cause fractures. Sites commonly affected are the hip, wrist, and vertebrae.

Two major factors in the development of osteoporosis are the bone mass developed from birth to age 30 and rate of loss of bone mass in later life. Usually osteoporosis is caused by several genes and their interaction with the environment, including nutritional and other lifestyle factors. Identifying genetic causes may aid in assessment of fracture risk and individualizing drug treatment (Albagha and Ralston, 2003).

Osteoporosis is most common in postmenopausal, fair-complexioned white women. A woman loses 2 to 5 percent of bone tissue per year immediately before and for about 8 years after menopause. The most rapid loss of bone occurs in the first 5 years after menopause. Intuitively, then, treatment with estrogen might be beneficial, but a trial of estrogen plus progestin was stopped early because overall health risks exceeded benefits (Rossouw et al, 2002), and Follin and Hansen state that estrogen should not be used for the sole purpose of osteoporosis prevention (2003). Men and black women lose bone mass also, but because their skeletons are generally heavier, they are at lower risk of osteoporosis. Blacks have higher bone mineral density than whites and Asians, a difference that is noted beginning in early childhood (Krall and Dawson-Hughes, 1999). Figure 8–4 shows a sketch of normal and osteoporotic cancellous bone. Lacking a direct test of bone strength, clinicians use bone mineral density as a surrogate measure accounting for about 70 percent of bone strength (NIH Consensus Development Panel, 2001). Figure 8–5 shows an x-ray of a normal bone and an x-ray of an osteoporotic bone. Dual-energy x-ray absorptiometry (DEXA) is the

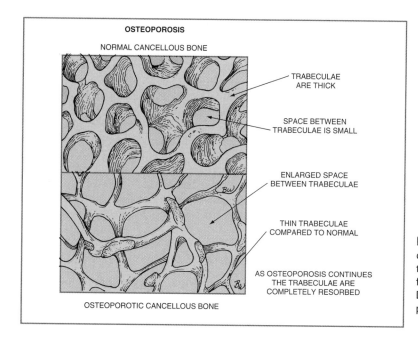

OSTEOPOROSIS

NORMAL CANCELLOUS BONE

TRABECULAE ARE THICK

SPACE BETWEEN TRABECULAE IS SMALL

ENLARGED SPACE BETWEEN TRABECULAE

THIN TRABECULAE COMPARED TO NORMAL

AS OSTEOPOROSIS CONTINUES THE TRABECULAE ARE COMPLETELY RESORBED

OSTEOPOROTIC CANCELLOUS BONE

Figure **8–4** Sketch of normal and osteoporotic cancellous bone showing enlarged spaces and thinner bony structure in the latter. (Reprinted from Venes, D [ed]: Taber's Cyclopedic Medical Dictionary, ed 19. FA Davis, Philadelphia, 2001, p 1469, with permission.)

best predictor of fractures, but ultrasonography is often used as a screening device. Two tools to identify candidates for screening are available at the University of Washington's OsteoEd Web site at http://www.osteoed.org/faq/screening/orai.html and http://www.osteoed.org/tools/tools_score.html. (Clinical Application 8–3 outlines recommendations for diagnosis and treatment of osteoporosis.)

Additional lifestyle factors impacting bone include smoking and alcohol consumption. Smokers absorbed less calcium than nonsmokers (Need, 2002). Current smokers had lower bone mineral density (BMD) in hips and total body (Gerdhem and Obrant, 2002) and a higher prevalence of vertebral deformities after adjustment for age and body weight than never-smokers (Szulc et al, 2002). Smoking had a dose-response effect on ankle fractures so that smoking more than 20 cigarettes per day nearly tripled the risk (Valtola et al, 2002). Alcohol consumption has been reported to have varying effects on bone health. Alcohol has been shown to reduce bone formation in healthy humans and to produce low bone mass, decreased bone formation rate, and increased fracture incidence in individuals who abuse alcohol. Chronic alcohol abuse is detrimental to men's skeletons, but light to moderate drinking has been associated with neutral or positive effects on women's bone health (Turner, 2000), possibly caused by changes in calcitonin and estrogen balance (New, 2003a). In men with chronic alcoholism, osteopenia was mainly attributed to malnutrition (Santolaria et al, 2000).

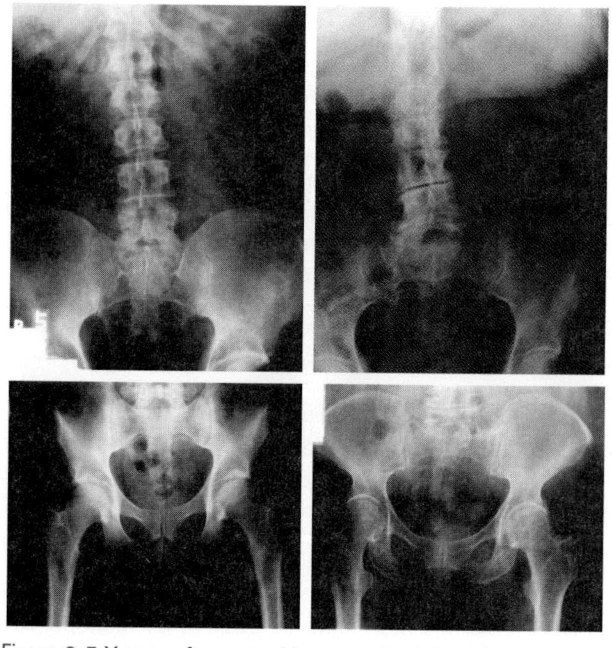

Certain minor risk factors for osteoporosis (alcohol, caffeine, fiber, high protein intake unopposed by adequate fruits and vegetables, phytic acid-containing and oxalic acid-containing foods, sodium, and smoking), although not considered in the protocol described in Clinical Application 8–3, when combined, and especially when coupled with low calcium and vitamin D intake, might make a difference in bone health for an individual. Because of the complexity of osteoporosis, no single intervention, whether pharmacologic or nutritional, can be reasonably expected to solve the problem (Heaney, 2000).

TETANY. Despite the hormonal control of serum calcium and the large reservoir in the bones, serum calcium sometimes falls below normal. An actual lack of calcium or a lack of ionized calcium may cause tetany. A serum calcium level that is too low is called **hypocalcemia.** If the signs and symptoms described here appear, the condition is called **tetany.** Causes include parathyroid deficiency, vitamin D deficiency, and alkalosis.

Parathyroid deficiency has been caused by accidental removal of the parathyroid glands during thyroidectomy

Figure **8–5** X-rays of a normal bone on the left and an osteoporotic bone on the right. (Courtesy of Dr. Russell Tobe.)

Clinical Application 8-3

Osteoporosis Prevalence, Diagnosis, and Treatment

Prevalence:

- An estimated 10 million people in the United States, 80 percent of them women, have osteoporosis, the major factor in fractures in the elderly.
- Annually in the United States, osteoporotic fractures occur at the hip (300,000), at the spine (700,000), or at the forearm (250,000), totaling approximately $17 billion in direct costs (National Osteoporosis Foundation, 2003).
- One-half of postmenopausal women will have an osteoporosis-related fracture in their lifetimes, including 25 percent who will develop vertebral deformities and 15 percent who will fracture a hip.
- By age 80, when bone mineral density is measured at hip, spine, and wrist, 70 percent of white women have osteoporosis in at least one site (U.S. Preventive Services Task Force, 2002).

Diagnosis:

- Assessment of risk factors: female sex, increased age, estrogen deficiency, white race, low weight and body mass index (BMI), family history of fractures, long-term use of drugs affecting bone, such as anticonvulsants or corticosteroids
- Personal history of fracture after age 45. Forearm fractures are "sentinel events" that should trigger assessment for osteoporosis but frequently do not (Cuddihy et al, 2002).
- History and physical examination including assessment for height loss and posture changes

- Measurement of bone mineral density (BMD) if post menopause. Until 30 to 40 percent of bone mass is lost, it is not detectable on x-ray (Figure 8–5), but dual-energy x-ray absorptiometry (DEXA) permits earlier diagnosis.

Treatment:

- Adequate nutrition, including vitamin D and calcium at RDA and AI levels. Calcium via food is primary, and supplements should be absorbable and carry the U.S. Pharmacopoeia designation (NIH Consensus Development Panel, 2001).
- Exercise. Weight training stimulates skeletal accrual of bone mineral. Walking has minimal effect on BMD, but improvement in balance and other areas is beneficial (NIH Consensus Development Panel, 2001). Among women who did no other exercise, however, walking for at least 4 hours per week was associated with a 41 percent lower risk of hip fracture compared with walking for less than 1 hour per week (Feskanich, Willett, and Colditz, 2002).
- Medications. In cases marked by increased osteoclastic resorption, calcitonin or bisphosphonates (to suppress osteoclast formation or activity) may be helpful. In cases with decreased osteoblastic activity, selective estrogen receptor modulators (SERMs), fluoride, or parathyroid hormone may be prescribed (Davidson, 2003). Natural estrogens, especially plant-derived phytoestrogens, have shown no reduction in fracture risk in humans (NIH Consensus Development Panel, 2001).

---

but more often is caused by edema following thyroid surgery or by disease of the gland. One recent study reported 4.6 percent of 109 patients developed tetany following subtotal thyroidectomy, all on the first postoperative day (Yamashita et al, 1999). Tetany related to vitamin D deficiency can result from inadequate sunlight, malnutrition, or impaired kidney function.

In **alkalosis,** because of the excessive alkalinity of body fluids, a greater number of calcium ions are bound to serum proteins, effectively inactivating the calcium. Therefore, nerve and muscle function is impaired. Alkalosis may be caused by the loss of acid (due to vomiting or gastric suction) or by the ingestion of alkalis (for example, sodium bicarbonate). Alkalosis can even be caused by breathing too rapidly, either in response to fear or through mechanical ventilation. The result is excessive loss of carbon dioxide. In the blood, carbon dioxide is transported as carbonic acid. Thus, when too much carbon dioxide is exhaled, the alkalinity of the blood increases and produces tetany.

Early symptoms of tetany are nervousness, irritability, numbness, tingling of the extremities and around the mouth, and muscle cramps. Diagnostic signs are Trousseau's sign and Chvostek's sign. In **Trousseau's sign,** inflation of the blood pressure cuff above systolic pressure for 3 minutes causes ischemia of the peripheral nerves,

increasing their excitability. What the examiner sees is muscle spasms of the forearm and hand. In **Chvostek's sign,** a tap over the facial nerve in front of the ear causes a twitch of the facial muscles on that side. Figure 8–6 depicts these diagnostic signs.

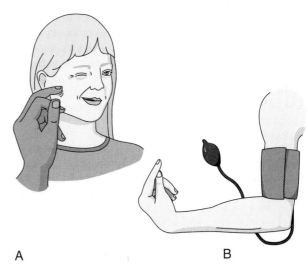

A   B

Figure **8–6** Indications of hypocalcemia: A, positive Chvostek's sign; B, positive Trousseau's sign.

Because of the many functions of calcium, tetany is a medical emergency. Untreated, it can progress to respiratory paralysis, seizures or coma, heart dilatation, and blood clotting problems.

Calcium Toxicity

A serum calcium level that is too high, above 11 milligrams per 100 milliliters of serum in adults, is called **hypercalcemia.** It can be caused by **hyperparathyroidism** and other diseases, vitamin D poisoning, or antacids, but almost never by ingestion of foods. Idiopathic hypercalcemia associated with vitamin D toxicity is seen most frequently in infants. Kidney stones are not usually caused by dietary calcium but by malfunctioning kidneys that permit too much calcium to be spilled into the urine (Weaver and Heaney, 1999).

In a series of 100 clients with hypercalcemia, the most common causes were malignancy and hyperparathyroidism. The third most common cause was milk-alkali syndrome, a group that included three people who underwent surgery for parathyroid disease before the diagnosis was established (Beall and Scofield, 1995).

Milk-alkali syndrome, a condition caused by ingestion of excessive absorbable alkali and milk, is characterized by high blood calcium and urine more alkaline than normal that predisposes to the formation of calcium deposits in the kidney. It was associated with the milk and cream antacid treatment of peptic ulcers that was common years ago. Recent cases, in which some clients required hemodialysis for renal failure, resulted from self-prescribed calcium carbonate tablets (Abreo et al, 1993; Beall and Scofield, 1995; Vanpee et al, 2000). Individuals reported taking 2 to 18 grams daily, usually for indigestion. (Package instructions caution not to take more than 8 grams per day and not to use that dose for more than 2 weeks without consulting a physician.) Some concern is raised about the use of calcium carbonate to prevent osteoporosis (George and Clark, 2000; Vanpee et al, 2000). These cases emphasize the importance of a careful dietary and medication history and of client teaching regarding over-the-counter as well as prescription medications.

Phosphorus

Phosphorus occurs in bones and teeth as calcium phosphate. The body of a 154-pound man contains about 700 grams of phosphorus, 85 percent in bone, 14 percent in soft tissue, and 1 percent in body fluids (Gropper, Smith, and Groff, 2005). Phosphorus is closely associated with calcium both in foods and in interrelated metabolic functions in the body. See Clinical Application 8–4 for information on phosphorus intake and calcium balance.

Phosphorus is a component of DNA and RNA. The storage forms of energy, **adenosine diphosphate (ADP)** and **adenosine triphosphate (ATP),** contain phosphorus. Phosphorus is an essential mineral in **phospholipids,** which are structural components of cells. Lecithin, a part of cell membranes, and myelin, the insulating covering of many nerves, are phospholipids. Phosphorus is contained in almost all enzymes, and phosphorus compounds are used as a buffer system to maintain the pH of the blood between 7.35 and 7.45.

Phosphorus Intake and Calcium Balance

In the past, the ratio of calcium to phosphorus was considered to be crucial to proper calcium balance. Now authorities believe that the calcium-to-phosphorus ratio is less important than the adequacy of calcium intake for adults, however infants and children are believed to need correctly balanced intakes. Calcium to phosphorus ratios no less than 1.1 nor more than 2.0 are recommended for infant formulas (Appendix D, 2004). On the other hand, athletes and others with high energy expenditure often consume amounts of phosphorus greater than the UL with no apparent ill effects (Institute of Medicine, 2003).

Control Mechanism for Phosphorus

Between 50 and 70 percent of dietary phosphorus is absorbed primarily in the **duodenum** and **jejunum** (Gropper, Smith, and Groff, 2005). That which is not absorbed is eliminated in the feces. The same factors that affect calcium absorption are at work for phosphorus.

Low levels of serum phosphorus stimulate the kidney to produce more active vitamin D (calcitriol). The vitamin D then increases the absorption of phosphorus from the intestinal tract and enhances phosphate resorption from the bones. Excess phosphorus is excreted by the kidney in response to parathyroid hormone.

Dietary Reference Intakes and Sources of Phosphorus

The RDA for phosphorus is 700 milligrams for men and women aged 19 and older. The UL is 4000 milligrams for 19- to 70-year-old men and women and 3000 milligrams for persons older than 70. Phosphorus, essential in plant and animal cells, is widespread in foods. Animal protein, especially lean meat, is the best source of phosphorus. Good plant sources include nuts and legumes. In many plants, much of the phosphorus is found as phytate which limits its bioavailability to 50 percent. Depending upon a person's habits, cola beverages (that contain phosphoric acid) can contribute significantly to intake (Gropper, Smith, and Groff, 2005).

Deficiency of Phosphorus

Although calcium and magnesium impair phosphorus absorption, deficiency is unlikely in healthy persons consuming a normal diet. Certain diseases or medications, however, can produce **hypophosphatemia,** as has occurred in persons ingesting a diet low in phosphorus while also taking a phosphate-binding drug, such as the antacid aluminum hydroxide. Malabsorption disorders, severe burns, or uncontrolled diabetes mellitus have precipitated hypophosphatemia. In addition, a condition called **refeeding syndrome,** related to imbalances in phosphorus, occurs when wasted or starved clients are given nutrients in excess of what their bodies can handle (Chapter 24). In the client with alcoholism, the clinical picture of severe hypophosphatemia could be mistaken for delirium tremens because the client may suffer from hallucinations (Knochel, 1999).

Hyperparathyroidism is a disease that causes excess excretion of phosphorus. In this disease, parathyroid hormone causes withdrawal of calcium from the bones. Because the two are combined in the bones, phosphorus is lost along with calcium. Chronic kidney disease often produces the same result.

Phosphorus Toxicity

Hyperphosphatemia caused by dietary overload is unusual. Cases have occurred in infants during the first few weeks of life when they were given only cow's milk which has twice the phosphorus content of human milk and infant formula. The cow's milk diet, too much for an infant's immature kidneys, overtaxes the infant's ability to maintain homeostasis.

Other cases of hyperphosphatemia in previously healthy persons have occurred following excessive or chronic administration of sodium phosphates used as a saline laxative or as an enema. Clients with conditions that would increase the permeability of the intestine are at special risk when using these ordinarily harmless products.

Sodium

The body of a 154-pound adult contains about 105 grams (3.5 ounces) of sodium. Approximately 70 percent of the sodium in the body is in the blood and other extracellular fluids and in nerve and muscle tissue. The other 30 percent is on the surface of the bone crystals where it is available for release to counteract a low serum sodium level (Gropper, Smith, and Groff, 2005).

Sodium, which has a major role in maintaining fluid balance in the body, is also necessary for the transmission of electrochemical impulses along nerve and muscle membranes and is a component of two phosphate buffers.

The intestine readily absorbs sodium. At most, 5 percent of dietary sodium travels within the intestine to remain in the feces. All the remaining 95 percent of ingested sodium is absorbed into the bloodstream. To maintain a normal level of sodium in the blood, the kidney either reabsorbs sodium and returns it to the bloodstream or allows it to be spilled in the urine. A hormone from the adrenal cortex, **aldosterone,** stimulates the kidney to return sodium to the bloodstream (see Chapter 9).

Dietary Reference Intakes for and Sources of Sodium

The AI for sodium 1.5 grams per day for adults through age 49, 1.3 grams for those 50 to 70 years of age, and 1.2 grams for those 71 years of age and older. The AI would not apply to individuals who are highly active and lose large amounts of sweat on a daily basis. The UL for sodium is 2.3 grams per day, again not applicable to unacclimatized persons exercising in a hot environment (Institute of Medicine, 2004).

Table salt, the major dietary source of sodium, is 40 percent sodium and 60 percent chloride. One teaspoonful (5 grams) of salt contains about 2 grams of sodium, nearly the UL. Many foods, such as milk, milk products, and several vegetables, are naturally high in sodium. Most dietary sodium is derived from the salt or sodium-containing additives in processed foods, despite the fact that salt is not so necessary to maintaining year-round food stocks as it was years ago, when, for instance, meat was salted to preserve it. Table 8–3 compares the sodium content of relatively unprocessed foods with processed versions.

Deficiency of Sodium

Deficiency of sodium is associated primarily with increased sodium loss. Conditions such as diarrhea, vomiting, heavy sweating, or kidney disease may cause low serum sodium. The technical name for low serum sodium, less than 135 milliequivalents per liter in adults, is **hyponatremia.** A serum sodium that is low, not because of an absolute lack of sodium but because of an excess of water, is called **dilutional hyponatremia.** One condition producing this effect, the syndrome of inappropriate secretion of antidiuretic hormone (SIADH), is detailed in Chapter 9.

Sodium Toxicity

The reported 4 to 6 grams of sodium in the average American diet is probably an underestimate. Frequently such surveys do not account for all sources of sodium. Healthy people excrete excess sodium without immediate adverse effects. Because of the previously mentioned loss of calcium with high sodium intake, long-range adverse effects may accrue for individuals at risk for osteoporosis. For people with hypertension, heart disease, or kidney disease, the control of sodium balance becomes an important issue, as explained in Chapters 20 and 21. An excess of sodium in the blood, greater than 145 milliequivalents per liter in adults, is called **hypernatremia.** Signs and symptoms of low and high serum sodium levels appear in Table 9–2.

Potassium

The body of a 154-pound adult contains about 245 grams of potassium, approximately 8 ounces. Over 90 percent of ingested potassium is absorbed probably from the small

Table 8–3 **Comparison of Sodium Content in Fresh and Processed Foods**

FRESH FOOD	SODIUM (mg)	PROCESSED FOOD	SODIUM (mg)
Natural Swiss cheese, 1 oz	74	Pasteurized, processed Swiss cheese, 1 oz	388
Lean roast pork, 3 oz	65	Lean ham, 3 oz	930
Whole raw carrot, 1	25	Canned carrots, 1/2 cup	176
Tomato juice, canned without salt, 1 cup	24	Tomato juice, canned with salt, 1 cup	881

intestine and colon (Gropper, Smith, and Groff, 2005). From 95 to 98 percent of the body's potassium is inside the cells, where it helps to control fluid balance.

In addition to fluid balance, potassium is essential for the conduction of nerve impulses and the contraction of muscles, including one vital muscle, the heart. It also helps to maintain the **electrolyte** and pH balance in the body (see Chapter 9). The potassium in fruits and vegetables, but not in supplements or food additives, acts to neutralize diet-derived acids in high-protein foods and thus prevents bone demineralization. Increased bone turnover and kidney stones are adverse consequences of bone titration of excess diet-derived acids (Institute of Medicine, 2004).

The kidney responds to systemic alkalosis by excreting potassium to conserve hydrogen. Retaining the hydrogen will make the blood more acidic and help to correct the alkalosis. Conversely, in acidosis, the body responds by excreting hydrogen and retaining potassium. Similarly, when aldosterone stimulates the kidney to retain sodium, potassium is excreted to maintain electrolyte balance (see Chapter 9).

Dietary Reference Intakes

The AI for potassium is 4.7 grams for adults, an amount expected to lower blood pressure, blunt the effects of sodium chloride on blood pressure, reduce the risk of kidney stones, and possibly reduce bone loss. No UL has been determined. The median intake in the United States ranges from 2.9 to 3.2 grams for men and 2.1 to 2.3 grams for women. In Canada, intake is slightly better, 3.2 to 3.4 grams for men and 2.4 to 2.6 grams for women (Institute of Medicine, 2004).

Sources of Potassium

Potassium is present in all plant and animal cells but the best sources are unprocessed foods. Only fats, oils, and white sugar have negligible amounts of potassium. Legumes are high in potassium as are green leafy vegetables, winter squash, baked potato with skin, bananas, cantaloupe, watermelon, and orange juice. Potassium might also be obtained from salt substitutes that often replace the sodium with potassium.

Deficiency of Potassium

A potassium deficiency is related to diet only in cases of severe protein-energy malnutrition. **Hypokalemia,** a serum potassium less than 3.5 **milliequivalents** per liter, can be fatal if prolonged or severe. Hypokalemia may be caused by diarrhea, vomiting, laxative abuse, alkalosis, protein-energy malnutrition, and overhydration with plain water by perspiring athletes. Deficiency symptoms include fatigue, muscle weakness, irregular heart rhythm, nausea, vomiting, decreased reflexes, and mental disorientation. To convert milligrams to milliequivalents, see Clinical Calculation 9–1.

Potassium Toxicity

A potassium level greater than 5.0 milliequivalents per liter is **hyperkalemia.** The normal kidney excretes potassium effectively so that excessive dietary intake rarely causes hyperkalemia. Intravenous intake is a different matter, so that a client's urine output should be verified before administering an infusion containing potassium. Serum levels of 10 to 12 milliequivalents per liter usually produce cardiac arrest (Brensilver and Goldberger, 1996).

Potassium toxicity is most often the result of diabetic acidosis, kidney failure, adrenal insufficiency, or severe dehydration. Hyperkalemia may also be caused by excessive destruction of cells in burns, crushing injuries, or severe infections. Vague muscle weakness usually appears first, followed by flaccid paralysis beginning in the legs and moving up the body. The heart's rhythm is affected, and characteristic changes appear on the electrocardiogram. The muscles supplied by the cranial nerves are usually spared. The client remains alert and apprehensive (Brensilver and Goldberger, 1996). See Clinical Application 9–7 to relate hyperkalemia to blood transfusion. Signs and symptoms of low and high serum potassium levels appear in Table 9–2.

Magnesium

The body of a 154-pound adult contains about 35 grams (1.2 ounces) of magnesium. About 55 to 60 percent of the magnesium is combined with calcium and phosphorus in the bones, 20 to 25 percent of it is located in soft tissue, and 1 percent is in body fluids (Gropper, Smith, and Groff, 2005).

Absorption, Elimination, and Functions

Magnesium is absorbed throughout the small intestine, mostly in the distal jejunum and ileum and may be absorbed in the colon if disease has impaired small intestine absorption. Of usual intakes, from 40 to 60 percent is absorbed, but a smaller percentage is absorbed at high intakes and a larger percentage at low intakes (Gropper, Smith, and Groff, 2005). Serum magnesium concentration is maintained within a narrow range by the small intestine and kidney which both increase their magnesium absorption when necessary. If even greater amounts are required, the bones can release some magnesium into the extracellular fluid. Excess magnesium is eliminated by the kidneys. Such excretion can be increased by protein, alcohol, and caffeine consumption (Gropper, Smith, and Groff, 2005).

Magnesium is involved in more than 300 essential metabolic reactions (Gropper, Smith, and Groff, 2005). Magnesium is necessary for the transmission of nerve impulses and the relaxation of skeletal muscles after contraction. It activates enzymes for the metabolism of carbohydrates, fats, and proteins, including protein synthesis. Magnesium activates the enzymes that add the third phosphate group to ADP to form ATP. It also aids in the release of energy from muscle glycogen. As a cofactor in calcium utilization, magnesium not only aids bone formation but also helps to hold calcium in tooth enamel, thus preventing tooth decay.

Dietary Reference Intakes and Sources of Magnesium

The RDA for magnesium is 400 to 420 milligrams for adult males and 310 to 320 milligrams for adult females. The UL is 350 milligrams for adults considering supplemental mineral only and not food and water. Focusing on magnesium status by assessing dietary intake may mislead the health-care provider because of questions about the accuracy of the tables of food composition. The data on magnesium are inadequate or missing for some foods (Shils, 1999).

Magnesium is widely distributed in foods, especially plant foods, because it is part of the chlorophyll molecule. Green vegetables are good sources of magnesium, as are as carrots and corn. Other good sources are seeds, nuts, legumes, seafood, chocolate, and whole-grain cereals, especially oats and barley. On the other hand, removing the germ and outer layers of the wheat kernel can remove 80 percent of its magnesium content. Beverages such as coffee, tea, and cocoa are also rich in magnesium (Gropper, Smith, and Groff, 2005).

Interfering Factors and Deficiency of Magnesium

Calcium and phosphorus can inhibit magnesium absorption. High zinc intake may be a health concern for individuals consuming less than recommended amounts of magnesium (Nielsen and Milne, 2004). In addition, calcium and magnesium compete with one another in the kidney for reabsorption. These effects are most apparent when magnesium intake is low and that of the other minerals is high (Gropper, Smith, and Groff, 2005).

Inadequate diets do not generally cause magnesium deficiency. Deficiency may accompany protein-energy malnutrition, but it is usually the result of increased magnesium excretion or decreased magnesium absorption. Excessive excretion of magnesium can result from major surgery, vomiting, diarrhea, or diuretic therapy. Magnesium absorption is decreased in malabsorption syndromes and chronic alcoholism.

Magnesium deficiency may exacerbate the increased neuroirritability in cases of acute alcohol withdrawal. The association of magnesium with the nervous system is also being studied in relation to migraine headaches (Demirkaya et al, 2001; Trauninger et al, 2002).

Magnesium deficiency is a common occurrence, especially in older people with poor diets, clients with chronic alcoholism, and those who use diuretics (Santinelli et al, 1999). In a study of emergency department clients on whom serum magnesium was determined, 31 percent had low magnesium levels, statistically associated only with pregnancy and diabetes mellitus (Stainikowicz, 2003). Insufficient magnesium impairs central nervous system activity and increases muscular excitability. Because magnesium metabolism is intricately linked to calcium metabolism, magnesium-deficient clients display the signs of tetany. Other signs include disorientation, convulsions, and psychosis. Relief of signs and symptoms may take 60 to 80 hours after treatment begins (Brensilver and Goldberger, 1996).

Magnesium Toxicity

Ordinarily, magnesium levels do not build up in the blood except as a result of kidney disease. In fact, oral magnesium can cause diarrhea—Epsom salt is magnesium sulfate. A person with magnesium toxicity displays lethargy, sedation, hypotension, slow pulse, depressed respirations, and loss of patellar reflex. Respiratory or cardiac arrest may ensue. Because of magnesium's close link to calcium, the effects of magnesium toxicity can be blocked by administering calcium.

Sulfur

The adult body contains approximately 175 grams of sulfur, a component of the cytoplasm of every cell. It is especially notable in hair, skin, and nails, where the **disulfide linkages** help to hold the amino acids in their distinct shapes. Sulfur is a component of thiamin, biotin, insulin, and heparin and of the amino acids methionine and cysteine. A protective function of sulfur is that of combining with toxins to neutralize them.

The major source of sulfate for humans is provided through the amino acid pool (see Figure 5–2) by catabolism of the sulfur-containing amino acids, methionine and cysteine (Institute of Medicine, 2004). Dietary intake of foods containing these amino acids helps to replenish the supply, but no AIs or ULs have been established. Important sources of sulfur are meat, fish, poultry, eggs, milk, and cheese. Cases of deficiency of sulfur alone are unknown. Only people with a severe protein deficiency lack this mineral. Toxicity is related to environmental causes such as air pollution with sulphur dioxide (Komarnisky, Christopherson, and Basu, 2003).

Chloride

Whenever an industrial accident involving chlorine occurs, such as the derailment of a chlorine tanker car, the surrounding area is quickly evacuated because of the chemical's toxic effects. A harmless form of chlorine, chloride, far from being poisonous, is a required nutrient. The body of a 154-pound adult contains approximately 105 grams of chloride. Of the body's chloride, 88 percent is found in extracellular fluids such as the hydrochloric acid in the stomach and 12 percent is found in intracellular fluids (Gropper, Smith, and Groff, 2005). It plays a major role in maintaining normal fluid balance and correct acid-base balance. It also is released by white blood cells as they fight substances foreign to the body (Gropper, Smith, and Groff, 2005). Chloride is almost completely absorbed through the small intestine and is excreted primarily by the kidney as result of sodium regulation.

The AI for chloride is 2.3 grams for younger adults, a level established proportionate to the AI for sodium because nearly all dietary chloride is derived from salt. Table salt, which is 60 percent chloride, contains about 3 grams of chloride per teaspoon (5 grams). Foods high in chloride include eggs, meat, seafood, salty snacks, and processed foods.

Normally, most chloride is excreted by the kidney; however, loss of gastrointestinal fluids through severe vomiting, nasogastric suctioning, or diarrhea is a common cause of chloride deficiency. Chloride deficiency occurred in infants because chloride was omitted from the formula they received. Long-term sequelae in some of these children included cognitive impairments, visual-motor difficulties, and attention deficit disorder (Kaleita, Kinsbourne, and Menkes, 1991).

See Table 8–4 for a summary of the major minerals.

Table 8-4 Major Minerals

MINERAL	ADULT RDA/AI AND FOOD PORTION CONTAINING IT	FUNCTIONS	SIGNS AND SYMPTOMS OF DEFICIENCY	SIGNS AND SYMPTOMS OF EXCESS	BEST SOURCES
Calcium	1000–1200 mg 3.3–4 cups milk	Structure of bones and teeth Nerve conduction Muscle contraction Blood clotting	Tetany Osteoporosis Rickets (Premature infants)	Renal calculi Calcification of soft tissue	Milk Cheese Yogurt Sardines Oysters Clams Salmon
Phosphorus	700 mg 2.2 cups chili with beans	Structure of bones and teeth Component of DNA and RNA Component of buffers and almost all enzymes Component of ADP and ATP Component of phospholipids (i.e., myelin)	Increased calcium excretion Bone loss Muscle weakness	Tetany Convulsions Renal insufficiency	Lean meat Fish Poultry Milk Eggs Nuts Legumes
Sodium	1.2 to 1.5 grams 0.6 to 0.75 tsp salt	Fluid balance Transmission of electrochemical impulses along nerve and muscle membranes	Hyponatremia	Hypernatremia	Table salt Processed foods Milk and milk products
Potassium	4.7 grams 4 cups white baked beans	Conduction of nerve impulses Muscle contraction	Hypokalemia (not usually dietary)	Hyperkalemia (not usually dietary)	Legumes Green leafy vegetables Winter squash Baked potato with skin Canteloupe Banana Watermelon Orange juice Salt substitutes
Magnesium	310–320 mg (female) 400–420 mg (male) 1 to 1.4 cups All Bran cereal	Transmission of nerve impulses Relaxation of skeletal muscle Bone formation Stability of tooth calcium	Impaired CNS function Tetany	Weakness Depressed respirations Cardiac arrest	Green vegetables Nuts Legumes Seafood Whole grains Chocolate
Sulfur	None	Component of amino acids methionine and cysteine Gives shape to hair, skin, and nails	None known due solely to sulfur	None known due solely to sulfur	Complete protein foods
Chloride	2.3 grams 0.75 tsp salt	Component of hydrochloric acid Fluid and acid base balance	In infants: failure to thrive, lethargy, muscle weakness	None known	Table salt Snacks Processed foods Seafood Meat Eggs

Trace Minerals

Trace minerals are present in the body in amounts of less than 5 grams and have a recommended intake of less than 100 milligrams per day. Many trace minerals occur in such small amounts that they are difficult to measure and analyze; thus their physiological functions and possible roles in nutrition are not completely understood. For example, lead and mercury are found in body tissue but only, as far as is known, as the result of environmental contamination; see Clinical Application 8–5 and Chapters 11 and 14. Aluminum is a toxic metal frequently found in the environment. Concern has been raised about aluminum toxicity through ingestion in pharmaceuticals, food, and water, through injections of contaminated intravenous or total parenteral nutrition solutions or kidney dialysis solutions, and through inhalation in the workplace (Greger and Sutherland, 1997), leading to a call for establishment of threshold values for aluminum contamination of parenteral products (Wilhelm et al, 2001).

Ten trace minerals have well-known bodily functions, and nine of them have been assigned RDAs or AIs. Four of them are commonly recognized for their relationship with health: iron, iodine, fluoride, and zinc. The other six are selenium, chromium, copper, manganese, cobalt, and molybdenum. These 10 minerals are detailed individually in the sections below, starting with iron.

Five additional trace minerals, sometimes termed ultratrace minerals, arsenic, boron, nickel, silicon, and vanadium, appear in the DRI tables, but with RDAs or AIs not determinable. These five are included in the final section on trace minerals.

Iron

For a nutrient with functions as vital as those of iron, the amount in body is very slight—approximately 38 milligrams per kilogram of body weight for women and 50 milligrams per kilogram for men (Gropper, Smith, and Groff, 2005). Thus our 154-pound male would have 3.5 grams of iron, less than the weight of a penny, in his body.

The body conserves its supply of iron by recycling the mineral released from the catabolism of worn-out red blood cells. In adult men, about 95 percent of the iron needed for RBC production comes from this source and only 5 percent from the diet. Infants who are rapidly growing, however, derive 70 percent of their need from recycled iron and 30 percent from the diet (Centers for Disease Control, 1998b).

Functions of Iron

Iron is essential to the formation of hemoglobin, the component of the red blood cell that transports approximately 98.5 percent of the oxygen in the blood. **Hemoglobin** is composed of **heme,** the nonprotein portion that contains iron, and globin, a simple protein. Iron is also a component of **myoglobin,** a protein located in muscle tissue. Myoglobin stores oxygen within the muscle cells. When the body needs an immediate supply of oxygen, such as during strenuous exercise, myoglobin releases its stored oxygen. Iron is also present in enzymes that permit the oxidation of glucose to produce energy.

Because the brain has the highest metabolic rate of any organ, it requires high levels of iron and oxygen. Iron is required for the synthesis of myelin and of the neurotransmitters serotonin and dopamine. Areas of the brain related to movement contain relatively high amounts of iron. The concentrations in the **basal ganglia** are similar to those in the liver (Connor and Beard, 1997).

About 80 percent of the iron in a healthy body is available for carrying oxygen: hemoglobin contains 65 percent, myoglobin 10 percent, and iron-containing enzymes 3 percent. The remainder is stored. The main storage form of iron in the body is a protein-iron compound called **ferritin.** It is kept in the liver, spleen, and bone marrow for future use. When surplus iron accumulates in the blood because of the rapid destruction of red blood cells, the excess is stored in the liver in another compound, **hemosiderin.**

Absorption of Iron

The body tightly conserves its supply of iron. Dietary iron is absorbed throughout the small intestine, most efficiently in the duodenum. When red blood cells are destroyed after their usual life span of 120 days, their iron is stored for reuse. Once iron is absorbed, there is no effective mechanism for excreting the excess. Fortunately, under normal conditions, the body is selective about absorbing iron.

FACTORS AFFECTING AMOUNTS. As the body's need for iron increases, so does the proportion absorbed. In a healthy person, up to 15 percent of the iron in foods is absorbed. A person who is iron deficient, however, absorbs as much as 35 percent (Gropper, Smith, and Groff, 2005).

The amount of dietary iron that is absorbed is determined by the amount of ferritin present in the intestinal mucosa. The iron obtained from ingested food is bound to a protein called **apoferritin** in the intestinal mucosa to form ferritin. When the total supply of apoferritin has been bound to iron, any additional iron in the gut is rejected and eliminated in the feces. Similarly, iron within the apoferritin that is not needed remains in the intestinal cell to be sloughed off and excreted in the feces (Gropper, Smith, and Groff, 2005). Absorbed iron combines with a protein in the blood, **transferrin,** which transports iron to the bone marrow for hemoglobin synthesis, to the liver or spleen for storage, or to the body cells for use. Hemoglobin synthesis requires many other substances, including adequate protein and traces of copper, in addition to iron.

FACTORS AFFECTING RATES OF ABSORPTION. Two types of iron are found naturally in food: heme iron and nonheme iron. **Heme iron** is bound to the hemoglobin and myoglobin in meat, fish, and poultry. Fifty to 60 percent of the total iron in these animal sources is heme iron. Because heme iron is composed of ferrous iron (Fe^{2+}), it is rapidly transported and absorbed intact. The other 40 to 50 percent of the total iron in meat, fish, and poultry, and all the iron in plant sources, is **nonheme** iron (Gropper, Smith, and Groff, 2005). Heme iron is two to three times more absorbable than nonheme iron (Centers for Disease Control, 1998b).

The absorption of nonheme iron is slow because it is closely bound to organic molecules in foods as **ferric iron**

Lead Poisoning (Plumbism)

Lead is a contaminant in the human body. The effects of lead toxicity, such as neurological damage and retardation, can be devastating and permanent. Lead abatement programs have been successful in the U.S. The prevalence of a blood lead level (BLL) of 10 micrograms per 100 milliliters of blood in 1- to 5-year-old children fell from 88.2 percent in 1976–1980 to 2.2 percent in 1999–2000, but this still represents an estimated 434,000 children. The goal of Healthy People 2010 is to eliminate BLLs of 10 micrograms per deciliter or more in children younger than 6 years of age (Meyer et al, 2003). No level of lead has been declared safe, however, and BLLs below 10 micrograms per deciliter are inversely associated with IQ scores at 3 and 5 years of age (Canfield et al, 2003). Black children and Hispanic children are at greater risk of lead poisoning than white children, as are all low-income children.

Food is not the chief source of lead. Years ago, "painters' colic" or chronic lead poisoning was a fairly common occupational hazard. Today, lead-based paint in older homes is the primary source of poisoning in inner-city children, as was the case of a 2-year-old child who died from acute lead poisoning (Centers for Disease Control, 2001a). Other children with elevated BLLs may not actually be eating paint chips. A principal mode of ingestion is that of lead dust on hands, toys, and household objects. Lead was banned for residential use in 1978, but homes built before then, especially those built before 1950, pose a particular risk for children.

Other sources of lead are automobile emissions from leaded gasoline, solder in metal food and beverage cans, and lead in or lead glazes on serving utensils that leaches out of the container, particularly into acidic juices and wine (Hackley and Katz-Jacobson, 2003). The first has been drastically reduced since 1973 by the use of unleaded gasoline and the second since the 1980s by the elimination of lead solder in cans packaged in the U.S. Reports of ingestion of lead from dishware or foreign packaging materials still appear sporadically.

Cases of childhood lead poisoning have been discovered by astute clinicians:

- After the family pets were affected by exterior renovations in the neighborhood (Dowsett and Shannon, 1994).
- By candy packaged in lead-containing wrappers from Mexico (Centers for Disease Control, 2002a), by candy in ceramic jars from Mexico, and by a spice purchased in Iraq (Centers for Disease Control, 1998a).
- Involving ingested curtain weights or fishing sinkers (Mowad, Haddad, and Gemmel, 1998).
- From retained shrapnel from gunshot wounds (Farrell et al, 1999; Raymond et al, 2002).
- In toddlers who ingested pool cue chalk (Miller et al, 1996).
- To be transferred to the home from a furniture refinishing workplace (Centers for Disease Control, 2001b).

Although fetuses and children are the most susceptible to damage from lead poisoning, adults can be affected also. About 90 percent of total body lead is accumulated in the bones, where it remains for decades. The U.S. Occupational Safety and Health Administration permits a lead-exposed worker to return to work when BLLs drop to 40 micrograms per deciliter (Roscoe et al, 2002). Of special concern among adults are pregnant and lactating women whose bone turnover releases sequestered lead into the bloodstream that readily crosses the placenta. Lastly, moonshine whiskey ingestion is a source of high-dose lead exposure in adults that can be fatal (Kaufmann, Staes, and Matte, 2003).

Concern about the lead content in aging municipal water pipes prompted the Environmental Protection Agency (EPA) to lower the permissible lead level from 50 parts per billion to 15 parts per billion. Older homes also may have plumbing that could contaminate drinking water. Ten infants were poisoned from formula reconstituted with lead-contaminated water (Shannon and Graef, 1992). Since boiling increases the concentration of lead in water, the need to boil water for infant formula needs individual evaluation. To decrease the chance of lead leaching into drinking or cooking water, (1) flush the system for 2 minutes in the morning before drawing water and (2) use cold water. Local health departments should be able to direct people to appropriate laboratories if they wish to have their water tested.

Early diagnosis and treatment of lead poisoning are essential. Foremost is the avoidance of further exposure through environmental control. Several nutritional tactics can be used in addition. Iron and calcium supplementation can be started so these minerals will compete with lead for absorption. A reduced-fat diet and frequent meals also decrease gastrointestinal absorption of lead. Use of chelating agents that will bind with lead are recommended if the blood lead level is greater than 45 micrograms per 100 milliliters, and a BLL of 70 micrograms or higher is a medical emergency (Meyer et al, 2003). Even children successfully treated and kept away from further intake showed lasting brain damage in 25 percent of cases.

Universal screening is recommended in communities with inadequate local data on blood lead levels and in communities with 27 percent or more of housing units built before 1950. Targeted screening is recommended in communities where 12 percent or fewer children have blood lead levels of 10 micrograms per 100 milliliters or higher or where fewer than 27 percent of the houses were built before 1950. Selecting children to screen focuses on such risk factors as the housing or day care facilities, family history of lead poisoning, birth country's prevalence of lead poisoning, likelihood of folk remedies being used, and the family's financial resources (American Academy of Pediatrics, 1998).

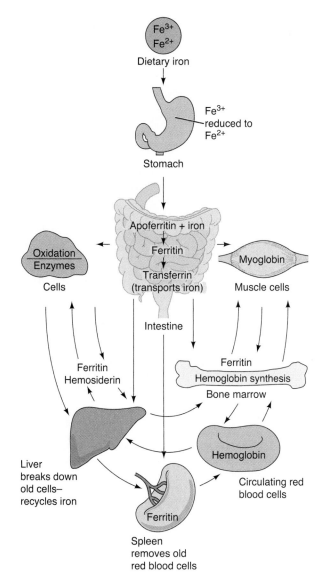

Figure **8–7** In the process of dietary iron absorption, iron is absorbed primarily in the small intestine and may be transported or stored to meet the body's needs.

(Fe^{3+}). In the acidic medium of the stomach, the oxygen is removed from ferric iron during a chemical reaction called reduction. The end product is **ferrous iron,** which is more soluble and bioavailable. See Figure 8–7 for an overview of the steps involved in the process of iron absorption.

FACTORS ENHANCING ABSORPTION. Several factors increase the absorption of iron through very different mechanisms. Consumption of large amounts of alcohol damages the intestine, which then permits absorption of increased amounts of iron. A high calcium intake increases iron absorption because the calcium combines with phosphates and phytates so that they are not available to inhibit iron absorption. Vitamin C forms a soluble compound with iron, negating the effect of phytates (see below) and increasing the absorption of iron. Finally, an MFP (meat, fish, poultry) factor increases the absorption

of iron. Nonheme iron absorption is increased when meat, fish, or poultry is consumed at the same time. Adding 1.8 or 2.6 ounces of pork to a phytate-rich vegetarian test meal increased absorption of nonheme iron by 44 and 57 percent, respectively (Bch et al, 2003).

FACTORS INTERFERING WITH ABSORPTION. When less gastric acid is present, whether because of antacid medications or gastric resection, less iron is absorbed. Phytic acid from cereals (wheat, rice, and maize) and nuts (walnuts, peanuts, and hazelnuts) and oxalic acid from certain vegetables both combine with iron, reducing its availability. Other minerals compete with iron for binding sites. Excesses of copper, zinc, or manganese decrease absorption of each other and of iron. Calcium, in foods or in supplements, decrease iron absorption (Gropper, Smith, and Groff, 2005).

Nonheme iron can be locked out of the absorption process by substances called **tannates,** which are found in coffee and tea. Coffee may reduce iron absorption by 40 percent, and tea may reduce iron absorption by 60 percent. Tea consumption does not influence iron status in Western populations in which most people have adequate iron stores; however, in populations of individuals with marginal iron status, there does seem to be a negative association between tea consumption and iron status (Temme and Van Hoydonck, 2002). Table 8–5 summarizes the factors that affect iron absorption. People who consume vegetarian diets should be especially careful to construct optimal menus. Practical suggestions to enhance iron and zinc nutrition in vegetarian diets are given in Table 8–6.

Excretion of Iron

No known mechanism exists to regulate the excretion of iron. Small amounts of iron are lost daily via the gastrointestinal tract, shed skin cells, and urine. Blood and mucosal cells are lost from the gastrointestinal tract even in healthy people. Certain medications and diseases increase the losses. Physiologic status also influences iron loss. Post menopausal women lose an average of 0.8 milligrams of iron per day, men lose about 1 milligram per day, whereas women of reproductive age lose an average of 1.3 to 1.4 milligrams per day, depending on menstrual flow (Gropper, Smith, and Groff, 2005). Blood contains about 0.5 milligram of iron per milliliter, so a blood donor would lose 250 milligrams per unit donated. Someone who donates every 2 months, then, would have losses amounting to 4 milligrams of iron per day all year long, which necessitates a fourfold increase in iron intake to replace (Fairbanks, 1999).

Table 8–5 **Factors Affecting Iron Absorption**

INCREASE	DECREASE
Large alcohol intake	Less gastric acid
High calcium intake	Coffee or tea (tannates)
Vitamin C	Phytic or oxalic acids
Meat, fish, or poultry	Excessive copper, manganese, or zinc intake

Table 8–6 **Improving Iron and Zinc Nutrition With Vegetarian Diets**

GOAL	STRATEGY	RATIONALE
Increase the total amount of iron and zinc consumed.	Select foods rich in iron and zinc at all meals. Consume cereals and pasta fortified with these nutrients.	Obtaining sufficient iron and zinc without animal products requires careful planning.
Make use of contamination iron.	Use cast iron cookware or steel woks for vegetable casseroles or curries, spaghetti sauces, or stewed fruits.	Moist, acidic foods have increased iron content when thus cooked for a long period. Even 20 minutes has shown an effect (Fairweather-Tait, Fox, and Mallilin, 1995).
Expand the intake of absorption enhancers.	Consume fermented foods such as yogurt and oriental soy products (tempeh, miso, natto, and soy sauce).	Certain organic acids (citric, lactic, malic, and tartaric) prevent the formation of insoluble iron and zinc phytates.
	Include a good source of vitamin C at every meal.	Ascorbic acid is the most effective enhancer of nonheme iron absorption when consumed with the nonheme iron. It reduces ferric to ferrous iron that is more soluble at the pH of the duodenum and small intestine. Vitamin C also forms a stable complex with iron, thus preventing iron from complexing with phytates and tannins (Lubin et al, 1997).
Reduce the intake of absorption antagonists.	Consumption of both sprouted whole-grain cereals and legumes and yeast-leavened baked products can potentially reduce the phytic acid content of a meal.	Microbial fermentation can enhance bioavailability of iron and zinc via hydrolysis induced by microbial phytase enzymes derived from microflora on the surface of cereal grains or from yeast.
	Soak legumes before cooking.	Soaking reduces the phytic acid of most legumes since it is relatively water-soluble.
	Delay drinking coffee and tea until at least 2 hours after meals.	These beverages reduce nonheme iron absorption 40 to 60 percent.
Avoid taking high doses of mineral supplements.	Dietary sources alone are unlikely to compromise iron and zinc status.	Antagonistic interactions between copper and zinc and between nonheme iron and zinc are most likely when high doses of supplemental zinc and nonheme iron are ingested without food.

SOURCE: Primarily adapted from Gibson, Donovan, and Heath, 1997.

Dietary Reference Intakes for Iron

The RDAs for iron are 8 milligrams for men and for women over the age of 50 years and 18 milligrams for 19- to 50-year-old women. Because the authors of the RDAs assume that 75 percent of iron intake is derived from heme iron sources, they suggest that vegetarians double the RDA amounts (Institute of Medicine, 2003). The UL for adults is 45 milligrams.

Sources of Iron

The Western diet contains an estimated 5 to 7 milligrams of iron per 1000 kilocalories. In the United States, one-third of dietary iron is supplied by grains, one-third by meats, and one-third by other sources. Good sources of iron include liver, other red meats, oysters, clams, lima and navy beans, dark green leafy vegetables, and dried fruits. Absorption also varies among the sources of iron. Ten to 30 percent of iron is absorbed from liver and other meats; less than 10 percent is absorbed from eggs; and less than 5 percent is absorbed from grains and most vegetables.

Many foods are fortified with iron, but its bioavailability depends on the compounds used. If the added iron is metallic iron, very little can be absorbed (Fairbanks, 1999). Iron from spinach, iron supplements, and contamination iron are absorbed at a 2 percent rate. Clinical Application 8–6 describes one way iron becomes available from nonfood sources. To show that all foods are not equal in nutrient content, the labeled percentages of iron and calcium in ready-to-eat cereals popular with children are compared in Figure 8–8. Manufacturers sometimes change these amounts. People who are trying to maximize their nutritional intake must read labels.

Deficiency of Iron

Iron is the most common nutrient deficiency in the United States. Iron deficiency can be determined by laboratory tests such as serum ferritin and transferrin saturation before the person's hemoglobin value drops sufficiently to diagnose **anemia** that occurs when iron stores are severely depleted (Gropper, Smith, and Groff, 2005). A person who is anemic has insufficient hemoglobin to provide oxygen to

Clinical Application 8–6

Contamination Iron

Cooking in iron pots can increase the iron content of foods. This source of dietary iron is called **contamination iron.** Significant transfer occurs during simmering of acidic foods, especially tomatoes. For instance, 3 1/2 oz of spaghetti sauce cooked for 3 hours in a cast iron pot contains almost 90 mg of iron, compared to less than 5 mg of iron when cooked in a glass container (Zhou and Brittin, 1994). The East Indian practice of cooking curries in cast iron woks also was shown to increase iron content 4- to 12-fold (Fairweather-Tait, Fox, and Mallillin, 1995). The absorption rate of contamination iron is the same as that of supplements, 2 percent.

the cells of the body. The features of the red blood cells are characteristic of various anemias. In iron-deficiency anemia, the red blood cells are **microcytic** (smaller than normal) and **hypochromic** (contain less hemoglobin, giving the cell less color than normal).

Insufficient intake of iron, excessive blood loss, malabsorption, or lack of gastric hydrochloric acid can lead to **iron-deficiency** anemia, but iron is not the only nutrient required for adequate blood formation. Some of the other nutrients needed include protein, the vitamins C, E, B$_6$, and B$_{12}$, riboflavin, folic acid, and the mineral copper.

Longitudinal studies have linked poorer cognitive skills in school with anemia in infancy, but to what extent socioeconomic status affects the outcome is uncertain (Grantham-McGregor and Ani, 2001). In a study of 11- to 14-year-old children in Costa Rica, however, those with severe, chronic anemia in infancy scored lower in mental and motor functioning than those with good iron status in infancy (Lozoff et al, 2000). In Thailand, a dose-response relationship was found between hemoglobin levels and cognition in iron-deficient school children but not in iron-sufficient children (Sungthong, Mo-suwan, and Chong-suvivatwong, 2002).

OCCURRENCE. Iron deficiency is the most common single-nutrient-deficiency disease in the world. In tropical countries where intestinal **helminthiasis** is common, prevalence of iron deficiency is especially high. In India, where hookworm disease is prevalent and vegetarianism is mandated by religion, iron deficiency is nearly universal (Fairbanks, 1999). Iron deficiency also affects an estimated 94 million people in the Americas (Darnton-Hill et al, 1999).

In 1999 to 2000, 12 percent of 12- to 49-year-old females were iron deficient, including 16 percent of 16- to 19-year-olds. Iron deficiency was found in 22 percent of Mexican-American 12- to 49-year-old females compared with 19 percent of black, non-Hispanic females and 10 percent of white non-Hispanic females (Centers for Disease Control, 2002b). More information on anemia in children is included in Chapter 12. Fortunately, the number of children in the United States with iron deficiency is decreasing, due largely to fortification of cereals and infant formulas.

RISK OF IRON DEFICIENCY. Individuals at greatest risk of iron deficiency are young children and women of childbearing age, especially low-income minority women, who have 12 or fewer years of education or have had four or more children (Looker et al, 1997). Children 4 months to 3 years old, adolescents, and pregnant women should be monitored carefully for signs of iron deficiency because of their increased needs. All women in their menstrual years are at risk, a risk that increases with use of an intrauterine contraceptive device, which increases blood loss.

ASSESSMENT DATA. Although no single test is diagnostic for iron deficiency, a common test to determine the

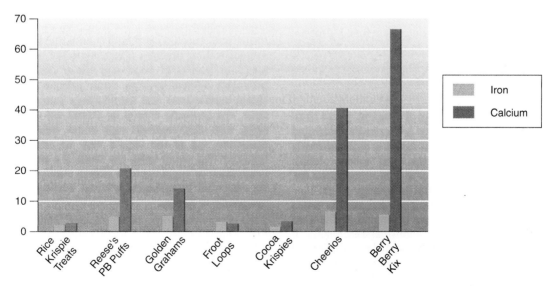

Figure **8–8** Three-fourths of a cup of each of these cereals supplies the indicated content of iron and calcium. Iron varies from 1.8 to 6 milligrams and calcium from 2 to 66 milligrams. Serving the usual way with milk would increase the amount of calcium obtained. (Data source: USDA Table 9 Nutritive Value of the Edible Part of Foods, 2002.)

hemoglobin level of the blood delivers valuable assessment data. The normal level for men is 14 to 18 grams per 100 milliliters of blood; for women it is 12 to 16 grams. A second common laboratory test is the **hematocrit.** This test measures the percentage of red blood cells in a volume of blood. Normal hematocrit levels are 40 to 54 percent for men and 36 to 46 percent for women. Low hemoglobin and hematocrit levels are late indicators of iron deficiency.

In early iron deficiency, before hemoglobin and hematocrit readings drop, **serum transferrin** levels rise. The person with early iron deficiency will, providing the body is attempting to compensate, manufacture more transferrin to increase iron-carrying capacity. Because serum ferritin is usually proportional to the amount of iron stored as ferritin and hemosiderin in body tissues, it is used as a measure of iron stores (Schnell, Van Leeuwen, and Kranpitz, 2003) but can be falsely high due to infection and inflammation (Gropper, Smith, and Groff, 2005).

TREATMENT PRECAUTIONS. After a person has been treated for iron deficiency, iron therapy should be continued for several months after hemoglobin and hematocrit levels return to normal. This prolonged therapy will enable the body to rebuild iron stores.

Oral iron supplements can cause side effects such as nausea and constipation and have been blamed for noncompliance with therapy. Suggestions to increase acceptance of a supplement include delayed-release preparations and intermittent dosing along with moderate dosages (Beard, 2000).

In developing countries with high levels of infectious diseases, iron administration for anemia has been followed by increased morbidity from infections. Bacteria also require iron, and when the body's supply increases, they thrive. This refers to free iron, not protein-bound iron (Gropper, Smith, and Groff, 2005). In Sri Lanka, however, 5- to 10-year-old children supplemented with iron had fewer and shorter upper respiratory infections than children receiving placebos (de Silva et al, 2003). Because the children receiving iron significantly increased their hemoglobin and serum ferritin levels, both containing protein, perhaps there was limited free iron for bacteria to utilize, thus decreasing morbidity.

Iron Toxicity

For most people, there is little risk of developing iron overload from the diet. Iron absorption is effectively controlled in healthy people even when meat intake is high and foods are fortified (Hallberg, Hulthen, and Garby, 1998). Nevertheless, iron toxicity is seen in iron metabolism disorders, chronic alcoholism, or iron poisoning.

Surplus iron is stored in the liver as hemosiderin. When large amounts of hemosiderin are deposited in the liver and spleen, a condition called **hemosiderosis** results. If prolonged, it can lead to **hemochromatosis,** a disease of iron metabolism in which iron accumulates in and damages the tissues. A person with this autosomal-recessive disease is unable to cease iron absorption despite high iron stores and as a result accumulates iron deposits in the liver, heart, pancreas, and other organs. Signs and symp-

toms include impaired liver function, blood sugar disturbances, joint pain, and skin discoloration. Eventually organ failure may lead to cardiac failure and death. An estimated 5 per 1,000 whites in the United States have the disease, most common in males, that becomes symptomatic around the age of 20 (Gropper, Smith, and Groff, 2005).

A different cause involving a genetic mutation that may contribute to iron overload in Africans and African Americans is under investigation (Gordeuk et al, 2003). High dietary iron from traditional beers brewed in nongalvanized steel drums (Gordeuk et al, 1992) along with the alcohol content of the beers had been considered causative. Such beers contain 21 to 52 milligrams of iron per liter compared with 0.1 to 3.6 milligrams in commercial beers (Saungweme et al, 1999).

Clients with alcoholism, although often lacking many other nutrients, sometime suffer from iron overload. Some alcoholic beverages themselves contain a significant amount of iron. For example, inexpensive red wines contain 10 to 350 milligrams of iron per liter. The problem may be more complex than just oversupply. Most alcoholic cirrhosis clients with iron overload have hereditary hemochromatosis whereby alcohol abuse increases the risk of cirrhosis but does not cause the iron overload (Fairbanks, 1999).

Toxicity from supplemental iron tablets is a major threat to children. The body's absorptive controls for dietary iron are circumvented by the large amounts of soluble iron in pharmaceutical preparations. Iron is the most common cause of pediatric poisoning deaths reported to poison control centers in the United States. As few as five or six tablets of a high-potency product could prove fatal for a 22-pound child. During 1991, of 5144 ingestions of iron supplements reported to poison control centers in the United States, 11 were fatal. An additional two deaths were caused by prenatal multivitamin preparations with iron. Between June 1992 and January 1993, five toddlers in the Los Angeles area died from ingesting iron supplements (Centers for Disease Control, 1993).

The Consumer Product Safety Commission requires child-resistant packaging for iron preparations in certain forms and specified strengths, and the Food and Drug Administration requires a warning label on solid dosage forms of iron (U.S. Food and Drug, 2003). Health-care providers should impress upon parents the enormous threat medications and supplements pose for small children. The products should be stored out of reach, out of sight, with child-resistant caps intact. Adults should take medicines out of the child's view to avoid modeling a behavior that could harm the child. If a child ingests any medication or supplement, a poison control center should be consulted immediately without waiting for signs and symptoms to appear.

Iodine

Iodine can be found in the muscles, thyroid gland, skin, and skeleton typically as iodide. The body of the average adult contains about 15 to 20 milligrams of iodide. The thyroid gland in the neck contains 70 to 80 percent of the total body iodide and takes up approximately 120 micrograms of iodide per day (Gropper, Smith, and Groff, 2005).

Function of Iodine and Control of the Thyroid Gland

The thyroid gland secretes **thyroxine (T$_4$)** and **triiodothyronine (T$_3$)** in response to the **thyroid-stimulating hormone (TSH)** from the anterior pituitary gland. Both T$_3$ and T$_4$ increase the rate of oxidation in cells, thereby increasing the rate of metabolism. The only known function of iodine is its participation in the synthesis of T$_4$ and T$_3$. When serum levels of T$_3$ and T$_4$ are adequate, secretion of TSH ceases. This is called a **negative feedback cycle:** TSH stimulates T$_4$ and T$_3$ production until a sufficient level of those hormones stops the secretion of TSH; when T$_4$ and T$_3$ levels drop, more TSH is secreted.

Absorption and Excretion of Iodine

Iodine is easily absorbed from all portions of the intestinal tract, including the stomach. Of the absorbed iodine, 33 percent is used by the thyroid cells for the synthesis of T$_4$ and T$_3$, and the remaining 67 percent is excreted by the kidneys, which have no mechanism to conserve iodine. After performing their functions, T$_4$ and T$_3$ are degraded by the liver, and the iodine content is excreted in bile. Some iodine is lost in sweat, which may be important in hot climates if intake is low (Gropper, Smith, and Groff, 2005).

Dietary Reference Intakes and Sources of Iodine

The RDA for iodine is 150 micrograms for adult men and women. The UL is 1100 micrograms. Iodine can come from foods, either naturally present or fortified, or from incidental sources.

IODINE IN FOODS. Foods that are naturally high in iodine include saltwater fish, shellfish, and seaweed. The iodine content in plants varies with the mineral content of the soil in which they are grown. The amount of iodine present in eggs and dairy products depends on the animals' diets. Using food tables to calculate iodine intakes has resulted in erroneous estimates of intake, because the regions producing the food analyzed would vary significantly in the iodine content of the soil. Table salt fortified with iodine (1 milligram of iodine in 10 grams of salt) has been available in the United States since 1924.

INCIDENTAL IODINE. Sometimes iodine is present as a side effect of processing. For example, iodine solutions are used to sterilize milk pasteurization vats; some iodine may remain on the vat and be mixed into the next batch of milk to be processed. Iodine is also used to improve the texture of bread dough.

Deficiency of Iodine

Because the normal function of the thyroid gland depends on an adequate supply of iodine, a deficiency may result in goiter, cretinism, or myxedema. Since the introduction of iodized salt, these deficiency diseases are rarely encountered in North America. Between 1922 and 1927, with the implementation of a statewide prevention program, the goiter rate in Michigan declined from 38.6 percent to 9.0 percent (Centers for Disease Control, 1999a). At particular risk of iodine deficiency are vegans who consume sea salt,

containing virtually no iodine, rather than iodized salt. In a group of North American strict vegetarians, 12 percent developed hypothyroidism (Remer, Neubert, and Manz, 1999). Diagnosis of thyroid malfunction can be readily evaluated by measuring protein-bound iodine and the serum levels of T$_4$ and T$_3$.

LOCAL EFFECTS. When the thyroid gland does not receive sufficient iodine, it increases in size, attempting to increase production. The gland may reach 1 to 1.5 pounds (about 500 to 700 grams). This enlargement of the thyroid is called **goiter** (see Figure 8–9). Sometimes the gland may attain sufficient size to impede breathing (Tsukada et al, 1999). Unfortunately, in rare cases, replacement of iodine does not reduce the goiter and surgery or radiotherapy may be needed. It is also possible in some cases for prolonged deficiency to short circuit the negative feedback control system, resulting in thyroid tissue that produces T$_3$ and T$_4$ in response to dietary iodine rather than to TSH. Iodine given to these people may cause **hyperthyroidism** (Corvilain et al, 1998).

Goiter has been known as a disease entity since 3000 BC. Because of iodine-poor soil, the Great Lakes States and the Rocky Mountain States once were considered the "goiter belt." Now that food is distributed nationwide and iodized salt is readily available, goiter is less common in this country. In contrast, worldwide, 211 million people have goiter, and 1.6 billion people are at risk for iodine deficiency, particularly in mountainous areas or those with eroded soil. When a population's prevalence of goiter is 10 percent or more, it is termed endemic goiter (Gropper, Smith, and Groff, 2005).

SYSTEMIC EFFECTS. Iodine deficiency is the most common cause of preventable mental defect in the world (Hetzel and Clugston, 1999). Severe **hypothyroidism** during pregnancy results in **cretinism** in the newborn. As a consequence of the mother's thyroid deficiency, the infant exhibits mental and physical retardation. Cretinism is a congenital condition (present at birth). About 20 million people in developing countries are at risk for overt cretinism

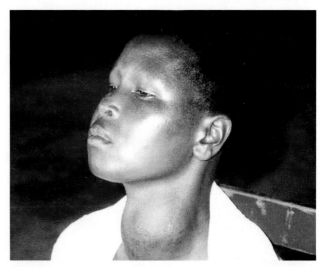

Figure **8–9** Woman with a goiter. (Reprinted from Kenya Medical Mission Web site, with permission.)

due to iodine deficiency. **Endemic** cretinism affects up to 10 percent of the people living in severely iodine-deficient areas of India, Indonesia, and China (Hetzel and Clugston, 1999). Prevention must focus on treating the iodine deficiency in the mother.

Hypothyroidism due to iodine deficiency occurring in older children and adults is called **myxedema.** In areas where food fortification is difficult to implement, treatment may consist of iodized oil administered by injection, which can suffice for 3 to 4 years, or oral iodized walnut, soybean, or peanut oils, which last 1 to 2 years (Hetzel and Clugston, 1999).

Factors Interfering with Iodine

Substances called **goitrogens** may block the body's absorption or utilization of iodine. Goitrogens are found in vegetables belonging to the cabbage family, including cauliflower, broccoli, Brussels sprouts, rutabaga, and turnips. The only food linked to goiter is cassava, a starchy root eaten in developing countries (recall konzo in Chapter 5). The persistence of goiter in Greece despite correction of iodine deficiency suggests a possible role for a naturally occurring goitrogen (Doufas et al, 1999).

Iodine Toxicity

Toxicity has been reported with intakes of 2000 to 3200 micrograms, but normal diets of natural foods are likely to supply just 1000 micrograms per day (Hetzel and Clugston, 1999). The exception would be a diet containing large quantities of marine fish, seaweed, or contamination iodine. Toxicity from iodine has occurred in parts of Japan from the ingestion of large amounts of seaweed. Too much iodine can cause either hypothyroidism or hyperthyroidism. In autoimmune thyroid disease, high dietary iodine may induce hypothyroidism or "iodine goiter" and may also cause skin lesions similar to acne. The opposite effect, iodine-induced hyperthyroidism, results from the thyroid gland becoming autonomous and ignoring the controlling attempts by thyroid-stimulating hormone.

Fluoride

In body fluids, fluorine exists as fluoride, a salt of hydrofluoric acid, or as an ion. About 99 percent of the body fluoride accumulates as fluorapatite in the bones and teeth. It seems to make bone mineral less soluble and hence less likely to be reabsorbed. Nearly 100 percent of soluble fluoride such as is found in fluoridated water and toothpaste is rapidly absorbed from the stomach and small intestine. Absorption diminishes to 50 to 80 percent when fluoride is consumed with solid foods or with calcium-containing beverages (Gropper, Smith, and Groff, 2005). Increased gastric secretion increases its rate of absorption, and aluminum hydroxide (an antacid) inhibits absorption (Nielsen, 1999). Approximately 90 percent of excess fluoride is rapidly excreted in the urine with most of the remainder in the feces and only minor losses in sweat (Gropper, Smith, and Groff, 2005).

Function of Fluoride

In addition to its function in bone, fluoride in plaque and saliva inhibits demineralization and enhances remineral-ization of early carious lesions. Drinking fluoridated water and using fluoride toothpaste and other dental products can raise the concentration of fluoride in saliva 100- to 1000-fold for 1 to 2 hours. Adults as well as children can benefit from these interventions. Nationally, the prevalence of any dental caries among children 12 to 17 years of age declined from 90 percent in 1971 to 1974 to 67 percent in 1988 to 1991, and the mean number of missing, decayed, or filled teeth fell from 6.2 to 2.8 (Centers for Disease Control, 2001c). A study in Louisiana showed that Medicaid-eligible children 1 to 5 years old in communities without fluoridated water were three times more likely to require dental treatment in a hospital operating room, inferring greater severity of disease, than Medicaid-eligible children in communities with fluoridated water. The resulting costs of dental treatment were approximately twice as much for the first group as for the second (Centers for Disease Control, 1999b).

Dietary Reference Intakes and Sources of Fluoride

The AI for fluoride has been set at 4 milligrams for men and 3 milligrams for women. The UL is 10 milligrams for both. Recommendations for dietary supplements of fluoride are based on the age of the child and the concentration of fluoride in the child's drinking water (Centers for Disease Control, 2001c).

One of the main sources of fluoride is drinking water that has been fluoridated at a cost of approximately 72 cents per person per year. Recommended concentrations are 0.7 to 1.2 parts per million (ppm) depending on the average maximum daily air temperature of the area. The U.S. Environmental Protection Agency (EPA), which is responsible for the safety and quality of drinking water in the United States, sets a maximum allowable limit for fluoride in community drinking water at 4 ppm (Centers for Disease Control, 2001c). A concentration of one part per million provides 1 milligram of fluoride per liter. The goal for Healthy People 2010 is to give 75 percent of people served by community water supplies access to optimally fluoridated water, a level that had been achieved by 26 states and the District of Columbia in 2000 (see Figure 8–10). The issue still evokes controversy (Coggon and Cooper, 1999). In England and Wales, less than 10 percent of the population receives fluoridated water.

Concern has been raised regarding the substitution of bottled water for fluoridated tap water. In Australia the practice was linked to increased decayed, missing, or filled baby teeth (Sidney Morning Herald, 2003). Infant formula prepared with bottled water contained less than optimal amounts of fluoride (Indiana University, 2000). The Food and Drug Administration regulates the amount of fluoride in the water but requires labeling of fluoride content only if fluoride is added by the bottler; however, the manufacturer should supply the information upon request (Centers for Disease Control, 2001c). The American Dental Association supports the labeling of bottled water with its fluoride concentration and the inclusion of information on the effect on fluoride of home water treatment systems (2002). Steam distillation removes all the fluoride and reverse osmosis units remove 65 to 95 percent, but water softeners and charcoal/carbon filters generally do not

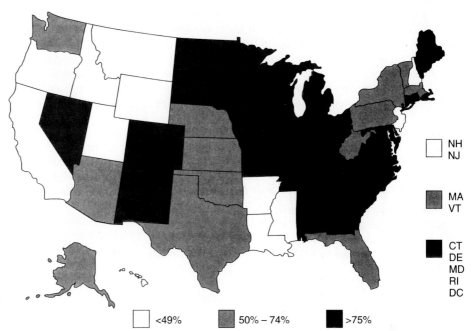

Figure **8–10** Percentage of state populations with access to fluoridated water through public water systems in the year 2000. (Source: Centers for Disease Control, 2001C.)

	NH NJ
	MA VT
	CT DE MD RI DC

☐ <49%   ▦ 50% – 74%   ■ >75%

remove significant fluoride from water (American Dental Association, undated).

Food sources of fluoride include fish, fish products, and tea that accumulates fluoride in the leaves so that brewed tea contains 1 to 6 milligrams per liter with decaffeinated varieties containing the larger quantities (Gropper, Smith, and Groff, 2005). Also, foods and beverages prepared with fluoridated water have increased levels of fluoride. Additional sources of fluoride are supplements and fluoride-containing dental products.

Fluoride Toxicity

Excessive, prolonged ingestion of fluoride results in **fluorosis,** a condition that can cause mottled discoloration of the teeth in children up to 8 years of age as well as bone and kidney dysfunction. Fluorosis has been observed when the concentration of fluoride in water has reached 2 parts per million. The fluorosis produced by this dose may be cosmetically unacceptable, but the teeth are sound. Just as an excess of iodine can cause the same symptoms as deficiency (i.e., goiter), a fluoride concentration of 4 parts per million is associated with increased dental caries.

Toxicity can also occur after ingestion of supplements and dental products containing fluoride. Children who begin using fluoride toothpaste when younger than 2 years of age are at higher risk of enamel fluorosis than children who begin later or do not use fluoridated toothpaste, because young children tend to swallow toothpaste (Centers for Disease Control, 2001c). Package labeling directs caregivers to limit the amount of fluoridated toothpaste for children younger than 6 years of age to "a pea-sized amount" and to consult a dentist or physician before using such toothpaste for a child under 2 years of age. Death may occur with intake as low as 5 milligrams of fluoride per kilogram of body weight (Gropper, Smith, and Groff, 2005).

Zinc

Estimated content of zinc in adult humans is 1.5 to 2.5 grams, over 95 percent of it within the cells. Zinc is a component of all body tissues. As much as 20 percent of total body zinc is found in the skin (Andrews and Gallagher-Allred, 1999), five to six times more concentrated in the epidermis as in the dermis (Rostan et al, 2002). Greater concentrations are found in the eyes, hair, bone, and male reproductive organs than in other tissues. Zinc is essential for the growth and repair of tissues because it is involved in the synthesis of DNA and RNA. Zinc is incorporated into the structure of at least 70 and perhaps more than 200 enzymes some of which can release zinc when needed for other more essential functions (Gropper, Smith, and Groff, 2005). Zinc is associated with insulin and is a component of a protein involved in taste acuity. The production of active vitamin A for the visual pigment rhodopsin requires zinc. It is integral to the formation of collagen, which is necessary for wound healing. Zinc also protects against disease through its role in providing immunity and is the subject of research with the common cold.

Whether zinc is effective in warding off or minimizing symptoms of the common cold is still unproved (Jackson, Lesho, and Peterson, 2000), but a retrospective chart analysis found zinc decreased duration and number of colds in school children (McElroy and Miller, 2002). In 1999, however, in answer to charges by the Federal Trade Commission, two companies agreed not to make unsubstantiated claims for their zinc products (Federal Trade Commission, 1999).

Absorption and Control of Zinc

Zinc is released from foods in the acid environment of the stomach and absorbed from the small intestine through the same absorption sites as iron. Control of zinc levels is achieved through limitations on absorption and excretion into intestinal waste. Gastric acidity facilitates zinc absorption, and conditions or medications that decrease gastric acidity impede it (Gropper, Smith, and Groff, 2005). As the concentration of zinc in the intestinal lumen increases, the percentage absorbed decreases, but the total amount absorbed increases. The body does not store zinc.

Most zinc is excreted in the feces. Small amounts are lost in the urine, in exfoliated skin cells, in sweat, in semen, and in menstrual flow. Because hair contains 0.1 to 0.2 milligrams of zinc per gram, hair loss is also a route for zinc depletion (Gropper, Smith, and Groff, 2005).

Dietary Reference Intakes and Sources of Zinc

The RDAs for zinc are 11 milligrams for men and 8 milligrams for women. The UL is 40 milligrams for both. The DRIs contain a suggestion that vegetarians consume twice as much as persons consuming a mixed diet (Institute of Medicine, 2003).

The best dietary sources of zinc are fortified cereals, shellfish, especially oysters, red meat, and cheese. Animal products are estimated to provide 40 to 70 percent of the zinc in diets in the United States. Zinc is also recovered from pancreatic and biliary secretions in the gastrointestinal tract for reuse (Gropper, Smith, and Groff, 2005).

Interfering Factors for Zinc

Iron and zinc compete for the same absorption sites. Zinc and iron interact when ingested together in solution but not always when taken with a meal however, supplements are problematic. Vitamin and mineral supplements with a ratio greater than 2 to 1 of iron to zinc inhibit zinc absorption (Gropper, Smith, and Groff, 2005). Decreased absorption of zinc has been noted when a 30-milligram supplement of iron is taken. Pregnant women taking 60 milligrams of iron daily should also take supplemental zinc (King and Keen, 1999).

Fiber, phytates, oxalates, tannins, and **chelating agents** all reduce the absorption of zinc. Zinc itself is a chelating agent protecting the body from poisoning from lead and cadmium.

Deficiency of Zinc

Clinical zinc deficiency is not commonly diagnosed in the United States. In other parts of the world, zinc deficiency is widespread, especially where the population subsists on cereal grains. The possibility of subclinical zinc deficiency in the United States exists, because the U.S. food supply provides only 12.3 milligrams per person per day. Zinc intake correlates directly with protein consumption. Groups at risk because of limited meat intake include the poor, the elderly, and vegetarians. A reliable, sensitive laboratory index is needed to identify people at risk of zinc deficiency (King and Keen, 1999).

In Colorado, a group of healthy children, short for their ages, were supplemented with 5 milligrams of zinc daily and gained more height than an unsupplemented control group of comparable children. In contrast, zinc supplementation in children who had normal height for age did not increase their growth (King and Keen, 1999).

Zinc deficiency in adults can also occur as a result of diseases that either hinder zinc absorption or cause excessive amounts of zinc to be excreted in the urine. Some of the clinical conditions that may precipitate zinc deficiency include alcoholism, chronic illness, stress, trauma, surgery, and diseases causing malabsorption. A rare autosomal recessive disease, **acrodermatitis enteropathica,** causes zinc deficiency through an unknown defect in absorption and is fatal if untreated. Oral zinc sulfate rapidly alleviates the symptoms.

Less severe deficiency of zinc produces the symptoms of abnormal fatigue, decreased alertness, impaired night vision, anorexia, and diminished sense of taste. Signs of severe zinc deficiency include skin lesions, hypopigmentation of the hair (giving it a reddish cast), patchy **alopecia,** diarrhea, and corneal edema. Other signs are retarded growth (dwarfism), delayed sexual maturation (if deficiency occurs during critical growth periods), low sperm counts, and delayed healing of wounds and burns.

Zinc deficiency impairs wound healing as the result of decreased collagen synthesis. Oral zinc supplementation has not been shown to be generally beneficial in the healing of chronic venous or arterial leg ulcers, but limited evidence found it helpful for individuals with low serum zinc levels (Wilkinson and Hawke, 2000). Similarly, zinc supplementation was credited with curing recalcitrant viral warts in clients with low serum zinc levels (Al-Gurairi, Al-Waiz, and Sharquie, 2002). Because serum zinc levels greater than 400 milligrams per deciliter may inhibit wound repair, supplemental zinc should be given only to clients who are deficient.

Zinc Toxicity

Because zinc can be toxic if consumed in excessive amounts, it should be obtained from foods in the diet and not from routine or long-term supplementation. Supplemental doses only two to three times the RDA can interfere with copper absorption and lead to copper deficiency. Adverse effects associated with chronic intake of supplemental zinc include suppression of immune response, decrease in high-density lipoprotein (HDL) cholesterol, and reduced copper status (Institute of Medicine, 2001). Men who took zinc supplements for longer than 10 years or in daily doses greater than 100 milligrams had more than twice the risk of advanced prostate cancer as other men (Leitzmann et al, 2003).

Copper

The healthy adult body contains less than 150 milligrams of copper, located in the liver (the main storage site), kidney, brain, heart, bone, muscle, skin, intestine, spleen, hair, and nails (Gropper, Smith, and Groff, 2005). Copper is a cofactor for enzymes involved in hemoglobin and collagen formation. It helps to incorporate iron into hemoglobin and to transport iron to the bone marrow. As a component of Factor V, copper is necessary for blood clotting. Copper is required for melanin pigment formation and for maintaining myelin sheaths.

Gastric secretions aid in the release of bound copper in foods. Although some absorption is possible in the stomach, most copper is absorbed from the small intestine, chiefly the duodenum. Typically, 50 percent of ingested copper is absorbed but may be more than 50 percent if intake is less than 1 milligram per day and may be 20 percent if intake exceeds 5 milligrams per day. The major route of excretion is via the liver and biliary tract into the feces. The amount excreted increases as body stores increase and vice versa but at intakes of as low as 0.38 milligrams per day, this mechanism is no longer adequate to prevent depletion of copper (Gropper, Smith, and Groff, 2005).

Dietary Reference Intakes and Sources of Copper

The RDA for copper for adults is 900 micrograms. The UL is 10,000 micrograms. In the United States, adult intake averages 1 to 2 milligrams. The World Health Organization has proposed a limit of 2 milligrams per liter for drinking water (Olivares et al, 1998). Unfortunately, data are missing on the copper content of many foods listed in or programmed into databases for nutritional analysis. Also, a food's copper content depends on its handling. The best sources of copper are organ meats, shellfish, nuts, seeds, chocolate, and dried fruits. The body may also recycle copper from digestive secretions (Gropper, Smith, and Groff, 2005).

Interfering Factors and Deficiency of Copper

High intakes of zinc, iron, calcium, phosphorus, and phytate interfere with copper absorption. The recommended iron-to-copper ratio is 10 to 17:1, but 80 percent of infant formulas examined were found to have ratios exceeding 20:1 (Johnson, Smith, and Edmonds, 1998). As little as 18.5 milligrams of zinc per day was shown to impair copper absorption. Overt signs of copper deficiency developed in people taking 150 milligrams (10 times the RDA) of zinc daily for 2 years (King and Keen, 1999).

Phytates hinder absorption by forming more stable complexes with copper than with calcium or iron. An alkaline medium also inhibits copper absorption so that a dose of 15 antacid tablets per day may precipitate copper and induce deficiency. Vitamin C has the opposite effect with copper as it has with iron because it makes reduces copper to a less absorbable form (Gropper, Smith, and Groff, 2005).

Copper deficiency is not known to occur in adults under normal conditions, but it has occurred as a result of the administration of total parenteral nutrition (TPN) solutions deficient in copper. Copper deficiency has also occurred in premature infants exclusively fed cow's milk; the result is an anemia that does not respond to iron supplementation. In a more unusual case, copper deficiency was caused by swallowed coins that released zinc into the body (Hassan, Netchvolodoff, and Raufman, 2000).

Because of its link with iron utilization, copper deficiency produces a hypochromic, microcytic anemia. Other manifestations of copper deficiency are skeletal demineralization, impaired immune function, and depigmentation of the skin and hair. A hereditary abnormality that blocks the absorption of copper from the gastrointestinal tract causes **Menkes' disease.** It is an X-linked recessive trait occurring in 1 in 50,000 to 100,000 live births. The natural history of the disease involves cerebral degeneration, retarded growth, and death by the age of 3 years. Intravenous administration of copper corrects the blood levels but does not improve brain function or slow the progressive deterioration (Turnlund, 1999).

Copper Toxicity

Clients treated with an artificial kidney that used copper tubing, others who consumed acidic foods stored in copper vessels, and infants fed water high in copper have experienced toxicity. A defect in the excretion of copper into the bile causes **Wilson's disease.** It is inherited as an autosomal recessive trait, occurring in 1 of 200,000 people in the United States (Turnlund, 1999). As a result, copper accumulates in various organs, particularly the liver, kidneys, brain, spleen, and cornea of the eye. Chelation therapy may be augmented by a dietary prescription to avoid foods high in copper.

Selenium

Most selenium occurs in proteins as a component of amino acids. It can substitute for sulphur in methionine and cysteine (Gropper, Smith, and Groff, 2005). The mineral selenium is part of an enzyme that works with vitamin E to protect cellular compounds from oxidation. In this role, selenium functions as an antioxidant. Selenium and vitamin E have a reciprocal sparing relationship (each spares the other). Selenium is part of many enzymes in the body and is necessary for iodine metabolism. It contributes to the work of drug-metabolizing enzymes and plays a role in preventing heavy metal poisoning from mercury, cadmium, and silver (Burk and Levander, 1999). In addition, a possibly unique selenoprotein occurring in the sperm mitochondrial capsule is vital to the integrity of sperm flagella (Holben and Smith, 1999).

The highest concentrations of this mineral occur in the liver, kidneys, and heart. About 50 to 100 percent of selenium is absorbed in the small intestine without regard to nutritional status. Rather, urinary excretion maintains homeostasis of the nutrient. Further data are needed on which to base more reliable estimates for intakes and plasma selenium levels that are protective (Thomson, 2004). Selenium is excreted almost equally in urine and feces but some is also lost via the lungs and skin (Gropper, Smith, and Groff, 2005).

The RDA for selenium for adults is 55 micrograms. The UL is 400 micrograms. Adolescence, pregnancy, and lactation increase the need for selenium, whereas a high intake of vitamin E reduces it. The amount of selenium present in plant foods depends on the selenium content of the soil and water where the foods are grown. The selenium in the British diet fell from 65 to 31 micrograms per day after switching from North American wheat to European wheat (Burk and Levander, 1999). In Finland, selenium is added to the soil to increase the selenium content of the plants and in other countries, selenium is added to animal feed.

Seafood, organ meats, poultry skin, eggs, nuts, and some fortified cereals are the best dietary sources of selenium. Selenium from fish, especially that contaminated with mercury, may have low bioavailability because of unabsorbable mercury-selenium complexes (Gropper, Smith, and Groff, 2005).

Selenium deficiencies have been produced in animals but are unlikely in humans who eat meat on a regular basis. Nevertheless, there are some exceptions. Clients being maintained long-term on special formulas, such as that used to treat phenylketonuria, should have the formula checked for adequacy of trace nutrients. Several clients being maintained on TPN have developed heart disease that responded to selenium treatment. A deterioration of the heart due to selenium deficiency has occurred in residents of the province of Keshan, China. The fatality rate of **Keshan disease** is as high as 80 percent, and once heart failure occurs, supplementation does not reverse it. Researchers have linked selenium deficiency in mice to a mutation of an avirulent virus to a virulent one producing myocardial disease. Significantly, the virulent strain then caused heart disease in non-selenium-deficient mice, an unusual situation in which a host's nutritional status affected the genetic composition of a microorganism (Burk and Levander, 1999). Signs and symptoms of selenium deficiency include poor growth, muscle pain and weakness, depigmentation of hair and skin, and whitening of nail beds (Gropper, Smith, and Groff, 2005).

Toxicity from selenium occurs in animals grazing on selenium-rich land. In humans, selenium toxicity has occurred in miners or due to industrial accidents and when the amount in a supplement was 125 times the correct dose. Signs and symptoms of selenium toxicity include fatigue, nausea and vomiting, garlic or sour-milk breath odor, and nail and hair loss. Animals that consume excessive selenium exhibit nervous system impairment and die of respiratory failure.

Chromium

The adult body contains approximately 4 to 6 milligrams of chromium. High concentrations are found in the kidney, liver, muscle, spleen, heart, pancreas, and bone. Only about 0.3 to 2.5 percent of dietary chromium is absorbed probably throughout the small intestine. More chromium is absorbed at low levels of daily dietary intake (less than 40 micrograms) than for higher levels (Garcia et al, 2001). The chief organ of excretion is the kidney. Chromium potentiates the action of insulin but the mechanism of action is uncertain. A meta-analysis of randomized clinical trials showed chromium had no effect on glucose or insulin concentrations in nondiabetic subjects and showed inconclusive results in individuals with diabetes (Althuis et al, 2002). Chromium may also influence cholesterol metabolism because supplementation has produced improvements in blood lipid profiles (Gropper, Smith, and Groff, 2005).

The AI for chromium for 19- to 50-year-old men is 35 micrograms and for 19- to 50-year-old women is 25 micrograms. For those older than 50, the AI is 30 micrograms for men and for 20 micrograms for women. The UL is not determinable. Severe trauma and stress, through related elevated secretion of glucagon and cortisol, may increase the need for chromium (Gropper, Smith, and Groff, 2005). Vitamin C may enhance absorption, but antacids decrease it.

Meats, especially organ meats, poultry, whole grains, cheese, mushrooms, tea, beer, and wine, as well as seasonings such as thyme and black pepper. are good sources of chromium. Population studies of quantifiable chromium intake reported a daily intake of 60 micrograms in Poland (Marzec, 2004) and 16 to 117 micrograms in southern Spain (Garcia et al, 2001). Although cooking utensils have been suggested to add to chromium intake, extensive testing has shown that, apart from new pans on first use, the contribution made by stainless steel cooking utensils to chromium and nickel in the diet is negligible (Flint and Packirisamy, 1997).

Signs of deficiency, including impaired glucose utilization, peripheral neuropathy, and high plasma levels of free fatty acids, occurred in individuals receiving TPN without chromium (Gropper, Smith, and Groff, 2005). In some clients receiving TPN, chromium, not insulin, successfully lowered blood sugar levels.

Chromium toxicity occurs rarely and under unusual circumstances. A 33-year-old white woman ingested of chromium picolinate, 1200–2400 micrograms per day, to enhance weight loss. After 4–5 months she did achieve weight loss along with anemia, liver dysfunction and kidney failure (Cerulli et al, 1998). Dietary chromium toxicity usually occurs as a result of eating contaminated foods; the characteristic symptom is a disagreeable metallic taste in the mouth. A more common cause is absorption of a different form of chromium through the skin or lungs in an industrial setting. Stainless steel welding may be the most common source of this contamination (Stoecker, 1999).

Manganese

The body contains only 10 to 20 milligrams of manganese, which is found in highest concentrations in the bones, liver, pancreas, and kidneys. Manganese is a cofactor of enzymes involved in energy metabolism and is required for bone formation. Absorption throughout the small intestine varies from 1 percent to 14 percent and is inhibited by iron, copper, oxalates, phytates, and fiber (Gropper, Smith, and Groff, 2005). Excretion is via the bile primarily with small losses through sweat and skin desquamation. Unlike nutrients that fulfill unique functions, manganese's roles can sometimes be filled by other minerals. One such mineral is magnesium.

The AI for manganese is 2.3 milligrams for men and 1.8 milligrams for women. The UL is 11 milligrams. The best sources of manganese are wheat bran, legumes, nuts, and green leafy vegetables. Deficiency is unlikely except when manganese is deliberately eliminated from the diet. The client displays hypocholesterolemia, nausea, vomiting, dermatitis, and changes in hair color. The best-documented case involved a child on TPN whose bone demineralization was cured by manganese supplements (Nielsen, 1999).

Toxicity due to dietary intake has not been reported in healthy people, but miners exposed to manganese dust over prolonged periods have suffered liver and central nervous system damage (including severe psychiatric symptoms), muscle spasms, and monotone voice. Those at risk for manganese toxicity are clients receiving parenteral nutrition and those with decreased liver function or **cholestasis.** Whole-blood manganese levels do not necessarily correlate with the accumulated mineral in the brain (Iinuma et al, 2003; Masumoto et al, 2001). The clinical picture of manganese toxicity resembles that of Parkinson's disease. Two children receiving long-term parenteral nutrition at home showed manganese in the basal ganglia on magnetic resonance imaging (MRI) without overt clinical signs. Over time the deposited manganese was removed by the body, indicating a good prognosis in the absence of neurological signs and liver disease (Kafritsa et al, 1998).

Cobalt

As an essential component of the vitamin B$_{12}$ molecule, cobalt is necessary for red blood cell formation, but a role for the ionic form of cobalt has not been demonstrated (Gropper, Smith, and Groff, 2005). DRIs for cobalt have not been established. Foods that provide vitamin B$_{12}$ are good sources of cobalt; these foods are meats, poultry, fish, shellfish, and milk. Cobalt deficiency has not been reported in humans or animals.

Molybdenum

Molybdenum, a cofactor for enzymes involved in catabolism of sulfur-containing amino acids and purines, is found primarily in the liver, kidneys, and bone. It is absorbed in the stomach and small intestine and is mainly excreted in urine, but also via bile in the feces, and in sweat and hair (Gropper, Smith, and Groff, 2005).

The RDA for molybdenum is 45 micrograms for adults, and the UL is 2000 micrograms. Daily intake from the average diet provides 200 to 500 micrograms. Sources of molybdenum are legumes, meat, fish, poultry, grains, potatoes, cabbage, and carrots. Content varies depending on soil conditions. Because molybdenum is a copper antagonist, high levels of copper decrease the absorption of molybdenum.

Molybdenum deficiency is not found in free-living humans, but deficiency has been reported in a client receiving prolonged TPN who displayed tachycardia, headache, mental disturbances, and coma (Sardesai, 1993). A client on TPN was treated as molybdenum deficient with signs and symptoms caused by an inability to process sulfur-containing amino acids. He exhibited increased pulse and respiratory rates, visual defects, night

blindness, irritability, and coma. After discontinuing his intake of sulfur-containing amino acids and supplementation with molybdenum, the symptoms disappeared (National Research Council, 1989).

No definite molybdenum toxicity has been documented in humans. In Russia, intakes of 10 to 15 milligrams of molybdenum per day (222 times the U.S. AI) have been associated with hyperuricemia and gout.

A summary of the main food sources of each of the trace minerals detailed thus far appears in Table 8–7. The food groups contributing to the intake of major and the above-mentioned trace minerals is illustrated in Figure 8–11.

Arsenic, Boron, Nickel, Silicon, and Vanadium

All of these minerals appear in the DRI tables, but none of them have RDAs or AIs nor have clear biological functions in humans been identified. Boron, nickel, and vanadium have been assigned ULs of 20, 1, and 1.8 milligrams, respectively.

Arsenic, a notorious poison often used in detective stories, is mostly found in human skin, hair, and nails. Environmental sources of arsenic are pesticides and fallout from pesticides, smelters, and coal-fired power plants (Gropper, Smith, and Groff, 2005). Most humans acquire it from food, where arsenic is in an organic form, but individuals most severely affected with overdoses receive it from drinking water, where arsenic is found in a more toxic inorganic form and in higher amounts. The maximum level for drinking water is 10 micrograms per liter (Abernathy, Thomas, and Calderon, 2003).

Boron is found mainly in the bones, teeth, hair, and nails and is a major ingredient in some antibiotics, antacids, and cosmetics. It was used to preserve fish, meat, cream, and butter from the 1870s to the 1920s when it was deemed dangerous for humans but essential for plants (Gropper, Smith, and Groff, 2005).

Nickel is found in highest concentrations in the thyroid and adrenal glands, hair, bone, lungs, heart, kidneys, and

Table 8–7 **Trace Minerals**

MINERAL	ADULT RDA/AI AND FOOD PORTION CONTAINING IT	FUNCTIONS	SIGNS AND SYMPTOMS OF DEFICIENCY	SIGNS AND SYMPTOMS OF EXCESS	BEST SOURCES
Iron	8–18 mg (female) 8 mg (male) 3–6.8 oz Braun-schweiger	Component of hemoglobin	Fatigue, listlessness Impaired cognition Hypochromic, microcytic anemia	Hemosiderosis Hemochromatosis	Liver, other red meats Clams Oysters Lima and navy beans Green leafy vegetables Dried fruit
Iodine	150 mcg 0.3 tsp iodized salt	Component of thyroid hormones	Goiter Cretinism Myxedema	Acne-like lesions Goiter	Iodized salt Saltwater seafood
Fluoride	3–4 mg 3–4 L fluoridated water	Hardens teeth	Dental caries	Mottled teeth Increased caries	Fluoridated water Seafood Brewed tea

(Continued on the following page)

Table **8–7** **Trace Minerals** *(Continued)*

MINERAL	ADULT RDA/AI AND FOOD PORTION CONTAINING IT	FUNCTIONS	SIGNS AND SYMPTOMS OF DEFICIENCY	SIGNS AND SYMPTOMS OF EXCESS	BEST SOURCES
Zinc	8 mg (female) 11 mg (male) 2.6 to 3.5 oz beef chuck roast, lean only	Involved in DNA and RNA synthesis Required for the formation of active vitamin A Component of 70 enzymes Serves role in immunity Associated with insulin Necessary for collagen formation Essential role in sexual maturation	Growth failure Hypogonadism Delayed wound healing Impaired night vision Impaired taste Delayed sexual maturation	Copper deficiency Decreased HDL cholesterol Suppressed immune response	Shellfish, especially oysters Red meat Cheese Fortified cereals
Copper	900 mcg 1.5 oz lobster	Cofactor for enzymes involved in hemoglobin and collagen formation Component of Factor V in clotting sequence Necessary for melanin formation and maintenance	Anemia Demineralization of skeleton Depigmentation of skin and hair Impaired immune function	Copper deposits in liver, kidneys, brain, spleen, and cornea	Shellfish Organ meats Nuts Seeds Dried fruit Chocolate
Selenium	55 mcg 0.5 oz oil-roasted mixed nuts	Antioxidant Interchangeable with vitamin E for some functions Necessary for iodine metabolism Part of many enzymes	Keshan cardiomyopathy	Nail and hair loss Nervous system impairment Sour milk or garlic breath odor	Seafood Organ meats Poultry skin Eggs Nuts
Chromium	20–35 mcg 0.6–1.1 egg yolks	Cofactor in enzymes used in fat and cholesterol metabolism	Glucose intolerance Elevated blood lipids	Rare related to food Metallic taste	Meats, especially organ meats Poultry Cheese Whole grains Mushrooms Black pepper Thyme Tea Beer Wine
Manganese	1.8 to 2.3 mg 3 to 4 tsp blanched hazelnuts or filberts	Cofactor of enzymes involved in energy metabolism Required for bone formation Magnesium may substitute for manganese in some functions	Hypercholesterolemia Dermatitis Changes in hair color	Accumulated mineral in brain In miners: liver damage and Parkinson-like syndrome—monotone voice, CNS impairment	Wheat bran Legumes Nuts Green, leafy vegetables
Cobalt	None	Component of vitamin B$_{12}$	Not reported	Polycythemia	Meat Fish Poultry Shellfish Eggs Milk
Molybdenum	45 mcg 2.3 cups raw shredded cabbage	Cofactor for enzymes involved in protein catabolism of sulfur-containing amino acids and purines	TPN clients only: tachycardia, headache, mental disturbances, coma	Hyperuricemia Gout	Legumes Meat Fish Poultry Grains Potatoes Cabbage Carrots

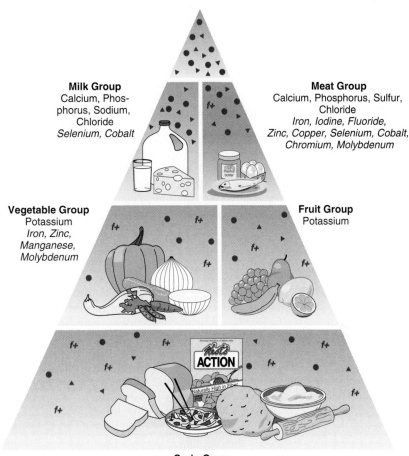

Milk Group
Calcium, Phos-
phorus, Sodium,
Chloride
Selenium, Cobalt

Meat Group
Calcium, Phosphorus, Sulfur,
Chloride
*Iron, Iodine, Fluoride,
Zinc, Copper, Selenium, Cobalt,
Chromium, Molybdenum*

Vegetable Group
Potassium
*Iron, Zinc,
Manganese,
Molybdenum*

Fruit Group
Potassium

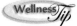

Grain Group
Magnesium
*Zinc, Copper, Chromium,
Manganese, Molybdenum*

Figure **8–11** This pyramid illustrates the food groups supplying the various minerals. Italics indicate trace minerals.

liver. Its industrial uses include the manufacture of stainless steel and of nickel-cadmium batteries. Nickel is released into the environment with the combustion of nickel-containing products (Gropper, Smith, and Groff, 2005).

Silicon is second only to oxygen in abundance in the earth. Quartz, the most abundant mineral in the earth's crust, is crystallized silica. The tissues with the greatest concentrations of silicon are bone, tendons, and skin (Gropper, Smith, and Groff, 2005).

Vanadium is found mainly in bone, spleen, and liver. Toxicity of the mineral produces a green tongue due to vanadium deposits as well as gastrointestinal disturbances, mental dysfunction, hypertension, and renal toxicity (Gropper, Smith, and Groff, 2005).

A summary DRI table of most of the minerals included in the chapter can be found at http://www.iom.edu/file.asp?id=7294. Information on sodium, potassium, sulfur, and chloride is available at http://www.nap.edu/openbook/0309091691/html/1.html.

Supplementation

Excessive intake of nutrients can be as harmful as insufficient intake. For most healthy people, foods are the preferred source of minerals rather than medicinal supplementation (Wellness Tips 8–1). People who take supplements should not take more than the RDAs or AIs for each mineral. In the case of some minerals, toxicity is possible at levels slightly above the recommended intake amounts. In addition, an excess of one mineral may cause a deficiency of another.

Wellness Tip **8–1** • Implement MyPyramid. Keep score to identify goals to emphasize.

- Attempt to restrain your taste for salt. It is a learned preference and can be unlearned.
- If you choose to use a mineral supplement, select a balanced one at RDA/AI levels, not individual minerals, unless under your professional health-care provider's direction.
- If you choose to use a mineral supplement, select a pharmaceutical one, not one of raw materials.
- Be extremely cautious and skeptical of remedies or foods privately imported into the United States.
- Consult your health-care provider if it has been necessary to make daily use of over-the-counter medicines such as antacids for more than 2 weeks.
- Treat dietary supplements as medicine. Lock them in childproof cupboards. Do not take medicines in front of children lest they imitate you.

SUMMARY

Minerals are inorganic substances that are necessary for good health. Like vitamins, they help to regulate body functions without providing energy. Unlike vitamins, minerals become part of the body's structure and enzymes.

In human nutrition, minerals are classified as major or trace. Major minerals are present in the body in amounts of 5 grams (1 teaspoonful) or more; the daily recommended intake is 100 milligrams or more. Trace minerals are those present in amounts smaller than 5 grams; the daily recommended intake is less than 100 milligrams.

People can be adversely affected by either insufficient or excessive intakes of minerals. Strangely, some miner-

als produce the same symptoms in both cases. When a client is nourished only by a very restrictive diet or by intravenous feedings for a long time, deficiencies of trace minerals may become apparent. In the United States, increasing the intake of iron and calcium has the potential to improve the health of millions of people.

Food is the safest source of nutrients. To prevent possible toxicity, people who take mineral supplements should limit intake to RDA or AI levels. Pharmaceutical preparations are preferred to "natural" supplements, whose strengths may be uncertain and that may contain possible contaminants.

CASE STUDY 8–1

Mrs. B is a 34-year-old woman who has related her fear of osteoporosis to the nurse. A recent visit to a 75-year-old aunt crystallized this fear. The aunt has become stooped and recently broke her hip. Mrs. B is especially concerned because she has often been told she resembles this aunt. Mrs. B asks, "Is there anything I can do to prevent this from happening to me?"

A 24-hour recall of dietary intake revealed a total of 1 cup of milk and no other dairy products. Mrs. B did consume two 3-oz servings of meat. Mrs. B has three small children and stated that they are exercise enough for her. She sits outside and watches them play on every nice day.

Mrs. B is 5 ft 3 in tall and weighs 110 lb. She is white with fair skin.

NURSING CARE PLAN

SUBJECTIVE DATA Fear of osteoporosis
Family history positive for osteoporosis
Less than AI for calcium previous 24 hours
Met MyPyramid guideline for meat group previous 24 hours
No planned exercise program

OBJECTIVE DATA Height: 5 ft, 3 in
Weight: 110 lb
White, fair, slight build

NURSING DIAGNOSIS NANDA: Health-seeking behavior (NANDA, 2003, with permission) regarding preventive measures for osteoporosis related to fear of repeating aunt's experience as evidenced by request for information

DESIRED OUTCOMES EVALUATION CRITERIA	NURSING ACTIONS/INTERVENTIONS	RATIONALE
NOC: Health-seeking behavior (Moorhead, Johnson, and Maas, 2004, with permission)	NIC: Self-modification assistance (Dochterman and Bulechek, 2004, with permission)	
Client will list appropriate actions to maintain a strong skeleton after teaching session.	Teach client how to consume 1000 mg of calcium daily: 3 cups of milk or equivalent.	One cup of milk contains approximately 300 mg of calcium +100 mg from other sources.
	Teach client factors favoring calcium absorption: moderate protein intake.	High protein intake causes increased calcium excretion by the kidneys.
	Teach client role of exercise in strengthening bones.	Weight-bearing exercise stimulates the osteoblasts to build bone.

C T Q CRITICAL THINKING QUESTIONS

1. What additional dietary information would you need before recommending good sources of calcium for Mrs. B?

2. Suppose Mrs. B implements the suggested interventions.

What other assessment data would be helpful to broaden the scope of preventing osteoporosis?

3. Is the problem described in the Case Study a significant one for a 34-year-old woman? Why or why not?

⟫⟫⟫ CHAPTER REVIEW

1. Like vitamins, minerals give no energy to the body. Unlike vitamins, minerals:
   a. Are completely absorbed from the intestinal tract
   b. Become part of the structure of the body
   c. Cause few clinical problems because of their great abundance in foods
   d. Cannot accumulate to the extent that they cause problems
2. Calcium is necessary for strong bones and teeth. It is also necessary for:
   a. Maintaining stomach acidity
   b. Enabling muscle contraction
   c. Preventing blood clots
   d. Assisting with the production of insulin
3. From which of the following sources of iron is the greatest percentage of iron absorbed by the average person?
   a. Eggs
   b. Ferrous sulfate tablets
   c. Meat
   d. Vegetables
4. Which of the following individuals would be at greatest risk for a mineral deficiency?
   a. Someone who consumes no dairy products
   b. Someone who consumes no shellfish
   c. Someone who consumes no red meat
   d. Someone who drinks tea or coffee with every meal
5. The most common mineral deficiency in the United States is that of:
   a. Calcium
   b. Iodine
   c. Iron
   d. Zinc

✚ CLINICAL ANALYSIS

Mrs. H is a 30-year-old mother of three children all under 5 years of age. On her 6-week postpartum visit, her hemoglobin level was 10 grams per 100 milliliters of blood. She is given a prescription for ferrous sulfate and referred to the office nurse for nutrition counseling regarding her iron intake.

Mrs. H tells the nurse that she eats what the children eat: cold cereal and milk for breakfast, peanut butter and jelly sandwiches and maybe a banana for lunch, and casseroles of tuna or hamburger for dinner. Mrs. H is a heavy coffee drinker, consuming 10 cups per day, two with each meal and a total of four others during "coffee breaks."

The H family is lower-middle class. Mr. H is a long-distance truck driver and is away from home for long intervals. Mrs. H has some knowledge of iron needs and sources because of her three pregnancies. She is reluctant to continue the ferrous sulfate she has been taking throughout her pregnancy. "It binds me up," she tells the nurse. Also, Mrs. H maintains she cannot eat liver: "It gags me."

1. To maximize Mrs. H's iron intake with as little change in her habits as possible, the nurse would want to know:
   a. Whether Mrs. H drinks regular or decaffeinated coffee
   b. What kinds of cereal Mrs. H consumes
   c. At what time of day the H family eats
   d. Whether or not Mrs. H has tried veal liver

2. Which of the following statements by Mrs. H would indicate she understood the nurse's instructions correctly?
   a. "I should eat a little meat, fish, or poultry with every meal containing grain, fruit and vegetable sources of iron."
   b. "I should increase the fiber in my diet because it will increase the absorption of iron."
   c. "If I want an alcoholic beverage, beer contains the most iron in a readily absorbable form."
   d. "Since I am taking an iron supplement, it is not important how I eat."

3. To meet the safety needs of the H children, the nurse instructs Mrs. H to keep her ferrous sulfate in a locked cupboard. The reason for this is:
   a. Interactions of iron tablets with vitamin supplements intended for children can cause deficiencies of water-soluble vitamins.
   b. The human body has no effective means of excreting an overload of iron.
   c. Iron poisoning, although rare, can occur if a child ingests more than 30 tablets of ferrous sulfate.
   d. Because iron binds with calcium, an overdose of iron would cause rickets.

REFERENCES

Abernathy, CO, Thomas, DJ, and Calderon, RL: Health effects and risk assessment of arsenic. J Nutr 133:1536S, 2003.

Abreo, K, et al: The milk-alkali syndrome. Arch Intern Med 153:1005, 1993.

Al-Gurairi, FT, Al-Waiz, M, and Sharquie, KE: Oral zinc sulphate in the treatment of recalcitrant viral warts: Randomized placebo-controlled clinical trial. Br J Dermatol 146:423, 2002.

Albagha, CM, and Ralston, SH: Genetic determinants of susceptibility to osteoporosis. Endocrinol Metab Clin North Am 32:65, 2003.

Althuis, MD, et al: Glucose and insulin responses to dietary chromium supplements: A meta-analysis. Am J Clin Nutr 76:148, 2002.

American Academy of Pediatrics Committee on Environmental Health: Screening for elevated blood lead levels. Pediatrics 101:1072, 1998.

American Dental Association: ADA policy on bottled water, home water treatment systems and fluoride exposure, 2002. Accessed December 8, 2003 at http://www.ada.org/prof/resources/positions/statements/bottledwater.asp.

American Dental Association: Home water treatment systems. Accessed December 8, 2003 at http://www.ada.org/public/topics/documents/art_water_home.pdf.

Andrews, M, and Gallagher-Allred, C: The role of zinc in wound healing. Adv Wound Care 12:137, 1999.

Appendix D. In Kleinman, RE (ed): Pediatric Nutrition Handbook, 5 ed. American Academy of Pediatrics, Elk Grove Village, IL, 2004.

Bch, SB, et al: Nonheme iron absorption from a phytate-rich meal is increased by the addition of small amounts of pork meat. Am J Clin Nutr 77:173, 2003.

Beall, DP, and Scofield, RH: Milk-alkali syndrome associated with calcium carbonate consumption. Medicine 74:89, 1995.

Beard, JL: Effectiveness and strategies of iron supplementation during pregnancy. Am J Clin Nutr 71:1288S, 2000.

Brensilver, JM, and Goldberger, E: A Primer of Water, Electrolyte, and Acid-Base Syndromes, ed 8. FA Davis, Philadelphia, 1996.

Burk, RF, and Levander, OA: Selenium. In Shils, ME, et al (eds): Modern Nutrition in Health and Disease, ed 9. Lippincott Williams & Wilkins, Philadelphia, 1999.

Canfield, RL, et al: Intellectual impairment in children with blood lead concentrations below 10 micrograms per deciliter. N Engl J Med 348:1517, 2003.

Centers for Disease Control: Childhood lead poisoning associated with tamarind candy and folk remedies—California, 1999–2000. MMWR 51:684, 2002a. Accessed November 26, 2003 at http://www.cdc.gov/mmwr/preview/mmwrhtml/mm5131a3.htm.

Centers for Disease Control: Iron deficiency—United States, 1999–2000. MMWR 51:897, 2002b. Accessed April 29, 2004 at http://www.cdc.gov/mmwr/preview/mmwrhtml/mm5140a1.htm.

Centers for Disease Control: Fatal pediatric lead poisoning—New Hampshire, 2000. MMWR 50:457, 2001a. Accessed June 7, 2001 at http://www.cdc.gov/mmwr/preview/mmwrhtml/mm5033a1.htm.

Centers for Disease Control: Occupational and take-home lead poisoning associated with restoring chemically stripped furniture—California, 1998. MMWR 50:246, 2001b. Accessed October 26, 2003 at http://www.cdc.gov/mmwr/preview/mmwrhtml/mm5013a2.htm.

Centers for Disease Control: Recommendations for using fluoride to prevent and control dental caries in the United States. MMWR 50:1, 2001c. Accessed December 4, 2003 at http://www.cdc.gov/mmwr/PDF/RR/RR5014.pdf.

Centers for Disease Control: Achievements in public health, 1900–1999. MMWR 48:905, 1999a. Accessed March 23, 2000 at http://www.cdc.gov/epo/mmwr/preview/mmwrhtml/mm4840a1.htm.

Centers for Disease Control: Water fluoridation and costs of Medicaid treatment for dental decay—Louisiana, 1995–1996. MMWR 48:753, 1999b. Accessed September 6, 1999 at http://www.cdc.gov/epo/mmwr/preview/mmwrhtml/mm4834a2.htm.

Centers for Disease Control: Lead poisoning associated with imported candy and powdered food coloring—California and Michigan. MMWR 47:1041, 1998a. Accessed March 23, 2000 at http://www.cdc.gov/epo/mmwr/preview/mmwrhtml/00055939.htm.

Centers for Disease Control: Recommendations to Prevent and Control Iron Deficiency in the United States. MMWR 47:1, 1998b. Accessed March 26, 2000 at http://www.cdc.gov/epo/mmwr/preview/mmwrhtml/00051880.htm.

Centers for Disease Control: Toddler deaths resulting from ingestion of iron supplements—Los Angeles, 1992–1993. MMWR 42:111, 1993. Accessed November 27, 1999 at http://www.cdc.gov/epo/mmwr/preview/mmwrhtml/00019593.htm

Cerulli, J, et al: Chromium picolinate toxicity. Ann Pharmacother 32:428, 1998.

Chiu, KM, et al: Changes in bone resorption during the menstrual cycle. J Bone Miner Res 14:609, 1999.

Christensen, NK, et al: Juniper ash as a source of calcium in the Navajo diet. J Am Diet Assoc 98:333, 1998.

Coggon, D, and Cooper, C: Fluoridation of water supplies. Br Med J 319:269, 1999. Accessed March 27, 2000 at http://www.bmj.com/cgi/content/full/319/7205/269.

Cohen, AJ, and Roe, FJ: Review of risk factors for osteoporosis with particular reference to a possible aetiological role of dietary salt. Food Chem Toxicol 38:237, 2000.

Connor, JR, and Beard, JL: Dietary iron supplements in the elderly: To use or not to use? Nutr Today 32:102, 1997.

Corvilain, B, et al: Autonomy in endemic goiter. Thyroid 8:107, 1998.

Cuddihy, MT, et al: Osteoporosis intervention following distal forearm fractures: A missed opportunity? Arch Intern Med 152:421, 2002.

Darnton-Hill, I, et al: Iron and folate fortification in the Americas to prevent and control micronutrient malnutrition: An analysis. Nutr Rev 57:25, 1999.

Davidson, MR: Pharmacotherapeutics for osteoporosis prevention and treatment. J Midwifery Womens Health 48:39, 2003.

Dawson-Hughes, B: Interaction of dietary calcium and protein in bone health in humans. J Nutr 133:852S, 2003.

Dawson-Hughes, B, and Harris, SS: Calcium intake influences the association of protein intake with rates of bone loss in elderly men and women. Am J Clin Nutr 75:773, 2002.

Demirkaya, S, et al: Efficacy of intravenous magnesium sulphate in the treatment of acute migraine attacks. Headache 41:171, 2001.

de Silva, A, et al: Iron supplementation improves iron status and reduces morbidity in children with or without upper respiratory tract infections: A randomized controlled study in Colombo, Sri Lanka. Am J Clin Nutr 77:234, 2003.

Dochterman, J, and Bulechek, G (eds): Nursing Interventions Classification (NIC), ed 4. Mosby, St. Louis, 2004.

Doufas, AG, et al: The predominant form of non-toxic goiter in Greece is now autoimmune thyroiditis. Eur J Endocrinol 140:505, 1999.

Dowsett, R, and Shannon, M: Childhood plumbism identified after lead poisoning in household pets [Letter]. N Engl J Med 331:1661, 1994.

Fairbanks, VF: Iron in medicine and nutrition. In Shils, ME, et al (eds): Modern Nutrition in Health and Disease, ed 9. Lippincott Williams & Wilkins, Philadelphia, 1999.

Fairweather-Tait, SJ, Fox, TE, and Mallilin A: Balti curries and iron. Br Med J 310:1368, 1995.

Farrell, SE, et al: Blood lead levels in emergency department patients with retained lead bullets and shrapnel. Acad Emerg Med 6:208, 1999.

Federal Trade Commission: QVC Cable Network and maker of Cold-eeze zinc lozenges agree to settle FTC charges. November 23, 1999. Accessed March 4, 2000 at http://www.ftc.gov/opa/1999/9911/qvcquig.htm.

Feskanich, D, Willett, W, and Colditz, G: Walking and leisure-time activity and risk of hip fracture in postmenopausal women. JAMA 288:2300, 2002.

Flint, GN, and Packirisamy, S: Purity of food cooked in stainless steel utensils. Food Addit Contam 14:115, 1997.

Follin, SL, and Hansen, LB: Current approaches to the prevention and treatment of postmenopausal osteoporosis. Am J Health Syst Pharm 60:883, 2003.

Garcia, E, et al: Estimation of chromium bioavailability from the diet by an in vitro method. Food Addit Contam 18:601, 2001.

George, S, and Clark, JD: Milk alkali syndrome—an unusual syndrome causing an unusual complication. Postgrad Med J 76:422, 2000.

Gerdhem, P, and Obrant, KJ: Effects of cigarette-smoking on bone mass as assessed by dual-energy x-ray absorptiometry and ultrasound. Osteoporos Int 13:932, 2002.

Gibson, RS, Donovan, UM, and Heath, A-LM: Dietary strategies to improve the iron and zinc nutriture of young women following a vegetarian diet. Plant Foods Hum Nutr 51:1, 1997.

Gordeuk, VR, et al: Iron overload in Africans and African-Americans and a common mutation in the SLC40A1 (ferroportin 1) gene. Blood Cells Mol Dis 31:299, 2003.

Gordeuk, VR, et al: Iron overload in Africa. N Engl J Med 326:95, 1992.

Grantham-McGregor, S, and Ani, C: A review of studies on the effect of iron deficiency on cognitive development in children. J Nutr 131:649S, 2001.

Greger, JL, and Sutherland, JE: Aluminum exposure and metabolism. Crit Rev Clin Lab Sci 34:439, 1997.

Gropper, SS, Smith, JL, and Groff, JL: Advanced Nutrition and Human Metabolism, ed 4. Wadsworth, Belmont, CA, 2005.

Hackley, G, and Katz-Jacobson, A: Lead poisoning in pregnancy: A case study with implications for midwives. J Midwifery Womens Health 48:30, 2003.

Hallberg, L, Hulthen, L, and Garby, I: Iron stores in man in relation to diet and iron requirements. Eur J Clin Nutr 52:623, 1998.

Hassan, HA, Netchvolodoff, C, and Raufman, JP: Zinc-induced copper deficiency in a coin swallower. Am J Gastroenterol 95:2975, 2000.

Heaney, RP: Effects of caffeine on bone and the calcium economy. Food Chem Toxicol 40:1263, 2002.

Heaney, RP: Calcium, dairy products, and osteoporosis. J Am Coll Nutr 19:83S, 2000.

Hetzel, BS, and Clugston, GA: Iodine. In Shils, ME, et al (eds): Modern Nutrition in Health and Disease, ed 9. Lippincott Williams & Wilkins, Philadelphia, 1999.

Holben, DH, and Smith, AM: The diverse role of selenium within selenoproteins: A review. J Am Diet Assoc 99:836, 1999.

Iinuma, Y, et al: Whole-blood manganese levels and brain manganese accumulation in children receiving long-term home parenteral nutrition. Pediatr Surg Int 19:268, 2003.

Indiana University Purdue University Indianapolis: Formula may not provide babies with adequate fluoride. News Release, July 7, 2000. Accessed December 3, 2003 at http://www.iupui.edu/news/formula.htm.

Institute of Medicine: Dietary Reference Intakes for Water, Potassium, Sodium Chloride, and Sulfate. National Academies Press, Washington, DC, 2004. Accessed March 31, 2004 at http://www.nap.edu/openbook/0309091691/html/1.html.

Institute of Medicine: Dietary Reference Intakes: Elements. National Academy of Sciences, Washington, DC. Accessed November 5, 2003 at http://www.eds.od.nih.gov/showpage.aspx?pageid=89.

Institute of Medicine Food and Nutrition Board: Dietary Reference Intakes for Vitamin A, Vitamin K, Arsenic, Boron, Chromium, Copper, Iodine, Iron Manganese, Molybdenum, Nickel, Silicon, Vanadium, and Zinc. National Academies Press, Washington, DC, 2001.

Jackson, JL, Lesho, E, and Peterson, C: Zinc and the common cold: A meta-analysis revisited. J Nutr 130:1512S, 2000.

Johnson, MA, Smith, MM, and Edmonds, JT: Copper, iron, zinc, and manganese in dietary supplements, infant formulas, and ready-to-eat breakfast cereals. Am J Clin Nutr 67:1035S, 1998.

Kafritsa, Y, et al: Long-term outcome of brain manganese deposition in patients on home parenteral nutrition. Arch Dis Child 79:262, 1998.

Kaleita, TA, Kinsbourne, M, and Menkes, JH: A neurobehavioral syndrome after failure to thrive on chloride-deficient formula. Dev Med Child Neurol 33:626, 1991.

Kaufmann, RB, Staes, CJ, and Matte, TD: Deaths related to lead poisoning in the United States, 1979–1998. Environ Res 91:78, 2003.

King, JC, and Keen, CL: Zinc. In Shils, ME, et al (eds): Modern Nutrition in Health and Disease, ed 9. Lippincott Williams & Wilkins, Philadelphia, 1999.

Knochel, JP: Phosphorus. In Shils, ME, et al (eds): Modern Nutrition in Health and Disease, ed 9. Lippincott Williams & Wilkins, Philadelphia, 1999.

Komarnisky, LA, Christopherson, RJ, and Basu, TK: Sulfur: Its clinical and toxicologic aspects. Nutrition 19:54, 2003.

Krall, EA, and Dawson-Hughes, B: Osteoporosis. In Shils, ME, et al (eds): Modern Nutrition in Health and Disease, ed 9. Lippincott Williams & Wilkins, Philadelphia, 1999.

Lau, EM, and Woo, J: Nutrition and osteoporosis. Curr Opin Rheumatol 10:368, 1998.

Leitzmann, MF, et al: Zinc supplement use and risk of prostate cancer. J Natl Cancer Inst 95:1004, 2003.

Looker, AC, et al: Prevalence of iron deficiency in the United States. JAMA 277:973, 1997.

Lozoff, B, et al: Poorer behavioral and developmental outcome more than 10 years after treatment for iron deficiency in infancy. Pediatrics 105:E51, 2000.

Lubin, BH, et al: Nutritional anemias. In Walker, WA, and Watkins, JB (eds): Nutrition in Pediatrics, ed 2. BC Decker, Hamilton, Ontario, 1997.

Martini, L, and Wood, RJ: Relative bioavailability of calcium-rich dietary sources in the elderly. Am J Clin Nutr 76:1345, 2002.

Marzec, Z: Alimentary chromium, nickel, and selenium intake of adults in Poland estimated by analysis and calculations using the duplicate portion technique. Nahrung 48:47, 2004.

Masumoto, K, et al: Manganese intoxication during intermittent parenteral nutrition: Report of two cases. JPEN J Parenter Enteral Nutr 25:95, 2001.

McElroy, BH, and Miller, SP: Effectiveness of zinc gluconate glycine lozenges (Cold-Eeze) against the common cold in school-aged subjects: A retrospective chart review. Am J Ther 9:472, 2002.

Meyer, PA, et al: Surveillance for elevated blood lead levels among children—United States, 1997–2001. MMWR 52:SS10, 2003. Accessed November 30, 2003 at http://www.cdc.gov/mmwr/PDF/ss/ss5210.pdf.

Miller, MB, et al: Pool cue chalk: A source of environmental lead. Pediatrics 97:916, 1996.

Moorhead, S, Johnson, M, and Maas, M (eds): Nursing Outcomes Classification (NOC), ed 3. Mosby, St. Louis, 2004.

Mowad, E, Haddad, I, and Gemmel, DJ: Management of lead poisoning from ingested fishing sinkers. Arch Pediatr Adolesc Med 152:485, 1998.

NANDA International: Nursing Diagnoses: Definitions and Classification 2003–2004. NANDA International, Philadelphia, 2003.

National Osteoporosis Foundation: Disease statistics, Fast Facts. 2003. Accessed November 17, 2003 at http://www.nof.org/osteoporosis/stats.htm.

National Research Council: Diet and Health: Implications for Reducing Chronic Disease Risk. Report of the Committee on Diet and Health, Food and Nutrition Board, Commission on Life Sciences. National Academy Press, Washington, DC, 1989.

Need, AG, et al: Relationships between intestinal calcium absorption, serum vitamin D metabolites and smoking in postmenopausal women. Osteoporos Int 13:83, 2002.

New, SA: Alcohol and bone health. Medscape Ob/Gyn & Women's Health 8(2), 2003a. Accessed November 19, 2003 at http://www.medscape.com/viewarticle/460433.

New, SA: Fruit and vegetables and bone health. Medscape Ob/Gyn & Women's Health 8(2), 2003b. Accessed October 12, 2003 at http://www.medscape.com/viewarticles/460440_print.

Nielsen, FH: Ultratrace minerals. In Shils, ME, et al (eds): Modern Nutrition in Health and Disease, ed 9. Lippincott Williams & Wilkins, Philadelphia, 1999.

Nielsen, FH, and Milne, DB: A moderately high intake compared to a low intake of zinc depresses magnesium balance and alters indices of bone turnover in postmenopausal women. Eur J Clin Nutr 58:703, 2004.

NIH Consensus Development Panel on Osteoporosis Prevention, Diagnosis, and Therapy, March 7–29, 2000: Highlights of the Conference. South Med J 94:569, 2001.

Olivares, M, et al: Copper in infant nutrition: Safety of World Health Organization provisional guideline value for copper content of drinking water. J Pediatr Gastroenterol Nutr 26:251, 1998.

Parcell, S: Sulfur in human nutrition and application in medicine. Alter Med Rev 7:22, 2002.

Raymond, LW, et al: Maternal-fetal lead poisoning from a 15-year-old bullet. J Matern Fetal Neonatal Med 11:63, 2002.

Remer, T, Neubert, A, and Manz, F: Increased risk of iodine deficiency with vegetarian nutrition. Brit J Nutr 81:45, 1999.

Roscoe, RJ, et al: Adult blood lead epidemiology and surveillance—United States, 1998–2001. MMWR 51:1, 2002. Accessed November 30, 2003 at http://www.cdc.gov/mmwr/preview/mmwrhtml/ss5111a1.htm.

Ross, EA, Szabo, NJ, and Tebbett, IR: Lead content of calcium supplements. JAMA 284:1425, 2000.

Rossouw, JE, et al: Risks and benefits of estrogen plus progestin in healthy postmenopausal women: Principal results from the Women's Health Initiative randomized controlled trial. JAMA 288: 321, 2002.

Rostan, EF, et al: Evidence supporting zinc as an important antioxidant for skin. Int J Dermatol 41:606, 2002.

Santinelli, et al: Magnesium deficiency and dizziness: A case of electrolyte imbalance. Geriatrics 54:67, 1999.

Santolaria, F, et al: Osteopenia assessed by body composition analysis is related to malnutrition in alcoholic patients. Alcohol 22:147, 2000.

Sardesai, VM: Molybdenum: An essential trace element. Nutr Clin Pract 8:277, 1993.

Saungweme, T, et al: Iron and alcohol content of traditional beers in rural Zimbabwe. Cent Afr J Med 45:136, 1999.

Scelfo, GM, and Flegal, AR: Lead in calcium supplements. Environ Health Perspect 108:309, 2000.

Schnell, AB, Van Leeuwen, AM, and Kranpitz, TR: Davis's Comprehensive Handbook of Laboratory and Diagnostic Tests with Nursing Implications. FA Davis, Philadelphia, 2003.

Shannon, M, and Graef, J: Hazard of lead in infant formula [Letter]. N Engl J Med 326:137, 1992.

Shils, ME: Magnesium. In Shils, ME, et al (eds): Modern Nutrition in Health and Disease, ed 9. Lippincott Williams & Wilkins, Philadelphia, 1999.

Sidney Morning Herald: Bottled water linked to child tooth decay. April, 16, 2003. Accessed December 4, 2003 at http://www.smh.com.au/articles/2003/04/16/1050172643083.html.

Stainikowicz, R: The significance of routine serum magnesium determination in the ED. Am J Emerg Med 21:444, 2003.

Stoecker, BJ: Chromium. In Shils, ME, et al (eds): Modern Nutrition in Health and Disease, ed 9. Lippincott Williams & Wilkins, Philadelphia, 1999.

Sungthong, R, Mo-suwan, L, and Chongsuvivatwong, V: Effects of haemoglobin and serum ferritin on cognitive function in school-children. Asia Pac J Clin Nutr 11:117, 2002.

Sunyer, T, et al: Estrogen's bone-protective effects may involve differential IL-1 receptor regulation in human osteoclast-like cells. J Clin Invest 103:1409, 1999.

Szulc, P, et al: Increased bone resorption in moderate smokers with low body weight: The Minos study. J Clin Endocrinol Metab 87:666, 2002.

Temme, EH, and Van Hoydonck, PG: Tea consumption and iron status. Eur J Clin Nutr 56:379, 2002.

Thomson, CD: Assessment of requirements for selenium and adequacy of selenium status: A review. Eur J Clin Nutr 58:391, 2004.

Trauninger, A, et al: Oral magnesium load test in patients with migraine. Headache 42:114, 2002.

Tsukada, H, et al: Intrathoracic retroesophageal goiter causing tracheal stenosis. Jpn J Thorac Cardiovasc Surg 47:174, 1999.

Turner, RT: Skeletal response to alcohol. Alcohol Clin Exp Res 24:1693, 2000.

Turnlund, JR: Copper. In Shils, ME, et al (eds): Modern Nutrition in Health and Disease, ed 9. Lippincott Williams & Wilkins, Philadelphia, 1999.

United States Department of Agriculture: Results for USDA's 1994–96 Diet and Health Knowledge Survey: Table Set 19, 2000. Accessed November 17, 2003 at http://www.barc.usda.gov/bhnrc/foodsurvey/home.htm.

United States Food and Drug Administration: Iron-containing supplements and drugs: Label warning statements and unit-dose packaging requirements; removal of regulations for unit-dose packaging requirements for dietary supplements and drugs. Final rule; removal of regulatory provisions in response to court order. Fed Regist 68:59714, 2003. Accessed May 20, 2004 at http://www.gpoaccess.gov/fr/index.html.

United States Preventive Services Task Force: Screening for osteoporosis in postmenopausal women: Recommendations and rationale, 2002. Accessed November 17, 2003 at http://www.ahrq.gov/clinic/3rduspstf/osteoporosis/osteorr.htm.

Valtola, A, et al: Lifestyle and other factors predict ankle fractures in perimenopausal women: A population-based prospective cohort study. Bone 30:238, 2002.

Vanpee, D, et al: Ingestion of antacid tablets (Rennie) and acute confusion. J Emerg Med 19:169, 2000.

Venes, D (ed): Taber's Cyclopedic Medical Dictionary, ed 19. FA Davis, Philadelphia, 2001.

Weaver, CM, and Heaney, RP: Calcium. In Shils, ME, et al (eds): Modern Nutrition in Health and Disease, ed 9. Lippincott Williams & Wilkins, Philadelphia, 1999.

Wilhelm, M, et al: Aluminum balance in intensive care patients. J Trace Elem Med Biol. 14:223, 2001.

Wilkinson, EA, and Hawke, CI: Oral zinc for arterial and venous leg ulcers. Cochrane Database Syst Rev 2000(2), 2000.

Yamashita, H, et al: Postoperative tetany in Graves disease: Important role for vitamin D metabolites. Ann Surg 229:237, 1999.

Zhou, Y, and Brittin, HC: Increased iron content of some Chinese foods due to cooking in steel woks. J Am Diet Assoc 94:1153, 1994.

Water and Body Fluids

After completing this chapter, the student should be able to:

1. Describe the locations and functions of water in the body.
2. Discuss the body's control mechanisms for maintaining fluid and electrolyte balance.
3. Recognize how buffer systems maintain acid-base balance.
4. List amounts of water recommended for young adults and situations that would increase the amounts.
5. Differentiate insensible from sensible water loss.
6. Identify methods of assessing water balance in the body.
7. Distinguish between heat exhaustion and heat stroke as to signs and symptoms and first-aid treatment.

Water is the largest single constituent of the human body, and the need for water is more urgent than the need for any other nutrient. Human beings can live 1 month without food but only 6 days without water. This chapter explains why water is so important in the body and details ways in which water balance is achieved. The assessment and treatment of deficient fluid volume and excess fluid volume are also included.

The distribution and movement of water in the body are intricately bound to certain elements. Understanding this relationship requires knowledge of the essentials of atomic structure. This chapter begins, then, with a brief explanation of how atoms interact with one another.

Interactions Between Atoms

An element is a primary, simple substance that cannot be broken down by ordinary chemical methods into any other substance. There are 110 named elements. Oxygen is an element, as are sodium, chlorine, and the other minerals considered in the previous chapter.

Atoms

Elements are composed of smaller parts called **atoms.** In the center of an atom is the nucleus, which contains protons and neutrons and gives an atom its weight and mass. Circling around the nucleus like satellites are electrons. These electrons are arranged in a consistent manner: a maximum of two in the orbit or shell closest to the nucleus, and a maximum of eight in each of the outer shells. The ability of an atom to react chemically depends on the number of "empty slots" in the outermost electron shell.

Chemical Bonding

A **compound** is a substance created by the chemical bonding (joining) of two or more different kinds of atoms (elements). A chemical bond is the force that binds atoms together. A compound is formed when atoms share electrons or when one atom donates one or more electrons to another atom. For example, water (a liquid) is formed when two atoms of hydrogen (a colorless, odorless gas) are joined with one atom of oxygen (another colorless, odorless gas).

Similarly, sodium chloride (table salt) is a compound of sodium (an unstable, silvery white, waxy, soft metal) and chlorine (a greenish yellow poisonous gas). Sodium and chlorine are so chemically active that in nature they are always found bound to each other or to other elements (Fig. 9–1).

A sodium atom has only one electron in its outer shell; a chlorine atom has seven. In close proximity, the sodium atom donates the electron in its outer shell to the outer shell of the chlorine atom. With the loss of its electron, the sodium now has an electrical charge of $+1$ and is called a sodium **ion** (Na^+). Ions with positive charges are referred to as **cations.** The chlorine atom, which gained an electron, now has a charge of -1 and is called a chloride ion (Cl^-). Ions with negative charges are referred to as **anions.**

Because these ions have opposite charges ($+$ and $-$), they are attracted to one another and unite, forming sodium chloride (NaCl). The chemical bond that holds the

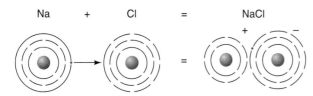

Figure **9–1** Formation of an ionic bond. An atom of sodium loses an electron to an atom of chlorine. The two ions formed have unlike charges, are attracted to one another, and form a molecule of sodium chloride. (Reprinted from Scanlon and Sanders, 2003, p 24, with permission.)

sodium and chloride ions together is called an **ionic bond.** There are other types of chemical bonds (not elaborated upon here). Sodium can donate its single electron to other elements beside chlorine, and other elements can form ionic bonds as well.

An **electrolyte** is an element or compound that, when dissolved in water, separates (dissociates) into ions capable of conducting an electrical current. These electrically charged particles are then available to take part in other chemical reactions. Clinical Application 9–1 gives examples of uses and hazards related to electrolytes in the body.

Distribution of Water in the Body

More than half of body weight is water, which is found in and around the cells, within the blood and lymph vessels, and in various body cavities. Some tissues have significantly more water than others: muscle tissue is 70 percent water, fat tissue is 30 percent water, and bone tissue is 10

Clinical Application 9–1

Diagnostic Uses and Potential Hazards of Electrolytes

Skin sensors attached to an electrocardiograph can trace the electrical activity of the heart. The resulting graphic record is called an **electrocardiogram (ECG)**. The machine's sensors on the skin can detect the electric current because the blood is an electrolyte solution and thus capable of conducting electricity. The same principle applies to the use of an electroencephalograph, a device that traces brain-wave activity. The record obtained from this machine is called an **electroencephalogram (EEG)**.

The same characteristic of electrolyte solutions that allows these machines to sense electrical activity can also be hazardous. A fluid-filled tube, such as a nasogastric tube or catheter, can conduct stray electricity from faulty electrical devices to the client's heart, which could result in dysrhythmias. The amount of electricity in the shock may be minuscule but enough to be fatal if it happens at the wrong time in the cardiac cycle. The health-care worker should be particularly vigilant for defective electrical equipment in the clinical setting. Such equipment should be tagged for repair and replaced immediately.

percent water. A man's body is 60 to 65 percent water, and a woman's body is 50 to 54 percent water. Men have higher water content than women because of their greater muscle mass. The body of a 70-kg (154-lb) man would contain about 42 liters of water.

Age also affects the proportion of water in a body. Compared with the 50 to 65 percent for women and men, an infant's body is 75 percent water. Premature infants may be 80 percent water by weight. Infants, especially premature infants, are at high risk of fluid imbalances because of the proportion and distribution of water in their bodies. The adult proportion of water to body weight is reached at about 3 years of age (Gropper, Smith, and Groff, 2005). The proportion of intracellular or extracellular water to total body water was found to be similar in younger adults and in those over the age of 60. The same finding was true for the proportion of intracellular water to fat-free mass, leading to the conclusion that hydration of fat-free mass and cellular hydration are not affected in healthy aging. This does not negate the risk of dehydration in diseased elderly persons (Ritz, 2000).

Fluid Compartments

Body fluids are contained in intracellular and extracellular compartments (see Fig. 9–2). These compartments are separated by semipermeable membranes, which allow some substances to pass through and prevent the passage of other substances. Water passes freely through the membranes. Eleven water transport proteins, called aquaporins, have been identified, each with a distinct distribution throughout the body (Yasui, 2004). Aquaporins are membrane proteins that function as water-selective channels in the plasma membranes of many cells and help to explain the speed at which water moves across cell membranes (Dibas, Mia, and Yorio, 1998; Knoers and Deen, 1998). They are intimately involved in the production of cerebrospinal fluid and the control of water movement at the blood-brain barrier (Griesdale and Honey, 2004). Specifically, aquaporin-4 was increased in human brains after traumatic brain injury, within brain-derived tumors, and around brain tumors (Hu et al, 2005). At least 5 aquaporins are found in the eye that may lead to new treatments for glaucoma, corneal edema, and other diseases of the eye involving abnormalities in intraocular pressure or tissue hydration (Verkman, 2003). As more is learned about aquaporins in health, it may be possible to develop new drug treatments to target specific areas of malfunction in disease.

Intracellular Fluid

The fluid inside the cells is called intracellular. In adults, intracellular water constitutes 65 percent of body water. In infants, 46 percent of the body water is intracellular.

Extracellular Fluid

All fluid outside the cells is extracellular. In adults, 35 percent of the body's water is extracellular; in infants, 54 percent is extracellular. Figure 9–3 illustrates the proportions of intracellular to extracellular fluid in men, women, and infants. The difference is important, because extracellular fluid is more easily and rapidly lost to the outside of the

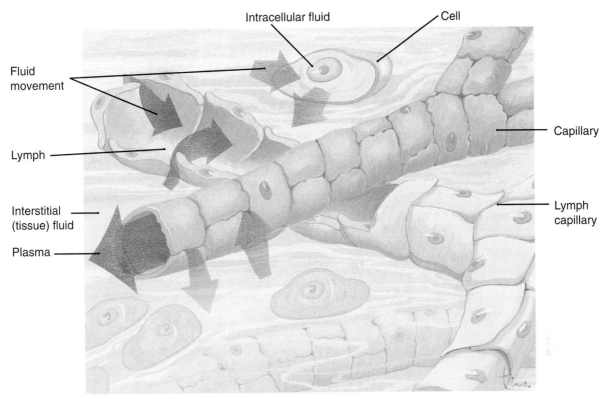

Figure **9–2** Water compartments, showing the names water is given in its different locations and the ways in which water moves between compartments. (Reprinted from Scanlon and Sanders, 2003, p 27, with permission.)

body than is intracellular fluid. **Extracellular fluid** includes interstitial, intravascular, lymph, and transcellular fluids.

INTERSTITIAL FLUID

Located between the cells or surrounding the cells, **interstitial fluid** assists in transporting substances between the cells and the blood and lymph vessels.

INTRAVASCULAR FLUID

Intravascular fluid is found within the blood vessels, arteries, arterioles, capillaries, venules, and veins. The liquid part of the blood is called **plasma;** minus the clotting elements, the liquid part of the blood is called **serum.** As is illustrated in Figure 9–4, 91.5 percent of the plasma is water.

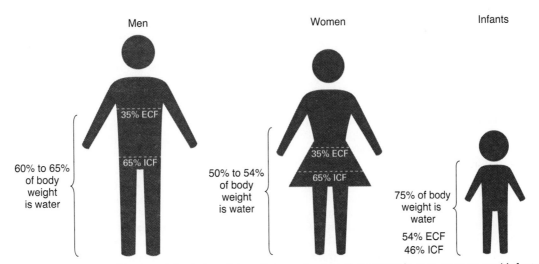

Figure **9–3** The relative amounts of body weight that are intracellular and extracellular water in men, women, and infants.

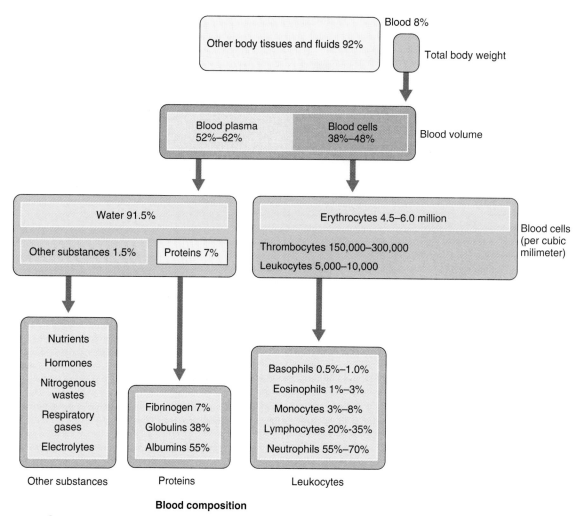

Blood composition

Components of blood and relationship of blood to other body tissues

Figure **9–4** The blood constitutes 8 percent of the body weight. The largest single component of the blood is water. (Reprinted from Venes, 2001, p 251, with permission.)

LYMPHATIC FLUID

The venous system cannot collect and return all the fluid from the tissues to the heart. The **lymph,** via the lymphatic vessels, assists in returning the fluid part of the blood to the heart.

TRANSCELLULAR FLUID

The **transcellular fluids** include cerebrospinal fluid, pericardial fluid, pleural fluid, synovial fluid, intraocular fluids, and gastrointestinal secretions. The transcellular fluids are constantly being secreted into their spaces and reabsorbed into the vascular system.

Functions of Water

Water has important functions in the body. As a component of cells, water helps give the body shape and form, and as the major constituent of blood, it helps to maintain blood volume and blood pressure. It is part of the struc-

ture of many of the body's large molecules, such as protein and glycogen. Some body water also serves as a lubricant, as in mucus secretions and joint fluid.

Water helps to regulate body temperature. It absorbs the heat produced by fever and the heat resulting from metabolic processes. On average, tissue metabolism generates 100 kilocalories per hour. The blood carries excess heat to the skin, where it is dissipated by sweating or radiation. (Clinical Calculation 9–4 gives an example involving evaporative water loss in fever.)

Water is a **solvent** for minerals, vitamins, glucose, and other small molecules. (The substance that is dissolved in a solvent is called a **solute.**) As a solvent, water is able to transport nutrients to the cells and carry waste products away from the cells. In addition, it becomes a medium for chemical reactions and participates in chemical reactions, as may be seen in many of the digestive processes, such as the breakdown of proteins to amino acids. See Box 9–1 for a summary of the functions of water in the body.

Functions of Water

- Gives shape and form to cells
- Helps form the structure of large molecules
- Serves as a lubricant
- Helps to regulate body temperature
- Serves as a solvent
- Transports nutrients to cells
- Carries waste products away from cells
- Is a medium for chemical reactions
- Participates in chemical reactions

Absorption, Metabolism, and Storage of Water

No storage tanks for water exist in the body. Water continually moves from one body compartment to another and is often reused by the body to perform different tasks. A small amount of water can be absorbed into the bloodstream from the stomach but a liter of water can be absorbed from the small intestine in an hour.

The metabolism of the energy nutrients produces water. Each energy nutrient produces a different amount of metabolic water: 1 gram of carbohydrate produces 0.60 gram, 1 gram of fat produces 1.07 grams, and 1 gram of protein produces 0.41 gram. One ounce of pure alcohol requires 8 ounces of water for its metabolism. Alcohol also blocks antidiuretic hormone (ADH) activity, thus permitting more water to be spilled in the urine (Klotz, 1998). Alcohol, rather than quenching thirst, can cause dehydration and increased thirst.

Under conditions that have disrupted the individual's automatic adaptive mechanisms, water may be retained. The accumulation of excessive amounts of fluid between the cells (in the interstitial compartments) is called **edema.** Hypothyroidism, congestive heart failure, severe protein deficiency, and some kidney conditions may cause such water retention. Excessive water also can be dispersed throughout the body. This condition is called **water intoxication.** It can be caused by excessive water intake (either by the intravenous or gastrointestinal route), cerebral concussion, or hormonal disorders. Many of the symptoms are caused by diluting the concentration of the electrolytes in the body's fluid compartments.

Water Balance

For optimum health, the water lost through the kidneys, skin, lungs, and large intestine must be continually replaced. The electrolyte content of all body fluids must also be maintained within narrow limits. The body has automatic monitoring and regulating mechanisms to achieve this balance or homeostasis.

The Effect of Electrolytes on Water Balance

Each fluid compartment has an electrolyte composition that best serves its needs. Each of the fluid compartments has automatic mechanisms that are designed to keep it electrically neutral or balanced. The positive ions within a compartment must equal the negative ones. When shifts and losses occur, compensating shifts and gains take place to reestablish electroneutrality.

Regulation of Fluid Balance

Fluid balance is regulated by electrolytes because cells have no mechanism for holding onto water molecules, which pass freely through all membranes. However, cells can control the movement of electrolytes, and water tends to remain wherever the concentration of electrolytes is highest. Except in some tubules of the kidney, water will follow high concentrations of electrolytes such as sodium, the ion most closely associated with water balance.

Important Body Electrolytes

Major mineral ions strongly influence not only water balance but also osmotic pressure, blood pressure, and acid-base balance, which will be covered later in this chapter. Cations of importance in body fluids are sodium, potassium, calcium, and magnesium. Anions of importance include chloride, bicarbonate, phosphate, and sulfate. Sodium (Na^+) is the main electrolyte in extracellular fluid (ECF). Potassium (K^+) is the main electrolyte in **intracellular fluid** (ICF). Ionized sodium, potassium, and chloride are the solutes that maintain the balance between the intracellular and extracellular compartments. See Table 9–1 for a summary of the major body electrolytes.

Measurement of Electrolytes

Electrolytes are measured by the total number of particles in solution rather than their total weight, because chemical activity is determined by the concentration of electrolytes in any given solution. The unit of measure used in the United States is the **milliequivalent** expressed as milliequivalents per liter. The concentration of a pharmaceutical electrolyte in solution is also measured in milliequivalents per liter. Clinical Calculation 9–1 shows the conversion of milligrams of sodium chloride to milliequivalents.

Osmotic Pressure

Osmosis is the movement of water (or another solvent) across a semipermeable membrane from an area with fewer particles to one with more particles. The result, as long as the difference is reasonable, is an equalization of concentration on either side of the membrane. Clinical Application 9–2 describes an experiment to demonstrate osmosis.

Osmosis is a passive process. The movement of some substances, however, is active. Some substances require active transport mechanisms to push them through a membrane. Two such transport mechanisms are the sodium pump and the potassium pump. Located in cell membranes, these pumps are actually proteins that can move ions. **Sodium pumps** move sodium ions out of the cells (and the water follows). **Potassium pumps** move potassium ions into the cells. In this manner, the electrolyte

Table 9–1 Major Body Electrolytes

ELECTROLYTE	FLUID COMPARTMENT*	FUNCTIONS
CATIONS		
Sodium (Na$^+$)	Extracellular	Major cation in ECF. Na$^+$ concentration in fluids determines the distribution of H$_2$O by osmosis. With Cl$^-$ and HCO$_3^-$, Na$^+$ regulates acid-base balance.
Potassium (K$^+$)	Intracellular	Major cation in ICF. K$^+$ with Na$^+$ maintains water balance. With Na$^+$ and H$^+$, K$^+$ regulates acid-base balance.
Calcium	Extracellular†	Participates in permeability of cell membranes, transmission of nerve impulses, muscle action.
Magnesium (Mg^{2+})	Intracellular	Regulates nerve simulation and normal muscle action.
ANIONS		
Chloride (Cl$^-$)	Extracellular	Major anion in ECF. Helps maintain water balance and acid-base balance.
Bicarbonate (HCO$_3^-$)	Extracellular	Most important ECF buffer.
Phosphate (HPO$_4^{2-}$)	Intracellular	Within the ICF, phosphates and proteins buffer 95 percent of the body's carbonic acid and 50 percent of other acids.

*ECP and ICF both contain all the cations and anions listed in this table but are labeled as either ECP or ICF according to the concentration. For example, sodium ions make up 142 of the total 155 milliequivalents per liter (of the cations) in the ECF.
†Of the cations, 3 percent in ECF and 1 percent in ICF.

concentrations of the intracellular and extracellular fluid compartments are maintained. Active transport requires energy.

DETERMINATION OF OSMOTIC PRESSURE

When two solutions on either side of a semipermeable membrane have different concentrations, pressure develops. This pressure, which is exerted on the semipermeable membrane, is called **osmotic pressure.** Osmotic pressure causes a solvent such as water to cross the membrane, while the solutes (particles) that are outside the membrane cannot go through.

The size of the molecule and its ability to ionize determines the number of particles in a given concentration. Electrolytes readily ionize in solution. Disaccharides and monosaccharides do not ionize. Without the appropriate enzymes to split the disaccharide into its component monosaccharides, the disaccharide molecule remains intact. Just as there are more tacks in a pound than there are spikes in a pound, there are more particles in a given volume containing 100 kilocalories of a monosaccharide such as glucose compared with 100 kilocalories of a disaccharide such as lactose. The larger number of particles per unit volume exerts more osmotic pressure.

 Clinical Calculation 9–1

Converting Milligrams to Milliequivalents

Milligram is a measure of weight. Milliequivalent is a measure of the concentration of electrolytes (number of particles) per volume of solution. The usual amount of solution on which electrolytes are reported is 1 L.

To convert milligrams to milliequivalents, it is necessary to know the number of milligrams per liter, the molecular weight of the substance, and its valence. Valence, a number indicating the combining power of an atom, is found in many dictionaries.

A teaspoonful of table salt in 1 L of water will produce a 0.5-percent solution. (Isotonic sodium chloride is 0.9 percent.) How would the electrolytes be reported in milliequivalents? A teaspoonful is roughly 5 g. Since table salt is 40 percent sodium and 60 percent chloride, the liter of 0.5 percent salt water would contain 2 g (2000 mg) of sodium and 3 g (3000 mg) of chloride.

Two other values are needed: atomic or molecular weights, and valences. The atomic weight for sodium is 22.9898. Sodium has a valence of 1. The formula for converting milligrams to milliequivalents is:

$$mEq/L = \frac{(mg/L) \times valence}{molecular\ weight}$$

Filling in the sodium values we know for this case, we have:

$$mEq/L = \frac{2000\ (mg/L) \times 1}{22.9898} = 87\ mEq/L\ of\ sodium$$

Continuing, we can use the same formula with different values to calculate the milliequivalents of chloride. The atomic weight for chlorine is 35.453. Chlorine has a valence of 1.

Filling in the values for chloride, we have:

$$mEq/L = \frac{3000\ (mg/L) \times 1}{35.453} = 85\ mEq/L\ of\ chloride$$

Then, adding the sodium and chloride, we have:

$$87 + 85 = 172\ mEq/L\ in\ the\ 0.5\text{-}percent\ solution.$$

Osmosis in the Kitchen

To make sauerkraut, the cabbage is sliced very fine and placed in the bottom of a crock. Salt is then added to the dry cabbage. This is repeated, layer after layer, until the crock is full. At this point, much liquid already will have gathered, pulled from the cabbage pieces by the concentrated salt. After the cabbage ferments for 5 or 6 weeks, the crock is full of "extra" juice.

To try a tiny batch of sauerkraut, use 2 tsp of canning salt per pound of cabbage.

OSMOLARITY OF BODY FLUIDS

The measure of the osmotic pressure exerted by the number of particles per volume of liquid is referred to as its **osmolarity.** The unit of measure for osmotic activity is the **milliosmole.** Clinically, osmolarity is usually reported in milliosmoles per liter.

Osmolality, in contrast, is the measure of the osmotic pressure exerted by the number of particles per weight of solvent. Clinically, osmolality is usually reported in milliosmoles per kilogram. It has the advantage over osmolarity of being unaffected by temperature but is less convenient to measure (Gropper, Smith, and Groff, 2005). The normal value for osmolality of human blood serum is about 275 to 295 milliosmoles per kilogram. Critical values are those less than 265 or more than 320 milliosmoles per kilogram (Schnell, Leeuwen, and Kranpitz, 2003). In the extracellular fluid, sodium is the primary determinant of osmolality.

OSMOLALITY AND NUTRITION

Fluids are designated **isotonic** if they approximate the osmolality of the blood plasma, for example, 5 percent glucose in water and 0.9 percent sodium chloride. Fluids exerting less osmotic pressure than plasma are labeled **hypotonic.** Those exerting greater osmotic pressure than plasma are called **hypertonic.**

Achieving the correct osmolality of fluids administered intravenously (by needle or tube into the vein) is very important. A solution that is too concentrated pulls water out of the red blood cells, and the cells shrivel and die. A solution that is too weak allows water to be pulled into the red blood cells until the cells burst. For these reasons, isotonic sodium chloride is given with red blood cell products to avoid shrinking or bursting the red blood cells.

Solutions containing sufficient nutrients to provide all a person's known needs are so hypertonic that they must be infused into a very large vein so that they are diluted quickly by the liberal volume of blood flowing past the infusion port or catheter. This procedure is described in Chapter 15.

Oral fluids also can be categorized by osmotic pressure. Plain water is hypotonic. Whole milk at 275 milliosmoles per liter is close to isotonic but is not recommended for infants for another reason (see Clinical Application 12–2). Ginger ale with 510 milliosmoles per liter and 7-Up with 640 are both hypertonic. The significance of these differences will become apparent in the later section on treatment of deficient fluid volume.

SERUM ELECTROLYTES

The electrolyte content of blood can also be reported in milliequivalents per liter. Normal serum sodium is 135 to 145 milliequivalents per liter. In most cases, because sodium is the most influential extracellular ion, osmolarity of the extracellular fluid can be estimated clinically by doubling the serum sodium value. Normal serum sodium doubled would be 270 to 296 milliosmoles per liter. Normal osmolality of the serum is about 300 milliosmoles per kilogram. This simple method gives a close approximation.

The other ion that health-care providers monitor carefully in clients with potential fluid and electrolyte imbalances is potassium. Most of the potassium in the body is inside the cells, at a concentration of 150 milliequivalents per liter. By contrast, potassium concentration in the blood is only 3.5 to 5.0 milliequivalents per liter. Even slight variations above or below these values can produce severe consequences. The heart muscle is particularly sensitive to high or low levels of potassium; abnormal levels can produce cardiac arrest.

Electrolyte Imbalances

Table 9–2 lists the normal values for serum sodium and serum potassium, along with the technical names and some of the signs and symptoms for deviations from normal. Many other signs, including the direct measurement of serum electrolytes and the results of electrocardiograms, assist in the diagnosis. Dire consequences can result from any of these four imbalances. If the nurse recognizes and reports early signs and symptoms, the need for drastic treatment measures may be averted. Unfortunately, older clients may display fewer signs and symptoms than younger ones do. The clinical chapters in Unit III present more information about electrolyte imbalances that commonly accompany various disease conditions.

The Effect of Plasma Proteins on Water Balance

The body has highly developed mechanisms that maintain the constant flow of water and nutrients to the cells and the flow of water and waste materials from the cells. Adequate blood pressure is necessary for this transport system to function. Blood pressure is the force exerted against the walls of the arteries by the beating heart. It is reported in two numbers, 120/80, for example (measured in millimeters of mercury). The top number is the pressure when the heart beats, called **systolic pressure.** The bottom number is the pressure between beats, called the **diastolic pressure.** One of the factors necessary to maintain blood pressure is a sufficient volume of blood in the arteries and veins.

Water and nutrients in the blood are pushed out through the thin walls of the capillaries into the interstitial fluid by **hydrostatic pressure** (blood pressure) supplied by the heart. From the interstitial compartment, the water and nutrients cross cell membranes to bathe and nourish the cell. Plasma proteins, including **albumin,** remain in the capillaries because they are too large to squeeze through

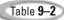

Table 9–2 **Signs and Symptoms of Abnormal Serum Sodium and Potassium Levels**

	LOW	NORMAL	HIGH
SODIUM			
Lab value	Less than 135 mEq/L	135–148 mEq/L	Greater than 148 mEq/L
Condition	Hyponatremia		Hypernatremia
Symptoms	Irritability		Thirst
	Anxiety		Fatigue
Signs	Muscle twitching		Flushed skin
	Fingerprinting over the sternum		Sticky mucous membranes
	Seizures		Agitation
	Coma		Coma
POTASSIUM			
Lab value	Less than 3.5 mEq/L	3.5–5.0 mEq/L	Greater than 5.0 mEq/L
Condition	Hypokalemia		Hyperkalemia
Symptoms	Nausea and/or vomiting		Irritability
	Paresthesias, especially lower extremities		Abdominal cramps
			Weakness, especially lower extremities
Signs	Decreased bowel sounds		Irregular pulse
	Weak, irregular pulse		Cardiac arrest if greater than 8.5 mEq/L
	Coma		

the capillary wall. Inside the blood vessels, the plasma proteins exert **colloidal osmotic pressure** (COP). The COP, now greater than the hydrostatic pressure, pulls water and waste materials from the interstitial fluid back into the blood capillaries. Thus, the volume of fluid within the blood vessels is maintained. Clinical Application 9–3 describes a condition in which a low serum protein is the cause of water imbalance.

Body Regulation of Water Intake and Excretion

The body has mechanisms that regulate both the intake and the excretion of water. Normally, thirst governs water

Protein-Energy Malnutrition and Water Balance

Starving children often look plump (see Fig. 5–4). They are not fat but edematous. These children are victims of **kwashiorkor,** a disease of protein-energy malnutrition. It occurs most often in children just after weaning when there is not enough protein in their diets to replace that in their mothers' milk.

Protein plays a crucial role in maintaining the volume of fluid in the blood vessels. These children develop edema because they do not have enough plasma proteins remaining in the capillaries to pull water back into the circulatory system. Thus, it accumulates in the interstitial spaces. Once treatment begins, the plasma proteins will pull the retained water into the blood and the children will appear emaciated. This is a reminder that appearances can be deceiving. Malnutrition occurs in this country also. A thorough assessment may identify problem areas that on first glance are not apparent.

intake. The excretion of water is controlled mainly by two hormones: antidiuretic hormone causes the body to reabsorb (retain) water; aldosterone causes the body to retain sodium.

Thirst Mechanism

Thirst is the desire for fluids, especially water. Thirst normally occurs when 10 percent of the intravascular volume is lost or when cellular volume is reduced by 1 to 2 percent. When there is too little water in the blood (or, put another way, when the solutes are too concentrated), there is an increase in the osmotic pressure of the blood. Special sensors in the **hypothalamus** monitor the osmotic pressure of the blood as it circulates in the brain. When the hypothalamus detects an increase in the osmotic pressure, it triggers the desire to drink. Sometimes the thirst mechanism goes awry. In such cases, because the precise neural control of thirst is unknown, conscious control of fluid intake is the mode of treatment (McKenna and Thompson, 1998).

Antidiuretic Hormone

If thirst is not alleviated, the sensors in the hypothalamus increase the secretion of **antidiuretic hormone (ADH)** from the posterior pituitary gland. ADH, also named **vasopressin,** causes the kidneys to return more water to the bloodstream rather than spill it into the urine.

Antidiuretic hormone has an additional effect of arterial vasoconstriction that increases blood pressure. (When someone places a finger over the end of a garden hose and partly blocks the opening, the amount of water flowing is the same as before, but the smaller outlet increases the pressure.)

Sometimes the ADH mechanism goes awry. In **diabetes insipidus,** the hypothalamus does not secrete ADH or the kidneys do not respond appropriately. Diabetes insipidus can be caused by brain tumor, surgery, trauma, infection, radiation injury, or congenital conditions. If the hypothalamus is not secreting ADH, a pharmaceutical preparation can be given. Clinical Application 9–4 provides information about a condition called syndrome of inappropriate secretion of antidiuretic hormone (SIADH).

Aldosterone

The release of **aldosterone,** a hormone secreted by the adrenal glands, is another water-balancing mechanism in the body. It causes sodium ions to be returned to the

Syndrome of Inappropriate Secretion of Antidiuretic Hormone (SIADH)

Normally, increased osmolality of the blood stimulates the posterior pituitary gland to release ADH. When enough water is returned to the bloodstream by the kidney, the ADH secretion stops.

Several situations cause ADH to be released inappropriately. Certain lung tumors produce an ADH-like substance, and lung conditions such as pneumonia, tuberculosis, and asthma have caused SIADH. Other cancers, stress, pain, surgery, some anesthetics, and morphine have been implicated in increased release of ADH. Medications such as chlorpropamide and oxytocin as well as various antidepressants, anticonvulsants, and cancer chemotherapeutic agents have precipitated SIADH. Even paradoxical reactions to thiazide diuretics have been reported (van Assen and Mudde, 1999; Wierzbicki, Ball, and Singh, 1998). Diseases directly affecting the brain (including the hypothalamus and the pituitary gland) such as meningitis, brain tumors, and subarachnoid hemorrhage have been linked to SIADH.

The signs and symptoms of SIADH are those of hyponatremia. In this case it is dilutional hyponatremia. The client has enough sodium, but it is diluted in too much retained water. Initially, the client becomes apprehensive. When the serum sodium drops to 120 to 125 mEq per liter, neurological signs appear, owing to edema of the brain cells. The client becomes irritable, apathetic, and displays personality changes. Other signs of hyponatremia include tremors, hyperactive reflexes, muscle spasms, and convulsions. Fingerprints remain over the sternum due to the excess intracellular fluid. Urine osmolality is typically higher than serum osmolality (Brensilver and Goldberger, 1996). When the serum sodium drops to less than 115 mEq per liter, seizures, coma, and permanent neurological damage can occur.

Effective treatment of SIADH is based upon discovering and removing the cause of the condition. Beyond that, or in the instance of a postoperative or stress reaction, treatment involves diuretic therapy and fluid restriction. The client is given precisely prescribed amounts of fluids throughout the day. Over a period of several days, through obligatory excretion, the client's body will excrete the extra water.

bloodstream by the kidneys rather than to be spilled into the urine. Sodium, the most influential extracellular ion, pulls water along with it.

The stimulus for the release of aldosterone is decrease in the pressure of the blood supplying kidney tissue. In response, the kidneys produce **renin** which then acts as an enzyme to split angiotensinogen, a serum globulin secreted by the liver, to form angiotensin I. Enzymes in the lungs convert angiotensin I to **angiotensin II.** Angiotensin II constricts the body's blood vessels, which increases blood pressure, and also stimulates the secretion of aldosterone and ADH. Aldosterone then increases sodium retention, which retains water along with it. ADH also increases water retention, and thus the blood volume is increased (Figure 9–5).

Another side of sodium retention is potassium loss. Within fluid compartments, positively charged particles must equal negatively charged ones. When sodium is retained, to maintain electroneutrality, the kidney excretes more potassium, also under the influence of aldosterone.

Acid-Base Balance

The body is well equipped to digest and metabolize acidic and basic foods without jeopardizing its acid-base balance. The use of substances such as baking soda to treat an upset stomach should be discouraged, however, because the baking soda can be absorbed into the blood, thereby affecting the total body systems. Antacids designed to treat stomach upsets, used according to directions, are a better choice than baking soda.

Electrolytes play an important role in maintaining the correct acidity or alkalinity of various body fluids. Acids are compounds that yield hydrogen ions when dissociated in solution. The more hydrogen ions a solution contains, the more concentrated the acid. Bases, or alkalis, are substances that accept hydrogen ions. The acidity or alkalinity of a substance is measured according to a scale called **pH** for *potential of hydrogen*. The pH scale ranges from 0 to 14: acids are rated 0 to 6.999; 7.0 is neutral; bases (alkalis) are greater than 7. One on the scale would indicate a strong acid, and 14 a strong base. Figure 9–6 illustrates the pH scale showing placement of acid, neutral, and alkaline fluids. There is a 10-fold difference between units. Thus, lemon juice at a pH of 2 is 10 times as acidic as orange juice with a pH of 3.

The balance between too much and too little acid in body fluids is maintained by the action of the lungs, the kidneys, and the buffer systems of the body. The purpose of buffer systems is to minimize significant changes in the pH of the body fluids by controlling the hydrogen ion (H^+) concentration. **Buffers** are substances that can neutralize both acids and bases. **Bicarbonate** (HCO_3^-) is the most important buffer in the extracellular fluid. Phosphate (HPO_4^{2-}) and proteins are two important buffers in the intracellular fluid.

Extracellular Fluid

The normal pH of the extracellular fluid (including the blood and interstitial fluid) is 7.35 to 7.45. It is slightly alkaline despite the acidity of the waste products of metabolism.

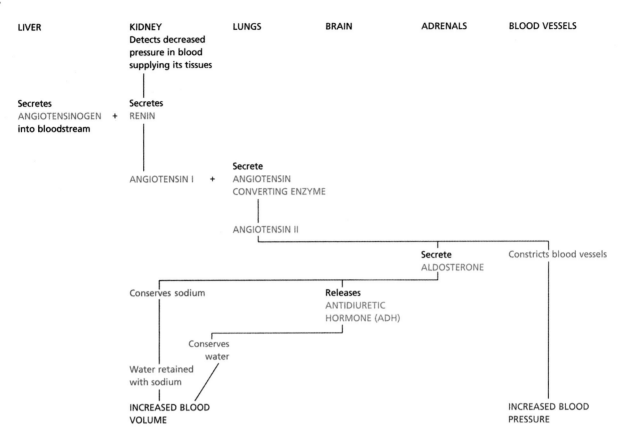

Figure **9–5** Hormonal control of water balance. Although the kidneys do most of the work, the complex process also involves the liver, lungs, brain, adrenal glands, and blood vessels.

The body is continually working to maintain the pH within this narrow range. If the serum pH drops below 6.8 or rises above 7.8, death usually results.

Extracellular fluid contains both positive sodium ions (Na^+) and negative bicarbonate ions (HCO_3^-). When a strong acid is introduced into the fluid, a chemical reaction takes place. The end products of this reaction are sodium chloride (a salt), which is neutral, and carbonic acid (a weak acid). The **carbonic acid** breaks down to carbon dioxide and water. The carbon dioxide is excreted by the lungs (exhaled), and the water is excreted by the kidneys.

Another chemical reaction takes place when a strong base (alkali) is introduced into the fluid system. When a strong base enters the system, carbon dioxide and water (the two main waste products of cellular metabolism) react to form carbonic acid to counteract the alkaline effect of the base. The end products of this reaction are water and a weak base that does not drastically affect the pH.

Respiratory System

The lungs help maintain pH by varying the amount of carbon dioxide (CO_2) exhaled. Excess carbon dioxide makes the body fluids more acidic because it reacts to form **carbonic acid,** a source of hydrogen ions. Too much carbonic acid, or too much of any acid, results in **acidosis,** a condition that causes the lungs to automatically increase the rate and depth of breathing, eliminating more carbon dioxide and water.

This respiratory response to acidosis begins within minutes of an increase in acidity. Respiratory compensation for acidosis is 50 to 75 percent effective and is an extremely important component in the regulation of pH. Normally, the respiratory system has one or two times the buffering power of all chemical buffers in the body.

Renal System

The respiratory system acts quickly but can eliminate only carbonic acid. Other acids, as well as excess carbonic acid, must be eliminated in the urine. The kidney spills or retains hydrogen, sodium, and bicarbonate ions as necessary to maintain an acceptable pH in the blood. For example, in response to acidosis, the kidneys excrete hydrogen ions and reabsorb sodium and bicarbonate ions. Conversely, in response to alkalosis, the kidneys conserve hydrogen ions and excrete sodium and bicarbonate ions. The kidneys initiate these actions within 24 hours but require 3 to 4 days to compensate for changes in blood pH.

Intracellular Fluid

The normal pH of the intracellular fluid is 6.8 to 7.0, slightly acid to neutral. Within the intracellular fluid, organic phosphates and proteins are the most important buffers. These substances buffer 95 percent of the body's carbonic acid and 50 percent of other acids. Protein is the most powerful and plentiful buffer system in the body. Of the body's proteins, hemoglobin has the largest buffering capacity. Thus,

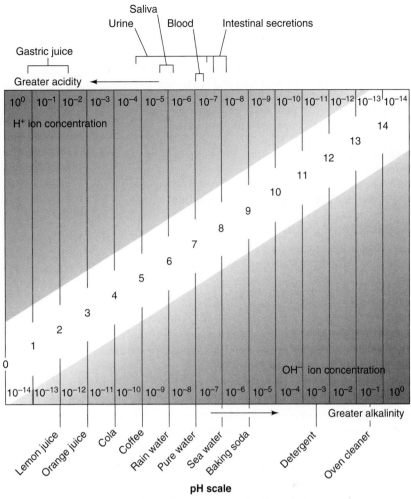

Figure **9–6** Representation of the pH scale with usual readings for body fluids, beverages, and household products. (Reprinted from Venes, 2001, p 1567, with permission.)

the red blood cells have 70 percent of the buffering power of the blood. This buffering capacity allows large quantities of carbon dioxide to be transported from the tissues to the lungs with only a small change in venous pH compared with arterial pH.

When the blood contains excessive hydrogen ions, they move into the cells to be buffered. Then, to maintain electroneutrality, potassium moves from the intracellular compartment to the extracellular (intravascular), raising serum potassium levels.

Dietary Reference Intakes

To prevent deleterious effects of dehydration, AIs for water for 19- to 30-year-old adults have been set at 3.7 liters for men and 2.7 liters for women. Approximately 80 percent of those amounts should come from fluids and 20 percent from foods. Larger intakes will be required by people who are physically active or are exposed to hot environments. The previously publicized negative effects of caffeine and alcohol on water balance have been refuted by evidence showing the diuretic effects of those substances to be transient. No UL has been established, although note was made of the hazard of acute water toxicity in individuals rapidly con-

suming much more than the kidneys' maximal excretion rate of 0.7 to 1.0 liters per hour (Institute of Medicine, 2004).

Those outside of the age range specified will have to have their intake monitored individually. Infants have a greater need for water than adults. Their basal heat production per kilogram is twice that of adults. To rid their bodies of the heat and waste products, they need 1.5 milliliters of water per kilocalorie ingested. Infants must drink 10 to 15 percent of their body weight daily to maintain health. Breast milk alone can supply the infant's needed water even in a desert environment. Older adults often have a blunted sense of thirst and may have their water needs impacted by disease and medication. As is described later, a good day-to-day measure of hydration status is the color of urine.

Sources of Water

Much of our water is consumed in other beverages. Skim milk is 91 percent water, and whole milk is 88 percent water. Water itself may contain other nutrients. Hard water has calcium, magnesium, and often iron. Water conditioners used to soften water replace the calcium, magnesium, and iron with sodium. Drinking softened water increases some people's sodium intake excessively. In fact, most experts recommend that the cold water at the kitchen sink be unsoftened.

We obtain about 4 cups of water per day in foods. Some foods that are solids also have a high water content: a head of lettuce is 96 percent water, celery is 95 percent water, and raw carrots are 88 percent water. Other foods that contain a large percentage of water include apples (84 percent), grapes (81 percent), bananas (74 percent), hard-cooked eggs (75 percent), drained tuna (61 percent), and chicken breast or thigh (52 percent). Whole wheat bread is 38 percent water; its water content drops to 29 percent when the bread is toasted.

Water is also a product of metabolism. The average person acquires 1 cup of water per day from this process.

Applicable Regulation

Municipal water systems serving more than 25 people are subject to the federal Safe Drinking Water Act that requires big cities to test for coliform bacteria 100 or more times a month compared to once a week for bottled-water plants. An estimated 60 to 70 percent of bottled waters are exempt from FDA regulation entirely because they are bottled and sold within a state. Forty states have some regulation, but 12 do not (Natural Resources Defense Council, 1999). See Box 9–2 for facts about bottled water.

Losses of Water

We lose water in obvious ways, such as in perspiration and urine. These means are called **sensible water losses.** We also lose water in less obvious ways, such as through breathing, which are called **insensible water losses.**

Sensible Water Losses

Sensible water losses include losses of the major extracellular ions, sodium and chloride. Three important routes commonly account for sensible water losses: through the skin as perspiration, through the kidney as urine, and through the gastrointestinal tract in the feces.

Perspiration

Evaporation of sweat from the skin is the main means of dissipating the heat produced in the body by exercise. To produce 1 liter of perspiration requires 600 kilocalories. In extreme cases, a person may perspire at the rate of 2 liters per hour. For example, during a marathon race, runners may lose 6 to 7 percent of their body weight, primarily as perspiration. A 150-pound person could then lose 9 to 10 1/2 pounds, or 4.3 to 5 liters, of fluid. To the extent that sweat drops from the body, it is not useful for evaporative cooling.

Sweat is not pure water. It is salty to the taste and is hypotonic. One liter of perspiration contains approximately 45 milliequivalents of sodium, 5 milliequivalents of potassium, and 58 milliequivalents of chloride. In this instance, the milliosmole value is the same as the milliequivalent value (because all the ions are monovalent), so the milliequivalents can be added to obtain an osmolarity of about 108 milliequivalents per liter of perspiration.

For a sweat loss of less than 5 or 6 liters, rehydration with water suffices (Gropper, Smith, and Groff, 2005). See Clinical Application 9–5 to learn about conditions resulting from exposure to extreme heat.

Box 9–2 **Bottled Water**

In 1991, Americans consumed 5 billion gallons of bottled water (Bullers, 2002). The cost of bottled water is $7 billion per year, 120 to 7500 times as much per gallon as for tap water (Shermer, 2003). Whether the price guarantees quality is debatable.

Sources of Bottled Water

An estimated 25 percent of bottled water is bottled tap water (Natural Resources Defense Council, 1999). If it is labeled "from a municipal source" or "from a community water system," the bottle contains tap water (Shermer, 2003). If the water has been treated by distillation, reverse osmosis, or other suitable processes that meet the definition of "purified water" in the U.S. Pharmacopeia, it can be so labeled. Other sources recognized by the FDA are artesian well water, mineral water, spring water, and well water (Bullers, 2002).

Evidence in Water Samples

The Natural Resources Defense Council concluded that most bottled water is safe but that 17 percent contained more bacteria than allowed under unenforceable guidelines. A study in Cleveland found substantially more bacteria in bottled water than in tap water, in some

samples 370 to 1800 times more (Lalumandier and Ayers, 2000).

Reusing plastic bottles raises another concern. One-third of those used by elementary children in Calgary were contaminated with bacteria, most likely from the children themselves if the bottles were not washed and dried between uses. Sanitation efforts could produce another hazard, because frequent washing might accelerate the breakdown of the plastic, possibly adding chemicals to the water (Canadian Press, 2003).

Labels can mislead as well as inform. One such label pictured a lake and mountains while the source of the water actually was a well in an industrial facility's parking lot, near a hazardous waste dump, and periodically contained chemicals exceeding FDA standards (Natural Resources Defense Council, 1999).

Decision Making

The consumer should obtain as much information as possible. Undoubtedly, taste and convenience, as well as price, contribute to the use of bottled water. As with many other nutritional and life choices, however, the advice to "let the buyer beware" applies to this market equally as much as to any other.

Heat-Related Illnesses

Exposure to extreme heat may overtax the body's adaptive capabilities. Between 1979 and 1999, hot weather caused an average of 182 deaths annually in the United States. Advanced age and inability to care for oneself are major risk factors for heat-related deaths (Centers for Disease Control, 2003a). Figure 9–7 depicts the average annual rate of heat-related deaths by age group. Because time spent in air conditioned places prevents heat-related mortality, communities have begun opening emergency cooling shelters when weather conditions warrant. Table 9–3 shows heat index values derived from the combined effect of temperature and humidity and projects the likelihood of heat disorders as the index rises.

A particularly difficult situation occurs in a crowd. Individuals in the center of a mass of bodies are unable to cool themselves through normal physiological mechanisms. This phenomenon is called the "Penguin Effect" after the practice of penguins to huddle together, ostensibly to conserve heat (Blows, 1998). In certain crowds, moreover, heat production is increased, as in pop concerts where the audience cheers and dances. If the people are shoulder-to-shoulder as in an audience or on a commuter train, a person may faint but remain upright, thwarting the normal mechanism of restoring circulation to the brain.

Heat Edema

In heat edema, unacclimatized people experience swelling in the feet and ankles and other dependent areas of the body during hot summer months, caused by transient peripheral vasodilation and orthostatic pooling when they sit or stand for a long time. Elevating the legs and exercising periodically may improve the condition until the person becomes acclimatized (Barrow and Clark, 1998).

Heat Cramps

Heat cramps, brief, intermittent and often severe muscular cramps that frequently occur in muscles fatigued by heavy work or exercise, are believed to be caused by a rapid change in the extracellular fluid osmolarity resulting from sodium and water loss (Weinmann, 2003). Treatment involves stretching the muscle and replacing fluid and salt. An oral rehydration solution using 1 teaspoon of salt to 1 quart of water can be helpful (Barrow and Clark, 1998). Caution is necessary, because overhydrating with hypotonic intravenous fluids has led to hyponatremia (Herfel et al, 1998). In a year-long investigation of deep underground miners, dehydration but not hyponatremia was associated with heat cramps (Donoghue, Sinclair, and Bates, 2000).

Heat Syncope

Heat syncope is an episode of heat-related fainting that usually follows rising from a sitting or lying position. The skin blood vessels have dilated to promote cooling, leaving insufficient blood circulating to the brain. Once the person falls down, his or her brain is reperfused, and the person recovers consciousness. To treat heat syncope, have the client lie down in a cooler location and replace the water deficit (Barrow and Clark, 1998).

Heat Exhaustion

In heat exhaustion, the client suffers the loss of water and sodium chloride in sweat. The client's temperature is usually less than 102.2°F (39°C). He or she suffers from dizziness, weakness, and fatigue but remains coherent. The pulse is weak, thready, and rapid. Respirations are shallow and quiet. The skin is cool, clammy, and sweaty. First-aid treatment consists of moving the client to a cooler environment. The client should lie down with the

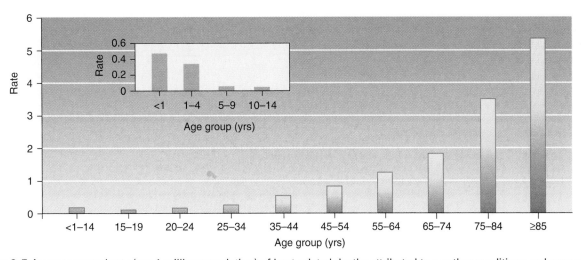

Figure **9–7** Average annual rate (per 1 million population) of heat-related deaths attributed to weather conditions and exposure to excessive natural heat by age group, United States, 1979–1999. (From Centers for Disease Control, 2002.)

(Continued on the following page)

feet elevated, and clothing should be loosened. If the person can drink it, 1/2 teaspoon of salt in 1/2 glass of water will begin to replace the water and sodium chloride lost. The salt-in-water treatment should be repeated every 15 minutes, and the client's temperature should be monitored until the emergency team arrives.

In underground miners, the incidence of heat exhaustion increased in summer and at deeper locations. It would be less likely with improved ventilation and air cooling (Donoghue, Sinclair, and Bates, 2000).

Heat Stroke

Heat stroke is characterized by a core body temperature greater than 40°C (104°F) and central nervous system dysfunction that results in delirium, convulsions, or coma. Heat stroke is a life-threatening medical emergency that can progress to multiorgan dysfunction syndrome (Bouchama and Knochel, 2002). Even when treated promptly, the death rate is 15 percent (Centers for Disease Control, 2002), but studies have shown that cooling the client to a temperature of less than 39.9°C (103.8°F) within 30 minutes improves survival (Dematte et al, 1998). Up to 17 percent of survivors suffer permanent neurologic damage (Centers for Disease Control, 2001).

The client with heat stroke fails to perspire because the body can no longer regulate body temperature and also has impaired regulation of inflammatory and stress responses (Bouchama and Knochel, 2002). When the client has an extremely elevated temperature, 105°F (40.6°C) or above, many body enzymes become denatured so that chemical reactions cannot occur (Curtis, 1997). The client's mental state goes from lethargy to disorientation, delirium, and coma. The skin is flushed, hot, and typically dry but could be wet if the client's condition has just progressed to heat stroke from heat exhaustion (Curtis, 1997) or has resulted from exertion (Wexler, 2002). The pulse is full and bounding as the body shunts blood to the surface for cooling. Breathing is difficult and respirations are loud. The first-aid treatment of heat stroke includes resting with the head elevated, removal of clothing, application of ice bags to neck, axillae, and groin, and dousing with water while fanning. Airway, breathing, and circulation should be monitored until the medical team arrives (Wexler, 2002).

Heat stroke ranks third behind head and neck trauma and cardiac disorders as a cause of death among United States high school athletes (Barrow and Clark, 1998). Hyperthermia and dehydration caused the deaths of three collegiate wrestlers within 33 days in 1997. Those young men were attempting to dehydrate themselves before the official weigh-in in order to compete in desired weight classes (Centers for Disease Control, 1998).

Table 9–3   **Heat Index Chart**

Exposure to direct sunlight can increase the heat index by up to 15°F

DEGREES F	RELATIVE HUMIDITY								
	10%	20%	30%	40%	50%	60%	70%	80%	90%
120	118	132	148	169	193	220	250	283	319
115	112	122	136	152	171	193	218	245	275
110	106	114	124	137	152	169	189	211	235
105	100	106	114	123	135	148	163	181	200
100	94	99	104	111	120	130	141	154	169
95	89	92	96	101	107	114	122	131	142
90	84	87	89	92	96	101	106	112	119
85	80	82	84	86	88	90	93	97	101
80	76	77	79	80	82	83	84	86	88

Heat Index	Possible Heat Disorder
80 to 90	**Fatigue possible with prolonged exposure and physical activity**
90 to 105	**Sunstroke, heat cramps, and heat exhaustion possible**
105 to 130	**Sunstroke, heat cramps, and heat exhaustion likely, and heat stroke possible**
130 or greater	**Heat stroke likely with continued exposure**

Urine

In the normal, healthy person, with average exertion throughout the day, urine output is roughly equal to liquid intake. A well-hydrated individual produces light yellow or straw-colored urine. A minimum amount of urine must be excreted each day to carry away the waste products resulting from metabolic processes. This function, called **obligatory excretion,** eliminates 400 to 600 milliliters per day.

The hourly urine output of seriously ill clients must be monitored. The amounts must be interpreted in relation to the client's whole situation. Even if a person is losing massive amounts of fluid through the gastrointestinal tract, such losses do not rid the body of metabolic wastes as efficiently as the kidney does. Adults should excrete 40 to 80 milliliters per hour—although the amount varies throughout the day and night. Clinical Calculation 9–2

Clinical Calculation 9–2

Hourly Urine Output in Children

Children should excrete between 0.5 and 2 milliliters of urine per kilogram of body weight per hour. What would be a normal hourly urine output for a child who weighs 50 pounds?

First convert pounds to kilograms. There are 2.2 pounds per kilogram.

$$\frac{50\ lb}{2.2\ lb/kg} = 22.7\ kg$$

To find the desirable range of output, multiply the child's weight in kilograms by the desired factors of 0.5 to 2 mL per kilogram.

$$22.7 \times 0.5 = 11.4\ mL/h$$
$$22.7 \times 2 = 45.4\ mL/h$$

Thus, the 50-lb child normally should excrete between 11 and 45 mL/h of urine.

shows a method of determining a desirable hourly urine output for children.

Gastrointestinal Secretions

Abnormal gastrointestinal function can cause extensive fluid loss. When the secretion occurs from a point high in the gastrointestinal tract, the resulting symptoms differ from those that occur when the secretion is from a point lower in the tract. Gastric juice is acid, whereas intestinal juices are alkaline. Therefore, conceptually, gastrointestinal losses are divided into those lost above the outlet of the stomach, the pylorus, and those lost below it.

ABOVE THE PYLORUS

The common causes of losses above the pylorus are vomiting or stomach suctioning. Two organs secrete digestive juices above the pylorus, the salivary glands in the mouth and the gastric glands in the stomach. Both of these secretions are isotonic, so their loss threatens electrolyte balance to a greater extent than loss of an equal amount of perspiration would. The ions lost in secretions above the pylorus are sodium, potassium, chloride, and hydrogen.

About 1 liter of saliva per day is mixed with food or just swallowed. The stomach secretes about 1.5 to 2.5 liters of gastric juice per day. If gastric juices are lost, hydrogen ions in the hydrochloric acid are also lost, putting the person at risk for alkalosis.

BELOW THE PYLORUS

The usual causes of losses below the pylorus are diarrhea and intestinal suctioning. Gastrointestinal secretions below the pylorus also are isotonic. They contain sodium, potassium, and bicarbonate. About 2 to 3 liters of intestinal secretions per day flow into the bowel to digest food. Normally, bile is released from the gallbladder into the small intestine at the rate of 1 liter per day. The total gastrointestinal secretions amount to 6.5 to 8.5 liters per day. Yet, because water is absorbed back into the blood from the large intestine, normal feces from an adult contain only 100 to 200 milliliters of water.

Insensible Water Losses

An invisible amount of water is lost through the lungs and the skin. These are insensible losses. An amount between 800 and 1000 milliliters of water is lost each day via the lungs and skin. Breath is visible only in very cold weather. Even in warmer weather and indoors, people lose 400 milliliters of water per day in exhaled air. Deep respirations or a dry climate increase the amount of water lost.

The insensible loss of water through the skin is evaporative. It is almost pure water and nearly electrolyte-free. This insensible water loss amounts to 6 milliliters per kilogram of body weight in 24 hours, which is a baseline amount.

Environmental conditions influence the amount of water lost. Greater losses occur at high temperatures, at high altitudes, and in low humidity (Kleiner, 1999). Clinical Calculation 9–3 gives a client an example of insensible water loss. Burns, phototherapy, radiant warmers, or fever will increase the amount of insensible water loss. Fever increases evaporative losses by about 12 percent per Celsius degree of temperature elevation. Clinical Calculation 9–4 shows how **evaporative water losses** are calculated. Table 9–4 lists average fluid gains and losses for 24 hours.

Assessment of Water Losses

Gathering data on water losses is quite straightforward. Because water is more than 50 percent of body weight,

Clinical Calculation 9–3

Insensible Water Loss Through the Skin

The rule of thumb for insensible water loss through the skin is 6 mL/kg per 24 hours. Let us look at a 154-lb client to see what his or her amount of water loss would be in a 24-hour period. First, convert pounds to kilograms:

$$\frac{154\ lb}{2.2\ lb/kg} = 70\ kg$$

Then multiply the client's weight (in kilograms) by the amount of water loss per kilogram:

$$70\ kg \times 6\ mL/kg = 420\ mL$$

Thus, this client's insensible water loss in a 24-hour period is expected to be 420 mL

Clinical Calculation 9–4

Evaporative Water Loss in Fever

Fever increases the amount of evaporative loss by 12 percent for every degree Celsius of fever. If the 154-lb client in Clinical Calculation 9–3 had a fever of 102.2°F, how much additional evaporative loss would he or she sustain?

Temperatures can be reported in Fahrenheit or Celsius degrees, and the conversion formulas account for the fact that the Celsius scale sets freezing at zero and the Fahrenheit sets it at 32 degrees.

To convert Fahrenheit to Celsius, subtract 32 and multiply by 5/9.

$$102.2 - 32 = 70.2 \times 5/9 = 39°C$$

Normal body temperature on the Celsius scale is 37 degrees.

To convert Celsius to Fahrenheit, multiply by 9/5 and add 32.

$$37 \times 9/5 = 66.6 + 32 = 98.6°F$$

The client had insensible losses of 420 mL.

The client has an elevation of 2°C, which would increase evaporative loss by 24 percent.

$$420 \text{ mL} \times 0.24 = 100.8 \text{ mL additional evaporative water loss.}$$

$$420 \text{ mL} + 100.8 \text{ mL} = 520.8 \text{ total insensible water loss through the skin.}$$

---

with few exceptions a loss of water is reflected in the client's weight. Recording the liquid a client takes in and puts out (Intake and Output or I&O) is a second common means of tracking water balance.

Weight

Rapid weight changes usually reflect fluid balance. Daily weight is the single most important indicator of fluid status. An easy way to relate volume to weight is to remember "a pint is a pound the world around." One liter is 1 kilogram or 2.2 pounds. Acute weight loss in adults is rated as fol-

lows: mild volume deficit, 2 to 5 percent loss; moderate volume deficit, 5 to 10 percent loss; severe volume deficit, 10 to 15 percent loss.

Fluid balance in the infant is much more precarious. Because a greater proportion of their body water is in the extracellular space, infants can lose it more rapidly than can adults. Therefore, a loss of 5 percent of body weight in an infant merits medical attention.

Sudden weight changes are not always due to fluid shifts. If a client receives no oral, enteral, or parenteral nutrition, the loss of body tissue may amount to 0.3 to 0.5 kilogram per day.

Intake and Output

In addition to monitoring weight, recording liquid intake and output is a common nursing action. In the healthy person, liquid intake and output should be approximately equal. Measuring intake is easier than measuring output, but it still is frequently inaccurate. Most institutions post the amounts that food and beverage containers hold. Amounts remaining should be measured and subtracted from the total liquid served.

Rather than assume that clients have consumed everything missing from the pitcher or tray, the nurse should ask if they drank the fluid (as opposed to, for instance, giving it to a visitor). Updating the intake form throughout the day rather than at the end of a shift is likely to produce a more complete record. Record the amount of water from ice chips as one-half of their volume. One cup of ice chips yields only 1/2 cup of water.

Fluid that is lost into a dressing or a diaper can be estimated by weighing it. Subtract the dry material's weight from the total. One gram of weight equals 1 milliliter of water. **Specific gravity** is the weight of a substance compared with that of distilled water. Normal specific gravity of urine is 1.010 to 1.025 but lower value is common in newborns. So, although the weight of a diaper wet with urine is not exactly the same as if it were wet with water, this method of recording incontinent urine is adequate in most situations.

In a sick person, intake and output totals may not balance every day. The client's intake and output should be assessed over a period of several days, because a 1-day evaluation could prove misleading. Of utmost importance is the ability to see the big picture. See Charting Tips in Box 9–3 for teaching and documentation tips.

Table 9–4 **Average Fluid Gains and Losses in Adults in 24 Hours**

FLUID GAINS		FLUID LOSSES*	
Energy metabolism	300 mL	Kidneys	1200–1500 mL
		Skin	500–600 mL
Oral fluids	1100–1400 mL	Lungs	400 mL
Solid foods	800–1000 mL	Intestines	100–200 mL
Total	2200–2700 mL	Total	2200–2700 mL

*Includes sensible and insensible losses.

- Be specific when teaching clients.
- Record both the content and the client's response to the material.
- One client was told to "drink a lot of fluid" when he was discharged from the hospital. He interpreted this to be 3 to 4 gallons per day! His kidneys did their best, but kidneys cannot produce plain water. In a few days, the client was back in the hospital for correction of electrolyte imbalance. This outcome could have been prevented if the client had been taught to drink a specific amount of fluid rather than "a lot."

Water Imbalances

Two common imbalances are deficient fluid volume and excess fluid volume.

Deficient Fluid Volume

In deficient fluid volume, the individual experiences vascular, interstitial, or cellular dehydration. Loss of 2 percent of body weight strains the cardiovascular and thermoregulatory systems of the body. For each 1 percent decrease in body weight, plasma volume typically decreases by 2.5 percent, muscle water decreases by 1 percent, and rectal temperature increases by 0.4°C to 0.5°C (Hultman, Harris, and Spriet, 1999). In the body's effort to compensate, fluid moves from one compartment to another, so the client's situation is constantly changing.

Losses of Fluid

Fluid losses can be external or internal. Treatments may differ, but the signs and symptoms of deficient fluid volume are similar whatever the cause.

EXTERNAL LOSSES

Fluids lost to the outside of the body are called **external fluid losses;** gastrointestinal losses are the most common. Vomiting or diarrhea are just two of the ways in which gastrointestinal fluids are lost. But medical treatments such as gastrointestinal suctioning or surgical rerouting of intestinal contents also can produce fluid deficits. Hemorrhage causes not only fluid loss but also the loss of blood cells.

INTERNAL LOSSES

It may be hard to imagine, but fluids can be "lost" inside the body. Edema is excessive fluid accumulation in the interstitial fluid compartment. Although the fluid remains inside the body, it is outside the blood vessels and lost to the circulation. As a result of injury or trauma, capillary permeability increases so that more fluid and cells can travel to the site of the injury to begin repairs or healing. This process also causes the swelling, or edema, at the site

of an injury—blisters at the site of burns, for example. Fluid leaves the vessels and accumulates in the skin. Correct fluid replacement is a high priority for severely burned clients.

There are also several places in the body where vast amounts of fluid can accumulate. These losses are called **third-space losses.** Several liters of fluid can accumulate in the bowel when a person has a bowel obstruction. Certain diseases can cause **ascites,** the accumulation of fluid (often amounting to several liters), not within the bowel but around it in the abdominal cavity. Other third-space losses involve internal bleeding or the collection of fluid in the chest cavity. An alert nurse can spot an early clue to third-space losses. Decreasing urine output despite seemingly adequate fluid intake demands further assessment.

Assessment of Deficient Fluid Volume

Loss of fluid may be mild and corrected easily if the client has and obeys the body's thirst command to drink. On the other hand, the client's life may be threatened if the fluid loss is severe or sudden.

SYMPTOMS

The thirst response is triggered when 10 percent of intravascular volume is lost or when cellular volume is reduced by 1 to 2 percent. Thus, thirst is a symptom of deficient fluid volume. The client may also suffer a loss of appetite or be nauseated because of decreased blood flow to the intestines. Other symptoms of fluid deficit are headache, light-headedness, and fatigue (Kleiner, 1999).

SIGNS

Clients who have a deficient fluid volume are less able to maintain their blood pressure immediately after rising from a lying or sitting position. This sign is called **orthostatic hypotension.** The nurse measures the blood pressure with the client lying or sitting, asks the client to stand, and immediately retakes the blood pressure. A drop of 15 millimeters or mercury in either systolic or diastolic blood pressure upon standing suggests deficient fluid volume. A narrowing of **pulse pressure** (the difference between systolic and diastolic readings) also occurs with deficient fluid volume.

In an effort to maintain perfusion of the tissues, the body compensates for a lowered blood pressure by an increase in pulse rate. Taking a pulse when lying or sitting and immediately after rising is another method of assessing deficient fluid volume. An increase of 20 beats per minute upon standing merits further assessment.

Decreased skin **turgor** or elasticity is a sign of deficient fluid volume associated with sodium loss. To assess skin turgor, pinch the skin on the forearm, over the sternum, or on the back of the hand. If the skin stays pinched, suspect deficient fluid volume. This is a less reliable sign in the elderly because their skin loses elasticity.

Another sign of deficient fluid volume can be found in the client's mouth. Besides dry mouth, many longitudinal furrows of the tongue are visible instead of the single one in the well-hydrated adult.

Delayed filling of hand veins is a sign of deficient fluid volume. To assess vein filling, raise the hand above the heart. Normally, the veins will collapse in 3 to 5 seconds. Then lower the hand below the heart. The veins should refill in 3 to 5 seconds. The veins of a person with deficient fluid volume require more than 5 seconds to refill.

The symptoms of loss of appetite and nausea attributable to fluid deficit may progress to the sign of vomiting caused by decreased blood flow to the intestines.

Deficient fluid volume produces changes in certain laboratory readings. The deeper color of concentrated urine is easily observed, and urine's specific gravity can be measured at the bedside. Clients also show increases in hemoglobin and hematocrit levels unless they have lost red blood cells through hemorrhage.

Special attention must be given to the assessment of infants. Because 75 percent of the infant's body weight is water and 54 percent of the water is extracellular, dehydration from fluid loss can occur rapidly. Signs to assess in the infant, in addition to poor skin turgor and dry mucous membranes, are depressed fontanel ("soft spot" in skull), sunken eyes, and lack of tears when crying.

SHOCK

If deficient fluid volume continues, the client goes into shock. The loss of 20 to 25 percent of intravascular volume produces shock. **Shock** is an acute peripheral circulatory failure due to loss of circulatory fluid or derangement of circulatory control. Signs of shock are decreased blood pressure and increased pulse. The person's skin is pale, cool, and clammy from perspiration. Urine output may be less than 15 milliliters per hour.

Treatment of Deficient Fluid Volume

It is essential to correct the cause of the fluid depletion. Hypotonic fluids are given to replace fluid volume and correct electrolyte imbalances (Clinical Application 9–6). If possible, use the oral route. Be aware that oral electrolyte solutions, although effective in maintaining hydration, do not necessarily reduce stool volume or the duration of diarrhea. In 2002, the World Health Organization lowered the osmolarity of the solution it recommends from 311 to 245 mOm/L to reduce vomiting and stool output. Other possible future changes are under investigation (Centers for Disease Control, 2003b; Duggan et al, 2004).

Thickened hydration solutions are also available for clients who have difficulty swallowing thin liquids. A dietitian should be consulted before using food thickeners, inasmuch as some of them bind with water, making water less available for absorption.

An alternative to intravenous rehydration in selected clients is the use of hypodermoclysis. In this technique, fluid is introduced into the subcutaneous tissue, in the thighs or abdomen, for instance, usually by means of a pair of long needles. A drug may be used to aid in dispersal of

Clinical Application 9–6

Oral Electrolyte Solutions

Originally, oral electrolyte solutions were designed to combat diarrheal diseases in developing countries. They proved so useful that they have since been modified for use in Western nations.

One commonly used oral electrolyte solution is Pedialyte. It is available over the counter without a prescription. One liter of Pedialyte contains:

ELECTROLYTES
45 mEq sodium
20 mEq potassium
35 mEq chloride
30 mEq citrate, a base
The total osmolarity of Pedialyte is mildly hypotonic, about 269 milliosmoles per liter. Pedialyte also illustrates electroneutrality. The sodium and potassium are cations carrying positive charges. The chloride and citrate are anions carrying negative charges.

45 mEq Na^+	35 mEq Cl^-
+20 mEq K^+	+30 mEq citrate$^-$
65 mEq cations	65 mEq anions

Pedialyte is designed for maintenance of an infant or child experiencing vomiting or diarrhea. If the client becomes dehydrated, as evidenced by loss of 5 percent of body weight, medical attention is needed. Intravenous fluids or an oral rehydration solution of different composition from Pedialyte may be prescribed for the dehydrated client.

Pedialyte also has a concentration of glucose that promotes sodium and water absorption, 25 g/L. In contrast, athletic beverages contain concentrated sweeteners to mask the bitter taste of the electrolytes (Brensilver and Goldberger, 1996).

---

the solution. Hypodermoclysis may be appropriate if the client has an adequate blood pressure and requires hypotonic or isotonic solutions of 2 or 3 liters per day (Abdulla and Keast, 1997).

If hypertonic solutions are given orally to correct fluid loss, the concentrated solution would remain in the stomach longer than water, providing satiety and restraining water intake (Brensilver and Goldberger, 1996). Additionally, hypertonic solutions draw fluid from the bowel wall into the lumen; the result would be osmotic diarrhea. Some commercial laxatives and enemas are hypertonic solutions that work in this way.

Maximal sodium and water absorption is thought to occur with a glucose concentration of 10 to 25 grams per liter. Higher concentrations allow less sodium and water to be absorbed, in addition to causing osmotic diarrhea. Cola beverages, ginger ale, and apple juice are poor choices for rehydration in prolonged diarrhea, owing to their high glu-

Hyperkalemia Following Blood Transfusion

A person who has hemorrhaged may need blood replacement. Red blood cells do not live as long in the blood bank as they do in the human body. Potassium is the major cation in red blood cells (intracellular). When the red blood cells die and their cell walls rupture, potassium is spilled into the serum.

Blood that has been stored for a prolonged period may contain up to 30 mEq per liter of potassium due to the destruction of the red blood cells. This may not sound like a lot, but potassium is usually administered intravenously at a concentration of 40 mEq per liter to a person who is potassium depleted. The person receiving a blood transfusion may have a serum potassium level that is nearly normal, and the old blood containing a higher concentration of potassium may push him or her into hyperkalemia. The nurse should be aware of the age of fresh blood products to be given and identify clients at risk of hyperkalemia. A potassium-adsorption filter to reduce hyperkalemia following blood transfusion is in clinical trials (Inaba et al, 2000).

cose and low electrolyte concentrations. In contrast, attempts to rehydrate with large volumes of plain water inhibit thirst and produce a diuretic response (Maughan, Leiper, and Shirreffs, 1997).

Another situation that causes electrolyte imbalance can occur if a client in shock requires blood transfusions. Clinical Application 9–7 covers hyperkalemia following blood transfusion.

Excess Fluid Volume

The opposite of deficient fluid volume is excess fluid volume. The individual is retaining fluid intracellularly or extracellularly. Fluid compartments do not operate in isolation: if one is out of balance, the other compartments eventually will be affected as the body attempts to equalize osmotic pressure across the compartments.

Gains of Fluid

If the kidney and the hormones from the adrenal and pituitary glands are functioning normally, excess water is excreted from the body in the urine. When a person becomes ill and these control mechanisms stop working, fluids shift from the intravascular and interstitial spaces to the intracellular space so as to equalize osmotic pressure. A person can overwhelm his own physiological mechanisms with voluntary water consumption. Such cases were reported in 17 military trainees who were hospitalized to treat overhydration (O'Brien et al, 2001) and in hyponatremic Boston Marathon runners (Almond et al, 2005).

Inflammation increases the fluid in interstitial space, causing edema. In most cases, localized edema is not life threatening. The accumulation of fluid in the brain (cerebral edema) or in lung tissue (pulmonary edema), however, is a life-threatening condition. Cerebral edema may result from tumors, toxic chemicals, or infection. Pulmonary edema can be a consequence of a failing heart or irritation of the lung, as in a client who inhales toxic gases.

Assessment of Excess Fluid Volume

Many of the presenting signs and symptoms of excess fluid volume are opposite those of deficient fluid volume. One symptom common to both is loss of appetite.

SYMPTOMS

The client with excess fluid volume complains of loss of appetite and nausea. In this case, the symptoms are due to edema of the gastrointestinal tract rather than decreased blood flow as in deficient fluid volume.

SIGNS

The same edema of the gastrointestinal tract causing the anorexia and nausea causes the sign of vomiting. Because the brain cells are extremely sensitive to changes in the internal environment, a person with excess fluid volume exhibits deteriorating consciousness. Increased fluid in the blood decreases the proportion of red blood cells to total volume. Consequently, the hematocrit reading is decreased. The increase in blood volume causes an increased pulse pressure. The same technique described under deficient fluid volume is used to assess hand veins. With excess fluid volume, the veins will not empty 3 to 5 seconds after raising the hand above the heart.

Increased blood flow to the kidneys causes increased urine output if the kidneys are functioning. The increased systolic blood pressure due to the excessive fluid pushes more fluid into the interstitial space, causing edema. Firm pressure over a bone, the ankle, or the top of the foot forces some of the fluid aside. If the indentation remains visible for 5 seconds, it is called **pitting edema.** Table 9–5 lists signs and symptoms for deficient fluid volume and excess fluid volume.

Treatment of Excess Fluid Volume

As with deficient fluid volume, the remedy for excess fluid volume is to treat the cause. Osmotic diuretic drugs such as mannitol remain in the plasma. By increasing the osmotic pressure there, these drugs pull excess fluid from the cells to be excreted by the kidney.

Nutritionally, the client may be on a restricted fluid regimen. The physician may prescribe an intake of no more than 1000 milliliters in 24 hours. This amount compensates for insensible losses through the skin and lungs. It is essential for the nurse to supply fluid as prescribed and to teach the client the reason for the restriction. Over a period of several days, the obligatory urine output and any diuretic therapy will help the client's body to excrete the excess fluid.

Table 9–5 **Signs and Symptoms of Abnormal Fluid Volume**

	DEFICIENT FLUID VOLUME	EXCESS FLUID VOLUME
SYMPTOMS		
Gastrointestinal	Thirst	Nausea
	Loss of appetite (decreased blood to intestines)	Loss of appetite (edema of the bowel)
SIGNS		
General	Weight loss	Weight gain
	Depressed fontanel (infant)	Edema
	Sunken eyes (infant)	
	Lack of tears when crying (infant)	
Skin and mucous membranes	Dry mucous membranes	Skin stretched and shiny
	Decreased skin turgor	
Cardiovascular system	Orthostatic hypotension (pressure decrease of 15 mmHg in systolic or diastolic)	Decreased hematocrit values
	Increased pulse rate upon standing	Increasing pulse pressure
	Increased hematocrit values (unless red blood cells also lost)	Emptying of hand veins takes longer than 5 seconds
	Narrowing pulse pressure	
	Filling of hand veins takes longer than 5 seconds	
Urinary	Decreased urine output	Polyuria
	Concentrated urine	Dilute urine
Gastrointestinal	Vomiting (decreased blood to intestines)	Vomiting (edema of intestines)
	Longitudinal furrows on tongue	
Central nervous system	Confusion, disorientation	Deteriorating consciousness

SUMMARY

Water is our most essential nutrient. It constitutes at least half of everyone's body weight. The amount of water varies with the type of tissue, with sex, and with age. Body fluids are held in two compartments: intracellular fluid is the water within the cells; extracellular fluid is the water outside the cells. The latter includes intravascular fluid, lymph, interstitial, and transcellular fluids.

Water has many vital functions in the body. It gives shape and form to the cells, helps form the structure of large molecules, serves as a lubricant, and helps regulate body temperature. As a solvent, water transports solutes to and from the cells, is a medium for chemical reactions, and participates in chemical reactions. Because of its vital importance, everyone should take care to stay well hydrated (Wellness Tip 9–1).

The human body has no storage tanks for water. When necessary, the body can absorb water rapidly. Although some water can be absorbed from the stomach, 1 liter per hour can be absorbed from the small intestine.

The movement, distribution, and composition of body fluids are influenced and controlled by electrolyte and plasma protein concentrations. In the extracellular fluid, sodium is the major cation and chloride is the major anion. The major cation in the intracellular fluid is potassium. Ionized sodium, potassium, and chloride are the solutes that maintain the balance between the extracellular and intracellular compartments.

Wellness Tip **9–1** • Tally your intake of fluids for a day. If it is less than optimum, consciously decide to drink fluids at specified intervals. Select trigger events (before meals, after a bathroom break) to consume a healthful beverage.

- Establish modest goals to be achieved. When those are met, increase the amount of fluids you will try to consume.
- Enter any exercise period well hydrated. Consume moderate amounts of fluid (6 to 12 fluid ounces) at 15–20 minute intervals during exercise (American College of Sports Medicine, 2000).
- If you know you have lost electrolytes in sweat, consume fruit or vegetable juice with a salty snack food along with plain water.
- Before prolonged or heavy exercise, obtain advice from a health-care provider.

A complex system regulates the amount of water retained or excreted by the kidney. Aldosterone and ADH are hormones that cause retention of sodium and water, respectively. The hypothalamus stimulates the thirst mechanism when fluids inside the cells become too concentrated (with solutes).

Acid-base balance is maintained in the body by the action of the lungs, the kidneys, and chemical buffers. Bicarbonate is the most important buffer in the extracellular fluid. Phosphate and protein are two important buffers in the intracellular fluid.

The body's sources of water include beverages, foods, and water from the metabolism of the energy nutrients (except pure alcohol). Water can be lost through the skin, lungs, kidneys, and intestinal tract. Although still present in the body, fluid can be lost to circulation through third spacing. The single most important measure of fluid balance is daily weight.

Since most fluid losses are hypotonic, the fluids usu-ally used to correct deficient fluid volumes and elec-trolyte imbalances are hypotonic. The use of hypertonic fluids would have the opposite effect, pulling more water out of the tissues and into the bowel or bloodstream.

Excess fluid volume can be local or generalized. The most dangerous sites for local edema are the brain and the lungs. Generalized excess fluid volume can make exorbitant demands on the heart. Common treat-ments for excess fluid volume are diuretics and fluid restriction.

CASE STUDY 9-1

Mr. N, a 75-year-old retired office worker, recently arrived from his summer home in the North to his winter home in Florida. He had anticipated enjoying the 85°F weather. He left temperatures in the forties. Although Mr. N had hired someone to care for his small yard while he was away from Florida, there were still a number of chores to be done, which he tackled with a vengeance.

After 1 1/2 hours, Mr. N began to get a headache. He felt a bit weak and dizzy but continued his work. He was nearly finished with the outside tasks.

Half an hour later, Ms. N found her husband lying on the ground and called to their neighbor, a retired nurse, who was reading in her lanai.

The nurse noted that Mr. N's skin was pale and cool but that he was perspiring profusely. He was conscious and coherent but said he felt weak. The nurse took Mr. N's pulse. It was 90 beats per minute, regular but weak. His respira-tions were 12 per minute and shallow.

The nurse provided the emergency care described in the following nursing care plan. (Of course, she did not write it all out before helping Mr. N.)

NURSING CARE PLAN

SUBJECTIVE DATA   Has worked outside in 85°F heat 2 hours
Headache, weakness, dizziness
Recently arrived from colder climate

OBJECTIVE DATA   Conscious, coherent
Skin pale, cool, wet with perspiration
Pulse 90, regular and weak
Respirations 12 and shallow

NURSING DIAGNOSIS   NANDA: Deficient fluid volume (NANDA, 2003, with permission) related to excessive loss of hypo-tonic fluid (sweat) as evidenced by wet, pale skin and weak, rapid pulse.

DESIRED OUTCOMES EVALUATION CRITERIA	NURSING ACTIONS/ INTERVENTIONS	RATIONALE
NOC: Thermoregulation (Moorhead, Johnson, and Maas, 2004, with permission)	NIC: Fluid/Electrolyte Management (Dochterman and Bulechek, 2004, with permission)	
Client will remain conscious and oriented, with a pulse no greater than 90, until the emergency team arrives.	Instruct Ms. N to call emergency medical services and return to help.	In an emergency situation, the nurse stays with the client. Potential electrolyte imbalance requires medical care.
	Loosen Mr. N's clothing.	Mr. N is already in a state of shock. Loosening the clothing will allow maxi-mum air exchange and permit relaxation.
	With Ms. N, move client to shade or provide shade where he lies.	Mr. N must get out of the sun. Depending on the situation, he might be moved indoors, but perhaps the two women could not manage to move him.

(Continued on the following page)

CASE STUDY *(Continued)*

DESIRED OUTCOMES EVALUATION CRITERIA	NURSING ACTIONS/ INTERVENTIONS	RATIONALE
	Keep client lying down with legs elevated slightly.	Lying down permits maximum blood circulation to the brain. Raising the legs increases the return of blood to the heart. The head should not be lowered because this causes venous congestion in the brain.
	Ask Ms. N to prepare a 1/2 glass water with 1/2 teaspoonful of salt in it. Administer salty water to Mr. N.	Although this is a hypertonic solution, sodium is readily absorbed by the intestine, so it is unlikely to cause osmotic diarrhea. Only 5 percent of consumed sodium remains in the feces. Sodium levels in the blood are controlled by the kidneys. This client has lost water and sodium chloride in perspiration.

CTQ CRITICAL THINKING QUESTIONS

1. What would you include in a presentation on preventing heat-related illnesses for an audience of elderly residents such as Mr. N, who follow the sun for the winter?
2. Reread the narrative. At what points in the narrative or in your expansion of the story could you envision Mr. N avoiding this incident?
3. The case study narrative does not discuss Mr. N's usual dietary intake. What dietary modifications can you think of that would make Mr. N's situation of overworking in the heat more critical?

⟫ CHAPTER REVIEW

1. Which of the following people has the greatest percentage of body weight as water?
   a. A 154-pound man
   b. A 120-pound woman
   c. An 8-pound girl, 4 days old
   d. An 18-pound boy, 14 months old
2. Which of the following is the AI for water for healthy young adults?
   a. 800 to 1000 milliliters
   b. 1200 to 1800 milliliters
   c. 2000 to 2300 milliliters
   d. 2700 to 3700 milliliters
3. Heat exhaustion is caused by:
   a. Insufficient secretion of ADH
   b. Loss of water and salt in sweat
   c. Inability to perspire
   d. Retention of excessive water
4. When aldosterone secretion is increased, _____ is retained by the kidney and _____ is excreted to maintain electroneutrality.
   a. Sodium, potassium
   b. Potassium, sodium
   c. Calcium, hydrogen
   d. Hydrogen, potassium
5. If a person's body is too acid, the automatic response of the body is to:
   a. Increase sweat production
   b. Retain water
   c. Decrease rate and depth of breathing
   d. Increase rate and depth of breathing

CLINICAL ANALYSIS

Baby I, a 4-month-old boy, has developed diarrheal stools within the past 2 days. At birth he weighed 7 pounds 8 ounces. Since then he has gained steadily. Three days ago he weighed 12 pounds 8 ounces. Baby I's present weight is 12 pounds 2 ounces.

Mrs. I has been feeding the baby his usual formula. He drinks eagerly but then has an explosive bowel movement with loud crying. Baby I has had six bowel movements per day instead of his usual two.

1. With this history, what physical assessment measures would the nurse include initially?
   a. Skin turgor, fontanel fullness, moisture of mucous membranes
   b. Condition of hair, strength of grasp, presence of sucking reflex
   c. Heart sounds, lung sounds, blood pressure
   d. Urine specific gravity, observation of diaper rash

2. Which of the following recommendations by the nurse would show understanding of supportive care of this client?
   a. Give Baby I whole milk to maintain nutrition.
   b. Continue, as Mrs. I has been doing, to allow the bowel to empty itself.
   c. Substitute orange juice for the formula for 3 days.
   d. Start Baby I on an oral electrolyte solution.

3. The nurse instructs Mrs. I to return for additional care for Baby I if one of the following events takes place. Which one would indicate the need for reassessment of Baby I?
   a. The baby sleeps soundly and has to be awakened for a night feeding.
   b. The baby has three loose bowel movements the day after beginning treatment.
   c. The baby continues to lose weight or passes blood in the stool.
   d. The baby gains more than 2 ounces per day.

REFERENCES

Abdulla, A, and Keast, J: Hypodermoclysis as a means of rehydration. Nurs Times 93:54, 1997.

Almond, CSD, et al: Hyponatremia among runners in the Boston Marathon. N Engl J Med 352:1550, 2005.

American College of Sports Medicine, American Dietetic Association, and Dietitians of Canada: Joint Position Statement: nutrition and athletic performance. Med Sci Sports Exerc 32: 2130, 2000.

Barrow, MW, and Clark, KA: Heat-related illnesses. Am Fam Physician. 58:749, 1998.

Blows, WT: Crowd physiology: The "penguin effect." Accid Emerg Nurs 6:129, 1998.

Bouchama, A, and Knochel, JP: Heat stroke. N Engl J Med 346:1978, 2002.

Brensilver, JM, and Goldberger, E: A Primer of Water, Electrolyte, and Acid Base Syndromes, ed 8. FA Davis, Philadelphia, 1996.

Bullers, AC: Bottled water: Better than tap? FDA Consumer July-August 2002. Accessed December 8, 2003 at http://www.fda.gov/fdac/features/2002/402_h2o.html.

Canadian Press: People who frequently reuse water bottles may be risking their health. Sunday, January 26, 2003.

Centers for Disease Control: Heat-related deaths—Chicago, Illinois, 1996–2001, and United States, 1979–1999. MMWR 52:610, 2003a. Accessed December 20, 2003 at http://www.cdc.gov/mmwr/PDF/wk/mm5226.pdf.

Centers for Disease Control: Managing acute gastroenteritis among children. MMWR 52:1, 2003b.

Centers for Disease Control: Heat-related deaths—Four states, July-August 2001, and United States, 1979–1999. MMWR 51:567, 2002. Accessed December 31, 2003 at http://www.cdc.gov/mmwr/PDF/wk/mm5126.pdf.

Centers for Disease Control: Heat-related deaths—Los Angeles County, 1999–2000, and United States, 1979–1998. MMWR 50:623, 2001. Accessed December 31, 2003 at http://www.cdc.gov/mmwr/PDF/wk/mm5029.pdf.

Centers for Disease Control: Hyperthermia and dehydration-related deaths associated with intentional rapid weight loss in three collegiate wrestlers—North Carolina, Wisconsin, and Michigan, November-December 1997. MMWR 47:105, 1998. Accessed August 24, 1999 at http://www.cdc.gov/epo/mmwr/preview/mmwrhtml/00051388.htm.

Curtis, R: OA guide to heat related illnesses and fluid balance. Accessed September 6, 1999 at http://www.princeton.edu/~oa/safety/heatill.html.

Dematte, JE, et al: Near-fatal heat stroke during the 1995 heat wave in Chicago. Ann Intern Med 129:173, 1998.

Dibas, AI, Mia, AJ, and Yorio, T: Aquaporins (water channels): Role in vasopressin-activated water transport. Proc Soc Exp Biol Med 219:183, 1998.

Dochterman, J, and Bulechek, G (eds): Nursing Interventions Classification (NIC), ed 4. Mosby, St. Louis, 2004.

Donoghue, AM, Sinclair, MJ, and Bates, GP: Heat exhaustion in a deep underground metalliferous mine. Occup Environ Med 57:165, 2000.

Duggan, C, et al: Scientific rationale for a change in the composition of oral rehydration solution. JAMA 291:2628, 2004.

Griesdale, DE, and Honey, CR: Aquaporins and brain edema. Surg Neurol 61:418, 2004.

Gropper, SS, Smith, JL, and Groff, JL: Advanced Nutrition and Human Metabolism, ed 4. Wadsworth, Belmont, CA, 2005.

Herfel, R, et al: Iatrogenic acute hyponatremia in a college athlete. Br J Sports Med 32:257, 1998.

Hu, H, et al: Increased expression of aquaporin-4 in human traumatic brain injury and brain tumors. J Zhejiang Univ Sci B 6:33, 2005.

Hultman, E, Harris, RC, and Spriet, LL: Diet in work and exercise performance. In Shils, ME, et al (eds): Modern Nutrition in Health and Disease, ed 9. Lippincott Williams & Wilkins, Philadelphia, 1999.

Inaba, S, et al: Potassium-adsorption filter for RBC transfusion: A phase III clinical trial. Transfusion 40:1469, 2000.

Institute of Medicine: Dietary Reference Intakes for Water, Potassium, Sodium Chloride, and Sulfate. National Academies Press, Washington, DC, 2004. Accessed March 31, 2004 at http://www.nap.edu/openbook/0309091691/html/1.html.

Kleiner, SM: Water: An essential but overlooked nutrient. J Am Diet Assoc 99:200, 1999.

Klotz, RS: The effects of intravenous solutions on fluid and electrolyte balance. J Intraven Nurs 21:20, 1998.

Knoers, NV, and Deen, PM: Aquaporin molecular biology and clinical abnormalities of the water transport channels. Curr Opin Pediatr 10:428, 1998.

Lalumandier, FA, and Ayers, LW: Fluoride and bacterial content of bottled water vs tap water. Arch Fam Med 9:246, 2000.

Maughan, RJ, Leiper, JB, and Shirreffs, SM: Factors influencing the restoration of fluid and electrolyte balance after exercise in the heat. Br J Sports Med 31:175, 1997.

McKenna, K, and Thompson, C: Osmoregulation in clinical disorders of thirst appreciation. Clin Endocrinol 49:139, 1998.

Moorhead, S, Johnson, M, and Maas, M (eds): Nursing Outcomes Classification (NOC), ed 3. Mosby, St. Louis, 2004.

NANDA International: Nursing Diagnoses: Definitions and Classification 2003–2004. NANDA International, Philadelphia, 2003.

Natural Resources Defense Council: Bottled water: Pure drink or pure hype? Executive Summary, 1999. Accessed January 4, 2004 at http://www.nrdc.org/water/drinking/bw/execsum.asp

O'Brien, KK, et al: Hyponatremia associated with overhydration in U.S. Army trainees. Mil Med 166:405, 2001.

Ritz, P: Body water spaces and cellular hydration during healthy aging. Ann N Y Acad Sci 904:474, 2000.

Scanlon, VC, and Sanders, T: Essentials of Anatomy and Physiology, ed 4. FA Davis, Philadelphia, 2003.

Schnell, ZB, Van Leeuwen, AM, and Kranpitz, TR: Davis's

Comprehensive Handbook of Laboratory and Diagnostic Tests. FA Davis, Philadelphia, 2003.

Shermer, M: Bottled twaddle. Sci Am 289:33, 2003.

van Assen, S, and Mudde, AH. Severe hyponatremia in an amiloride/hydrochlorthiazide-treated patient. Neth J Med 54:108, 1999.

Venes, D (ed): Tabor's Cyclopedic Medical Dictionary, ed 19. FA Davis, Philadelphia, 2001.

Verkman, AS: Role of aquaporin water channels in eye function. Exp Eye Res 76:137, 2003.

Weinmann, M: Hot on the inside. Emerg Med Serv 32:34, 2003.

Wexler, RK: Evaluation and treatment of heat-related illnesses. Am Fam Physician 11:2307, 2002.

Wierzbicki, AS, Ball, SG, and Singh, NK: Profound hyponatremia following an idiosyncratic reaction to diuretics. Int J Clin Pract 52:278, 1998.

Yasui, M: Molecular mechanisms and drug development in aquaporin water channel diseases: structure and function of aquaporins. J Pharmacol Sci 96:260, 2004.

CHAPTER 10

Digestion, Absorption, Metabolism, and Excretion

After completing this chapter, the student should be able to:

1. List the anatomic structures that make up the gastrointestinal tract.
2. Describe the processes of digestion, absorption, metabolism, and excretion.
3. Discuss how cells use nutrients.
4. Describe appropriate dietary treatments for lactose intolerance, lipid malabsorption, food allergies, and gluten-sensitive enteropathy.
5. List the ways the body eliminates waste.

Every part of the human body requires nutrients for energy, maintenance, and growth. Food supplies the necessary nutrients. Food is composed of complex substances that must be broken down to simpler forms that the cells can use.

The **cell** is the ultimate destination for the nutrients found in food. Digestion, absorption, and metabolism are the three interrelated processes that act on food to prepare it for use by the body. A fourth process, excretion, is the elimination of undigestible or unusable substances. This chapter discusses all the bodily activities, organs, and systems involved in these major processes.

Overview of the Major Processes

The first step in preparing food for use by the cells is digestion. **Digestion** is the process by which food is broken down mechanically and chemically in the gastrointestinal tract into forms small enough for absorption to occur. The end products of digestion move from the gastrointestinal tract into the blood or lymphatic system in a process called **absorption.**

After absorption, the nutrients usually are transported to the liver, where they may be adjusted to suit the needs of the body. **Metabolism,** the sum of all physical and chemical changes that take place in the body, determines the final use of the individual nutrients as well as medications. What the cells have no use for becomes waste that is eliminated through **excretion.**

Digestion

Digestion takes place in the alimentary canal and the accessory organs.

Alimentary Canal

The **alimentary canal** is a long, muscular tube that extends through the body from the mouth to the anus. It includes the oral cavity, pharynx, esophagus, stomach, small intestine, and large intestine. Muscle rings, called **sphincters,** separate segments of the alimentary canal. They act as valves to control the passage of food. When the muscles contract, the passageway closes; when the muscles relax, the passageway opens. **Mucosa** lines the alimentary canal. It secretes **mucus,** which lubricates the canal and helps facilitate the smooth passage of food. The mucosa secretes the digestive enzymes of the stomach and small intestine.

Accessory Organs

Three **organs** located outside of the alimentary canal are considered part of the digestive system—the liver, gallbladder, and pancreas. They make important contributions to the digestive process.

Liver

The **liver** is the second largest single organ in the body (skin is the largest). The liver performs many functions, but its primary digestive function is the production of bile. **Bile** is important in breaking down dietary fats. Bile exits the liver by the hepatic duct (a **duct** is a narrow tube that permits the movement of fluid from one organ to another). A later section in this chapter discusses some of the tasks the liver performs after the absorption of nutrients.

Gallbladder

The **gallbladder** is a 3- to 4-inch sac that concentrates and stores bile until it is needed in the small intestine. Bile is delivered to the small intestine through the common bile duct. About 2 to 3 cups of bile are secreted each day into the alimentary canal.

Pancreas

The **pancreas** secretes enzymes that are involved in the digestion of all the energy nutrients. These secretions are collectively known as pancreatic juice. Pancreatic juice is carried to the small intestine via the pancreatic and common bile ducts.

Digestive Action

Mechanical and chemical digestion occur simultaneously throughout the alimentary canal. **Mechanical digestion** is the physical breaking down of food into smaller pieces. **Chemical digestion** involves the splitting of complex molecules into simpler forms.

Mechanical Digestion

Examples of mechanical digestion include chewing or **mastication,** swallowing, peristalsis, and emulsification. **Peristalsis** is a wavelike movement that propels food through the entire length of the alimentary canal. This one-way movement is caused by the alternate contraction and relaxation of the circular and longitudinal muscles that make up the external muscle layer of the alimentary canal. Other muscular activity churns the food, reducing it to successively smaller particles and mixing it with digestive secretions. All of these muscular actions are regulated by a network of nerves within the wall of the alimentary canal. Emulsification is discussed later in this chapter.

Chemical Digestion

Many **chemical reactions** are involved in digestion. For example, the conversion of starch to maltose, of fat to glycerol and fatty acids, and of protein to amino acids all involve the process of **hydrolysis.** The hydrolysis of nutrients is achieved mostly through the action of digestive enzymes, which are present in saliva, gastric juice, pancreatic juice, and intestinal juice.

Each enzyme is specific in its action; it acts only upon a particular substance and no other. Enzymes sometimes require the presence of additional substances such as activators, coenzymes, or hormones to make them active. More than 500 are enzymes involved in the digestive process; this chapter discusses a few of the major ones.

In addition to enzymes, other secretions and chemicals are used in the chemical digestion of food, including mucus, electrolytes, and water. Mucus lubricates passages and facilitates the movement of food. It also protects the inside walls of the alimentary canal from acidic solutions. **Electrolytes** are substances that conduct an electric current in solution (see the previous chapter). One example of an electrolyte is the **hydrochloric acid (HCl)** the stomach secretes. HCl performs many functions necessary to the digestive process, discussed later in this chapter.

CONTROL OF SECRETIONS

The amount of mucus, electrolytes, water, and enzymes released during the digestive process depends on several factors. Hormones frequently initiate a given secretion. For example, the acid content of the food mixture in the stomach causes the release of a hormone called **secretin.** The release of secretin in the small intestine causes the pancreas to send pancreatic juices into the small intestine.

Emotions and conditioned responses can affect the amount of a secretion released. For example, the smell of a roasting turkey on Thanksgiving day causes the release of hydrochloric acid in the stomach. Stress and tension can also produce this effect, sometimes with deleterious results.

The presence of food in the gastrointestinal tract can influence the release of alimentary canal secretions. Coffee drinking, for instance, causes a hormone to be released into the stomach that in turn causes the secretion of hydrochloric acid. Another trigger for the release of bile from the gallbladder is the presence of fat in the small intestine. A chain of reactions whereby one event causes another and then another is very common in all biological **systems.**

END PRODUCTS OF DIGESTION

Four to 6 hours after a meal, the body has broken down the food into some trillion molecules. Each of the energy nutrients is broken down into simpler molecules. Carbohydrates are digested into monosaccharides. Fats are broken down into molecules of glycerol, fatty acids, and monoglycerides. The end products of protein digestion are amino acids and small peptides. It is thought that as much as one-third of dietary protein is absorbed into mucosal cells as dipeptides and tripeptides. Vitamins, minerals, and water are also released during digestion.

The Food Pathway

Food passes through the mouth into the oral cavity, where it is chewed and exposed to chemicals in the saliva. The tongue voluntarily forces the mass of food, called a **bolus,** into the pharynx, which is responsible for the reflex action of swallowing. When swallowed, the bolus enters the esophagus, a muscular, mucus-lined tube, and is propelled downward by peristalsis to the stomach. Both mechanical and chemical digestion occur in the stomach, reducing the food to a semifluid mass that is then released into the small intestine. Further digestion takes place in the small intestine, and most of the absorption of nutrients occurs there as well. Any food remaining after digestion and absorption passes into the large intestine and is excreted as fecal matter.

Oral Cavity

The **oral cavity,** the hollow space in the skull directly behind the mouth, includes the roof of the mouth, the cheeks, and the floor of the mouth. Within the oral cavity are the teeth, tongue, and openings of the ducts of the salivary glands.

DIGESTIVE ACTION

Food entering the oral cavity is chewed and thus broken into smaller particles. This mechanical action increases the surface area of the food for exposure to saliva, a digestive secretion produced by the **salivary glands.** Saliva moistens and softens the food for swallowing and contains the digestive enzyme known as **salivary amylase.** Salivary amylase converts starch to maltose (a disaccharide) or to shorter chains of glucose. Because simple sugars (monosaccharides) require no digestion, some absorption of them may occur in the mouth. A few medications such as nitroglycerin are absorbed in the mouth. The chemical digestion of carbohydrates (starch) continues until the hydrochloric acid in the stomach halts the action of the salivary amylase. After being chewed, the bolus (food mass) is maneuvered backward by the tongue into the pharynx. Box 10–1 introduces the dietary treatment of dysphagia.

Pharynx

The **pharynx** is a muscular passage between the oral cavity and the esophagus. No digestive action occurs there. The pharynx continues the movement of the bolus by the reflexive action of swallowing. The bolus then enters the esophagus.

Esophagus

The **esophagus** is a muscular tube about 10 inches long that takes food from the pharynx to the stomach. No digestive action occurs there. Peristalsis forces the bolus into the stomach with the help of mucous secretions. Between the esophagus and the stomach is the **cardiac sphincter** (the first portion of the stomach is called the cardia), which opens to permit passage of the food. The sphincter closes after the passage of food to prevent the backup of stomach contents.

Stomach

The **stomach** is a J-shaped sac that extends from the esophagus to the small intestine. Folds in the mucous

---

Box 10–1 **Dietary Treatment for Dysphagia**

One in 17 people, including 6.2 million Americans over 60, have a swallowing disorder called dysphagia, literally meaning difficulty swallowing (Galvani, 2001). Although a swallowing disorder may prompt a cough, this does not always occur. Many times swallowing disorders go unnoticed because of short hospital stays. Food particles may pass into the lungs (aspiration), allowing bacteria to multiply. For example, aspiration occurs in 43 to 54 percent of patients who have had strokes. Of these patients, 37 percent develop pneumonia and 3.8 percent die of it (Galvani, 2001). Diets for dysphagia that safely meet nutrient needs range from nothing by mouth (NPO) to total oral feedings. Candidates for oral feedings should demonstrate the ability to perform a safe swallow by a bedside evaluation or a modified **barium swallow,** be alert and able to follow directions, and be oriented to self and the task of eating.

Dysphagia diets provide graduated steps from the most easily managed food to the ones most difficult to manage:

- Liquids range from thick to thin.
- Solids range from pureed to regular.
- The most conservative starting point is thickened liquids and pureed textures.
- Liquids and solids may be progressed independently.
- High-protein high-calorie between-meal feedings as necessary.

The most precise diet orders specify both the texture of solid foods and the consistency of liquids as well as other therapeutic modifications. In order to address the multiplicity of dysphagia diet terminology and practices, a multi-disciplinary task force developed The National Dysphagia Diet (NDD) based on existing scientific evidence (McCallum, 2003). The NDD has four levels:
Level 1: Dysphagia Pureed
- homogenous, cohesive, pudding like
- requires minimum chewing

Level 2: Dysphagia Mechanically altered
- cohesive, moist, semi-solid
- requires some chewing ability
Level 3: Dysphagia Advanced
- semi-solid, easy to cut meats, vegetables, and fruits
- requires some chewing ability
Level 4: Regular
- any solid texture

Hydration is a challenge for clients with dysphagia and thickening agents are commonly used to increase fluid intake. The use of thickening agents to modify the consistency of beverages, soups, and pureed foods is both an art and a science. Commercial thickening agents, instant potato flakes, unflavored gelatin, and dehydrated baby foods and cereals can all be used to thicken foods. The nurse should recognize that thickening agents may:

- Become thicker with time
- Add significant carbohydrate kcalories to clients' diets
- React differently in various foods
- Affect palatability of the thickened item

Staff need to be trained to follow recipes and mix complementary flavors. For example, tomato juice can be used to thin spaghetti sauce.

Some foods change their consistency at body temperature, such as ice cream and gelatin. Foods with mixed consistency such as vegetable soups with "chunks" and cereal with milk may not be appropriate for a given individual because he or she may not be able to swallow a food of mixed consistency. For individuals who have problems forming a food bolus, foods such as rice, scrambled eggs, corn, peas, and legumes may cause a problem. These foods do not form a cohesive bolus. For other patients, foods that crumble, such as crackers, cornbread, and unmoistened ground meats, may not be appropriate. Thus, each patient needs his or her diet highly individualized.

(Continued on the following page)

Box 10–1 **Dietary Treatment for Dysphagia** *(Continued)*

A preprinted sheet of dos and don'ts is of limited usefulness for many of these clients. A nurse, speech therapist, occupational therapist, and registered dietitian may collectively devote many sessions to the development of an individualized diet plan and to determine the best position for the client during feeding times. Usually the patient should be sitting upright with hips at a 90-degree angle, shoulder slightly forward, and feet flat on the floor or firmly supported (American Dietetic Association, 2000). Poorly functioning institutional systems may lack the resources and sometimes delay evaluation and treatment for these clients. The nurse can do much to help these clients by referring them to healthcare providers who can spend the time to work with them.

Signs and symptoms that indicate dysphagia include:

- "Gurgly" voice
- Coughing or choking with food and fluid intake
- Nasal regurgitation
- Pocketing of food in cheeks
- Drooling
- Difficulty in initiating a swallow
- Excessive chewing
- Poor tongue control
- Poor lip closure

- Lack of body position control
- Slurred speech
- Refusal to eat
- Absence of gag reflux
- Excessive time spent eating
- Multiple swallows required to clear a single bolus of food
- Pain upon swallowing
- Verbal complaints of food stuck in the throat
- Lack of attention to eating

Upon observation, these patients may have a documented weight loss, edema, poor skin turgor, and open wounds. These are all signs of poor nutrition.

Tips for safe swallowing include:

- Eat slowly
- Avoid distractions while eating
- Do not talk while eating
- Remove loose dentures
- Sit up while eating
- Position head correctly
- Use a teaspoon and take only one-half teaspoon of food or liquids at a time
- Swallow completely between bites or sips
- Select foods and fluids of appropriate consistency

membrane, called **rugae,** smooth out when the stomach is full. They allow the stomach to expand. There is no need to eat constantly, partly because the stomach serves as a reservoir for food—it takes 4 to 6 hours for food to pass completely through to the small intestine. Gastric juice, the collective secretions of the stomach, consists of hydrochloric acid, mucus, and the enzymes pepsin, **rennin,** and **gastric lipase.**

DIGESTIVE ACTION

In the stomach, the chemical digestion of protein begins and further mechanical digestion takes place. Some water and minerals, certain drugs, and alcohol are absorbed in the stomach. Even before food enters the mouth, the sight or smell of food can cause the gastric mucosa to excrete the hormone **gastrin.** This hormone stimulates the secretion of gastric juice so that there is some present in the stomach when the food arrives. The stomach's lining is partially protected from the corrosive effects of gastric juice by mucus.

The hydrolysis of protein is initiated when hydrochloric acid activates and then converts **pepsinogen** to its active form, **pepsin.** A protein molecule consists of as many as hundreds of amino acids joined together by **peptide bonds.** Such chains of amino acids linked by peptide bonds are called **polypeptides.** Pepsin breaks down large polypeptides into smaller polypeptides. In infants, the milk protein casein is broken down by the enzyme rennin. The action of rennin coagulates (curdles) the milk. In addition

to activating pepsin, hydrochloric acid destroys harmful bacteria, makes certain minerals such as iron and calcium more absorbable, and maintains the pH (1 to 2) of the gastric juice.

Some butterfat molecules of milk are also broken down into smaller molecules in the stomach. The enzyme that accomplishes this breakdown is gastric lipase. This enzyme is most active in infants; the more alkaline environment of the infant's stomach enables gastric lipase to work more effectively than in adults.

The mechanical digestion that occurs in the stomach is a result of the churning action of the muscular walls. This muscular activity agitates the contents of the stomach, thoroughly mixing the food with gastric juice. In this way, the food is reduced to a semifluid mass of partially digested material called **chyme.** Peristaltic waves push the chyme toward the **pyloric sphincter,** the valve separating the stomach from the small intestine. With each peristaltic wave, a small amount of chyme is forced through the pyloric sphincter into the small intestine.

Gastroparesis is defined as delayed gastric emptying and can be caused by a variety of pathologies including Diabetes Mellitus, neuropathic disorders, connective tissue diseases, infiltrating diseases, and as a post-surgical complication. Symptoms include nausea, vomiting, early satiety, bloating or fullness, and abdominal discomfort. Many clients are asymptomatic (no symptoms). Complications include fluid and electrolyte abnormalities, inadequate nutritional intake, weight loss, and difficult blood glucose control. Dietary treatment includes small feedings, low-fat foods, low-residue foods, and frequent feedings. Gastric motor and sensory function is complex and the care of clients with gastroparesis is a challenge.

Small Intestine

The **small intestine** is the longest portion of the alimentary canal, approximately 20 feet (610 cm) in length. It extends from the pyloric sphincter of the stomach to the large intestine. The small intestine is looped and coiled in the central part of the abdominal cavity, surrounded by the large intestine. It consists of three parts: the **duodenum** is the first 10 inches, the **jejunum** is the middle 8 feet, and the **ileum** is the last 11 feet. Ninety percent of the digestive action in the alimentary canal and nearly all absorption of the end products of digestion occur in the small intestine. Its anatomy is discussed further in the section on absorption.

The entry of chyme into the duodenum stimulates the secretion of two hormones, secretin and cholecystokinin. Collectively, these hormones are responsible for the secretion and release of bile and the secretion of pancreatic juice. Secretin stimulates the production of bile by the liver and the secretion of sodium bicarbonate juice by the pancreas. The bile salts in bile emulsify fats, and sodium bicarbonate juice (which is alkaline) neutralizes the gastric juice that enters the duodenum. This neutralization is necessary to prevent damage to the lining of the duodenum. Mucus secreted by intestinal glands also provides some measure of protection against such damage.

Cholecystokinin stimulates the contraction of the gallbladder, an action that forces stored bile into the duodenum. It also stimulates the secretion of pancreatic enzymes, which are essential for the breakdown of carbohydrates, fats, and proteins. Intestinal juice is also secreted in response to the presence of chyme in the duodenum. Peristaltic action of the small intestine mixes together the bile, the pancreatic juice, and the intestinal juice with the chyme as it moves toward the colon. The collective action of these juices yields the final end products of the digestive process.

DIGESTION OF CARBOHYDRATES

Carbohydrate digestion is completed through the action of pancreatic and intestinal enzymes. Pancreatic **amylase** breaks down any remaining starch into maltose. The disaccharides maltose, sucrose, and lactose are reduced to monosaccharides by the action of three enzymes located in the walls of the small intestine. Each of these enzymes is specific for a given disaccharide: **maltase** breaks down maltose to glucose and glucose, **sucrase** breaks down sucrose to glucose and fructose, and **lactase** breaks down lactose to glucose and galactose. Often, low levels of these enzymes can lead to intolerances for the respective disaccharides.

In fact, approximately 70 percent of the world's population has some degree of lactose intolerance. This intolerance is the result of a lack of the intestinal enzyme lactase. Clinical Application 10–1 discusses carbohydrate intolerances, including lactose intolerance. Table 10–1 lists food

Clinical Application 10–1

Carbohydrate Intolerances

Some individuals are deficient in one or more of the enzymes lactase, maltase, or sucrase. They are unable to digest these disaccharides into monosaccharides. The resulting disease is called a lactose intolerance, maltose intolerance, or sucrose intolerance.

Lactose intolerance, the most common of these diseases, may occur in 60 to 100 percent of Hispanics, blacks, and southeast Asians. The condition can be hereditary or can be secondary to other disease processes involving the small intestine. Symptoms of a lactose intolerance include abdominal cramping and pain, loose stools, and flatulence (gas) after eating or drinking milk products.

Dietary treatment of a lactose intolerance involves three steps: (1) identifying food items that contain lactose; (2) eliminating all sources of lactose from the diet; and (3) establishing an individual tolerance level for the client on a trial-and-error basis. The tolerance levels for lactose vary widely among individuals.

The lactose content of cheeses varies. One gallon of milk is required to produce 1 lb of cheese. During cheese making, the **whey** is separated from the curd. The whey is the liquid and the **curd** is the solid material (similar to the curd in cottage cheese). Most of the lactose in cheese is contained in the whey. In ripened cheese, the small amount of lactose entrapped in the curd is transformed into lactic acid, which does not require lactase for absorption.

Generally, cheese must age for more than 90 days to be lactose free. The following cheeses are considered hard ripened (low in lactose): blue, brick, Brie, Camembert, Cheddar, Colby, Edam, Gouda, Monterey, Muenster, Parmesan, Provolone, and Swiss. The following cheeses are considered soft cheeses and thus contain more lactose: cream cheese, Neufchatel, ricotta, mozzarella, and cottage cheese.

Clients on a lactose-free diet should read all labels carefully to see if milk or milk solids, lactose, or whey have been added to the products. Many toothpastes and over-the-counter medications contain a small amount of lactose. Generally, the amount is very small and is tolerated well.

Lactaid is an over-the-counter product specially designed for individuals with a lactose intolerance. Lactaid is a natural enzyme that is available in liquid or tablet form. The liquid form is typically added to milk, whereas the tablet form is chewed before consumption of a food product containing lactose. Some grocery stores also sell milk that has been pretreated with Lactaid. This product will digest 70 percent of the lactose in a product into glucose galactose. As a result, most lactose-intolerant persons can drink Lactaid-treated milk or eat foods that contain lactose and digest it comfortably. Milk treated with Lactaid is slightly sweeter than regular milk. The sweeter taste results naturally when lactose is broken down into glucose and galactose.

A lactose-restricted diet may be low in calcium, riboflavin, and vitamin D. Clients should be instructed in alternative sources of these nutrients or advised to take supplements.

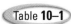

Table 10–1   **Lactose Content of Foods**

LACTOSE-FREE FOODS

Broth-based soups
Plain meat, fish, poultry, peanut butter
Breads that do not contain milk, dry milk solids, or whey
Cereal, crackers
Fruit, plain vegetables
Desserts made without milk, dry milk solids, or whey
Tofu and tofu products, such as tofu-based ice cream substitute
Nondairy creamers

LOW-LACTOSE FOODS (0–2 g/serving)

Milk treated with lactase enzyme, 1/2 cup
Sherbet, 1/2 cup
Aged cheese, 1–2 oz
Processed cheese, 1 oz
Butter or margarine
Commercially prepared foods containing dry milk solids or
    whey
Some medications and vitamin preparations may contain a
    small amount of lactose. Generally, the amount is very small
    and is tolerated well.

HIGH-LACTOSE FOODS (5 TO 8 g/serving)

Milk (whole, skim, 1 percent, 2 percent, buttermilk, sweet
    acidophilus), 1/2 cup
Powdered dry milk (whole, nonfat, buttermilk—before reconsti-
    tuting), 1/8 cup
Evaporated milk, 1/4 cup
Sweetened condensed milk, 3 tbsp
Party chip dip or potato topping, 1/2 cup
White sauce, 1/2 cup
Creamed or low-fat cottage cheese, 3/4 cup
Dry cottage cheese, 1 cup
Ricotta cheese, 3/4 cup
Cheese food or cheese spread, 2 oz*
Sour cream, 1/2 cup
Heavy cream, 3/4 cup
Ice cream or ice milk, 3/4 cup
Half and half, 1/2 cup
Yogurt, 1/2 cup†

*Lactose content is higher than that of aged cheese and of processed
    cheese because of the addition of whey powder and dry milk solids.
†Yogurt may be tolerated better than foods with similar lactose content
    because of hydrolysis of lactose by bacterial lactase found in the cul-
    ture. Tolerance may vary with the brand and processing method.
SOURCE: Nelson JK et al: Mayo Clinic Diet Manual, with permission.

items that are lactose-free, low in lactose, and high in lactose. Table 10–2 contains a lactose-restricted diet with a
sample menu.

DIGESTION OF FATS

Fats are emulsified by bile salts in the small intestine
before they are digested further. **Emulsification** is the
physical breaking up of fats into tiny droplets. In this way,
more surface area of the fat is exposed to the chemical
action of the enzyme pancreatic lipase. Pancreatic lipase
completes the digestion of fats by reducing triglycerides to
diglycerides and monoglycerides, fatty acids, and glycerol.
Lingual lipase is an important enzyme in infants, although
not in adults.

DIGESTION OF PROTEIN

Although hundreds of enzymes are involved in protein
digestion, this text reviews only a few of the major ones.
The shorter polypeptides resulting from the digestive
action in the stomach are broken down even further by the
action of pancreatic and intestinal enzymes. Two of the
major pancreatic enzymes that are responsible for this
additional protein splitting are **trypsin** and **chymotrypsin.**
Both trypsin and chymotrypsin have inactive precursors
that are activated by other enzymes.

The intestinal wall also secretes a group of enzymes
known as peptidases. The **peptidases** act on the smaller
molecules produced by the pancreatic enzymes, reducing
them to single amino acids and small peptides, the final
end products of protein digestion.

Table 10–3 summarizes the digestion of carbohydrates,
fats, and proteins by body organ (mouth, stomach,
and small intestine). The Table 10–3 subcategories
identify whether the digestive action is mechanical or
chemical.

Absorption

The end products of digestion move from the gastrointestinal tract into the blood or lymphatic system in a
process called **absorption.** The **lymphatic system** transports **lymph** from the tissues to the bloodstream. This system is technically part of the circulatory or cardiovascular
system. Eventually, all fluid in the lymphatic system enters
the blood. It is only after nutrients have been absorbed
into either the blood or lymphatic system that the cells of
the body can use them.

The end products of digestion include the monosaccharides from carbohydrate digestion, the fatty acids and
glycerol (and often monoglycerides) from fats, and small
peptides and amino acids from protein digestion.
Absorption occurs primarily in the small intestine.

Small Intestine

The inner surface of the small intestine has mucosal folds,
villi, and microvilli to increase the surface area for maximum absorption (Fig. 10–1). The mucosal folds are like
pleats in fabric. On each fold ("pleat") are millions of
finger-like projections, called **villi.** Each villus has hundreds of microscopic, hair-like projections (resembling
bristles on a brush), called **microvilli,** on its surface. The
large surface area resulting from this arrangement fosters
the movement of nutrients into the blood or lymphatic system. The structure of the mucosa serves as a unit that
accomplishes the absorption of nutrients.

Within each villus is a network of blood capillaries and
a central lymph vessel called a **lacteal.** The villi absorb
nutrients from the chyme by way of these blood and lymph
vessels. Monosaccharides, amino acids, glycerol (which is
water soluble), minerals, and water-soluble vitamins are
absorbed into the blood in the **capillary** network. Because
short- and medium-chain fatty acids have fewer carbons in
their chain length, they are more water soluble than long-
chain fatty acids. Thus, they are absorbed directly into the
blood as well.

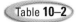 **Table 10–2** **Lactose-Restricted Diet**

Description: This diet restricts foods that contain lactose. Soy milk substitutes are used as a milk replacement. Individual tolerances should be taken into consideration, because some clients may tolerate foods low in lactose (see Table 10–1).

Note: All labels should be read carefully for the addition of milk, lactose, or whey.

Indications: This diet is used for the management of patients exhibiting the signs and symptoms of lactose intolerance, Crohn's disease, short bowel syndrome, or colitis. Persistent diarrhea and excessive amounts of gas may be lessened by decreasing lactose intake.

Nutritional adequacy: This diet is low in calcium, riboflavin, and vitamin D. Supplementation is recommended.

FOOD GROUP	ALLOWED	AVOIDED
Milk	Hard, ripened cheese Ensure Sustacal Ensure Plus Soy milk Lactaid-treated milk Coffee Rich	Unripened cheese Fluid milk Powdered milk Milk chocolate Cream Most chocolate drink mixes Most coffee creamers
Breads and cereals	Most water-based bread (French Italian, Jewish) Graham crackers Ritz crackers without cheese	Bread to which milk or lactose has been added (check label)
Fruits	Any	None
Vegetables	Fresh, frozen, or canned without milk	Creamed, buttered, or breaded vegetables
Meats	Those not listed under "Avoided" Kosher prepared meat or milk products	Breaded or creamed meat, fish, poultry Most luncheon meats Sausage Frankfurters
Desserts and miscellaneous items	Angel food cake Gelatin desserts Milk-free cookies Popcorn (with milk-free margarine) Pretzels Mustard, catsup Pickles	Most commercially made desserts Sherbet Ice cream Toffee Cream candies Caramels Most chewing gums

SAMPLE MENU

BREAKFAST	LUNCH/DINNER
1/2 cup orange juice 1/2 cup cream of wheat 2 slices whole grain milk-free bread 2 tsp milk-free margarine Jelly Coffee 1/2 cup nondairy "creamer"	3 oz baked chicken Baked potato 1/2 cup carrots Sliced tomato 1 slice milk-free bread 2 tsp milk-free margarine Angel food cake with fresh fruit topping Coffee

These water-soluble nutrients, including short- and medium-chain fatty acids, eventually enter into hepatic portal circulation (via the portal vein) and travel to the liver. **Hepatic portal circulation** is a subdivision of the vascular system by which blood from the digestive organs and spleen circulates through the liver before returning to the heart. In the liver, the nutrients are modified according to the needs of the body.

Because long-chain fats are not soluble in water and the blood is chiefly water, the fat-soluble nutrients cannot be absorbed directly into the blood. Instead, fat-soluble nutrients—including long-chain fatty acids, any monoglycerides remaining from fat digestion, and fat-soluble vitamins—are first combined with bile salts as a carrier. Then, this complex of fat-soluble materials is absorbed into the cells lining the intestinal wall.

Once the fat is absorbed, the bile separates from it and returns to recirculate. Within the intestinal cells, any remaining monoglycerides are reduced to fatty acids and glycerol by an enzyme. Glycerol, fatty acids, and absorbed long-chain fatty acids are recombined (within the intestinal cells) to form human triglycerides in a process called triglyceride synthesis.

The newly formed triglycerides and any other fat materials present (such as cholesterol) are covered with special proteins, forming lipoproteins called **chylomicrons**. The chylomicrons are released into the lymphatic system via the lacteals. Remember that the lymphatic system is connected

Table **10–3** **Summary of Digestion**

NUTRIENT	MOUTH AND ESOPHAGUS	STOMACH	SMALL INTESTINE
CARBOHYDRATES			
	Mechanical	Mechanical	Mechanical
	Mastication	Peristalsis	Peristalsis
	Swallowing	Mucus	Mucus
	Peristalsis		
	Mucus		
	Chemical	Chemical	Chemical
	Salivary amylase	None	Pancreatic enzymes: Pancreatic amylase
			Intestinal enzymes:
			Maltase
			Sucrase
MONOSACCHARIDES			Lactase
Fats yield	Mechanical	Mechanical	Mechanical
	Mastication	Peristalsis	Peristalsis
	Swallowing	Mucus	Mucus
	Peristalsis		Gallbladder: Bile*
	Mucus		
	Chemical	Chemical	Chemical
	None	Gastric lipase†	Pancreatic enzymes: Pancreatic lipase
	Lingual lipase in infants		
GLYCEROL, FATTY ACIDS, AND MONOGLYCERIDES			
Proteins yield	Mechanical	Mechanical	Mechanical
	Mastication	Peristalsis	Peristalsis
	Swallowing	Mucus	Mucus
	Peristalsis		
	Mucus		
	Chemical	Chemical	Chemical
	None	Rennin	Pancreatic enzymes: Trypsin
			Chymotrypsin
		Pepsin	
		Hydrochloric acid	
Amino acids and small peptides			Intestinal enzymes: Peptidases

*Emulsifies fat.
†Digests butterfat only.

to the blood system. The protein "wrapping" these packages of fat enables the chylomicrons to move into the blood via the **thoracic** lymphatic duct (and hence into portal blood). In the liver, lipids are also modified to suit the needs of the body before distribution to body cells. Table 10–4 describes some of the nutrient modifications that are made in the liver.

Further passage of undigested food is controlled by the **ileocecal valve,** which relaxes and then closes with each peristaltic wave. This valve prevents backflow and ensures that chyme remains in the small intestine long enough for sufficient digestion and absorption.

Large Intestine

The **large intestine,** also called the **colon,** extends from the ileum (last part of the small intestine) to the anus. When the chyme leaves the small intestine, it enters the first portion of the large intestine, the **cecum** (the appendix, an organ with no known function, is attached to the cecum).

Chyme leaves the cecum and travels slowly through the remaining parts of the large intestine: the ascending colon, the transverse colon, the descending colon, the sigmoid colon, the **rectum,** and the anal canal.

Water is the main substance absorbed by the large intestine. However, the absorption of some minerals and vitamins also occurs in the colon. Most of the water, up to 80 percent, is extracted in the cecum and the ascending colon and returned to the bloodstream. Vitamins synthesized by intestinal bacteria, including vitamin K and some of the B-complexes, are absorbed from the colon. After absorption and digestion have taken place, the remaining waste products are eliminated in the feces through the rectum.

Elimination of Unabsorbed Materials

Absorption of water into the bloodstream slowly reduces the water content of the material left inside the large intestine, and the waste product has a solid consistency. This solid material is the feces. Mucus, the only secretion of the

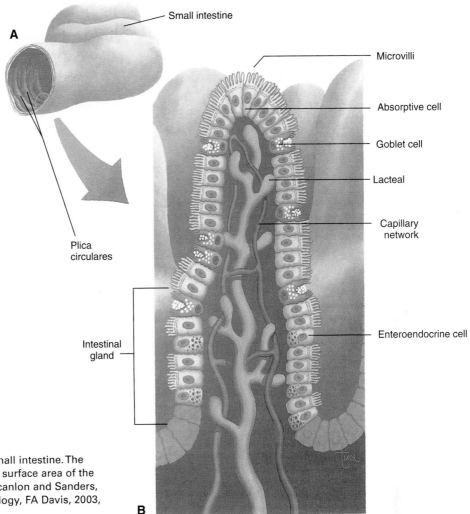

Figure **10–1** Cross-section of the small intestine. The multiple folds greatly increase the surface area of the small intestine. (Reprinted from Scanlon and Sanders, Essentials of Anatomy and Physiology, FA Davis, 2003, with permission.)

large intestine, provides lubrication for the smooth passage of the feces. By the time feces reach the rectum, it consists of 75 percent water and 25 percent solids. The solids include cellular wastes, undigested dietary fiber, undigested food, bile salts, cholesterol, mucus, and bacteria.

Indigestible Carbohydrates

The body cannot digest some forms of carbohydrates because it lacks the necessary enzyme to split the appropriate molecule. Some vegetables and legumes contain these indigestible sugars and fibers. Intestinal gas is formed in the colon by the decomposition of undigested materials. Examples of gas-forming foods are beans, onions, radishes, and vegetables of the cabbage family.

Factors Interfering with Absorption

Malabsorption is the inadequate movement of digested food from the small intestine into the blood or lymphatic system. Malnutrition can be caused by malabsorption. Table 10–5 lists factors that interfere with the absorption of nutrients. Note in the table that many diseases, medications, and some medical treatments have a negative impact on the absorption of nutrients. Clinical Applications 10–2 discusses surgical removal of all or part

Table 10–4	Metabolic Modifications in the Liver
ENERGY NUTRIENT	**MODIFICATION**
Carbohydrates	Fructose and galactose changed to glucose, excess glucose converted to glycogen
Lipids	Lipoproteins formed, cholesterol synthesized, triglycerides broken down and built
Amino acids	Nonessential amino acids manufactured, excess amino acids deaminated and then changed to carbohydrates or fats, ammonia removed from the blood, plasma proteins made
Other	Alcohol, drugs, and poisons detoxified

Table **10–5**	Factors Decreasing Absorption
Medications	Antacids
	Laxatives
	Birth control pills
	Anticonvulsants
	Antibiotics
Parasites	Tapeworm
	Hookworm
Surgical procedures	Gastric resections
	Any surgery on the small intestine
	Some surgical procedures on the large intestine
Disease states	Infection
	Tropical sprue
	Gluten-sensitive enteropathy
	Hepatic disease
	Pancreatic insufficiency
	Lactase deficiency
	Sucrase deficiency
	Maltase deficiency
	Circulatory disorders
	Cancers involving the alimentary canal
Medical complications	Effects of radiation therapy
	Chemotherapy

Note: Most of these conditions will be discussed in later chapters.

of the alimentary canal and the effect on absorption. Clinical Applications 10–3 discusses inadequate absorption.

The cells lining the inside layer of the small intestine have a very short life. The smallest structures are replaced every 2 to 3 days. Although this rapid cell turnover helps to promote healing after injury, it also allows vulnerability to any nutritional deficiency or process that might interfere with cell reproduction.

Gut failure is a term used to describe a situation in which the small intestine fails to absorb nutrients properly. Symptoms include diarrhea, malabsorption, and a poor response to oral feedings. A vicious cycle starts when the cells lining the small intestine fail to reproduce because they do not have the necessary nutrients for cell replace-

Surgical Removal of All or Part of the Alimentary Canal

Clients may need to have a portion of the small intestine surgically removed for a variety of reasons. These clients are frequently at a nutritional risk because they are either permanently or temporarily unable to absorb essential nutrients. In such cases, a nutritional assessment is indicated. In the past, some clients elected to have a portion of the alimentary canal removed to lose weight. This procedure is discussed in the weight-control chapter.

Clinical Applications 10–3

Inadequate Absorption

Visually inspecting a client's feces can confirm a suspicion of poor digestion or poor absorption. Large chunks of food indicate a problem with digestion. A large amount of liquid or near-liquid stools suggests poor absorption. A simple question directed to the client, such as "Are your stools formed?" can provide some information. Sometimes, however, client's concept of normal may be different from the health-care provider's.

ment. The result is chronic diarrhea caused by malabsorption. In turn, the malabsorption leads to malnutrition, which prevents cell reproduction. Figure 10–2 diagrams this cycle.

Steatorrhea

Some diseases and medications result in the malabsorption of fat. In these conditions, clients have **steatorrhea,** or fat in the stools. Frequently the condition is caused by the inhibition of pancreatic lipase, an enzyme necessary for the digestion of fats. Clinical Applications 10–4 discusses lipid malabsorption and dietary treatment.

Nontropical Sprue

Nontropical **sprue** is a disorder of the small intestine. This disease is commonly referred to as **celiac disease** or **gluten-sensitive enteropathy.** Celiac disease is an inherited condition that affects approximately 1 of every 3000

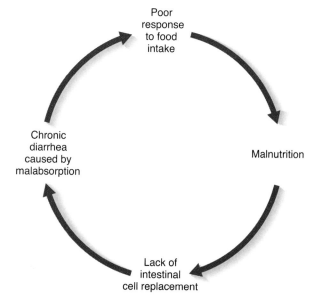

Figure **10–2** "Gut failure." Gut failure is a self-perpetuating cycle. Poor response to food intake leads to poor intestinal cell regeneration, which leads to chronic diarrhea caused by malabsorption.

Clinical Applications 10–4

Lipid Malabsorption

Some clients for a variety of reasons are unable to digest and absorb long-chain fatty acids. For these clients, the use of medium-chain triglyceride (MCT) oil is indicated. MCT oil can provide a kilocalorie source for patients with a fat malabsorption problem.

Any food that contains fat must be fitted into the diet of any client who suffers from a lipid malabsorption. The American Dietetic and Diabetes Associations' Exchange Lists for Menu Planning can be used as a guide in planning this type of diet. Usually the physician will order a specified number of grams of fat high in long-chain fatty acids. A typical low-fat diet order may read "40-g fat diet." Such a diet may be planned as follows:

EXCHANGE	NUMBER OF EXCHANGES/DAY	GRAMS OF FAT
Skim milk	Unlimited	0
Starches	8	4 (0.5 g of fat/exchange
Fruits	Unlimited	0
Vegetables	Unlimited	0
Meat, lean	7	21 (7 × 3 g/exchange)
Fat	3	15 (3 × 5 g/exchange)
		40 g fat/day

The MCT oil is then added to the diet as necessary to bring the kilocalories up to meet the client's kilocalorie requirement.

Some physicians prefer to treat a lipid disorder with medication. Pancrease is one of the medications indicated for steatorrhea secondary to pancreatic insufficiency, as in cystic fibrosis or chronic alcoholic pancreatitis (discussed in Gastrointestinal chapter). Pancrease is an enzyme that digests nutrients.

Americans and is due to an unknown genetic defect (IFIC, 2003). Gluten-sensitive enteropathy results from the toxic effects that occur from the ingestion of **gluten,** a protein present in the following grains: wheat, rye, oats, and barley. Individuals with this disease suffer from a wide variety of nutritional problems.

The result of the toxic effect of gluten is the direct destruction of intestinal cells. This may be related to an allergic reaction and can be either severe or mild. In the severe form, the loss of the intestinal mucosa causes malnutrition. The damaged intestine results in an impaired ability to absorb nutrients, including carbohydrates, proteins, fats, and fat-soluble vitamins. Lactose intolerance is commonly seen. The potential risks extend further: premature osteoporosis, colon cancer, autoimmune disorders (including thyroid disease and type 1 diabetes), arthritis, miscarriage, and birth defects (Duyff, 2002).

Treatment in this situation would involve the use of medium-chain triglycerides to increase the kilocaloric content of the diet and a lactose-free, gluten-free diet. This is a complex diet for the health-care professional to plan and for the client to follow. Usually frequent consultations with the physician regarding the status of the client's intestinal cells are necessary. These clients are often malnourished. As such, the client benefits from being kept on this severe a diet only until intestinal cell regeneration is completed. Once the client is able to tolerate both lactose and long-chain triglycerides, these should be included in the diet. This will increase the client's compliance in maintaining a high kilocalorie intake and assist in treating the malnutrition.

In milder forms, only a gluten-restricted diet is indicated (Table 10–6). Gluten is present in several prepared foods that contain thickened sauces. Extensive client teaching is necessary for a positive client outcome. Removal of all forms of wheat, rye, oats, and barley from the diet frequently results in remission or improvement within weeks.

Table 10–6 Gluten-Restricted Diet

Description: The diet is free of cereals that contain gluten: wheat, oats, rye, and barley.
Indications: This diet is used to treat the primary intestinal malabsorption found in celiac disease.
Adequacy: Unless an effort is made to increase kilocalories, the energy intake may be inadequate to replace previous weight loss. This diet may not meet the RDA for B-complex vitamins, especially thiamin. Iron intake may be inadequate for the premenopausal woman.

FOOD GROUPS	FOODS THAT CONTAIN GLUTEN	FOODS THAT MAY CONTAIN GLUTEN	FOODS THAT DO NOT CONTAIN GLUTEN
Beverage	Cereal beverages (e.g., Postum), malt, Ovaltine, beer and ale	Commercial* chocolate milk, cocoa mixes, other beverage mixes, dietary supplements	Coffee, tea, decaffeinated coffee, carbonated beverages, chocolate drinks made with pure cocoa powder, wine, distilled liquor
Meat and meat substitutes		Meat loaf and patties, cold cuts and prepared meats, stuffing, breaded meats, cheese foods and spreads; commercial soufflés, omelets, and fondue; soy protein meat substitutes	Pure meat, fish, fowl, egg, cottage cheese, peanut butter
Fat and oil		Commercial salad dressing and mayo, gravy, white and cream sauces, nondairy creamer	Butter, margarine, vegetable oil

(Continued on the following page)

Table **10–6** **Gluten-Restricted Diet** *(Continued)*

FOOD GROUPS	FOODS THAT CONTAIN GLUTEN	FOODS THAT MAY CONTAIN GLUTEN	FOODS THAT DO NOT CONTAIN GLUTEN
Milk	Milk beverages that contain malt	Commercial chocolate milk	Whole, low-fat, and skim milk; buttermilk
Grains and grain products	Bread, crackers, cereal, and pasta that contain wheat, oats, rye, malt, malt flavoring, graham flour, durham flour, pastry flour, bran, or wheat germ; barley; millet; pretzels; communion wafers	Commercial seasoned rice and potato mixes	Specially prepared breads made with wheat starch,† rice, potato, or soybean flour or cornmeal; pure corn or rice cereals; hominy grits; white, brown, and wild rice; popcorn; low-protein pasta made from wheat starch
Vegetable		Commercially seasoned vegetable mixes; commercial vegetables with cream or cheese sauce; canned baked beans	All fresh vegetables; plain commercially frozen or canned vegetables
Fruit		Commercial pie fillings	All plain or sweetened fruits; fruit thickened with tapioca or cornstarch
Soup	Soup that contains wheat pasta; soup thickened with wheat flour or other gluten-containing grains	Commercial soup, broth, and soup mixes	Soup thickened with cornstarch, potato rice or soybean flour; pure broth
Desserts	Commercial cakes, cookies, and pastries	Commercial ice cream and sherbet	Gelatin; custard; fruit ice; specially prepared cakes, cookies, and pastries made with gluten-free flour or starch; pudding and fruit filling thickened with tapioca, cornstarch, or arrowroot flour
Sweets		Commercial candies, especially chocolates	
Miscellaneous		Ketchup, prepared mustard, soy sauce, commercially prepared meat sauces and pickles, vinegar, flavoring syrups (syrups for pancakes or ice cream)	Monosodium glutamate, salt, pepper, pure spices and herbs, yeast, pure baking chocolate or cocoa powder, carob, flavoring extracts, artificial flavoring

SAMPLE MENU

BREAKFAST	LUNCH/DINNER
1/2 cup orange juice	Chicken breast
Cocoa Puffs, Sugar Pops, Puffed Rice	Baked potato
2 slices gluten-free bread	1/2 cup broccoli
1 poached egg	Lettuce/tomato salad
1 cup milk	French dressing
2 tsp margarine	Sour cream
Jelly	1/2 cup milk
	Cornstarch pudding

*The terms *commercially prepared* and *commercial* are used to refer to partially prepared foods purchased from a grocery or food market and to prepared foods purchased from a restaurant.

†Wheat starch may contain trace amounts of gluten. Avoid if not tolerated.

Note: Medications may contain trace amounts of gluten. A pharmacist may be able to provide information on the gluten content of medications.

SOURCE: Mayo Clinic Diet Manual, 1994.

Table **10–7**	Substitutions for 2 Tablespoons of Wheat Flour

3 tsp cornstarch
3 tsp potato starch
3 tsp arrowroot starch
3 tsp quick-cooking tapioca
3 tbsp white or brown rice flour

Table 10–7 lists products that can be substituted for flour in many recipes.

Food Allergies

A food **allergy** is a sensitivity to a food that does not cause a negative reaction in most people. Clients often use the term **food allergy** as a generic term that encompasses a broad range of symptoms triggered by certain foods. The medical community reserves the term to immunologically mediated abnormal reactions to foods that are life threatening. A true allergy requires meticulous avoidance of food implicated to minimize the risk of potentially life-threatening reactions (Sheikh, 2002; Taylor, Hefle, and Munoz-Furlong, 1999). Individuals may be genetically predisposed to a food allergy. Common triggers for food allergies include eggs, milk, peanuts, and fish. Less common triggers include fruit, vegetables, tree nuts, and wheat. Some food allergies may be due to an alteration in absorption. The susceptible person absorbs a part of a food before it has been completely digested. The incomplete digestion of protein in particular is responsible for many allergic reactions.

The body does not recognize the sequence of amino acids (because the protein was absorbed partly undigested) and therefore treats the protein as a foreign substance and tries to destroy it. This attempt produces the symptoms of food allergy, including skin rash, nausea, vomiting, diarrhea, intestinal cramps, swelling in various parts of the body, and spasm of the small intestine. An allergen may also be inhaled into the body. For example, the smell of peanuts may cause an allergic reaction in susceptible people.

Once diagnosed, the treatment for a food allergy is to avoid the offending food. This is difficult even with the current U.S. labeling laws and especially challenging when eating away from home or in foreign countries.

Food allergies are frequently diagnosed in children. One approach used to treat these clients is the Allergy I and Allergy II diets. The Allergy I diet is limited to rice, lamb, and a few fruits and vegetables and therefore eliminates most common food allergens, including wheat, eggs, and milk. The Allergy II diet includes a few meats, potatoes, and a few more fruits and vegetables. This second diet is completely free of cereal, milk, and eggs. These diets are typically used for 1 to 2 weeks. If symptoms are relieved, selected foods are gradually added back into the diet one at a time. Chewing gum, vitamin pills, and certain medications such as antibiotics and antihistamines should be discontinued during the test period. These diets are often prescribed for any apparent allergic response with a multitude of varying and individual symptoms, including rash, sinus congestion, headache, wheezing, and cough.

The Allergy I and II diets are not nutritionally adequate. Both diets are deficient in calcium, riboflavin, thiamin, folic acid, vitamin B_6, magnesium, and possibly vitamin C for all ages. In addition, iron is inadequate for teenagers and premenopausal women. For this reason, these diets are not recommended for long-term use. Allergy I and II diets are presented in Table 10–8.

Metabolism

After digestion and absorption, nutrients are carried by the blood (usually after being modified in the liver cells) to all cells of the body. After entry into the cells, the nutrients from food undergo many chemical changes, which result in either the release of energy or the use of energy. **Metabolism** is the sum of all chemical and physical processes continuously going on in living organisms, comprising both anabolism and catabolism. Catabolic reactions usually result in the release of energy. Anabolic reactions require energy. The next section describes how cells utilize the end products of digestion to meet the energy needs of the body.

Catabolic Reactions

Glucose, glycerol, fatty acids, and amino acids can be broken down even further. These nutrients are held together by bonds that require energy to form and that, when broken, release energy. The breakdown of the fuel-producing nutrients yields carbon dioxide, water, heat, and other forms of energy. The carbon dioxide is eventually exhaled, and the water becomes part of the body fluids or is eliminated in the urine. Fifty percent or more of the total potential energy usually is lost as heat. The remaining available energy is temporarily stored in the cells as adenosine triphosphate (ATP).

ATP, a high-energy compound that has three phosphate groups in its structure, is thus available in all cells. Practically speaking, ATP is the storage form of energy for the cells, because each cell has enzymes that can initiate the hydrolysis (breakdown through the addition of water) of ATP. In this reaction, one or more phosphate groups split off and subsequently release energy. If one phosphate group is removed, the result is ADP (adenosine diphosphate) plus phosphate.

Many steps are involved in the catabolic process responsible for the release of this energy. These steps require one or more of the following agents: enzymes, coenzymes, and/or hormones. Some vitamins and minerals act as coenzymes. Oxygen is also necessary for the full release of any potential energy. This addition of oxygen to the reaction is called **oxidation.** During the many steps that occur, the energy is released little by little and stored as ATP. The breakdown process includes the formation of intermediate chemical compounds such as **pyruvate** (pyruvic acid) and **acetyl CoA.** Acetyl CoA can be broken down further by entering a series of chemical reactions known as the **Krebs cycle** or the TCA (tricarboxylic acid)

Table 10–8 **Allergy I and II Diets**

ALLERGY I

FOOD GROUP	ALLOWED FOODS
Bread, cereal, rice, and pasta group	Rice, rice wafers, rice biscuits, Rice Chex, puffed rice, rice flakes, cream of rice, tapioca, white rice
Vegetable group	Beets, carrots, chard, lettuce, sweet potatoes, yams
Fruit group	Apricots, cranberries, peaches, pears, juice of allowed fruit (unsweetened or sweetened with sucrose)
Meat, poultry, fish, dry beans, eggs, and nut group	Lamb
Milk, yogurt, and cheese group	None
Fats, oils, and sweets group	Any vegetable oil or shortening, margarine without milk solids
	Cane or beet sugar
	Salt
	White vinegar
	Tapioca

SAMPLE MENU

BREAKFAST	LUNCH/DINNER
Hot cream of rice cereal	Lamb chop or ground lamb patty
2 rice biscuits	1/2 cup cooked white rice
1/2 cup peaches	Baked sweet potato
2 tsp apricot preserves	1/2 cup canned pears
1/2 cup peach juice (drained from canned peaches)	Cranberry juice

ALLERGY II

FOOD GROUP	ALLOWED FOODS
Bread, cereal, rice, and pasta group	Tapioca, soy flour, potato flour, white and sweet potatoes
Vegetable group	Soybean sprouts, lettuce, spinach, chard, carrots, beets, artichoke, squash, asparagus, peas, string beans, lima beans
Fruit group	Sucrose-sweetened and unsweetened apricots, cranberries, peaches, pears, pineapple, prunes, and the juices of these fruits
Meat, poultry, fish, dry beans, eggs, and nuts group	Lamb, beef, chicken, bacon, veal, soybeans
Milk, yogurt, and cheese group	None
Fats, oils, and sweets	Any vegetable oil and shortening, margarine without milk solids
	Cane or beet sugar (sucrose)
	Salt, white vinegar, tapioca

SAMPLE MENU

BREAKFAST	LUNCH/DINNER
1/2 cup pineapple chunks	4 oz lamb, beef, chicken, veal or 1/2 cup soybeans
2 slices of bacon	Boiled potatoes
1/2 cup potatoes fried in oil	2 tsp milk-free margarine
1 cup pineapple juice	1/2 cup of cooked carrots
	Lettuce wedge with oil and vinegar
	Stewed prunes
	1 cup cranberry juice

cycle. Figure 10–3 is a simplified schematic of the steps involved in the release of energy by the cells.

Storage of Excess Nutrients

If the cells do not have immediate energy needs, the excess nutrients are stored. Glucose is stored as glycogen in liver and muscle tissue; surplus amounts are converted to fat. Glycerol and fatty acids are reassembled into triglycerides and stored in adipose tissue. Amino acids are used to make body proteins; any excess is deaminated (stripped of

nitrogen) and ultimately used for glucose formation or stored as fat. If energy is not available from food, the cells will seek energy in body stores.

Anabolic Reactions

Once immediate energy needs have been met, the cells utilize the nutrients as needed for growth and repair of body tissue. The cellular supply of ATP is used first. When this instant energy source is exhausted, glycogen and fat stores are used. In addition to building up body protein, other

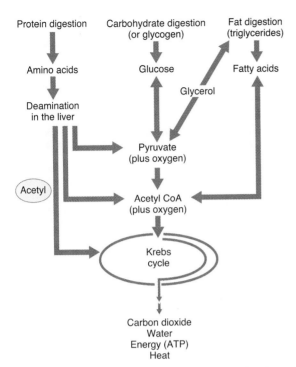

Figure **10–3** Energy production in the cells. Energy is released bit by bit during the further breakdown of amino acids, glucose, glycerol, and fatty acids.

anabolic reactions include the recombination of glycerol and fatty acids to form triglycerides and the formation of glycogen from glucose.

Excretion of Waste Products

Materials of no use to the cells become waste that is eliminated through excretion. Solid waste and some liquid is disposed of in the feces. The digestive system needs assistance from other body systems in the disposal of nonsolid waste. The lungs dispose of gaseous waste. Most liquid waste is sent first to the kidneys and then to the **bladder** to be eliminated in the urine. Some liquid waste is disposed of by the skin through perspiration.

Carbon dioxide (CO_2) is a gas that is eliminated through the lungs each time one exhales. The amount of carbon dioxide exhaled depends on the type of fuel (lipid, protein, or carbohydrate) and/or the source of fuel that the body is currently burning for energy. For example, more CO_2 is produced when carbohydrates are being utilized than with protein or fat.

The skin removes some of the liquid waste in the form of perspiration or water, and some is excreted in the feces. The kidneys eliminate most of the excess water, sodium, hydrogen, and urea. **Urea** is synthesized in the liver from the nitrogen resulting from the breakdown of amino acids. Some water is also removed from the body each time one exhales.

SUMMARY

The cell is the ultimate destination for the nutrients in food. For food to be of use to the cells, it must first be broken down into many tiny particles and then absorbed into the body. Digestion is the process whereby food is broken down into a form usable by the cell: carbohydrates are broken down to monosaccharides, fats are reduced to glycerol and fatty acids, and proteins are split to yield amino acids. This is accomplished by both mechanical and chemical means. Secretions from the salivary glands, stomach, small intestine, liver, and pancreas assist in chemical digestion. Absorption refers to the movement of food from the gastrointestinal tract into the blood and lymphatic system. Metabolism involves the two processes of anabolism and catabolism. The liver plays a major role in metabolism.

After absorption, water-soluble nutrients go directly to the liver for further processing. The liver releases the nutrients into the bloodstream for delivery to the cells. Most of the fat-soluble nutrients are absorbed into the lymphatic system before entering the bloodstream. Short- and medium-chain triglycerides are absorbed differently than long-chain triglycerides. The cells remove the nutrients from the bloodstream as needed for energy and growth. Energy is released little by little from the end products of digestion in a series of chemical reactions. Energy nutrients not needed immediately by the cells are placed in storage as glycogen and adipose tissue.

The metabolism of food produces waste. Waste products are released from the body in the feces, urine, perspiration, and exhaled air.

Many ailments and diseases are related to the structure and function of the gastrointestinal system. Many forms of malabsorption, including disaccharide intolerances and gluten-sensitive enteropathy, are related to structural damage of the small intestine.

CASE STUDY 10–1

Mr. H is a 25-year-old man, 6 ft tall and weighing 170 lb (dressed without shoes). He has a medium frame, as determined by measuring his wrist circumference. Mr. H has just been admitted to the hospital on your service for an elective arthroscopic (surgical procedure) on his right knee. During the nursing admission process, Mr. H complained of gas pains and frequent loose stools. He stated that he does not avoid any particular foods and has a healthy appetite. He claims to drink about 3 cups of milk each day. The client complains of a loss of 5 lb during the prior month. Mr. H needs to use the restroom twice during the interview to "move his bowels." The second time you inspect the stool. The client's stool is loose and unformed.

(Continued on the following page)

CASE STUDY (Continued)

The next day you note that a diagnosis of lactose intolerance has been made. A lactose-restricted diet is ordered. The following nursing care plan originates on the day the client is admitted. The physician uses the information collected from the nurse in making his or her diagnosis. Please note that the client has already met the first desired outcome and part of the second; they have been charted. The client has not met the third desired outcome.

NURSING CARE PLAN

SUBJECTIVE DATA Client complains of gas pains and loose stools. Client states that he does not avoid any particular foods. He drinks milk.

OBJECTIVE DATA Client observed to use the restroom twice in 10 minutes to defecate. Visual inspection shows stool to be loose and unformed

NURSING DIAGNOSIS Nursing Diagnosis NANDA: Diarrhea (NANDA, 2003, with permission) related to client's complaints of loose unformed stools as evidenced by the client's need to use the restroom twice in a 10-minute period and by direct observation of one loose and unformed stool.

DESIRED OUTCOMES EVALUATION CRITERIA	NURSING ACTIONS/INTERVENTIONS	RATIONALE
NOC: Bowel Continence (Moorhead, Johnson, and Maas, 2004, with permission)	NIC: Diarrhea Management (Dochterman and Bulechek, 2004, with permission)	
The client will assist in ruling out causes for his loose stools and report his signs and symptoms to the nurse.	Teach the client to observe and record the pattern, onset, frequency, characteristics, amount, time of day, and precipitating events related to occurrence of diarrhea. Refer client to the dietitian to determine usual food intake and nutritional status.	Observation and documentation of the client's response to these factors will assist in determining the cause of his loose stools.
	Determine exposure to recent environmental contaminants, such as drinking water, food-handling practices, and proximity to others who are ill.	
	Review drug intake for medications affecting absorption (see Table 10–5, Factors Decreasing Absorption).	
The client will eliminate causative factors at once after these factors have been determined.	Follow through with the elimination of causative factors, restrict intake if necessary, note change in drug therapy, if any.	Elimination of the causative factors should decrease the frequency of loose, unformed stools. The client needs to be instructed on the relationship of his diarrhea to causative factors.
The client will have formed stools within 24 hours after the causative factors have been eliminated.	Document stool consistency.	Whenever possible, an objective measure should be used to evaluate the success of any client intervention. Stool consistency is an objective measure for treatment response to diarrhea and malabsorption.

CTQ CRITICAL THINKING QUESTIONS

1. The client asks you how long he will need to follow this diet and whether he will ever be able to reintroduce milk into his diet. What do you tell him?

2. What would you tell the client if the diet were only partially effective in controlling the diarrhea?

CHAPTER REVIEW

1. An appropriate snack for a child on a gluten-free diet would be:
   a. Crackers and peanut butter
   b. Half of a cheese sandwich
   c. Potato chips and an oatmeal cookie
   d. Rice cakes and a banana

2. Solid body waste is stored in the:
   a. Large intestine
   b. Gallbladder
   c. Small intestine
   d. Stomach

3. Gaseous waste is expelled:
   a. In the urine
   b. In the feces
   c. Through the lungs
   d. Through the skin

4. The end products of protein digestion are:
   a. Glycerol and fatty acids
   b. Amino acids
   c. Fatty acids
   d. Monosaccharides

5. A food commonly responsible for an allergic reaction is:
   a. Chicken
   b. Peanuts
   c. Rice
   d. Carrots

CLINICAL ANALYSIS

1. The nurse is visiting Mr. D, who is receiving home health care. His caregiver is concerned that Mr. D chokes on liquids but swallows semisolid food well. Which of the following actions by the nurse would be the most appropriate?
   a. Observe Mr. D's efforts to swallow liquids.
   b. Recommend a fluid restriction
   c. Refer Mr. D to a speech therapist
   d. Contact Mr. D's physician

2. Brenda, a 3-year-old, has been admitted to the pediatric unit with a diagnosis of celiac disease. She has a gluten-free diet ordered. Which of the following meals would be compatible with the diet order?
   a. Goulash, green beans, and milk
   b. Hamburger on bun, French fries, and a chocolate shake
   c. Tomato soup, grilled cheese, applesauce, and a cookie
   d. Baked chicken, baked potato, sour cream, green beans, peaches, and milk

3. Mr. P is on a low-fat diet (20 grams) to control his steatorrhea. An appropriate snack would be:
   a. Fruit
   b. Nuts
   c. Cheese
   d. Cookies

REFERENCES

American Dietetic Association: Manual of Clinical Dietetics, ed 6. American Dietetic Association, Chicago, 2000.

Dochterman, JC, and Bulechek, GM: Nursing Interventions Classification (NIC), ed 3. Mosby, Philadelphia, 2004.

Duyff, RL: American Dietetic Association Complete Food and Nutrition Guide, ed 2. Hoboken, NY, 2002.

Galvan, TJ: Dysphagia: Going down and staying down. Am J Nurs 101:37, 2001.

IFIC Foundation: Food sensitivities, allergies, and intolerance: Separating fact from fiction. Food Insight. IFIC Foundation, Washington, DC, 2003.

McCallum, SL: The National Dysphagia Diet: Implementation at a regional rehabilitation center and hospital system. J Am Diet Assoc. 103:285, 2003.

Moorhead, S, Johnson, M, and Maas, M: Nursing Outcomes Classification (NOC), ed 3. Mosby, Philadelphia, 2004.

NANDA International: Definitions and Classification, 2003–2004. NANDA International, Philadelphia, 2003.

Nelson, JK, et al: Mayo Clinic Diet Manual: A Handbook of Dietary Practice, ed 7. Elsevier Health Science, Philadelphia, 1994.

Scanlon, VC, and Sanders, T: Essentials of Anatomy and Physiology, ed 4. FA Davis, Philadelphia, 2003.

Sheikh, A: Food Allergy. BMJ. 335:1337, 2002.

Taylor, SL, Hefle, SL, and Munoz-Furlong, A: Food allergies and avoidance diets. Nutr Today 34:15, 1999.

The National Dysphagia Diet Task Force: The national dysphagia diet standardization for optimal care. Chicago, Il; The American Diet Assoc, 2002.

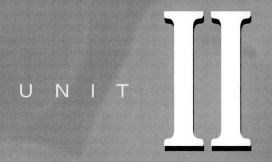

UNIT **II**

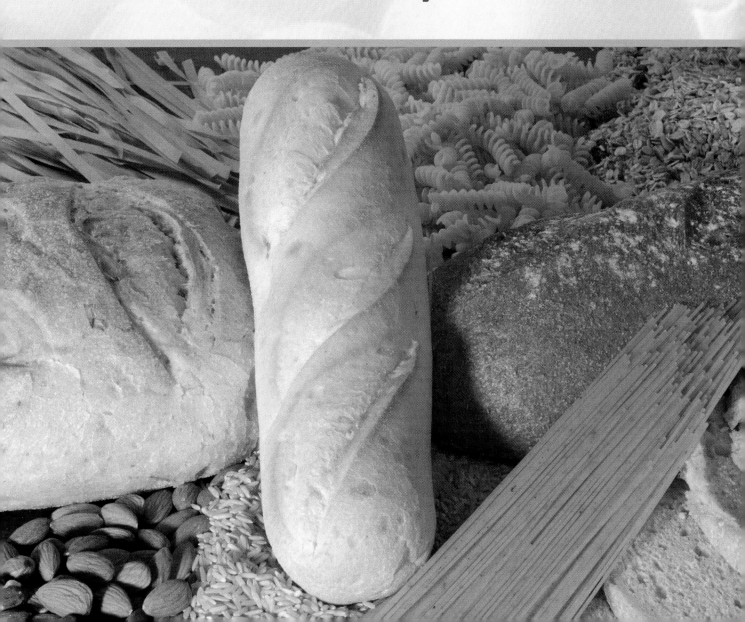

Family and Community Nutrition

11

Life Cycle Nutrition:
Pregnancy and Lactation

After completing this chapter, the student should be able to:

1. Compare the nutritional needs of a pregnant woman with those of a nnpregnant woman of the same age.
2. Contrast the nutritional needs of a pregnant adolescent with those of a pregnant adult.
3. Explain why folic acid intake is critical in pregnancy.
4. Identify substances to be avoided by pregnant and breast-feeding women.
5. Discuss the dietary treatment of common problems of pregnancy.
6. List three advantages that breast-feeding confers on the mother.

The needs for many nutrients change at different stages of life. Social, economic, and psychological circumstances also influence nutritional status. Human beings are most vulnerable to the impact of poor nutrition during periods of rapid growth. If the essential nutrients are not present to support growth, permanent damage to tissues and organs can occur. This chapter focuses on the period of most rapid growth, that of the unborn child.

Nutrition During Pregnancy

An expectant mother's nutritional status can affect the outcome of pregnancy. For example, during the first month of **gestation,** it is crucial that the mother be well nourished so that the **placenta** that forms will be healthy. As well, within 2 to 3 months of conception, all the major body organs are formed in the **embryo.** From the beginning of the third month until birth, the developing child is called a **fetus.** Because the fetus obtains nutrients from the mother's diet or body stores, its health depends on her nutritional intake.

The placenta is not just a passive conduit for nutrients, however. It can selectively extract nutrients of the appropriate form, for instance long-chain essential fatty acids

and alpha-tocopherol (vitamin E), suited to the needs of the fetus (James, 1997; Dutta-Roy, 2000).

After the birth and weaning of the child, the mother needs time to rebuild her nutrient stores. Occurrence of a second pregnancy within 6 months of delivery is associated with adverse outcomes (Kitzman, 2000).

Poor outcomes of pregnancy include spontaneous abortion (miscarriage), premature delivery, a **low-birth-weight (LBW) infant,** a **small-for-gestational-age (SGA) infant,** and mental and physical abnormalities in the newborn. These complications are not evenly distributed throughout the population. Black women are twice as likely as white women to give birth to a LBW infant (Centers for Disease Control, 2002e).

The best action an expectant mother can take for her unborn child is to enter the pregnancy with good nutrient stores and to consume a well-balanced diet while pregnant. She must also avoid harmful substances, such as alcohol and contraindicated drugs, including over-the-counter and prescription preparations.

From **implantation** to birth, the fertilized **ovum** (which weighs less than 100 micrograms) develops into an infant who weighs about 3.4 kilograms (7.5 pounds) on the average. During this period of rapid growth and development, the mother needs additional nutrients, including kilocalories, protein, and certain vitamins and minerals.

Energy Needs

Increased energy is needed to sustain the mother and for the development of the fetus and the placenta. From the third through the sixth month, the second trimester, much of this energy supports the growth of the uterus (womb) and other maternal tissues. During the seventh through ninth months, the third trimester, much of the energy supports the fetus and the placenta. To meet this increased metabolic workload and to spare protein for tissue building, a pregnant woman needs an additional energy intake (see Table 6–4). Energy costs of pregnancy also vary by BMI. In women with normal BMIs, energy requirements increased negligibly in the first trimester, by 350 kcal/d in the second trimester, and by 500 kcal/d in the third trimester (Butte et al, 2004). Intake should be distributed throughout the day. Maintaining blood glucose levels in the mother is vital because glucose is the fetus's preferred fuel and because the fetus's blood glucose level is always lower than the mother's (Brown, 2005; McGanity, Dawson, and Van Hook, 1999).

Protein Needs

Protein is required to build fetal **tissue.** The mother also needs adequate protein for growth of her tissues. Her blood volume increases in anticipation of blood loss at delivery. Her breasts develop in preparation for lactation. Her uterus enlarges and fills with a sac containing **amniotic fluid.** For these reasons, the RDA for protein for pregnant women is 71 grams per day, compared to 46 grams for nonpregnant women. Translating this need to the exchange system, 2 extra cups of milk (16 grams of protein) and 1.5 additional ounces of meat (10.5 grams of protein) would more than meet the increased protein requirement.

A complication arises if a woman with phenylketonuria (PKU) consumes a regular diet during pregnancy. The high level of phenylalanine in such a woman's bloodstream can cross the placenta and cause fetal malformations and defects. Careful monitoring of blood levels of phenylalanine and provision of a special medical food (see Clinical Application 5–3) are begun before conception and continued throughout the pregnancy. When women with PKU do not adhere to their diets before and during pregnancy, their infants have a 93 percent risk for mental retardation and a 72 percent risk for microcephaly (Centers for Disease Control, 2002b). In a 15-year study, 27 percent of the offspring had microcephaly and 7 percent had serious congenital heart disease. These outcomes occurred most frequently in women with mean IQ scores of 83 associated with low socioeconomic status and decreased educational achievement as well as unplanned pregnancies in women off dietary treatment with phenylalanine-restricted products (Koch et al, 2000).

All women should be asked directly if they have ever had a special diet prescription. It may be difficult to convince even known clients with PKU to change their diets, but it is even harder if the person's medical history is vague. Because women of childbearing age with PKU may have been taken off the special diet after age 4 to 6, they may have little memory of this part of their medical history. The health-care worker should investigate further when a woman cites a history of troubled pregnancies, congenital abnormalities, a mentally retarded infant, spontaneous abortion, or stillbirth. Women needing careful screening for PKU include those born before 1967, those who immigrated to the United States, those with a history of seizures, and those who have low IQs (Acosta and Wright, 1992).

Vitamin Needs

Pregnant women have an increased need for some vitamins. They must avoid taking excessive amounts of others because of potential hazard to the fetus.

Water-Soluble Vitamins

Increased amounts of certain B vitamins, especially folic acid, and vitamin C are needed during pregnancy. Vitamin C is needed to (1) convert folic acid to an active form, (2) enhance the absorption of iron, and (3) help to form connective tissues. Women who have been using oral contraceptives have been found to have lower blood levels of folate, vitamin C, vitamins B_6 and B_{12}, and beta-carotene that may take 4 months to return to normal after the drugs have been discontinued (Hally, 1998). Increased metabolic demands make intake of some of the other B vitamins necessary in additional amounts; they include thiamin, riboflavin, niacin, and vitamin B_6. These B vitamins are all coenzymes involved in the metabolism of the energy nutrients.

VITAMIN B_{12}

The cobalamin RDA is only slightly increased for pregnant and lactating women, to 2.6 and 2.8 micrograms per day. Vegetarians particularly should be knowledgeable about the cobalamin content of their food or seek nutritional advice, because neurological impairment has occurred in their infants (Centers for Disease Control, 2003b). Fortified food and supplements made from cobalamin provide a physiologically active form of the vitamin, whereas products that list only vitamin B_{12} might include nonbioavailable sources. If it is not possible to obtain the RDA of cobalamin through food, pregnant and lactating women should take a daily supplement containing a reliable source.

FOLIC ACID

The RDA for folic acid for all women of childbearing potential is 400 micrograms of synthetic folic acid daily from fortified foods or a supplement in addition to food folate from a varied diet. For pregnant women, the RDA for folate is 600 micrograms that would include 400 micrograms of synthetic folic acid from fortified foods or a supplement. A CDC guideline recommends that a woman who has previously borne a child with a neural tube defect take 4 milligrams of folic acid per day from 1 month before conception through the first trimester (Centers for Disease Control, 1992). The objective of Healthy People 2010 to increase the median RBC folate level (a better measure of long-term folate status than serum folate) to 220 nanograms per milliliter (ng/mL) has been met for non-Hispanic white women and Mexican Americans but not for non-Hispanic black women (Centers for Disease Control, 2002c).

Since January 1, 1998, 43 to 140 micrograms of folic acid per pound have been added to all enriched foods in an attempt to reduce the occurrence of NTDs. Breakfast cereals can be fortified with up to 400 micrograms per serving, and the FDA permits the labels of foods containing sufficient amounts of folate to claim that the products may reduce the risk of having a pregnancy affected with NTD (Centers for Disease Control, 1996). Following fortification, in 1999–2000, the occurrence of NTD-affected live births and stillbirths declined by 26 percent (Centers for Disease Control, 2004b). Food fortification may help but is not designed to completely meet the preconception and first-trimester needs of fertile women, hence the revised RDA for folate, specifying synthetic sources. Box 11–1 contains a brief explanation of the pathophysiology, occurrence, and prevention of neural tube defects.

Women are slowly becoming aware of the need for sufficient folic acid. In 2004, 40 percent of 18- to 45-year old women reported daily consumption of a vitamin containing folic acid but that meant that 60 percent were not taking such a vitamin. Moreover, 25 percent of the women surveyed had dieted in the preceding 6 months. Almost half of the dieters used a low-carbohydrate diet that could reduce their intake of folate-fortified foods (Centers for Disease Control, 2004c). Health-care providers need to increase their efforts to promote adequate folic acid intake among fertile women. Although 88 percent of women of reproductive age indicated they would take a folic acid-containing supplement if their health-care providers recommended it, only 37 percent reported having received such advice (Centers for Disease Control, 2004c).

Opportunities to educate clients abound. Pediatric nurses should counsel adolescent girls as well as mothers of younger children. Nurses caring for women of reproductive age in any setting can help to decrease their clients' risks of NTDs by making this subject a priority for teaching.

In addition to general education, populations with high rates of NTD can be targeted for specific interventions. A project in the Texas counties bordering Mexico recruited women who had given birth to an infant with NTD. In 14 border counties, the rate of NTD-affected pregnancies was 13.8 per 10,000 live births for Hispanic women compared with 8.8 per 10,000 live births for white women. Counseling and folic acid supplements were provided, the dose dependent on whether contraception was practiced. Women who used no contraception were given 4 milligrams, compared to 400 micrograms for women using contraception. Early results indicate the folic acid to be effective in reducing the risk for NTD among Hispanic women. Even this carefully aimed intervention was not perfectly received by the 36 percent of the women eligible for the program who refused enrollment, dropped out, or were lost to follow-up (Centers for Disease Control, 2000c).

Fat-Soluble Vitamins

For pregnant women older than 25 years of age, an adequate diet usually provides the needed additional vitamins D, E, and K. Vitamin A as retinol or retinoic acid in excess of 10,000 IU per day or treatment with isotretinoin during the first trimester increase the risk of **retinoic acid syndrome.** The characteristic fetal deformities include small

---

Box 11–1 Neural Tube Defects: Pathophysiology, Occurrence, Prevention

Neural tube defects (NTDs), resulting from failure of the neural tube to close during the fourth week of embryogenesis, are the most common severely disabling birth defects in the United States, with a frequency of approximately 1 in every 2000 births (Northrup and Volcik, 2000). The neural tube is embryonic tissue that develops into the brain and spinal cord. A critical time in the development of this structure is from conception through the fourth week of pregnancy. Interference with normal development produces major congenital defects, including **anencephaly, meningoencephalocele, spina bifida,** and **meningocele.**

The identification of a gene producing an abnormality in an enzyme necessary to folate metabolism bolsters the argument for genetic susceptibility in this multifactorial condition. Genetic and environmental influences are likely causative factors, because a higher incidence of NTD occurs in Newfoundland, Quebec, northern China, parts of India, Scotland, and Ireland. Almost half the Irish population is either **heterozygous** or **homozygous** for the affected thermolabile gene, but its low rate of detectable effects has led researchers to search for additional mechanisms producing NTDs (James, 1997).

Autoantibodies against folate receptors have been found in women who experienced NTD-affected pregnancies, but determination of causality awaits further investigation (Rothenberg et al, 2004). Researchers have also found an abnormal folate metabolism in some mothers of infants with Down's syndrome (Barkai et al, 2003; O'Leary et al, 2002) also necessitating further study.

In the United States, approximately 4000 pregnancies are affected by NTDs each year; 50 to 70 percent of them could be prevented with daily intake of 400 micrograms of folic acid throughout the period before and after conception (Centers for Disease Control, 1999a). The effectiveness of folic acid was demonstrated in a large randomized trial conducted in seven countries. Women with a history of NTD pregnancy were given 4 milligrams of folic acid per day. Control groups received placebos or other vitamins. The study was stopped early to permit treatment of all participants because the folic acid reduced the risk of a subsequent child with NTD by 70 percent (MRC Vitamin Study Research Group, 1991). Women with a history of a previous NTD pregnancy have 10 to 30 times the risk of women without such a history (Centers for Disease Control, 2002d).

Unfortunately, the neural tube develops when many women are unaware they are pregnant. In addition, approximately 50 percent of all pregnancies in the United States are unplanned. Preconception health counseling is the ideal but not the norm.

One potential hazard of fortification is the masking of vitamin B_{12} deficiency. No reports of delayed diagnosis have been published since 1973 (Oakley, Adams, and Dickinson, 1996) however, and neurological signs and symptoms of pernicious anemia do occur without anemia (Dickinson, 1995). An additional concern is that of folic acid interfering with anticonvulsant medications, but numerous controlled trials have demonstrated no effect by oral folic acid at doses up to 20 milligrams daily (Romano et al, 1995).

ears or no ears, abnormal or missing ear canals, brain malformation, and heart defects. Therefore a maximum of 5000 IU from supplements is recommended (Brown, 2005). Three ounces of beef liver may contain 30,000 IU; and of chicken liver 14,000 IU. A pregnant woman who eats liver regularly may consume enough vitamin A to pose risk to her baby (March of Dimes, 2002), and the United Kingdom lists liver as contraindicated during pregnancy (McLaren and Frigg, 2001).

Table 11–1 lists the vitamin A RDAs and ULs for pregnancy and lactation. Remember the conversion to IUs depends upon the source. Supplements usually list the percentage of vitamin A from betacarotene that requires more provitamin per IU that the body may not convert to preformed vitamin A anyway.

Vitamin A, sometimes used to treat acne, could pose a risk to the fetus of a teenager who unintentionally becomes pregnant. The risk of a major congenital abnormality in a child exposed to isotretinoin, a vitamin A metabolite, in utero during the first trimester appears to be increased about 25 times (Futoryan and Gilchrest, 1994). Despite a pregnancy prevention program started by the manufacturer of isotretinoin in 1988, approximately 900 pregnancies occurred between 1989 and 1998 in women enrolled in the Boston University Accutane Survey. CDC follow-up of isotretinoin-exposed pregnancies in California revealed that all the respondents knew the drug should not be used during pregnancy, but only 7 percent followed the contraceptive protocol and 57 percent reported having intercourse without contraception at the time of the exposed pregnancy. None of the respondents reported being referred for the free contraceptive counseling that is part of the prevention program (Centers for Disease Control, 2000a). Consequently, the FDA is strengthening the program to monitor physicians, pharmacies, and clients, including a requirement for repeated negative pregnancy tests, so that no pregnant woman begins isotretinoin therapy and no woman taking the drug becomes pregnant (United States Department of Health and Human Services, 2004). Women of childbearing age taking isotretinoin should adhere to strict contraceptive protocols, including simultaneous use of two methods. Furthermore, no one should donate blood during or for 30 days after cessation of therapy with isotretinoin (Nursing 2004).

In contrast, vitamin A deficiency is a greater problem than toxicity in developing countries. Either preformed vitamin A or provitamin A (beta carotene) was shown to reduce mortality related to pregnancy by 40 to 49 percent in Nepal (West et al, 1999), a country in which night blindness is considered an annoyance of pregnancy reportedly affecting 16 percent of women (Christian et al, 1998).

See Table 11–2 for the specific amounts recommended for selected vitamins during pregnancy.

Mineral Needs

Minerals become part of the structure of the body, whereas vitamins do not. Both the mother and the fetus require minerals to build new tissues.

Iron

During pregnancy, the mother's blood volume increases about 35 percent, and her volume of red blood cells increases by 21 to 26 percent. Additional iron is needed for the red blood cells in the fetus, placenta, and umbilical cord. Iron is transported to the fetus regardless of the mother's iron status. The total iron need for a single-fetus pregnancy is estimated to be 0.8 to 1 gram. During the third trimester, 3 to 4 milligrams of iron per day is transferred to the fetus (Fairbanks, 1999).

Iron-deficiency anemia during the first two trimesters of pregnancy is associated with twice the risk for preterm delivery and three times the risk for producing a LBW infant. Since 1979, **anemia** prevalence among low-income pregnant women in the United States has been fairly stable. In 1993, it was 9 percent, 14 percent, and 37 percent for the first, second, and third trimesters (Centers for Disease Control, 1998b). Participants in the Women, Infants, and Children supplemental nutrition (WIC) program in 12 states had a prevalence of postpartum anemia of 27 percent but 48 percent among non-Hispanic black women (Bodnar et al, 2001).

Fortunately, the body adjusts to limited or abundant sources of iron. Absorption of iron is enhanced in the second and third trimesters of pregnancy. In women who are not taking an iron supplement, iron absorption increases from 6.5 percent early in pregnancy to 14.3 percent at term. This rate drops to 8.6 percent with an iron supplement.

The Centers for Disease Control recommends educating clients about iron-rich foods and those that enhance iron absorption as well as prescribing a daily 30-milligram supplement beginning when clients enter prenatal care (1998b). If iron needs are not met, a pregnant woman may develop iron deficiency anemia. Even when she takes supplements, the woman's hemoglobin and hematocrit should be monitored every 2 to 3 months. Lower values are

Table 11–1   **DRIs for Vitamin A During Pregnancy and Lactation**

	RDA		UL	
	MICROGRAMS	**INTERNATIONAL UNITS**	**MICROGRAMS**	**INTERNATIONAL UNITS**
PREGNANCY				
<19 y	750	2475	2800	9240
19–50 y	770	2541	3000	9900
LACTATION				
<19 y	1200	3960	2800	9240
19–50 y	1300	4290	3000	9900

Table **11–2**   **RDAs and AIs for Selected Vitamins**

LIFE STAGE GROUP	VITAMIN A (ug/d)	VITAMIN C* (mg/d)	VITAMIN D (ug/d)	VITAMIN E (mg/d)	THIAMIN (mg/d)	NIACIN (mg/d)	VITAMIN B_6 (mg/d)	FOLATE† (ug/d)	VITAMIN B_{12} (ug/d)
Pregnancy									
<19 y	750	80	5	15	1.4	18	1.9	600	2.6
19–50 y	770	85	5	15	1.4	18	1.9	600	2.6
Lactation									
<19 y	1200	115	5	19	1.4	17	2.0	500	2.8
19–50 y	1300	120	5	19	1.4	17	2.0	500	2.8

*Smokers require an additional 35 mg/d of vitamin C.

†Women able to become pregnant should consume 400 μg of synthetic folic acid from fortified foods/supplements besides food folate.

SOURCE: Adapted from http://www.iom.edu/file.asp?id=7296, accessed July 26, 2004.

expected during the first and second trimesters because of expanding blood volume. Among women who do not take iron supplements, the hemoglobin and hematocrit levels remain low during the third trimester, but in women with adequate iron intake, the values gradually rise toward prepregnancy levels (Centers for Disease Control, 1998b).

Prescribing an iron supplement does not necessarily mean the woman will take it. Side effects or economic factors may influence the extent to which a woman takes her supplements. A randomized, double-blind, placebo-controlled trial of a low dose (20 mg) daily iron supplement (ferrous sulfate) beginning at week 20 of gestation showed significant reduction in iron deficiency and iron-deficiency anemia at delivery with no difference in gastrointestinal side effects (Makrides, 2003). Clinical Application 11–1 illustrates the principles of knowing the client as well as the subject matter and seeking feedback on one's teaching.

Calcium

Calcium is the chief mineral in the adult body, with the bones serving as a storage depot. When serum calcium is low, the bones demineralize to restore the serum level; however, no long-term detrimental effect of pregnancy or breast-feeding on bone mineral measures was found in a study of 2516 twins (Paton et al, 2003). As with iron, intestinal absorption of calcium increases during pregnancy. In a longitudinal study, the average proportion of calcium absorbed increased from 32.9 percent at prepregnancy to 49.9 percent during the second trimester and to 53.8 percent during the third trimester (Ritchie et al, 1998). One reason for this increased absorption is the ability of the placenta to convert inactive vitamin D to the active form. Chapters 7 and 8 describe the effects and interactions of calcium and vitamin D.

Pregnancy-associated osteoporosis, a rare complication, has been recognized for 40 years but is still not well understood. Poor general nutrition, low calcium intake, and a positive family history of osteoporosis seem to be strong risk factors for pregnancy- and lactation-associated osteoporosis (Di Gregorio et al, 2000). The bone mass of 15 **first-degree relatives** of five women with pregnancy osteoporosis, most of whom suffered vertebral fractures in their first pregnancy, revealed osteoporosis in 53 percent of the relatives versus 15 percent of the controls, suggesting a genetic component to pregnancy osteoporosis (Peris et al, 2002). The literature shows that most women are not affected in their subsequent pregnancies (Liel, Atar, and Ohana, 1998).

The Adequate Intake (AI) for calcium for pregnant and lactating women 19 years of age and older is 1000 milligrams. For women 18 years of age and younger, the amount is 1300 milligrams. These amounts can be obtained from 3.3 to 4.3 servings of milk or milk products equivalent in calcium. (Treatment of lactose intolerance is covered in Chapter 10.)

Phosphorus and Magnesium

In addition to calcium, two other minerals involved in skeletal formation are also in great demand during

---

Clinical Application 11–1

Effective Teaching

Often the facts presented by a health-care provider who is educating a client are misunderstood by the client or perceived as counter to the client's goals. The following incidents illustrate the point (Galloway and McGuire, 1996).

1. When anemic pregnant women were give iron tablets, they took the supplement until they felt better and then stopped, thinking they were cured. Prevention is a new concept to people in many countries.
2. Anemic pregnant women accepted the notion of iron supplements to correct "too little blood" but were fearful that too much iron would give them too much blood so that they would bleed more extensively at delivery.
3. Presenting the idea that iron would produce bigger babies was a disincentive for anemic pregnant women who thought they then would face a more difficult labor.

Teaching is more than just presenting facts, especially when the goal is changed behavior. Local knowledge and cultural perspective are essential to the health-care provider who is promoting a new health practice. For instance, it would help to know that some Puerto Rican women would avoid iron as a "hot" food during pregnancy (Purnell and Paulanka, 2003).

Table 11–3 RDAs and AIs for Selected Minerals and Energy Nutrients

LIFE STAGE GROUP	CALCIUM (mg/d)	FLUORIDE (mg/d)	IODINE (ug/d)	IRON (mg/d)	ZINC (mg/d)	DIGESTIBLE CARBOHYDRATE (g/d)*	PROTEIN (g/d)
Pregnancy							
<19 y	1300	3	220	27	12	175	71
19–50 y	1000	3	220	27	11	175	71
Lactation							
<19 y	1300	3	290	10	13	210	71
19–50 y	1000	3	290	9	12	210	71

*Based on its role as primary energy source for the brain.
SOURCE: Adapted from http://www.iom.edu/file.asp?id=7296, accessed July 26, 2004.

pregnancy: phosphorus and magnesium. For pregnant or lactating women younger than 19 years of age, the RDA for phosphorus is 1250 milligrams per day. For those 19 to 50 years old, the RDA is 700 milligrams. These are the same amounts recommended for nonpregnant women. The RDA for magnesium is 350 to 400 milligrams per day for pregnant and 310 to 360 milligrams per day for lactating women, in both instances slightly higher amounts than recommended for nonpregnant women.

Iodine

As part of thyroid hormones, iodine is essential to the control of metabolism. During the second half of pregnancy, resting energy expenditure increases by as much as 23 percent. The RDAs for iodine are 220 micrograms for pregnant women and 290 micrograms for lactating women, an increase of 46 to 93 percent over those of other women. In the United States, a pregnant woman's usual need for iodine is met, like that of other adults, by the use of iodized salt. In parts of the world with endemic cretinism, supplementation is beneficial (Mahomed and Gulmezoglu, 1999).

Fluoride and Zinc

The fetus begins to develop teeth at the tenth to twelfth week of pregnancy. One might expect that fluoride supplementation of pregnant women would prevent dental caries, but it was found to be ineffective at mitigating caries in their offspring (Centers for Disease Control, 2001b) because only trace amounts of the mineral pass through the placenta (Brown, 2005). The AI for pregnancy and lactation is the same as for nonpregnant women, 3 milligrams per day.

Zinc is not mobilized from the mother's tissues. To provide for the fetus, the mother needs constant intake. Zinc deficiency has been associated with abnormally long labors and delivery of small and malformed infants. Zinc supplementation was associated with fewer preterm deliveries and less perinatal mortality (McGanity, Dawson, and Van Hook, 1999). African American women with low plasma zinc levels who took a zinc supplement delivered heavier infants than did the control group. The greatest increase occurred in women with prepregnant body mass indices (BMIs) of less than 26 (Goldenberg et al, 1995). Many studies failed to correlate plasma zinc levels with pregnancy outcomes, but a reliable, sensitive laboratory index is not yet available.

The RDA for zinc is 11 to 12 milligrams for pregnant women and 12 to 13 milligrams for lactating women. These values are about 50 percent higher than those for other women. Lean meat from beef chuck roast, 3.5 to 4 ounces, would provide these RDAs. Table 11–3 summarizes selected mineral and energy nutrient needs for pregnancy and lactation.

Clinical Calculation 11–1

Determining Recommended Weight Gain During Pregnancy

Body mass index (BMI) = Weight in kilograms/Height in meters^2

Suppose a woman is 5 ft, 4 in tall and weighs 125 lb.

$$5 \text{ ft, } 4 \text{ in} = 64 \text{ in}$$

$$1 \text{ m} = 39.371 \text{ in}$$

$$\frac{64}{39.371} = 1.6 \text{ m}$$

$$\frac{125 \text{ lb}}{2.2 \text{ lb/kg}} = 56.8 \text{ kg}$$

$$\text{BMI} = \frac{56.8}{(1.6)^2} = \frac{56.8}{2.56} = 22.2$$

Looking at the table below, we see that 22.2 is in the normal category. Recommended weight gain for this woman is 25 to 35 lb.

Recommended Weight Gain for Pregnancy

BMI CATEGORY	KILOGRAMS	POUNDS
<19.8 = Low	12.5–18	28–40
19.8–26 = Normal	11.5–16	25–35
26–29 = High	7–11.5	15–25
>29 = Obese	6.8	15

Young adolescents and black women should strive for gains at the upper end of the recommended range. Women whose height is less than 157 cm (62 in) should strive for gains at the lower end of the range.

SOURCE: Reprinted with permission from Nutrition During Pregnancy. © 1990 by the National Academy of Sciences. Published by National Academy Press, Washington, DC.

The Weighting Game Weight Graph

Your Beginning Weight _ _ _ _ _ _ lbs.

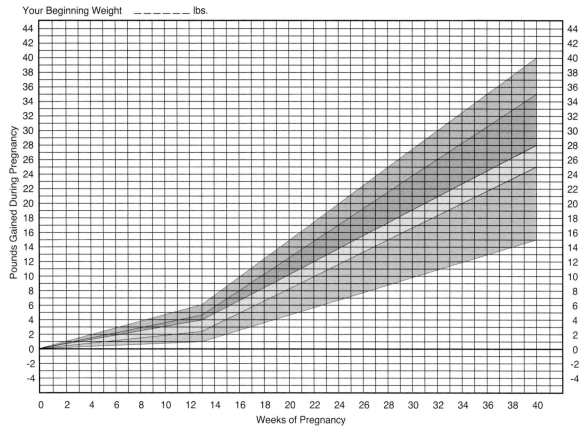

Adapted from the National Academy of Science's Nutrition during Pregnancy, 1990.

HERE'S HOW IT ALL ADDS UP

Baby	7–8 1/2 pounds
Amniotic fluid	2 pounds
Placenta	2–2 1/2 pounds
Increased blood volume	4–5 pounds
Tissue fluid	3–5 pounds
Increased weight of uterus	2 pounds
Body changes for breast-feeding	1–4 pounds
Mother's stores*	4–6 pounds
Total	25–35 pounds

*Mother's stores are reserves of extra fat and probably a little protein. These serve as a source of energy to support the work of pregnancy. These stores also supply energy for labor and delivery and for milk production after birth.

Figure **11–1** Great Beginnings: The Weighting Game Weight Graph. This is an example of a chart on which a woman can plot her weight gain during pregnancy. Goals are shown in pink/orange for women who begin pregnancy underweight, in orange/yellow for normal weight women, and in blue for overweight women. (Reprinted from the Great Beginnings Calendar, ed 2, 1991. Courtesy of National Dairy Council, with permission.)

Water and Weight Gain

Plasma volume during pregnancy expands by about 50 percent that necessitates a fluid intake of about 9 cups daily (Brown, 2005). Because some women fear excessive weight gain, the nurse should reinforce the need for adequate fluid intake.

The amount of weight a woman is advised to gain during pregnancy has varied over the years. The current recommendation is based on a BMI that incorporates the woman's height and weight before pregnancy. Clinical Calculation 11–1 shows the procedure to determine a goal for weight gain in pregnancy based on prepregnancy body weight. On average, a woman of normal weight should gain 2 to 4 pounds during the first trimester, followed by 1 pound per week for the remainder of the pregnancy. Figure 11–1 is a graph on which the woman can plot her weight gain.

Obese women (a BMI >29 before pregnancy) have increased risk of complications such as hypertension and diabetes and of surgical delivery by Caesarean section. Those with a prepregnancy BMI over 28 run twice the risk of NTD-affected fetuses, independent of folate status and supplement use. Weight gain during pregnancy is not perfectly correlated with birth weight, but it is inversely related to perinatal mortality (McGanity, Dawson, and Van Hook, 1999).

Meal Pattern

Relatively few modifications in MyPyramid recommendations for adults are needed for mature women who become pregnant. They can meet their basic needs and those of the fetus by consuming one additional cup of milk, an additional 1/2 ounce of meat, and an additional 1/2 cup of fruit or vegetable rich in vitamin C each day. Additional foods should be consumed to attain the desirable weight gain.

Pregnant teenagers need nutrients to provide for their own growth as well as that of the fetus. They should have additional milk, meat, vegetables, grains, and oils over and above the intake recommended for mature pregnant women. Clinical Application 11–2 relates the particular hazards of teenage pregnancy.

Moderation is suggested in implementing the meal pattern. For instance, overfeeding of protein to pregnant women may be counterproductive. Giving high-protein supplements to pregnant women, many of whom were adolescents, seems to have reduced birth weight. Similar effects have been seen by animal breeders (James, 1997). Table 11–4 can be used as a starting point to plan a balanced food intake for pregnant adult women and adolescents during pregnancy and lactation.

Careful food selection is critical for pregnant vegetarian women. Strict vegetarians, particularly, may be prescribed a vitamin and mineral supplement that at a minimum provides folate, cobalamin, iron, and zinc (McGanity, Dawson, and Van Hook, 1999).

Food Assistance

Supplemental food assistance is available for families in the Food Stamp Program and for women and children in the Supplemental Feeding Program for **Women, Infants, and Children (WIC).** The latter program serves 7.6 million people annually (United States Department of Agriculture, 2003).

Substances to Avoid

Women are urged to eliminate certain substances from their diets while they are pregnant or nursing. Alcohol, caffeine, soft cheeses, ready-to-eat meats, and certain species and amounts of fish are such substances. Tobacco and cocaine use also affect fetal nutrition.

Serious allergies to nuts and seeds affect less than 1 percent of the population. But women with personal or family histories of allergies may be advised to avoid peanuts while pregnant or breast-feeding to prevent sensitization of the fetus. This is more likely if close relatives have allergies, not only to nuts and seeds, but also those producing asthma, eczema, or hay fever (Food Standards Agency, 2004).

Alcohol

First recognized in 1973, **fetal alcohol syndrome (FAS)** is the major cause of mental retardation in the Western world (Murphy-Brennan and Oei, 1999) because alcohol readily crosses the placenta but the fetus has inadequate enzymes to detoxify it. Approximately 40 percent of fetuses born to women who drink heavily early in pregnancy will develop FAS (Brown, 2005). The fetus is most vulnerable to FAS during the first trimester when basic structural development occurs. Often, the woman does not know that she is pregnant until late in the first trimester.

Children with FAS, a completely preventable condition, are malformed and suffer from mental retardation (Fig. 11–2). Because researchers have not been able to determine how much alcohol is safe to ingest during pregnancy, women who are planning a pregnancy should be encouraged to abstain from alcohol for the good of the fetus. An intervention to reduce alcohol-exposed pregnancies that provided a maximum of four motivational counseling sessions and one visit to a family planning provider found 69%

Clinical Application 11–2

Teenage Pregnancy

In the United States, 9 percent of women aged 15 to 19 years become pregnant each year: 5 percent give birth, 3 percent have induced abortions, and 1 percent have miscarriages or stillbirths—rates much higher than those in other developed countries (Darroch, 2001). The teen birth rate declined by 30 percent over the past decade to an all-time low, and the rate for black teens was down by more than 40 percent. For young black teens (15 to 17 years), the results were even more striking—the rate was cut in half since 1991 (Centers for Disease Control, 2003c).

The average girl does not reach her full height or attain gynecologic maturity until age 17. When pregnant before that age, she herself is still growing and has a fetus to nourish as well.

Nutrients most often lacking in the pregnant teenager's diet are folate, vitamins A, E, and B_6, calcium, iron, zinc, and fiber. In addition, kilocaloric intake is usually insufficient to meet daily needs. The 11- to 14-year-old expectant mother requires 2700 kilocalories per day; the 15- to 18-year old, 2400 kilocalories. The criterion for adequacy, however, is the adequate weight gain throughout pregnancy.

Teenage mothers are at increased risk of complications of pregnancy, such as preeclampsia and premature delivery. Infants born to mothers under the age of 16 are twice as likely to be of low birth weight as infants born to mothers age 20 and older and three times more likely to die in the first month of life as infants of older mothers (Story, 1997).

The cause is not solely age-related, however. Complications of pregnancies are more strongly associated with poor nutrition than with maternal age. Because teenage pregnant girls tend to enter prenatal care later than older pregnant women, improving access to prenatal care and focusing on nutritional needs when providing that care are important steps toward reducing the poor outcomes of teenage pregnancy (Story, 1997).

Table 11–4   **Basic Food Guide for Pregnancy and Lactation**

	PREGNANT ADULT*	PREGNANT ADOLESCENT*	LACTATION
Milk, cups	4	5	4
Meat and Beans, oz	6	6 1/2	6 1/2
Fruit, cups			
High vitamin C	1	1	1 1/2
Other	1	1	1
Vegetable, cups			
High vitamin A	1/2	1/2	1
Other	2 1/2	3	2 1/2
Grains (1/2 Whole), oz	7	9	8 1/2
Oils, teaspoons	6	8	1/2
Additional foods	To meet kilocaloric needs	To meet kilocaloric needs	To meet kilocaloric needs

*Meets RDA/AIs except for iron and folic acid.

of the women in the study reduced their risk for an alcohol-exposed pregnancy. The women with the lowest baseline drinking achieved the highest rates of outcome success, primarily by choosing effective contraception (Centers for Disease Control, 2003a).

The task of protecting the unborn is formidable. One of the goals of Healthy People 2010 is to increase to 94 percent the percentage of pregnant women abstaining from alcohol use (Centers for Disease Control, 2002a), but a recent survey indicated approximately 10 percent of pregnant women used alcohol, and approximately 2 percent engaged in binge drinking or frequent use of alcohol. Moreover, more 55 percent of the women not using birth control reported alcohol use and 12 percent reported binge drinking (Centers for Disease Control, 2004a).

Caffeine

The effects of caffeine consumption during pregnancy have been studied with inconsistent results. In a prospective, population-based cohort study of 873 women, there were no associations between moderate caffeine consumption and birth weight, gestational age, and birth weight ratio (Clausson, 2002). In another study, mean birth weight was reduced by 28 grams per 100 milligrams of caffeine consumed daily, but the researchers concluded that this small decrease in birth weight is unlikely to be clinically important except for women consuming 600 milligrams or more of caffeine daily. Decaffeinated coffee did not increase risk for any perinatal outcome (Bracken et al, 2003).

In some studies, caffeine consumption during pregnancy has been associated with spontaneous abortion. Compared with a maternal caffeine intake of less than 151 milligrams per day, caffeine consumption greater than 300 milligrams per day doubled the risk of miscarriage (Bracken et al, 2003). In the United Kingdom, women are advised to limit their caffeine intake to less than 300 milligrams of caffeine a day (Food Standards Agency, 2001).

Caffeine intake has also been associated with delays in achieving pregnancy (Bolumar et al, 1997; Jensen et al, 1998). Changes in fetal heart rate and breathing patterns have been observed even with moderate caffeine intake that apparently gave the mother no noticeable signs. Moreover, caffeine is secreted in breast milk and has a half-life of up to 100 hours in infants (Eskenazi, 1999). Therefore, limiting caffeine intake is prudent advice for pregnant or lactating women and for women desiring to become pregnant.

Soft Cheeses and Ready-to-Eat Meats

Listeriosis is a bacterial infection that is particularly virulent for fetuses, with a case-fatality rate of 30 percent in newborns and almost 50 percent if the onset occurs in the first 4 days of life (Heymann, 2004). The causative organism, *Listeria monocytogenes,* is transmitted from the mother (who may be asymptomatic) to the fetus in utero or through the birth canal. The infection may result in abortion or septicemia or meningitis in the newborn. Other individuals at risk are the elderly, those with impaired immune systems, and farm workers.

Outbreaks of listeriosis have been associated with raw or contaminated milk, soft cheeses, contaminated vegetables, and ready-to-eat meats. The reservoir of the organism is soil, forage, water, mud, and silage (Heymann, 2004). An

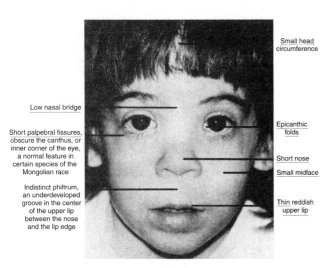

Figure **11–2** Specific facial signs of fetal alcohol syndrome include microcephaly or small head size, small eyes and/or short eye openings, and an underdeveloped upper lip with flat upper lip ridges. (Reprinted from Feldmen, 1988, p 164, with permission.)

outbreak from August 1998 through January 6, 1999 sickened at least 50 people in 11 states, resulting in six adult deaths and two spontaneous abortions (Centers for Disease Control, 1999b). The mode of transmission in this case was hot dogs traced to a single packing plant. An outbreak in 2000 involved 8 perinatal and 21 nonperinatal cases in 10 states, causing four deaths and three spontaneous abortions. A case-control study implicated eating deli turkey meat as the probable source of infection (Centers for Disease Control, 2000b). An outbreak in North Carolina in 2001 involved a soft Mexican cheese made with raw milk. The clients, 11 women and 1 70-year-old immunocompromised man, were Hispanic. Ten of the women were pregnant, and infection with *L. monocytogenes* resulted in five stillbirths, three premature deliveries, and two infected newborns. The eleventh woman was 5 months postpartum when she was hospitalized with meningitis caused by *L. monocytogenes*. The male client, who presented with a brain abscess, was receiving corticosteroid therapy after brain tumor surgery (Centers for Disease Control, 2001a). In addition to those usually affected products, the FDA issued a health warning after finding *L. monocytogenes* in cold-smoked fish products (United States Department of Health and Human Services, 2000).

Listeria infections during pregnancy can cause influenza-like symptoms, with fever and chills. Illness may not appear until 2 to 8 weeks after a person has eaten the contaminated food (Centers for Disease Control, 1999b). If the infection is diagnosed, antimicrobial therapy may prevent fetal infection and the associated high mortality (Yonekura and Mead, 1999).

In addition to the general rules for safe food handling, pregnant women and immunocompromised individuals should:

1. Avoid soft cheeses (feta, Brie, Camembert, blue-veined, and Mexican-style cheese). Hard cheeses, processed cheeses, cream cheese, cottage cheese, and yogurt may be eaten safely.
2. Cook leftover foods or ready-to-eat foods (hot dogs) until steaming hot (165°F).
3. Although the risk for listeriosis associated with foods from deli counters is low, pregnant women and immunocompromised individuals may avoid these foods altogether or thoroughly reheat cold cuts before eating (Centers for Disease Control, 1998a).

Certain Species and Amounts of Fish

Nearly all fish and shellfish have traces of mercury from the environment. Because of high levels of mercury in some species of fish (those that grow larger and live longer), the Food and Drug Administration and the Environmental Protection Agency have advised pregnant women and women who may become pregnant, nursing mothers, and young children to avoid eating shark, swordfish, King mackerel, and tilefish. If chosen as the week's seafood meals, albacore tuna or tuna steak should be limited to 6 ounces per week, whereas up to 12 ounces per week may be consumed of species of seafood with lower amounts of mercury (shrimp, canned light tuna, salmon, pollock, and catfish). Fish sticks and fish sandwiches at fast food restaurants generally contain species with lower amounts of mercury. Local advisories should be sought to determine the safety of recreationally caught fish. If no local advice is available, a general rule is to limit local seafood to 6 ounces per week (U.S. Department of Health and Human Services, 2004).

Over time, the body can eliminate mercury, but it can accumulate in the body faster than it can be eliminated. As an example, blood mercury levels of 1709 women were almost 4-fold higher among women who ate three or more servings of fish in the previous 30 days compared with women who ate no fish in that period. Approximately 8 percent of the women had concentrations higher than the U.S. Environmental Protection Agency's recommended reference dose of 5.8 micrograms per liter, below which exposures are considered to be without adverse effects (Schober, 2003). Developing nervous tissue is at particular risk, hence the warning regarding pregnant women and young children.

Undercooked Meat and Cat Litter

Health-care providers should reinforce the principles of food hygiene to pregnant women. An infection with *Toxoplasma gondii* causes an estimated 400 to 4000 cases of congenital toxoplasmosis annually, producing mental retardation, blindness, and epilepsy. The wide range of the estimate occurs because the disease is not nationally reportable or widely recognized as a threat by pregnant women. Only 48 percent of mothers of affected infants recognized risk factors of the disease, a situation that possibly could have been prevented by education however, only systematic serologic screening of all pregnant women at prenatal visits or of all newborn infants at birth would prevent or detect a higher proportion of these congenital infections (Boyer et al, 2005). Treatment of acute infection in pregnancy has reduced fetal infection by about 50 percent (Centers for Disease Control, 2000d). The protozoan is spread by undercooked meat, unwashed fruits and vegetables, contaminated soil, and cat feces. To prevent the infection, the pregnant woman should:

- Cook meat, poultry, and seafood thoroughly
- Clean items that those raw foods have contacted with hot soapy water
- Peel or meticulously wash raw fruits and vegetables before eating
- Keep cats indoors and feed them only cooked food or prepared cat food
- Avoid changing cat litter or, if not possible, use mask and gloves and wash hands carefully afterwards.

Tobacco

Pregnant women who smoke one or more packs of cigarettes per day deliver infants weighing about one-half pound less than those delivered by nonsmoking women. Exposure to tobacco smoke in utero was associated with double the risk of stillbirth, and infant mortality was increased by 80 percent in women who had smoked during pregnancy compared with children of nonsmokers. Among children of women who stopped smoking during the first trimester, stillbirth and infant mortality was comparable with that in children of women who had been nonsmokers from the beginning of pregnancy (Wisborg et al, 2001). Physiologically, smoking causes a decrease in the oxygen-carrying capacity of the blood of up to 10 percent and vasoconstriction of the blood vessels of the placenta. To maintain normal blood levels, smokers need three times the intake of folic acid and twice the intake of vitamin C as nonsmokers. Lower vitamin C levels are associated with weakened amniotic membranes containing less collagen leading to premature rupture of the membranes and early delivery. Limiting cigarette use to fewer than five per day reduces the ill effects on the fetus to a statistically insignificant level (McGanity, Dawson, and Van Hook, 1999).

Cocaine

Cocaine crosses the placenta and can be detected in the infant's intestinal waste for up to 8 weeks. Chronic cocaine addiction causes a weight deficit in the fetus of as much as 500 grams (1.1 pounds). In addition, the infant usually suffers from immature mental development that may be related directly to the drug or to malnutrition of the mother, which has been likened to wartime intrauterine starvation (McGanity, Dawson, and Van Hook, 1999).

Problems and Complications of Pregnancy Affecting Nutrition

The physiological changes that take place in a woman's body during pregnancy may cause a variety of possible medical conditions. Some of the more common problems such as morning sickness and leg cramps are usually annoying but only occasionally require medical intervention. Other conditions, such as hypertensive disorders of pregnancy and gestational diabetes, are more complicated and hazardous and require medical treatment.

Common Problems

Four of the most common problems of pregnancy are morning sickness, leg cramps, constipation, and heartburn. Pica is a regional practice that is mainly influenced by culture.

MORNING SICKNESS

Hormonal changes, some of which produce relaxed gastrointestinal muscle tone, cause the nausea and vomiting of pregnancy. About 70 to 85 percent of pregnant women feel nauseated, and about half experience vomiting (Jewell and Young, 2003). The occurrence and duration of these events vary widely, and they are not confined to mornings. Control of the problem without medication is the goal. Eating dry crackers before getting out of bed is the classic preventive. Other suggestions are to (1) avoid fatty foods in favor of fruits and complex carbohydrates taken in small, frequent meals; (2) consume cold foods rather than hot foods; (3) drink liquids between rather than with meals; and (4) eat a high-protein snack at bedtime. In most cases, morning sickness subsides after the first trimester. One double-blind randomized placebo-controlled trial found ginger extract significantly reduced nausea but not vomiting in pregnant women (Willetts, Ekangaki, and Eden,

2003), and another determined that ginger was equivalent to pyridoxine in reducing nausea and vomiting of pregnancy (Smith et al, 2004). A larger review of randomized controlled trials concluded that, aside from antiemetic medication (which was effective but produced side effects with little information available on fetal effects), pyridoxine (vitamin B_6) was effective in reducing the severity of nausea (Jewell and Young, 2003). An algorithm for medication use for nausea and vomiting of pregnancy based on safety and efficacy was developed by the College of Family Physicians of Canada (Levichek et al, 2002) and current information is available at http://www.motherisk.org.

LEG CRAMPS

Pregnant women often complain of leg cramps. One possible cause may be neuromuscular irritability due to low serum calcium, but the evidence that supplemental calcium reduces cramping is weak. Because of its close link to calcium metabolism, magnesium deficiency has been postulated to cause leg cramps. If a woman finds cramping troublesome in pregnancy, the best evidence is for magnesium lactate or citrate taken twice a day (Young and Jewell, 2002).

Advice directed to athletes may also be applicable to pregnant women suffering from leg cramps. Staying well hydrated is of prime importance, followed by maintaining adequate intakes of potassium, sodium, calcium, and magnesium. A noninvasive procedure to prevent muscle cramps is to stretch the muscles before exercise and, for night time cramps, before bedtime.

CONSTIPATION

The growing uterus presses on the intestines, causing constipation. Adequate fluid intake, regular exercise, and a high-fiber diet should relieve this condition. Ideally, the suggested amount of fiber intake, 30 grams per day, should be achieved with food rather than pharmaceutical preparations. Foods high in fiber but relatively low in kilocalories are listed in Table 11–5. If needed, dietary supplements of bran or wheat fiber are likely to help women experiencing constipation in pregnancy (Jewell and Young, 2001).

HEARTBURN

A burning sensation beneath the breastbone is called heartburn. Hormonal changes cause relaxation of the cardiac sphincter, located between the esophagus and the stomach. That and the upward pressure on the diaphragm from the enlarging uterus cause reflux of gastric contents into the esophagus and the burning sensation.

Heartburn can be controlled by avoiding spicy or acidic foods and taking small, frequent meals. Sitting up for an hour after a meal may help. Pregnant women should not self-medicate with sodium bicarbonate or antacids. The bicarbonate can be absorbed, producing alkalosis. Antacids decrease iron absorption by decreasing gastric acids, thus increasing the risk of anemia.

PICA

The compulsive ingestion of nonfood items, usually dirt, clay, laundry starch, or ice, is called **pica.** It is an ancient

Table 11–5 Nutrient-Dense Foods High in Fiber

FOOD	QUANTITY	GRAMS OF DIETARY FIBER	KILOCALORIES
Grains			
All bran	1/3 cup	10	70
Bran buds	1/2 cup	11.5	109
100% Bran	1/2 cup	10	89
Fruits			
Applesauce, unsweetened	1 cup	4	106
Orange sections, raw	1 cup	4	85
Pear, d'Anjou raw with skin	one	6	120
Prunes, cooked, unsweetened	1/2 cup	4.5	114
Strawberries, fresh	1 cup	4	45
Vegetables			
Baked beans, in tomato sauce with pork	1/2 cup	7	129
Lima beans, cooked from frozen	1/2 cup	8	94
Broccoli, raw	one spear	6	42
Brussels sprouts, cooked from raw	1 cup	6	60
Kidney beans, canned	1/2 cup	8.5	108
Navy beans, cooked from dry	1/2 cup	8	130
Black-eyed peas, cooked from dry	1/2 cup	10.5	99

behavior. Most notable in some regions of the southern United States, pica occurs in conjunction with inadequate diets due to poverty, but it also occurs in women at other socioeconomic levels. Of 128 women who sought prenatal care from two rural community health agencies, 38 percent practiced pica, with African American women practicing pica more often than other ethnicities (Corbett, Ryan, and Weinrich, 2003). Many women with pica have it only during pregnancy, believing it cures the annoyances of pregnancy or ensures a beautiful baby. Others contend that the substances they ingest taste good to them.

Health concerns about pica include inadequate nutrition due to substitution of nonfood items for nutritious foods, iron-deficiency anemia, constipation, and lead poisoning. Laundry starch interferes with iron absorption. A study in Texas showed significantly lower hemoglobin levels at delivery for women who admitted to having pica than for women who did not (Rainville, 1998). Ingestion of clay may lead to fecal impaction. Sometimes the substance ingested contains lead, as occurred in 15 women, 70 percent Hispanic, with lead poisoning caused by pica. Because lead freely crosses the placenta, their infants had higher blood levels than the women (Shannon, 2003).

Women who have migrated to an area where pica is uncommon may continue the custom. A caring, nonjudgmental assessment on the nurse's part may encourage a woman to reveal that she has a craving for and is eating nonfood items and could lead to a teaching opportunity.

Complications of Pregnancy

Three complications of pregnancy with nutritional ramifications are hyperemesis gravidarum, the hypertensive disorders of pregnancy, and gestational diabetes.

HYPEREMESIS GRAVIDARUM

Severe nausea and vomiting persisting after the fourteenth week of pregnancy is called **hyperemesis gravidarum.** Its cause is unknown but is thought to be multifactorial (Philip, 2003). It develops most often in Western countries and in first pregnancies. Estimated to occur in 2 percent of pregnancies, it can be life threatening, causing dehydration, electrolyte imbalance, weight loss, and, rarely, esophageal rupture (Eroglu et al, 2002; Liang et al, 2002) and renal failure (Hill, Yost, and Wendel, 2002). Because of the physiological increase in blood volume that occurs in pregnancy, hypovolemia can become severe without clinical signs. The body's adaptive response causes vasoconstriction of uterine vessels, reducing its blood supply up to 20 percent without notable change in the woman's blood pressure (Wagner et al, 2000). Loss of more than 5 percent of prepregnancy weight has been used as a criterion for steroid therapy (Moran and Taylor, 2002). Vitamin K deficiency has produced a bleeding disorder (Robinson, Banerjee, and Thiet, 1998), deficiencies of vitamins B_6 and B_{12} can result in peripheral neuropathy, and deficiency of thiamine has caused Wernicke's encephalopathy in these clients (Wagner et al, 2000). See Chapters 7 and 22 for information on the latter.

Hyperemesis gravidarum warrants treatment for the health of the woman and the fetus. Many approaches have been used to treat it: pyridoxine, ginger, rehydration, enteral and parenteral nutritional support, antiemetics (without teratogenic effects), and corticosteroid therapy. The onset of ketonuria often triggers aggressive hydration and nutritional support, because ketones readily cross the placenta and may impair fetal development (Wagner et al, 2000). Treatments are used that will not harm the fetus.

HYPERTENSIVE DISORDERS OF PREGNANCY

This group of disorders includes chronic hypertension, gestational hypertension, preeclampsia, and eclampsia. Hypertension is defined as blood pressure greater than 140 mmHg systolic or greater than 90 mmHg diastolic (see Chapter 20). Hypertensive disorders of pregnancy account for nearly 15 percent of maternal mortality in the United States and more than 33 percent worldwide. Fetal complications include growth restriction, prematurity, and stillbirth. Distinctions among the categories and a summary of risks, pathophysiology, and treatment of preeclampsia follow.

• Chronic hypertension existed before pregnancy or in retrospect when gestational hypertension or the hypertension of preeclampsia do not resolve after delivery. Preeclampsia develops in 25 percent of these women compared to 5 percent of normotensive women.

• Gestational hypertension is first detected in midpregnancy without proteinuria.

• Preeclampsia occurs after the 20th week of pregnancy with proteinuria. It affects 5 to 8 percent of pregnant women in the United States, a rate that increased 33 percent in the 1990s likely due to pregnancy among older women and multiple-fetus gestations (National Heart, Lung, and Blood Institute, 2001).

• Eclampsia is the occurrence in preeclamptic women of seizures not attributable to another cause. It is an obstetrical emergency that occurs in 1 of 200 cases of preeclampsia. The mother is in immediate danger of convulsing. She requires intensive nursing care because she is at high risk of cerebral hemorrhage, circulatory collapse, and kidney failure. The fetus, too, is in grave danger.

Preeclampsia produces vasospasms and abnormal clotting mechanisms that produce ischemia of the placenta, kidney, liver and brain that even with mild hypertension can result in serious complications in the mother and fetus (Zamorski, 2001). Supporting the role of vasculature in preeclampsia is its link to decreased urinary placental growth factor which is a protein that supports blood vessel development (Levine et al, 2005). Evidence of causal links between oxidative stress, depletion of vitamin C, and low levels of the endogenous vasodilator nitric oxide support the need for further research in this area (National Heart, Lung, and Blood Institute, 2001).

The possibility of genetic factors contributing to preeclampsia is suggested by increased risk associated with personal or family histories of preeclampsia, diabetes, hypertension, or vascular or renal diseases. Women who conceive multiple fetuses through assisted reproductive technologies have twice the risk of preeclampsia as those who conceive multiple fetuses spontaneously (Lynch et al, 2002). Increased risk in women who used condoms during a short period of cohabitation suggests the possibility of an immune reaction to paternal proteins as a contributing factor (Einarsson, Sangi-Haghpeykar, and Gardner, 2003), as does the increased risk to women who were normotensive in a first pregnancy and then develop preeclampsia after conceiving with different partners (Lenfant, 2001).

Definitive treatment of preeclampsia, aside from delivery of the fetus, awaits elucidation of its cause. Eclampsia may occur even 12 days after delivery (Brown, 2005). Without question, careful monitoring of pregnant women and early intervention is crucial. Calcium supplementation appears to be beneficial for women at high risk of gesta-

tional hypertension and in communities with low dietary calcium intake. Supplementation with calcium reduced the risk of preeclampsia by 32 percent overall, but by 79 percent in in women at high risk of hypertension and by 68 percent in those with low baseline calcium intake (Atallah, Hofmeyr, and Duley, 2002). Magnesium sulfate is the drug of choice to treat severe preeclampsia or eclampsia during labor and delivery (Zamorski, 2001). Treating preeclampsia with magnesium sulfate cut the risk of eclampsia by more than half (Duley, Gulmezoglu, and Henderson-Smart, 2003) but was not effective in preventing preeclampsia and also is hazardous in women with severe renal failure (Lenfant, 2001).

GESTATIONAL DIABETES

The appearance of diabetes in pregnancy, **gestational diabetes** is considered to be a form of type 2 diabetes (see Chapter 19). It appears to develop in women with a predisposition to insulin resistance and type 2 diabetes that becomes apparent due to physiological changes of pregnancy. Among these changes is the production of hormones by the placenta that decrease insulin sensitivity and increase insulin resistance both of which insure a constant supply of glucose to the fetus (Brown, 2005). A woman's risk for gestational diabetes is usually assessed at the first prenatal visit. It affects approximately 7 percent of pregnant women in the United States who then have a 45 percent risk of recurrence with the next pregnancy and a 63 percent risk of developing type 2 diabetes later in life (Luerssen and Winsch, 2005). Treatment of gestational diabetes, requiring an aggressive team approach, is included in Chapter 19. If medication is needed, insulin is prescribed rather than oral antiglycemic agents that cross the placenta and stimulate fetal insulin production.

The Breast-Feeding Mother

One of the goals of Healthy People 2010 is to increase to 75 percent the proportion of mothers who breast-feed in the early postpartum period, to 50 percent those who breast-feed until the infant is 6 months old, and to 25 percent those who breast-feed until the infant is 1 year old. In 2001, 65 percent of infants had received some breast milk. At 6 months, 27 percent of infants received some breast milk, and at 12 months, 12 percent. Non-Hispanic blacks had the lowest rates of breast-feeding initiation and continuation but also showed the greatest increases between 1996 and 2001 (Ryan, Wenjun, and Acosta, 2002). Only 8 percent of infants were exclusively breast-fed at 6 months of age (Li et al, 2003). Figure 11–3 shows breast-feeding rates in the United States from 1970 through 2000. The following chapter covers the advantages of breast milk for the infant. In the next section, the nutritional implications of breast-feeding for the mother are considered.

Nutritional Needs

The recommended meal plan for breast-feeding women is the same as for pregnant women, with the stipulation of 120 milligrams of vitamin C or 1 1/2 cups of foods rich in vitamin C daily. The meat-bean group should provide 6 1/2

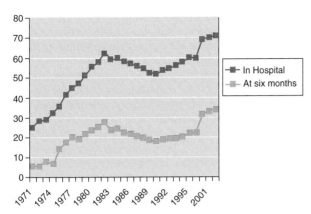

Figure **11–3** U.S. breast-feeding rates, 1971–2002: all infants receiving any breast milk in the hospital and at 6 months of age. The rates in 2002, 70.1 percent and 33.2 percent, are all-time highs. (Data from Ross Products Division, 2002, with permission.)

ounces per day. While exclusively breast-feeding their infants for 6 months, lactating women preserved their lean body mass by consuming 55 percent more protein than a nonlactating control group (Motil et al, 1998). A total intake of 3.8 liters of fluid is the AI for lactating women but adequate intake to produce a sufficient output of pale yellow urine should be the standard.

The AI for calcium for lactating women is the same as for other women of their same age, 1000 to 1300 milligrams per day. Women experience a transient loss of approximately 3 to 7 percent of their bone density during lactation, which is rapidly regained after weaning. Additional calcium intake neither prevents bone loss during lactation nor enhances remineralization after weaning, but the recovery of bone is complete for most women even with shortly spaced pregnancies. Furthermore, epidemiologic studies have found that pregnancy and lactation are not associated with an increased risk of osteoporotic fractures (Kalkwarf and Specker, 2002).

Energy

A breast-feeding mother requires an additional 500 kilocalories per day from food. Although 750 kilocalories are required, the remainder should be derived from fat stores. The calculation is as follows. Thirty ounces of breast milk a day at 20 kilocalories per ounce equals 600 kilocalories total. Another 150 kilocalories are needed to produce the milk.

Effect of Maternal Deficiencies

In the developing world, severe malnutrition in mothers has caused stunted growth in their infants (Umeta et al, 2003), but if a healthy mother lacks some nutrients in her current diet, her milk usually contains the correct level of nutrients with two notable exceptions, vitamins C and B_{12}. If the mother's diet is low in vitamin C, her milk also will be deficient in the vitamin. Mothers with cobalamin deficiency also can adversely affect their nursing infants. Cases of growth failure and neurologic impairment occurred in breast-feeding infants of vegetarian mothers

(Centers for Disease Control, 2003b). Supplemental cobalamin provides a physiologically active form of the vitamin compared with some other forms of vitamin B_{12}. In an otherwise well-nourished mother, the use of a vitamin supplement does not increase the vitamin content of her milk.

Benefits to the Mother

Several advantages to the mother are associated with breast-feeding. It helps the uterus return to its nonpregnant state more quickly. Breast-feeding is convenient and less costly than bottle feeding and may be protective against later breast cancer.

Aids Uterine Involution

During breast-feeding, the sucking of the infant stimulates the release of **oxytocin** from the posterior pituitary gland in the brain. Oxytocin causes the uterine muscles to contract and helps return the uterus to its nonpregnant size.

Convenience at Less Cost

Breast milk is always ready at the correct temperature. There is no formula to make or contamination to worry about. The additional foods the mother consumes are less expensive than infant formula.

Lessens Risk of Breast Cancer

Over the long term, breast-feeding has been associated with a decreased risk of breast cancer later in life. An analysis of 47 epidemiological studies in 30 countries including 50,302 women with invasive breast cancer and 96,973 controls found that the relative risk of breast cancer decreased by 4.3 percent for every 12 months of breast-feeding in addition to a decrease of 7.0 percent for each birth. The size of the decline in the relative risk of breast cancer associated with breast-feeding did not differ significantly for women in developed and developing countries (Collaborative Group on Hormonal Factors in Breast Cancer, 2002). These are statistical proportions for the group, not an individual guarantee. Some of the factors in cancer's complex etiology are described in Chapter 23.

Techniques of Breast-Feeding

The medical and nursing staff will assist the mother to start breast-feeding her infant. Even mothers of twins and premature babies can successfully breast-feed with additional education and support. Some general principles to aid in breast-feeding have been established.

The mother and infant should be permitted to spend as much time together as possible during the first 24 hours after birth. This practice permits bonding of infant and mother. Some areas encourage fathers to "room in" also to bond with the baby.

One correct position for breast-feeding is shown in Figure 11–4. It is tummy to tummy. The infant should face the breast squarely. If the breast is very large, the mother must take care to prevent it from blocking the infant's nose lest it impede infant's breathing. When nursing, the infant should grasp the entire areola (the colored portion around the nipple) to prevent the nipples from becoming sore.

Most infants will take 80 to 90 percent of the milk from each breast in the first 4 minutes of nursing. Because nursing stimulates further milk production, the mother should alternate which breast is first offered to the infant. This method allows the infant to vigorously stimulate milk production in the first breast offered and to finish feeding on the other breast if it is still hungry or is just enjoying the experience. At the next feeding, the mother should start with the breast the infant finished on the time before.

Encouraging Breast-Feeding

Pediatricians are encouraged to provide information on the benefits and methods of breast-feeding so that the mother can make an informed choice (American Academy of Pediatrics, 2005). Prenatal encouragement increases breast-feeding rates and identifies potential problem areas. A prospective study showed women were less likely to be still fully breast-feeding at 6 to 10 weeks postpartum if they thought they needed more breast-feeding information before delivery or had experienced breast-feeding problems. Women were less likely to be fully breast-feeding at 4 months postpartum if they had experienced breast-feeding problems (McLeod, Pullon, and Cookson, 2002).

Hospital practices should focus on rooming in, early and frequent breast-feeding, skilled support and avoidance of artificial nipples, pacifiers, and formula. Infants should be assessed while nursing at 2 to 4 days after discharge, with liberal use of referral and support groups, including lactation consultants and peer counselors (Moreland and Coombs, 2000). There is clear evidence for the effectiveness of professional support on the duration of any breast-feeding and of lay support on the promotion of exclusive breast-feeding (Sikorski et al, 2003). First-time, low-income

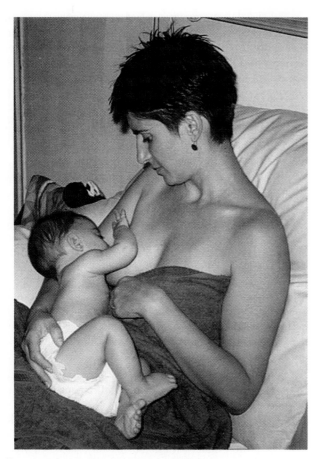

Figure **11–4** One correct breast-feeding position, tummy-to-tummy. The infant takes the entire areola in its mouth. Notice how focused the mother is on the baby.

Box 11–2 **The Baby-Friendly Hospital Initiative**

The Baby-Friendly Hospital Initiative (BFHI) is a global UNICEF/WHO-sponsored effort to promote breast-feeding. During the 8 years since the initiative began, more than 15,000 hospitals in 136 countries have been inspected and designated as Baby Friendly (Naylor, 2001). More than 34 of these officially designated institutions are in the United States (National Center for Chronic Disease Prevention, 2003).

The WHO and UNICEF recommend that the following practices be implemented in every facility providing maternity services and care for newborn infants:

Ten Steps to Successful Breast-Feeding

1. Have a written breast-feeding policy that is routinely communicated to all health-care staff.
2. Train all health-care staff in skills necessary to implement this policy.
3. Inform all pregnant women about the benefits and management of breast-feeding.
4. Help mothers initiate breast-feeding within a half-hour of birth.
5. Show mothers how to breast-feed and how to maintain lactation even if they should be separated from their infants.
6. Give newborn infants no food or drink other than breast milk unless *medically* indicated.
7. Practice rooming-in: allow mothers and infants to remain together 24 hours a day.
8. Encourage breast-feeding on demand.
9. Give no artificial teats or pacifiers (also called dummies or soothers) to breast-feeding infants.
10. Foster the establishment of breast-feeding support groups and refer mothers to them on discharge from the hospital or clinic (Centers for Disease Control, 2003d).

In addition, Baby-Friendly institutions are expected to abide by the International Code of Marketing of Breast Milk Substitutes that forbids accepting free formula or other gifts and grants from formula producers. Distributing sample packs of formula is also not permitted (Naylor, 2001).

black mothers younger than 18 years of age living in multi-generational households who received mentoring were more likely than the control group to provide breast milk, formula, or water as their infants' sole nourishment until the age of 3 months (Black et al, 2001). Box 11–2 summarizes a program to increase breast-feeding worldwide. Structured education and behavioral counseling programs led by specially trained nurses or lactation specialists using face-to-face sessions are recommended by the U.S. Preventive Services Task Force (2003), which found that incidental counseling in the clinical setting alone was not effective in promoting breast-feeding.

Adoptive mothers have successfully breast-fed their infants by using physical stimulation and breast pumps to establish a milk supply. A breast-feeding supplementer system, the Lact-Aid Nursing Trainer System, is available to provide additional milk while the infant is nursing at the breast. Compelling stories of women who have breast-fed adopted infants can be found on an adoptive breast-feeding resource at http://www.fourfriends.com/abrw. The Web site is maintained by an adoptive mother who breast-fed two children.

On the other hand, overselling of the benefits and ease of breast-feeding has resulted in starvation deaths of infants (see Chapter 12). Not only should the mother's choice be respected and supported, but the infant's condition should be monitored carefully regardless of the feeding method chosen.

Maternal Contraindications to Breast-Feeding

Most women can feed their infants at breast. There are a few contraindications to breast-feeding, including the mother's exposure to toxic chemicals, the mother's use of illegal drugs and certain medications, and certain illnesses in the mother. Galactosemia, a contraindication due to a metabolic defect in the infant, is covered in Chapter 12.

Exposure to Toxic Chemicals

Certain chemicals, such as DDT and PCB, have been shown to be **teratogenic,** causing congenital defects. Concern has been raised about the transmission of toxic chemicals to the infant through breast milk. Once ingested, if the body has no means of excreting the chemicals, the contaminants are stored in adipose tissue. When the lactating mother's fat stores are mobilized to produce milk, it, too, contains the chemicals.

Some experts believe that the risk to the infant is minimal unless the mobilization of the mother's fat is due to inadequate intake. Others say that there is no hazard unless the woman has had occupational exposure to the chemicals or has consumed a large amount of fish from contaminated waters. Women with concerns about the issue should discuss them with their health-care providers.

Medication Use

Mothers are sometimes counseled to interrupt breast-feeding or to wean the infant when there is no compelling medical reason to do so (Crenshaw, 2005). Although many medications the mother takes are secreted in breast milk, most do not affect the milk supply or the infant when taken in recommended doses. Particularly if the medication can be administered directly to infants, the amount received in breast milk is unlikely to be harmful, but the capabilities of the livers and kidneys of premature and young infants as well as the characteristics of the medication should be considered (Marks and Spatz, 2003). Radioactive compounds require temporary cessation of breast-feeding. Cytotoxic drugs, drugs of abuse, psychotropic drugs, some anticonvulsants, salicylates, and ergot derivatives all have had significant effects on nursing infants or raise concerns because of their modes of action (American Academy of Pediatrics, 2001). The physician should be consulted about both prescription and nonprescription drugs the mother takes.

Substances that are often not thought of as drugs may also affect the breast-fed infant. These include alcohol and caffeine. The American Academy of Pediatrics recommends against the use of alcohol by breastfeeding mothers except for an occasional small drink as long as a two-hour delay until the next feeding is instituted (2005). Decreased milk consumption and poorer quality sleep have been documented in infants following alcohol ingestion by their mothers (Mannella, 2001; Manella and Garcia-Gomez, 2001).

Altered Physiology or Pathology

In the United States, absolute contraindications to breast-feeding include active untreated tuberculosis and AIDS. Acute or chronic diseases in the mother also may preclude breast-feeding. Some are heart disease, severe anemia, and nephritis. If the woman with these diseases becomes pregnant again, she will have to stop breast-feeding.

In the United States, maternal infection with human immunodeficiency virus (HIV) is a contraindication. If an uninterrupted supply of safe, nutritionally adequate breast milk substitute is available (as is possible in industrialized countries), HIV-infected women should be counseled not to breast-feed their infants (Weinberg, 2000). In developing countries, the risks of malnutrition and other infectious diseases may be more immediate than the risk of HIV. Preventive strategies supported by WHO/UNICEF and charitable agencies in some centers in Africa include routine antenatal voluntary counseling and testing, testing of infants of seropositive mothers at 6 weeks of age, various combinations of a shortened period (3 to 6 months) of exclusive breast-feeding, perinatal administration of anti-retroviral drugs, and provision of affordable and safe infant formulas, presently given free by UNICEF in some centers. For women in poor countries with the benefit of the above services, continued promotion of exclusive breast-feeding for at least 6 months, irrespective of HIV status, followed by a properly prepared, high-energy, nutritious complementary diet, with the possibility of early weaning to an animal milk formula, still appears appropriate. While a longer period of breast-feeding would probably increase the risk of mother-to-child transmission, shorter duration would certainly increase infant morbidity and mortality from other causes (Ogundele and Coulter, 2003).

The use of breast-feeding as a method of birth spacing has been shown to be 98 percent successful for 4 to 6 months under certain conditions: if the infant feeds frequently, if no supplementary feedings are given, and so long as the woman remains amenorrheic (Tommaselli et al, 2000; van Unnik and Roosmalen, 1998; World Health Organization, 2004). Because estrogen inhibits lactation, means of contraception other than those containing estrogen are advised beyond 6 months postpartum.

Nursing Makes a Difference

In a replication of an earlier study, home visits by nurses to pregnant women and to the mother and child after hospital discharge improved the subsequent life choices made by the woman. The nursing visits focused not only on immediate needs but also on clarifying goals, identifying barriers, and planning the women's futures related to education, employment, and child bearing. Compared with a control group, the women visited by the nurses had fewer subsequent pregnancies, fewer closely spaced pregnancies, and longer intervals between the births of first and second children. The visits continued over 2 years, but the improvements in lifestyles were maintained for 5 years (Kitzman et al, 2000). Nursing does make a difference in clients' lives. Wellness Tips 11–1 summarizes key information nurses can use in client education.

Wellness Tip **11–1** • Women of reproductive age should maximize their nutritional status before pregnancy, including optimizing their weight and nutrient stores.

- Obtaining prepregnancy counseling and seeking prenatal care early in the pregnancy are means to focus on wellness and the prevention of complications.
- Those who have been using oral contraceptives should delay 4 months before attempting pregnancy to permit blood levels of folate, vitamins B_6 and B_{12}, and beta-carotene to return to normal after discontinuing the oral contraceptive. An alternative method of contraception should be used in the interim.
- All women capable of becoming pregnant should consume 400 micrograms of synthetic folic acid daily. This amount is in addition to food folate. Although synthetic folic acid is used to fortify grains, the surest means to obtain this amount of folic acid is with a multivitamin supplement.
- It is best to avoid consuming large amounts (>10,000 IU/day) of preformed vitamin A during the first trimester because of its teratogenic potential. The medication isotretinoin, a vitamin A metabolite, is prescribed for intractable acne and bears specific warnings pertaining to contraception that must be heeded.
- Substances to avoid for 8 weeks before and during pregnancy include alcohol and foods related to the transmission of *Listeria monocytogenes* (soft cheeses and ready-to-eat meats), certain species and amounts of fish, undercooked meats, as well as tobacco, cocaine, and cat litter.

SUMMARY

To support her own and the fetus's growth, a pregnant woman requires increased intake of kilocalories, protein, B and C vitamins, iron, iodine, and zinc. Recent efforts to prevent neural tube defects in the embryo have included revision of the RDA for folic acid and fortification of grains with folic acid. The pregnant woman should avoid ingesting alcohol, soft cheeses, ready-to-eat meats, certain species and amounts of fish, undercooked meats, and immoderate amounts of preformed vitamin A. Other substances to avoid are tobacco, cocaine, and cat litter.

A pregnant teenage client is at especially high nutritional risk. Her own body still needs adequate nutrients for growth, and she also has a fetus to nourish.

Nutritional interventions are sometimes helpful for common complaints of pregnancy: morning sickness, leg cramps, constipation, and heartburn. Tact and diplomacy may be required to counsel women who have pica. Medical intervention and nutritional support are indicated for clients with hyperemesis gravidarum, hypertensive disorders of pregnancy, or gestational diabetes.

Breast-feeding offers benefits to the mother. It aids uterine involution and offers convenience since the milk is constantly ready-to-feed. Some maternal contraindications to breast-feeding are exposure to toxic chemicals, ingestion of certain medications and drugs, and some illnesses, including AIDS and tuberculosis.

CASE STUDY 11-1

Ms. T is a 21-year-old sexually active woman who has been followed in a family planning clinic for three years. She has been faithful about keeping appointments and taking her oral contraceptives. She also takes the multi-vitamin/multi-mineral supplement containing 400 micrograms of folic acid about four times a week "when she remembers and eats breakfast." She is taking no other medications. There are no known allergies in herself or her immediate family. Now she relates that she is seriously considering becoming pregnant. Her boyfriend proposed at her 21st birthday celebration. The couple has no pets but they do enjoy outdoor sports. Ms. T denies knowledge of means to minimize fetal risk and states she drinks a beer or a glass of wine on Saturdays and Sundays. She does not smoke. She received the standard measles, mumps, and rubella (MMR) vaccination as a child.

Ms. T is a 5-ft 3-in woman and weighs 136 lb. Her elbow breadth measures 2.5 in. Her hemoglobin was 14 g/dL and hematocrit was 42 percent last month.

(Continued on the following page)

CASE STUDY *(Continued)*

NURSING CARE PLAN

SUBJECTIVE DATA Expressed interest in becoming pregnant
Regular moderate alcohol intake
History of compliance with medical regimen
Immunized against measles, mumps, and rubella

OBJECTIVE DATA 115 percent of healthy body weight
Hemoglobin 14 g/dL, within normal limits (WNL)
Hematocrit 42 percent, within normal limits (WNL)

NURSING DIAGNOSIS NANDA: Risk for injury, fetal (NANDA, 2003, with permission) related to lack of knowledge of measures to decrease risk to embryo

DESIRED OUTCOMES EVALUATION CRITERIA	NURSING ACTIONS/INTERVENTIONS	RATIONALE
NOC: Risk Control (Moorhead, Johnson, and Maas, 2004, with permission)	NIC: Health Education (Dochterman and Bulechek, 2004, with permission)	
Will affirm today her intention to abstain from alcohol when attempting to achieve a pregnancy and throughout gestation.	Teach Ms. T about fetal alcohol syndrome. Use photographs of affected children.	No amount of alcohol is presumed to be safe in pregnancy. "A picture is worth 1,000 words." Photographs introduce visual learning and impact feelings.
Will take multivitamin, multimineral supplement every day beginning tomorrow.	Reiterate that vitamin preparation should contain 400 micrograms of folic acid. Review the value of a varied diet and good sources of food folate.	This is the RDA for all women capable of becoming pregnant. The RDA also emphasizes the importance of food folate.
Will eat breakfast or equivalent morning nourishment every day beginning tomorrow.	Review Dietary Guidelines with Ms. T. Explore means to take nourishment in morning.	This is a good habit to acquire. Once Ms. T achieves pregnancy, supplying the embryo/ fetus with a steady supply of nutrients is critical.
Will recount the limits to vitamin A intake during pregnancy by next visit.	Inform Ms. T of RDA for vitamin A in pregnancy. Alert Ms. T to the large amounts of preformed vitamin A in liver and liver products. Caution against supplements of vitamin A in addition to the multivitamin, multimineral tablet. Discuss the safety of beta-carotene (provitamin A) in pregnancy.	Teratogenic effects usually occur during the first trimester. Beta-carotene has not been associated with birth defects. Supplements containing provitamin A are considered safe for pregnant women at the RDA level.
Will list actions to take to minimize exposure to Listeria infection by 8 weeks before attempted conception.	Provide Ms. T with a list of cheeses to avoid and those that are considered safe. Review rules for safe handling of ready-to-eat meats. Alert her to report flu-like symptoms promptly to her primary health-care provider.	Because the incubation period of Listeria is up to 8 weeks, avoidance of possibly contaminated food should begin well before conception. Antimicrobial therapy may prevent fetal infection and the associated high mortality.

DESIRED OUTCOMES EVALUATION CRITERIA	NURSING ACTIONS/INTERVENTIONS	RATIONALE
Will monitor own intake of fish to remain within recommended limits by conception.	Emphasize complete abstinence from shark, swordfish, King mackerel, and tilefish. If available, use food models showing the weekly limits of 12 ounces or 6 ounces of fish.	These advisories from the FDA and the EPA to minimize the exposure of the fetus to methylmercury are not to be taken lightly.
Will discuss discontinuing oral contraceptive therapy and attempting conception with the primary health-care provider before changing her regimen.	Advise Ms. T about the possibility of birth defects with some oral contraceptives. To maximize chances of a favorable outcome, she may want to delay conception attempts and use alternate means of contraception for 4 months.	Progestins may cause birth defects if taken early in pregnancy. It may take 4 months for blood levels of folate, vitamin C, vitamins B_6 and B_{12}, and beta-carotene to return to normal after discontinuation of oral contraceptives.

CTQ CRITICAL THINKING QUESTION

1. If Ms. T were to achieve a pregnancy, what would her month-by-month recommended weight gain be? If she expresses concern about "gaining too much weight" when within the recommended amounts, how would you counsel her?

2. What additional assessment data would you obtain to design a comprehensive, personalized nursing care plan with her?

3. Are there other issues you believe ought to be raised with Ms. T before she attempts to become pregnant? Are they more or less important than the ones addressed in the Nursing Care Plan? Why?

⟫⟫ CHAPTER REVIEW

1. A pregnant woman should consume one more cup of milk daily than she consumed when not pregnant and which of the following?
   a. Two additional cups of deep green leafy or yellow vegetables and two ounces of liver weekly
   b. One-half additional ounce of meat-beans and one extra 1/2 cup of a good source of vitamin C
   c. Three additional ounces of whole-grains and three additional ounces of meat/beans
   d. Two extra cups of fresh fruit and at least four total servings of "free" vegetables from the ADA Exchange Lists

2. Which of the following substances are contraindicated during pregnancy?
   a. Alcohol and swordfish
   b. Cocoa and peanut butter
   c. Coffee and well-done beef
   d. Tea and cheddar cheese

3. Which of the following principles is not recommended by the Baby-Friendly Hospital Initiative?

   a. Feeding on demand
   b. Keeping mother and infant together 24 hours a day
   c. Hydrating the infant with sterile water until the mother's milk supply is established
   d. Putting the infant to breast within a half-hour of birth

4. The RDA for folic acid specifies 400 micrograms of synthetic folic acid from fortified foods or supplements for:
   a. All women capable of becoming pregnant
   b. Women taking oral contraceptive medications
   c. Women of northern European descent
   d. Breast-feeding mothers

5. If a pregnant woman complains of heartburn, she should be instructed to:
   a. Increase her intake of milk products
   b. Decrease her overall food intake
   c. Rest in bed after eating
   d. Avoid spicy or acidic foods

CLINICAL ANALYSIS

Ms. T is a 15-year-old girl who thinks that she is 2 months pregnant. She confides to the school nurse that she is not sure if she should have an abortion. She has not told anyone else of the pregnancy. Her purpose in disclosing the information to the school nurse is to obtain assistance with weight control so she has more time to make up her mind.

1. Based on the above information, which one of the following interventions would be of highest priority at this time?
   a. Designing a weight-control program that is high in calcium
   b. Giving information on the desirability of breast-feeding the infant
   c. Instructing the girl regarding substances that are likely to harm the fetus
   d. Scheduling a visit with a social worker to help the girl decide on a course of action

2. Knowing that adolescents are often lacking in certain nutrients, the nurse would want to assess the girl's intake of:
   a. Cola, coffee, and tea
   b. Fruits, vegetables, milk, and red meat
   c. Fried foods and pastries
   d. Poultry, seafood, and white bread

3. Ms. T complains of morning sickness. The nurse instructs her to:
   a. Eat breakfast later in the morning
   b. Drink at least two glasses of liquid with every meal
   c. Increase her intake of whole-grain breads and cereals to two ounces per meal
   d. Drink a large glass of skim milk at bedtime

REFERENCES

Acosta, RB, and Wright, L: Nurses' role in preventing birth defects in offspring of women with phenylketonuria. J Obstet Gynecol Neonatal Nurs 21:270, 1992.

American Academy of Pediatrics Committee on Drugs: The transfer of drugs and other chemicals into human milk. Pediatrics 108:776, 2001. Accessed April 28, 2005 at http://aappolicy.aappublications.org/cgi/content/full/pediatrics;108/3/776.

American Academy of Pediatrics Section on Breastfeeding: Breastfeeding and the use of human milk. Pediatrics 115:496, 2005.

Atallah, AN, Hofmeyr, GJ, and Duley, L: Calcium supplementation during pregnancy for preventing hypertensive disorders and related problems. Cochrane Database Syst Rev 1:CD001059, 2002.

Barkai, G, et al: Frequency of Down's syndrome and neural tube defects in the same family. Lancet 361:1331, 2003.

Black, MM, et al: Home and videotape intervention delays early complementary feeding among adolescent mothers. Pediatrics 107:E67, 2001.

Bodnar, LM, et al: High prevalence of postpartum anemia among low-income women in the United States. Am J Obstet Gynecol 186:438, 2001.

Bolumar, F, et al: Caffeine intake and delayed conception: A European multicenter study on infertility and subfecundity. European Study Group on Infertility Subfecundity. Am J Epidemiol 145:324, 1997.

Boyer, KM, et al: Risk factors for Toxoplasma gondii infection in mothers of infants with congenital toxoplasmosis: Implications for prenatal management and screening. Am J Obstet Gynecol 192:564, 2005.

Bracken, MB, et al: Association of maternal caffeine consumption with decrements in fetal growth. Am J Epidemiol 157:456, 2003.

Brown, JE: Nutrition Through the Life Cycle, ed 2. Thomson Wadsworth, Belmont, CA, 2005.

Butte, NF, et al: Energy requirements during pregnancy based on total energy expenditure and energy deposition. Am J Clin Nutr 79:1078, 2004.

Centers for Disease Control: Accutane-exposed pregnancies—California, 1999. MMWR 49:28, 2000a. Accessed April 12, 2000 at http://www.cdc.gov/epo/mmwr/preview/mmwrhtml/mm4902a.htm.

Centers for Disease Control: Alcohol consumption among pregnant and childbearing-aged women—United States, 1991–1999. MMWR 51:273, 2002a. Accessed April 21, 2002 at http://www.cdc.gov/epo/mmwr/preview/mmwrhtml/mm5113a2.htm.

Centers for Disease Control: Alcohol Consumption Among Women Who Are Pregnant or Who Might Become Pregnant—United States, 2002. MMWR 53:1178, 2004a. Accessed April 28, 2005 at http://www.cdc.gov/mmwr/preview/mmwrhtml/mm5350a4.htm.

Centers for Disease Control: Barriers to dietary control among pregnant women with phenylketonuria—United States, 1998–2000. MMWR 51:117, 2002b. Accessed April 28, 2002 at http://www.cdc.gov/mmwr/preview/mmwrhtml/mm5106a1.htm.

Centers for Disease Control: Folate Status in women of childbearing age, by race/ethnicity—United States, 1999–2000. MMWR 51:808, 2002c. Accessed September 12, 2002 at http://www.cdc.gov/mmwr/preview/nnwrhtml/mm5136a2.htm.

Centers for Disease Control: Folic acid awareness and use among women with a history of a neural tube defect pregnancy—Texas, 2000–2001. MMWR 51:16, 2002d. Accessed November 22, 2002 at http://www.cdc.gov/mmwr/preview/mmwrhtml/rr5113a5.htm.

Centers for Disease Control: Infant Mortality and Low Birth Weight Among Black and White Infants—United States, 1980–2000. MMRW 51:589, 2002e. Accessed January 18, 2004 at http://www.cdc.gov/mmwr/PDF/wk/mm5127.pdf.

Centers for Disease Control: Knowledge about folic acid and use of multivitamins containing folic acid among reproductive-aged women—Georgia. MMWR 45:793, 1996. Accessed September 13, 1999 at http://www.cdc.gov/epo/mmwr/preview/mmwrhtml/00043735.htm.

Centers for Disease Control: Knowledge and use of folic acid by women of childbearing age—United States, 1995–1998. MMWR 48:325, 1999a. Accessed September 13, 1999 at http://www.cdc.gov/epo/mmwr/preview/mmwrhtml/00056982.htm.

Centers for Disease Control: Motivational Intervention to Reduce Alcohol-Exposed Pregnancies—Florida, Texas, and Virginia, 1997–2001. MMWR 52:441, 2003a. Accessed January 25, 2004 at http://www.cdc.gov/mmwr/preview/mmwrhtml/mm5219a4.htm.

Centers for Disease Control: Multistate outbreak of listeriosis—United States, 1998. MMWR 47:1085, 1998a. Accessed September 19, 1999 at http://www.cdc.gov/epo/mmwr/preview/mmwrhtml/00056024.htm.

Centers for Disease Control: Multistate outbreak of listeriosis—United States, 2000. MMWR 49:1129, 2000b. Accessed January 27, 2004 at http://www.cdc.gov/mmwr/preview/mmwrhtml/mm4950a1.htm.

Centers for Disease Control: Neural tube defect surveillance and folic acid intervention—Texas-Mexico border, 1993–1998. MMWR 49:1, 2000c. Accessed April 12, 2000 at http://www.cdc.gov/epo/mmwr/preview/mmwrhtml/mm4901a1.htm.

Centers for Disease Control: Neurologic impairment in children associated with maternal dietary deficiency of cobalamin—Georgia, 2001. MMWR 52:61, 2003b. Accessed January 22, 2004 at http://www.cdc.gov/mmwr/preview/mmwrhtml/mm5204a1.htm.

Centers for Disease Control: Outbreak of listeriosis associated with homemade Mexican-style cheese—North Carolina, October 2000–January 2001. MMWR 50:560, 2001a. Accessed

January 27, 2004 at http://www.cdc.gov/mmwr/preview/mmwrhtml/mm5026a3.htm.

Centers for Disease Control: Preventing congenital toxoplasmosis. MMWR 49:57, 2000d. Accessed November 8, 2000 at http://www.cdc.gov/mmwr/preview/mmwrhtml/rr4902a5.htm.

Centers for Disease Control: Recommendations for the use of folic acid to reduce the number of cases of spina bifida and other neural tube defects. MMWR 41 (No. RR-14):1, 1992.

Centers for Disease Control: Recommendations for using fluoride to prevent and control dental caries in the United States. MMWR 50:1, 2001b. Accessed December 4, 2003 at http://www.cdc.gov/mmwr/PDF/RR/RR5014.pdf.

Centers for Disease Control: Recommendations to prevent and control iron deficiency in the United States. MMWR 47:1, 1998b. Accessed September 13, 1999 at http://www.cdc.gov/epo/mmwr/preview/mmwrhtml/00051880.htm.

Centers for Disease Control: Spina bifida and anencephaly before and after folic acid mandate—United States, 1995—1996 and 1999—2000. MMWR 53:362, 2004b. Accessed April 28, 2005 at http://www.cdc.gov/mmwr/preview/mmwrhtml/mm5317a3.htm.

Centers for Disease Control: Teen Birth Rate Continues to Decline. Fact Sheet, 2003c. Accessed January 26, 2004 at http://www.cdc.gov/od/oc/media/pressrel/fs031217.htm.

Centers for Disease Control: Update: Multistate outbreak of listeriosis—United States, 1998–1999. MMWR 47:1117, 1999b. Accessed September 19, 1999 at http://www.cdc.gov/epo/mmwr/preview/mmwrhtml/00056169.htm.

Centers for Disease Control: Use of Vitamins Containing Folic Acid among women of childbearing age—United States, 2004. MMWR 53:847, 2004c. Accessed October 1, 2004 at http://www.cdc.gov/mmwr/preview/mmwrhtml/mm5336a6.htm.

Centers for Disease Control: WHO/UNICEF Baby-Friendly Hospital Initiative, 2003d. Accessed February 8, 2004 at http://www.cdc.gov/breastfeeding/compend-babyfriendlywho.htm tensteps.

Christian, P, et al: An ethnographic study of night blindness "ratauni" among women in the Terai of Nepal. Soc Sci Med 46:879, 1998.

Clausson, B, et al: Effect of caffeine exposure during pregnancy on birth weight and gestational age. Am J Epidemiol 155:429, 2002.

Collaborative Group on Hormonal Factors in Breast Cancer: Breast cancer and breastfeeding: Collaborative reanalysis of individual data from 47 epidemiological studies in 30 countries, including 50302 women with breast cancer and 96973 women without the disease. Lancet 360:187, 2002.

Corbett, RW, Ryan, C, and Weinrich, SP: Pica in pregnancy: Does it affect pregnancy outcomes? MCN Am J Matern Child Nurs 28:183, 2003.

Crenshaw, J: Breastfeeding in nonmaternity settings. Am J Nurs 105(1):40, 2005.

Darroch, JE: Adolescent pregnancy trends and demographics. Curr Womens Health Rep 1:102, 2001.

Dickinson, CJ: Does folic acid harm people with vitamin B_{12} deficiency? Q J Med 88:357, 1995.

Di Gregorio, S, et al: Osteoporosis with vertebral fractures associated with pregnancy and lactation. Nutrition 16:1052, 2000.

Dochterman, J, and Bulechek, G (eds): Nursing Interventions Classification (NIC), ed 4. Mosby, St. Louis, 2004.

Duley, L, Gulmezoglu, AM, and Henderson-Smart, DJ: Magnesium sulphate and other anticonvulsants for women with preeclampsia. Cochrane Database Syst Rev 2: CD000025, 2003.

Dutta-Roy, AK: Transport mechanisms for long-chain polyunsaturated fatty acids in the human placenta. Am J Clin Nutr 71:312S, 2000.

Einarsson, JI, Sangi-Haghpeykar, H, and Gardner, MO: Sperm exposure and development of preeclampsia. Am J Obstet Gynecol 188:1241, 2003.

Eroglu, A, et al: Spontaneous esophageal rupture following severe vomiting in pregnancy. Dis Esophagus 15:242, 2002.

Eskenazi, B. Caffeine—filtering the facts. N Engl J Med 341:1688, 1999.

Fairbanks, VF: Iron in medicine and nutrition. In Shils, ME, et al (eds): Modern Nutrition in Health and Disease, ed 9. Lippincott Williams & Wilkins, Philadelphia, 1999.

Food Standards Agency (UK): Agency issues caffeine advice to pregnant women, 2001. Accessed January 27, 2004 at http://www.foodstandards.gov.uk/news/newsarchive/caffeine pregnancy.

Food Standards Agency (UK): Should I avoid peanuts while I'm breastfeeding? 2004. Accessed February 6, 2004 at http://www.foodstandards.gov.uk/healthiereating/asktheexpert/allergyintolerance/peanutsbreastfeeding.

Futoryan, T, and Gilchrest, BA: Retinoids and the skin. Nutr Rev 52:299, 1994.

Galloway, R, and McGuire, J: Daily versus weekly: How many iron pills do pregnant women need? Nutr Rev 54:318, 1996.

Goldenberg, RL, et al: The effect of zinc supplementation on pregnancy outcome. JAMA 274:463, 1995.

Hally, SS: Nutrition in reproductive health. J Nurse Midwifery 43:459, 1998.

Heymann, DL (ed): Control of Communicable Diseases Manual, ed 18. American Public Health Association, Washington, DC, 2004.

Hill, JB, Yost, NP, and Wendel, GD: Acute renal failure in association with severe hyperemesis gravidarum. Obstet Gynecol 100:1119, 2002.

James, WPT: Long-term fetal programming of body composition and longevity. Nutr Rev 55:S31, 1997.

Jensen, TK, et al: Caffeine intake and fecundability: A follow-up study among 430 Danish couples planning their first pregnancy. Reprod Toxicol 12:289, 1998.

Jewell, D, and Young, G: Interventions for nausea and vomiting in early pregnancy. Cochrane Database Syst Rev 4:CD000145, 2003.

Jewell, DJ, and Young, G: Interventions for treating constipation in pregnancy. Cochrane Database Syst Rev 2:CD001142, 2001.

Kalkwarf, HJ, and Specker, BL: Bone mineral changes during pregnancy and lactation. Endocrine 17:49, 2002.

Kitzman, H, et al: Enduring effects of nurse home visitation on maternal life course. JAMA 283:1983, 2000.

Koch, R, et al: Maternal phenylketonuria: An international study. Mol Genet Metab 71:233, 2000.

Lenfant, C: Working group report on high blood pressure in pregnancy. J Clin Hypertens 3:75, 2001.

Levichek, Z, et al: Nausea and vomiting of pregnancy. Canadian Family Physician 48:267, 2002.

Levine, RJ, et al: Urinary placental growth factor and risk of preeclampsia. JAMA 293:77, 2005.

Li, R, et al: Prevalence of breastfeeding in the United States: The 2001 National Immunization Survey. Pediatrics 111:1198, 2003.

Liang, SG, et al: Pneumomediastinum following esophageal rupture associated with hyperemesis gravidarum. J Obstet Gynaecol Res 28:172, 2002.

Liel, Y, Atar, D, and Ohana, N: Pregnancy-associated osteoporosis: Preliminary densitometric evidence of extremely rapid recovery of bone mineral density. South Med J 91:33, 1998.

Lynch, A, et al: Preeclampsia in multiple gestation: The role of assisted reproductive technologies. Obstet Gynecol 99:445, 2002.

Luerssen, MA, and Winsch, AL: Identifying and treating gestational diabetes mellitus. Am J Nurs 105(4):65, 2005.

Mahomed, K, and Gulmezoglu, AM: Maternal iodine supplements in areas of deficiency. [Computer software]. The Cochrane Library, Oxford, 1999, issue 2. Abstract accessed through CINAHL, accession no. 1999040422.

Makrides, M, et al: Efficacy and tolerability of low-dose iron supplements during pregnancy: A randomized controlled trial. Am J Clin Nutr 78:145, 2003.

Mannella, JA: Regulation of milk intake after exposure to alcohol in mothers' milk. Alcohol Clin Exp Res 25:590, 2001.

Mannella, JA, and Garcia-Gomez, PL: Sleep disturbances after acute exposure to alcohol in mothers' milk. Alcohol 25:153, 2001.

March of Dimes: Food-borne risks in pregnancy. Quick Reference and Fact Sheets, 2002. Accessed January 26, 2004 at http://www.modimes.org/professionals/681_1152.asp.

Marks, JM, and Spatz, DL: Medications and lactation: What PNPs need to know. J Pediatr Health Care 17:311, 2003.

McGanity, WJ, Dawson EB, and Van Hook, JW: Maternal nutrition. In Shils, ME, et al (eds): Modern Nutrition in Health and Disease, ed 9. Lippincott Williams & Wilkins, Philadelphia, 1999.

McLaren, DS, and Frigg, M: Sight and Life Manual on Vitamin A

Deficiency Disorders (VADD), ed 2. Sight and Life, Basel, Switzerland, 2001.

McLeod, D, Pullon, S, and Cookson, T: Factors influencing continuation of breastfeeding in a cohort of women. J Hum Lact 18:335, 2002.

Moorhead, S, Johnson, M, and Maas, M (eds): Nursing Outcomes Classification (NOC) ed 3. Mosby, St. Louis, 2004.

Moran, P, and Taylor, R: Management of hyperemesis gravidarum: The importance of weight loss as a criterion for steroid therapy. Q J Med 95:153, 2002.

Moreland, J, and Coombs, J: Promoting and supporting breastfeeding. Am Fam Physician 61:2093, 2000.

Motil, KJ, et al: Lean body mass of well-nourished women is preserved during lactation. Am J Clin Nutr 67:292, 1998.

MRC Vitamin Study Research Group: Prevention of neural tube defects: Results of the Medical Research Council Vitamin Study. Lancet 338:131, 1991.

Murphy-Brennan, MG, and Oei, TP: Is there evidence to show that fetal alcohol syndrome can be prevented? J Drug Educ 29:5, 1999.

NANDA International: Nursing Diagnoses: Definitions and Classification, 2003–2004. NANDA International, Philadelphia, 2003.

National Center for Chronic Disease Prevention and Health Promotion. Baby-friendly USA. 2003. Accessed February 5, 2004 at http://www.cdc.gov/breastfeeding/compend-babyfriendly.htm.

National Heart, Lung, and Blood Institute: Report of the Working Group on Research on Hypertension During Pregnancy. April 27, 2001. Accessed May 1, 2005 at http://www.nhlbi.nih.gov/resources/hyperten_preg/

Naylor, AJ: Baby-Friendly Hospital Initiative: Protecting, promoting, and supporting breastfeeding in the twenty-first century. Pediatr Clin North Am 48:475, 2001.

Northrup, H, and Volcik, KA: Spina bifida and other neural tube defects. Curr Probl Pediatr 30:313, 2000.

Nursing 2004 Drug Handbook, ed 24. Lippincott, Williams & Wilkins, Philadelphia, 2004.

Oakley, GP, Adams, MJ, and Dickinson, CM: More folic acid for everyone, now. J Nutr (Suppl)126:251S, 1996.

Ogundele, MO, and Coulter, JB: HIV transmission through breastfeeding: Problems and prevention. Ann Trop Paediatr 23:91, 2003.

O'Leary, VB, et al: MTRR and MTHFR polymorphism: Link to Down syndrome? Am J Med Genet 107:151, 2002.

Paton, LM, et al: Pregnancy and lactation have no long-term deleterious effect on measures of bone mineral in healthy women: A twin study. Am J Clin Nutr 77:707, 2003.

Peris, P, et al: Pregnancy associated osteoporosis: The familial effect. Clin Exp Rheumatol 20:697, 2002.

Philip, B: Hyperemesis gravidarum: Literature review. WMJ 102:46, 2003.

Purnell, LD, and Paulanka, BJ: Transcultural Health Care, ed 2. FA Davis, Philadelphia, 2003.

Rainville, AJ: Pica practices of pregnant women are associated with lower maternal hemoglobin level at delivery. J Am Diet Assoc 98:293, 1998.

Ritchie, LD, et al: A longitudinal study of calcium homeostasis during human pregnancy and lactation and after resumption of menses. Am J Clin Nutr 67:693, 1998.

Robinson, JN, Banerjee, R, and Thiet, MP: Coagulopathy secondary to vitamin K deficiency in hyperemesis gravidarum. Obstet Gynecol 92:673, 1998.

Romano, PS, et al: Folic acid fortification of grain: An economic analysis. Am J Public Health 85:667, 1995.

Ross Products Division: Mothers' Survey. Abbott Laboratories, Columbus, OH, 2002.

Rothenberg, SP, et al: Autoantibodies against folate receptors in women with a pregnancy complicated by a neural tube defect. N Engl J Med 350:134, 2004.

Ryan, AS, Wenjun, Z, and Acosta, A: Breastfeeding continues to increase into the new millennium. Pediatrics 110:1103, 2002.

Schober, SE, et al: Blood mercury levels in US children and women of childbearing age, 1999–2000. JAMA 289:1667, 2003.

Shannon, M: Severe lead poisoning in pregnancy. Ambul Pediatr 3:37, 2003.

Sikorski, J, et al: Support for breast feeding mothers. Cochrane Database Syst Rev 2:CD001141, 2003.

Smith, C, et al: A randomized controlled trial of ginger to treat nausea and vomiting in pregnancy. Obstet Gynecol 103:639, 2004.

Story, M: Promoting healthy eating and ensuring adequate weight gain in pregnant adolescents: Issues and strategies. Ann N Y Acad Sci 817:321, 1997.

Tommaselli, GA, et al: Using complete breastfeeding and lactational amenorrhoea as birth spacing methods. Contraception 61:253, 2000.

Umeta, M, et al: Factors associated with stunting in infants aged 5–11 months in the Dodota-Sire District, rural Ethiopia. J Nutr 133:1064, 2003.

United States Department of Agriculture: WIC Funding and Program Data, 2003. Accessed January 29, 2004 at http://www.fns.usda.gov/wic/fundingandprogramdata/.

United States Department of Health and Human Services: FDA announces enhancement to isotretinoin risk management program. FDA Talk Paper November 23, 2004. Accessed April 28, 2005 at: http://www.fda.gov/bbs/topics/ANSWERS/2004/ANS01328.html

United States Department of Health and Human Services: FDA issues nationwide health warning about Royal Baltic cold-smoked fish products. HHS News March 10, 2000. Accessed March 12, 2000 at http://www.fda.gov/bbs/topics/NEWS/NEW00719.html.

United States Department of Health and Human Services and United States Environmental Protection Agency: What you need to know about mercury in fish and shellfish. March 2004. Accessed July 22, 2004 at http://www.cfsan.fda.gov/~dms/admehg3.html.

United States Preventive Services Task Force: Behavioral interventions to promote breastfeeding. AHRQ Publication No. APPIP03-0016, July 2003. Accessed July 22, 2004 at http://www.ahrq.gov/clinic/3rduspstf/brstfeed/brfeedwh.pdf.

van Unnik, GA, and van Roosmalen, J: Lactation-induced amenorrhea as birth control method [in Dutch]. Ned Tijdschr Geneeskd 142:60, 1998.

Wagner, BA, et al: Nutritional management of hyperemesis gravidarum. Nutr Clin Pract 15:65, 2000.

Weinberg, GA: The dilemma of postnatal mother-to-child transmission of HIV: To breastfeed or not? Birth 27:199, 2000.

West, KP, Jr, et al: Double blind, cluster randomized trial of low dose supplementation with vitamin A or beta carotene on mortality related to pregnancy in Nepal. BMJ 318:570, 1999.

Willetts, KE, Ekangaki, A, and Eden, JA: Effect of a ginger extract on pregnancy-induced nausea: A randomised controlled trial. Aust NZ J Obstet Gynaecol 43:139, 2003.

Wisborg, K, et al: Exposure to tobacco smoke in utero and the risk of stillbirth and death in the first year of life. Am J Epidemiol 154: 322, 2001.

World Health Organization. Lactational amenorrhoea method (LAM). Accessed January 5, 2004 at http://www.who.int/reproductive-health/publications/RHR_00_2_medical_eligibility_criteria_second_edition/rhr_00_02_lam.html.

Yonekura, ML, and Mead, PB: Protocols: OB/GYN infection. Listeria infection in pregnancy. Contemp OB/GYN 44:16, 1999.

Young, GL, and Jewell, D: Interventions for leg cramps in pregnancy. Cochrane Database Syst Rev 1:CD000121, 2002.

Zamorski, MA: NHBPEP Report on high blood pressure in pregnancy: A summary for family physicians—National High Blood Pressure Education Program. Am Fam Physician 64:263, 2001.

CHAPTER 12

Life Cycle Nutrition: Infancy, Childhood, and Adolescence

Learning Objectives

After completing this chapter, the student should be able to:

1. Describe normal growth patterns and corresponding nutritional needs for a full-term infant, a toddler, a school-age child, and an adolescent.
2. Explain why breast milk is uniquely suited to the human infant's capabilities.
3. Discuss the rationale for the sequence in which semi-solid foods are introduced into an infant's diet.
4. List causes and treatments of five common nutritional problems of infancy.
5. Summarize common nutritional problems of the pre-school child.
6. Relate ways in which a child can be encouraged to establish good nutritional habits.
7. Identify areas of concern regarding the typical adolescent's diet.
8. Devise a comprehensive plan to prevent obesity in a target population of children or adolescents.

Good nutrition is of paramount importance for both infants and children. Because of public health efforts, U.S. infant mortality rates decreased significantly between 1915 and 1997. Of every 1000 infants born alive in 1915, approximately 100 died before the age of 1 year (Centers for Disease Control, 1999a). Between 1980 and 2000, the U.S. infant mortality rate declined from 10.9 to 5.7 for white infants and from 22.2 to 14.0 for black infants, but the goal of Healthy People 2010 to reduce the infant mortality rate to 4.5 or less for all racial/ethnic groups is a formidable task when the rate in 2000 was 6.9 (Centers for Disease Control, 2002b). Infants of very low birth weight (<1500 grams or 3.3 pounds) account for approximately two-thirds of the black-white gap in infant mortality (Centers for Disease Control, 2002b) but 90 percent of these infants survive long term compared with 50 percent in the 1970s (Hofman et al, 2004). American Indian/Alaska Native infants and Hispanics of Puerto Rican origin also have

higher death rates than white infants (Centers for Disease Control, 1999a).

This chapter focuses on periods of rapid **growth** during infancy, childhood, and adolescence. In addition to nutritional needs for all periods of growth, the stages of physical and **psychosocial development** are considered for these ages, noting ways in which food relates to psychosocial development.

Psychosocial Development

American psychoanalyst **Erik Erikson** formulated a theory of psychological development based on an individual's interactions with other people. Erikson divided life into eight stages, each of which involves a psychosocial developmental task to be mastered and an opposite negative trait that emerges if the task is not mastered. Even if a developmental task is successfully mastered, a new situation may arise, challenging the person to reaffirm his or her mastery.

Erikson's developmental tasks through adolescence are listed in Table 12–1. This chapter and the next consider ways that nutrition and food can influence psychosocial development.

Nutrition in Infancy

Growth, the progressive maturation and increase in size of a living thing, entails the synthesis of new protoplasm and multiplication of cells. Infancy, the first year of life, is a

Table 12–1 Erikson's Theory of Psychosocial Development

STAGE OF LIFE	DEVELOPMENTAL TASK	OPPOSING NEGATIVE TRAIT
Infancy	Trust	Distrust
Toddler	Autonomy	Doubt
Preschooler	Initiative	Guilt
School-age child	Industry	Inferiority
Adolescent	Identity	Role confusion

critical period for the growth of essential organs. Health-care workers use certain milestones to judge the adequacy of a baby's growth.

Growth

The only time human beings grow faster than in infancy is the 9 months before they are born. A baby's birth weight should double by age 4 to 6 months and triple by 1 year. An infant who weighs 7 pounds at birth, for example, should weigh 14 pounds at 6 months and 21 pounds at 1 year. From a birth length of about 20 inches, a baby grows to about 30 inches by age 1.

The infant's *rate of growth* is more significant than absolute values. Is the infant progressing at a reasonable pace? A gain of 5 to 8 ounces per week is expected during the first 4 or 5 months. Thereafter, a gain of 4 to 5 ounces per week until the first birthday is reasonable.

The growth charts in Appendix D reflect growth patterns of all children in the United States. A British foundation has published growth charts for breast-fed infants showing that initially they gain weight more rapidly than formula-fed infants, but at 2 to 3 months of age their weight gain decreases and they begin to move downward across centiles. The specific charts purportedly could prevent mothers and health professionals from becoming anxious and changing the infant from breast to formula milk when growth begins to slow (Fry, 2003).

During the first few days after birth, a baby loses weight as it adjusts to its new environment and food supply. Among its adaptations is learning to feed compared to receiving a continuous supply of nutrients in utero. To feed successfully, the infant has to be calm but alert and has to learn to display cues to its needs to the caregiver (Chatoor, 2002). The amount of weight lost in these first few days should not exceed 10 percent of the birth weight. The newborn (or neonate, as a baby is called during its first 28 days after birth) usually returns to its birth weight within 14 days.

The period most critical to brain development extends from conception into the second year of life. Brain cells increase most rapidly before birth and during the first 5 or 6 months after birth. To attain maximum brain growth, the baby needs optimal nutrition. Severe protein-calorie malnutrition in the last trimester of pregnancy or the first 6 months of life may decrease the number of brain cells by as much as 20 percent.

Development

Development is the gradual process of changing from a simple to a more complex organism. Becoming a mature individual involves psychosocial and physical changes, not only an increase in size.

Psychosocial Development of the Infant

The psychosocial developmental task of the infant is to learn to **trust** (Table 12–1). The parent who responds promptly and lovingly to the infant's cries is teaching the baby to trust, laying the foundation for future human relationships. If the caregiver handles the infant inconsistently—gently one time and roughly the next—however, the baby learns to mistrust. If the psychosocial task of trust is not accomplished, it lays a groundwork of mistrust and suspicion in the individual's personality.

In situations where physical care is provided but a tender relationship does not develop, infants may actually suffer stunted physical growth. Feeding problems and growth deficiencies can also occur within secure child-parent relationships, but insecure attachment relationships may intensify feeding problems and may lead to more severe malnutrition (Chatoor et al, 1998). **Failure to thrive (FTT)** is a medical diagnosis for severely underweight infants, and weight itself is the most reasonable marker for failure to thrive and associated problems (Raynor and Rudolf, 2000). Some researchers suggest that the role of deprivation and neglect has been overstated and that undemanding behavior, low appetite, and poor feeding skills may contribute to the onset and persistence of failure to thrive (Wright and Birks, 2000). Among 6-year-olds, FTT in infancy was associated with lower weight and BMI but was not related to cognitive abilities, suggesting that the adverse effects of early malnutrition on cognitive functioning seem to diminish over time (Boddy, Skuse, and Andrews, 2000).

An infant can explore the world through feeding and foods. New foods encourage experimentation. Babies like to poke their fingers into the food. When attempting to feed themselves, they may turn the spoon upside down on the way to their mouths. Consistent acceptance from parents teaches the infant to trust his or her world. Parents should not, for example, laugh at a particular behavior of their child one time and scold the next.

Physical Development

Development proceeds at a different pace in various tissues and organs. Proper feeding practices are based on the maturation rate of body organs.

GASTROINTESTINAL SYSTEM

The infant's gastrointestinal system is very different from the adult's. For several months, an infant's salivary and pancreatic amylases are inadequate to easily digest complex carbohydrates, but infants have lingual lipase for the digestion of fat, an enzyme that adults lack.

An infant's intestinal tract is also immature. It resembles a chain-link fence rather than a sieve, allowing whole proteins to be absorbed into the bloodstream. The more mature intestine permits absorption of amino acids but not whole proteins. This is one reason many foods that often cause allergies are not offered to the infant younger than 1 year of age.

Infants have to be fed often. A newborn's stomach holds about 1 ounce. By 1 year of age, the stomach holds about 8 ounces. An adult's stomach, by comparison, can hold about 2 quarts.

NERVOUS SYSTEM

Development of nervous tissue, bile, and hormones requires fat and cholesterol. Because of the rapid growth of the brain and the nervous system, the infant requires adequate fat and cholesterol in its diet.

A **term infant** does have some well-developed reflexes. One of these is the **rooting reflex.** When the infant's cheek is stroked, the head turns toward that side to nurse. For the first 3 or 4 months, the infant suckles by using an up-and-down motion of the tongue. If semisolid food is offered at this time, the natural motion of the tongue tends to spit it out.

After 4 months, the infant can suck using orofacial muscles. The tongue moves back and forth instead of up and down. At this point, semisolid food is more likely to be swallowed than spit out. By 6 months of age, the infant has enough hand-to-eye coordination to put food and other objects into its mouth. A 7-month-old infant can chew appropriate foods.

URINARY SYSTEM

An infant's kidneys are immature and have limited capacity to filter solutes. Not until the end of the second month can the infant's kidneys excrete the waste of semisolid foods. As indicated later, however, feeding of semisolids often is delayed another 2 to 4 months. By the infant's first birthday, the kidneys have reached full functional capacity.

Nutritional Needs of the Term Infant

A normal pregnancy is 38 to 42 weeks. Breast milk is the species-specific food for human infants. Its characteristics are the standard for infant formulas, which replicate many of the components of breast milk but which cannot supply all of its desirable qualities.

Protein

Because of the extensive tissue building that occurs, an infant's AI for protein is 9.1 grams per day for the first 6 months and its RDA is 13.5 grams for the second 6 months of life. By comparison, the RDA for protein is 56 grams for adult males and 46 grams for adult females.

The protein in breast milk is easy for the infant to digest. Human milk contains 70 percent whey and 30 percent **casein,** compared with 18 percent whey and 82 percent casein in cow's milk. The **whey** portion of milk consists of soluble proteins that are easily digested. The major whey protein in breast milk is alpha-**lactalbumin,** with an amino acid pattern much like that of the body tissues. The infant's body can absorb it easily and, without much processing, can use it for building tissue. Thus, gastric emptying is faster with human milk than cow's milk formula.

Energy

Infants need much higher relative energy intakes than do adults, primarily because the resting metabolic rates of infants and their needs for growth and development are so high. Normal pulse rate is 120 to 150 beats per minute; normal respiratory rate is 30 to 50 breaths per minute. Because of the large proportion of skin surface to body size, temperature regulation takes significant energy. An activity such as crying may double the infant's energy expenditure.

During the first 6 months, an average infant requires 108 kilocalories per kilogram of body weight per day. If a 154-pound (70-kilogram) man consumed energy at this rate, he would take in 7560 kilocalories per day. By the end of the

first year of life, the average infant requires only 98 kilocalories per kilogram of body weight (Brown, 2005).

CARBOHYDRATE

The carbohydrate in breast milk is easily digested by the infant. Breast milk contains amylase that is 40 to 60 times more active than that of cow's milk (Lo, 1997). The lactose in milk provides galactose, which is necessary for brain cell formation.

One source of carbohydrate an infant must not be given is honey (see Clinical Application 12–1).

FAT

An infant needs 30 to 55 percent of kilocalories from fat as a concentrated source of energy because of his small stomach capacity. Since breast milk contains the necessary lipase to begin digestion for the infant, about 95 to 98 percent of the fat in human milk is absorbed. The developing nervous system also requires fat, particularly *arachidonic* and *docosahexaenoic* (very-long-chain) *fatty acids,* the main omega-6 and omega-3 fatty acids of the central nervous system. These two fatty acids are essential for retinal

---

Clinical Application 12–1

Honey Is a Danger to Infants

No honey should be given to an infant until after the first birthday because it frequently contains organisms that the infant cannot fight off. Bees may contaminate honey with botulism **spores** acquired from plants or the soil. Up to 25 percent of honey products have been found to contain spores, but in only 15 percent of botulism cases reported to the CDC was honey ingested (Cox and Hinkle, 2002). Processing the honey does not destroy these spores. Other foods and even dust contain botulism spores. Since the late 1970s, more than 1000 cases of infant botulism (now called intestinal botulism) have been reported in the United States (Tanzi and Gabay, 2002), and in 2001, powdered infant formula contaminated with spores, presumably from raw ingredients, was recalled in Great Britain (Hilton, 2001).

If ingested by the infant, the spores become active in its intestinal tract and produce a neurotoxin that irreversibly binds to acetylcholine receptors on motor nerve terminals. Symptoms include constipation, weakness, an altered cry, poor feeding, and a striking loss of head control (Heymann, 2004). Unrecognized, the condition can quickly progress to respiratory failure. More than 70 percent of these infants will require mechanical ventilation, but the case-fatality rate of infant botulism is less than 2 percent (Cox and Hinkle, 2002). The nerve terminals regenerate as the child recovers. In adults and older children, natural defenses prevent the growth of the organism unless the person has abnormal gastrointestinal anatomy and microflora (Heymann, 2004).

Physicians are required to report all cases of infant botulism promptly to state and local health departments (Centers for Disease Control, 2003a).

Box 12–1 Research Linking Cognitive Abilities to Breast-Feeding

Breast milk contains arachidonic and docosahexaenoic (DHA) fatty acids, which accumulate during the brain growth spurt from the third trimester until age 2 (Fats and fatty acids, 2004). Breast-feeding has been associated with slightly enhanced performance on tests of cognitive development (American Academy of Pediatrics, 2005). For instance, a meta-analysis found significantly higher levels of cognitive function in breast-fed compared with formula-fed children at 6 to 23 months of age, with low-birth-weight infants showing larger differences than normal-birth-weight infants (Anderson, Johnstone, and Remley, 1999). Maternal intake of very-long-chain n-3 PUFAs, DHA and eicosapentaenoic acid, during pregnancy and lactation correlated significantly

with their children's mental processing scores at 4 years of age (Helland et al, 2003). Duration of breast-feeding was significantly associated with higher IQ scores in young adults, after consideration of potential confounding factors (Mortensen et al, 2002). A long-term study found breast-feeding was significantly and positively associated with reading ability at 53 years, an effect that was independent of early social background, educational attainment, and adult social class (Richards, Hardy, and Wadsworth, 2002). Similar effects were found for exclusive breast-feeding of small for gestational age infants (Rao et al, 2002), and for both cognitive and motor development in premature infants (Bier et al, 2002).

and neural development and are found in human milk but not in cow's milk (Breastfeeding, 2004). In healthy full term infants, dietary omega-3 intake was associated with improved visual acuity tasks at 2, and possibly, 4 months of age but long term advantage still questionable (SanGiovanni et al, 2000). Box 12–1 identifies some research linking cognitive development to breast-feeding.

EVALUATION

The best indicator of adequate kilocaloric intake is a normal growth rate according to standard growth charts. Measurements should be made every 3 months; they can be graphed on growth charts such as those that appear in Appendix D.

Vitamins

The RDA tables (Appendix F) specify vitamin intake for infants aged 0 to 6 months and 6 to 12 months. Infants need all the vitamins that other humans need but in different amounts.

Cow's milk contains nine times the vitamin B_{12} of breast milk from white women consuming a mixed diet, but vegan women produce milk containing only one-fourth to one-third as much vitamin B_{12} as women consuming a mixed diet (Weir and Scott, 1999). Cases of growth failure and neurologic impairment due to cobalamin deficiency occurred in breastfeeding infants of vegetarian mothers (Centers for Disease Control, 2003c). Human breast milk contains more vitamin C but less vitamin D than cow's milk. Breast-fed infants should be supplemented with vitamin D. A minimum intake of 5 micrograms of vitamin D from formula, fortified milk, or supplements is advised from the age of 2 months through adolescence, because adequate sunlight exposure is not easily determined for a given individual (Gartner et al, 2003).

In adults, intestinal bacteria produce some vitamin K. Until the infant's intestine becomes colonized with *Escherichia coli*, he or she is at risk for bleeding problems. In this regard, formula-fed infants have an advantage over breast-fed babies, because breast milk supports proliferation of lactobacilli rather than *E. coli* (Lo, 1997). This fact contributes to the infant morbidity and mortality caused

by vitamin K deficiency seen worldwide in breast-fed infants (Olson, 1999). The American Academy of Pediatrics recommends that all newborns be given a single intramuscular dose of vitamin K after the first breast-feeding and within 6 hours of birth (2005). A case report of intracranial hemorrhage in a 3-month-old infant was attributed to vitamin K deficiency even though the infant received oral vitamin K but also was treated with antibiotics that could reduce the intestinal flora. The authors recommend vitamin K prophylaxis for breast-fed infants and for those receiving antibiotics (Suzuki et al, 1999).

Special situations that warrant vitamin supplementation are included later in this chapter.

Minerals

Infants need the same minerals as other human beings. Breast milk contains only one-third the sodium, potassium, and chloride and one-eighth the phosphorus of cow's milk, an amount that accommodates the limited function of the infant's kidneys. Breast milk also contains less iron than cow's milk, but the infant absorbs 49 percent of it compared with 10 percent from cow's milk. Several factors in breast milk promote iron absorption: less protein and phosphorus, more lactose and ascorbate (Lo, 1997).

Breast milk contains about one-sixth to one-quarter of the calcium of cow's milk. The infant is able to absorb 67 percent of the calcium in breast milk compared with 25 percent of the calcium in cow's milk, possibly because the high phosphorus content of cow's milk produces decreased absorption and increased excretion of calcium (Lo, 1997).

The bioavailability of zinc in breast milk is 60 percent, compared with 43 to 50 percent in cow's milk and 27 to 32 percent in infant formulas (Lo, 1997).

These differences in mineral content affect the osmolality of the milk. See Clinical Application 12–2 for additional information on the extra minerals' effect on the workload of the kidneys. It is clear that unmodified cow's milk is inappropriate for young infants.

Fluoride should not be administered to infants until after 6 months of age. Even then, supplementation is recommended for all children over 6 months of age only if the water supply contains less than 0.3 ppm of fluoride and for

Clinical Application 12–2

Renal Solute Loads

When selecting a formula, it is important to distinguish two measures of osmotic pressure. One is the osmotic pressure the formula presents to the gut. The other examines what remains to be excreted by the kidney after digestion, absorption, and metabolism have taken place. These leftovers are excess electrolytes and byproducts of protein metabolism. The osmotic pressure of these leftovers presented to the kidney for disposal is called the renal solute load. It varies considerably among preparations. When dealing with an infant's immature digestive and urinary systems, selecting an appropriate formula may be crucial to health. Below, common infant feedings' intestinal osmolality and renal solute loads are compared. Because infant formulas are often changed in response to new scientific information, the following chart is offered as an example only. The agency's dietitian or pharmacist should be consulted for the latest information. As always, the standard of comparison is human breast milk. Clearly, unmodified cow's milk would place the greatest burden on the infant's immature renal system.

MILK FORMULA	INTESTINAL OSMOLALITY (mOsm/kg)	RENAL SOLUTE LOAD (mOsm/L)
Human breast milk	300	101
Milk-based formula		
Similac with iron	300	125
Soy-based formula		
Isomil with iron	200	152
3.3 percent cow's milk	275	275

SOURCES: Klish and Montandon, 1987; Ross Laboratories, 2004; Thorp, Pierce, and Deedwanea, 1987.

children older than 3 years if the water supply contains less than 0.6 ppm (Appendix W, 2004).

Water

The infant's body is about 75 percent water. By the age of 3, the body has developed so it has the adult proportion of about 60 percent water (Gropper, Smith, and Groff, 2005). The daily turnover of water in the infant is approximately 15 percent of body weight.

Breast milk contains more water than cow's milk. Even in desert climates, an infant can be adequately hydrated on breast milk alone. An infant will regulate its intake of formula to obtain sufficient energy. If the formula is dilute, the baby will take more of it; if concentrated, less. This self-regulating mechanism is not perfect, however, because the infant may consume excess formula to quench its thirst.

The Breast-Fed Infant

Breast milk is designed for human infants and is the standard against which substitute milks are measured. Breast-feeding rates in the United States are at an all-time high (Fig. 11–3), but compared with other countries, they are still low. Even in this country, breast-fed infants are 21 per-

cent less likely to die between 1 month and 1 year of age than those who never breast-fed; however, the effects of breast milk and breast-feeding cannot be segregated completely from the family context (Chen and Rogan, 2004). Another analysis of infant mortality indicated that breast-feeding accounts for the race difference in infant mortality in the United States at least as well as low birth weight does (Forste, Weiss, and Lippincott, 2001). Human breast milk banks make milk available for infants whose mothers do not produce enough milk. One of the goals of Healthy People 2010 is to increase to 75 percent the proportion of mothers who breast-feed in the early postpartum period, to 50 percent those who breast-feed until the infants are 6 months old, and to 25 percent those who breast-feed until the infants are 1 year old (U.S. Department of Health and Human Services, 2000). The American Academy of Pediatrics section on Breastfeeding recommends exclusive breast feeding (nothing but breast milk and vitamins, minerals, and medications) for the first six months of life (2005).

Practices conducive to breast-feeding and lactation are covered in Chapter 11. Care of ill or frail infants must be individualized. An additional benefit to the infant is the analgesia provided by breast-feeding during painful procedures such as heel-sticks, but such procedures on healthy term infants should be delayed until after the initial breast-feeding with skin-to-skin contact has been achieved (American Academy of Pediatrics, 2005).

The need for increased follow-up of breast-feeding by health-care providers was shown in a study in Cincinnati. Mothers who called someone about breast-feeding problems turned to family or friends 34.7 percent of the time, to the lactation consultant 16.5 percent, to the pediatrician 8.8 percent, to the obstetrician or midwife 8.2 percent, to a breast-feeding support group 5.9 percent, and to the birth hospital 2.5 percent of the time (Kuan et al, 1999). Of the 522 women in that study, 29 percent had stopped breast-feeding by 8 weeks postpartum.

Clinical Application 12–3 explains the procedures for storing human milk.

Composition of Breast Milk

All breast milk is not alike; its composition adjusts to the infant's needs during the weeks an infant is nursing, even during the course of a single feeding. Breast milk varies from mother to mother and even in one mother with the time of day. It also varies with the lactation cycle, as elaborated below.

COLOSTRUM

The milk secreted for the first 2 to 4 days after the birth of the baby is called *colostrum*. It is a thin, yellow, cloudy fluid. Colostrum is high in proteins such as immunoglobulins, in fat-soluble vitamins, and in minerals and low in fat.

TRANSITIONAL MILK

Transitional milk follows colostrum and continues through the second week after delivery. Transitional milk contains lactose, fat, and water-soluble vitamins at the level of mature milk. It is produced in larger quantities than is colostrum.

Storage of Human Milk

Care must be taken when breast milk is expressed and stored for later feeding. Contamination by skin bacteria is a major problem. Overall, glass is the container that preserves the milk best. Milk can be safely refrigerated for 72 hours with little change. Freezing destroys cellular activity and reduces vitamin B_6 and C content. Boiling, in addition, destroys lipase and reduces the effect of IgA. The nutrient value of human milk is essentially unchanged, but the immunological properties are reduced by various storage techniques (Lawrence, 1999). Antioxidant activity at both refrigeration and freezing temperatures was significantly decreased, more so for longer duration and at colder temperatures (Hanna et al, 2004). Although the bactericidal action of refrigerated breast milk diminished rapidly, up to two-thirds of the original activity was maintained after freezing for up to 3 months (Ogundele, 2002). Amylase and bile salt-dependent lipase were stable for 24 hours even at the undesirable storage temperatures of 15°C and 25°C, equivalent to 59°F and 77°F (Hamosh et al, 1997). Human milk banks in North America abide by national guidelines to screen and test donors and pasteurize the milk (American Academy of Pediatrics, 2005).

MATURE MILK

As breast-feeding becomes established, the mother produces mature milk, which varies in composition. At 3 months, for instance, immunoglobulins make up a smaller portion of the proteins than when the baby is younger.

During a feeding, the constituents of the milk change. Mature breast milk contains less fat at the beginning of a feeding (fore-milk) and more fat at the end (hind-milk). Fat provides satiety, or a feeling of fullness or satisfaction. If the infant receives high-fat milk at the beginning of a feeding, it might become contented and stop nursing. Mother's milk adapts to the needs of the infant over time in that fat content of the milk decreases by month 2 of lactation and increases at 9 months. Similarly, protein content decreases over the first 6 months of lactation and then remains steady (Mitoulas et al, 2002). The variation in content also offers the infant a variety of taste experiences.

A case was reported of a baby nursing as usual and then crying apparently from abdominal pain after breast-feeding following his mother's five-mile run. This occurred three times. Testing the breast milk for lactic acid before and after running revealed no differences. The mother was a competitive runner who solved the dilemma by pumping her breasts and discarding the milk after running and feeding the baby formula for this feeding only (Duffy, 1997). In contrast, an experiment involving 24 women showed that moderate or even high-intensity exercise during lactation did not hinder infant acceptance of breast milk consumed 1 hour after exercise (Wright, Quinn, and Carey, 2002).

Exercise may decrease immunologic factors, but the effect is transient. Breast milk contains significantly lower amounts of IgA for 10 to 30 minutes after exhaustive exercise but recovers in 1 hour (Gregory et al, 1997). In contrast, moderate exercise during lactation does not affect levels of IgA, lactoferrin, or lysozyme in breast milk (Lovelady, Hunter, and Geigerman, 2003).

Unique Advantages of Breast-Feeding

Two well-documented advantages to breast-feeding have not been duplicated by formulas. The first is the protection against disease that a mother's milk provides. The second is a lowered risk of allergies in the infant. Even a few weeks of breast-feeding benefits the infant. Additional advantages may be a negative association with obesity and an enhancement of cognition (see Box 12–1).

PROTECTION AGAINST DISEASE

In both developing and industrialized countries, breast-feeding reduces the incidence of gastrointestinal and respiratory diseases and otitis media (middle ear infection). Among generally healthy infants in developed nations, formula-fed infants were hospitalized for severe respiratory tract illnesses more than three times as often as infants who were exclusively breast-fed for 4 months (Bachrach, Schwartz, and Bachrach, 2003).

Breast milk, through bifidus growth factors, promotes a particular kind of bacteria, *Lactobacillus bifidus*, in the baby's intestine rather than *E. coli*. Although the normal adult intestine harbors *E. coli*, it can cause diarrhea in children. The *L. bifidus* produces acids that retard the growth of organisms such as staphylococci, shigella, protozoa, and yeast, which can cause disease. Another component of breast milk, lactoferrin, an iron-binding protein, competes with any bacteria for iron and kills some organisms such as *Streptococcus mutans* and *Vibrio cholerae* (Goldman, Goldblum, and Schmalstieg, 1997).

Among the infection-fighting agents in breast milk are leukocytes or white blood cells (WBCs). The highest concentration of WBCs in human milk occurs in the first few days of lactation, 1 to 3 million per milliliter. About 35 to 55 percent of the WBCs are macrophages that kill microorganisms (Goldman, Goldblum, and Schmalstieg, 1997).

Breast-feeding may, in addition to the well-known passive protection against infections during lactation, have a unique capacity to stimulate the immune system of the offspring (Hanson, 1998). Because certain immune factors appear in infants in amounts that could not be merely transferred through breast milk, it is thought that breast-feeding stimulates the activity of the infant's own immune system (Goldman, Goldblum, and Schmalstieg, 1997). Human milk protects against infections in the breast-fed offspring mainly via the secretory IgA antibodies, but also most likely via several other factors (Hanson, 1998). Secretory IgA in breast-milk coats intestinal bacteria and blocks their translocation across the gut mucosa. This mechanism may protect the infant from septicemia of intestinal origin (Wold and Adlerberth, 2000).

PREVENTION OF ALLERGIES

The young infant's gastrointestinal tract can permit the passage of whole proteins into the bloodstream. These proteins can stimulate an allergic response in susceptible infants. Meta-analyses revealed that in infants from atopic families, exclusive breast-feeding for 3 months reduced atopic dermatis by 42 percent and asthma by 48 percent (Zeiger, 2003). If breast milk is unavailable or insufficient, extensively **hydrolyzed** formulas are preferable to unhydrolyzed or partially hydrolyzed formulas in terms of the risk of some atopic manifestations (van Odijk et al, 2003).

Cow's milk is the most commonly offending food, affecting about 2.5 percent of infants. The major risk factors are positive family history of **atopy** and early exposure to cow's milk proteins (Businco, Bruno, and Giampietro, 1999). Either gross or occult gastrointestinal bleeding may result from cow's milk allergy, and after an infant becomes allergic to cow's milk, the risk of other allergies developing increases. For instance, 47 percent of children with confirmed cow's milk allergy react to soymilk and 35 percent react to oranges (Brown, 2005).

Breast-feeding does not provide absolute protection from allergies. One-year-old infants developed cow's milk allergy significantly more often if there had been a low concentration of IgA antibodies in their breast milk between 6 days and 4 weeks postpartum. A low IgA content in human milk may lead to defective exclusion of food antigens and thus predispose an offspring to develop food allergies (Jarvinen et al, 2000). Contrary to earlier opinion, infants can be allergic to their own mother's milk. The successful treatment of infant allergy by having the mother avoid cow's milk protein and several other items suggests that food allergy during breast-feeding may be due to multiple foods (de Boissieu, Matarazzo, and Dupont, 1997).

Even diet during pregnancy seems to influence the development of allergy. Pregnant women who consumed peanuts more often than once a week were more likely to have a peanut-allergic child than mothers who consumed peanuts less frequently. In this study, exclusive breast-feeding did not prevent peanut sensitization (Frank et al, 1999). Dietary modification before week 22 of the pregnancy and throughout lactation has been recommended to prevent allergies in the infant born to a family with a history of allergies (Hampton, 1999). In Britain, women with personal or family histories of allergies may be advised to avoid peanuts while pregnant or breast-feeding to prevent sensitization of the fetus and infant (Food Standards Agency, 2004).

Sensitization to peanut protein may also occur in children through the application of peanut oil to inflamed skin (Lack et al, 2003). Allergies to cow's milk, egg, and soy frequently abate, whereas allergies to peanuts, nuts, and fish typically persist into adulthood, but exceptions are possible (Zeiger, 2000).

NEGATIVE ASSOCIATION WITH OBESITY

A study of 32,200 Scottish children, aged 39 to 42 months, found significantly less obesity in breast-fed children, after adjustment for socioeconomic status, birth weight, and sex (Armstrong and Reilly, 2002). In a review of 11 studies that examined prevalence of overweight in children older than 3 years of age and that had a sample size of at least 100 per feeding group, 8 studies showed a lower risk of overweight in children who had been breast-fed, after controlling for potential confounders. Suggested mechanisms include learned self-regulation of energy intake, metabolic programming in early life, and residual confounding by parental attributes; however, the authors concluded that if the association is causal, the effect of breast-feeding is probably small compared to other factors that influence child obesity, such as parental overweight (Dewey, 2003). Further evidence for the impact of circumstances other than breast milk itself is suggested in the protective effect of breast-feeding on non-Hispanic white children but not on black or Hispanic children (Grummer-Strawn and Mei, 2004), suggesting that breast-feeding may not be as effective as changing dietary habits and physical activities in preventing childhood obesity (Hediger et al, 2001). Long-term effect is unproved. In the 1958 British birth cohort of 12,857 children at age 7, breast-feeding and BMI were unrelated in childhood, and the association was not significant in adults after adjustment for confounding factors (Parsons, Power, and Manor, 2003).

Specific Genetic Abnormalities and Breast-Feeding

The infant's lack of an enzyme to metabolize galactose is an absolute contraindication to breast-feeding. This condition of **galactosemia** is inherited as an autosomal recessive trait and occurs once in every 40,000 to 50,000 live births. The infant is fed a substitute formula containing no lactose or galactose.

The mother of an infant with phenylketonuria (Clinical Application 5–3) often chooses to feed the child only the special formula. Breast-feeding the baby requires both limited amounts of breast milk and the special formula. To determine the amount of breast milk the child may consume to keep its blood levels within the therapeutic limits requires constant monitoring and consultations, but it has been done successfully. Every state has at least one medical center for treating metabolic defects. The maternal and child health division of the state health department can assist with locating such a facility.

The Formula-Fed Infant

As good as it is, exclusive breast-feeding is not possible for all mothers and infants. Infant formula is the only food that is regulated by its own law, the Infant Formula Act of 1980, which sets minimum levels of 29 nutrients and maximal levels of 9 nutrients (Formula feeding, 2004). Commercial formulas for full-term infants must contain 20 kilocalories per ounce. The formula osmolality may be no more than 400 milliosmoles per kilogram. Commercial formulas are designed to imitate human breast milk but differ from it in protein, fat, and mineral content.

Formulas contain more protein than breast milk. The cow's milk proteins do not contain the optimal amino acids for human infants, so enough protein is included in the formula to provide a sufficient distribution of amino acids. Because the saturated fats of cow's milk are poorly digested by the infant, the saturated fats in formulas are replaced by vegetable oils.

Formulas are treated to lower the sodium content of cow's milk, but most formulas nonetheless contain more sodium than breast milk, which has 7 milliequivalents per liter. The American Academy of Pediatrics strongly advocates iron-fortified formulas and recommended that the manufacture of infant formulas containing less than 4 milligrams of iron per liter be discontinued (1999). As of 2004,

Soy Protein Formulas

The isolated soy protein formulas being marketed today are all free of cow's milk protein and lactose and are iron-fortified. Prospective studies of high-risk infants suggest that soy protein-based formula is no better than cow's milk formula in preventing allergies. Nor have controlled trials shown soy protein-based formulas to be better than cow's milk formulas for treating colic. A side-effect of the manufacturing process is an aluminum content of 600 to 1300 ng/mL, compared with the 4 to 65 ng/mL of human milk. Aluminum, for which no function is known in humans, may contribute to the reduced skeletal mineralization seen in preterm infants.

The American Academy of Pediatrics recommends the following appropriate uses for soy protein-based formulas:

- For term infants whose nutritional needs are not being met from breast milk or cow's milk formulas
- For infants with galactosemia and hereditary lactase deficiency
- For term infants for whom the parents desire a vegetarian diet
- For documented cases of lactose intolerance following acute gastroenteritis
- For infants with documented IgE-mediated allergy to cow's milk protein

In contrast, the Academy *does not* recommend soy protein-based formula under the following circumstances:

- For routine treatment of colic
- For healthy or high-risk infants to prevent atopic disease
- For infants with documented cow's milk protein-induced enteropathy or enterocolitis, because such infants are often sensitive to soy protein
- For preterm infants weighing <1800 grams (4 lbs)

SOURCE: Summarized from American Academy of Pediatrics, 1998b, and Formula feeding, 2004.

---

only one product without added iron was available in the United States and one such preterm formula was available in the United Kingdom (International Association, 2004).

Formula Preparations

Commercial formulas come in three forms: powder (to mix with water), liquid concentrate, and ready-to-feed. Less waste occurs with the powdered formula, but the powder is unsterile and in some cases unsafe for premature infants (Clinical Application 12–5). A smaller amount can be mixed for the young term infant who is exposed to many microorganisms from many sources and at lower risk of infection than the premature infant. Opened cans of liquid formula may be stored covered in the refrigerator but must be used within 48 hours. Prepared bottles of formula should be discarded once they have been out of the refrigerator for 1 hour or have been offered to the infant.

The American Academy of Pediatrics (Formula feeding, 2004) recommends boiling **potable water** for 1 minute and

cooling it before mixing with infant formula preparations. (See Clinical Application 8–5 if lead pipes are a concern.) Unless bottled water is labeled "sterile," it should also be boiled. Sterilization of all equipment and water used in preparing infant formula is commonly recommended until a health professional decides it is unnecessary. To sterilize equipment, bottles, and nipples, they should be washed thoroughly in hot soapy water, rinsed well, covered with water in a pot and boiled for 5 minutes. Separate utensils should be kept for formula preparation. Parents should be cautioned that equipment cannot be adequately sanitized in a microwave oven. Extreme caution is required if a microwave oven is used for infant foods, because heat may be unevenly distributed and continues to build up in the food even after it is removed from the oven.

The importance of feeding the correct-strength formula must be impressed upon the parents. Following the directions of the manufacturer for the product at hand is essential. Either too concentrated or too dilute a formula can cause severe electrolyte imbalances. Some cases have been fatal.

Feeding Techniques

Contrary to the rigid feeding practices of some years ago, the current practice is to feed the infant when it is hungry. Most of the time the infant evolves a schedule whereby it demands a feeding approximately every 4 hours. By the age of 2 to 3 months, the baby probably will have eliminated one feeding so the schedule is five times a day. By 6 months, most infants are feeding four times a day.

The baby is positioned in the crook of the arm, almost as if breast-feeding. The parent's or caregiver's touch is important to the infant's development. The nipple hole should be large enough for milk to drip out on its own without the parent shaking the bottle. The bottle should be tipped so that the nipple is kept full of milk at all times to prevent the infant from swallowing air while feeding. "Propping" an infant with a bottle is never acceptable, because choking is a real hazard and the infant needs to be held to develop a closeness with the parent or caregiver.

The daily formula intake for an infant should be 1.5 to 2 ounces per pound of body weight. At this rate, a 7-pound baby would take 10.5 to 14 ounces a day. An infant of this size would be feeding six times a day, so it would take 1.75 to 2.3 ounces per feeding. A 14-pound baby would be taking 21 to 28 ounces in four feedings of 5.25 to 7 ounces. A single feeding should never exceed 8 ounces.

Ongoing observation of the infant's urinary output is used to confirm the adequacy of intake. The infant's urine should be light yellow and voided several times per day. Major changes in output merit medical attention.

Special Formulas

Manufacturers have devised formulas for special needs. Infants who are allergic to cow's milk, those with galactosemia or lactose intolerance, and those with fat-absorption problems all need special formulas. See Clinical Application 12–4 for a brief description of such formulas, which are often soy-based. Unfortunately, soy proteins may also cause allergies in as many as 10 percent of infants allergic to cow's milk, compared with 2 percent in those given extensively hydrolyzed formula (Klemola et al, 2002).

In the latter, whole proteins are broken into smaller components that may not stimulate an allergic response. Hydrolyzed formulas seem to be nutritionally adequate, and infants generally gain weight until they refuse the formula because of its bad taste, but none of the hydrolyzed formulas are nonallergenic (Cantani and Micera, 2000). Goat's milk is not an acceptable option for an infant allergic to cow's milk. Bellioni-Businco et al (1999) recommended a warning to that effect be placed on goat's milk formulas.

The full-term infant's digestive, nervous, and urinary systems are immature—even a greater issue for premature infants. Clinical Application 12–5 summarizes some of the nutritional problems and appropriate interventions used for premature infants. Box 12–2 categorizes commonly available infant formulas.

Clinical Application 12–5

Premature Infants

Premature infants are born before 37 weeks' gestation. A low-birth-weight (LBW) infant weighs less than 2500 g (5.5 lb) at birth, a very low-birth-weight (VLBW) infant less than 1500 g (3.3 lb), and an extremely low-birth-weight (ELBW) infant less than 1000 g (2.2 lb). An infant can be both premature and LBW or VLBW.

Not all premature infants weigh less than 2500 g. Nor are all LBW infants premature, but birth weight is the most powerful single predictor of an infant's future health status. Infants weighing less than 2500 grams are 20 times more likely to die before their first birthdays than normal-weight infants, and the mortality rates rise dramatically for VLBW and ELBW infants (Centers for Disease Control, 2002b).

Physiology Compared with full-term infants, premature infants have an even larger proportion of their bodies as water. The antidiuretic hormone and aldosterone mechanisms develop in the last weeks of gestation so VLBW infants have virtually no response to these hormones designed to conserve water (Yaseen, 1996). They have less protein and fat than babies born at term. Because the fetus accumulates about 80 percent of its calcium, phosphorus, and magnesium during the third trimester, premature infants' bones are poorly calcified and their muscles are poorly developed. There is almost no glycogen. The liver is immature in enzyme systems and in iron stores. The infant's ability to coordinate sucking, swallowing, and breathing is not developed prior to the 32nd or 34th week of gestation. As a result, premature infants often require tube feeding enterally or intravenously. Enteral tube feeding will conserve energy even in an infant who is able to suck but esophageal peristalsis is absent and the esophageal sphincter is weak, leading to increased danger of aspiration. Total parenteral nutrition for premature and sick newborn infants has great potential for dosage errors. A computerized order entry system reduced the number of potential calculation, osmolality, and knowledge errors by the providers (Lehmann, Connor, and Cox, 2004).

Macronutrients Fat digestion is limited by decreased activity of pancreatic lipase but the lipase in human milk compensates for this lack. Protein digestion and absorption functions are relatively intact. Intravenous amino acids should be given to VLBW infants within 24 hours of birth to preserve body protein stores (Nutritional needs, 2004). Carbohydrate absorption also is intact, but digestion is limited by decreased pancreatic and salivary amylase activity and delayed development of lactase. The proportion of carbohydrate and fat in the feedings is of particular concern in premature infants with immature lungs. Carbohydrate metabolism produces more carbon dioxide than fat metabolism does. Consequently, the carbon dioxide load may tax the infant's lung capacity and constant monitoring and adjusting of intake may be necessary.

Special formulas for premature infants are designed to provide for the infant's growth needs despite the immature digestive system. Glucose polymers, permitting a high energy, isotonic formula, and medium-chain triglycerides are used to construct a formula that will minimally strain the infant's digestive capabilities. The premature infant has high energy needs. A small study showed preterm infants to have lower energy expenditure when they are fed breast milk than when they are fed preterm infant formula (Lubetzky, 2003). If given 105 to 130 kcal/kg of body weight enterally, the infant will grow satisfactorily (Nutritional needs, 2004). Special growth grids for premature infants to 38-month gestational age are available (Appendix K-1, 2004). Premature infants should have their chronological age corrected by gestational age until age 18 months for head circumference, 24 months for weight, and 40 months for length (Failure to thrive, 2004).

Micronutrients Vitamin supplements are needed because the infant's intake is so small. Maximal transfer of vitamin E across the placenta occurs during the third trimester. Vitamin E supplementation reduced the risk of intracranial hemorrhage in preterm infants and reduced the risk of severe retinopathy and blindness in VLBW infants but increased the risk of sepsis in both. Consequently routine use of intravenous vitamin E at high doses is not advised (Brion, Bell, and Raghuveer, 2003). Preterm infants have low vitamin A status at birth and this has been associated with increased risk of developing chronic lung disease because Vitamin A is necessary for normal lung growth and the ongoing integrity of respiratory tract epithelial cells. Supplementing VLBW infants with vitamin A is associated with modest reductions in deaths or oxygen requirement at one month of age (Darlow and Graham, 2002) and has reduced bronchopulmonary dysplasia in ELBW infants without increasing mortality or neurodevelopmental impairment at 18 to 22 months (Ambalavanan et al, 2005). Because of its sensitivity to light, riboflavin has been depleted to deficiency by phototherapy for hyperbilirubinemia of newborns (Bohles, 1997). Premature infants are given higher doses of supplemental vitamins than are term infants because of their high protein intake and low vitamin reserves. They are also supplemented with vitamins not contained in the standard infant multivitamin supplements (Nutritional needs, 2004).

(Continued on the following page)

Premature infants may need to have their diets supplemented with the minerals calcium, phosphorus, and sodium. Rickets of prematurity can occur in the second postnatal month due not to the lack of vitamin D but to the lack of calcium and phosphorus. Sodium needs will increase as the infant grows. Monitoring serum and urine sodium levels will alert the physician to the infant's changing needs.

Breast Milk Human milk from the infant's mother is the feeding of choice. Compared to term mothers' milk, preterm milk has more protein, sodium, and host defense factors but less calcium, phosphorus, and magnesium. To better meet the premature infant's needs, human milk fortifiers have been developed. The fortifier adds protein, carbohydrate, vitamins, and minerals to the breast milk, and the mother's antibodies are still available to the baby. See Figure 12–1.

When infants are fed by stomach tube, the milk remaining in the stomach from the previous feeding is drawn out and measured. This is called a *gastric residual*. Depending upon the amount of the gastric residual, the scheduled feeding may be withheld to allow the stomach to empty, however there is little evidence to support the predictive value of gastric residual (Noerr, 2003). Nevertheless, in a study of 108 infants fed either fortified human milk or preterm formula, those receiving the human milk had fewer gastric residuals for which feedings were withheld, fewer major complications, and were discharged approximately 2 weeks earlier that those fed the preterm formula (Schanler, Shulman, and Lau, 1999). Administering the feeding over two to 25 minutes is recommended. Compared to continuous feeding, intermittently fed premature infants showed more growth and had less feeding intolerance (Nutritional needs, 2004).

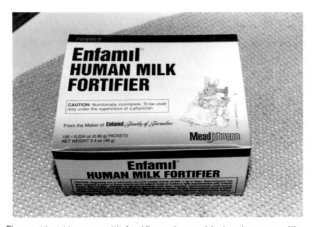

Figure **12–1** Human milk fortifier, when added to human milk, increases the amount of protein, carbohydrates, and selected vitamins and minerals available to meet the needs of rapidly growing low-birth-weight infants.

Formula Feeding Special formulas are available for preterm infants who cannot be fed human milk for many valid reasons. It is important to use ready-to-feed preparations rather than unsterile powders requiring reconstitution for these vulnerable infants. Meningitis caused by *Enterobacter sakazakii* resulted in the death of a VLBW infant and prompted a recall of formula powder (Centers for Disease Control, 2002a). Safe handling demands that prepared formula should not be at room temperature for more than four hours.

The placenta selectively and substantially extracts arachidonic acid (AA) and docosahexaenoic acid (DHA) from the mother and enriches the fetal circulation (Crawford, 2000). Infants born before term do not have the advantage of this selective delivery of AA and DHA for their use during the brain growth spurt. Preterm infants supplemented with AA and DHA showed better visual acuity and mental development than infants not receiving the supplements (O'Connor, 2001). Formulas with long-chain polyunsaturated fatty acids added in amounts similar to those in human milk have recently become available in the United States (Carver, 2003). Enfamil Lipil is one example. The addition of DHA to preterm formula remains controversial (Callen and Pinelli, 2005) because no long-term (24 month) benefits were demonstrated for healthy preterm infants receiving formula supplemented with long-chain PUFA (Simmer and Patole, 2004).

Necrotizing Enterocolitis The most serious gastrointestinal disorder of neonates is necrotizing enterocolitis (NEC), an acquired injury to the bowel that occurs in 7 percent of VLBW infants (Noerr, 2003). The cause of NEC is unknown, but its contributing factors include intestinal ischemia, small bowel bacterial colonization, formula feeding, and immunologic immaturity (Amin, et al, 2002). Levels of glutamine and arginine, amino acids necessary for gastrointestinal muscle cells, have been shown to be decreased ten days before the onset of symptoms (Noerr, 2003). In a study of arginine supplementation, 6.7 percent of infants weighing 1250 grams or less at birth developed NEC, compared to 27.3 percent of infants receiving placebo (Amin, et al, 2002). Encouraging breast milk feeding of premature infants for its immunologic properties is a practice currently available to decrease the incidence of NEC, however major reductions could be achieved by limiting preterm births (Noerr, 2003).

Feeding Techniques When the infant has matured to 32 to 34 weeks of gestation, he may be ready to begin to feed with a nipple, but nursing skill and care are needed as he learns to coordinate breathing and swallowing. Correctly interpreting the infant's cues is important to success. He also may be discharged home before mastering the feeding technique so that teaching the family is a vital nursing responsibility (Thoyre, 2003) and he still needs nutritional care. A preterm infants' discharge formula used until infants were nine months of age produced greater length, weight, and bone mineral content than a term infants' formula did (Nutritional needs, 2004).

Box 12–2 Infant Formulas for Special Purposes

The list below categorizes infant formulas for special purposes and gives the manufacturers and kilocalories per ounce of the formula.

Preterm Formulas for Use in Hospitals

- Similar Special Care with Iron (Ross Lab), 24 kcal/oz
- Enfamil Premature 24 with Iron (Mead Johnson), 24 kcal/oz

Preterm Formulas for Use After Discharge

- NeoSure (Ross Lab), 22 kcal/oz
- Enfamil 22 (Mead Johnson), 22 kcal/oz

Standard Cow's Milk-Based Formulas, all 20 kcal/oz

- Enfamil (Mead Johnson)
- Gerber (Gerber)
- Lactofree (Mead Johnson)
- Similac Lactose free (Ross)
- Similac Improved (Ross)
- Similac PM60/40 (Ross)

Soy Formulas, all 20 kcal/oz

- Isomil (Ross); Isomil DF & SF available
- Prosobee (Mead Johnson)

Specialized Pediatric Nutrition Products With Either Free Amino Acids or L-Amino Acids

- L-Emental (Nutrition Medical), 24 kcal/oz
- Elecare (Ross), 30 kcal/oz

- Neocate one + powder (SHS International), 30 kcal/oz
- Vivonex (Novartis), 24 kcal/oz

Formulas Consisting of Amino Acids and Small Peptides for Fat Malabsorption and Protein Allergies (Very Expensive and Used Only When Truly Needed)

- Pregestimil (Mead Johnson), 20 kcal/oz
- Nutramigen Lipil (Mead Johnson), 20 kcal/oz
- Similac Alimentum (Ross), 20 kcal/oz

Nutrient-Dense for the Older Child

- Nutren Junior with Fiber (Nestle Clinical Nutrition), 30 kcal/oz
- PediaSure (Ross), 30 kcal/oz
- PediaSure with fiber (Ross), 30 kcal/oz
- Resource Just for Kids (Novartis), 30 kcal/oz

INFANT'S WEIGHT	EXPECTED TOTAL DAILY INTAKE IN OUNCES	
Pounds	If 20 cal/oz	If 24 cal/oz
4.5	12	10
6	16	14
8	22	18
10	27	23
12	32	28

Hazards of Formula Feeding

On a few occasions, improperly manufactured formulas have been responsible for vitamin and mineral deficiencies in infants. This is an unacceptable, but fortunately rare, occurrence. A more common hazard, and one an individual nurse can monitor, is the improper preparation and use of formulas by the parent. Formulas can be (1) the wrong dilution, (2) prepared with contaminated water, equipment, or hands, or (3) kept at feeding temperature too long. Body temperature is "just right" for bacteria to multiply, whether in the body or in a formula bottle.

Choice of Breast or Bottle

In the United States, infants can be well nourished whether breast- or bottle-fed. To raise a child successfully takes more than simply supplying the correct ratio of nutrients. The mother's informed decision should be supported and appropriate teaching provided.

An estimated 5 percent of women may be unable to produce a full milk supply because of anatomic or medical reasons. Secondarily, because infants' sucking stimulates milk production, difficulty with the process may result in diminished milk supply. Tragically, infants have died from malnutrition and hypernatremic dehydration due to breastfeeding failures. Infants should be observed while suckling at 2 to 4 days of age by a knowledgeable health-care provider who also monitors the baby's weight. All parents should be taught to expect the infant to have at least four good-sized bowel movements and six saturated diapers per day. Most important, commitment to the benefits of breast-feeding should not deter the provision of adequate nutrition from infant formulas when medically indicated (Neifert, 2001).

Semisolid Foods

No proof exists of the folk wisdom that the early feeding of solid food to infants promotes their sleeping through the night. At 3 months, 75 percent of infants sleep all night, regardless of diet. If solid foods are introduced too early, the infant may develop allergies because of the permeability of the intestine. Additionally, solid foods, especially high-protein items, add to the renal solute load (Wharton, 1997). The American Academy of Pediatrics supports exclusive breast-feeding (nothing but breast milk and vitamins, minerals, and medications) for 6 months while recognizing that infants are often developmentally ready for complementary foods between 4 and 6 months of age (Complementary feeding, 2004).

The infant should achieve voluntary control of swallowing at about 3 to 4 months. Before being offered solid food, the infant should be able to control his or her head and trunk. With this ability, the baby can turn away when

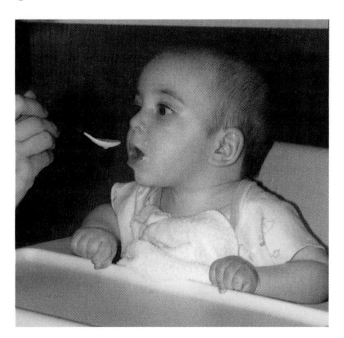

Figure **12–2** This 5-month-old baby is experiencing semisolid food for the first time. His readiness is clear. Notice how eager he is, how focused on the spoon.

satisfied. By this time, the infant has doubled its birth weight, is drinking 8 ounces of formula or a similar estimated amount of breast milk, and yet becomes hungry in less than 4 hours.

In introducing solid food, it is important to follow the infant's lead. To avoid later feeding problems, solid foods should be started when the baby is interested. Babies ready for solid food are hungry and not fussy about tastes (Fig. 12–2). Infants are more likely than children older than 2 years to accept a new food when it is first offered (Chatoor, 2002). Children learn from adults; parents should avoid showing distaste for particular foods.

Waiting too long to introduce solid foods may delay the infant's acquiring the skill to manipulate the tongue appropriately. Some infants who have not started spoon-feeding by 6 months of age show considerable delay in adapting from the milking action of the mouth to the chewing and tongue-rolling action needed to handle solid foods (Wharton, 1997).

How to Feed

New foods should be introduced one at a time and a week apart so that if a problem develops, it can be readily identified. A food should be tried for 3 to 5 days before the infant is permitted to reject it. Only a taste or two is sufficient for the first try. Even if the baby takes the food eagerly, small amounts should be given to keep a sufficient appetite for milk. Although traditional "wisdom" has advocated introducing vegetables before fruits because of humans' inborn preference for sweets, an experiment with formula-fed infants indicated that exposure to a variety of vegetables facilitated the acceptance of the novel food puréed chicken, and daily experience with fruit enhanced the infants' initial acceptance of carrots (Gerrish and Mennella, 2001).

The parent should heat a small amount to serve the infant. Food that has been heated and not consumed should be discarded because of possible contamination with salivary enzymes and bacteria. Food that has been opened but not heated can be stored in the covered jar in the refrigerator if it will be used in 2 to 3 days. A commonly used schedule for introducing new foods appears in Table 12–2. The baby's physician may modify it to meet individual needs, because evidence is lacking regarding benefits of a particular sequence in food introduction. In particular, infants might benefit from early introduction of infant meats containing iron and zinc (Complementary feeding, 2004). Care must be taken to offer only food that the infant can chew and swallow safely (Clinical Application 12–6).

This is a critical time in the infant's life. Eating adult foods is a skill that the babies must learn, but their culture affects the food choices they will be offered. Flavors from the mother's diet during pregnancy are transmitted to amniotic fluid and swallowed by the fetus. Some of the same flavors will later be experienced by infants in breast milk that reflects the foods, spices, and beverages consumed by the mother (Mennella, Jagnow, and Beauchamp, 2001). In this way, very early flavor experiences may provide the foundation for cultural and ethnic preferences in cuisine.

Weaning the Infant

Teaching the infant to use a cup is a gradual process. Often the baby will show an interest in the cup at 4 to 6 months. For these early experiments, and if the infant is not exclu-

---

Table 12–2 **Suggested Progression for Offering Foods to Infant at Low Risk of Allergies**

AGE OF INFANT	FOOD	RATIONALE/PRECAUTIONS
4 months	Infant cereal mixed with formula	Because of risk of allergies, rice offered first; wheat after age 12 months. Read labels: some mixed infant cereals contain wheat.
5 to 6 months	Strained vegetables	Less sweet than fruits; thought less likely to be rejected if offered before fruit.
6 to 7 months	Strained fruits	Will be well accepted; humans have strong preference for sweets.
6 to 8 months	Finger foods (bananas, crackers)	Encourages self-feeding. Different textures may aid speech development.
7 to 8 months	Strained meats	May be introduced earlier to add iron and zinc to the diet. Offer variety. (See Clinical Application 12–6.)
10 months	Strained or mashed egg yolk	Start with 1/2 tsp. Due to possible allergy, delay egg white until 1 year old.
10 months	Bite-sized cooked foods	Select appropriate foods. See Clinical Application 12–6.
12 months	Foods from adult table	Select suitable foods, prepared according to baby's abilities.

Avoiding Choking Accidents

Each year, several hundred infants are asphyxiated by food. This is a hazard for older children as well. On average, one death every 5 days is reported in children from infancy to 9 years of age.

Hot dogs, or frankfurters, are involved most often. Hot dogs, apples, cookies, and biscuits cause choking most often in infants. Peanuts and grapes are the most dangerous for 2-year-old children, while 3-year-olds still face a risk from hot dogs.

Other foods that are often implicated in choking accidents are listed below. Because there are many other foods the child can eat safely, the prudent course is to avoid all of the foods listed. If a choking incident occurs, any caregiver needs to be able to administer cardiopulmonary resuscitation (CPR) should it become necessary. Training in CPR should be sought by all parents or parents-to-be.

Small children should always be supervised while they are eating and they should be seated at a table to eat. Likewise, eating in a moving vehicle is discouraged. Special care is needed if local teething agents are used because of potential numbing of throat muscles (Feeding the child, 2004).

HARD FOODS	STRINGY FOODS	STICKY FOODS	PLUG-SHAPED FOODS
Apples	Beans	Bread	Grapes
Carrots	Celery	Chewing gum	Hot dogs
Cookies		Peanut butter	
Corn			
Hard candy			
Nuts			
Peanuts			
Popcorn			
Raisins			
Raw vegetables			
Seedy items (e.g., watermelon)			

sively breastfed, water can be offered. If the mother decides to wean the child from breast or bottle before its first birthday, the replacement should be infant formula, not unmodified cow's milk. The bottle-fed infant may not be ready to give up the bottle until 12 to 14 months of age. If bedtime bottles have not been used, weaning will proceed more rapidly. It is best to substitute the cup for the bottle for one feeding period at a time. Use the new schedule for 5 days or so, and then substitute the new method for a second feeding. Allowing the infant to set the pace will make the task easier.

Health-care providers face special challenges attempting to teach Western child-care methods to immigrants. Appropriate strategies include learning and respecting the mothers' beliefs, carefully monitoring the infants' progress, and adapting advice to cultural practices.

Nutritional Problems in Infancy

Iron deficiency anemia is the most prevalent nutritional deficiency in children in the United States. Other problems related to nutrition are allergies, cow's milk protein-sensitive enteropathy, colic, and diarrhea. Additional problems of nutrition in infancy are summarized in Table 12–3. The table includes some home remedies, but if an infant does not improve rapidly from a nutrition-related problem, medical attention should be sought.

Iron Deficiency Anemia

Iron deficiency, the lack of adequate iron stores in the body to meet physiological needs for growth, affects 9 percent of children under 2 years of age. Iron deficiency anemia, depletion of iron sufficient to impair red blood cell

Table 12–3 **Nutritional Problems in Infancy**

PROBLEM	INTERVENTION	COMMENTS
Regurgitation of milk	Handle baby gently. Burp well; sit up after feeding.	Very common for first 6 months; not serious unless vomiting is projectile or bile-tinged or baby has persistent respiratory symptoms or poor weight gain.
Hiccoughs	Offer water to drink. Continue regular feedings.	May be caused by swallowed air.
Constipation	1/2 oz prune juice with 1/2 oz water; or 1/2 tsp dark corn syrup per feeding.	Rare in breast-fed infants.
Burns to mouth	Shake formula after heating; test well.	Formula warmed in a microwave oven continues to increase in temperature after removal.
Nursing-bottle syndrome	Do not use milk or juice as bedtime bottle. Do not put sweetener on pacifier.	See Chapter 3.

production, affects 3 percent of children under 2 years of age (Carley, 2003). Longitudinal studies consistently indicate that children anemic in infancy continue to have poorer cognition, poorer school achievement, and more behavior problems into middle childhood, but the possible confounding effects of poor socioeconomic backgrounds preclude imputing causation. Treating anemic children younger than 2 years of age with short-term iron treatment has generally failed to benefit development. It therefore remains uncertain whether the poor development of iron-deficient infants is due to poor social backgrounds or irreversible damage or if it is remediable with iron treatment (Grantham-McGregor and Ani, 2001).

OCCURRENCE AND RISK FACTORS

Children from low-income families and black or Mexican-American children are at higher risk for iron deficiency than children from middle- or high-income families or white children (Centers for Disease Control, 1998). Other risk factors for iron deficiency include premature birth, low birth weight, malnutrition, adolescent parents, single mothers, absent fathers, maternal depression, low parental educational level, and parental psychiatric problems. Often many of these risk factors occur in a single family. Sometimes a child drinks so much milk that he or she does not take in enough iron-rich foods and becomes anemic. The type of milk is significant. In Great Britain, 33 percent of 18-month-old children receiving unmodified cow's milk were anemic, compared with 2 percent of those receiving an iron-supplemented formula (Williams et al, 1999). See Cow's Milk Protein-Sensitive Enteropathy below.

Cultural practices affect even the youngest members of a family. In Spain, preschool children showed better iron status if meat had been included in their diets during their eighth month or earlier compared with those who were given meat later (Requejo et al, 1999). East Indian mothers living in Great Britain did not feed their children beef if they were Hindu, or pork or meats not "halal" if they were Muslim, and often did not replace the nutrients in those items with equivalent foods (Wharton, 1997).

EARLY DIAGNOSIS

To be sure that iron deficiency anemia is diagnosed promptly in infants and toddlers, monitoring of the hemoglobin level is recommended through the infant's second birthday. Normal hemoglobin levels are 14 to 24 grams per 100 milliliters in the newborn and 10 to 15 grams per 100 milliliters in the infant. Tests of early iron deficiency (serum ferritin and iron-binding capacity) are not routinely performed, however, which is one reason that the American Academy of Pediatrics recommends universal use of iron-fortified formula.

PREVENTION AND TREATMENT

Exclusive breast-feeding for 4 to 6 months, without supplementary liquid, formula, or food, is a method of primary prevention of iron deficiency anemia. When exclusive breast-feeding ceases, iron-fortified formula should be given (Centers for Disease Control, 1998).

Treatment of iron deficiency anemia may include medication and ingestion of iron-fortified foods or foods naturally high in iron. Treatment should produce a normal hemoglobin level in 1 to 2 months (Deglin and Vallerand, 2005). Red meats, especially liver, are high in iron. The parent should offer the iron-rich foods at the beginning of the meal, when the infant is hungry. After the baby has eaten the strained or pureed foods, breast milk or formula may be given.

A number of special circumstances make vitamin or mineral supplementation desirable. Some of these situations appear in Table 12–4.

Table 12–4 Vitamin-Mineral Supplementation for Infants

SUPPLEMENT	PRESCRIBED FOR	SITUATION OR RATIONALE
VITAMIN		
D	Breast-fed infants	Beginning during 1st two months of life; continued until consuming 500 mL of fortified milk or formula daily (American Academy of Pediatrics, 2005)
E	Premature infants	See Clinical Application 12–5
K	All infants	Given immediately after birth
C	2-week-old formula-fed infants, if vitamin is not in formula	Synthetic preferable to juices Orange juice, especially, may be allergen
Folic acid	Evaporated milk formula-fed infant	Sterilizing heat destroys folic acid
B_{12} as cobalamin	Breast-fed infant, if mother is strict vegetarian	See Chapter 11
MINERAL		
Calcium	Premature infants	See Clinical Application 12–5
Phosphorus	Premature infants	See Clinical Application 12–5
Iron	Term infant, when birth weight has doubled	Iron-fortified formula is available
	Formula-fed premature, from onset	
	Fortified human milk-fed premature, when full enteral feeding established (Schanler, 1997)	
Fluoride	All >6 months of age	If drinking water contains <0.3 ppm
	Children over 3 years of age	If drinking water contains <0.6 ppm

Allergies

About 6 to 8 million children younger than 4 years old have food allergies that reflect the immaturity of the newborn's immune system (Sampson, 2002). Introducing certain foods too early increases the likelihood that the child will develop allergies. Special caution is needed for infants with a family history of allergies. If a parent or sibling has allergies, the infant's risk of developing allergies doubles (Wharton, 1997), but the specific allergens affecting the individuals in the family may differ (Taylor, Hefle, and Munoz-Furlong, 1999). Both exposure to allergens and a genetic predisposition probably involving multiple genes seem to interact to produce an allergy (Long, 2002).

COMMON FOOD ALLERGENS IN INFANCY

An **allergen** is a substance that provokes an abnormal individual hypersensitivity. Allergies develop, for the most part, when a person is exposed to an allergen, usually a protein, which sensitizes the individual to that item, causing the immune system to produce IgE antibodies. The most common allergenic foods are milk, eggs, peanuts, and wheat. Peanuts and peanut products are particularly hazardous (see Box 12–3). Clinical Application 12–7 summarizes a report on six fatal and seven near-fatal cases of **anaphylaxis** following ingestion of an allergen in which multiple errors of judgment are evident. The seriousness of food allergies should never be underestimated. The Food

Clinical Application 12-7

Anaphylactic Reactions to Food

Allergy to food can be fatal. An analysis of 13 anaphylactic reactions to food identifies points along the critical path that had the potential to alter the outcome. Of 13 cases identified, 6 were fatal. In all cases, the client was known to be asthmatic and to be allergic to some food. None of the clients was aware that the allergen was present in the foods consumed. The items were candy, cookies, and pastry. Symptoms began soon after ingestion but in some cases abated before becoming severe.

Of particular significance is the fact that fewer than half the children had self-injectable epinephrine prescribed, and only one of the six children used a dose. The average delay between ingestion of the allergenic food and receipt of a dose of epinephrine was two and a half times as long in the fatal cases as in the nonfatal cases. Also, more of the fatal cases occurred in public places than in a private home. These and other similarities and differences are tabulated below. Several recommendations came from this study:

- Epinephrine should be prescribed, kept available, and used for clients with IgE-mediated food allergies.
- Children and adolescents who have an allergic reaction to food should be observed for 3 to 4 hours after the reaction at a center capable of dealing with anaphylaxis.
- Parents of such children should be taught to ensure a rapid response by schools and other institutions.

SITUATIONAL FACTOR	FATAL CASES		NEAR-FATAL CASES	
Age of client (average and range)	11.5 years		12.4 years	
	2 to 16 years		9 to 17 years	
Gender	1 male		2 males	
	5 females		5 females	
Known to have asthma	6		7	
Cause of anaphylactic reaction	Peanuts	3	Filberts	2
	Cashews	2	Milk	2
	Eggs	1	Peanuts	1
			Brazil nuts	1
			Walnuts	1
Average number of foods identified as allergenic for each client	1.7		2	
Onset of symptoms	3 to 30 minutes		1 to 5 minutes	
Location	School	4	Home	2
	Fair	1	Relative's home	2
	Home	1	Friend's home	2
			Vacation home	1
Parent present at site	3		4	
Had a prescription for self-injectable epinephrine	3		3	
Used the self-injectable dose	0		1	
Number of minutes after ingestion that any epinephrine was given (average and range)	93.3		36.4	
	15 to 180		10 to 130	

SOURCE: Summarized from Sampson, Mendelson, and Rosen, 1992.

Box 12-3 **Peanut Allergy**

Peanut-induced anaphylaxis is an IgE-mediated condition that is estimated to affect 1.5 million people and cause 50 to 100 deaths per year in the United States (Leung et al, 2003). A registry of more than 5000 individuals allergic to peanuts or tree nuts revealed that the median age of reaction to peanut was 14 months and that for 74 percent of the individuals, that was the first known exposure to peanut. Also, 85 percent of the persons had been breast-fed (Sicherer et al, 2001a). Because allergies require previous exposure and IgE antibodies do not cross the placenta, it appears that the sensitizing dose of peanut was acquired in utero or through breast milk (Sampson, 2002). Peanut protein was demonstrated in the breast milk of almost half of a group of mothers after ingesting 50 grams of dry-roasted peanuts (Vadas et al, 2001).

Most clients with peanut allergies have lifelong clinical sensitivities to peanuts (Lee and Sheffer, 2003; Sampson, 2002), but a small number of clients with milder reactions can become tolerant to peanut (Spergel and Fiedler, 2001). Differences in cooking peanuts may contribute to its allergenicity. Frying or boiling peanuts,

as practiced in China, which has lower rates of peanut allergy than the United States, seems to reduce the allergenicity of peanuts compared with dry roasting, which uses higher temperatures, as practiced in this country (Beyer et al, 2001). Additional support for this theory is the fact that children of Chinese immigrants have similar rates of peanut allergy as native-born U.S. children (Sampson, 2002).

Currently, avoidance of the antigen is paramount and requires diligent label reading and monitoring of food intake. Children with family histories of allergies should not receive peanuts until after the age of 3 years. Infants who are allergic to milk or eggs should avoid peanuts, because one-third of such children develop other food allergies. Children younger than 5 years who are allergic to peanuts should avoid all nuts (Sampson, 2002).

Possible future treatments might include recombinant peanut protein immunotherapy and anti-IgE therapy (Lee and Sheffer, 2003). Work on the latter has been shown to decrease sensitivity to peanut by 18 times, offering potential protection against severe reactions to most accidental ingestions (Leung et al, 2003).

Allergy Network provides educational materials to assist in analyzing labels for ingredients with allergenic potential. It also has a model emergency plan that should be provided in writing to caregivers of at-risk clients (Sampson, 2002). Its Web site can be accessed at http://www.foodallergy.org. Unfortunately, even with preplanning, mistakes occur. One study found that an emergency plan was in place for 33 percent of reactions, but it was implemented only 73 percent of the time. Treatment was delayed due to failure to recognize the reaction, failure to follow the emergency plan, calling parents instead of administering emergency medication, and inability to administer self-injectable epinephrine (Sicherer et al, 2001b).

An area of technology that bears watching is genetically engineered foods. A project designed to improve the nutritional quality of soybeans by introducing a Brazil nut gene was stopped when most volunteers allergic to Brazil nuts reacted to the modified soybean (Seeds of Change, 1999).

The identification of allergies to orange juice inspired an important change in infant feeding. Formerly, infants were given orange juice as the first food to complement evaporated milk formulas. With modern formulas and breast-feeding, an infant receives sufficient vitamin C. Currently, if additional vitamin C is needed, a synthetic product is usually prescribed to avoid the allergens in orange juice.

The British government has advised women with close family members with allergic reactions, asthma, hay fever, or **eczema** to avoid eating peanuts when pregnant or breast-feeding (Food Standards Agency, 2004). Other authors conclude that the development of food allergies in high-risk infants (those with two parents with allergies) can be delayed but not prevented (Taylor, Hefle, and

Munoz-Furlong, 1999). For infants at high risk of allergies, the American Academy of Pediatrics advises:

- Breastfeeding for 1 year or longer
- Eliminating peanuts and tree nuts from the mother's diet
- Considering the elimination of eggs, cow's milk, and fish from the mother's diet (may necessitate a dietary consultation regarding adequacy of intake)
- Delaying the introduction of semisolid foods to the infant until 6 months of age
- Offering dairy products to the infant after the age of 1 year
- Introducing eggs to the infant's diet after the age of 2 years
- Serving peanuts, nuts, and fish only after the age of 3 years (Food sensitivity, 2004)

SIGNS AND SYMPTOMS

Food allergies may produce signs and symptoms in the gastrointestinal tract and other systems. They can cause skin and respiratory problems as well. An infant may have **hives,** eczema, or other rashes; asthma, bronchitis, wheezing; or a runny nose, called allergic rhinitis. Chronic recurring atopic eczema is the main sign of atopic disease in the first years of life (Kalliomaki, 2001).

The signs and symptoms of food allergies may appear as long as 5 days after exposure to the allergen. Thus, if at least 5 days are allowed to elapse between the introduction of each new food, chances are better that any allergens will be readily identified.

Allergens can be transferred by modes other than ingestion. Twenty clients reported allergic reactions following kissing, one life-threatening and four even after the partner had brushed his teeth (Hallett, Haapanen, and Tueber,

2002). Cooking vapors from legumes caused asthma in one report (Garcia-Ortiz et al, 1995). In Spain, weak associations were identified between asthma and unloading of soybeans from ships (Ballester et al, 1999). Inhalation of seafood allergens through occupational exposure or through visiting an open-air fish market prompted experiments to demonstrate fish allergen in the air is measurable (Taylor et al, 2000). Even more striking, a 60-year-old man with no history of nut allergy had an anaphylactic reaction to cashew nut after receiving the liver of a 15-year-old atopic boy who died of anaphylaxis after peanut ingestion, illustrating the transfer of IgE-mediated hypersensitivity through organ transplantation (Phan et al, 2003).

Allergens from dissimilar sources also can evoke an allergic response. Cautions pertaining to cross-sensitivity to latex among persons allergic to various foods appear in Clinical Application 12–8.

TREATMENT OF ALLERGIES

Soy formula has been used to treat children allergic to cow's milk protein, but soy also can cause allergies. Other special formulas contain hydrolyzed protein or amino acids in an attempt to break up the protein into small pieces so that the body does not recognize the antigen. For infants who develop symptoms of food allergy, the American Academy of Pediatrics recommends maternal restriction of cow's milk, egg, fish, peanuts, and tree nuts, or, if that is unsuccessful, extensively hydrolyzed or amino acid formula (Food sensitivity, 2004).

The normal gastrointestinal microorganisms contribute to the gut mucosal defense barrier. A strain of Lactobacillus promotes local antigen-specific immune responses, prevents permeability defects, and confers controlled antigen absorption. Lactobacillus GG given to children hospitalized for reasons other than diarrhea reduced their risk of (hospital-acquired) diarrhea by 80 percent compared with placebo (Szajewska et al, 2001), but another study failed to show an effect (Mastretta et al,

2002). Many infants outgrow food sensitivities by age 1 or 2. It is important not to permanently exclude foods from the diet on the basis of the first year's experience. In small infants, most allergic reactions to food are not IgE-mediated, whereas in older children they probably are (Vanderhoof and Young, 2003). The physician should be reminded of diet limitations so that an appropriate time can be chosen to reintroduce the offending foods. An exception is allergy to peanuts and other nuts, which is rarely outgrown (Box 12–3).

Although anaphylaxis guidelines suggest treatment with epinephrine, teaching about self-injectable epinephrine, and referral to an allergist, chart reviews of 678 clients treated for food allergies in 21 North American emergency departments found that only 16 percent received epinephrine, 16 percent were given prescriptions for self-injectable epinephrine (Epi-pen), and 12 percent were referred to an allergist. Among patients with severe reactions, just 24 percent received epinephrine (Clark et al, 2004). A diagram for the use of the Epi-pen can be found at http://www.foodallergy.org/anaphylaxis.html.

Cow's Milk Protein-Sensitive Enteropathy

Approximately 1 percent of infants incur intestinal injury from cow's milk protein that usually begins in the first year of life and may last 2 years. Initial symptoms are diarrhea, emesis, and irritability. Continued consumption of the causative food worsens the intestinal inflammation, resulting in bloody diarrhea, anemia, dehydration, and failure to thrive. The offending antigen is usually cow's milk protein or soy protein (Lake, 2001). Treatment involves soy or extensively hydrolyzed formula. Exclusive breast-feeding for more than 4 months can postpone the onset of cow's milk protein-sensitive enteropathy (Yimyaem, 2003).

Colic

Although the cause of colic is unknown, the condition is named for the presumed manifestation, spasms of the muscles of the colon. The abdomen is tense and the infant draws its legs up to its belly. He or she may cry for hours, starting late in the afternoon, just when caregivers are also tired and cranky. The classic definition of colic is the rule of threes: crying for more than 3 hours a day, more than 3 days per week, for more than 3 weeks. Infantile colic occurs in 10 to 25 percent of infants and usually improves by 3 to 4 months of age (Duro et al, 2002).

POSSIBLE CAUSES

Suggested causative factors fall into two main groups: gastrointestinal and nongastrointestinal. Food protein hypersensitivity or allergy is the leading candidate in the first group, and parental or maternal-child interaction problems in the second. The various factors act together, leading to disturbances in infant gastrointestinal motility that manifests clinically as colic (Gupta, 2002).

Other physiological causes have been proposed. Abdominal distention may result from swallowing air, because passage of flatus seems to relieve the pain. If the baby is bottle-fed, it may be that the nipple holes are too big or too small, increasing the amount of air swallowed.

| Clinical Application 12–8 |

Latex Alleries and Food Hypersensitivity

Individuals allergic to latex have demonstrated hypersensitivity to foods botanically unrelated to latex but that may share allergenic components. Authors of one study concluded that in most cases, sensitization to latex occurs via pollen or food (Ganglberger et al, 2001). Among the fruits and nuts identified as allergens are avocado, banana, chestnut, fig, kiwi, mango, melon, papaya, passion fruit, peach, peanut, pineapple, and tomato (Brehler et al, 1997; SaraOclar et al, 1998). Anaphylaxis occurred in many of those cases (Blanco et al, 1994; Cinquetti et al, 1995; Llatser, Zambrano, and Guillaumet, 1994). Researchers have identified components common to latex and some of the fruits (Delbourg et al, 1996; Latasa et al, 1995). Latex allergy should be ruled out in individuals allergic to any of those foods before performing clinical procedures using latex gloves.

The breast-fed infant might be swallowing air because of incorrect nursing position.

Carbohydrate metabolism may be immature. Transient lactose intolerance, resulting from inadequate production of the lactase, is one possibility. Studies have shown a reduced crying time when lactase is added to formula or breast milk (Buckley, 2000). A history of colic was associated with laboratory-tested carbohydrate malabsorption from apple juice (Duro et al, 2002).

Breast-fed infants may react to flavors such as garlic and onion in the mother's milk but in general, the consumption of gas-producing foods by the mother should not directly affect the infant. Neither the fiber from which intestinal bacteria produce gas nor the gas enter breast milk. Nonetheless, some infants are bothered by garlic, onions, cabbage, turnips, broccoli, beans, rhubarb, apricots, or prunes (Brown, 2005). If a mother notes an undesirable effect on her infant following ingestion of certain foods, she probably would thereafter avoid those foods.

Parental-child interaction difficulties may play a role in colic. The infant may sense parental anxiety, or the infant cannot give clear cues about its needs to the caregiver (Ellett, 2003). It is easy for either situation to worsen as the frustration grows.

TREATMENT OF COLIC

Holding the baby upright, burping, or giving it some warm water sometimes helps. Diluting the formula or offering cold formula has been successful with some babies. Other interventions reported to soothe colicky infants are swaddling, carrying the infant, rocking, and soft repetitive sounds.

Even though their baby's condition is stressful for them, the parents should try not to be overly concerned. Most infants grow and gain weight despite colic. Infantile colic generally resolves by the time the baby is 4 to 6 months old (American Academy of Pediatrics, 1998b).

Diarrhea

Passage of more than three loose, watery stools a day distinguishes acute diarrhea. Among children in the United States, acute diarrhea accounts for more than 1.5 million outpatient visits, 200,000 hospitalizations, and approximately 300 deaths per year. In developing countries, diarrhea is a common cause of mortality among children younger than 5 years old, with an estimated 2 million deaths annually (Centers for Disease Control, 2003b). Seventy-five percent of an infant's body weight is water, 54 percent of it extracellular. For this reason, an infant is at high risk of rapid dehydration from diarrhea.

CAUSES

Infants are subject to osmotic diarrhea. Overfeeding and food intolerances are common causes of diarrhea. Apple juice may produce diarrhea in infants because of carbohydrate malabsorption (see colic).

The most common cause of infectious **enteritis** in human infants is **rotavirus.** Worldwide, rotavirus is associated with about one-third of the cases of diarrhea requiring hospitalization in children younger than 5 years old

(Heymann, 2004). Severe vomiting may accompany the diarrhea. Children between 6 months and 2 years of age are most susceptible; by age 3, most individuals have antibodies against the virus. The fecal-oral route is its probable mode of transmission, but the virus survives for long periods on hard surfaces, in contaminated water, and on hands. Breast-feeding does not affect infection rates but may reduce the severity of the illness (Heymann, 2004). Protection of infants against rotavirus is associated with the glycoprotein lactadherin in human milk, which binds specifically to rotavirus and inhibits its replication (Newburg et al, 1998).

PATHOPHYSIOLOGY

As a result of diarrhea, the wall of the intestine may become inflamed. The inflammation diminishes the amount of lactase produced, so the infant may exhibit a temporary lactose intolerance. Distension, cramps, and osmotic diarrhea ensue. In diarrhea caused by rotavirus, the virus damages the villous brush border, causing osmotic diarrhea, and also produces an enterotoxin that causes a secretory diarrhea (Centers for Disease Control, 2003b).

TREATMENT

Treatment should begin at home at the onset of the diarrhea. Caregivers should be instructed regarding signs and symptoms of dehydration and other parameters of treatment failure. The usual protocol is:

- Oral rehydration solutions (ORS) should be used for rehydration, which should be accomplished in 3 to 4 hours.
- An age-appropriate, unrestricted diet should be given as soon as dehydration is corrected.
- For breast-fed infants, nursing should be continued.
- For formula-fed infants, diluted formula is not recommended and special formula usually is not necessary.
- Additional ORS should be administered for ongoing losses through diarrhea.
- No unnecessary laboratory tests or medications should be administered (Centers for Disease Control, 2003b).

ORSs (see Chapter 9) are life-saving not only in developing countries but also in North America. Most infants who are vomiting can be rehydrated with oral fluids. They may have to be given 5 mL of ORS every 5 minutes, gradually increasing the amount (Centers for Disease Control, 2003b).

In an emergency room study, oral rehydration therapy (ORT) obtained better results than intravenous therapy on length of stay, staff time, and satisfaction expressed by parents (Atherly-John, Cunningham, and Crain, 2002). Rehydration via a nasogastric tube may be used in an emergency room to rapidly correct dehydration (Centers for Disease Control, 2003b).

Ceralyte, Pedialyte, and Oralyte are available at nearly all drug stores and grocery stores. The Centers for Disease Control (1999b) advises parents to keep two bottles or packages of these products on hand to use when the child develops diarrhea, following the package instructions according to the child's age. Sports drinks are not adequate substitutes for these solutions. Large amounts of fluids containing simple sugars, such as carbonated soft drinks, juice, and gelatin desserts, should be avoided because they might increase osmotic diarrhea. Liquids at room temperature are often better tolerated than warm or cold beverages.

Zinc supplementation has been effective in preventing and treating diarrhea in developing countries. Currently, the Centers for Disease Control does not recommend its use in the United States (2003b).

Assessment of parents' knowledge and sources of information on home care is advised. Often information obtained from Internet web sites is erroneous and out of date. For instance, only 20 percent of traditional medical sources identified by Web searches offered advice congruent with the guidelines by the American Academy of Pediatrics on treatment of diarrhea. The source of the information, even if a major academic medical center, did not guarantee correct advice, and various departments within an institution sometimes offered conflicting recommendations (McClung, Murray, and Heitlinger, 1998). More specifically, original misdiagnosis and later incorrect advice from an emergency room physician, reinforced by information found on an Internet site, caused a 1-year-old infant to continue to suffer from diarrhea for 9 days. Referral by his family physician to a pediatric enterologist and hospitalization under the ORS protocol for 2 days cured his diarrhea (Crocco, Villasis-Keever, and Jadad, 2002). The authors conclude that the best protection for clients is the courage to challenge any advice, regardless of source, when it does not produce the desired results.

WHEN TO CALL THE PHYSICIAN

Parents should be instructed to call the primary healthcare provider regarding an infant's diarrhea under the following conditions:

- Young or small infant (e.g., aged <6 months or weight <8 kg)
- History of premature birth, chronic medical conditions, or concurrent illness
- Fever >38°C (100.4°F) for infants aged <3 months or >39°C (102.2°F) for children aged 3 to 36 months
- Visible blood in stool
- High output, including frequent and substantial volumes of diarrhea
- Persistent vomiting
- Signs of dehydration (e.g., sunken eyes or decreased tears, dry mucous membranes, or decreased urine output)
- Change in mental status (e.g., irritability, apathy, or lethargy)
- Suboptimal response to oral rehydration therapy already administered or inability of the caregiver to administer oral rehydration therapy (Centers for Disease Control, 2003b)

Risk factors for increased mortality from acute diarrhea in the United States are prematurity, young maternal age, black race, and rural residence. Decision to hospitalize an infant should also consider these factors (Centers for Disease Control, 2003b).

Nutrition in Childhood

Childhood covers the growth periods of the toddler (1 to 3 years), the preschool child (3 to 6 years), and the school-age child (6 to 12 years). The child's nutritional needs become more like those of adults after the first birthday. A Food Guide Pyramid from the U.S. Department of Agriculture for 2- to 6-year-old children is illustrated in Figure 12–3. Suggestions for implementing the Food Pyramid for 2- to 6-year old children are described in Table 12–5. A measure of diet quality devised by the U.S. Department of Agriculture, the **Healthy Eating Index (HEI),** is explained in Chapter 2. The data gathered on children and adolescents ages 2 to 18 years in 1999 and 2000 using the HEI are graphed in Figure 12–4.

Nutrition of the Toddler

During the toddler years, growth is slower than during infancy, and although activity increases, the proportional need for kilocalories decreases compared with infancy. So the child's appetite slackens.

Nevertheless, the child has to eat. How and what the family eats will influence the child's habits and tastes for many years. How family members treat one another and the toddler at mealtimes and at other times is more important than the precise amount of food the toddler swallows at each meal. Being forced to eat a distasteful food because "it's good for you" has imprinted permanent avoidance behaviors on some individuals. Conversely, some parents expand their repertory of menu choices to set good examples for their children.

Psychosocial Development

According to Erikson, the psychosocial developmental task of the toddler is to build **autonomy,** or independence. Every 2-year-old knows the word "No." One way parents can assist the toddler to achieve autonomy is to encourage choices from acceptable alternatives (Fig. 12–5). If the parents insist that the child eat certain items or amounts, he or she may learn to use food rejection as a means of gaining attention. Later, more serious eating problems may result from such interactions. The parent can, however, create structure in the child's day by insisting the child remain at the table during mealtime whether or not items are consumed.

Physical Growth and Development

During the toddler years, growth slows. The expected weight gain in the second year may be just 4 to 6 pounds. Height may increase by about 4 inches. By age 2, however, head circumference reaches two-thirds of its adult size.

The toddler is aptly named. One of the skills being acquired during this time is walking upright. As this skill is being perfected, the child's muscles of the back, buttocks, and thighs are enlarging. The bones are becoming more mineralized, and baby fat is disappearing. Along with the gross motor skill of walking, the toddler's fine motor control improves. He or she is able to use eating utensils with more finesse. The spoon is likely to reach the mouth still filled with food. The toddler's mouth is more sensitive than an adult's mouth. Foods are eaten better at lukewarm

**Food Guide Pyramid for Young Children: A Daily
Guide for 2- to 6-Year-Olds**

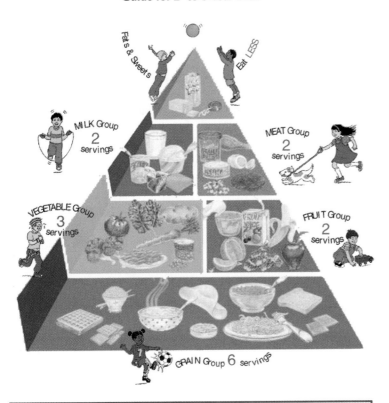

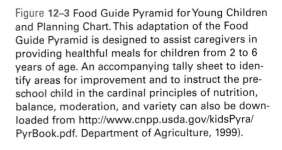

WHAT COUNTS AS ONE SERVING?

GRAIN GROUP
1 slice of bread
$\frac{1}{2}$ cup of cooked rice or pasta
$\frac{1}{2}$ cup of cooked cereal
1 ounce of ready-to-eat cereal

VEGETABLE GROUP
$\frac{1}{2}$ cup of chopped raw
or cooked vegetables
1 cup of raw leafy vegetables

FRUIT GROUP
1 piece of fruit or melon wedge
$\frac{3}{4}$ cup of juice
$\frac{1}{2}$ cup of canned fruit
$\frac{1}{4}$ cup of dried fruit

MILK GROUP
1 cup of milk or yogurt
2 ounces of cheese

MEAT GROUP
2 to 3 ounces of cooked lean
meat, poultry, or fish
$\frac{1}{2}$ cup of cooked dry beans, or
1 egg counts as 1 ounce of lean
meat
2 tablespoons of peanut
butter count as 1 ounce of meat

FATS AND SWEETS
Limit calories from these.

Four- to six-year-olds can eat these serving sizes. Offer 2- to 3-year-olds less, except for milk.
Two-to six-year-olds need a total of 2 servings from the milk group each day.

Figure **12–3** Food Guide Pyramid for Young Children and Planning Chart. This adaptation of the Food Guide Pyramid is designed to assist caregivers in providing healthful meals for children from 2 to 6 years of age. An accompanying tally sheet to identify areas for improvement and to instruct the preschool child in the cardinal principles of nutrition, balance, moderation, and variety can also be downloaded from http://www.cnpp.usda.gov/kidsPyra/ PyrBook.pdf. Department of Agriculture, 1999).

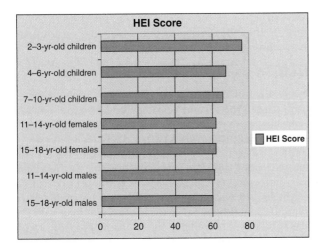

Figure **12–4** This Healthy Eating Index graph illustrates the steady decline in overall mean scores of diet quality from 2- and 3-year-olds to 15- to 18-year-olds. (Constructed from data in Basiotis et al, 2002.)

temperatures rather than hot. Thus, dawdling at the table may have a physiological basis.

Nutrition Fundamentals

The toddler needs all the essential nutrients. The need for many nutrients increases proportionately with body size throughout the growth years. These needs, coupled with the toddler's poorer appetite, stretch the parents' ingenuity and patience. Despite the toddler's poorer appetite, according to the American Academy of Pediatrics, vitamin supplements are probably unnecessary for healthy children older than 1 year (Vitamins, 2004).

FOOD LIKES

Toddlers like finger foods. From a variety of finger foods, the child learns about texture. Toddlers prefer plain foods to most mixtures such as casseroles. Familiar combinations, however, may be relished. Some popular dishes are macaroni and cheese, spaghetti, and pizza. The parent

Table 12–5 **Food Pyramid for 2- to 6-Year-Olds**

FOOD GROUP	NUMBER OF SERVINGS	SERVING SUGGESTIONS
Bread/Cereal	Six or more	Select whole-grain breads and iron-fortified cereals.
Fruit	Two or more	Include 4 oz of orange juice or other food high in vitamin C.
Vegetable	Three or more	Include one vegetable high in vitamin A. Crisp-cooked, warm rather than hot, vegetables preferred.
Meat	Two	Child-size servings of red meat are essential for RBC synthesis.
Milk	Two	Not to be overdone at expense of blood-forming nutrients. Low-fat milks are now permissible.

should serve favorite foods occasionally but not all the time so that new foods are given a fair trial (Cathey and Gaylord, 2004). Neither should the parent, in an effort to entice a child to eat, become a short-order cook, catering to each family member's particular tastes.

MEALTIMES

Toddlers are learning social skills as well as good nutritional habits. Eating is a social experience for adults most of the time; toddlers appreciate company also. Visiting other homes might introduce food items and experiences not encountered at home.

Keeping to a regular schedule will help maintain the child's food intake. A 1-year-old's stomach holds just 1 cup.

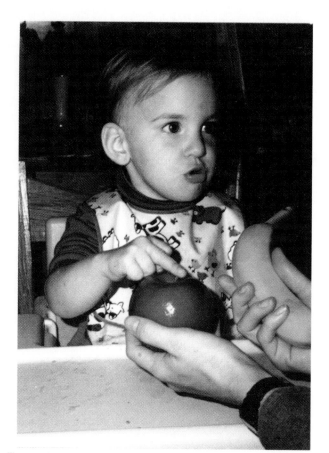

Figure **12–5** Autonomy is achieved in small steps. This 19-month-old girl is choosing her dessert.

Eating regular meals and nutritious snacks helps to prevent fatigue and control the appetite. If high-sugar snacks are used to assuage hunger before a meal, however, the more nutritious foods at the meal may be taken poorly.

NEW FOODS

After the pureed foods of infancy, parents will be pleased to offer more attractive plates of food to the toddler. Brightly colored foods are appealing. Nevertheless, chewing may not be well developed. Tough meat or very fibrous vegetables are not for the toddler.

All of the foods that were not recommended until after the first birthday can be gradually introduced if family history of allergies is not a concern. These include unmodified cow's milk, egg white, wheat, citrus fruits, seafood, chocolate, and nut butters. The careful parent will continue to introduce foods one at a time and watch for reactions.

Eight to 15 exposures to a new food are needed to effect behavior change, but a group of children followed through age 8 were only offered a new food fewer than three times. These same children liked 60.2 percent of 196 foods at age 2 to 3 but only an additional 3.7 percent by age 8. The younger children disliked 11.5 percent of the foods and had never tasted 28 percent compared to 17 and 19 percents when they were 8 years old. These data indicate that food preferences are formed early in life (Skinner et al, 2002).

Because of the toddler's small stomach capacity, small servings are all that can be tolerated. A serving is one-fourth to one-fifth the size of an adult serving. A good rule of thumb is to serve 1 tablespoonful for each year of age. Even very young children make their wishes known through body movements, pushing food away, closing their mouths, and turning away from the feeder. The astute parent will respond to these cues before the child resorts to crying to communicate distress.

Daily intake should include one serving of a vitamin C-rich fruit or vegetable and one serving of a green leafy or yellow vegetable. Difficult as it may be, the parent should limit sugar and encourage consumption of fiber in cereals as well as in other foods. Beginning at age 2, an amount of fiber in grams equal to the child's age + 5 is recommended. Thus, a 2-year-old should consume foods containing 7 grams of fiber with sufficient fluid to permit optimal passage through the intestinal tract. Current dietary guidelines for fiber are based on assumptions and data extrapolated from studies in adults, so research is needed to base recommendations on data collected in appropriate age groups (Edwards and Parrett, 2003). Iron-fortified cereals with at least 5 grams of fiber and no more than 3 grams of fat per serving are the best choices. In addition, cereals made from at least 51 percent whole grain can carry a health claim that in a low-fat diet, the cereals may reduce the risk of heart disease (Separating, 1999).

Offering three meals and three nutritious snacks daily will increase the likelihood that the toddler will obtain sufficient nourishment. The wise parent will avoid hazardous foods (review Clinical Application 12–6). Sometimes chopping the food into very tiny pieces eliminates a choking hazard. Nevertheless, a toddler should not be left alone while eating.

Because the kidneys become mature at about age 1, the toddler can tolerate salt in moderation. The liking for salty foods is an acquired taste. Because of the association between salt and high blood pressure later in life, the prudent parent will discourage the consumption of heavily salted foods.

Problem Areas

Toddlers are still at risk for iron-deficiency anemia. Balancing a diet of a child with a waning appetite can be a challenge.

IRON-DEFICIENCY ANEMIA

The Centers for Disease Control (1998) recommends that milk intake be limited to 24 ounces per day for children aged 1 to 5 years to maintain the appetite for iron-enriched cereals, meats, and iron-rich fruits and vegetables. The term *milk anemia* refers to iron deficiency anemia caused by overconsumption of milk and underconsumption of iron-rich foods. Whether due to excessive milk (or juice) consumption or to lack of iron-rich foods, iron deficiency is found in 7 percent of 1- to 2-year-old children and iron deficiency anemia in an estimated 2 percent (Centers for Disease Control, 2002c). Juice for toddlers should not exceed 4 to 6 ounces per day (Box 12–4).

A more proactive stance regarding prevention of iron deficiency in toddlers is taken by Eden (2003), who recommends routine iron supplementation for 1- to 2-year-old children because of rapid brain growth and vulnerability to psychomotor and mental impairment from iron deficiency.

In a small pilot study involving a poor and minority population, prophylactic daily iron supplementation was estimated to reduce the incidence of iron deficiency anemia by 72 percent. Likewise, studies of transferrin saturation have shown that iron deficiency in most subpopulations of children has decreased to such an extent that screening by hemoglobin concentration no longer efficiently predicts iron deficiency (Centers for Disease Control, 1998).

Vegetarian diets may pose a risk for iron deficiency in toddlers. The position of the American Dietetic Association and Dietitians of Canada is that *well-planned* vegan diets are appropriate for all ages (italics added). Extremely restrictive diets such as fruitarian and raw foods diets, however, have been associated with impaired growth and are not recommended for infants and children (American Dietetic Association, 2003).

INADEQUATE FAT INTAKE

Also, to support brain growth and development, the American Academy of Pediatrics recommends that between ages 2 and 5, the proportion of energy from fat be reduced to 30 percent of a child's intake (Feeding the child, 2004). Therefore, 1- to 2-year-old children should drink whole milk to provide adequate fat for the still-growing brain. Cases of kwashiorkor and rickets have been reported in toddlers given a rice beverage and a soy beverage not formulated for children in place of milk (Carvalho et al, 2001).

The Quality of Toddlers' Diets

In 1999 to 2000, toddlers' HEI scores averaged 75.7, which, although the highest children's score, is still below the level of 80 used to define a good diet. The children's diets were scored above 8.0 in grains, cholesterol, sodium, and variety. None of the components were scored below the 5.1 that signifies a poor diet. The lowest scores were 5.7 for saturated fat and 6.3 for meat (Basiotis et al, 2002).

Nutrition of the Preschool Child

The preschool child requires all the nutrients necessary for other human beings. This is a delightful time of enthusiastic learning, including food preferences. Because food

---

Box 12–4 **Recommendations for Juice Consumption**

For Infants
- No juice before 6 months of age
- No juice from bottles or covered cups that permit consumption throughout the day
- No juice at bedtime
- No unpasteurized juice

For Children and Adolescents
- Ages 1 to 6: Limit juice to 4 to 6 ounces per day
- Ages 7 to 18: Limit juice to 8 to 12 ounces per day

- Encourage consumption of whole fruits
- No unpasteurized juice

Assessment and Interventions
- Determine amount of juice intake for children with overnutrition or undernutrition and those with chronic diarrhea or abdominal symptoms
- Determine the amount and means of juice intake for children with dental caries
- Teach parents the difference between juice and juice drinks

SOURCE: Summarized from American Academy of Pediatrics, 2001.

is consumed every day, opportunities to teach good nutritional practices abound.

Psychosocial Development

Erikson's theory postulates **initiative** as the psychosocial task to be mastered by the preschool child. Within their capabilities, children should be encouraged to set and achieve some goals of their own. Children can participate in planning and preparation of meals. They should be prompted to help in the kitchen, not just with the cleanup. Preschool children love to make fancy cookies and showy relishes. Making even simple things like gelatin desserts gives the child a sense of accomplishment.

By making the meal a social time and eating slowly themselves, parents can encourage the same behavior in the child. Exemplifying good manners will be more productive than criticizing the child's manners. It is helpful for children to have company their own age. Children have been observed to stay at the table longer and to eat more in the company of their peers. Exchanging visits with a friend's child will begin to broaden the child's horizons.

Physical Growth and Development

From the third to the sixth year, a child continues to gain 4 to 5 pounds per year. A gain in height of about 2 inches per year is average so that by age 4, birth length will have doubled. Adequacy of growth should be assessed every 6 to 12 months. Growth charts remain the standard against which a given assessment is judged.

Nutrition Fundamentals

Preschool children are very active. A 3-year-old may need 1300 to 1500 kilocalories per day. But the child may have little appetite. Serving sizes for 4- to 6-year-old children are the same as those for adults.

DEVELOPING GOOD HABITS

The preschool child responds best to regular mealtimes. When the adult meal will be served late, the parents have to decide if it would be better to allow the child to socialize with adults at a late meal or to feed the child early.

Preschoolers, like toddlers, cannot eat enough in only three meals to meet their needs. By age 3, a child is able to verbalize hunger. A good supply of wholesome snacks will serve the conscientious parent well. Such items as cottage cheese, low-fat yogurt, fresh fruit, raw vegetables, milk, fruit juices, graham crackers, or fig bars all are nutrient dense and low in fat. So long as the parent still has control over the child's world, concentrated sweets such as candy and soda pop should be strictly limited.

Tableware appropriate for the preschool child will ease tensions during mealtimes. Unbreakable dishes that are designed for stability, with deep sides to permit scooping the food onto a spoon or fork, are practical choices. Small glasses and cups, also unbreakable, with a squat design and low center of gravity, will serve the child's and the parents' needs well.

It is not too early to emphasize the importance of cleanliness. Regularly washing hands before meals and brushing teeth after meals will cultivate good health habits.

NEW FOODS

Parents should offer new foods one at a time in small amounts. Trying something new is most acceptable at the beginning of the meal when the child is hungriest. A taste or two is sufficient if new foods are offered at regular intervals.

Parents have the advantage over their children of being able to select the food offered. Items the parents dislike will not grace the family table regularly, if at all. Children, too, should be permitted their preferences. This advice is not permissive, just practical. If an argument over food develops into a power struggle, as sometimes happens, the child will not admit to liking the food, even when it turns out to be quite tasty.

Nutritional Problems and Concerns

Preschool children should be monitored for problems such as iron-deficiency anemia and dental caries and general nutritional concerns. Their environment should also be scrutinized, particularly if they spend a significant amount of time in the care of others.

IRON-DEFICIENCY ANEMIA

In 1999 and 2000, 5 percent of 3- to 5-year-old children were iron deficient (Centers for Disease Control, 2002c). Children aged 2 to 5 years of age should be assessed annually for risk factors for iron deficiency anemia: a low-iron diet, limited access to food because of poverty or neglect, or special health-care needs (Centers for Disease Control, 1998).

DENTAL HEALTH

The destruction of tooth enamel by dental caries (Chapter 3) is a problem for all economic groups. The "baby" teeth, as well as the permanent teeth, deserve care and professional attention. In order for teeth to be correctly brushed, the parent may have to do it. Fluorosis (Chapter 8) has occurred as a result of the overuse of supplements and the ingestion of toothpaste. Children younger than 6 years are likely to swallow rather than to expectorate toothpaste. A pea-sized portion of toothpaste is sufficient. Regular dental checkups should be a part of the preschool child's routine.

Adequate dentition supports good nutrition and vice versa. Children with caries had lower median intakes of milk at 2 and 3 years of age and higher median intakes of regular (sugared) soda pop at 2, 3, 4, and 5 years than subjects without caries (Marshall et al, 2003).

CHILD-CARE PROGRAMS

In 1999, 60 percent of the nation's children (13 million preschoolers, including 6 million babies and toddlers) were regularly receiving care from people other than their parents or guardians. The American Dietetic Association

(1999) has addressed the means of meeting children's nutrition and nutrition education needs in a safe, sanitary, supportive environment. Some of the specific recommendations follow.

- If the child is in the program 4 to 7 hours per day, the child-care program should be responsible for meeting one-third of the child's daily nutrition needs; if the child is in the program 8 or more hours per day, it should be responsible for meeting one-half to two-thirds of the child's daily nutrition needs.
- The program should offer food at least every 3 hours but not force it on the child or withhold it when the child fails to consume other food.
- Caregivers should not add extra salt or sugar to food.
- Good institutional food management practices should be implemented, including good hand washing, service with plates and utensils (rather than foam cups and plates, which pose a choking hazard), adequate refrigeration, and proper storage of supplies.

- Nutrition education can include food preparation, identification of colors and shapes, counting, field trips, and keeping parents informed.

Satter emphasizes a division of responsibilities for feeding. Adults are responsible for "what, when, and where" and children for "whether and how much." Explanation of such a feeding policy for child-care facilities and additional information is available at http://www.ellynsatter.com. Some preschool programs specify acceptable foods for parents to provide as snacks for the class.

SPECIAL ASSESSMENT TECHNIQUES

A nutrition screening tool, the PEACH Survey, for use with children up to 6 years old appears as Box 12–5. The questionnaire is completed by the primary caregiver to help identify potential nutrition problems. A score of 4 or more indicates a probable problem that should be assessed further.

Box 12-5 **A Nutrition Screening Tool for Young Children**

The PEACH Survey consists of 17 yes or no questions carrying weights from 1 to 4. It is designed to be self-administered by a child's primary caregiver. The tool was validated on children from birth to age 5 years against a pediatric dietitian's assessment. A score of 4 or more indicates a probable nutrition problem.

PEACH* Survey

Agency: _____ Date: _____
Child's Name: _____ Date of Birth: _____
Address: _____ Phone #: _____

Please circle YES or NO for each question as it applies to your child.

Does your child have a health problem (do not include colds or flu). If yes, what is it?	YES	NO	1
Is your child: Small for age: _____ Too thin? _____ Too heavy? _____ (If you check any of the above, please circle YES)	YES	NO	3
Does your child have feeding problems? If yes, what are they?	YES	NO	3
Is your child's appetite a problem? If yes, describe:	YES	NO	1
Is your child on a special diet? If yes, what type of diet?	YES	NO	2
Does your child take medicine for a health problem? (Do not include vitamins, iron, or fluoride.) Name of medicine(s):	YES	NO	1
Does your child have food allergies? If yes, to what foods?	YES	NO	1
Does your child use a feeding tube or other special feeding method? If yes, explain:	YES	NO	4
Circle YES if your child does not eat any of these foods: Milk _____ Meats _____ Vegetables _____ Fruits _____ (Check all that apply)	YES	NO	1
Circle YES if your child has problems with: Sucking _____ Swallowing _____ Chewing _____ Gagging _____ (Check all that apply)	YES	NO	3
Circle YES if your child has problems with: Loose stools _____ Hard stools _____ Throwing up _____ Spitting up _____ (Check all that apply)	YES	NO	3
Does your child eat clay, paint chips, dirt, or any other things that are not food? If yes, what?	YES	NO	2
Does your child refuse to eat, throw food, or do other things that upset you at mealtime? If yes, explain:	YES	NO	2
For infants **under 12 months** who are bottle-fed: Does your child drink less than 3 (8-ounce) bottles of milk per day?	YES	NO	1
For children **over 12 months:** (Check if applies and circle YES) Is your child not using a cup? _____ Is your child not finger feeding? _____	YES	NO	1
For children **over 18 months:** Does your child still take most liquids from a bottle?	YES	NO	2
Circle YES if your child is not using a spoon.	YES	NO	2

*Parent Eating and Nutrition Assessment for Children with Special Health Needs

Total =

SOURCE: Campbell and Kelsey, 1994.

The Quality of Preschool Children's Diets

As an overall score, 4- to 6-year-old children received a mean of 66.9 on the HEI in 1999 to 2000. Their best scores were 9.1 for cholesterol, which would be rated "good," and 7.8 for sodium and variety. Their worst scores, which all would be categorized as "poor," were 4.9 for fruits and meat and 5.0 for vegetables (Basiotis, 2002).

More than half of all 3-year-olds in the United States (54.4 percent) were given some vitamin and mineral supplement. Among other characteristics, their mothers tended to be non-Hispanic white, older, more educated, married, and insured, whereas children in the opposite demographic groups may actually be at greater risk of nutritional deficiencies (Yu, Kogan, and Gergen, 1997).

Nutrition of the School-Age Child

Few modifications in foodstuffs are necessary to accommodate the school-age child. A balanced diet suitable for healthy adults, emphasizing intake of protein, vitamins, and minerals, will also be good for a school-age child. Overemphasis on limiting foods is not advised. Diets should not be restricted because of the energy, fat, or sugar content of any one food, nor should foods be labeled "good" or "bad." In the first case, food may be regarded as medicine, and in the second, as "forbidden fruit." Neither viewpoint fosters positive attitudes. For instance, the more mothers of 5-year-old girls restricted their food, the more likely the girls were to eat when they were not hungry at ages 7 and 9 (Birch, Fisher, and Davison, 2003).

The total diet is key: does it provide variety, balance, and moderation? Severely curbing intake of meat and milk may result in undersupplying energy, iron, zinc, and calcium. After the age of 5 years, the child's fat intake should amount to no more than 30 percent and no less than 20 percent of energy (American Academy of Pediatrics, 1998a). Some fat is needed to supply essential fatty acids and to aid in absorption of fat-soluble vitamins.

Psychosocial Development

According to Erikson, the developmental task of the school-age child is **industry.** The school years are the years to build competence in many different skills. School work, sports, hobbies, and chores at home permit the child to recognize the worth of work. Making and keeping commitments is part of developing industry.

School-age children can participate in planning menus, shopping for food, preparing the meals, as well as cleaning up afterwards (Fig. 12–6). As with younger children, limiting the child to washing the dishes or taking out the garbage will be more likely to foster a sense of inferiority than habits of industry. In addition, working with the parents or siblings on food preparation and clean-up can foster teamwork and togetherness.

Nutrition education continues in school. Interactions with other children and school experiences expose a child to new foods and different cultures. Approximately 60 percent of school children in the United States participate in school lunch programs. Comprehensive demonstration projects were successful in reducing fat content of lunches from 40 to 30 percent of kilocalories, assisting teachers

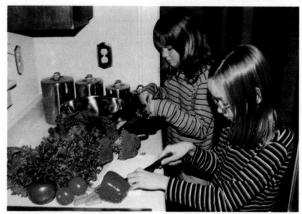

Figure **12–6** A dinner invitation to a friend can involve culinary practice.

with nutrition education projects, and increasing opportunities for the children to be physically active (Harris et al, 1997). Educational messages directed at children should be focused on foods, not nutrients.

Fourth graders whose nutrition curriculum included gardening projects reported significantly greater preference for snow peas and zucchini than students receiving only classroom instruction on nutrition and a control group without nutrition instruction. The gardening group maintained the difference 6 months after the intervention (Morris and Zidenberg-Cherr, 2002).

Growth and Health

By age 6, a child should weigh twice as much as at age 1. Suppose that a 7-pound infant who weighed 21 pounds at 1 year gained 5 pounds in the second year and 4 pounds per year through age 6. At age 6, the child would weigh 42 pounds, or twice the 1-year weight.

By school age, the effects of good or poor nutrition will begin to be apparent. The well-nourished child will display most of the qualities listed in Table 12–6. The poorly nourished child will be lacking in a significant number of these qualities.

Nutrition Fundamentals

School-age children, especially those 8 to 10 years old, generally have good appetites and like almost all foods. Vegetables are the least liked of the food groups.

Breakfast is very important. The child needs energy and other nutrients to last until lunch. Breakfast can improve cognitive function, although not universally found, and is most evident in young and nutritionally vulnerable children (Gibson and Green, 2002). Breakfast should contain one-fourth to one-third of the day's nutrients. The School Breakfast Program, subsidized by the U.S. Department of Agriculture, serves over 6 million children a meal that provides one-fourth to one-third of the children's RDAs for energy and selected nutrients. It is available even in schools without kitchen facilities. Participation is higher in rural areas and among boys, children in the lower grades, African American and Hispanic children, and those in low-income households (Kennedy and Davis, 1998).

Table 12–6	Indications of Good Nutrition in the School-Age Child
General appearance	Alert, energetic
	Normal height and weight
Skin and mucous membranes	Skin smooth, slightly moist; mucous membranes pink, no bleeding
Hair	Shiny, evenly distributed
Scalp	No sores
Eyes	Bright, clear, no fatigue circles
Teeth	Straight, clean, no discoloration or caries
Tongue	Pink, papillae present, no sores
Gastrointestinal system	Good appetite, regular elimination
Musculoskeletal system	Well-developed, firm muscles; erect posture, bones straight without deformities
Neurological system	Good attention span for age; not restless, irritable, or weepy

The school-age child needs adequate protein intake for developing muscle and laying down bone matrix. Calcium is necessary to build dense bones. The body anticipates the adolescent growth spurt; the greatest retention of calcium and phosphorus precedes the rapid growth of adolescence by 2 years or more. Therefore, a liberal intake of milk and milk products before the age of 10 gives a child a great advantage.

Exercise

Exercise can help the school-age child achieve growth and development in several areas. Weight-bearing exercise stimulates the osteoblasts, the bone-building cells. Exercise and activity balance energy intake to achieve weight control. Exercise, especially team sports, fosters interactions with peers. Activities that are likely to become lifetime interests should be especially encouraged. Unlike sports such as football that are played by few adults, skill at tennis or similar sports may provide an outlet for a lifetime.

The Centers for Disease Control (2003d) surveyed children aged 9 to 13 years and their parents, finding that 61.5 percent do not participate in any organized physical activity during their nonschool hours and that 22.6 percent do not engage in any free-time physical activity. Non-Hispanic black and Hispanic children were significantly less likely than non-Hispanic white children to report involvement in organized activities, as were children with parents who had lower incomes and education levels. Regardless of race/ethnicity, age, and sex, the three organized physical activities engaged in most often by the children were baseball/softball, soccer, and basketball. Overall, regardless of age or sex, children reported that their most frequent free-time activities were riding bicycles and playing basketball. In 2002, the CDC started a 5-year effort to promote physical activity through research, media, partnership, and community efforts. Its Web site for children is at http:// www.verbnow.com and for parents at http:// www. verbparents.com

Problem Areas

School-age children are generally so active that they may have trouble sitting still. Requiring them to spend 15 to 20 minutes at the table for meals will increase the likelihood that they will eat a complete meal.

Some children are bothered by caffeine. Eight ounces of hot chocolate or 12 ounces of cola contains 50 milligrams of caffeine. Two such beverages in a 60-pound child are the equivalent of 8 cups of coffee in a 175-pound man. If the child has difficulty sleeping or has an irregular pulse, the first factor to investigate is caffeine intake.

Drinking more than 12 ounces of sweetened drinks daily displaced milk from 6- to 13-year-old children's diets, resulting in lower protein, calcium, magnesium, phosphorus, and vitamin A intakes. Those children gained 2.5 pounds over the 4- to 8-week study compared with the gain of 0.9 pounds by children who drank less than 12 ounces of sweetened drinks daily (Mrdjenovic and Levitsky, 2003).

In contrast, little scientific evidence exists to link sugar consumption to hyperactivity. Twelve double-blind, placebo-controlled studies of sugar challenges failed to provide any evidence that sugar ingestion leads to untoward behavior in children with attention-deficit hyperactivity disorder (ADHD) or in normal children. Likewise, none of the studies testing candy or chocolate found any negative effect of these foods on behavior (Krummel, Seligson, and Guthrie, 1996). Another nutrient associated with ADHD is iron, suggesting that low iron stores contribute to ADHD and that some such children may benefit from iron supplementation. Abnormal serum ferritin levels were found in 84 percent of children with ADHD but in only 18 percent of children without it (Konofal et al, 2004).

Middle-school teachers reported using food as a reward for students; however, the foods selected would not promote the development of healthy eating patterns. Candy was the item most often mentioned, followed by cookies, doughnuts, sweetened drinks, and pizza (Kubik et al, 2002).

Long-lasting effects of malnutrition have been demonstrated in Mauritius, a former British colony in the Indian Ocean. There, malnutrition at age 3 years was associated with poor cognition at age 11 years independent of psychosocial adversity (Liu et al, 2003). Extreme prematurity also has a negative effect on school performance. More than half of extremely low-birth-weight infants (ELBW, 500 to 1000 grams) studied in New Jersey, Ontario, Bavaria, and Holland had required special educational assistance and/or had repeated a grade by ages 8 to 11 (Saigal et al, 2003).

The Quality of School-Age Children's Diets

The mean overall score of 7- to 10-year-old children on the HEI was 66.0. The only areas that would have rated "good" were on the cholesterol component at 8.6 and the grains and variety components at 8.0. The lowest scores tallied were for fruit at 3.9 and vegetables at 5.0, both of which would be categorized as "poor" (Basiotis et al, 2002). The use of nutritional supplements for children was not included in those reports.

Eating dinner with the family was associated with improved diet quality for 9- to 14-year-old children. A survey of 16,202 children revealed that those eating family dinner oftener consumed more fruits and vegetables and less fried food and soda than those who ate dinner with the family less often. More than half of the 9-year-olds dined with the family every day, compared with about one-third of the 14-year-olds (Gillman et al, 2000).

Nutrition in Adolescence

Adolescence is the period that extends from the onset of **puberty** until full growth is reached. For most individuals, adolescence occurs between the ages of 12 and 20. Adolescence is second only to infancy in the nutritional requirements necessary for growth and development.

Psychosocial Development

Achieving their own **identity** is the developmental task Erikson identified for adolescents, including accepting their capabilities. In this process, teenagers "try on" various identities. Peers exert a major influence on a teenager's decisions. Adolescents pick up fads instantly and drop them just as suddenly. Food fads are part of the same pattern.

Knowledge may improve behavior but does not guarantee behavior change. In New Orleans, high school students averaged 39 percent on a test of knowledge about fruits and vegetables prepared by the National Cancer Institute, with white students scoring significantly higher than African American students (Beech et al, 1999).

Targeting knowledge and behavior were goals of an intervention project featuring a media campaign, classroom workshops, school meal modification, and parental support. Students at the intervention high schools showed a significant difference in knowledge scores and demonstrated a significant 14 percent increase in consumption of fruits and vegetables in the first 3 years. At follow-up, however, consumption of fruits and vegetables by students in the high schools used as a control group also increased to the point that the groups were equal (Nicklas et al, 1998), illustrating the difficulty of isolating influences on behavior in free-living people over a long period of time. The students at the control-group high schools no doubt received some of the same messages about healthy diets from other sources than those prepared for students at the intervention schools.

Oftentimes, modifying systems or communities offers the best chance of improving nutritional outcomes. A first step is understanding the client's perspective. A program in California aimed to improve nutrition and physical fitness in 10- to 14-year-old minority youth in low-income communities. Assessment indicated that adolescents in the target communities spent about 40 percent of the family food dollar and prepared about 13 meals per week for themselves or their families without the necessary knowledge or skills to plan, buy, or prepare food. Further, they avoided outdoor exercise for fear of crime, and many of them believed they would not live long enough to reap the benefits of reduced chronic disease should they even try to modify their lifestyles. Consequently, their leisure activ-

Table 12–7 Adolescent Growth Spurts

| | AGE IN YEARS | |
STATUS	BOYS	GIRLS
Begins	12 to 13	10 to 11
Peaks	14	12
Completed	19	15

ities focused on television and eating or meeting their friends at a fast-food restaurant, one of the few clean, brightly lit, safe places in the neighborhood (Hinkle, 1997).

Physical Growth and Development

The term *growth spurt* is accurate. A teenager who may seem not to grow as much as others the same age will suddenly sprout like a weed, seemingly overnight. Boys and girls differ in the timing and completion of the growth spurt. Table 12–7 summarizes the ages of typical adolescent growth spurts. Growth is not completed at ages 15 to 19, only the growth spurt. Growth of the skeleton during adolescence contributes to about 45 percent of the adult skeletal mass (Heald and Gong, 1999).

Nutrient Needs of the Adolescent

Because of their growing and developing bodies, adolescents need more energy, vitamins, minerals, and protein than younger children. To supply those additional nutrients and because one-fourth of the adolescent's kilocalories come from snacks, these "between-meal meals" should be nutritionally dense and chosen to balance the diet.

Energy

The adolescent may require 60 to 80 kilocalories per kilogram of body weight per day, that is, 2700 to 3600 kilocalories for a 100-pound teenager. Boys need more kilocalories than girls. A 15-year-old girl requires 2100 kilocalories, whereas a 15-year-old boy requires 3000 kilocalories. The boy may be in a growth spurt, whereas the girl has probably completed hers. In addition, the gender differences in body composition become apparent. Boys' bodies develop more metabolically active muscle tissue, whereas girls' bodies naturally increase fat stores that use less energy to maintain.

Vitamins and Minerals

At least 25 percent of adolescents reported intakes of vitamins A, B_6, C, and E as well as of calcium and zinc that were below 75 percent of the RDAs regardless of vitamin-mineral supplementation. Only one-third of the adolescents used supplements, and just half of those used them every day. Furthermore, the users of supplements also consumed better diets containing less fat than nonusers (Stang et al, 2000). Of adolescents attending a Boston clinic, 24 percent had deficient serum levels of vitamin D, with the highest prevalence of deficiency in African American teenagers and during the winter (Gordon et al, 2004). To build bone, calcium is needed along with vitamin D. If nearly the entire

RDA for calcium of 1300 milligrams is desired to be obtained from dairy products without considering other foods, four cups of milk or the equivalent would give this assurance.

The adolescent athlete may need up to 6000 kilocalories per day. Thiamin and niacin are related to energy expenditure, and riboflavin is needed for protein utilization; the need for these B-vitamins is increased in the athlete. A training table laden with extra whole-grain bread and milk should meet these vitamin needs.

Emotional or physical stress can increase the utilization of vitamin C by three or four times, so fruits and vegetables are important components of the diet in adolescents undergoing multiple changes in their lives and their bodies. As covered in Chapter 8, zinc is necessary for DNA and protein synthesis, and overt deficiency produces retarded growth and delayed sexual maturation. Before an adolescent eliminates red meat from the diet, he or she should consider the best sources of zinc—shellfish and red meat. On the other hand, vegetarian adolescents were significantly more likely than nonvegetarian adolescents to meet the Healthy People 2010 objectives, reporting the consumption of less fat and more fruits and vegetables than nonvegetarians, but the vegetarians also had lower intakes of vitamin B_{12} (Perry et al, 2002).

Problem Areas

Two common nutritional problems of teenagers are overenthusiastic weight control and poor choices of foods. Overweight and obesity, tremendous problems throughout childhood and adolescence with momentous consequences for health, are detailed in the next section. Adolescents with BMIs greater than 30 should be referred for medical diagnosis and follow-up.

Overenthusiastic Weight Control

Perceptions of body image may not be realistic. Female adolescents, regardless of ethnic background, were more likely to identify themselves as overweight than were males, 33.5 percent versus 22.2 percent. Female students were significantly more likely than male students to be trying to lose weight, 59.7 percent versus 23.1 percent, again, regardless of ethnic background. White and Hispanic female students (62.2 percent and 61.1 percent, respectively) were significantly more likely than black female students (50.7 percent) to be trying to lose weight. The percentage of students nationwide who had taken laxatives or had vomited either to lose weight or to keep from gaining weight during the 30 days preceding the survey was 4.5 percent, 7.5 percent of the females and 2.1 percent of the males, a significant difference (Kann et al, 1998). These undesirable strategies are covered in Chapter 18.

Many dieting teens, however, are not overweight. Self-prescribed weight-reduction diets are common among American women and girls. Of the psychosocial factors investigated in 2536 normal-weight and underweight female adolescents, the strongest contributing factor differentiating dieters from nondieters was low self-esteem (Pesa, 1999). To prevent unhealthy dieting, nutritional education programs should incorporate activities to build self-esteem. Unfortunately, Americans are lured by the "quick fix," promising instant results. Most often the diet consultants who promise quick results do so with an unbalanced diet.

Some adolescents may adopt vegetarianism as a means to control weight and body shape rather than for ecological or spiritual reasons. Regardless of the reason they have become vegetarians, these adolescents need special assessment of their nutritional status and dietary intakes.

Athletes who compete in events in which lower body weight is an advantage may adopt unhealthy dieting practices. Adolescent vegetarians are at greater risk than others for unhealthy and extreme weight-control behaviors. A study in Minnesota showed vegetarian males to be at particularly high risk. Vegetarianism among adolescents may indicate a need for preventive intervention and instruction on a healthy vegetarian diet (Perry et al, 2001). On the positive side, implementation of a minimal weight program for Wisconsin high school wrestlers resulted in significantly fewer weight-cutting practices and bulimic behaviors (Opplinger et al, 1998). The danger of weight cutting though dehydration is included in Chapter 9, and principles of safe weight reduction as well as **bulimia** and **anorexia nervosa** are covered in Chapter 18.

Poor Food Choices

Some fast-food restaurant chains offer salads, light salad dressings, and reduced-fat milks. There are some healthy choices possible. However, the old standbys on the fast-food menus are generally higher in kilocalories, fat, sugar, and sodium than are similar items prepared at home.

The percentage of girls drinking milk falls from 78 percent at age 12 years to 36 percent at age 19 years, with a corresponding increase in consumption of soda from 276 to 423 grams. Those not drinking milk had inadequate intakes of vitamin A, folate, calcium, phosphorus, and magnesium (Bowman, 2002). Carbonated beverage consumption is associated with bone fractures in ninth- and tenth-grade girls. Among physically active girls, cola beverages, in particular, are highly associated with bone fractures (Wyshak, 2000). Mean intake of soft drinks by 14- to 17-year-olds is reported to be 22 ounces per day for boys and 14 ounces for girls. In those same age groups, 73 percent of the boys and 62 percent of the girls consume soft drinks on any given day, with the primary source of soft drinks (48.6 percent) the home (French, Lin, and Guthrie, 2003). The American Academy of Pediatrics (2004) is concerned that sales of soft drinks in schools encourage consumption and contribute to potential health problems: overweight or obesity, osteoporosis and fractures due to lower milk intake, and dental caries.

In the United Kingdom, lack of cooking skills was suggested as contributing to unhealthy eating, and a comprehensive curriculum revision was recommended (Caraher and Lang, 1999). In Georgia, a survey revealed the percentage of adolescents who usually ate a healthy breakfast was related to the family living situation: 43 percent with two parents, 32 percent with a single parent, 24 percent with other family members, and 12 percent with a foster family. Similarly, the consumption of one or more fruits and vegetables per day fell from 75 percent in two-parent homes to 68 percent in single-parent homes, 61 percent when living with other family members, and 44 percent in foster homes (Young and Fors, 2001).

Dermatologists are reexamining the relationship of diet to acne, the nearly universal skin disease afflicting 79 to 95 percent of the adolescent population, which even persists into middle age in 12 percent of women and 3 percent of men (Cordain et al, 2002). Acne is caused by sex hormones stimulating the sebaceous glands. The skin becomes oilier and the ducts to the glands sometimes plug up, permitting the accumulation of harmful bacteria. The possibility has been suggested that hyperinsulinemia initiates an endocrine sequence, affecting sebaceous glands (Thiboutot and Strauss, 2002). In addition to those related to hyperinsulinemia (specifying high-glycemic-load carbohydrates or insulinotropic dairy products), theories linking diet to acne postulate etiologic factors such as *trans*-fatty acids and a high dietary omega-6 to omega 3 fatty acid ratio, but at present all those theories lack empirical data (Cordain, 2003).

The Quality of Adolescents' Diets

The overall HEI scores for 11- to 14-year-olds are 60.8 for males and 61.4 for females. For those 15 to 18 years of age, the scores are 59.9 for males and 61.7 for females. The only component scores above 8.0 were recorded for cholesterol by girls and the younger boys. Mean scores under 5.1 indicating a poor diet were recorded for vegetables and fruits by 11- to 14-year-olds, for fruits and sodium by 15- to 18-year-old males, and for fruits and milk by 15- to 18-year-old females (Basiotis et al, 2002).

The mean HEI scores for meat would not reveal iron deficiency in adolescents consuming poor diets. The estimated prevalence of iron deficiency is 9 percent of 12- to 15-year-old nonpregnant girls and 16 percent of 16- to 19-year-old nonpregnant girls. By comparison, 5 percent of 12- to 15-year-old boys and 2 percent of 16- to 19-year-old males are estimated to be iron deficient. Iron-deficiency sufficient to cause anemia has an estimated prevalence of 2 percent in 12- to 19-year old females (Centers for Disease Control, 2002c).

Overweight Children and Adolescents

A widespread problem is the increasing prevalence of overweight children throughout the world. Box 12–6 provides the U.S. data, including the variations associated with gender and ethnicity. Because of the increased occurrence of overweight and obesity in children, pediatricians are seeing more hypertension, dyslipidemia, and non-insulin-dependent diabetes mellitus in obese children. Diabetes complications (heart disease, stroke, gangrene, blindness, and kidney failure) in ever-younger clients do not bode well for the health of the world (see Chapter 19). Between 1979–1981 and 1997–1999, the percentage of youths aged 6 to 17 years discharged from hospitals with diagnoses of diabetes doubled, of gallbladder disease tripled, and of sleep apnea increased fivefold. Obesity-associated hospital costs (in constant dollars) tripled over those years (Wang and Dietz, 2002). Overweight does not necessarily mean well nourished. The prevalence of iron deficiency in 2- to 16-year-olds increased as BMI increased, so that children at or above the 85th percentile were approximately twice as likely to be iron-deficient as those who were not overweight. The highest prevalences of iron deficiency were 6.2 percent for overweight 2- to 5-year-olds and 9.1 percent for overweight 12- to 16-year-olds (Nead et al, 2004). The estimated risk of obesity persisting into adulthood ranges from 20 percent for a 4-year-old to 80 percent for adolescents (American Academy of Pediatrics, 2003).

Weight control is the subject of Chapter 18, so its implications for children and adolescents will only briefly be considered here. Basically, as was stated in Chapter 6, to maintain a stable weight, energy output must equal energy input. Many factors enter the equation, some of which are enumerated next.

Contributing Factors

Children with one obese parent run a 40 percent risk of obesity, whereas children with two obese parents have double the risk (Nichols and Livingston, 2002). Twin, adoption, and family studies indicate that inheritance can account for 25 to 40 percent of adiposity, but genes contribute susceptibility to fat gain in a particular food environment and do not guarantee obesity; however, parents

---

Box 12–6 **Overweight in Childhood and Adolescence**

Overweight has a significant prevalence in young people as well as in adults. There are no universally accepted definitions of overweight and obesity for youths. Either term is used by researchers to define children and adolescents above the 85th, 90th, or 95th percentiles of a reference group for their age and sex. Thus, comparison of prevalence figures from various sources becomes difficult.

The 85th percentile on weight-for-height standardized growth charts corresponds to 120 percent of ideal body weight, a traditional benchmark for obesity (Nichols and Livingston, 2002), but Morgan et al (2002) use the 85th percentile to define overweight and the 95th to define obesity. Technically, obesity refers to fatness, often measured by skinfold thickness, not weight; however BMI is used as a surrogate measure of obesity because its components, height and weight, are readily available data and the growth charts for comparison are easily obtained (see Appendix D).

also select the food provided in the home (Maffeis, 2000). Predisposition to obesity may involve more than 250 genes (Ebbeling, Pawlak, and Ludwig, 2002). Whether due to their own weight problems or other interfering factors, 66 percent of caregivers failed to recognize their obese children's health risks, but health providers also failed these children, because only 8 percent had received treatment for weight problems and 6 percent had received dietary services (Young-Hyman et al, 2000).

The influence of a sedentary lifestyle cannot be overstated. Low-income, preschool children were 30 percent more likely to have a BMI >85th percentile if they had television sets in their bedrooms (Dennison, Erb, and Jenkins, 2002). Children between the ages of 6 and 11 years spend as much time watching TV as they do attending school, an average of 26 hours per week (McWhorter, Wallmann, and Alpert, 2003). Besides TV entertainment, many children play computer or video games in their leisure time rather than outdoor games. Additional factors may lead to a sedentary lifestyle, such as apartment living, unsafe neighborhoods, lack of time for parents to engage their children in sports, and the cost of recreational activities. Our culture's emphasis on competitive and spectator sports often excludes those students most in need of physical activity. Mastery of skills and self-improvement for all should be emphasized, but in 2003, only 56 percent of high school students were enrolled in a physical education class, 28 percent attended daily, and only 39 percent were physically active *during the class* (Centers for Disease Control, 2004). Prevention of weight gain is key, because once overweight or obese, increasing activity requires more effort and dedication than it does in a normal-weight person.

Ability to regulate intake may be impaired by social and physiological factors. Overcontrolling parents seem to decrease a child's self-regulation of energy intake (American Academy of Pediatrics, 2003). Effective monitoring of one's internal cues of hunger and satiety seems to be extinguished early in life to be replaced by external cues. When portion sizes of macaroni and cheese were varied, 3 1/2-year-olds ate the same amount of energy regardless of portion served, whereas 5-year-olds consumed more energy when served large portions than when given small ones (Rolls, Engell, and Birch, 2000). Parents should not encourage children to eat beyond satiety to avoid leftovers or wasted food. Neither should they promote a "clean your plate" policy (Hoppin, 2004). Not only is it easier and quicker to drink than to eat, but also the body may process the input differently. Over 2 academic years, 57 percent of sixth- and seventh-grade children increased their intake of sugar-sweetened beverages, so that the risk of becoming obese increased by 60 percent for each additional glass of those drinks taken per day. The authors suggest the physiological mechanism involved relates to the body's imprecise and incomplete compensation for energy consumed in liquid form (Ludwig, Peterson, and Gortmaker, 2001).

Selection of food items has a major impact on energy intake. Fruits and vegetables, low-fat items, fewer empty calories, essentially the implementation of MyPyramid, would go a long way in stemming the tide of obesity. More

servings per day of dairy products were associated with lower body fat in 2- to 5-year-old children (Carruth and Skinner, 2001). In a very large survey, 41.7 percent of 2- to 9-year-old children and 50.3 percent of 10- to 19-year-olds consumed fast food on one or both of the survey days. Those eating fast food had higher intakes of energy, fat, saturated fat, sodium, and carbonated soft drinks and lower intakes of vitamins A and C, milk, fruits, and vegetables than those not eating fast food on those days (Paeratakul et al, 2003). Another study showed that adolescents overconsumed fast food regardless of body weight but that lean subjects ate less and later adjusted other intake to compensate for the large meal, whereas the overweight individuals ate more and made no such accommodation (Ebbeling et al, 2004).

Successful Interventions

Adequate evidence suggests that public programs to increase physical activity in children are likely to be helpful in preventing obesity (Hoppin, 2004). Two studies focused on promoting single clear lifestyle changes. A 6-month, 18-lesson classroom curriculum to reduce screen-time for elementary students produced significant reductions in BMIs and anthropometric measures, but there were no differences in high-fat food intake, moderate-to-vigorous activity, or cardiorespiratory fitness (Robinson, 1999). A focused classroom curriculum to decrease consumption of carbonated beverages among 7- to 11-year-olds in England resulted 12 months later in a reduction of 0.2 percent in the number of overweight and obese children in the intervention group but an increase of 7.5 percent of the number of overweight and obese individuals in the control group (James et al, 2004).

To prevent overweight and obesity, the American Academy of Pediatrics (2003) recommends the following:

- Calculate and plot BMIs yearly on all children and adolescents
- Encourage healthy eating
- Routinely promote physical activity
- Limit screen time to 2 hours per day
- Help parents, teachers, coaches, and others to discuss health habits in efforts to control overweight and obesity
- Advocate for social marketing to promote healthful food choices and increased physical activity

The conditions permitting or encouraging overweight among youth have evolved over a period of years and have become embedded in the dominant culture that involves the food industry and marketing. No single change is going to reverse the trend. Multiple interventions and strategies are needed at all levels: individuals, families, schools, communities, and the nation.

Data collected by the Centers for Disease Control Center for Health Statistics in the 1999 to 2000 **NHANES surveys** are shown in Table 12–8. The prevalence is based on measured height and weight and varies markedly by ethnicity, gender, and age. Comparing prevalence data from NHANES surveys, Figure 12–7 illustrates the increasing prevalence of overweight since 1976 in both sexes and in all age groups.

Table 12–8 **Percentages of Overweight Children At or Above the 95th Percentile for Their Age and Sex, NHANES 1999–2000**

ETHNIC GROUP	MALES			FEMALES		
	2–5 YEARS	6–11 YEARS	12–19 YEARS	2–5 YEARS	6–11 YEARS	12–19 YEARS
Non-Hispanic White	8.8	12.0	12.8	11.5	11.6	12.4
Non-Hispanic Black	5.9	17.1	20.7	11.2	22.2	26.6
Mexican American	13.0	27.3	27.5	9.2	19.6	19.4

SOURCE: Adapted from Ogden, 2002.

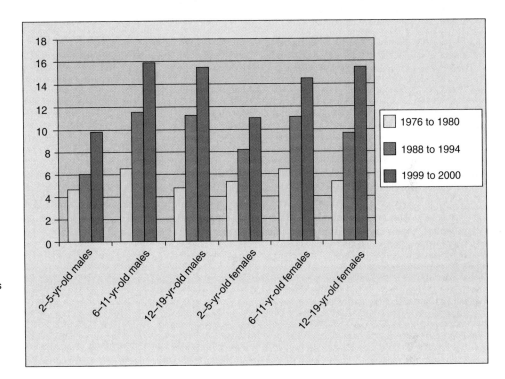

Figure **12–7** From 1976 through 2000, the percentages of males and females at or above the 95th percentile of BMI for age increased steadily in both sexes and in all age groups. (Constructed from data in Ogden, 2002.)

SUMMARY

During periods of rapid growth, the need for nutrients is critical. The lack of nutrients or the excessive intake of certain substances during such periods may cause serious, permanent damage in the individual. Both infancy and adolescence are characterized by rapid growth.

While infants require the same nutrients as adults, they need them in different amounts. Breast milk is especially suited to the human infant, because the protein, fat, and carbohydrate in breast milk are tailored to the infant's digestive capabilities. After the age of 4 to 6 months, semisolid and then solid foods are added to the diet gradually. Nutritional problems in infancy include iron deficiency anemia, allergies, colic, and diarrhea.

Childhood includes the growth periods of the toddler, the preschool child, and the school-age child. Growth

and development during childhood are not as rapid as during infancy. Nevertheless, the total amounts of nutrients recommended continue to increase with age to meet body needs. Toddlers and preschoolers should be assessed for iron deficiency anemia.

During adolescence, the final growth spurt of childhood occurs. Physical growth and development are rapid, and sexual maturity is attained. Energy, protein, vitamins, and minerals are needed in increasing amounts. Adolescent girls often lack enough calcium and iron in their diets. Major problems in adolescents are self-prescribed reduction diets and poor choices of food.

Some experts characterize pediatric obesity as the primary childhood health problem in the United States and the industrialized world, with the potential to spread in developing countries. Wellness Tips 12–1 summarizes healthy practices for the nutrition of infants, children, and adolescents.

(Continued on the following page)

SUMMARY *(Continued)*

 12–1 • Habits and attitudes formed in children and youths may last a lifetime. Healthy practices are worth pursuing and may prevent obesity and its attendant disease risks.

- Eating should be pleasurable, but portions may need to be limited to achieve moderation, balance, and variety.
- For infants, resist proceeding too fast with new foods. Watching the baby's response to new foods may be entertaining, but long-range effects may be less desirable, such as allergies.
- Ensure the toddler's safety by avoiding any food that might cause choking. Provide sufficient iron-rich foods to prevent anemia.

- Preschoolers need frequent healthy snacks to complement the usual three-meals-a-day pattern.
- Drinking milk with meals would improve the nutrition of many children. Carbonated beverages or fruit drinks should not displace milk in a healthy diet.
- School-age and adolescent individuals should have enough exercise to permit them the pleasures of eating a healthy diet without incurring overweight or obesity.
- Adolescents need individualized assessment for eating disorders or inappropriate dieting and obesity, both of which are more prevalent in females than in males. Females, particularly, should consume the recommended servings of milk.
- For most children, increasing their intakes of fruit and milk would greatly improve their nutritional state.

CASE STUDY 12-1

Ms. S is a public health nurse whose assignment includes an inner-city high school. The principal asked for Ms. S's assistance in improving the students' nutritional and fitness states. A committee was formed that included students, teachers (classroom, home economics, and physical education), cafeteria and kitchen staff, parents, a dietitian from a nearby hospital, YMCA staff, neighborhood business owners, and city officials. The following nursing care plan reflects the program they devised after many meetings.

NURSING CARE PLAN

SUBJECTIVE DATA Focus groups with students revealed their opinions of food and physical activity. A school-wide survey solicited suggestions for classroom content, menu items, and physical activities.

OBJECTIVE DATA Analysis of school lunch menus revealed an average fat content of 38 percent of kilocalories. Vending machines in and around school offered only high-fat snacks or those with empty kilocalories. Inspection of building usage identified 2 days after school when the gym was empty but other parts of the building were in use.

NURSING DIAGNOSIS NANDA: Readiness for Enhanced Community Coping (NANDA International, 2003, with permission).

DESIRED OUTCOMES EVALUATION CRITERIA	NURSING ACTIONS/INTERVENTIONS	RATIONALE
NOC: Community Health Status (Moorhead, Johnson, and Maas, 2004, with permission)	NIC: Environmental Management: Community (Dochterman and Bulechek, 2004, with permission)	
Students will have increased opportunities to choose healthful foods in and around school.	Analyze lunch menus periodically to select areas to improve and to note progress.	Prioritizing changes is important to budget resources. Feedback to cafeteria staff will help maintain their interest and effort to improve.
	Include fresh fruit and vegetables on every lunch menu.	Fresh fruits and vegetables can offer vitamins, minerals, and fiber as well as decrease the dominance of high-fat items on the menu.
	Use student tasters to develop low-fat versions of popular dishes.	Palatability is critical in devising dishes the students will eat.
	Diversify contents of vending machines to include dairy products, fruit juices, cereal-and-dried-fruit snacks.	Items must be available to give students the opportunity to choose.
	Collaborate with biology teacher on fruit or vegetable growing as student projects.	Producing food items can stimulate interest in eating their own produce.

DESIRED OUTCOMES EVALUATION CRITERIA	NURSING ACTIONS/INTERVENTIONS	RATIONALE
Students will demonstrate higher goals for their physical fitness.	Evaluate the place of physical education in the curriculum and campaign for needed changes.	To effectively prepare students for life requires offering skill development for an active life.
	Institute fitness testing in physical education classes.	Feedback to students allows them to track their progress.
	Ensure that 75 percent of time in physical education class is active.	Inactivity is a major contributor to overweight. PE class should not add to the problem.
	Institute activities students suggest, such as ethnic dances and games other than major sports in the United States.	Capitalizing on students' interests will recognize the value of their ideas. Later activities might broaden the scope to activities from other cultures.
	Arrange for supervised activities in the gym after school on the days the building would be open for other events. Vary the activities.	If community or volunteer leaders could be recruited, the cost would be minimized for the school and the students. A variety of activities would attract students other than the usual athletes who are active anyway.
Students will increase knowledge of healthful eating practices within time and budgetary constraints.	Design and promote a practical course in skills of modern life for both genders.	Practical courses will attract a different student than strictly academic courses do.
	Devise short instructional units on planning, purchasing, and preparing healthful food for classroom or after-school activity sessions.	Short units would give immediate feedback on the value of the information. Consuming the day's lesson is a bonus.
	Incorporate field trips to grocery stores as appropriate.	Expanding the students' perception of the choices open to them would offer the opportunity to increase variety in their diets.

CTQ CRITICAL THINKING QUESTIONS

1. What additional interventions might be used to improve nutritional intake and increase physical activity in these students?
2. Identify possible barriers to implementing the outlined program. Suggest strategies to overcome them.
3. It is possible that the committee's goals are not compatible with those of many of the students in this high school. How could the students be persuaded to value a more healthful lifestyle?

⟫⟫ CHAPTER REVIEW

1. A nurse in a clinic would identify which of the following infants as needing additional assessment of growth?
   a. Baby girl A, 4 months old, birth weight 7 pounds 6 ounces, present weight 14 pounds 14 ounces
   b. Baby boy B, 2 weeks old, birth weight 6 pounds 10 ounces, present weight 6 pounds 11 ounces
   c. Baby boy C, 6 months old, birth weight 8 pounds 8 ounces, present weight 14 pounds 8 ounces
   d. Baby girl D, 2 months old, birth weight 7 pounds 2 ounces, present weight 9 pounds 10 ounces

2. Which of the following are advantages of breast milk that formula does not provide
   a. Less fat and cholesterol
   b. More antibodies and less risk of allergy
   c. More fluoride and iron
   d. More vitamin C and vitamin D

3. Which of the following foods would be appropriate for a 6-month-old infant?
   a. Cocoa-flavored wheat cereal, orange juice, and strained chicken
   b. Graham crackers, strained prunes, and stewed tomatoes
   c. Infant rice cereal, mashed banana, and strained squash
   d. Mashed potatoes, strained beets, and chopped hard-cooked egg

4. If a family is following the dietary guidelines of the American Academy of Pediatrics, which of the following is it important not to eliminate from the school-age child's diet?
   a. Caffeine
   b. Fat
   c. Salt
   d. Sugar

5. Which of the following individuals is at greatest nutritional risk?
   a. 3-month-old infant being fed commercial formula
   b. 3-year-old child who drinks 3 cups of milk a day
   c. 8-year-old child who eats four chocolate chip cookies and drinks 2 glasses of milk after school
   d. 16-year-old girl who is pregnant and attempting weight loss

✚ CLINICAL ANALYSIS

1. Mrs. T is having her 2-month-old son checked in the well-baby clinic. She tells the nurse that the baby is not sleeping through the night yet. Mrs. T's mother advised her to start the infant on cereal to "fill him up" at bedtime. Despite the nurse's instructions, Mrs. T says she is going to try her mother's idea. Which of the following would be most important if Mrs. T chooses to start the cereal?
   a. Following the cereal with a bedtime bottle to wash it down
   b. Making cream of wheat very thin and feeding the baby with an eyedropper
   c. Putting infant cereal into a bottle and enlarging the nipple hole
   d. Using infant rice cereal mixed with formula

2. Ms. C has given a 24-hour dietary recall for her 18-month-old son. The nurse is alert to identify common causes of choking. To avoid choking accidents, which of the following groups of foods would be considered safest for a toddler?
   a. Apple quarters, green beans, and chicken noodle casserole
   b. Grapes, carrot strips, and macaroni and cheese
   c. Diced peaches, mashed potatoes, and spaghetti
   d. Watermelon chunks, cheese-stuffed celery, and sliced frankfurters

3. Ms. K has delivered a 3-pound 8-ounce premature infant. She had planned to breast-feed. Upon which of the following statements should the nurse base her teaching?
   a. Human breast milk can be specially fortified for premature infants to increase its nutritive value.
   b. Because of their larger proportion of body weight as water, premature infants need supplemental water after every feeding.
   c. Formula feeding is advisable because room temperature feedings are better absorbed than those at body temperature.
   d. Breast-feeding a premature infant offers no advantage to the infant and is difficult for the mother because of the necessary supplements.

REFERENCES

Ambalavanan, N, et al: Vitamin A supplementation for extremely low birth weight infants: outcome at 18 to 22 months. Pediatrics 115:e249, 2005.

American Academy of Pediatrics Committee on Nutrition: Cholesterol in childhood. Pediatrics 101:141, 1998a.

American Academy of Pediatrics Committee on Nutrition: Iron fortification of infant formulas. Pediatrics 104:119, 1999.

American Academy of Pediatrics Committee on Nutrition: Prevention of pediatric overweight and obesity. Pediatrics 112:424, 2003.

American Academy of Pediatrics Committee on Nutrition: Soy protein-based formulas: Recommendations for use in infant feeding. Pediatrics 101:148, 1998b.

American Academy of Pediatrics Committee on Nutrition: The use and misuse of fruit juice in pediatrics. Pediatrics 107:1210, 2001.

American Academy of Pediatrics Committee on Pediatric AIDS: Human milk, breastfeeding, and transmission of human immunodeficiency virus in the United States. Pediatrics 96:977, 1995.

American Academy of Pediatrics Committee on School Health: Soft drinks in schools. Pediatrics 113:152, 2004.

American Academy of Pediatrics Section on Breastfeeding: Breastfeeding and the use of human milk. Pediatrics 115:496, 2005.

American Dietetic Association: Position of the American Dietetic Association and Dietitians of Canada: Vegetarian diets. J Am Diet Assoc 103:748, 2003.

American Dietetic Association: Position of the American Dietetic Association: Nutrition standards for child-care programs. J Am Diet Assoc 99:981, 1999.

Amin, HJ, et al: Arginine supplementation prevents necrotizing enterocolitis in premature infants. J Pediatr 140:425, 2002.

Anderson, JW, Johnstone, BM, and Remley, DT: Breast-feeding and cognitive development: A meta-analysis. Am J Clin Nutr 70:525, 1999.

Appendix K-1. In Kleinman, RE (ed): Pediatric Nutrition Handbook, ed 5. American Academy of Pediatrics, Elk Grove Village, IL, 2004.

Appendix W. In Kleinman, RE (ed): Pediatric Nutrition Handbook, ed 5. American Academy of Pediatrics, Elk Grove Village, IL, 2004.

Armstrong, J, and Reilly, JJ: Breastfeeding and lowering the risk of childhood obesity. Lancet 359:2003, 2002.

Atherly-John, YC, Cunningham, SJ, and Crain, EF: A randomized trial of oral vs intravenous rehydration in a pediatric emergency department. Arch Pediatr Adolesc Med 156:1240, 2002.

Bachrach VR, Schwarz E, and Bachrach LR: Breastfeeding and the risk of hospitalization for respiratory disease in infancy: A meta-analysis. Arch Pediatr Adolesc Med 157:237, 2003.

Ballester, F, et al: Asthma visits to emergency rooms and soybean unloading in the harbors of Valencia and A Coruna, Spain. Am J Epidemiol 149:315, 1999.

Basiotis, PP, et al: The Healthy Eating Index: 1999–2000. U.S. Department of Agriculture, Center for Nutrition Policy and Promotion, Washington, DC, 2002.

Beech, BM, et al: Knowledge, attitudes, and practices related to fruit and vegetable consumption of high school students. J Adolesc Health 24;244, 1999.

Bellioni-Businco, B, et al: Allergenicity of goat's milk in children with cow's milk allergy. J Allergy Clin Immunol 103:1191, 1999.

Beyer, K, et al: Effects of cooking methods on peanut allergenicity. J Allergy Clin Immunol 107:1077, 2001.

Bier, JB, et al: Human milk improves cognitive and motor development of premature infants during infancy. J Hum Lact 18:361, 2002.

Birch, LL, Fisher, JO, and Davison, KK: Learning to overeat: maternal use of restrictive feeding practices promotes girls' eating in the absence of hunger. Am J Clin Nutr 78:215, 2003.

Blanco, C, et al: Latex allergy: Clinical features and cross-reactivity with fruits. Ann Allergy 73:309, 1994.

Boddy, J, Skuse, D, and Andrews, B: The developmental sequelae of nonorganic failure to thrive. J Child Psychol Psychiatry 41:1003, 2000.

Bohles, H: Antioxidative vitamins in prematurely and maturely born infants. Int J Vitam Nutr Res 67:321, 1997.

Bowman, SA: Beverage choices of young females: Changes and impact on nutrient intakes. J Am Diet Assoc 102:1234, 2002.

Breastfeeding. In Kleinman, RE (ed): Pediatric Nutrition Handbook, ed 5. American Academy of Pediatrics, Elk Grove Village, IL, 2004.

Brehler, R, et al: "Latex-fruit syndrome": Frequency of cross-reacting IgE antibodies. Allergy 52:404, 1997.

Brion, LP, Bell, EF, and Raghuveer, TS: Vitamin E supplementation for prevention of morbidity and mortality in preterm infants. Cochrane Database Syst Rev 3:CD003665, 2003.

Brown, JE: Nutrition Through the Life Cycle, ed 2. Thomson Wadsworth, Belmont, CA, 2005.

Buckley, M: Product focus: Some new and important clues to the causes of colic. Br J Community Nurs 5:462, 2000.

Businco, L, Bruno, G, Giampietro, PG: Prevention and management of food allergy. Acta Paediatr Suppl 88:104, 1999.

Callen, J, and Pinelli, J: A review of the literature examining the benefits and challenges, incidence and duration, and barriers to breastfeeding in preterm infants. Adv Neonatal Care 5:72, 2005.

Campbell, MK, and Kelsey, KS: The PEACH survey: A nutrition screening tool for use in early intervention programs. J Am Diet Assoc 94:1156, 1994.

Cantani, A, and Micera, M: Immunogenicity of hydrolysate formulas in children (part 1): Analysis of 202 reactions. J Investig Allergol Clin Immunol 10:261, 2000.

Caraher, M, and Lang, T: Can't cook, won't cook: A review of cooking skills and their relevance to health promotion. Int J Health Promot Educ 37:89, 1999.

Carley, A: Anemia: When is it iron deficiency? Pediatr Nurs 29:127, 2003.

Carruth, BR, and Skinner, JD: The role of dietary calcium and other nutrients in moderating body fat in preschool children. Int J Obes Relat Metab Disord 25:559, 2001.

Carvalho, NE, et al: Severe nutritional deficiencies in toddlers resulting from health food milk alternatives. Pediatrics 107:E46, 2001.

Carver, JD: Advances in nutritional modifications of infant formulas…Breast milk and breastfed infants: implications for improving infant formula: proceedings of the symposium Innovaciones en Fórmulas Infantiles (Innovations in Infant Formula) held in Cancun, Mexico, May 23–24, 2002. Am J Clin Nutr 77:1550S, 2003.

Cathey, M, and Gaylord, N: Picky eating: A toddler's approach to mealtime. Pediatr Nurs 30:101. 2004.

Centers for Disease Control. Achievements in public health, 1900–1999: Healthier mothers and babies. MMWR 48:849, 1999a. Accessed October 1, 1999 at http://www.cdc.gov/epo/mmwr/preview/mmwrhtml/mm4838a2.htm.

Centers for Disease Control. Childhood diarrhea: Messages for parents. 1999b. Accessed October 29, 1999 at http://www.cdc.gov/od/oc/parents.

Centers for Disease Control: *Enterobacter sakazakii* infections associated with the use of powdered infant formula—Tennessee, 2001. MMWR 51:298, 2002a. Accessed April 17, 2002 at http://www.cdc.gov/mmwr/preview/mmwrhtml/mm5114a1.htm.

Centers for Disease Control: Infant botulism—New York City, 2001–2002. MMWR 52:21, 2003a. Accessed February 25, 2004 at http://www.cdc.gov/mmwr/preview/mmwrhtml/mm5202a1.htm.

Centers for Disease Control: Infant mortality and low birth weight among black and white infants—United States, 1980–2000. MMWR 51:589, 2002b. Accessed February 18, 2004 at http://www.cdc.gov/mmwr/preview/mmwrhtml/mm5127a1.htm

Centers for Disease Control: Iron deficiency—United States, 1999–2000. MMWR 51:897, 2002c. Accessed March 7, 2007 at http://www.cdc.gov/mmwr/preview/mmwrhtml/mm5140a1.htm.

Centers for Disease Control: Managing acute gastroenteritis among children: Oral rehydration, maintenance, and nutritional therapy. MMWR 52:1, 2003b. Accessed May 10, 2005 at http://www.cdc.gov/mmwr/PDF/RR/RR5216.pdf

Centers for Disease Control: Neurologic impairment in children associated with maternal dietary deficiency of cobalamin—Georgia, 2001. MMWR 52:61, 2003c. Accessed January 22, 2004 at http://www.cdc.gov/mmwr/preview/mmwrhtml/mm5204a1.htm.

Centers for Disease Control: Participation in high school physical education—United States, 1991—2003. MMWR 53:844, 2004. Accessed October 1, 2004 at http://www.cdc.gov/mmwr/preview/mmwrhtml/mm5336a5.htm

Centers for Disease Control: Physical activity levels among children aged 9–13 years—United States, 2002. MMWR 52:785, 2003d. Accessed April 2, 2004 at http://www.cdc.gov/mmwr/preview/mmwrhtml/mm5233a1.htm.

Centers for Disease Control: Recommendations to prevent and control iron deficiency in the United States. MMWR 47:1, 1998. Accessed May 10, 2005 at http://www.cdc.gov/epo/mmwr/preview/mmwrhtml/00051880.htm

Chatoor, I: Feeding disorders in infants and toddlers: Diagnosis and treatment. Child Adolesc Psychiatr Clin N Am 11:163, 2002.

Chatoor, I, et al: Attachment and feeding problems: a reexamination of nonorganic failure to thrive and attachment insecurity. J Am Acad Child Adolesc Psychiatry 37:1217, 1998.

Chen, A, and Rogan, W: Breastfeeding and the risk of postneonatal death in the United States. Pediatrics 113:e435, 2004.

Cinquetti, M, et al: Latex allergy in a child with banana anaphylaxis. Acta Paediatr 84:709, 1995.

Clark, S, et al: Multicenter study of emergency department visits for food allergies. J Allergy Clin Immunol 113:347, 2004.

Complementary feeding. In Kleinman, RE (ed): Pediatric Nutrition Handbook, ed 5. American Academy of Pediatrics, Elk Grove Village, IL, 2004.

Cordain, L: In reply [letter]. Arch Dermatol 139:942, 2003.

Cordain, L, et al: Acne vulgaris: A disease of Western civilization. Arch Dermatol 138:1584, 2002.

Cox, N, and Hinkle, R: Infant botulism. Am Fam Physician 65:1388, 2002.

Crawford, M: Placental delivery of arachidonic and docosahexaenoic acids: Implications for the lipid nutrition of preterm infants. Am J Clin Nutr 71:275S, 2000.

Crocco, AG, Villasis-Keever, M, and Jadad, AR: Two wrongs don't make a right: Harm aggravated by inaccurate information on the Internet. Pediatrics 109:522, 2002.

Darlow, BA, and Graham, PJ: Vitamin A supplementation for preventing morbidity and mortality in very low birthweight infants. Cochrane Database Syst Rev 4:CD000501, 2002.

de Boissieu, D, Matarazzo, P, and Dupont, C: Allergy to extensively hydrolyzed cow milk proteins in infants: Identification and treatment with an amino acid-based formula. J Pediatr 131:744, 1997.

Deglin, JH, and Vallerand, AH: Davis's Drug Guide for Nurses, ed 9. FA Davis Company, Philadelphia, 2005.

Delbourg, MF, et al: Hypersensitivity to banana in latex-allergens of 33 and 37 kD. Ann Allergy Asthma Immunol 76:321, 1996.

Dennison, BA, Erb, TA, and Jenkins, PI: Television viewing and television in bedroom associated with overweight risk among low-income preschool children. Pediatrics 109:1028, 2002.

Dewey, KG: Is breastfeeding protective against child obesity? J Hum Lact 19:9, 2003.

Dochterman, J, and Bulechek, G (eds): Nursing Interventions Classification (NIC), ed 4. Mosby, St. Louis, 2004.

Duffy, L: Breastfeeding after strenuous aerobic exercise: A case report. J Hum Lact 13:145, 1997.

Duro, D, et al: Association between infantile colic and carbohydrate malabsorption from fruit juices in infancy. Pediatrics 109:797, 2002.

Ebbeling, CB, et al: Compensation for energy intake from fast food among overweight and lean adolescents. JAMA 291:2828, 2004.

Ebbeling, CB, Pawlak, DB, and Ludwig, DS: Childhood obesity: Public-health crisis, common sense cure. Lancet 360:473, 2002.

Eden, AN: Preventing iron deficiency in toddlers: A major public health problem. Contemp Pediatr 20:57, 2003.

Edwards, CA, and Parrett, AM: Dietary fibre in infancy and childhood. Proc Nutr Soc 62:17, 2003.

Ellett, MLC: What is known about infant colic? Gastroenterol Nurs 26:60, 2003.

Failure to thrive. In Kleinman, RE (ed): Pediatric Nutrition Handbook, ed 5. American Academy of Pediatrics, Elk Grove Village, IL, 2004.

Fats and fatty acids. In Kleinman, RE (ed): Pediatric Nutrition Handbook, ed 5. American Academy of Pediatrics, Elk Grove Village, IL, 2004.

Feeding the child. In Kleinman, RE (ed): Pediatric Nutrition Handbook, ed 5. American Academy of Pediatrics, Elk Grove Village, IL, 2004.

Feldman EB: Pregnancy and lactation. In Feldman, EB (ed): Essentials of Clinical Nutrition. FA Davis, Philadelphia, 1988.

Food sensitivity. In Kleinman, RE (ed): Pediatric Nutrition Handbook, ed 5. American Academy of Pediatrics, Elk Grove Village, IL, 2004.

Food Standards Agency (UK): Should I avoid peanuts while I'm breastfeeding? 2004. Accessed February 6, 2004 at http://www.foodstandards.gov.uk/healthiereating/asktheexpert/allergyintolerance/peanutsbreastfeeding.

Formula feeding of term infants. In Kleinman, RE (ed): Pediatric Nutrition Handbook, ed 5. American Academy of Pediatrics, Elk Grove Village, IL, 2004.

Forste, R, Weiss, J, and Lippincott, E: The decision to breastfeed in the United States: Does race matter? Pediatrics 108:291, 2001.

Frank, L, et al: Exposure to peanuts in utero and in infancy and the development of sensitization to peanut allergens in young children. Pediatr Allergy Immunol 10:27, 1999.

French, SA, Lin, B-H, and Guthrie, JF: National trends in soft drink consumption among children and adolescents age 6 to 17 years: Prevalence, amounts, and sources, 1977/1978 to 1994/1998. J Am Diet Assoc 103:1326, 2003.

Fry, T: The new "breast from birth" growth charts: An updated version of the paper given at the Primary Care Conference and Exhibition, May 2003. J Fam Health Care 13:124, 2003.

Ganglberger, E: Hev b 8, the Hevea brasiliensis latex profilin, is a cross-reactive allergen of latex, plant foods and pollen. Int Arch Allergy Immunol 125:216, 2001.

Garcia-Ortiz, JC, et al: Bronchial asthma induced by hypersensitivity to legumes. Allergol Immunopathol Madr 23:38, 1995.

Gartner, LM, et al: Prevention of rickets and vitamin D deficiency: new guidelines for vitamin D intake. Pediatrics 111:908, 2003.

Gerrish, CJ, and Mennella, JA: Flavor variety enhances food acceptance in formula-fed infants. Am J Clin Nutr 73:1080, 2001.

Gibson, EL, and Green, MW: Nutritional influences on cognitive function: mechanisms of susceptibility. Nutr Res Rev 15:169, 2002.

Gillman, MW, et al: Family dinner and diet quality among older children and adolescents. Arch Fam Med 9:235, 2000.

Goldman, AS, Goldblum, RM, and Schmalstieg, FC: Protective properties of human milk. In Walker, WA, and Watkins, JB (eds): Nutrition in Pediatrics, ed 2. BC Decker, Hamilton, Ontario, 1997.

Gordon, CM, et al: Prevalence of vitamin D deficiency among healthy adolescents. Arch Pediatr Adolesc Med 158:531, 2004.

Grantham-McGregor, S, and Ani, C: A review of studies on the effect of iron deficiency on cognitive development in children. J Nutr 131:649S, 2001.

Gregory, RL, et al: Effect of exercise on milk immunoglobulin A. Med Sci Sports Exerc 29:1596, 1997.

Gropper, SS, Smith, JL, and Groff, JL: Advanced Nutrition and Human Metabolism, ed 4. Wadsworth, Belmont, CA, 2005.

Grummer-Strawn, LM, and Mei, Z: Does breastfeeding protect against pediatric overweight? Analysis of longitudinal data from the Centers for Disease Control and Prevention Pediatric Nutrition Surveillance System. Pediatrics 113:e81, 2004.

Gupta, SK: Is colic a gastrointestinal disorder? Curr Opin Pediatr 14:588, 2002.

Hallett, R, Haapanen, LAD, and Teuber, SS: Food allergies and kissing. N Engl J Med 346:1833, 2002.

Hamosh, M, et al: Digestive enzymes in human milk: Stability at suboptimal storage temperatures. J Pediatr Gastroenterol Nutr 24:38, 1997.

Hampton, SM: Prematurity, immune function and infant feeding practices. Proc Nutr Soc 58:75, 1999.

Hanna, N, et al: Effect of storage on breast milk antioxidant activity. Arch Dis Child Fetal Neonatal Ed 89:F518, 2004.

Hanson, LA: Breastfeeding provides passive and likely long-lasting active immunity. Ann Allergy Asthma Immunol 81:523, 1998.

Harris, KJ, et al: Reducing elementary school children's risks for chronic diseases through school lunch modifications, nutrition education, and physical activity interventions. J Nutr Educ 29:196, 1997.

Heald, FP, and Gong, EJ: Diet, nutrition, and adolescence. In Shils, ME, et al (eds): Modern Nutrition in Health and Disease, ed 9. Lippincott Williams & Wilkins, Philadelphia, 1999.

Hediger, ML, et al: Association between infant breastfeeding and overweight in young children. JAMA 285:2453, 2001.

Helland, IB, et al: Maternal supplementation with very-long-chain N-3 fatty acids during pregnancy and lactation augments children's IQ at 4 years of age. Pediatrics 111:e39, 2003.

Heymann, DL(ed): Control of Communicable Diseases Manual, ed 18. American Public Health Association, Washington, DC, 2004.

Hilton, J: SMA infant formula product recall of specific batches. Food Standards Agency, August 15, 2001.

Hinkle, AJ: Community-based nutrition interventions: Reaching adolescents from low-income communities. Ann NY Acad Sci 817:83, 1997.

Hofman, PL, et al: Premature birth and later insulin resistance. N Engl J Med 351:2179, 2004.

Hoppin, AG: Assessment and management of childhood and adolescent obesity. Medscape CME. June 25, 2004. Accessed July 28, 2004 at http://www.medscape.com/viewprogram/3221.

International Association of Infant Food Manufacturers: Iron deficiency, part 3. September 2004. Accessed May 11, 2005 at http://www.ifm.net/industry/iron_deficiency3.htm.

James, J, et al: Preventing childhood obesity by reducing consumption of carbonated drinks: Cluster randomised controlled trial. BMJ 328:1237, 2004.

Jarvinen, KM, et al: Does low IgA in human milk predispose the infant to development of cow's milk allergy? Pediatr Res 48:457, 2000.

Kalliomaki, M, et al: Probiotics in primary prevention of atopic disease: A randomised placebo-controlled trial. Lancet 357:1076, 2001.

Kann, L, et al: Youth risk behaviour surveillance—United States, 1997. J Sch Health 68:355, 1998.

Kennedy, E, and Davis, C: US Department of Agriculture School Breakfast Program. Am J Clin Nutr 67(Suppl):798S, 1998.

Klemola, T, et al: Allergy to soy formula and to extensively hydrolyzed whey formula in infants with cow's milk allergy: A prospective, randomized study with a follow-up to the age of 2 years. J Pediatr 140:219, 2002.

Klish, WJ, and Montandon, CM: Nutrition and upper gastrointestinal disorders. In Halpern, SL (ed): Quick Reference to Clinical Nutrition, ed 2. JB Lippincott, Philadelphia, 1987.

Konofal, E, et al: Iron deficiency in children with attention-deficit/hyperactivity disorder. Arch Pediatr Adolesc Med 158:1113, 2004.

Krummel, DA, Seligson, FH, and Guthrie, HA: Hyperactivity: Is candy causal? Crit Rev Food Sci Nutr 36:31, 1996.

Kuan, LW, et al: Health system factors contributing to breastfeeding success. Pediatrics 104:e28, 1999. Accessed October 24, 1999 at http://www.pediatrics.org.

Kubik, MY, et al: Food-related beliefs, eating behavior, and classroom food practices of middle school teachers. J Sch Health 72:339, 2002.

Lack, G, et al: Factors associated with the development of peanut allergy in childhood. N Engl J Med 348:977, 2003.

Lake, AM: Dietary protein enterocolitis. Curr Allergy Rep 1:76, 2001.

Latasa, M, et al: Fruit sensitization in patients with allergy to latex. J Investig Allergol Clin Immunol 5:97, 1995.

Lawrence, RA: Storage of human milk and the influence of procedures on immunological components of human milk. Acta Paediatr Suppl 88:14, 1999.

Lee, CW, and Sheffer, AL: Peanut allergy. Allergy Asthma Proc 24:259, 2003.

Lehmann, CU, Conner, KG, and Cox, JM: Preventing provider errors: Online total parenteral nutrition calculator. Pediatrics 113:748, 2004.

Leung, DY, et al: Effect of anti-IgE therapy in patients with peanut allergy. N Engl J Med 348:986, 2003.

Liu, J, et al: Malnutrition at age 3 years and lower cognitive ability at age 11 years: Independence from psychosocial adversity. Arch Pediatr Adolesc Med 157:593, 2003.

Llatser, R, Zambrano, C, and Guillaumet, B: Anaphylaxis to natural rubber latex in a girl with food allergy. Pediatrics 94:736, 1994.

Lo, CW: Human milk: Nutritional properties. In Walker, WA, and Watkins, JB: Nutrition in Pediatrics, ed 2. BC Decker, Hamilton, Ontario, 1997.

Long, A: The nuts and bolts of peanut allergy. N Engl J Med 346:1320, 2002.

Lovelady, CA, Hunter, CP, and Geigerman, C: Effect of exercise on immunologic factors in breast milk. Pediatrics 111:E148, 2003.

Lubetzky, R, et al: Energy expenditure in human milk- versus formula-fed preterm infants. J Pediatr 143:750, 2003.

Ludwig, DS, Peterson, KE, and Gortmaker, SL: Relation between consumption of sugar-sweetened drinks and childhood obesity: A prospective, observational analysis. Lancet 357:505, 2001.

Maffeis, C: Aetiology of overweight and obesity in children and adolescents. Eur J Pediatr 159(Suppl):S35, 2000.

Marshall, TA, et al: Dental caries and beverage consumption in young children. Pediatrics 112:e184, 2003.

Mastretta, E, et al: Effect of Lactobacillus GG and breast-feeding in the prevention of rotavirus nosocomial infection. J Pediatr Gastroenterol Nutr 35:527, 2002.

McClung, HJ, Murray, RD, and Heitlinger, LA: The Internet as a source for current patient information. Pediatrics 101:e2, 1998. Accessed May 3, 2000 at http://www.pediatrics.org/cgi/content/full/101/6/e2.

McWhorter, J, Wallman, HW, and Alpert, PT: The obese child: Motivation as a tool for exercise. J Pediatr Health Care 17:11, 2003.

Mennella, JA, Jagnow, CP, and Beauchamp, GK: Prenatal and postnatal flavor learning by human infants. Pediatrics 107:E88, 2001.

Mitoulas, LR, et al: Variation in fat, lactose and protein in human milk over 24 h and throughout the first year of lactation. Br J Nutr 88:29, 2002.

Moorhead, S, Johnson, M, and Maas, M (eds): Nursing Outcomes Classification (NOC), ed 3. Mosby, St. Louis, 2004.

Morgan, CM, et al: Childhood obesity. Child Adolesc Psychiatr Clin N Am 11:257, 2002.

Morris, JL, and Zidenberg-Cherr, S: Garden-enhanced nutrition curriculum improves fourth-grade school children's knowledge of nutrition and preferences for some vegetables. J Am Diet Assoc 102:91, 2002.

Mortensen, EL, et al: The association between duration of breastfeeding and adult intelligence. JAMA 287:2365, 2002.

Mrdjenovic, G, and Levitsky, DA: Nutritional and energetic consequences of sweetened drink consumption in 6- to 13-year-old children. J Pediatr 142:604, 2003.

NANDA International: Nursing Diagnoses: Definitions and Classification 2003–2004. NANDA International, Philadelphia, 2003.

Nead, KG, et al: Overweight children and adolescents: A risk group for iron deficiency. Pediatrics 114:104, 2004.

Neifert, MR: Prevention of breastfeeding tragedies. Pediatr Clin North Am 48:273, 2001.

Newburg, DS, et al: Role of human-milk lactadherin in protection against symptomatic rotavirus infection. Lancet 351:1160, 1998.

Nichols, MR, and Livingston, D: Preventing pediatric obesity: assessment and management in the primary care setting. J Am Acad Nurse Pract 14:55, 2002.

Nicklas, TA, et al: Outcomes of a high school program to increase fruit and vegetable consumption: Gimme 5—a fresh nutrition concept for students. J Sch Health 68:348, 1998.

Noerr, B: Current controversies in the understanding of necrotizing enterocolitis. Adv Neonatal Care 3:107, 2003.

Nutritional needs of the preterm infant. In Kleinman, RE (ed): Pediatric Nutrition Handbook, ed 5. American Academy of Pediatrics, Elk Grove Village, IL, 2004.

O'Connor, DL, et al: Growth and development in preterm infants fed long-chain polyunsaturated fatty acids: A prospective, randomized controlled trial. Pediatrics 108:359, 2001.

Ogden, C: Prevalence and trends in overweight among US children and adolescents, 1999–2000. JAMA 288:1728, 2002.

Ogundele, MO: Effects of storage on the physicochemical and antibacterial properties of human milk. Br J Biomed Sci 59:205, 2002.

Olson, RE: Vitamin K. In Shils, ME, et al (eds): Modern Nutrition in Health and Disease, ed 9. Lippincott Williams & Wilkins, Philadelphia, 1999.

Opplinger, RA, et al: Wisconsin minimum weight program reduces weight-cutting practices of high school wrestlers. Clin J Sport Med 8:26, 1998.

Paeratakul, S, et al: Fast-food consumption among US adults and children: Dietary and nutrient intake profile. J Am Diet Assoc 103:1332, 2003.

Parsons, TJ, Power, C, and Manor, O: Infant feeding and obesity through the lifecourse. Arch Dis Child 88:793, 2003.

Perry, CL, et al: Adolescent vegetarians: How well do their dietary patterns meet the healthy people 2010 objectives? Arch Pediatr Adolesc Med 156:431, 2002.

Perry, CL, et al: Characteristics of vegetarian adolescents in a multiethnic urban population. J Adolesc Health 29:406, 2001.

Pesa, J: Psychological factors associated with dieting behaviors among female adolescents. J Sch Health 69:196, 1999.

Phan, TG, et al: Passive transfer of nut allergy after liver transplantation. Arch Intern Med 163:237, 2003.

Rao, MR, et al: Effect of breastfeeding on cognitive development of infants born small for gestational age. Acta Paediatr 91:267, 2002.

Raynor, P, and Rudolf, MC: Anthropometric indices of failure to thrive. Arch Dis Child 82:364, 2000.

Requejo, AM, et al: The age at which meat is first included in the diet affects the incidence of iron deficiency and ferropenic anaemia in a group of pre-school children from Madrid. Int J Vitam Nutr Res 69:127, 1999.

Richards, M, Hardy, R, and Wadsworth, ME: Long-term effects of breast-feeding in a national birth cohort: Educational attainment and midlife cognitive function. Public Health Nutr 5:631, 2002.

Robinson, TN: Reducing children's television viewing to prevent obesity: A randomized controlled trial. JAMA 282:1561, 1999.

Rolls, BJ, Engell, D, and Birch, LL: Serving portion size influences 5-year-old but not 3-year-old children's food intakes. Am J Diet Assoc 100:232, 2000.

Ross Laboratories: Pediatric products. Accessed July 28, 2004 at http://www.ross.com/productHandbook/default.asp.

Saigal, S, et al: School-age outcomes in children who were

extremely low birth weight from four international population-based cohorts. Pediatrics 112:943, 2003.

Sampson, HA: Clinical practice: Peanut allergy. N Engl J Med 346:1294, 2002.

Sampson, HA, Mendelson, L, and Rosen, JP: Fatal and near-fatal anaphylactic reactions to food in children and adolescents. N Engl J Med 327:380, 1992.

SanGiovanni, JP, et al: Dietary essential fatty acids, long-chain polyunsaturated fatty acids, and visual resolution acuity in healthy fullterm infants: a systematic review. Early Hum Dev 57:165, 2000.

SaraOclar, Y, et al: Latex sensitivity among hospital employees and atopic children. Turk J Pediatr 40:61, 1998.

Schanler, RJ: The low-birth-weight infant. In Walker, WA, and Watkins, JB: Nutrition in Pediatrics, ed 2. BC Decker, Hamilton, Ontario, 1997.

Schanler, RJ, Shulman, RJ, and Lau, C: Feeding strategies for premature infants: Beneficial outcomes of feeding fortified human milk versus preterm formula. Pediatrics 103:1150, 1999.

Seeds of change. Consumer Reports 64:41, 1999.

Separating the wheat from the chaff. Consumer Reports 64:30, 1999.

Sicherer, SH, et al: A voluntary registry for peanut and tree nut allergy: Characteristics of the first 5149 registrants. J Allergy Clin Immunol 108:128, 2001a.

Sicherer, SH, et al: The US Peanut and Tree Nut Allergy Registry: Characteristics of reactions in schools and day care. J Pediatr 138:560, 2001b.

Simmer, K, and Patole, S: Longchain polyunsaturated fatty acid supplementation in preterm infants. Cochrane Database Syst Rev 3:CD000375, 2004.

Skinner, JD, et al: Children's food preferences: A longitudinal analysis. J Am Diet Assoc 102:1638, 2002.

Spergel, JM, and Fiedler, JM: Natural history of peanut allergy. Curr Opin Pediatr 13:517, 2001.

Stang, J, et al: Relationships between vitamin and mineral supplement use, dietary intake, and dietary adequacy among adolescents. J Am Diet Assoc 100:905, 2000.

Suzuki, K, et al: Intracranial hemorrhage in an infant owing to vitamin K deficiency despite prophylaxis. Childs Nerv Syst 15:292, 1999.

Szajewska H, et al: Efficacy of Lactobacillus GG in prevention of nosocomial diarrhea in infants. J Pediatr 138:361, 2001.

Tanzi, MG, and Gabay, MP: Association between honey consumption and infant botulism. Pharmacotherapy 22:1479, 2002.

Taylor, AV, et al: Detection and quantitation of raw fish aeroallergens from an open-air fish market. J Allergy Clin Immunol 105:166, 2000.

Taylor, SL, Hefle, SL, and Munoz-Furlong, A: Food allergies and avoidance diets. Nutr Today 34:15, 1999.

Thiboutot, DM, and Strauss, JS: Diet and acne revisited. Arch Dermatol 138:1591, 2002.

Thorp, FK, Pierce, P, and Deedwania, C: Nutrition in the infant and young child. In Halpern, SL (ed): Quick Reference to Clinical Nutrition, ed 2. JB Lippincott, Philadelphia, 1987.

Thoyre, S: Techniques for feeding preterm infants. Am J Nurs 103(9):69.

United States Department of Agriculture. The Food Guide for Young Children. March 25, 1999. Accessed August 8, 2005 at http://www.cnpp.usda.gov/kidsPyra/Pyrbook.pdf

United States Department of Health and Human Services. Healthy People 2010. Accessed April 14, 2000 at http://web.health.gov/healthypeople/document/html/volume2/16mich.htm#_TOC471 971365.

Vadas, P, et al: Detection of peanut allergens in breast milk of lactating women. JAMA 285:1746, 2001.

Vanderhoof, JA, and Young, RJ: Role of probiotics in the management of patients with food allergy. Ann Allergy Asthma Immunol 90(Suppl 3):99, 2003.

van Odijk, J, et al: Breastfeeding and allergic disease: a multidisciplinary review of the literature (1966–2001) on the mode of early feeding in infancy and its impact on later atopic manifestations. Allergy 58:833, 2003.

Vitamins. In Kleinman, RE (ed): Pediatric Nutrition Handbook, ed 5. American Academy of Pediatrics, Elk Grove Village, IL, 2004.

Wang, G, and Dietz, WH: Economic burden of obesity in youths aged 6 to 17 years: 1979–1999. Pediatrics 109:e81, 2002.

Weir, DG, and Scott, JM: Vitamin B_{12} "Cobalamin." In Shils, ME, et al (eds): Modern Nutrition in Health and Disease, ed 9. Lippincott Williams & Wilkins, Philadelphia, 1999.

Wharton, B: Weaning: Pathophysiology, practice, and policy. In Walker, WA, and Watkins, JB: Nutrition in Pediatrics, ed 2. BC Decker, Hamilton, Ontario, 1997.

Williams, J, et al: Iron supplemented formula milk related to reduction in psychomotor decline in infants from inner city areas: Randomised study. Br Med J 318:693, 1999.

Wold, AE, and Adlerberth, I: Breast feeding and the intestinal microflora of the infant: Implications for protection against infectious diseases. Adv Exp Med Biol 478:77, 2000.

Wright, C, and Birks E: Risk factors for failure to thrive: A population-based survey. Child Care Health Dev 26:5, 2000.

Wright, KS, Quinn, TJ, and Carey, GB: Infant acceptance of breast milk after maternal exercise. Pediatrics 109:585, 2002.

Wyshak, G: Teenaged girls, carbonated beverage consumption, and bone fractures. Arch Pediatr Adolesc Med 154:610, 2000.

Yaseen, H: Fluid, electrolyte and nutritional requirements of extremely premature infants during the first days of life: Pathophysiology and guidelines. Neonatal Intensive Care 9:39, 1996.

Yimyaem, P, et al: Gastrointestinal manifestations of cow's milk protein allergy during the first year of life. J Med Assoc Thai 86:116, 2003.

Young, EM, and Fors, SW: Factors related to the eating habits of students in grades 9–12. J Sch Health 71:483, 2001.

Young-Hyman, D, et al: Care giver perception of children's obesity-related health risk: A study of African American families. Obes Res 8:241, 2000.

Yu, SM, Kogan, MD, and Gergen, P: Vitamin-mineral supplement use among preschool children in the United States. Pediatrics 100:e4, 1997. Accessed April 23, 2000 at http://www.pediatrics.org/cgi/content/full/100/5/e4.

Zeiger, RS: Dietary aspects of food allergy prevention in infants and children. J Pediatr Gastroenterol Nutr 30:S77, 2000.

Zeiger, RS: Food allergen avoidance in the prevention of food allergy in infants and children. Pediatrics 111:1662, 2003.

CHAPTER **13**

Life Cycle Nutrition: The Mature Adult

Learning Objectives

After completing this chapter, the student should be able to:

1. Identify the foods and food groups most likely to be lacking or excessive in the diets of adults.
2. Describe the changes in the older adult's body that affect nutritional status.
3. Explain how a nutritional assessment of an older adult differs from that of a younger one.
4. Illustrate ways in which food can be used to aid in the developmental tasks of adulthood.
5. List several suggestions to improve food intake for older people in a variety of living situations.

The life cycle of human growth and development continues throughout the adult years. Both psychosocial and physical developments continue as a person matures. This chapter considers the impact on nutrition of the physiological and psychosocial changes that occur during young, middle, and older adult years. Because much of this book emphasizes the nutritional needs of young and middle-aged adults, the main focus of this chapter is the older adult.

Overall food consumption of American adults poorly matches the Food Guide Pyramid recommendations, as Figure 13–1 illustrates. Even so, a major threat to health in adulthood is inactivity (Box 13–1). It can lead to overweight and obesity, the subject of Chapter 18.

Young Adulthood

Young adulthood spans ages 18 through 39. Not all 18-year-olds are adults, developmentally speaking; nor are all 40-year-olds middle-aged in thought or behavior. Chronological age is a convenient means of grouping people but may have limited applicability to a given individual.

Psychosocial Development

For identifying the client's stage of psychosocial development, chronological age is not as important as a person's life situation. During the early years of young adulthood, the individual may be completing the adolescent task of identity. According to Erik Erikson, the developmental task of young adulthood is **intimacy** (Table 13–1). For example, people who delay commitment to a life partner until their 30s and 40s will probably be working at achieving intimacy; other 40-year-olds may be tackling the next task of generativity.

To achieve intimacy, the individual strives to build reciprocal, caring relationships. The word *intimacy* may suggest sexuality, but intimate relationships are not necessarily sexual. Solid friendships are based on intimacy, the revealing of oneself to another at a special, quiet dinner, perhaps. Failure at the task of intimacy could result in isolation. At this stage, perhaps more than with other developmental tasks, it is apparent that a person chooses what he or she is to become.

Nutrition in the Young Adult

Throughout this book, the RDAs and AIs for individual nutrients, as well as dietary guidelines, have been specified. Often the age categories in the literature differ from source to source. Any division into young, middle, and older adulthood is somewhat arbitrary. The reported compliance with the Food Guide Pyramid for 20- to 39-year-old men and women is shown in Table 13–2. More men than women reported consuming recommended intakes of all food groups except fruit, where 30- to 39-year-old women tied with the men. The best intake was reported by the 71 percent of 20- to 29-year-old men who met the recommended intake for grains.

Although 24-hour recall data are insufficient to evaluate an individual's nutritional status, recall data from large groups can serve to identify problem areas. Of 19- to 50-year olds, females achieved a mean Healthy Eating Index (HEI) score of 63.2. They scored 3.3 in fruits, a poor rating, but 8.1 in cholesterol, which is rated good. The males achieved a mean total score 61.3, poor scores of 2.7 for fruits and 4.2 for sodium, and no good scores. All other areas for both genders need improvement.

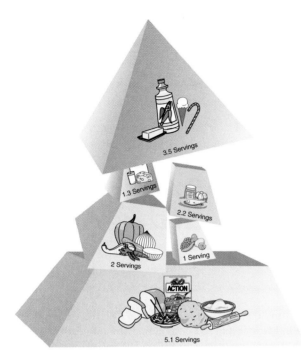

Figure **13–1** The Tumbling Pyramid. Actual consumption of foods in the United States shows the meat group as the only food group for which intake corresponds with recommendations. (Reprinted from Eating in America Today, ed 2, National Live Stock and Meat Board, 1995, courtesy of National Cattlemen's Beef Association, with permission.)

As mentioned in Chapter 2, acculturation into the mainstream society seems to stimulate deterioration in diet quality. When the survey was conducted in Spanish, taken to indicate less acculturation, the mean HEI composite score for those over age 18 was 65.1, compared with 62.7 for Hispanic persons who were interviewed in English (Aldrich and Variyam, 2000).

Middle Adulthood

The middle adult years are those between ages 40 and 65. Mandatory retirement rules in the past designated age 65 as the beginning of old age. Now the age range for middle age is more flexible as the Social Security retirement age has edged upward and more seniors are remaining active in old or new careers.

Psychosocial Development

Erikson's task of **generativity** involves serving the next generation as a mentor and guiding it to adopt one's values.

Box 13–1 **The Prevalence of Inactivity in Adults**

In 2002, 22.3 percent of men and 27.5 percent of women reported no leisure-time physical activity. This represents a decrease of 7 percentage points for men and 4.1 percentage points for women from 1988. Individuals older than 70 years are the most sedentary, but they reported an even greater change: from 40.6 percent of men in 1988 to 29.7 percent in 2002 reporting no leisure-time physical activity. Women over 70 years were the most inactive in both time periods, with 47.3 percent reporting no leisure-time physical activity in 1988 compared with 39.2 percent in 2002 (Centers for Disease Control, 2004a). These were all noninstitutionalized adults, so presumably most would be able to participate in some physical activities.

A greater percentage of Hispanic women reported no leisure-time physical activity in 2002 (40.1 percent) than in 1988 (39.6 percent). For all other groups the percentages reporting no physical activity declined in 2002 compared to 1988:

• White non-Hispanic women—23.2 percent from 29.0 percent
• Non-Hispanic black women—36.0 percent from 46.5 percent
• White non-Hispanic men—19.2 percent from 27.9 percent
• Black non-Hispanic men—27.7 percent from 36.0 percent
• Hispanic men—35.2 percent from 37.0 percent (Centers for Disease Control, 2004a).

In this way, middle-aged adults can attain a measure of immortality by influencing not only their own children but also their students or protégés at work. Teaching family members to prepare traditional foods, for example, may help a person achieve generativity.

Nutrition in Middle Adulthood

The reported compliance with the Food Guide Pyramid for 40- to 50-year-old men and women is shown in Table 13–3. More men than women claimed recommended intakes of all food groups except fruit, but 68 percent was the largest group in compliance again for the younger men consuming the recommended grains.

The average HEI score for 45- to 64-year olds was 63.4. Of this group, 13 percent achieved good HEI scores of 81 or

Table 13–1 **Erikson's Theory of Psychosocial Development in Maturity**

STAGE OF LIFE	DEVELOPMENTAL TASK	OPPOSING NEGATIVE TRAIT	USE OF FOOD TO ACHIEVE TASK
Young Adult	Intimacy	Isolation	Arranging candlelight dinner
Middle Adult	Generativity	Stagnation	Teaching someone to prepare family favorite or ethnic dishes
Older Adult	Integrity	Despair	Using food fragrances or memories of food to reminisce

Table 13–2 Reported Compliance With Food Guide Pyramid Recommendations by Men and Women 20 to 39 Years of Age

	20- TO 29-YEAR-OLD MEN	30- TO 39-YEAR-OLD MEN	20- TO 29-YEAR-OLD WOMEN	30- TO 39-YEAR-OLD WOMEN
At least 6 servings of grains	71 percent	70 percent	41 percent	41 percent
At least 3 servings of vegetables	67 percent	69 percent	43 percent	44 percent
At least 2 servings of fruit	23 percent	23 percent	20 percent	23 percent
At least 5 ounces of meat equivalents*	63 percent	66 percent	25 percent	27 percent
At least 2 servings of dairy products	30 percent	30 percent	17 percent	19 percent

*Tabulation includes meat, poultry, fish, simulated meat products, eggs, tofu, peanut butter, nuts, and seeds, but excludes dry beans and peas that were included with vegetables.

SOURCE: U.S. Department of Agriculture, February 1999.

above, 70 percent achieved scores needing improvement, and 18 percent tallied less than 51 or poor scores (U.S. Department of Agriculture, July 1999).

Older Adulthood

The population in the United States continues to change demographically. **Life expectancy** in 1900 was 45 years. By 2001, however, life expectancy at birth was 77.2 years: 80.2 for white females, 75.5 for black females, 75.0 for white males, and 68.6 for black males (Centers for Disease Control, 2004b). In 1900, 4.1 percent of the population was age 65 or older. By 1940, 5 years after Social Security was enacted, 6.8 percent of the population was 65 or older, and in 1970, 5 years after Medicare took effect, the proportion was 9.8 percent.

The proportion of the U.S. population aged 65 years and older is projected to increase from 12.4 percent in 2000 to 19.6 percent in 2030. By 2025, the proportion of Florida's population aged 65 years and older is projected to be 26 percent and to be more than 15 percent in all other states except Alaska and California (Centers for Disease Control, 2003b).

This aging of the population is attributed to improved sanitation, an increased concern for safety, and control of communicable diseases. The major causes of death in adults are heart disease, cancer, and stroke. All of them are linked to lifestyle, including a dietary component.

Distinctions Among Older Adults

As a group, older adults display a wide range of interests and abilities. Some are content to stay at home and work in the garden. Others travel extensively. Only 10 percent are confined in any serious way. In a roomful of 3-year-old children, individuals are more like each other than in a roomful of 70-year-old adults. In old age, people become "more like themselves," accentuating traits they have had all along. Many older people have difficulty changing their behavior patterns, including those related to food.

Commonly used categories for old age sort the population into

- Young-old—ages 65 to 75 years, the "go-go years"
- Aged—ages 75 to 85 years, the "slow-go years"
- Oldest-old—greater than 85 years, the "no-go years."

The stereotype of old folks in a nursing home is just that, a stereotype. Only 5 percent of older adults live in nursing homes. That 5 percent, however, represents more than 1 million clients, 51 percent of whom are 85-years-old or older. This subgroup of the older population has special nutrient needs. In 1997, 45 percent of nursing home residents needed help with eating (Sahyoun et al, 2001). Often they have very low calcium intakes and low intakes of vitamin A, vitamin C, thiamin, riboflavin, and iron. If they do not consume fortified dairy products and do not receive sufficient sun exposure appropriate to the diminished capacity of their skin to synthesize it, they are at increased risk for vitamin D deficiency.

Psychosocial Development

Erikson's developmental task for older adults to achieve is **integrity,** in the sense of being whole or complete. Those who accomplish this task will look back on their lives as

Table 13–3 Reported Compliance With Food Guide Pyramid Recommendations by Men and Women 40 to 59 Years of Age

	40- TO 49-YEAR-OLD MEN	50- TO 59-YEAR-OLD MEN	40- TO 49-YEAR-OLD WOMEN	50- TO 59-YEAR-OLD WOMEN
At least 6 servings of grains	68 percent	59 percent	39 percent	37 percent
At least 3 servings of vegetables	62 percent	67 percent	49 percent	50 percent
At least 2 servings of fruit	27 percent	30 percent	23 percent	31 percent
At least 5 ounces of meat equivalents*	65 percent	61 percent	27 percent	25 percent
At least 2 servings of dairy products	29 percent	20 percent	16 percent	14 percent

*Tabulation includes meat, poultry, fish, simulated meat products, eggs, tofu, peanut butter, nuts, and seeds, but excludes dry beans and peas that were included with vegetables.

SOURCE: U.S. Department of Agriculture, February 1999.

worthwhile. Although they may have suffered some failures and have some regrets, they are able to see their lives in perspective. They can forgive themselves for their faults because they know they did the best they could with what they had.

A technique to help the older person achieve integrity is reminiscence. Asking an older person to recall special foods can stimulate reminiscence. Familiar food odors oftentimes will evoke memories.

Socially, older adults often must adapt to the loss of friends and relatives. The death of a spouse demands a tremendous adjustment. The accompanying depression and new responsibility for tasks the spouse performed may significantly affect an older person's food intake.

Physical Changes of Aging

Just as adolescents have a changing body image, so do older adults. Even without frank disease, the physical abilities of older adults diminish. "Middle-age spread" gives way to dwindling bulk and waning strength. The clinical guidelines on overweight and obesity in adults set a BMI of 25 as the upper limit of ideal weight for all adults regardless of age. An analysis of the guidelines, however, determined that available data do not support the BMI range of 25 to 27 as a risk factor for all-cause and cardiovascular **mortality** among elderly persons, either in men or women (Heiat, Vaccarino, and Krumholtz, 2001).

Despite that, there are notable changes in organ function in the elderly. Among the body systems significantly affected are the integumentary, sensory, gastrointestinal, urinary, musculoskeletal, nervous, endocrine, and cardiovascular systems.

Integumentary System

Many changes take place in the skin as a person ages. As subcutaneous fat is lost, the skin becomes dry and wrinkled. Less elasticity is present to spring back after a pinch to the forearm, the usual site assessed for hydration status. The skin of the forehead or over the breastbone is a more reliable site in the elderly client than the forearm. The older adult also loses some of the ability to synthesize vitamin D from sunshine so that it may take twice as much sun exposure without sunscreens as necessary in a younger person to produce a given amount of vitamin D.

Sensory System

Four senses become markedly less acute as a person ages: vision, hearing, taste, and smell. Because the sense receptors do not deteriorate equally, some of the sense loss is attributed to changes in the central nervous system. Extensive variation exists among individuals.

EYES

Vision is reduced. The older person sees reds, oranges, and yellows better than blues and violets. Clouding of the lens of the eye—cataract formation—decreases overall vision. The fine-print labels on food items may be illegible to the elderly. Older eyes do not adjust well to glare.

Vision changes may make grocery shopping burdensome. Food preparation may become not only difficult but also hazardous if the person cannot see adequately. Compared to 60-year-old and 70-year-old Americans, 80-year-olds were less likely to read food labels, perhaps because of poor vision or limitations of activities such as grocery shopping (Elbon et al, 2000).

EARS

The sound receptors in the inner ear deteriorate. First to be lost is the ability to perceive high tones. The older person with poor hearing usually hears men's voices better than women's. Hearing aids do not fully compensate for the hearing loss. In fact, they often magnify sideline noise to the point of distracting the wearer. The result may be social isolation when it becomes too laborious to interact with others. Socializing at meals may become embarrassing or frustrating, and older people may avoid such interaction.

NOSE AND TONGUE

For the sense of taste to function well, the sense of smell must also be intact. Food tastes bland when a person has a head cold. Many, but not all, older adults have dulled senses of smell and taste that they begin to notice at about age 60. The sense of smell is frequently more impaired by aging than is the sense of taste, but both faculties are important to help protect the person from noxious elements in the environment. Blindfolded older subjects showed only half the ability of younger ones to recognize blended tastes, a loss attributed mainly to declining olfactory senses (Morley, 1997).

Taste receptors are concentrated on the tongue's surface but also are located at the base of the tongue, on the soft palate, and in other areas of the nasopharynx. The traditional taste receptors permit recognition of sweet, sour, salty, and bitter sensations, but receptors have been identified for umami, a sensation described as savory or rich. It is caused by the amino acid glutamine in its free form and is associated with monosodium glutamate (MSG); however, many people cannot identify umami as a distinct sensation (Taste sensation, 2002).

The sense of taste declines in most but not all aging clients. Usually salt receptors are most affected and sweet receptors least affected (Morley, 1997). Increasing the amounts of seasonings and condiments may be the older person's solution to diminishing taste sensations.

Gastrointestinal System

Particularly crucial to nutrition is gastrointestinal function. Hundreds of processes are required for the proper digestion, absorption, and metabolism of foods. Many functions of the gastrointestinal system decline significantly in older people.

Older individuals are not immune to dental caries. In fact, the risk for caries in individuals 70 years of age and older has increased. The tooth root, lacking enamel, is particularly vulnerable to caries, causing increased occurrence in the elderly population. Factors associated with increased risk of caries are reduced saliva flow, inadequate oral hygiene, frequent sugar intake, Asian ethnicity, and the use of partial dentures (Anusavice, 2002). In contrast, adults who were free of root caries consumed 50 percent more cheese and 25 percent more milk than persons with caries (DePaola, Faine, and Palmer, 1999).

Approximately 30 percent of individuals over the age of 65 have no permanent teeth or are **edentulous.** The major cause of tooth loss in the older adult is not dental caries but **periodontal disease,** which affects the gums (gingiva) and apparatus attaching the tooth to the jaw. Dentures, like hearing aids, only partially compensate, so that dentures are about 20 percent as efficient as natural teeth. Furthermore, a denture cannot be effective if the underlying tissue is in poor condition. Persons with upper dentures that cover the palate containing taste receptors lose some taste sensation and are also subject to impaired swallowing. Denture wearers select foods that they can manage. Thus, intake of carrots and tossed salads among denture wearers was shown to be 2.1 and 1.5 times less than for individuals with all their teeth (Nowjack-Raymer and Sheiham, 2003).

Box 13–2 illustrates a self-administered dental screening form designed to alert older people to their need for dental care. It was validated with a clinical dental examination on 165 people 65 to 94 years old, correctly identifying 82 percent of those with dental disease. Notice that not all of the items are weighted equally.

The production of saliva decreases sharply in older adults. This condition is called **xerostomia.** Chewing and swallowing become more difficult, and food intake may be affected. Also, with age, less mucus and smaller quantities of enzymes are secreted.

Atrophic gastritis, a chronic inflammation of the stomach lining with decreases in size of the glands and mucous membranes, occurs in 10 to 30 percent of the U.S. population over the age of 60 (Russell, Rasmussen, and Lichtenstein, 1999). An extreme case is **achlorhydria,** the absence of hydrochloric acid in the stomach. Either of these conditions may interfere with protein digestion and

with vitamin and mineral absorption. Vitamin B_{12} may remain locked to the food protein, and less iron will be absorbed in the more alkaline environment.

Intestinal **motility** decreases because of lessened muscle tone. Medications may interfere with electrolyte balance, also diminishing muscle tone. By the age of 70, the liver loses 18 percent of its weight and has reduced capabilities.

Urinary System

The kidneys lose about 10 percent of their weight by the time an adult reaches the age of 70. At age 80, the blood flow to the kidneys is half of what it was at age 35. By 90 years of age, the renal mass has fallen by 30 to 40 percent (Larson, 2003). Other changes observed in the aging kidney include the decreased ability to concentrate urine, the inability to conserve sodium, and the decreased excretion of potassium. Estimates of hyponatremia in elderly (that may double their mortality rate) are given as 7 percent of outpatients and 11.3 percent of inpatients, of which 73 percent of the latter cases were attributed to intravenous fluids and diuretics (Luckey and Parsa, 2003).

This compromised kidney function makes urine samples less reliable for nutrient analyses in the elderly. Two laboratory tests frequently are used to assess renal function: **blood urea nitrogen (BUN)** and serum creatinine. An increase in the BUN level usually indicates a decrease in kidney function. It may also be elevated in dehydration or if excessive protein is presented to the liver for breakdown, as with a high-protein diet or with gastrointestinal bleeding. Conversely, the BUN may be decreased in liver disease. Clients with even slightly elevated BUNs may not be able to excrete the waste products from protein metabolism. Caregivers must be judicious about giving high-protein nutritional supplements to older people with elevated BUNs.

Creatinine, an end product of creatine metabolism, is excreted very efficiently by the healthy kidney. The amount of creatinine produced is proportional to the individual's skeletal muscle mass and remains fairly constant in the absence of extensive muscle damage. The serum creatinine test has the advantage over the BUN of being little affected by dehydration, malnutrition, or liver function. Creatinine levels may not detect decreased kidney function, however, if a slow decline in renal function occurs simultaneously with a slow decrease in muscle mass, as happens in the aging process. Consequently, both tests may be performed to obtain a more complete diagnostic picture.

Musculoskeletal System

The major loss of body mass in the older adult involves muscle mass. By age 70, a person's skeletal muscle diminishes by 40 percent. Because muscle is a more metabolically active tissue than fat, energy needs decline with the diminished muscle mass.

Nutritional deprivation and catabolic states can affect the muscles of respiration in the chest and diaphragm. Because the older person relies more on the diaphragm than the chest muscles to breathe, a full stomach may impede breathing to a greater extent than in a younger

---

Box 13–2 **The D-E-N-T-A-L Screening Survey Form**

Certain dental conditions have been known to interfere with proper nutritional intake and possibly dispose a person to involuntary weight loss. Please answer the following questions regarding your dental health by placing a check before the conditions that apply to you.

	POINT VALUE
___ Dry mouth	(2)
___ Eating difficulty	(1)
___ No recent dental care (within 2 years)	(1)
___ Tooth or mouth pain	(2)
___ Alteration or change in food selection	(1)
___ Lesions, sores, or lumps in the mouth	(2)

If you have scored more than 2 points on this survey, you may have a dental problem that could be affecting your overall health and general well-being. We urge you to seek dental care as soon as possible for a check-up.

SOURCE: Bush et al, 1996, with permission.

person. The effect of respiratory disease on nutrition is covered in greater detail in Chapter 24.

Perhaps more noticeable than the overall loss of muscle is the loss of height in older people. The average lifetime loss of height amounts to 2.9 centimeters (1.16 inches) in men and 4.9 centimeters (1.93 inches) in women. A major cause of this loss of height is osteoporosis. The bone loss amounts to about 8 percent per decade after age 35, so that by the age of 70, 25 percent of the bone structure is gone.

Joint surfaces are roughened by arthritis. By age 50, half of all adults have some osteoarthritis. Arthritis impairs the use of the hands for opening jars, chopping raw foods, and cutting cooked foods at the table. Arthritis also impairs the operation of the mandibular joint of the jaw for chewing.

Nervous System

By the time a person reaches old age, the brain has endured a lifetime of stressors. Blood flow to the brain decreases because of narrowing of the arteries. Thirst sensation becomes less operative, increasing the risk of uncompensated dehydration. Adaptation to stress is less effective as people age. For instance, mortality from heat stroke rises sharply in people older than 60 years (Fig. 9–7).

The brain shrinks with age as well as with alcohol abuse. Age is the most powerful factor promoting shrinkage, however, with an odds ratio of 2.8 for each 10 years of age (Kubota et al, 2001). One theory for the decrease in brain volume is a decrease in brain water content other than cerebrospinal fluid (Pfefferbaum et al, 1999).

Various nutrients have been tested in relation to cognitive performance. For instance, because glucose is the brain's preferred fuel, numerous studies have tested its effect on cognition with mixed results. When tested against aspartame as the control substance, a healthy, non-food-deprived adult population showed no consistent effect of glucose on task performance (Green, Taylor, and Elliman, 2001).

Special concerns of nourishing clients with dementia are covered in Clinical Application 13–1. One type of dementia, Alzheimer's disease, affected approximately 4.5 million persons in the United States in 2000 and is predicted to affect 13.2 million by 2050 unless new preventive techniques are found (Hebert et al, 2003).

Another neurological disease that occurs more commonly in older than younger people is Parkinson's disease. In the United States, at least 500,000 people are believed to suffer from Parkinson's disease, and about 50,000 new cases are reported annually, with an average age at onset of 60 years (Parkinson's disease, 2004). Box 13–3 details nutritional ramifications of the disease.

Endocrine System

The average older person is slowing down. Resting energy expenditure (REE) decreases, especially in the brain, skeletal muscle, and heart. The older adult's REE may be 10 to

---

Clinical Application 13–1

Nutrition and Dementia

Care of clients with dementia challenges family and health-care providers. Clients progressively lose the ability for self-care, including feeding. A simple tool to assess the client's level of functioning is the Eating Behavior Scale, reproduced on page 271. The six items assessed direct the caregivers to an appropriate strategy to assist the client without taking over a task the client still can perform.

Managing the client's environment is a major part of the care of the client with dementia. Dining rooms should be quiet and have adequate lighting. Having the same seat gives the client a familiar experience at each meal. Offering one course at a time and providing appropriate but limited utensils, large-handled if necessary, are strategies that have been effective. Dishes with high sides to enable the client to scoop up the food onto a spoon or fork may prove useful. Offering finger foods that are within the client's capabilities to manage also may increase nutritional intake with minimal staff assistance. A very small study showed clients with dementia consumed more food by weight when served on orange rather than white plates (VanDusen and London, 2003).

Clients with dementia must be reminded of the steps involved in self-feeding: putting the food on the spoon, directing it to the mouth, swallowing. Verbal cues or guiding the client's hand can get him or her started or keep the process going. Despite the surroundings, common

courtesies can be effective in reminding clients of social expectations. Introducing the client to the other people at the table, providing a cup rather than a carton for milk, and offering foods separately rather than mixing them all together can contribute to maintaining a person's dignity (Kayser-Jones and Schell, 1997; Tully et al, 1997).

The effect of quiet music in the dining room on client behavior has been researched in various settings. Selections with a slow tempo—at or below the human heart rate—have usually been used to dampen environmental noises that might otherwise startle clients. Fewer incidents of agitated behaviors occurred during the weeks that music was played compared with weeks without music (Denney, 1997). Since staff members also heard the music, perhaps some of the effect was obtained by relaxing them also. Creating a pleasant environment at mealtime is an attempt at normalcy for demented clients.

A multidisciplinary project to improve nutrition in clients with late-stage dementia not only achieved that but also decreased the distress of clients and nursing staff caused by the clients' swallowing problems. Among the interventions used were thickened liquids, three levels of dysphagia diets, daylong snacks, and encouraging unbalanced diets if those were all that the clients would take, under the pragmatic principle that any food is better than no food (Biernacki and Barratt, 2001).

National Institutes of Health Warren G. Magnuson Clinical Center Nursing Department

Eating Behavior Scale (EBS)

Patient # _____   Admit date _____   Observation date _____
Observer initials _____   Meal start _____   Finished _____
Patient room _____   Day room _____   Time, minutes _____
Circle only one answer: Maximum score = 18   Total = _____

Observed Behavior	I.*	V.**	P.***	D.****
Was the patient:				
1. Able to initiate eating?	3	2	1	0
2. Able to maintain attention to meal?	3	2	1	0
3. Able to locate all food?	3	2	1	0
4. Appropriately using utensils?	3	2	1	0
5. Able to bite, chew, and swallow without choking?	3	2	1	0
6. Able to terminate meal?	3	2	1	0

Comments

_____

_____

_____

_____

*I. = Independent
**V. = Verbal prompts
***P. = Physical assistance
****D. = Dependent

Box 13–3 **Parkinson's Disease**

Parkinson's disease is a progressive neurological disorder characterized by degeneration of neurons in the area of the brain that controls movement. This degeneration causes a shortage of dopamine, a neurotransmitter or brain-signaling chemical (Parkinson's disease, 2004). Among the signs of the disease are tremors, rigidity, loss of facial expression, and gait disorders, all of which impact the ability to obtain, prepare, and consume food.

An extensive Swedish case study of 10 women with Parkinson's disease illustrates some of the difficulty encountered by these clients with a median age of 75 years and a median disease duration of 10 years. Five of the women lived with spouses; five lived alone.

	MARRIED, LIVING WITH SPOUSE	LIVING ALONE	ADAPTATION
Shopped for self	1 woman	2 women	Shopped in early morning and in small shops to avoid tiring crowds and distances
Cooked own meals	3 women	3 women	Simplified cooking and used ready-cooked foods
Difficulty feeding oneself	4 women	5 women	Took small portions, especially with guests Ate from packages Used spoon or fork to avoid spills Employed both hands to drink
Swallowing problems	3 women	3 women	Thickened liquids for better control
Deteriorated sense of smell	4 women	5 women	Imagined taste of familiar foods

Despite all of these problems, three of the married women were overweight and one was obese. Of the four single women reporting food intake, three were of normal weight and one was morbidly obese with a BMI of 40 (Andersson and Sidenvall, 2001).

It can be readily seen that providing for nutritional needs for individuals with Parkinson's disease can be a day-in-day-out, all-day process. Other impairments of movement may impact clients in similar ways.

An online forum, "Ask the Parkinson Dietitian," is available at:
http://www.parkinson.org/site/pp.asp?c=9dJFJLPwB&b=71418.

12 percent less than a younger person's. Lost muscle mass is replaced, if at all, by adipose tissue that is less active metabolically than muscle.

The pancreas often secretes inadequate amounts of insulin or the body loses its ability to utilize insulin, leading to diabetes mellitus (Chapter 19). Receptors in the kidney for antidiuretic hormone (ADH) may function poorly to produce a less-effective response. Levels of aldosterone also decrease with age. Both of these changes make maintaining correct fluid volume more difficult for an older person than a younger one.

Cardiovascular System

As the older adult continues to age, there is a decrease in cardiac output and a slower heart rate. In response to exercise, the heart rate does not increase as effectively as in youth, nor does it return to normal as rapidly. Because of these diminishments, the elderly are at risk for diseases of the heart. Dietary modifications for heart disease are included in Chapter 20.

The consequence of arriving at a stressful situation in a healthy state can be life-saving. For example, trauma victims older than 60 years with higher hemoglobin levels and greater oxygen delivery were more likely to survive than victims with lower cardiovascular functioning (Luckey and Parsa, 2003).

A part of the cardiovascular system, the immune system, is less effective in the older person than in the younger one. Certain white blood cells (WBCs), the lymphocytes, recognize and promote the body's response to foreign antigens. B lymphocytes or B cells are produced in the embryo's bone marrow and migrate to the spleen and lymph nodes, where, among other functions, they monitor foreign antigens and produce the appropriate antibodies to neutralize them, a mechanism called humoral immunity. T lymphocytes or T cells, originally produced in the embryo's bone marrow, mature in the thymus gland in the chest, and then are lodged in the spleen and lymph nodes until needed. T cells are important to the body's cellular immune response (that does not involve antibodies) to viruses, fungi, malignant cells, and foreign tissue grafts. Age-related impaired T cell functioning has been linked to chronic diseases such as arthritis, autoimmune diseases, and cancer and to increased susceptibility to infectious diseases (Serafini, 2000).

Nutrition in the Older Adult

MyPyramid or the one modified for adults older than 70 years can be used for assessment and counseling. The nutrition of older Americans has been investigated. Some of the findings regarding energy, vitamins, minerals, and water are presented next.

Food Pyramids

MyPyramid can serve the older adult well because age and activity level are two of the data fields required for computation. The older Food Guide Pyramid was the standard when the following surveys were conducted.

Adults over 65 years of age achieved a mean HEI score of 67.2. They tallied good median scores above 80 for total fat, saturated fat, cholesterol, sodium, and variety but poor scores below 51 for fruit and milk (U.S. Department of Agriculture, July 1999).

Table 13–4 lists the percentages of older men and women reporting consumption of food groups as recommended by the Food Guide Pyramid. It shows that in only 4 of the 20 categories did more than half the respondents consume the recommended servings and those respondents were all men.

A special Modified Food Guide Pyramid for People Over 70 Years of Age appears as Figure 13–2. Eight servings of water provide a foundation of the pyramid and symbols for fiber have been added to emphasize the food groups that are good sources of fiber. A pennant at the top of the pyramid signifies calcium, vitamin D, and vitamin B_{12} supplementation (Russell, Rasmussen, and Lichtenstein, 1999).

The approximate percentages of adult men and women, aged 20 and older, who consumed recommended servings from the major food groups are shown in Figure 13–3. In virtually every category, more men than women ate the recommended number of servings. With the exception of fruit and one slight reversal by the two younger groups of women in reporting vegetable intake, a greater proportion of younger people than older ones consumed the recommended number of servings.

With few exceptions, older people need the same intake of nutrients as do younger adults. Energy needs decrease with age. Thus, there is less leeway for indiscretions and empty kilocalories in the diet. Similarly, the AI for sodium is less for older persons than for younger ones. In contrast, the RDA/AIs for one mineral and three vitamins are

---

Table 13–4 **Reported Compliance With Food Guide Pyramid Recommendations by Men and Women 60+ Years of Age**

	60- TO 69-YEAR-OLD MEN	MEN 70 YEARS AND OLDER	60- TO 69-YEAR-OLD WOMEN	WOMEN 70 YEARS AND OLDER
At least 6 servings of grains	58 percent	49 percent	28 percent	28 percent
At least 3 servings of vegetables	61 percent	53 percent	46 percent	40 percent
At least 2 servings of fruit	36 percent	42 percent	34 percent	36 percent
At least 5 ounces of meat equivalents*	55 percent	37 percent	27 percent	17 percent
At least 2 servings of dairy products	23 percent	24 percent	12 percent	15 percent

*Tabulation includes meat, poultry, fish, simulated meat products, eggs, tofu, peanut butter, nuts, and seeds, but excludes dry beans and peas that were included with vegetables.

SOURCE: U.S. Department of Agriculture, February 1999.

Modified Food Pyramid for 70+ Adults

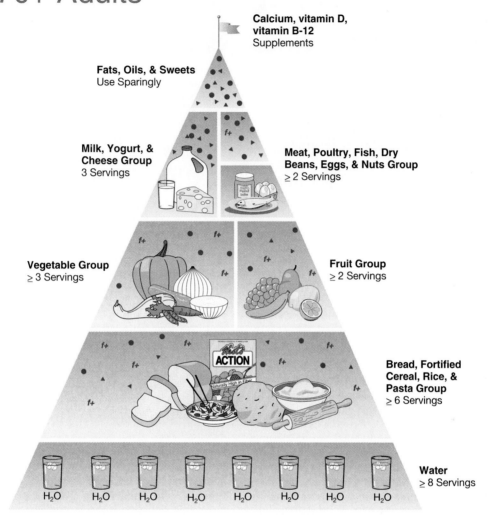

Calcium, vitamin D, vitamin B-12
Supplements

Fats, Oils, & Sweets
Use Sparingly

Milk, Yogurt, & Cheese Group
3 Servings

Meat, Poultry, Fish, Dry Beans, Eggs, & Nuts Group
≥ 2 Servings

Vegetable Group
≥ 3 Servings

Fruit Group
≥ 2 Servings

ACTION

Bread, Fortified Cereal, Rice, & Pasta Group
≥ 6 Servings

Water
≥ 8 Servings

● Fat (naturally occurring and added)
▲ Sugars (added)
f+ Fiber (should be present)
These symbols show fat, added sugars, & fiber in foods.

Figure **13–2** The Modified Food Guide Pyramid for People Over 70 Years of Age. (Reprinted from Russell, Rasmussen, and Lichtenstein, J Nutr 129:752, 1999, with permission of American Society for Nutritional Sciences.)

increased or more specific for older people than for younger ones.

Energy Nutrients and Energy Balance

It is estimated that older adults need about 5 percent fewer kilocalories per decade after the age of 40. Small changes have been recommended in intakes from carbohydrates, fats, and protein. As with younger people, the simplest criterion for the suitability of intake is the maintenance of a healthy body weight. There is much variation in energy expenditure within the elderly population. The proportion of energy to be obtained from carbohydrate, fat, and protein is changed slightly for older adults.

CARBOHYDRATES

Older people should derive 50 to 60 percent of their kilocalories from carbohydrates. The RDA for carbohydrate, based on its role as primary energy source for the brain, is 130 grams per day, the same as for younger adults.

FATS

Fats should contribute 20 to 30 percent of the day's kilocalories. Limiting fats should also increase comfort, because fat absorption is delayed in older people, leading to a feeling of fullness. Particularly among the elderly, rigid application of diet rules may be inappropriate. Restricting fat so as to eliminate whole milk and eggs, which are easily

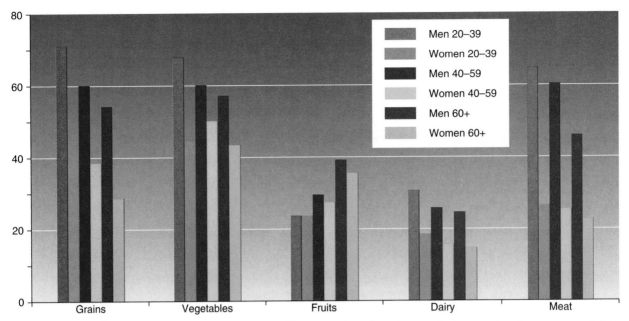

Figure **13–3** Approximate percentages of individuals, sorted by age and gender, who reported consuming the recommended servings from the major food groups. (Interpreted from U.S. Department of Agriculture, February 1999.)

eaten and relatively inexpensive, could endanger nutrition in the short term for uncertain long-term benefits.

PROTEIN

The RDA for protein for adults is 56 grams per day for men and 46 grams for women. Nothing different is specified for individuals older than 70 years in this category.

Although serum albumin levels are used as a measure of body protein stores, for a given individual, serum albumin levels can indicate nutritional status, pathology, or both. Protein status is an important component in the body's defense system. In seniors with protein-energy malnutrition (PEM), decreased functions in all aspects of immunity are strongly related to protein nutritional status. Refeeding can boost immune response in clients with inflammation but at a lower rate than in those without inflammatory responses (Lesourd, 2004).

A single laboratory measure is seldom the best predictor of clinical events. Regardless of illness severity, elderly hospitalized clients with a body mass index of less than 22 were almost three times as likely as other clients to suffer a life-threatening complication. Weight loss (more than 5 percent within 6 months), midarm circumference, and suprailiac skinfold thickness were also strong independent predictors of a life-threatening complication, whereas admission serum albumin, prealbumin, and cholesterol were not significantly correlated with the outcome after controlling for illness severity (Sullivan, Bopp, and Roberson, 2002).

EXERCISE

Older adults should have at least 30 minutes a day of moderate activity. It can be 30 minutes at one time or two 15-minute sessions or three 10-minute sessions. Progressive resistance training is feasible for many elderly individuals,

even the oldest old, to increase muscle mass and strength and decrease frailty (Vanitallie, 2003). An exercise routine should be introduced gradually. On average, physically active people live longer than inactive people do, even if exercise is started late in life. Exercise reduces the risk of chronic diseases and makes individuals feel healthier and look younger.

Vitamins

Fifty percent of older adults have a vitamin and mineral intake less than the RDA/AIs, and 10 to 30 percent have subnormal blood levels of vitamins and minerals (Johnson, Bernard, and Funderburg, 2002). Excesses are possible also, especially in people who self-medicate on megadoses of vitamins.

FAT-SOLUBLE VITAMINS

Because fat-soluble vitamins are stored in the body, it may take a long time for a deficiency to present clinical signs. Assessment of the individual's long-standing food habits might help to pinpoint a person's risks for either deficient or excessive intake.

Vitamin A may build to excessive levels in older persons because of reduced metabolic clearance and because of increased use of vitamin supplements (Lips, 2003). Retinol is involved in bone remodeling, but excessive intake has been linked to bone demineralization. In both sexes, increasing retinol was negatively associated with skeletal health at intakes not much more than the RDA. Higher intakes were reached predominantly by supplement users, suggesting a delicate balance exists between sufficient and excessive vitamin A for the elderly (Promislow et al, 2002). Women with retinol intakes greater than 1500 micrograms per day, twice the RDA, had a 64 percent greater risk of hip fracture compared with those consuming less than 500 microgams per day, 71 percent of the RDA (Feskanich et al, 2002).

Vitamin D may be problematic in older adults because of diminished intestinal absorption and impaired synthesis of it in the skin compared with that of younger adults. These physiological changes are reflected in the AIs of 10 micrograms for 51- to 70-year-olds and 15 micrograms for those older than 70. Milk is an excellent source of vitamin D because it is fortified. The elderly person who is most likely to be deficient in vitamin D is one who stays indoors, does not consume enough milk or milk products, and does not take a vitamin supplement. Vitamin D does not work alone, however. Randomized controlled trials have shown that a combination of vitamin D and calcium can prevent fragility fractures in the elderly, but in a study involving 51 nursing homes, supplementing residents with vitamin D alone did not prevent fractures (Meyer et al, 2002). In addition to its role in bone metabolism, vitamin D metabolites influence muscle cell maturation and functioning. Supplementing vitamin D-deficient elderly people improved their strength and walking distance and decreased their falls, but vitamin D did not prevent a decline in strength in healthy elderly people (Janssen, Samson, and Verhaar, 2002). In a meta-analysis of five randomized controlled trials involving 1237 participants, vitamin D reduced the risk of falling by 22 percent compared with calcium or placebo (Bischoff-Ferrari et al, 2004).

Vitamin E, besides functioning as a scavenger of free radicals, has been linked to immune and cognitive functions. Supplementation of the elderly with vitamin E has been shown to enhance immune response, delay onset of Alzheimer's disease, and increase resistance to oxidative injury associated with exercise (Meydani, 2002). Higher intake of vitamin E intake from food, not supplements, was related to decreased incidence of Alzheimer disease in community residents suggesting that various tocopherol forms rather than alpha-tocopherol alone may be important to the prevention of Alzheimer's disease (Morris et al, 2005). Vitamin E has also been related to another neurological condition, Parkinson's disease. Total intake of vitamin E was not related to the disease, but intake of foods high in vitamin E, particularly nuts, was associated with decreased risk of the disease, suggesting that other components of foods high in vitamin E might have a beneficial effect in preventing Parkinson's disease (Zhang et al, 2002).

Vitamin K can be depleted relatively more quickly than the other fat-soluble vitamins. Besides its role in the clotting of blood, vitamin K contributes to bone metabolism. Low dietary vitamin K intakes were associated with an increased incidence of hip fractures in elderly men and women (Booth et al, 2000) and with low bone mineral density in women (Booth et al, 2003). As a corollary, use of the vitamin K antagonist warfarin in some cases has been associated with fractures among older women. One study reported no association, but another reported a significantly higher risk for vertebral and rib fractures among warfarin users compared with nonusers (Booth and Mayer, 2000).

WATER-SOLUBLE VITAMINS

The RDAs for vitamin B_6 and vitamin B_{12} are different for older adults than for younger ones. In addition, persons in particular life situations are at risk for niacin and vitamin C deficiencies.

Vitamin B_6 has an increased RDA in the elderly over that for younger adults. The RDAs for vitamin B_6 are 1.5 milligrams for women older than 50 years and 1.7 milligrams for men older than 50 years, increases of 15 and 31 percent over those for younger adults.

Vitamin B_{12} in food may not be absorbed effectively by 10 to 30 percent of older persons. The RDAs stipulate that individuals older than 50 years should obtain it from fortified foods or supplements. The elderly are at increased risk for vitamin B_{12} deficiency because of inadequate dietary intake and age-related gastrointestinal abnormalities that limit absorption (Hamrick, 2003). Low serum vitamin B_{12} concentrations are found in more than 10 percent of older people, with a high prevalence reported among people with Alzheimer's disease, however no evidence has been found that vitamin B_{12} improves cognitive function of people with dementia (Malouf and Areosa Sastre, 2003).

Vitamin C status is generally better in older adults living at home than those living in institutions. The independent elderly may spend more money on fruits and vegetables than institutions do, or poor cooking and serving practices in institutions may destroy the vitamin C in foods. Scurvy most often occurs in disadvantaged groups: alcoholics with poor nutrition, the isolated elderly, and the institutionalized (Pimentel, 2003) as well as food faddists and the mentally ill (Stephen and Utecht, 2001). Widower's scurvy refers to the condition developing in a man after the death of his wife and subsequent poor dietary intake of vitamin C (Morrisson, 1997). See Chapter 7 for examples of recent cases of scurvy.

Niacin intake and utilization may be decreased in some elderly persons. Those who eat little meat and consume little milk or milk products containing tryptophan may be at risk for niacin deficiency. Higher risk occurs in clients with alcoholism, who may have multiple nutritional deficiencies, and clients with tuberculosis receiving isoniazid that interferes with tryptophan metabolism (Cervantes-Laurean, McElvaney, and Moss, 1999). See Chapter 17.

Minerals

Minerals of particular concern in the elderly are sodium, calcium, and iron but only calcium has been given an increased AI for older persons. Individuals older than 50 years should consume 1200 milligrams daily, an increase of 20 percent over the AI for younger adults. AIs for sodium are reduced compared to those for younger adults.

Calcium intake has been reported to be insufficient in individuals older than 60 years. Inadequate dietary intake of calcium was reported by 87 percent of women and 72 percent of men. Even with dietary supplements, two-thirds of the elderly adults had intakes below the calcium objective partly because their supplements contained low doses of calcium (Ervin and Kennedy-Stephenson, 2002). Over a 3-year period, community-dwelling residents in northern Europe given calcium and vitamin D supplements had 16 percent fewer osteoporotic fractures than the control group (Larsen, Mosekilde, and Foldspang, 2004). In elderly subjects, calcium was found to be equally bioavailable from skim milk, calcium-fortified orange juice, or calcium carbonate (Martini and Wood, 2002). Whether from food or supplements, calcium intake should be spread out throughout the day, with 500 milligrams or less being consumed at each meal to optimize absorption (Nieves, 2003).

Iron absorption is impaired by decreased gastric acidity, whether due to aging or to antacid use. Moreover, anemia is not always the result of physiological or nutritional deficits. Hidden blood losses should be suspected and their sources sought in the anemic elderly person, just as in younger clients. Sometimes, a clear-cut cause is illusive. Among 60 anemic nursing home residents, iron deficiency was the cause in 23 percent of the cases but 45 percent of the cases were **idiopathic** (Artz et al, 2004). Iron deficiency affects functions other than oxygen transport also. In 72 homebound elderly women, iron deficiency was associated with impairments in immunity that may render older adults more vulnerable to infections (Ahluwalia et al, 2004).

Sodium AIs are reduced compared to those for younger adults. due to decreased energy requirements, The AIs for sodium are 1.3 grams for individuals 50- to 70-years old and 1.2 grams for those 71 years of age and older. These represent reductions of 13 percent and 20 percent respectively.

Water

No AI for water has been established for individuals over the age of 30 years. Again, urine characteristics are the standard of comparison. Healthy older adults need enough fluid intake to produce about 1.5 liters of light yellow urine in 24 hours. Community-dwelling elders consume about 2100 milliliters of fluid per day, compared with 1100 to 1500 milliliters by residents of long-term care facilities, leading to an estimated prevalence of underhydration in the latter of 33 percent (Mentes and Iowa-Veterans, 2000). Loss of sphincter muscle tone in women and difficulty urinating in men may prompt older people to limit their fluid intake. Omitting fluids in the 2 hours before bedtime may help decrease the frequency of nocturia and night time incontinence.

One of the early signs of dehydration in the elderly is confusion, which may be difficult to ascertain in clients with dementia or altered consciousness, who are at the highest risk for dehydration and hypernatremia due to decreased fluid intake (Larson, 2003). If no one is alert to these mental changes, the person may compound his or her difficulties by forgetting to take medications or eat meals. Risk factors for fluid volume depletion are female gender, age greater than 85 years, bedridden state, more than four chronic conditions, chronic infections, more than four medications, or laxative abuse (Larson, 2003). Signs of dehydration in the elderly are listed in Table 13–5. The increase in pulse rate upon standing is an appropriate assessment technique for fluid volume status in the elderly except when heart disease and its treatments would block the physiological response.

Clients who are immobilized may need as many as 12 to 14 glasses of fluid per day. Immobility increases the calcium loss from bones, which then circulates in the blood until the kidney excretes the excess. A large fluid intake dilutes the urine so that the calcium does not form stones.

A project using colorful beverage carts and designated hydration assistants established a goal of increasing nursing home residents' fluid intake by 8 ounces each

Table 13–5   **Signs of Dehydration in the Elderly**

BODY SYSTEM	SIGN
Skin and mucous membranes	Skin warm and dry
	Decreased turgor; pinch test may be more accurate over the sternum or on the forehead than on the hand
	Furrowed tongue
	Elevated temperature
Cardiovascular	Elevated pulse
Urinary	Increased specific gravity
	Increased urinary sodium
Musculoskeletal	Weakness
Neurological	Confusion

midmorning and midafternoon. Providing choices of cold or hot beverages in colorful cups and assistance in drinking when needed increased the residents' total body water measured by bioelectrical impedance, decreased laxative use, increased the number of bowel movements, and decreased the number of falls during the 5-week program even though only 53 percent of residents consumed the desired 16 ounces every day. The 47 percent of the elders who had below normal total body water at the beginning of the project was reduced to just 6 percent at the end, all of whom were in the late stages of dementia and had much difficulty swallowing (Robinson and Rosher, 2002).

Common Problems Related to Nutrition

Although constipation, arthritis, osteoporosis, and protein-energy malnutrition are not unique to the elderly, they do represent special concerns for geriatric clients.

Constipation

A person may complain of acute constipation (lack of stool) or of chronic constipation (general difficulty passing bowel movements). Recommended methods to achieve bowel regularity include increasing fluid intake, consuming high-fiber foods, taking time for elimination, and exercising.

Doubling the person's water intake, medical conditions permitting, is the first step. Increasing fresh fruit and vegetable intake is the second. Helping the client determine his or her normal bowel evacuation pattern (after each meal, once a day, every other day, etc.) is the third step. Time should be set aside to have a bowel movement according to that pattern. Drinking a warm beverage often stimulates evacuation. In addition, exercise promotes regular bowel movements.

Many older individuals have the idea that they must have a bowel movement every day when that may not be their pattern. Sometimes older adults adopt the routine use of laxatives to correct bowel habits. For such people, the program mentioned above will not provide instant resolution. If they adhere to the regimen, however, it is possible to overcome even long-standing constipation. A special food-based recipe to control the symptom of constipation is given in Chapter 26.

Arthritis

This is a group of diseases characterized by inflammation of various joints often accompanied by pain, swelling, stiffness, and deformity. **Arthritis** prevalence increases with age, affecting approximately 60 percent of the U.S. population 65 years of age and older, and by 2030, an estimated 41 million persons in that age group will have arthritis or chronic joint symptoms (CJS) (Centers for Disease Control, 2003a).

Osteoarthritis, formerly called **degenerative joint disease (DJD),** also includes CJS and affects about 21 million individuals in the United States (Arthritis Foundation and CDC, 1999). Risk factors include aging, obesity, overuse or abuse of joints, and trauma. Osteoarthritis is characterized by progressive deterioration of cartilage in joints and vertebrae. Once believed to result only from "wear and tear" on the joints, osteoarthritis is increasingly believed to be the result of interactions between various biological and mechanical factors, including genetics and joint stress. Osteoarthritis results from an imbalance between the body's proteins that produce new cartilage and repair the old and the substances that break down cartilage (Habel, 2001). High doses of vitamins C and E have been reported to be beneficial in osteoarthritis (Darlington and Stone, 2001). Because the force exerted on the lower extremities may be up to six times the body weight, overweight people have a significantly increased risk of osteoarthritis of the knees (Habel, 2001). Thus, weight control has an important role in the prevention and treatment of osteoarthritis.

In contrast to osteoarthritis, which is a local disease, rheumatoid arthritis is a systemic disease generally thought to be of autoimmune origin affecting about 2.1 million people, mostly women (Arthritis Foundation and CDC, 1999). Because it is a systemic disease, efforts have been directed toward influencing the course of the disease through dietary or supplemental means. Omega-3 fatty acids have anti-inflammatory properties that could make them useful in treating inflammatory and autoimmune diseases (Simopoulos, 2002). Typically, human inflammatory cells contain high proportions of the omega-6 PUFA arachidonic acid and low proportions of omega-3 PUFA (Calder, 2002). A vegan diet is purported to improve symptoms by eliminating sources of arachidonic acid. Some supporting evidence was reported in a small study that found that a very low-fat (approximately 10 percent of kilocalories), vegan diet for 4 weeks decreased rheumatoid arthritis symptoms except for duration of morning stiffness (McDougall, 2002). Supplementation with long-chain omega-3 polyunsaturated fatty acids (PUFA) consistently demonstrates an improvement in rheumatoid arthritis symptoms and a reduction in nonsteroidal anti-inflammatory drug (NSAID) usage. Clients with rheumatoid arthritis should consume a balanced diet rich in long-chain omega-3 PUFA and antioxidants (Rennie et al, 2003).

Osteoporosis and Fractures

The pathophysiology and prevention of osteoporosis is covered in Clinical Application 8–3. This section examines only the risks of and results of hip fracture (actually a fracture of the femur), which although half as common as reported vertebral fractures, is much more likely to be diagnosed and treated. It is estimated that only one-third of vertebral fractures are clinically diagnosed. As an example, although vertebral fractures were identified in chest x-rays in 132 women, only 17 of their charts listed vertebral fractures as a discharge diagnosis (Gehlbach, 2000).

Approximately 250,000 hip fractures occur annually in the United States (Richmond et al, 2003). On a societal level, the lifetime cost for hip fractures in the United States in 1997 was estimated to be $20 billion (Braithwaite, Col, and Wong, 2003). On an individual level, one-half of all older adults hospitalized for hip fracture never regain their former level of function (Stevens and Olson, 2000). In the year after a hip fracture, functional abilities directly related to the hip fracture are projected to decline about 15 to 20 percent and those unrelated to hip fracture about 5 percent (Rosell and Parker, 2003). An estimated 10 percent of clients are disabled by hip fracture, and 19 percent require institutionalization (Melton, 2003). A hip fracture was shown to reduce life expectancy by 1.8 years with 17 percent of remaining life spent in a nursing facility (Braithwaite, Col, and Wong, 2003). Men were twice as likely as women to die during the first and second years after hip fracture, mainly due to septicemia and pneumonia (Wehren et al, 2003).

Among the risk factors for hip fractures are increasing age, female gender, white race, history of falls, insufficient exercise, low body mass index, being tall, and never having borne children. All these factors have been covered earlier or are self-explanatory, except height and **parity.** Engineering analysis of the hip indicates greater resistance to fracture in shorter femoral necks, which occur in shorter people (Slemenda, 1997), although lower-extremity length is proposed as a better predictor (Opotowsky, Su, and Bilezikian, 2003). Women who had never borne a child had a 44 percent increased risk of hip fractures, independent of hip bone mineral density, than women who had borne children, with each additional birth reducing hip fracture risk by 9 percent (Hillier et al, 2003). A proposed mechanism relates to changes produced in the pelvis by pregnancy. It can be readily seen that many clients have more than one of these risk factors.

Compared with clients not receiving supplements, clients with hip fractures receiving protein-rich nutritional supplements manifested lower rates of complications and death not only in the immediate postoperative period but also for 6 months afterward (Krall and Dawson-Hughes, 1999). A systematic review of 17 randomised trials involving 1266 participants however, concluded that the strongest evidence for the effectiveness of nutritional supplementation following hip fracture pertains to oral protein and energy feeds, but the evidence is still very weak (Avenell and Handoll, 2005). Many of the trials reviewed considered death as an outcome measure. Given the general benign character of balanced nutritional supplements, awaiting conclusive evidence of effect on mortality before proposing moderate use seems to be an overly strict interpretation of the evidence. Nonetheless, definitive treatment for existing osteoporosis is not dietary and sometimes is less than optimal.

Even after sustaining a hip fracture, only a minority of elderly clients receive treatment for osteoporosis to attempt to modify the risk of future fractures (Andrade et al, 2003; Juby and De Gues-Wenceslau, 2002; Harrington et al, 2002). Gardner et al (2002) reported similar low rates of treatment following hip fracture while finding improved rates between 1997 and 2000 but also noting only 6 percent of the overall group received a medication to actively prevent bone resorption and treat osteoporosis. The observation that osteoporosis drug treatment following hip fracture was associated with lower mortality than was true of those without treatment led to a proposal for randomized trials to test the efficacy of antiresorptive therapy for all clients after hip fracture (Cree, Juby, and Carriere, 2003).

Weight Loss and Protein-Energy Malnutrition

Some people in the United States simply do not get enough food to eat (Box 13–4). The main reason individuals do not consume enough protein or enough kilocalories is lack of money. To rectify the situation for older adults, the federal government, with an amendment to the Older Americans Act, established meal programs for senior citizens. Low-cost meals are offered at central gathering places and/or delivered to the homebound. Senior citizens participate in some 2200 such local meal programs (Fig. 13–4) that in

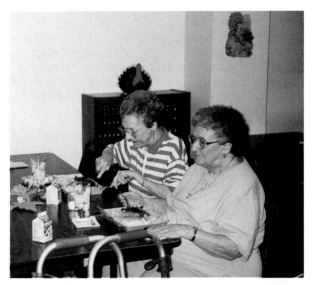

Figure **13–4** These women partake of an evening meal served at their place of residence under the auspices of the Older Americans Act and managed by a county agency.

Box 13–4 Food Insufficiency

Between 1988 and 1994, 4.1 percent of the people surveyed were designated "food insufficient" if the family respondent reported that the family sometimes or often did not have enough food to eat. Low income, low education, minority status, food assistance program participation, and social isolation were significantly related with food insecurity. In elderly persons, in addition to issues of affordability, availability, and accessibility, food insecurity is associated with functional impairments (Lee and Frongillo, 2001a).

In an apparent paradox, 58 percent of 19- to 55-year-old women in food-insufficient households were overweight compared with 47 percent in food-sufficient households. The former had significantly lower HEI scores than the latter, 58.8 versus 62.7, but both indicate diets that need improvement. Women in food-insufficient households also had significantly worse HEI scores for vegetables, fruits, milk, cholesterol, and variety (U.S. Department of Agriculture, 2002).

Assuming a client even has a household may be a mistake. Older women can be homeless, deriving most of their food at shelters. Such clients' food intake was found to be inadequate for most nutrients, with limited fruits, vegetables, dairy products, and whole grains (Johnson and McCool, 2003).

In New York state, regardless of food insecurity status, older people consumed less than the RDA for 8 nutrients, whereas food-insecure elderly persons had significantly lower intakes of 10 nutrients as well as lower skinfold thicknesses. In addition, food-insecure elderly persons were 2.3 times more likely to report fair or poor health status as food-secure elderly (Lee and Frongillo, 2001b).

2002 served about 250 million meals to 2.6 million older adults (Brown, 2005).

An analysis of recipients of home-delivered meals showed that lower intakes of specific nutrients were associated with subjects who were women, who were black, who reported a low income and limited education, and who did not usually eat breakfast. Intakes of less than the AIs for calcium were found in 96 percent of the people and for vitamin D in 99 percent, leading to the conclusion that home-delivered meals programs should target specific subgroups of participants with interventions, such as a breakfast meal or more-nutrient-dense meals (Sharkey et al, 2002).

A syndrome called **anorexia of aging** is described in Box 13–5. One of the most treatable psychological causes of weight loss in the older person is depression. Ninety percent of older depressed clients experience weight loss, compared with 60 percent of younger depressed people. SCALES, a rapid office practice screen for risk of protein-energy malnutrition, is shown in Box 13–6. Two components of the screen are serum albumin and cholesterol. Non-terminally ill hospitalized elderly who consumed less than 50 percent of their calculated energy requirements had average serum albumin levels of 2.9 g/dL and/or serum cholesterol levels of 154 mg/dL. They also had 8 times the risk of in-hospital death and 2.9 times the risk of death within 90 days as those whose nutrient intake exceeded 50 percent of requirements (Sullivan, Sun, and Walls, 1999). Malnutrition contributes to many complications of illness, such as pressure ulcers (Clinical Application 13–2). Nutritional status predicted nonelective hospital readmission following discharge of nutritionally compromised 65- to 92-year-old clients. Their 4-month nonelective readmission rate was 26 percent, and individuals with any amount of weight loss and no improvement in albumin concentrations during the first month after hospitalization had a much higher risk of readmission than were those who

Box 13–5 The Anorexia of Aging

Humans (and other animals) of advanced age have reduced food intake. Older humans become sated earlier than younger ones, the result of decreased enjoyment of food and of altered hormonal and neurotransmitter regulation of food intake (Morley, 1997).

Changes in the physiology of the aging body explain this phenomenon in the otherwise healthy individual. Diminished ability to smell and taste may make eating less enjoyable. Because gastric emptying is slowed, an older person feels full longer after a meal. Increased levels of circulating cholecystokinin, a hormone credited with satiating activity, occur in aged individuals. Animal and preliminary human studies indicate that aging is associated with increased satiety factors and a reduced feeding drive (Chapman et al, 2002).

In addition to physiologic causes of anorexia, social, psychological, and medical conditions impact the older person's appetite. Social causes include isolation, poverty, lack of transportation to obtain food, and unappealing environment or food selection, particularly for institutionalized clients. Companionship facilitates appetite. Women eat more when men are present, and both women and men eat more with family members present (Thomas and Morley, 2002). Psychological causes of anorexia include bereavement and depression. Recently widowed persons were shown to be at increased risk of weight loss compared with married individuals (Shahar et al, 2001). Preparing solitary meals and eating alone discourages balance and variety. Depression accounts for up to 30 percent of undernutrition in medical outpatients and up to 36 percent of nursing home residents who lose weight (Thomas and Morley, 2002). Some medical causes include drug side-effects, Parkinson's disease, and stroke (swallowing disorders, self-care deficit for feeding).

In a chronic-care hospital and a home for the aged, analysis of a 28-day cycle of menus revealed that, even if the 2000-kilocalorie diets were entirely consumed, they would not supply enough vitamins and minerals to provide recommended intakes. Whereas long-term care residents more consistently consume between 1000 and 1500 kilocalories per day, those authors recommend vitamin and mineral supplements for all older long-term care facility residents (Wendland et al, 2003).

Box 13–6 SCALES, A Rapid Office Practice Screen for Protein-Energy Malnutrition

S:	sadness
C:	cholesterol <4.14 mmol/L (160 mg/dL)
A:	albumin <40 g/L (4 g/dL)
L:	loss of weight
E:	eating problems (cognitive or physical)
S:	shopping problems or inability to prepare a meal

SOURCE: Morley, 1997. Reprinted with permission.

Clinical Application 13–2

Nutrition and Pressure Ulcers

The basic cause of **pressure ulcers** is impaired circulation from the weight of the body on a bony prominence or by shearing forces from pulling on the skin that damages the underlying tissue. Risk factors include immobility, inactivity, incontinence, impaired consciousness, and malnutrition. Progression of the ulcer from intact skin to an open, sometimes very deep sore increases the challenge to control infection, to replenish nutrient losses from the wound, and to promote healing. Copious wound drainage can result in a deficit of 100 grams of protein per day (Russell, 2001).

Data from 116 acute care facilities in 34 states indicated pressure ulcers developed in 7 percent of clients, with 73 percent occurring in persons older than 65 years. Fifty-seven percent of the ulcers were located over the coccyx or the sacrum (Whittington, Patrick, and Roberts, 2000). A similar overall prevalence of 8.5 percent was reported from 92 nursing homes in 22 states (Coleman et al, 2002). Most pressure ulcers develop within 2 weeks of admission to a facility (Ferguson et al, 2000), so early identification of individuals at risk is crucial.

The consumption of a diet high in protein and energy may promote pressure ulcer healing, but no single nutrient has proved to promote the healing of pressure ulcers in humans. Therefore, the key to effective treatment is early recognition of a depleted nutritional state and provision of adequate energy (35 kilocalories per kilogram of body weight) and protein (1.5 grams per kilogram of body weight) along with RDAs for micronutrients (Mathus-Vliegen, 2004). Specific vitamin (A and C) supplementation has aided healing in deficient clients but not in those without deficiencies. Moreover, excess vitamin E has impaired wound healing and blood clotting in animals (Scholl and Langkamp-Henken, 2001). Although zinc functions in collagen synthesis that contributes to wound healing, zinc supplementation has been shown to be beneficial only in clients with clinical zinc deficiency. Diagnosing deficiency is particularly problematic, because no consistent relationship between dietary zinc and plasma levels has been established. In addition, zinc supplementation has caused both stimulation and suppression of the immune system in elderly clients (Ausman and Russell, 1999).

Nutritional support is only a part of the overall strategy to combat pressure ulcers. The other risk factors must be controlled and diligent nursing care provided to effectively prevent or treat this serious complication.

maintained or increased their weight and had repleted their serum albumin levels (Friedmann et al, 1997).

Individual assessment and early intervention are keys to treating involuntary weight loss. From simple to complex, interventions are (1) modification of the environment, such as proper positioning, assistance, appropriate timing of medications; (2) administration of medical nutritional supplements, vitamins, and minerals; (3) medications such as the anabolic agent *oxandrolone* that decreases protein breakdown and increases protein synthesis; and (4) tube feeding if all efforts to provide adequate oral nutrition fail (Collins, 2001). For example, milk-based supplements that are both nutrient-dense and easy to consume might be a dietary recommendation for a person who is losing weight or one who cannot chew. Use of a nutrient-dense (120 kcalories and 5 grams of protein in 60 milliliters) supplement four times a day for 4 weeks as part of medication administration resulted in significant weight gain in residents of a long-term care facility. Contributing to the positive outcome was a 7 percent increase in intake at meals, including 16 percent at the evening meal (Welch, Porter, and Endres, 2003). As part of clinical guidelines to prevent and manage malnutrition in long-term care, Morley and Thomas (2003) recommend that liquid caloric supplements be administered between meals, because such supplements increased meal intake when given 1 hour before a meal but not when given with a meal.

To accommodate dentures, the person may reduce his or her intake of meats, fresh fruits, and vegetables and may need assistance selecting appropriate substitute items. A recommended procedure for learning to eat and drink with dentures is explained in Clinical Application 13–3.

The Nursing Process and the Elderly

Although elderly people are not all alike, often they do have some common problems (Box 13–7).

Assessment

Special care is necessary when assessing the elderly to ensure marginal deficiencies are detected before major problems occur. Body weight and its stability are critical data in nutrition screening, yet an investigation in three large medical centers revealed that just 65.7 percent of clients older than 18 years reporting being weighed at admission and only 67 percent of those not weighed had been asked about their weight. Over one-fourth (25.9 percent) of documented weights in the nursing records differed by 5 pounds (2.27 kg) or more compared with measurements by research personnel (Jensen et al, 2003).

A screening tool for geriatrics appear as Box 13–8. It has the advantage of incorporating alternative measures for

---

Clinical Application 13–3

Learning to Eat with Dentures

Persons need to learn to use dentures one step at a time. The steps are in exactly the same order as those used by infants learning to eat. The person should first practice swallowing liquids with the dentures in place. After this is mastered, soft foods can be chewed. Lastly, the person should learn to bite regular foods with the dentures. Splitting up the learning process into manageable units helps to make this process less frustrating for the new denture wearer.

Box 13–7 Topics to Be Assessed in the Elderly*

Oral Cavity Function
- Difficulty tasting, changes in taste perception
- Bleeding gums, dry mouth
- Difficulty chewing, toothaches, poorly fitting dentures
- Foods client is unable to eat

Meal Management
- Who shops? Where? Ease of making food decisions?
- Transportation problems?
- Budgeting a concern? Knowledge to make informed choices?
- Who cooks? Knowledge and skill level?
- Refrigeration, storage, and cooking facilities?
- Ability to manage containers: jars, cans, bottles

Psychosocial Factors
- Where are most meals eaten?
- Mealtime companions
- Recent change in living conditions?
- Satisfaction with situation?

*In addition to the normal assessment, that is, appetite or weight changes and bowel habits.

---

height if the person cannot stand and compensatory calculations for clients with missing limbs.

Nutritional assessment tools for use with older adults were developed by the Nutrition Screening Initiative, a joint project of the American Academy of Family Physicians, the American Dietetic Association, and the National Council on Aging, Inc. "Determine Your Nutritional Health" is a self-administered checklist with scoring directions to evaluate risk. The Level I Screening Tool is designed to be administered by professionals in health or social service programs and includes directions for appropriate referrals. These two instruments are reproduced in Appendix C. The Nutrition Screening Initiative also devised a Level II Screening Tool for use in physicians' offices and health-care institutions that includes a clinical examination, skinfold measurements, and laboratory tests (Quinn, 1997).

Implementation

Suggestions to increase the nourishment of elderly clients appear in Box 13–9. Oral supplementation resulted in a mean weight gain of 1.5 kilograms (3.3 pounds) in malnourished nursing home residents over a 60-day period (Lauque et al, 2000). Nutritional supplements may help maintain weight in individuals with poor appetites or eating problems, but a more economical choice may be a liquid breakfast preparation. Protein-energy malnutrition was reversed in one study by serving as much of a favorite food, ice cream, as the client wanted (Winograd and Brown, 1990).

When family members were asked for suggested nutritional interventions, however, liquid oral supplements were fifth of six possible choices. In order of most to least desirable, the family members preferred to (1) improve the quality of the food; (2) improve the quality and quantity of

Box 13–8 Geriatric Mini Nutrition Assessment

Assessment	Score
Has food intake declined over past 3 months due to loss of appetite, digestive problems, or chewing or swallowing difficulties? 0 = severe loss of appetite 1 = moderate 2 = no loss	
Weight loss during last 3 months 0 = >3 kg (6.6 lbs) 1 = unknown 2 = 1 to 3 kg (2.2 to 6.6 lbs) 3 = no weight loss	
Mobility 0 = bed or chair bound 1 = able to get out of bed/chair but does not go out 2 = goes out	
Psychological stress or acute disease in past 3 months 0 = yes 2 = no	
Neuropsychological problems 0 = severe dementia or depression 1 = mild dementia 2 = no psychological problems	
BMI (Weight in kg/Height in m^2) 0 = <19 1 = 19 – 20.9 2 = 21 – 22.9 3 = 23 or more	
Score (Max 14): 12 or more = normal; 11 or less = possible malnutrition, continue assessing	

Alternative Knee to Heel Height Calculation: with knee at 90-degree angle, measure from bottom of heel to top of knee.
Men = (2.02 × knee ht, cm) – (0.04 × age, yr) + 64.19 = ht, cm
Women = (1.83 × knee ht, cm) – (0.24 × age, yr) + 84.88 = ht, cm

Amputees' BMI Calculation: increase scale weight by percentage below.
Single below knee, 6.0%   Single at knee, 9.0%
Single above knee, 15%   Single arm, 6.5% Single below elbow, 3.6%

SOURCE: Rubenstein, 2001. Reprinted with permission.

Box 13–9 Increasing Food Intake in the Elderly

Get the Person Ready for Meals

- Provide oral hygiene before meals to freshen and moisten mouth.
- Suggest smokers refrain for 1 hour before a meal to increase appetite.
- Manage the environment by removing unsightly supplies or noxious waste.
- Allow 60 minutes to elapse after a significant amount of supplement before serving the next meal.

Promote Social Interaction

- Encourage potluck meals with friends for those who live alone.
- Combine meal at senior center with an activity of interest.
- Encourage alert nursing home residents to choose compatible mealtime companions.
- Control the noise in the dining room to avoid overstimulating those with hearing aids.

Serve Food Attractively

- Vary textures, colors, flavors.
- To increase vegetable intake, offer raw, crisp-cooked, or marinated vegetables as appetizers.
- Use "good" dishes and flatware, centerpieces, tablecloths, or placemats.

- Provide enough nonglaring light so food can be seen clearly.

Provide Nutrient-Dense Foods

- Add powdered milk or ice cream to appropriate beverages and foods.
- Increase the eggs, milk, or cheese in recipes.
- Help client to select satisfactory meal-replacer supplements, whether commercial canned products or instant-breakfast powders. When appropriate, offer 1 ounce every hour and use as "chaser" when administering medications.
- If additional kilocalories are needed, choose whole milk for beverages and cooking instead of reduced-fat varieties.
- If milk-based products are unpalatable for the client, explore the use of clear liquid supplements that offer nearly complete nutrition (see Chapter 15).

Obtain Outside Help

- Home health aide to shop, do basic fix-ahead preparations.
- Meals-on-Wheels for homebound.
- Food stamps, surplus commodity programs for those eligible.
- Instructional materials on food purchasing, storage, cooking from county extension services.

feeding assistance; (3) provide multiple small meals and snacks throughout the day; (4) place the resident in a preferred dining location; (5) provide an oral liquid nutritional supplement between meals; and (6) provide a medication to stimulate appetite (Simmons et al, 2003).

In 2003, Medicare and Medicaid rules were altered to permit long-term care facilities to use paid feeding assistants under certain conditions (Centers for Medicare, 2003). Health-care providers should plan occasions to bolster fluid intake in institutionalized elders. Establishing a minimum intake of a minimum of 180 milliliters of fluid with each medication pass or a program to give a resident 60 milliliters of fluid every time a provider enters the room are two such organized programs. Tea parties and serving liquid refreshments at all activities offer opportunities to increase fluid intake (Mentes and Iowa-Veterans, 2000). Increasing physical activity according to the client's ability offers benefits beyond weight control. Physical activity helps to prevent heart disease and hypertension, improves bone mineral density, enhances balance and strength for activities of daily living, and promotes restful sleep. Many individuals, however, report never having been advised to exercise by their health-care providers. An intervention to enable the client to see improvement (or the need for improvement) is the keeping of an activity log (Jones and Jones, 1997).

The nurse's role in nourishing the hospitalized older client undergoing diagnostic tests is elaborated upon in Clinical Application 13–4. Obtaining adequate food for such a client may tax the nurse's ingenuity because of both timing issues and the need to entice a fatigued and perhaps fearful client to eat.

Nutrition Education for Adults

Whether teaching individuals or groups, it is important to address the client's concerns. Designers of programs often use focus groups to shape the offering. Because none of the age groups of adults is remarkable for healthy eating, MyPyramid could be a basic starting point for many clients.

Knowledge is related to behavior and behavior change. Home-delivered meal clients reported positive changes in nutrition knowledge, attitude, and behavior after receiving a single-concept, monthly nutrition newsletter that was delivered with their meals (Fey-Yensan et al, 2002). Teaching clients about the benefits of lower-fat milks and about products to control lactose intolerance when appropriate could assist them in improving their health status. Because the true prevalence of lactose intolerance in the elderly is unknown (Ausman and Russell, 1999) and because dairy products are nutrient-dense, working with elderly clients to improve their intake is a good use of the health-care provider's expertise.

Clinical Application 13–4

Hospitalization of the Elderly

Except for obstetrical and pediatric clients, elderly clients dominate as consumers of health care. Eighty percent of the elderly, compared with 40 percent of individuals under the age of 65 years, have one or more chronic diseases. Frequently elderly clients are admitted to the hospital undernourished, but their situation also worsens during hospitalization. For instance, 21 percent of inpatients consumed less than 50 percent of their calculated maintenance energy requirements, for whom neither canned supplements nor nutritional support were used effectively (Sullivan, Sun, and Walis, 1999).

Serving no food to a client because of diagnostic tests is starvation. The conscientious nurse obtains meals or feedings for a client who is *nil per os*, or NPO (i.e., nothing by mouth) for breakfast and lunch. There is nothing magical about the times of 8 AM, 12 PM, and 6 PM for meals. The committed nurse will arrange for adequate nourishment for clients despite scheduling difficulties. Dietary personnel have no idea when an individual client is finished with tests for the day until notified by the nurse.

Use of a modified Nutrition Screening Initiative checklist identified 68 to 89 percent of elderly people served by congregate or home-delivered meal programs to be at moderate or high risk of malnutrition. The most frequent needs were nutrition counseling, drug/nutrient counseling, and dentition-related problems (Weddle, Wellman, and Bates, 1997). The tools provided in Appendix C can be used to identify learning needs of individual clients as well as to research the status of groups of clients. Recommending supplements for certain groups of people and instruction in the judicious use of those products might help clients modify their major risk factors. Vitamins D and B$_{12}$ and calcium supplements are recommended in the Modified Food Pyramid for 70+ Adults. In general, users of supplements are more likely to have healthier lifestyles than nonusers. Women who use multivitamin and multimineral supplements tend to be white, well-educated, middle-aged or older, with higher incomes, and living in the western states (Jasti, Siega-Riz, and Bentley, 2003).

Most adults could benefit from instruction in the key concepts of nutrition: balance, variety, and moderation. The alert nurse has an important contribution to make in identifying deficient knowledge and impaired health practices related to nutrition. This responsibility applies to all clients receiving nursing care, not only those with obvious nutrition-related medical diagnoses.

SUMMARY

As a group, adult men have better diets, although fewer than half of them consume the recommended number of servings of fruit and dairy products. Women's diets parallel men's except that 50 percent or fewer of women consume the recommended servings of any food group. Their lowest intake is from the dairy group, a fact that has important ramifications for prevention of osteoporosis.

Aging affects almost all body systems, but significant individual differences occur. Older skin is less capable of vitamin D synthesis than that of younger people. The senses deteriorate, leading to difficulty obtaining information from the environment. Loss of teeth, arthritis of the jaw, and slowing of gastrointestinal function may decrease intake and digestion of food and absorption of nutrients. The liver and kidneys become less capable of detoxifying and excreting wastes. Muscular strength diminishes, and in a significant minority of people the bones become osteoporotic. The nervous and endocrine controls become less effective, increasing the older client's risk for dehydration and diabetes mellitus. The cardiovascular and immune systems also are less likely to rebound quickly after stress than in a younger person.

Physical changes are not the only factors to be assessed. Changing social, economic, and physical circumstances affect the nutritional status of the elderly client. When a spouse dies, grief, depression, and poor appetite or lack of culinary skill often affect the survivor. Learning to live on Social Security benefits, a pension, and savings may place a strain on some elderly people.

Some of these factors may be difficult to elicit from the client during the history-taking. The multiple physiologic changes in the elderly client along with the occurrence of chronic diseases in this age group necessitates special care in assessment. Interaction of these many factors could exacerbate a marginal or subclinical deficiency or overdose into a major problem. Any of the cultural traditions associated with food could be important for psychosocial development. Enjoyment of food in the company of others offers opportunities to share one's knowledge and skill and to validate one's own life experiences.

Improving food intake in adults requires them to choose to upgrade their diets. Increasing their awareness and knowledge is the first step. Assisting them to set one or two achievable goals and to select acceptable strategies is likely to be more successful than simply dictating a plan to them (Wellness Tips 13–1).

Wellness Tip **13–1** **DAIRY PRODUCTS**

- To increase intake of calcium and vitamin D, use milk or cheese in sauces, desserts, casseroles, and beverages.
- Try flavored milk for an alternative taste experience.
- Experiment with drinking milk as part of a meal and with lactase products if intolerance is perceived.

- Choose low-fat products unless attempting to gain weight.
- Select calcium fortified foods such as orange juice and ready-to-eat cereals.
- If intake of calcium remains low, consult with health-care provider about supplementation.
- If client is housebound and consuming few vitamin D-fortified foods, consult with health-care provider about supplementation.

FRUITS AND VEGETABLES

- Tally the day's intake: 2 cups of fruit and 2 1/2 cups of vegetables are the minimums for a 2000 kilocalorie diet.
- Eat colorful vegetables: broccoli, spinach, carrots, sweet potatoes.
- Choose a variety of whole fruits rather than juices.
- Once the minimums are achieved, increase the amounts of fruits and vegetables consumed.
- Select fruit for dessert or between-meal snacks.
- Carry vegetables with you to work or play: snack packs of carrots, broccoli, etc.

MEAT AND BEANS

- Choose low-fat or lean meat, fish, and poultry.
- Cook meats, fish, and poultry with little fat: baked, broiled, or grilled.
- Substitute beans, peas, lentils, nuts, and seeds for some of the meat dishes.
- Add beans to dishes; for example, add some canned kidney beans to a tossed salad.
- Serve casseroles and combination dishes to keep meat equivalents to 5 1/2 ounces per day.
- Consult with health-care provider about advisability of vitamin B_{12} supplement if not consuming fortified foods and especially if regularly taking medications that alter gastric acidity.

WHOLE GRAINS

- Eat whole-grain cereals, breads, pastas, and baked products. Look for "whole grain" listed as the first ingredient on the package.
- If current intake is solely refined grains, begin by substituting one whole-grain product daily and increase to a minimum of 3 ounces daily.
- Experiment with various whole grain products to find ones you like.
- Sprinkle wheat germ on cereal, casseroles, salads, and desserts.
- Substitute wheat germ for some of the nuts or flour in a recipe.

CASE STUDY 13–1

Mr. E is a 70-year-old widower who relies on public transportation. His home is two blocks off the bus route and eight blocks from the nearest supermarket. Mr. E has moderately painful knees from arthritis. He has been taking the bus to the supermarket every other day so that he could manage one package on the way home. He has confided to the nurse in his doctor's office that he is ready to "just give up. It's too much trouble to eat anymore." Mr. E's weight today is 160 lb, 5 lb less than last month.

(Continued on the following page)

CASE STUDY (Continued)

NURSING CARE PLAN

SUBJECTIVE DATA   Dependent on public transportation
Painful knees
Verbalized discouragement with procuring food

OBJECTIVE DATA   Weight loss of 5 lb in past month

NURSING DIAGNOSIS   NANDA: Ineffective Health Maintenance (NANDA, 2003, with permission.) related to impaired mobility outside of home, as evidenced by verbalization to nurse and weight loss of 5 lb in past month.

DESIRED OUTCOMES EVALUATION CRITERIA	NURSING ACTIONS/ INTERVENTIONS	RATIONALE
NOC: Health Beliefs: Perceived Resources (Moorhead, Johnson, and Maas, 2004, with permission)	NIC: Health System Guidance (Dochterman and Bulechek, 2004, with permission)	
Mr. E will acknowledge need for assistance with meals to stop losing weight by end of visit today.	Discuss Mr. E's weight change with him. Determine what kind of assistance he would accept.	Clients are likely to change behaviors only if the new behavior is acceptable to them.
Given several options of community support, Mr. E will select one and begin to implement the change within 3 days.	Describe Senior Citizen Nutrition Program, Meals on Wheels, home health aide shopping service, and door-to-door Care-a-Van service.	Clients may know about these programs but prefer to remain independent. Allowing the client some time to choose makes the choice more his own.
	Explore social support available from family and less-restricted friends.	
	Nurse to follow up with telephone call in 3 days.	Following up with a telephone call shows the nurse is committed to working through this problem with Mr. E.

C T Q CRITICAL THINKING QUESTIONS

1. What additional data could be sought in a more comprehensive assessment?
2. What other areas could be investigated to help balance to Mr. E's need for assistance with his desire for independence?

3. As you read this case, how would you define the underlying problem?

⟫⟫ CHAPTER REVIEW

1. The RDA/AI for which of the following nutrients is increased for older adults compared to younger ones?
   a. Sodium
   b. Calcium
   c. Vitamin C
   d. Vitamin K

2. The decrease in gastric acid that accompanies aging causes concern for the absorption of which of the following nutrients?
   a. Carbohydrate and water
   b. Fat and cholesterol
   c. Vitamins A and E
   d. Vitamin B_{12} and iron

3. A nurse making a home visit routinely screens for dehydration in elderly clients. Which of the following would the nurse assess?
   a. Body temperature and urine-specific gravity
   b. Tongue condition, pulse rate, and muscle strength
   c. Skin turgor and heart and lung sounds
   d. Client's intake and output records

4. Which of the following conditions is likely to contribute to vitamin D deficiency in older adults
   a. Atrophied skin, dislike for milk, and indoor life
   b. Lack of exercise, failing hearing and vision
   c. Slowed peristalsis, diminished secretion of intrinsic factor
   d. Achlorhydria and inability to chew meats

5. Ms. P is a 58-year-old retired cook who tells the clinic nurse she regrets not having had children and grandchildren. Which of the following activities might assist Ms. P to attain generativity?
   a. Editing a cookbook for her church group
   b. Taking a class in ethnic cooking in preparation for her next trip
   c. Serving on the Meals-on-Wheels advisory board
   d. Volunteering to teach a special recipe at a local school

CLINICAL ANALYSIS

Ms. O is a 66-year-old retired schoolteacher who suffered a stroke 8 months ago. For the past 7 months she has resided in a nursing home. Ms. O has residual weakness on the right side. She has not mastered the use of tableware with her left hand. Her nurse is concerned because Ms. O weighs 125 pounds; she had weighed 135 pounds upon admission to the nursing home. The nursing assistants report that Ms. O takes a little of most foods but refuses to eat more than half of any of the foods.

1. The nurse discovers that a contributing factor in Ms. O's refusal to eat is embarrassment over her inability to control her lips. Which of the following outcomes would be appropriate in this case?

   a. Client will gain 5 pounds in the next 2 weeks

   b. Client will consume three-fourths of the food served within 1 week

   c. Client will feed herself with her left hand within the next 3 weeks

   d. Client will consent to tube feeding

2. Which of the following nursing actions is appropriate initially to minimize Ms. O's embarrassment?

   a. Allowing her to eat her meals alone in her room

   b. Ordering finger foods that she can eat with her left hand

   c. Assigning her to a table with other stroke clients who feed themselves

   d. Instructing the nursing assistants to feed Ms. O privately

3. Which of the following activities could reasonably be expected to increase Ms. O's appetite?

   a. Participating in a craft session before lunch

   b. Taking a nap before dinner

   c. Walking before lunch or dinner

   d. Watching television with her roommate after breakfast

REFERENCES

Ahluwalia, N, et al: Immune function is impaired in iron-deficient, homebound, older women. Am J Clin Nutr 79:516, 2004.

Aldrich, L, and Variyam, JN: Acculturation erodes the diet quality of U.S. Hispanics. Food Rev 23:51, 2000.

Andersson, I, and Sidenvall, B: Case studies of food shopping, cooking and eating habits in older women with Parkinson's disease. J Adv Nurs 35:69, 2001.

Andrade, SE, et al: Low frequency of treatment of osteoporosis among postmenopausal women following a fracture. Arch Intern Med 163:2052, 2003.

Anusavice, KJ: Dental caries: Risk assessment and treatment solutions for an elderly population. Compend Contin Educ Dent 23(Suppl):12, 2002.

Arthritis Foundation and Centers for Disease Control: National Arthritis Action Plan. Arthritis Foundation, Atlanta, 1999. Accessed April 22, 2004 at http://www.arthritis.org/resources/ActionPlanInterior.pdf.

Artz, AS, et al: Mechanisms of unexplained anemia in the nursing home. J Am Geriatr Soc 52:423, 2004.

Ausman, LM, and Russell, RM: Nutrition in the elderly. In Shils, ME, et al (eds): Modern Nutrition in Health and Disease, ed 9. Lippincott, Williams & Wilkins, Philadelphia, 1999.

Avenell, A, and Handoll, HHG: Nutritional supplementation for hip fracture aftercare in the elderly. Cochrane Database Syst Rev 1:CD001880, 2005.

Biernacki, C, and Barratt, J: Improving the nutritional status of people with dementia. Br J Nurs 10:1104, 2001.

Bischoff-Ferrari, et al: Effect of vitamin D on falls. JAMA 291:1999, 2004.

Booth, SL, et al: Dietary vitamin K intakes are associated with hip fracture but not with bone mineral density in elderly men and women. Am J Clin Nutr 71:1201, 2000.

Booth, SL, et al: Vitamin K intake and bone mineral density in women and men. Am J Clin Nutr 77:572, 2003.

Booth, SL, and Mayer, J: Warfarin use and fracture risk. Nutr Rev 58:20, 2000.

Braithwaite, RS, Col, NF, and Wong, JB: Estimating hip fracture morbidity, mortality, and costs. J Am Geriatr Soc 51:364, 2003.

Brown, JE: Nutrition Through the Life Cycle, ed 2. Thomson Wadsworth, Belmont, CA, 2005.

Bush, LA, et al: D-E-N-T-A-L: A rapid self-administered screening instrument to promote referrals for further evaluation in older adults. J Am Geriatr Soc 44:979, 1996.

Calder, PC: Dietary modification of inflammation with lipids. Proc Nutr Soc 61:345, 2002.

Centers for Disease Control: Prevalence of no leisure-time physical activity—35 states and the District of Columbia, 1988–2002. MMWR 53:82, 2004a. http://www.cdc.gov/mmwr/preview/mmwrhtml/mm5304a4.htm.

Centers for Disease Control: United States Life Tables, 2001. Natl Vital Stat Rep 52:1, 2004b.

Centers for Disease Control: Public health and aging: Projected prevalence of self-reported arthritis or chronic joint symptoms among persons aged ≥65 years—United States, 2005–2030. MMWR 52:489, 2003a. Accessed April 22, 2004 at http://www.cdc.gov/mmwr/preview/mmwrhtml/mm5221a1.htm.

Centers for Disease Control: Public health and aging: Trends in aging—United States and worldwide. MMWR 52:101, 2003b. Accessed April 15, 2004 at http://www.cdc.gov/mmwr/preview/mmwrhtml/mm5206a2.htm.

Centers for Medicare & Medicaid Services: Requirements for paid feeding assistants in long term care facilities final rule. Fed Regist 68:55528, 2003.

Cervantes-Laurean, D, McElvaney, NG, and Moss, J: Niacin. In Shils, ME, et al (eds): Modern Nutrition in Health and Disease, ed 9. Lippincott Williams & Wilkins, Philadelphia, 1999.

Chapman, IM, et al: The anorexia of ageing. Biogerontology 3:67, 2002.

Coleman, EA, et al: Pressure ulcer prevalence in long-term nursing home residents since the implementation of OBRA '87: Omnibus Budget Reconciliation Act. J Am Geriatr Soc 50:728, 2002.

Collins, N: Involuntary weight loss in the long-term care setting: a suggested nutritional intervention treatment algorithm. Wounds 13:32D, 2001.

Cree, MW, Juby, AG, and Carriere, KC: Mortality and morbidity associated with osteoporosis drug treatment following hip fracture. Osteoporos Int 14:722, 2003.

Darlington, LG, and Stone, TW: Antioxidants and fatty acids in the amelioration of rheumatoid arthritis and related disorders. Br J Nutr 85:251, 2001.

DePaola, DP, Faine, MP, and Palmer, CA: Nutrition in relation to dental medicine. In Shils, ME, et al (eds): Modern Nutrition in Health and Disease, ed 9. Lippincott Williams & Wilkins, Philadelphia, 1999.

Denney, A: Quiet music: An intervention for mealtime agitation? J Gerontol Nurs 23:16, 1997.

Dochterman, J, and Bulechek, G (eds): Nursing Interventions Classification (NIC), ed 4. Mosby, St. Louis, 2004.

Elbon, SM, et al: Demographic factors, nutrition knowledge, and health-seeking behaviors influence nutrition label reading behaviors among older American adults. J Nutr Elderly 19:31, 2000.

Ervin, RB, and Kennedy-Stephenson, J: Mineral intakes of elderly adult supplement and non-supplement users in the third national health and nutrition examination survey. J Nutr 132: 3422, 2002.

Ferguson, M, et al: Pressure ulcer management: the importance of nutrition. MEDSURG Nurs 9:163, 2000.

Feskanich, D, et al: Vitamin K intake and hip fractures among post-menopausal women. JAMA 287:47, 2002.

Fey-Yensan, N, et al: Evaluation of a nutrition education newsletter for home-delivered meal participants J Nutr Elderly 21:39, 2002.

Friedmann, JM, et al: Predicting early nonelective hospital read-mission in nutritionally compromised older adults. Am J Clin Nutr 65:1714, 1997.

Gardner, MJ, et al: Improvement in the undertreatment of osteo-porosis following hip fracture. J Bone Joint Surg Am 84-A:1342, 2002.

Gehlbach, SH, et al: Recognition of vertebral fracture in a clinical setting. Osteoporos Int 11:577, 2000.

Green, MW, Taylor, MA, and Elliman, NA: Glucose: Cognition: Placebo effect. Brit J Nutr 86:173, 2001.

Habel, M: Osteoarthritis: A new look at an old disease. Nurse Week Dec-Jan:8, 2000–2001.

Hamrick, I: Vitamin B$_{12}$ deficiency in the elderly: A new look at treatment. Fam Pract Recertif 25:16, 2003.

Harrington, JT, et al: Hip fracture patients are not treated for osteo-porosis: A call to action. Arthritis Rheum 47:651, 2002.

Hebert, LE, et al: Alzheimer disease in the US population: Prevalence estimates using the 2000 census. Arch Neurol 60:1119, 2003.

Heiat, A, Vaccarino, V, and Krumholz, HM: An evidence-based assessment of federal guidelines for overweight and obesity as they apply to elderly persons. Arch Intern Med 161:1194, 2001.

Hillier, TA, et al: Nulliparity and fracture risk in older women: The study of osteoporotic fractures. J Bone Miner Res 18:893, 2003.

Janssen, HCJ, Samson, MM, and Verhaar, HJJ: Vitamin D deficiency, muscle function, and falls in elderly people. Am J Clin Nutr 75:611, 2002.

Jasti, S, Siega-Riz, AM, and Bentley, ME: Dietary supplement use in the context of health disparities: Cultural, ethnic and demo-graphic determinants of use. J Nutr 133:2010S, 2003.

Jensen, GL, et al: Noncompliance with body weight measurement in tertiary care teaching hospitals. JPEN J Parenter Enteral Nutr 27:89, 2003.

Johnson, KA, Bernard, MA, and Funderburg, K: Vitamin nutrition in older adults. Clin Geriatr Med 18:773, 2002.

Johnson, LJ, and McCool, AC: Dietary intake and nutritional status of older adult homeless women: A pilot study. J Nutr Elderly 23:1, 2003.

Jones, JM, and Jones, KD: Promoting physical activity in the sen-ior years. J Gerontol Nurs 23:40, 1997.

Juby, AG, and De Geus-Wenceslau, CM: Evaluation of osteoporosis treatment in seniors after hip fracture. Osteoporos Int 13:205, 2002.

Kayser-Jones, J, and Schell, E: The mealtime experience of a cog-nitively impaired elder: Ineffective and effective strategies. J Gerontol Nurs 23:33, 1997.

Krall, EA, and Dawson-Hughes, B: Osteoporosis. In Shils, ME, et al (eds): Modern Nutrition in Health and Disease, ed 9. Lippincott Williams & Wilkins, Philadelphia, 1999.

Kubota, M, et al: Alcohol consumption and frontal lobe shrinkage: Study of 1432 non-alcoholic subjects. J Neurol Neurosurg Psychiatry 71:104, 2001.

Larsen, ER, Mosekilde, L, and Foldspang, A: Vitamin D and calcium supplementation prevents osteoporotic fractures in elderly community dwelling residents: A pragmatic population-based 3-year intervention study. J Bone Miner Res 19:370, 2004.

Larson, K: Fluid balance in the elderly: Assessment and interven-tion—Important role in community health and home care nurs-ing. Geriatr Nurs 24:306, 2003.

Lauque, S, et al: Protein-energy oral supplementation in malnour-ished nursing-home residents: A controlled trial. Age Ageing 29:51, 2000.

Lee, JS, and Frongillo, EA, Jr: Factors associated with food insecu-rity among U.S. elderly persons: Importance of functional impairments. J Gerontol B Psychol Sci Soc Sci 56:S94, 2001a.

Lee, JS, and Frongillo, EA, Jr: Nutritional and health consequences are associated with food insecurity among U.S. elderly persons. J Nutr 131:1503, 2001b.

Lesourd, B: Nutrition: A major factor influencing immunity in the elderly. J Nutr Health Aging 8:28, 2004.

Lips, P: Hypervitaminosis A and fractures. N Engl J Med 348:347, 2003.

Luckey, AE, and Parsa, CJ: Fluid and electrolytes in the aged. Arch Surg 138:1955, 2003.

Malouf, R, and Areosa Sastre, A: Vitamin B$_{12}$ for cognition. Cochrane Database Syst Rev 3:CD004326, 2003.

Martin, A, et al: Effects of fruits and vegetables on levels of vita-mins E and C in the brain and their association with cognitive performance. J Nutr Health Aging 6:392, 2002.

Martini, L, and Wood, RJ: Relative bioavailability of calcium-rich dietary sources in the elderly. Am J Clin Nutr 76:1345, 2002.

Mathus-Vliegen, EM: Old age, malnutrition, and pressure sores: An ill-fated alliance. J Gerontol A Biol Sci Med Sci 59:355, 2004.

McDougall, J, et al: Effects of a very low-fat, vegan diet in sub-jects with rheumatoid arthritis. J Altern Complement Med 8:71, 2002.

Melton, LJ, 3rd: Adverse outcomes of osteoporotic fractures in the general population. J Bone Miner Res 18:1139, 2003.

Mentes, JC, and Iowa-Veterans Affairs Research Consortium. Hydration management protocol. J Gerontol Nurs 26:6, 2000.

Meydani, M: The Boyd Orr lecture: Nutrition interventions in aging and age-associated disease. Proc Nutr Soc 61:165, 2002.

Meyer, HE, et al: Can vitamin D supplementation reduce the risk of fracture in the elderly? A randomized controlled trial. J Bone Miner Res 17:709, 2002.

Moorhead, S, Johnson, M, and Maas, M (eds): Nursing Outcomes Classification (NOC), ed 3. Mosby, St. Louis, 2004.

Morley, JE: Anorexia of aging: Physiologic and pathologic. Am J Clin Nutr 66:760, 1997.

Morley, JE, and Thomas, DR: Development of guidelines for the use of orexigenic drugs in long-term care. Cyberounds Continuing Education. Accessed April 13, 2004 at http://www.cyberounds. com/conf/geriatrics/2003-06-05/print.html.

Morris, MC, et al: Relation of the tocopherol forms to incident Alzheimer disease and to cognitive change. Am J Clin Nutr 81:508, 2005.

Morrisson, SG: Feeding the elderly population. Nurs Clin North Am 32:791, 1997.

NANDA International: Nursing Diagnoses: Definitions and Classi-fication, 2003–2004. NANDA International, Philadelphia, 2003.

National Live Stock and Meat Board: Eating in America Today, ed 2. Chicago, 1995.

Nieves, JW: Calcium, vitamin D, and nutrition in elderly adults. Clin Geriatr Med 19:321, 2003.

Nowjack-Raymer, RE, and Sheiham, A: Association of edentulism and diet and nutrition in US adults. J Dent Res 82:123, 2003.

Opotowsky, AR, Su, BW, and Bilezikian, JP: Height and lower extremity length as predictors of hip fracture: Results of the NHANES I Epidemiologic Follow-up Study. J Bone Miner Res 18:1674, 2003.

Parkinson's Disease Backgrounder. National Institute of Neuro-logical Disorders and Stroke. Accessed April 17, 2004 at http:// www.ninds.nih.gov/health_and_medical/pubs/parkinson's_ disease_backgrounder.htm.

Pfefferbaum, A, et al: In vivo brain concentrations of N-acetyl compounds, creatine, and choline in Alzheimer disease. Arch Gen Psychiatry 56:185, 1999.

Pimentel, L: Scurvy: Historical review and current diagnostic approach. Am J Emerg Med 21:328, 2003.

Promislow, JH, et al: Retinol intake and bone mineral density in the elderly: The Rancho Bernardo Study. J Bone Miner Res 17:1349, 2002.

Quinn, C: The Nutrition Screening Initiative: Meeting the nutri-tional needs of elders. Orthop Nurs 16:13, 1997.

Rennie, KL, et al: Nutritional management of rheumatoid arthritis: a review of the evidence. J Hum Nutr Diet 16:97, 2003.

Richmond, J, et al: Mortality risk after hip fracture. J Orthop Trauma 17:53, 2003.

Robinson, SB, and Rosher, RB: Can a beverage cart help improve hydration? Geriatr Nurs 23:208, 2002.

Rosell, PA, and Parker, MJ: Functional outcome after hip fracture: A 1-year prospective outcome study of 275 patients. Injury 34:529, 2003.

Rubenstein, LZ, et al: Screening for undernutrition in geriatric practice: Developing the short-form mini-nutritional assessment (MNA-SF). J Gerontol A Biol Sci Med Sci 56:M366, 2001.

Russell, L: The importance of patients' nutritional status in wound healing. Br J Nurs 10:S42, 2001.

Russell, RM, Rasmussen, H, and Lichtenstein, AH: Modified food guide pyramid for people over 70 years of age. J Nutr 129:751, 1999.

Sahyoun, NR, et al: The Changing Profile of Nursing Home Residents: 1985–1997. Aging Trends, No. 4. National Center for Health Statistics, Hyattsville, MD, 2001. Accessed May 5, 2005 at http://www.cdc.gov/nchs/data/agingtrends/04nursin.pdf.

Scholl, D, and Langkamp-Henken, B: Nutrient recommendations for wound healing. J Intravenous Nurs 24:124, 2001.

Serafini, M: Dietary vitamin E and T cell-mediated function in the elderly: Effectiveness and mechanism of action. Int J Devl Neuroscience 18:401, 2000.

Shahar, DR, et al: The effect of widowhood on weight changes, dietary intake, and eating behavior in the elderly population. J Aging Health 13:189, 2001.

Sharkey, JR, et al: Inadequate nutrient intakes among homebound elderly and their correlation with individual characteristics and health-related factors. Am J Clin Nutr 76:1435, 2002.

Simmons, SF, et al: Family members' preferences for nutrition interventions to improve nursing home residents' oral food and fluid intake. J Am Geriatr Soc 51:69, 2003.

Simopoulos, AP: Omega-3 fatty acids in inflammation and autoimmune diseases. J Am Coll Nutr 21:495, 2002.

Slemenda, C: Prevention of hip fractures: Risk factor modification. Am J Med 103:65S, 1997.

Stephen, R, and Utecht, T: Scurvy identified in the emergency department: A case report. J Emerg Med 21:2235, 2001.

Stevens, JA, and Olson, S: Reducing falls and resulting hip fractures among older women. MMWR Recomm Rep 49 (RR2): 3, 2000.

Sullivan, DH, Bopp, MM, and Roberson, PK: Protein-energy under-nutrition and life-threatening complications among the hospitalized elderly. J Gen Intern Med 17:923, 2002.

Sullivan, DH, Sun, S, and Walls, RC: Protein-energy undernutrition among elderly hospitalized patients: A prospective study. JAMA 281:2013, 1999.

Taste sensation. Nutrition News Focus, March 5, 2002. Accessed April 16, 2004 at http://www.nutritionnewsfocus.com/.

Thomas, DR, and Morley, JE: Regulation of appetite in older adults. Cyberounds Continuing Education. Accessed November 20, 2002 at http://www.cyberounds.com/conferences/geriatrics/conferences/current/conference.html.

Tully, MW, et al: The Eating Behavior Scale: A simple method of assessing functional ability in patients with Alzheimer's disease. J Gerontol Nurs 23:9, 1997.

U.S. Department of Agriculture Center for Nutrition Policy and Promotion: A focus on nutrition for the elderly: It's time to take a closer look. Nutrition Insights 14, July 1999.

U.S. Department of Agriculture Center for Nutrition Policy and Promotion: Food insufficiency and prevalence of overweight among adult women. Nutrition Insights 26, July 2002.

U.S. Department of Agriculture. Pyramid Servings Data: 1994–96 Continuing Survey of Food Intakes by Individuals. February 1999. Accessed October 5, 1999 at http://www.barc.usda.gov.

VanDusen, KC, and London, ML: Orange plates increase food intake of dementia patients: Poster presentation at American Dietetic Association Food and Nutrition Conference and Expo. San Antonio, TX, October 26, 2003.

Vanitallie, TB: Frailty in the elderly: Contributions of sarcopenia and visceral protein depletion. Metabolism 52(Suppl 2):22, 2003.

Weddle, DO, Wellman, NS, and Bates, GM: Incorporating nutrition screening into three Older Americans Act elderly nutrition programs. J Nutr Elderly 17:19, 1997.

Wehren, IE, et al: Gender differences in mortality after hip fracture: The role of infection. J Bone Miner Res 18:2231, 2003.

Welch, P, Porter, J, and Endres, J: Efficacy of a medication pass supplement program in long-term care compared to a traditional system. J Nutr Elderly 22:19, 2003.

Wendland, BE, et al: Malnutrition in institutionalized seniors: The iatrogenic component. J Am Geriatr Soc 51:85, 2003.

Whittington, K, Patrick, M, and Roberts, JL: A national study of pressure ulcer prevalence and incidence in acute care hospitals. J Wound Ostomy Continence Nurs 27:209, 2000.

Winograd, CH, and Brown, EM: Aggressive oral refeeding in hospitalized patients. Am J Clin Nutr 52:967, 1990.

Zhang, SM, et al: Intakes of vitamins E and C, carotenoids, vitamin supplements, and PD risk. Neurology 59:1161, 2002.

CHAPTER 14

Food Management

Learning Objectives

After completing this chapter, the student should be able to:

1. Describe the conditions under which microbiologic food illnesses can occur.
2. Discuss the information on food labels.
3. Identify foods that are likely to harbor disease-producing microbiologic organisms.
4. Describe one systematic approach to identify nutritional hazards in a person's diet.
5. Teach clients how to prevent food-borne illnesses.

Effective meal management requires knowledge about food safety, including microbiological hazards, environmental pollutants, natural food intoxicants, and nutritional hazards. How food is handled between the time it leaves the farm and the time it reaches the dinner table affects our health and well-being. Consumers also are concerned about methods used to grow crops and raise animals. As health care moves from institutions to home care, health-care workers need to understand the vital importance to human well-being of safe and nutritious food.

Each American eats more than 10,000 pounds of food each year. Considering the number of people involved in the growth, distribution, preparation, and service of food, our food safety record is excellent. The food supply in the United States is as safe, wholesome, and nutritious as any in the world.

Food safety is a concern not just here in the United States but also worldwide. Some food handling and consumption behaviors that were practiced 10 years ago are not considered safe today. New strains of pathogens or disease-producing organisms are continually evolving; in some cases, these organisms have proven resistant to antibiotics. The development of resistant food-borne pathogens has been attributed to increased use of antibiotics in hospitals, outpatient facilities, and veterinary applications (Wegener et al, 1999). See Figure 14–1 for food-borne disease outbreaks in the United States from 1993 to 1997 by reported contributing factor.

The Food and Drug Administration (FDA) has developed a list of food safety problems. Problems are ranked in descending order of importance, based on the number of people affected by the problem and its severity:

1. Microbiologic hazards
2. Nutritional hazards
3. Environmental pollutants
4. Natural food intoxicants
5. Food additives

The most common food-borne illnesses are caused when microbiological microorganisms that are naturally present in the environment contaminate food and are allowed to grow because of improper food handling. This chapter discusses each of the FDA's food safety concerns.

Microbiologic Hazards

Many organisms in our environment cause disease, including bacteria and parasites, viruses, and fungi. These microorganisms may be carried from one host to another by animals, humans, inanimate objects including food, and environmental factors, such as air, water, and soil. Many

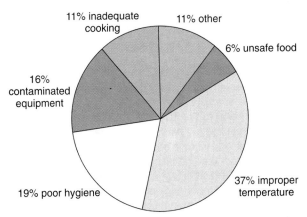

Figure **14–1** Food-borne disease outbreaks by contributing factor in the United States from 1993 through 1997.

microorganisms cause disease. Under certain conditions, food can become a vehicle for disease transmission.

Most food-borne diseases infect the tissues of the digestive tract and cause gastric distress; symptoms range from mild to severe. Mild symptoms include gastric and intestinal distress with abdominal pain, nausea, vomiting, diarrhea, and cramps. Severe symptoms include dehydration, bloody stools, and neurological disorders.

Prevalence and Costs

An estimated 76 million people contract food-borne diseases each year in the United States, resulting in 325,000 hospitalizations and 5000 deaths (Goldrick, 2003). Hospitalization is estimated to cost 3 billion dollars annually, with lost productivity costs estimated to range between 20 and 40 billion dollars per year (Food Safety, Healthy People 2010, 2004). Despite these large numbers and enormous costs, the U.S. government has reported that the incidence of several bacterial food-borne illnesses has decreased since 1976. These declines were attributed to increased government commitment to food safety (U.S. Department of Health and Human Services, 2002). Young, old, pregnant, and immunocompromised clients (YOPI)—25 percent of the U.S. population—are at the greatest risk. Clinical Application 14–1 discusses clients with suppressed immune systems.

Bacterial Food-Borne Disease

Bacteria are everywhere and account for 90 percent of all food-borne disease. Doorknobs, countertops, hands, eyelashes, mouths, some water supplies, and food are a few of the many places where bacteria can be found. Animal and human fluids and waste harbor bacteria and cause many food-borne illnesses.

Clinical Application 14–1

Food Safety and Immunosuppressed Clients

All clients receiving immunosuppressive agents need counseling on food safety and sanitation. These clients have an inability to fight infections, so a relatively small number of bacteria could cause illness. **Immunosuppressive agents** are drugs that interfere with the body's ability to fight infections. These drugs are used in tissue and organ transplantation procedures, such as a kidney transplant. They are also used in controlling certain diseases.

AIDS (acquired immune deficiency syndrome) is caused by a virus. This virus permits infections, malignancies, and nervous system disorders to develop out of control. According to the FDA, AIDS clients are 300 times more likely than healthy persons to contract a *Salmonella* infection if the organism is present. Preventing food illness from occurring in the first place will save these patients much expense and suffering. All clients with AIDS need instruction on the importance of good hand washing and personal hygiene. Proper instruction on food selection, storage, and preparation is also indicated.

On one square inch of our bodies live as many as 10,000 bacteria. Although a large number of bacteria cause disease, most are harmless and many are helpful. Bacteria that cause disease are called **pathogens,** and bacteria that are not harmful are called normal flora. Normal flora help keep pathogenic bacteria from multiplying as rapidly as they might otherwise.

Bacteria are hearty, and scientists have found colonies thriving 1600 feet below sea level with neither oxygen nor sunlight. Given sufficient time and the right conditions, most bacteria adapt to a new environment in 2 hours. For this reason, control of bacterial growth is vital.

Conditions for Growth

Bacterial growth refers to an increase in the number of organisms. Under ideal conditions, cell numbers can double every half hour: one cell becomes two, two become four, and four become eight (in an hour and a half). A single bacterium can multiply to 33 million after 12 hours. Bacteria cannot be eradicated from our environment. The growth of bacteria, however, can be controlled. For this reason, it is important to understand the conditions that are necessary for bacteria to grow. The following conditions are necessary for microbiological food illness to occur:

- Source of bacteria—The bacteria must come in contact with the food.
- Food—The food must permit the bacteria to grow and increase in number or produce a poisonous toxin.
- Temperature—The temperature must be favorable for the growth of bacteria. The temperature range in which most bacteria multiply rapidly is 40°F to 140°F, the range that includes room temperature and body temperature (Fig. 14–2).
- Time—Enough time must elapse for bacteria to grow, produce a toxin, or both.
- Moisture—Bacteria need water to dissolve and digest food. Foods that contain water support the growth of bacteria better than do dehydrated foods.
- Ingestion—An unsuspecting person must eat the food or drink the beverage that contains the toxin or bacteria.

Bacteria are frequently odorless, tasteless, and colorless. Without laboratory analysis, there is no way to tell whether a food will cause illness. Bacterial food-borne diseases are traditionally subdivided into two groups, food infections and food intoxication. Table 14–1 lists pathogens of both groups, foods linked to these organisms, and manifestations.

Food Infections

A **food infection** is an illness caused by eating a food containing a large number of disease-producing bacteria. Symptoms of food infections usually start 12 to 36 hours after consumption of the offending food. Probably the best-known genus of bacteria causing food-borne illness is *Salmonella.* The infection, called **salmonellosis,** is transmitted by the consumption of contaminated foods or contact with an infected person. One study found that 20 percent of samples of ground meat obtained in

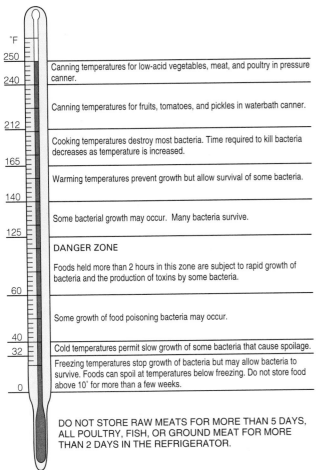

Figure **14–2** A temperature guide to food safety. (Source: USDA, 2000)

supermarkets were contaminated with *Salmonella* (White and Benbrook, 2001). Some foods support the growth of *Salmonella* better than others. See Clinical Application 14–2 for guidelines on the safe handling of eggs, a common vehicle for *Salmonella* transmission. Typhoid fever is caused by one type of *Salmonella bacteria*. This illness is

spread by food and water contaminated by feces and urine of clients and carriers. Figures 14–3 and 14–4 illustrate *Streptococci* and *Salmonella typhimurium*.

Other types of bacteria also cause food infections. *Campylobacter jejuni* should be a concern for consumers. This organism is carried in the intestinal tracts of cows, hogs, sheep, and poultry. Contaminated water or raw manure can spread the organism. For example, an animal can defecate on a vegetable garden and contaminate the produce. Foods found to be contaminated with *Campylobacter jejuni* include raw milk, fresh mushrooms, and raw hamburger. ***Campylobacter*** can be controlled by keeping food below 40°F or above 140°F and by maintaining good food-handling practices.

Another emerging pathogen is *Listeria*. This organism is problematic because the bacteria can grow slowly at refrigerator temperatures (32°F to 34°F) and on moist surfaces. Cooking facilities must be kept clean and dry to prevent the growth of this organism. One household compound effective in inhibiting or inactivating this organism is chlorine (bleach), one tablespoon per gallon of water. According to the Centers for Disease Control, pregnant women are 20 times more likely than other healthy adults to get listeriosis (www.cdc.gov. accessed January 2004). Hormonal changes during pregnancy have an effect on the mother's immune system that lead to an increased susceptibility to listeriosis in the mother. Listeriosis can be transmitted to the fetus through the placenta. This can lead to premature delivery, miscarriage, stillbirth, or serious health problems for the newborn. The USDA Food Safety and Inspection Service (FSIS) and the U.S. Food and Drug Administration provide the following guidelines for the pregnant woman:

- Do not eat hot dogs, luncheon meats, or deli meats unless they are reheated until steaming hot.
- Do not eat soft cheeses such as feta, Brie, Camembert, blue-veined cheeses, and Mexican-style cheeses such as queso blanco fresco. Hard cheeses, such as mozzarella, pasteurized processed cheese slices, and spreads, cream cheese, and cottage cheese may be safely consumed.

Table **14–1**   **Pathogens, Common Food Vehicles, and Symptoms**

PATHOGEN	COMMON FOOD VEHICLES	SYMPTOMS
Salmonella/Food Infection	Raw eggs, raw milk, poultry, red meat, ground beef	Sudden onset of headache, abdominal pain, diarrhea, nausea, and vomiting. Dehydration may be severe, and fever is usually present. May develop into septicemia.
Listeria/Food Infection	Soft cheeses, deli meats, pâté, burritos, ice cream	Meningoencephalitis and/or septicemia in newborns and adults and abortion in pregnant women.
Escherichia coli 0157:H7/ Food Infection	Ground beef, other beef, raw milk, unpasteurized apple juice	May lead to acute hemorrhagic colitis (cramps, bloody diarrhea, nausea, vomiting, and fever). May result in hemolytic uremic failure or kidney failure.
Campylobacter *jejuni*/ Food Infection	Poultry, beef, raw eggs, water	An acute gastroenteritis of variable severity characterized by diarrhea, abdominal pain, malaise, fever, nausea, and vomiting. Guillain-Barre syndrome or meningitis has been seen in severe cases.

(Continued on the following page)

Table **14–1** **Pathogens, Common Food Vehicles, and Symptoms** *(Continued)*

PATHOGEN	COMMON FOOD VEHICLES	SYMPTOMS
Norwalk Virus/Food Infection	Raw shellfish and salad ingredients in the United States; rehydrated cereals, grains, legumes, and nuts worldwide	Usually a self-limited mild to moderate disease with nausea, vomiting, diarrhea, abdominal pain, headache, malaise, and low-grade fever.
Staphylococcus aureus/ Food Intoxication	Poultry, processed meats, cheeses, ice cream, mixed dishes such as potato salad, spaghetti	Wide variety of syndromes with manifestations such as skin lesions, lung or brain abscess, and endocarditis. May lead to Ritter syndrome (an inflammatory skin disease seen in newborns, characterized by pustules that fill with a straw-colored fluid and become encrusted).
Clostridium botulinum/ Food Intoxication	Improperly processed canned food; large masses of food with air-free center	Acute bilateral cranial nerve impairment and descending weakness or paralysis. Double vision, dysphasia, and dry mouth may be present. Vomiting, diarrhea, or constipation may be present initially.

- Do not eat refrigerated pâté or meat spreads. Canned or shelf-stable pâté and meat spreads may be eaten.
- Do not eat refrigerated smoked seafood unless it is an ingredient in a cooked dish such as a casserole. Canned fish such as salmon and tuna or shelf-stable smoked seafood may be safely eaten.
- Do not drink raw (unpasteurized) milk or eat foods that contain unpasteurized milk.

Infection with **Clostridium perfringens** is characterized by intense abdominal cramps and diarrhea that usually begin 8 to 22 hours after consumption of the contaminated food or beverage. Careful control of a food's temperature and good personal hygiene help protect a person from infection.

Food Intoxication

Food intoxication is an illness caused by the consumption of a food in which bacteria have produced a poisonous toxin. One of the most common species of bacteria that produce a poisonous toxin is **Staphylococcus aureus**, often referred to simply as staph. Staph have been reported to be in the nasal passages of 30 to 50 percent of healthy people and on the hands of 20 percent of all healthy people. Infected cuts, boils, and burns harbor this organism. Heat destroys the bacteria but not the toxins the bacteria already have produced. Because heat does not

destroy the toxin, control of temperature alone will not provide protection. Prevention of staph poisoning must include good personal hygiene and keeping foods below 40°F or above 140°F.

Clostridium botulinum is another bacterium that produces a toxin. The resulting disease is **botulism.** The organism is found in soils throughout the world and can be found in the intestinal tracts of domestic animals. Vegetables grown in contaminated soil harbor this organism. Botulin, the toxin produced by *C. botulinum*, is so

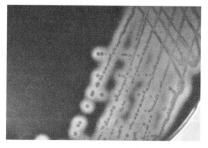

Figure **14–3** *Streptococci.* (Source: Venes, D [ed]: Taber's Cyclopedic Medical Dictionary, ed 19. FA Davis, Philadelphia, 2001, p 191.)

Clinical Application 14–2

Guidelines for the Safe Handling of Eggs

- Prepare eggs individually. For example, individually prepared and immediately served poached, soft-cooked, and over-easy eggs with a partially set yolk are a low-risk way to eat eggs.
- Serve eggs soon after preparation. Do not hold longer than necessary. Do not cook, chill, hold, and reheat unless temperature is tightly maintained (below 50°F or greater than 140°F).
- Refrigerate eggs. Keep eggs at less than 45°F, both shell eggs and mixtures. Egg should not remain out of refrigeration for more than 1 hour.
- Do not use eggs with cracks or leaks. Inspect each egg individually.
- Use a pasteurized egg product if procedures require pooling or undercooked/raw eggs. Pasteurized is safer, but be aware that pasteurized eggs must also be handled with care. Time/temperature abuse is still a factor: they must be thawed under refrigeration or kept refrigerated—the egg is still a perfect medium for bacteria.
- Cook eggs adequately. Cooking for any amount of time reduces the number of bacteria present. In general, cook eggs until the white is set and the yolk begins to thicken. The white coagulates between 144°F and 149°F and the yolk between 149°F and 158°F. Eggs are pasteurized at 140°F for 3 1/2 minutes.

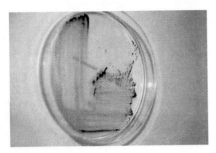

Figure **14-4** *Salmonella.* (Source: Venes, D [ed]: Taber's Cyclopedic Medical Dictionary, ed 19. FA Davis, Philadelphia, 2001, p 191.)

poisonous that a single ounce would be enough to kill the world's population. The spores of *C. botulinum* grow under anaerobic (without air) conditions. Canned foods are processed to be anaerobic; thus they provide an ideal medium for the growth of this bacterium. Home-canned, nonacid fruits and vegetables, faultily processed commercially canned tuna, and improperly packaged smoked fish all have transmitted botulism.

Outbreaks of botulism disease have been linked to changes is food preparation and processing. In botulism, the anaerobic organism secretes a toxin in airtight food packages. The source has classically been considered to be home-canned, nonacid fruits and vegetables. But other sources have been found. Years ago in Alaska, botulism was traced to the substitution of plastic bags for clay pots in the preparation of a Native American dish. Similarly, smoked fish packaged in plastic bags rather than in waxed paper and wooden crates was identified as the source of the disease in Michigan. More recently, in 1994, the largest outbreak of botulism in the United States since 1978 was documented in El Paso, Texas. Thirty people who ate a potato-based dip in a Greek restaurant became ill, four of whom required mechanical ventilation. The source of the type A botulism toxin was found to be baked potatoes wrapped in aluminum foil and stored at room temperature for several days before they were incorporated into the dip.

Botulism can be avoided by the proper processing and preparation of susceptible foods. Home canners should consult a reliable home-canning food guide regarding proper time, pressure, and temperature required to kill spores for each specific food. As an additional precaution, all home-canned foods should be boiled for at least 10 minutes before serving to destroy botulinal toxins.

Norwalk virus is another emerging pathogen that can withstand freezing temperatures and also chlorine solutions. This organism, however, is susceptible to high temperatures (above 140°F). The best insurance against this pathogen is to eat foods hot. Other control measures include good personal hygiene and the purchase of food and water from reliable sources.

Bacterial Food-Borne Disease

The following complicates the risk of food-borne illness:

- The worldwide overuse of antibiotics. Antibiotics kill not only pathogens but also normal flora, which help keep the disease-producing organisms in balance. If an antibiotic is overused, it loses its effectiveness in killing disease-producing bacteria, because in response to the antibiotics "attack," some of the bacteria undergo genetic mutations that make them strong enough to fight off the action of the drug. This leads to the emergence of antimicrobial resistance in human populations and is a public health problem of continually growing importance.

Some experts believe the overuse of antibacterial soap and sanitizing agents is leading to the development of bacteria that will be able to withstand the action of antibacterial agents. New strains of pathogens can evolve and become resistant to antibacterial agents in 90 days, yet it takes humans hundreds of thousands of years to build the immunity to fight them. For this reason, some experts do not recommend the use of antibacterial soaps in low-risk situations, such as daily household use. However, a review of many studies concludes that there is no evidence that the proper use of sanitizers in food manufacture will lead to resistant microorganisms. Some simple methods for overcoming the potential for development of an acquired resistance include using appropriate antimicrobials, avoiding use of sublethal concentrations of microbials, using combinations for environmental or process controls, and using microbials that have different mechanisms (David and Harrison, 2002).

- In the United States, the average age of the population continues to increase as life expectancy increases. Older people are more susceptible to pathogenic bacteria than younger people; fewer organisms are needed to produce symptoms in older people.
- Food production has become more centralized, an effect that has both good and bad ramifications. Food inspectors can more closely monitor the sanitation at food-processing plants, but a food-borne illness outbreak affects more people in wider geographical areas.
- Increased sensitivity of laboratory equipment has dramatically improved the ability to detect food-borne illness outbreaks and to trace the sources of these outbreaks.
- As the population becomes highly educated about food safety, illnesses that in the past might have been dismissed as "stomach flu" are increasingly being identified as food-borne illnesses.
- Many foods are imported from countries whose regulatory procedures are not as stringent as those in the United States.
- Consumers are eating more meals away from home and using more convenience foods. Both behaviors increase the number of individuals involved in food handling and the time food is held in the danger zones. For example, a frozen convenience food is held in the temperature danger zone (between 40°F and 140°F) twice, once during assembly in the food-processing factory and a second time when the consumer is reheating it.
- Consumers are eating more raw food and more lightly grilled and sautéed foods, which are sometimes not cooked to proper temperatures.

Infectious Agents

Mad cow disease, also known as **bovine spongeform encephalopathy (BSE),** is related to a disease in humans called Creutzfeldt Jakobs disease (vCJD). Humans acquire this disease by eating beef that contains an infective agent (called a prion). A **prion** is a small protein that is resistant to most traditional methods that destroy a protein. BSE has been found in infected brain, spinal cord tissue, retina, dorsal root ganglia (nervous tissue near the backbone), distal ileum, and bone marrow in cattle experimentally infected by the oral route. Cattle are believed to acquire the infection when fed ground-up carcasses of animals, both sheep and other cattle, that contain the infected prion. Both the United States and Canada banned this fed practice for cattle in 1997. This feed was not banned for poultry and hogs. Variant Creutzfeldt Jakob disease has been seen primarily in young adults and is characterized initially by psychiatric and sensory problems, followed by ataxia (defective muscular coordination), dementia, and myoclonus (caused by fungus). This disease is considered a fatal brain disorder (Am Diet Assoc, 2003).

Despite the ban against feeding cattle ground-up carcasses of other cattle and sheep, BSE was discovered in the United States in late 2003. The diseased animal was traced back to an older steer imported to the United States before the regulation banning this type of animal feed in cattle. The discovery in a nation of BSE has enormous consequences. For example, BSE was identified in the United Kingdom in November 1986. By 2003, more than 185,000 cases of the disease were confirmed worldwide. Studies suggest that more than 1 million animals were likely infected during this period. More than 94 human cases of vCJD in humans have been diagnosed in Britain, France, and Ireland. The European Union banned the export of British beef imports worldwide. The British agricultural economy was financially devastated.

Many critics and consumer advocates have recommended that the United States institute more extensive testing of cattle and require stringent regulations. For example, Japan tests every steer for BSE that enters the food chain. Europe tests every animal older than 30 months (Adler, 2004). The two critical steps recommended by the most vocal advocates include a total ban on rendered food for all animals and testing for BSE every cow that enters the food chain. The estimated cost to the consumer for enforcement of these proposals would be between 10 to 20 cents per pound (Adler, 2004). Available evidence suggests that if current measures are well enforced, then the risk if any, from US cattle, is very low, although further regulation to limit exposure to material from animals infected with chronic wasting disease would further reduce the potential risk. Consumers need not be overly anxious about the risks that they may have incurred by consuming beef, but they should press authorities to test more cattle, to strengthen the regulations on feed production, and to extend the ban on brain and spinal cord in food for human consumption to include cattle younger than 30 months of age (Donnelly, 2004). Consumers for the added cost may elect to purchase beef from suppliers than adhere to these standards. Consumers vastly underrate the economic power of food-purchasing decisions.

Parasitic Infections

A **parasite** is an organism that lives within, upon, or at the expense of a living host without providing any benefit to the host. Several parasites can live in animals that human beings use for food. When a person eats an animal infected with a parasite, he or she also consumes the parasite and the result is illness. Two common parasites are *Trichinella spiralis* and tapeworms.

Trichinella Spiralis

Trichinella spiralis is a worm that becomes embedded in the muscle tissue of pigs. A pig may be fed meat from an animal that harbors the worm in its muscle. Some farmers still feed hogs table scraps that contain meat. The worm produces larvae that are protected from animal (including human) digestion. The larvae mature in the animal's stomach in 5 to 7 days. The adult worms then invade the lining of the small intestine, where they reproduce. The larvae enter the bloodstream of the animal and are carried to all parts of the body. They then penetrate the muscles, form cysts, and remain alive and infective for months. The cycle is completed when another animal eats the muscle containing the live *Trichinella spiralis* larvae.

When a human eats the larvae, usually in undercooked pork, he or she develops **trichinosis.** The symptoms of trichinosis usually appear 9 days after the ingestion of the infected meat, but the time can vary from 2 to 28 days. This period of time is called the **incubation period—** the length of time it takes to show disease symptoms after exposure to the offending organism. The first symptoms, which mimic food poisoning, are nausea, vomiting, and diarrhea. When the larvae migrate into muscles, including the heart muscle, systemic symptoms develop that include fever, swelling of the eyelids, sweating, weakness, and muscular pain. Death due to heart failure may occur.

Tapeworms

Humans through the ingestion of raw seafood or undercooked beef and pork acquire **tapeworms.** Hogs and steers become intermediate hosts when they graze on sewage-polluted pastures. Tapeworm infestation can occur when human wastes contaminate freshwater streams and lakes, animal pastures, or feed. Symptoms of a tapeworm infection may be trivial or absent. In some people, the worms attach to the jejunum and hosts develop vitamin B_{12} deficiency, anemia, and massive infections with diarrhea. Obstruction of the bile duct or intestine can be another complication.

Viral Infections

A **virus** is a microscopic parasite that is entirely dependent on the nutrients inside host cells for its metabolic and reproductive needs. Viruses may invade the cells of people, animals, plants, and bacteria to survive and thereby cause disease. Food frequently serves as a vehicle for some viruses, including those that cause influenza and infectious hepatitis. Food can become contaminated in its growing environment or during processing, storage, distribution, or preparation. Partly for this reason, the federal government requires all food-service workers to wear plastic gloves when handling food.

Some viruses are found in the intestinal tract of infected humans. If an infected person neglects to wash his or her hands after defecation and then handles food, the virus can contaminate the food and be passed on to unsuspecting consumers. The disease varies from a mild illness lasting 1 to 2 weeks to a severely disabling disease lasting several months.

Hepatitis A Virus

The hepatitis A virus causes infectious hepatitis, a liver disease. This virus can be found in water that has been contaminated with raw sewage and in shellfish harvested from fecally contaminated water. During food processing, hepatitis A can be transmitted when polluted water is used or by fecal contamination from insects or rodents. Infected workers can transmit the virus through sandwiches, baked goods, or any other food that is handled. Thus there are three ways the virus can be spread: polluted water, insects and rodents, and infected food handlers. The onset of viral hepatitis A is abrupt, with fever, malaise, anorexia, nausea, and abdominal discomfort. A few days later, the client may develop jaundice.

Substances Made Poisonous by Other Organisms

The consumption of toxic fish and plants can cause illness. Some molds can also produce disease (others are beneficial).

Toxic Seafood

The tissue of fish and shellfish can be naturally toxic to humans, even when the fish is fresh. The fish may not show any outward signs of illness, and there is usually no way to tell whether the fish is toxic. Because most fish toxins are stable to heat, cooking does not destroy them. **Paralytic shellfish poisoning** outbreaks have been reported involving the consumption of poisonous clams, oysters, mussels, and scallops.

Ciguatera poisoning is a serious human intoxication caused by ingestion of any of over 400 species of marine fish (Shils, 1999). This intoxication results from eating certain fish that have consumed marine bacteria and algae associated with coastal reefs and nearby waterways. Fish eating the algae become toxic, and the effect is magnified through the food chain so that large predatory fish become the most toxic; this occurs worldwide in tropical areas. Coastal waters are routinely monitored for the presence of the organism that produces ciguatera. If excessive numbers of the organism are found, a "red tide" alert is made. The best prevention is to avoid eating fish caught during a red tide.

Scromboid fish poisoning is caused by the presence of undesirable bacteria. This poisoning occurs in fish such as tuna, mackerel, bonito, and skipjack. The bacteria produce a toxin on the flesh of fish after the fish have been caught. Scromboid fish poisoning can be prevented by the adequate refrigeration of freshly caught fish and the purchase of fish from reputable sources.

Molds

Molds are the most widely encountered microorganism. Molds are spread by air currents, insects, and rodents. Some molds are beneficial. For example, molds are used to manufacture several types of cheese and soy sauce. Like bacteria, molds are often involved in food spoilage and are a nuisance in the food industry. A number of molds grow well in cold storage but are easily destroyed by a mild heating process, at which temperatures of 140°F or higher are reached.

Molds grow on bread, cheese, fruits, vegetables, starchy foods, preserves, grains, and a wide variety of other products. ***Aspergillus*** molds produce a series of **mycotoxins** called **aflatoxins** that may be present in peanuts or peanut products, corn, and cottonseed meal (Shils, 1999). Many experts believe aflatoxins to be the most potent liver toxin and cancer-producing agent known.

The best advice is to discard moldy bread; even if no other mold is visible, mold may have penetrated the rest of the item. Mold on natural cheese can be safely removed and the remainder of the cheese eaten, because the mold is not as likely to have penetrated the rest of the cheese. Food-handling tips related to microbiological hazards are summarized in Table 14–2.

Avoiding Nutrition Hazards

Nutrition hazards are the number-two safety risk according to the FDA. Although problems associated with an unbalanced diet occur frequently, clinical symptoms of illness are not as acute and severe as those arising from microbiologic hazards. Illness from food infection or food intoxication poses an immediate danger. The following sections cover food-labeling laws and a method health-care workers can use to assist in the evaluation of a client's dietary status. Knowledge of these topics can help prevent the nutritional hazards associated with consumption of an unbalanced diet.

The Food Label

The Food and Drug Administration (FDA) requires food labeling under the Federal Food Drug and Cosmetic Act and its amendments. Most prepared foods, such as breads, cereals, canned fruits and vegetables, snacks, desserts, and drinks, require a food label. Nutrition labeling for raw produce (fruits and vegetables) and fish is voluntary. Figure 14–5 provides information on how to understand and use the Nutrition Facts panel. Figure 14–6 provides an opportunity to compare two food labels of similar products.

1. *Standardized Format:* Every label has the same layout and design; the nutrition information is entitled

Table 14–2 **Infective Agents, Susceptible Foods, and Food Handling Tips**

INFECTIVE AGENT AND SUSCEPTIBLE FOODS	FOOD-HANDLING TIPS
SALMONELLA SPECIES Meat, eggs, poultry, milk, and products made with these foods	Wash hands, especially after defecation and after preparing uncooked meat, poultry, and eggs. Wash all surfaces and utensils that come in contact with meat, eggs, and poultry thoroughly. Refrigerate prepared food in small containers. Thoroughly cook all foodstuffs from animal sources. Avoid recontamination within the kitchen after cooking. (For example, do not allow food that has been cooked to come into contact with utensils used in the preparation of raw meats.) Never serve raw eggs, fish, and undercooked meats (see Clinical Application 14–2). Do not allow infected people to handle food. Instruct children to wash their hands after handling pet turtles, ducklings, or chicks.
TYPHOID FEVER Any food or water	Wash hands after urination and/or defecation. Avoid contaminated water and ice.
STAPHYLOCOCCUS AUREUS Bruised poultry, processed meats, cheeses, ice cream, mixed dishes such as potato salad and spaghetti	Personal hygiene: hand washing, avoid handling food when you have infected cuts, boils, and burns. Temperature control: store food below 40°F or above 140°F (see Fig. 14–2); do not eat food held at room temperature for longer than 4 hours.
CLOSTRIDIUM PERFRINGENS Meats, stews, gravies, large masses of food	Cool food rapidly in shallow containers that are no more than 4 inches deep. Heat all leftovers to at least 165°F. Hold all hot food above 140°F.
CLOSTRIDIUM BOTULINUM Canned foods Large masses of food with an air-free center	Never taste food from a bulging container. Do not serve home-canned food to institutionalized clients. Follow manufacturer's directions when home canning and use only equipment that has been carefully cleaned. Avoid home-smoked fish. Do not store home-smoked fish in plastic bags.

"Nutrition Facts." Some very small packages may use a simplified format.

2. *Serving Sizes:* All serving sizes listed on similar products are stated in consistently used household and metric measures to allow comparison shopping.

3. *Daily Values:* The bottom half of the Nutrition Facts panel shows either the minimum or maximum levels of nutrients people should consume each day for a healthful diet. For example, the value listed for carbohydrates refers to the minimum level, whereas the value for fat refers to the maximum level.

4. *Percent Daily Values:* The figures for percentage of daily values are based on a 2000-kilocalorie diet; this schema makes it easier for consumers to judge the nutritional quality of a food.

5. *Health Claims:* The FDA regulates health claims on food labels. A **health claim** describes the relationship between a food or food component and a disease or health-related condition. To make a heath claim, a food must meet specific nutrient levels that are set by the government. For example, fruits, vegetables, and grain products that contain fiber have between shown to reduce the risk of coronary heart disease; calcium reduces the risk of osteoporosis; and fruits and vegetables can reduce the risk of cancer.

6. *A Structure/Function Claim:* The FDA also regulates these claims on food labels. A **structure/function claim** describes the role of a nutrient or dietary ingredient intended to affect the structure or function in humans or characterizes the documented mechanism by which a nutrient or dietary ingredient acts to maintain such structure or function, e.g., "helps promote a healthy heart" or "helps support the immune system."

7. *Descriptors:* Terms like *low, high,* and *free* used on food labels must meet legal definitions. *Free* means less than 0.5 gram of fat per serving and tiny or insignificant amounts of cholesterol, sodium, and sugar. *Low* indicates 3 grams of fat (or less) per serving; also low in saturated fat, cholesterol, and/or kilocalories. *Lean* signifies less than 10 grams of fat, 4 grams of saturated fat, and 95 milligrams of cholesterol per serving. (*Lean* is higher in fat than *Low.*) *Extra Lean* means 5 grams of fat, 2 grams of saturated fat, and 95 milligrams of cholesterol per serving. (*Extra Lean* is lower in fat than *Lean* but not as low in fat as *Low.*) *Light* (Lite) denotes one-third fewer kilocalories or one-half the fat of the original

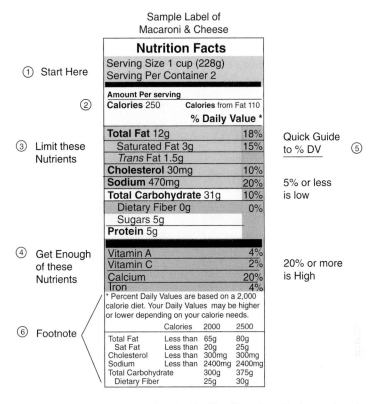

Sample Label of Macaroni & Cheese

① Start Here

②

③ Limit these Nutrients

④ Get Enough of these Nutrients

⑥ Footnote

Quick Guide to % DV ⑤

5% or less is low

20% or more is High

1. Start Here: The first place to start reading the Nutrition Facts Panel is the serving size and the number of servings in the package. Note how much you actually eat.

2. Calories: Displays the number of calories in the given serving size. The label also tells you how many calories are derived from fat.

3. Limit these nutrients: Eating too many of these nutrients may increase your risk of certain chronic diseases, such as heart disease, some cancers, and hypertension. Americans generally eat these nutrients in adequate amounts or too much.

4. Get enough of these nutrients: Americans often don't get enough of these nutrients.

5. Quick guide to % D.V.: % D.V. is based on 2000- and 2500-calorie diet.

6. Footnote: The D.V. are based on expert advice about some key nutrients that should be eaten daily.

Figure 14–5 Using the Nutrition Facts Panel on food labels. (Source: www.cfsan.fda.gov, accessed June 2004.)

or no more than one-half the sodium of the higher-sodium version. *Cholesterol Free* means the item has less than 2 milligrams of cholesterol and 2 grams (or less) of saturated fat per serving. In order for a food to be listed as *High* in a particular nutrient, it must contain 20 percent or more of the Daily Value for that nutrient. *Good Source Of* denotes that one serving of a food is considered to be a good source of a vitamin, mineral, or fiber, containing 10 to 19 percent of the Daily Value for that particular vitamin, mineral, or fiber.

8. Ingredients are listed in descending order by weight. The ingredients list is required on almost all foods, even some standardized ones like ice cream, mayonnaise, and bread.

Evaluation of Dietary Status

Reviewing a client's reported intake or actual food consumption and comparing this amount with the MyPyramid guide can assist in the identification of some nutrients that may be lacking in a person's diet. Table 14–3 lists recommended amounts of food from each of the major food groups for each day or week according to selected sex, age, and amount of physical activity. The following method of comparing a client's daily intake with the MyPyramid is suggested; answer these questions about the client.

1. Did the client consume at least the recommended amount of grains for his or her gender, age, and physical activity level? Were one-half of the grains eaten whole grains? Nutrients supplied by this group include carbohydrate, folic acid, thiamin, iron, and niacin. A person who does not eat enough grains may be deficient in these nutrients. In addition, this whole grains supply fiber.

2. Did the client consume recommended amount of fruits? After considering the amount of fruits eaten, check for a

REDUCED FAT MILK
2% Milkfat

Nutrition Facts

Serving Size 1 cup (236ml)
Servings Per Container 1

Amount Per Serving	
Calories 120	Calories from Fat 45

	0% Daily Value*
Total Fat 5g	8%
Saturated Fat 3g	15%
Trans Fat 0g	
Cholesterol 20mg	7%
Sodium 120mg	5%
Total Carbohydrate 11g	4%
Dietary Fiber 0g	0%
Sugars 11g	
Protein 9g	17%

Vitamin A 10% • Vitamin C 4%
Calcium 30% • Iron 0% • Vitamin D 25%

*Percent Daily Values are based on a 2,000 calorie diet. Your daily values may be higher or lower depending on your calorie needs.

CHOCOLATE NONFAT MILK

Nutrition Facts

Serving Size 1 cup (236ml)
Servings Per Container 1

Amount Per Serving	
Calories 80	Calories from Fat 0

	% Daily Value*
Total Fat 0g	0%
Saturated Fat 0g	0%
Trans Fat 0g	
Cholesterol Less than 5mg	0%
Sodium 120mg	5%
Total Carbohydrate 11g	4%
Dietary Fiber 0g	0%
Sugars 11g	
Protein 9g	17%

Vitamin A 10% • Vitamin C 4%
Calcium 30% • Iron 0% • Vitamin D 25%

*Percent Daily Values are based on a 2,000 calorie diet. Your daily values may be higher or lower depending on your calorie needs.

Figure **14–6** Comparison of two food labels. (Source: www.cfsan. fda.gov, accessed June 2004.)

reliable source of vitamin C (such as citrus, melons, and berries). It is difficult for a client to meet his or her vitamin C allowance without including fruits or some vegetables in the diet. Other nutrients in this group are fiber, iron, potassium, folic acid, carbohydrate, and other trace minerals. Remember that many fruits function as a "scrub brush" for the teeth and intestines.

If an individual's diet is low in fruits, ask about his or her **dentition,** the status of a person's teeth. Inspect the client's mouth and observe how many teeth are missing. Does the client have oral pain when chewing? Is the client able to tolerate all food textures? The client may avoid eating a particular fruit (especially raw) because

of chewing problems. The client may also have a problem with elimination.

3. Did the client consume the recommended amount of vegetables? After considering the amount of vegetables consumed, check for a reliable source of vitamin A (such as broccoli, carrots, or other dark green or yellow vegetable). It is difficult for an individual to meet his or her vitamin A allowance without including some dark green or yellow vegetables in the diet. Many of the comments listed under fruits also apply to the vegetable group. For example, elimination problems may be related to a poor dietary intake of fiber secondary to the exclusion of vegetables from the diet. A person may

Table **14–3**   **How Many Servings Do You Need Each Day Based on Age, Gender, and Activity Level?**

CALORIE LEVEL*	ABOUT 1600	ABOUT 1800	ABOUT 2800
Age, gender, activity	**55-yr; female; less than 30 minutes of daily physical activity**	**18 yr; female; 30 to 60 minutes of daily physical activity**	**18 yr male; 30 to 60 minutes of daily physical activity**
Grains	5 ounces total for day including 2 1/2 ounces whole grains	6 ounces total for day including 3 ounces whole grains	10 ounces for the day including 5 ounces whole grains
Vegetables	2 cups	2 1/2 cups	2 1/2 cups
Fruits	1 1/2 cups	1 1/2 cups	2 1/2 cups
Milk	3 cups	3 cups	3 cups
Meat and beans 1/4 cup cooked beans = 1 ounce	5 ounces	5 ounces	7 ounces
Oils	5 teaspoons	5 teaspoons	8 teaspoons
Discretionary Kcal	130	195	425

*These are the calorie levels if you choose low-fat and lean foods.
 These are the amounts needed for non-pregnant non-lactating healthy people.
 To determine the kilocalories and foods recommended for other age and activity levels go to: www.MyPyramid.gov (accessed April, 2005).

elect to omit raw vegetables from his or her diet because of poor dentition.

4. Did the client consume the appropriate amount of milk for his or her age, gender, and physical activity level? If not, the diet may be lacking in calcium, vitamin D, and riboflavin. Double-check for other reliable sources of calcium, such as cheese and foods made with milk.

5. Did the client consume the recommended amount from the meat and bean group for his or her age and physical activity level? If not, the diet may be lacking in protein, iron, and B-vitamins. Remember that the meat group also includes cheese, eggs, dried beans and legumes, and other protein-rich foods. Individuals who do not eat meat, poultry, and fish would count dry beans and peas in this group. One-fourth of a cup of cooked dry beans and peas or one egg are equivalent to 1 ounce of meat.

6. Did the client consume the recommended amount of oil? Most of the fat consumed should be either polyunsaturated (PUFA) or monounsaturated (MUFA). *Trans*-fatty acids should be avoided. Oils contain essential fatty acids and are the major source of vitamin E in the typical American diet. While some oil is needed for optimal health, too much can have a health detriment. All fats are high in kilocalories. The amount consumed needs to be limited to balance total kilocalorie intake (USDA, 2005).

Environmental Pollutants

Many people are concerned about environmental pollution. Although the problem is widespread, situations that pose a severe and immediate danger to health are uncommon. The U.S. Environmental Protection Agency (EPA) regulates the use of **pesticides** and sets tolerance levels to provide a high margin of safety in food. Issues in food preparation and processing are discussed in Box 14–1.

Box 14–1 **Food-Handling Guidelines**

Shop Carefully

Make meat, fish, poultry, eggs, and refrigerated and frozen foods the last items you pick up in the grocery store. (These foods support the growth of bacteria better than other foods.)

Do not buy containers or packages that leak, dented cans, or expired foods.

Wrap hazardous items in plastic bags before placing them in the grocery cart.

Wrap produce in plastic baggies.

Buy frozen items that are rock solid (not partially thawed).

Use a cooler to transport hazardous items when the temperature is above 80°F.

Insist that items to be eaten raw (bread and produce) are not bagged with hazardous items.

Buy only the amount of deli meat that can be eaten in 1 to 2 days.

If a prepared hot item is purchased, take it home and eat it or hold it above 140°F. Hold it for no longer than 2 hours.

Do not buy fish from unreliable sources.

Buy pasteurized fruit juices.

Storage

Keep the refrigerator, freezer, and storage cabinets clean.

Use pest-control measures.

Store cleaning supplies away from food.

Do not store home-smoked fish in plastic airtight bags.

Use thermometers.

Store raw meats on the bottom shelf of the refrigerator. Never store meats, fish, or poultry above fruits and vegetables.

Dispose of hazardous perishable items on a timely basis.

Cover and date food.

If the power goes out, keep the freezer closed except to add dry ice. Foods that contain ice crystals can be safely refrozen.

Use wraps and containers that are specifically manufactured for food use.

When in doubt, throw it out!

Food Preparation

Avoid hand-to-food contact; use utensils; wear disposable gloves.

Wash hands frequently.

Use a thermometer to check internal food temperatures:

- Meats and eggs, 160°F
- Leftovers and casseroles, 165°F
- Poultry, whole, 180°F; breast, 170°F
- Ground meats, 165°F (brown throughout)

Roast meats at oven temperatures of 300°F or above.

Cook with a constant heat source. Don't partially cook meat, fish, etc. at one time and then finish it later.

Clean work surfaces with soap and hot water before and after food preparation.

Carefully clean raw fruits and vegetables using warm water and a brush. Peel waxed fruit (wax makes it difficult to remove any residual pesticides).

Use roasting pans or covered containers to cook foods in the microwave to keep the steam in contact with the food. Rotate or stir food often; allow standing time and always use a thermometer when cooking foods in the microwave.

Cut mold from cheeses.

Food Display and Service

Serve food on clean platters.

Hold hot foods at 140°F or hotter if possible.

Hold cold foods at 40°F or colder.

If you cannot hold foods within these temperature ranges, display and serve food for no longer than 2 hours and then discard leftovers.

Do not taste leftovers until after you reheat them to an internal temperature of 165°F.

(Continued on the following page)

Box 14–1 **Food-Handling Guidelines** *(Continued)*

Use a thermometer.
Never serve raw eggs, fish, or undercooked meats.

Preventing Cross-Contamination

Keep work surfaces clean.
Think while cooking.
Never allow fresh bread, vegetables, and fruit to come in contact with hazardous items.
Clean chopping boards after the preparation of each menu item.
Use clean utensils to prepare each food item. Do not use the same utensil to both prepare and serve a hazardous food.
Always use a deep pan to store meats, fish, and poultry in the refrigerator to keep juices from dripping on other items.

Sanitation and Personal Hygiene

Do not smoke or eat while preparing food.
Wash hands especially after defecation and after preparing hazardous foods.

Avoid touching body parts.
Wear clean clothes.
Avoid handling foods when ill with diarrhea, sore throat, or cough or when you have infected fingers or other infectious signs.
Instruct children to wash their hands before touching food, especially after handling pet turtles, ducklings, or chickens.

Safe Cooling and Reheating

Thaw foods properly (in the refrigerator or under cold running water).
Use a microwave to thaw foods only as part of a continuous cooking process.
After thawing, cook food immediately.
Chill cooked foods rapidly in a shallow (2-inch-deep container).
Do not let foods cool off at room temperature.
Pack lunches in insulated containers and freeze sandwiches.
Reheat leftovers to an internal temperature of 165°F.

Chemical Poisoning

Chemical poisoning occurs when people eat toxic substances that may be intentionally or accidentally added to foods during growing, harvesting, processing, transporting, storing, or preparing foods. Two general types of chemical poisoning can occur. They are heavy metal and chemical-product contamination pesticides.

Heavy Metals

Several metals can be toxic. Sources of metals in the soil include parts of rocks and minerals that have weathered to produce soil, water erosion of soil particles, metals as added ingredients or impurities in fertilizers, pesticides containing metals, metals in manure and sludge, and metals in airborne dust. The origin of airborne dust is industrial and mining waste, fossil fuel combustion products, radioactive fallout, pollen, sea spray, and meteoric and volcanic material. Airborne dust eventually settles to the ground and becomes part of the soil. Plants may grow normally but contain levels of selenium, cadmium, molybdenum, or lead that are toxic to humans.

The toxic action of metals is believed to be important in enzyme poisoning. For example, mercury, lead, copper, beryllium, cadmium, and silver have been found to inhibit the enzyme **alkaline phosphatase.** One function of alkaline phosphatase is in the mineralization process of bone. Some disease states associated with the consumption of toxic minerals include rickets and bone tumors. Lead ingestion with a subsequent elevation of blood lead levels has been linked to a variety of toxic effects, including adverse neurologic, neurobehavioral, and developmental effects (Shils, 1999) (see Clinical Applications 8–5 in Chapter 8).

Mercury is extremely toxic and is widely distributed over the surface of the earth. Episodes of serious poisoning include those in Minamata (1953 to 1960) and the Niigata area (1965) in Japan (Shils, 1999), in which large chemical plants poured industrial waste containing mercury into nearby bays. Area residents who ate fish from the bays complained of numbness of the extremities, slurred speech, unsteady gait, deafness, and visual disturbances. Mental confusion and muscular incoordination were apparent in all the clients. Because mercury can damage the fetal nervous system, the Food and Drug Administration has issued a consumer alert for pregnant women and women of childbearing age not to eat large fish types in which mercury may accumulate: shark, swordfish, king mackerel, and tilefish (Am Diet Assoc, 2003).

Chemical Products

Chemical food-borne illness is also associated with chemical products such as detergents, sanitizers, pesticides, and other chemicals that may enter the food supply. After such toxins have been ingested, the symptoms of chemical poisoning appear in a few minutes to a few hours, but usually in less than 1 hour. Nausea, vomiting, abdominal pain, diarrhea, and a metallic taste are common complaints with chemical food-borne illnesses.

Consumers generally have many chemicals in their homes. When compounds such as detergents and cleaners are used for the wrong purpose or in excessive amounts, they can cause illness and death. Chemical poisoning can be prevented by:

1. Using each product for its intended use and in the amounts recommended
2. Reading the label before use
3. Keeping chemicals in their original containers
4. Never storing or transporting chemicals in containers

used to store food. They may be mistaken (especially by children) for food or beverages.

Pesticides are chemicals used to kill insects or rodents. Improperly used pesticides have caused poisonings when they were accidentally mixed with food. The use of pesticide-containing aerosols around foods and packaging materials and in food preparation areas can be dangerous. According to the Environmental Protection Agency (EPA), studies have linked pesticides to problems such as cancer, nerve damage, and birth defects (EPA, 2003).

Pesticide residues are of great concern to consumers. **Residues** are trace amounts of any substance remaining in a product at the time of sale. Three governmental agencies are involved in the regulation of products that enter the U.S. food supply:

- The Environmental Protection Agency (EPA)
- The Food and Drug Administration (FDA)
- The United States Department of Agriculture (USDA) Food Safety and Inspection Service (FSIS)

The EPA regulates the use of potentially harmful pesticides that are used in food production. Included among the duties of the EPA is the establishment of tolerance levels for pesticides.

The FDA, in addition to its other functions, regulates animal drugs, including food additives, herbicides, and environmental contaminants. The FSIS sets tolerance levels for these residues in edible foods. In setting a tolerance level, the FSIS determines the highest dose at which a residue causes no ill effects in laboratory animals, called the **tolerance level.** The tolerance level is then divided by a factor ranging from 100 to 1000 to account for possible differences between animals and humans.

The numbers used assume that humans are 10 times more sensitive than the most-sensitive animal species tested. In addition, a further assumption is made that children and the elderly are 10 times as sensitive as others. This is the 100-fold safety factor (multiplying 10 times 10). A large margin of safety is built into residue limits established for compounds involved in the production of human food.

The Food Safety and Inspection Service (FSIS) enforces the residue limits in meat and poultry. The FDA is responsible for foods other than meat and poultry. When an illegal residue is found, the FDA can conduct an investigation and the FSIS can detain future shipments from the violating producer.

Natural Food Intoxicants

Many foods (unprocessed or uncooked) contain natural components that can harm health. All foods are made up of chemicals, some of which can alter the way the body uses nutrients. For example, phytates contained in grains decrease the bioavailability of zinc, calcium, iron, and manganese (Shils, 1999). **Bioavailability** is defined as the rate and extent to which an active drug or nutrient or metabolite enters the general circulation, permitting access to the site of action (Venes, 2001).

Proteinase inhibitors found in many varieties of beans, peas, peanuts, and potatoes block the activity of enzymes such as trypsin and chymotrypsin (Shils, 1999). The literature on natural toxins in foods is extensive, and only a few examples can be discussed in this text.

Healthy people who eat well-balanced diets should not worry about natural food intoxicants. Illness from naturally occurring toxic compounds in foods is not common in this country. However, if an individual eats large amounts of a single food at one time, he or she may experience the effects of natural food intoxicants. The best protection against the effects of natural food intoxicants is to eat a wide variety of foods, thereby limiting exposure to any one toxic compound.

Food Additives

Additives may be introduced into food deliberately or accidentally. An **additive** is a substance added to food to increase its flavor, shelf life, characteristics such as texture, color, and aroma, and other qualities. In the United States, the Food and Drug Administration (FDA) regulates food additives under the authority of the Food, Drug, and Cosmetic Act of 1938 and amendments in 1958 and 1960. These amendments include the Delaney Clause, which bans the approval of an additive if it is shown to cause cancer in humans or animals. Before using a new food additive, a manufacturer must petition the FDA for approval. The manufacturer must prove the additive is not harmful to humans at expected consumption.

There are two categories of food additives that are not subject to testing and approval procedure: *prior-sanctioned* and *GRAS* substances. The FDA before the 1958 Food Additives Amendment approved substances appointed as prior sanctioned. GRAS (generally recognized as safe) additives have been used extensively in the past with no known harmful effect and are believed to be safe. Substances on the GRAS list have been under review since 1969. Some of the substances on the GRAS list are sugar, salt, and vinegar.

Intentional Use of Additives

Additives are intentionally added directly to food during processing for several reasons. For example, a preservative may be added to a bakery product to retard the growth of mold.

There are four reasons additives are intentionally used:

1. To maintain or enhance a food's nutritional value. Frequently, vitamins, minerals, and different forms of fiber are added to food.
2. To maintain a food's quality. Many additives are used to prevent the growth of microorganisms and extend a product's shelf life. Some additives, called antioxidants, are used to prevent fats in food from deteriorating. Antioxidants are substances that prevent chemical breakdown by preventing or inhibiting the uptake of oxygen. Selected antioxidants may be effective in delaying some cancers' proliferation, mainly those related to fat metabolism, such as breast and prostate cancer.
3. To assist in processing, transporting, or holding a food. One additive that helps facilitate the processing of food is an **emulsifier.** An emulsifier helps to evenly distribute the molecules of two liquids that normally do not mix.

Mayonnaise is an example of an emulsified product. Baking soda and baking powder are other commonly used additives. These substances cause such products as cakes to rise and improve their texture and volume.
4. To improve the way a food tastes, looks, or smells. Artificial colors, flavors, and sweeteners all fall into this category.

Types of common food additives are listed in Table 14–4.

Accidental Use of Additives

Some additives enter the food supply accidentally. For example, chemicals may enter food through contact with surfaces that have been cleaned with chemical solutions.

Food-Handling Guidelines

Food-handling guidelines that can help decrease the risks of food-borne disease are presented in Box 14–1.

FOOD SELECTION. The greater the variety of foods consumed, the less the likelihood of exposure to excessive amounts of contaminants from any single food item. Remember that contaminants of natural origin are present in foods.

FOOD STORAGE. Proper storage of food helps ensure that there will be minimal contamination of the food from any source. Clients should be instructed to use a refrigerator thermometer and check it daily.

SANITATION AND PERSONAL HYGIENE. The cleanliness of people involved in food handling and a clean working environment are essential to the prevention of

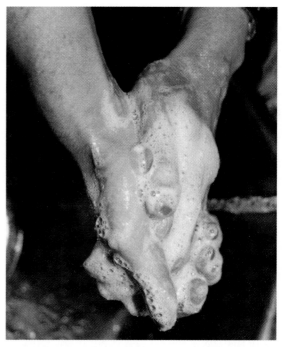

Figure **14–7** Amount of soap lather necessary to thoroughly cleanse the hands.

food-borne disease. An unclean person cannot handle food in a sanitary fashion. Smoking and eating while preparing food may result in food contamination. Personal practices such as scratching the head, placing fingers in or about the mouth or nose, and sneezing may contaminate food. Frequent hand washing with soap is the best

Table **14–4**	**Common Food Additives**	
Acidity control agents	Influence flavor, texture, and shelf life	Sodium bicarbonate Citric acid Hydrogen chloride Sodium hydroxide Acetic acid Phosphoric acid Calcium oxide
Antioxidants	Prevent discoloration Protect fats from rancidity	Vitamin C Vitamin E BHT and BHA
Flavors	Food enhancers	Hydrolyzed vegetable protein Black pepper Mustard Monosodium glutamate
Leavening agents	To make dough rise	Sodium acid phosphate Sodium aluminum phosphate Monocalcium phosphate Yeast
Preservatives	To extend shelf life	Sulfur oxide Benzoic acid Propionic acid EDTA
Stabilizers and thickeners	To enhance texture	Sodium caseinate Gum arabic Modified starch Pectin

insurance against food contamination. In fact, the most common way sources of disease are transmitted from a food handler to food is by the hands. Needless to say, it is essential to always wash your hands after using the toilet (Fig. 14–7).

PREVENTING CROSS-CONTAMINATION. Cross-contamination refers to the spreading of a disease-producing organism from one food to another. It can happen when a food preparer handles raw meat, eggs, or milk and then handles fruit, lettuce, or bread products that will be served uncooked. The cook transfers the offending substance or organism to the uncooked food item. Organisms can also be transferred to nonfood items such as a cooking utensil and then passed onto the food or a person.

SAFE FOOD PREPARATION. Food is least protected during actual food preparation because of necessary handling, possible contamination from the environment, and the room's temperature. Food should always be prepared with the least amount of hand contact. All work surfaces that come in contact with raw meats should be thoroughly cleaned using soap and hot water. Every attempt should be made to keep foods in the 40- to 140-degree temperature range for as short a time as possible.

SAFE COOLING AND REHEATING. Food should be thawed properly; it can be done in refrigerated units at a temperature that should not exceed 40°F. It can also be accomplished under running water at a temperature of 70°F or below. Using the microwave oven to thaw food is a safe method as long as the thawing is part of a continuous cooking process. After thawing, the food should be cooked immediately. All foods that have been cooked and then refrigerated should be reheated to a safe temperature of 165°F.

FOOD SERVICE AND DISPLAY. Foods should be served, displayed, and held on clean plates at correct temperatures and should be discarded if held for longer than recommended. Proper cleanliness, an awareness of time, and temperature regulation are the most important ways the consumers can control the growth of bacteria. If the temperature is above 90°F, foods should be held for no longer than 1 hour without refrigeration or heat. At cooler temperatures, hold the food for no longer than 2 hours. Hot foods should be held above 140°F and cold foods at 40°F or lower. Leftovers should be reheated to 165°F before they are tasted. Leftovers that are held outside these temperature ranges for longer than recommended times should be discarded.

SUMMARY

The U.S. food supply is as safe, wholesome, and nutritious as any in the world, but there are no guarantees that all food purchased and eaten in the country is safe. Thousands of substances besides nutrients are present in foods. Most of these substances are harmless in the amounts typically eaten if the food item is selected, stored, and prepared under recommended conditions. Many foods contain toxic substances naturally. Only in recent years have we been able to detect and measure these toxic substances. The human body appears able to safely handle small amounts of some toxic substances without injury.

The FDA ranks pathogenic (disease-causing) microorganisms as the most dangerous food-related public health threat. An individual is more likely to suffer from a food-borne illness due to microbiologic contamination than from any other source. Good food-handling methods can control most microbiologic hazards. Selecting a wide variety of foods, storing the foods appropriately, and preparing foods correctly all help prevent illness. Healthcare workers should teach their clients about the use of food labels and the risks of microbiologic and residual chemical hazards of foods.

CASE STUDY 14–1

Ms. N is a 95-year old woman who is 5 ft tall and weighs 122 lb. (dressed without shoes). She has just been admitted to the nursing home. During the routine nursing admission process, Ms. N requested an eggnog every night at 8:00 PM. She stated she dislikes packaged mixes and would prefer her eggnog made with whole milk, ice cream, and a raw egg. Ms. N's physician has ordered an eggnog at HS (Latin for hour of sleep, or just before bedtime) everyday. Ms. N stated she has always drunk a homemade eggnog every night for the past 50 years. The client's daughter has stated she makes her mother an eggnog from raw eggs.

(Continued on the following page)

CASE STUDY *(Continued)*

NURSING CARE PLAN

SUBJECTIVE DATA   Client stated she drinks an eggnog made with a raw egg each day. Client's daughter stated she makes her mother such a beverage.

OBJECTIVE DATA   Height: 5 ft, 0 in
Weight: adm 122 lb
100 percent RBW
Age: 95

NURSING DIAGNOSIS   NANDA: Risk for Infection (NANDA International, 2003, with permission) related to knowledge deficit as evidenced by client's statement, "I eat one raw egg each day," and the client's age.

DESIRED OUTCOMES EVALUATION CRITERIA	NURSING ACTIONS/ INTERVENTIONS	RATIONALE
NOC: Risk Control (Moorhead, S, Johnson, M, and Maas, M, 2004, with permission)	NIC: Nutrition Management (Dochterman and Bulechek, 2004, with permission).	
The client will state that raw eggs can make one ill.	Provide verbal and written information to the client and the client's daughter on the relationship between food illness and *Salmonella* infections.	Elderly clients are particularly at risk for salmonellosis.
	Have the client and the client's daughter state that raw eggs are hazardous.	Verbal recognition of a hazard is the first step in behavioral change.
The client will accept an eggnog made from pasteurized egg product.	Request the dietitian send an eggnog made from safe ingredients.	The risk of salmonellosis from pasteurized eggs is lower than from raw eggs.
	Chart acceptance or rejection of the beverage.	Acceptance of the modified eggnog will increase long-term compliance.

C T Q   CRITICAL THINKING QUESTIONS

1. What other areas of the home might you inspect to minimize the risk of a food-borne illness?
2. What clients need to take extra precautions to prevent a food-borne illness?
3. Do you think it is within the scope of practice for a nurse when making a home visit to discuss unsafe food practices?

⟫⟫ CHAPTER REVIEW

1. Cold foods should be stored:
   a. At less than 50°F
   b. At less than 0°F
   c. At less than 40°F
   d. For no more than 6 hours outside the recommended temperature range.

2. The term *low* on a food label means the product contains:
   a. Less than 3 grams of fat (or less) per serving; also low in saturated fat, cholesterol, or kilocalories
   b. _____ the fat of the original
   c. Less than 10 grams of fat, 4 grams of saturated fat, and 95 milligrams of cholesterol per serving
   d. More fat than a product labeled *Extra lean.*

3. Foods commonly contaminated with *Campylobacter* are:
   a. Hard-cooked scrambled eggs
   b. Raw vegetables
   c. Canned foods
   d. Raw poultry

4. The best method to control the spread of food-borne illness is by:
   a. Wearing gloves when handling food
   b. Proper hand washing
   c. Taking food supplements
   d. Avoiding certain foods

5. A person who excludes all vegetables from the diet is likely to lack adequate:
   a. Vitamin A
   b. Fat
   c. Riboflavin
   d. Zinc

CLINICAL ANALYSIS

1. Mr. P has brought his 35-year-old male companion who has a history of AIDS to the ambulatory care clinic for treatment for a sudden onset of headache, abdominal pain, diarrhea, nausea, and vomiting. The nurse should:
   a. Document all food consumed during the past 7 days
   b. Inquire about food practices in the home
   c. Inspect Mr. P's passport for foreign travel in the past month
   d. Document the client's immunization status

2. A nurse is on the planning committee for the annual hospital picnic. One employee volunteers to make Texas-style chili at home and serve it at the picnic. The nurse has a responsibility to:
   a. Inquire how the chili will be made, transported, and held at recommended temperatures

   b. Taste the chili upon arrival at the picnic for safety
   c. Check the temperature of the chili upon arrival at the picnic
   d. Review the recipe for the potential use of unsafe ingredients

3. Mr. J is an 85-year-old man recently discharged from the hospital for a partial bowel obstruction that he had surgically repaired. His wife is getting ready to serve him eggnog made with raw eggs. The nurse should:
   a. Ignore the situation because that is not the purpose of the visit
   b. Inquire about any gastrointestinal pain Mr. J may have had
   c. Instruct the wife about the safe preparation of eggs
   d. Assess the amount of sugar used in the beverage

REFERENCES

Adler, J: Mad Cow: What's safe now? Newsweek. 43–48. January 14, 2004.

American Dietetic Association: Position of the American Dietetic Association: Food and water safety. J Am Diet Assoc 103:1203, 2003.

Bailar, JC and Travers, K: Review of human health risk associated with the use of antimicrobial agents in agriculture. Clin Infect Dis 34(Suppl 3):874, 2002.

Centers for Disease Control. Accessed January, 2004 at www.cdc.gov/travel/madcow.

Centers for Disease Control. Accessed December 2003 at www.cdc.gov/mmwr/pdf/wk/mm5226.

Centers for Chronic Disease Control: Surveillance for foodborne-disease outbreaks-United States 1993–1997 CDC. Atlanta, GA.MMWR 49:1, 2000.

Davidson, PM and Harrison, MA: Scientific status summary: Resistance and adaptations to food antimicrobials, and other process controls. Food Technology 56:59, 2002.

Dochterman, J, and Bulechek, GM: Nursing Interventions Classification (NIC), 4 ed. Mosby, Philadelphia, 2004.

Donnelly, CA: Bovine spongiform encephalopathy in the United States—An epidemiologists view. N Eng J Med. 350:539, 2004

Food Safety Healthy People 2010. Accessed January 4, 2004 at http://www.health.gov/healthypeople/document//htm/volume1/.

Environmental Protection Agency: Pesticides and food: You and your family need to know health-related problems pesticides might pose. Accessed March 2003 at www.epa.gov/pesticides/food/risks.htm.

Goldrick, BA: Emerging infections: foodborne diseases. Am J Nurs 103:105, 2003.

Hightower, JM and Moore, D: Mercury levels in high-end consumers of fish. Environ Health Perspect 111:604, 2003.

Moorhead, S, Johnson, M, and Maas, M: Nursing Outcomes Classification (NOC), ed 3. Mosby, Philadelphia. 2004.

NANDA International: Nursing Diagnoses: Definitions and Classifications, 2003–2004. NANDA International, Philadelphia, 2003.

Shils, ME (ed): Modern Nutrition in Health and Disease, ed 9. Williams & Wilkins, Baltimore, 1999.

United States Department of Agriculture. Accessed April, 2000 at www.ars.usda.gov/dgac.

United States Department of Health and Human Services: Foodborne illness post dramatic six year decline (press release). Accessed April 18, 2002 at www.hhs.gov/news/2002press.

United States Department of Agriculture: Accessed April, 2005 at www.MyPyramid.gov

United States Department of Agriculture: Nutrition and Health: Dietary Guidelines for Americans. Washington DC. US Government Printing Office. 5th ed. Home and Garden Bulletin No. 232, 2000

Venes, CL (ed): Tabers Cyclopedic Medical Dictionary, ed 19. FA Davis, Philadelphia, 2001.

Wegener, HC, et al: Use of antimicrobial growth promoters in farm animals and Enterococcus faecium resistance to therapeutic antimicrobial drugs in Europe. Emerg Infect Dis 5:329, 1999.

White, DG, Benbrook, C, and Benbrook, KL: Hogging it: Estimates of antimicrobial abuse in livestock. Union of Concerned Scientists, Cambridge, MA, 2001.

CHAPTER **15**

Nutrient Delivery

Learning Objectives

After completing this chapter, the student should be able to:

1. Identify three routes used to deliver nutrients to clients and potential complications with two of these routes.
2. Discuss the kinds of commercial formulas available for oral and tube feedings.
3. Discuss why it is important to carefully control the concentration, rate of delivery, and volume of formula delivered to a client.
4. List at least five reasons for the high incidence of malnutrition in institutionalized clients and the interventions nurses can make to combat malnutrition.
5. Describe suggested procedures for administering medications through feeding tubes.

Food services in health-care facilities have two major functions: the preparation and delivery of meals to clients and the nutritional care of clients. The nutritional care of clients includes three areas:

1. Assessing the client's need for nutrients
2. Delivering nutrients to the client
3. Monitoring the client's nutrient intake
4. Counseling the client about nutritional needs

High-quality nutritional care saves the client and society health-care dollars and preventable hardship.

Food Service in Institutions

Nurses need to become familiar with some aspects of the food service in the organizations where they are employed. Specific duties of nurses are often related to meal-service schedules.

Meal Service Patterns

Most institutions serve three meals to clients each day as well as several between-meal feedings. Feedings between meals are available for clients in need of extra nutrients,

those who desire extra food, or those unable to consume sufficient kilocalories at the regular mealtimes.

It is important for nurses to know the times meals are served to clients. The dietary and nursing departments must coordinate their schedules so that clients receive their food while it is hot and attractive. The administration of medications sometimes must also be coordinated with meal-delivery schedules. Scheduling the client for diagnostic tests, blood work, and educational sessions should be coordinated with the meal-service schedule.

Nutritional Care Services

Institutions vary in the types of nutritional services they offer clients. A large teaching hospital or medical center frequently has nutrition professionals on staff who specialize in the treatment of particular types of clients. A critical-care dietitian, for example, has special training to assess, plan, implement, and counsel clients in high-risk stages of trauma, disease, and conditions that affect nutritional support. In such settings, other health-care workers can rely on the critical-care dietitian to provide technical support. At the other end of the spectrum, in a small community hospital or a long-term care facility, a dietitian may be present only part time or as a consultant. In such circumstances, other health-care workers must plan to make the best use of the dietitian's services when he or she is available. In this situation, the nursing staff assumes more responsibility for the nutritional care of clients.

Nutritional care services are also provided as a component of home- and community-based programs. Hospice, home-care programs, and some governmental agencies deliver nutritional care services. Frequently, a dietitian is available through any of these programs for consultation. Third-party payers increasingly cover medical nutritional care.

Assessment, Monitoring, and Counseling

Nutritional care is a joint responsibility of the dietary and nursing departments. Assessing, monitoring, and counseling activities are usually done in collaboration.

Assessment

Some dietary departments screen clients for nutritional problems during admission. Clients found to be at a nutritional risk have a complete nutritional assessment, which usually includes the following:

1. Height, weight, BMI, and weight history
2. Laboratory test values
3. Food intake information
4. Potential food-drug interactions
5. Mastication and swallowing ability
6. Client's ability to feed himself or herself
7. Bowel and bladder function
8. Evaluation for the presence of **pressure ulcers**
9. Food allergies and intolerances
10. Any other factors affecting nutritional status, such as food preferences and cultural and religious beliefs about food
11. Determination of body composition
12. Presence of severe burns, trauma, infection, or other physiological stress that increases nutrient needs and is likely to prolong hospital stay
13. Learning barriers such as hearing, mobility, language, need for interpreter, vision, speech, reading/writing skills, inability to follow instructions, cultural and religious barriers, learning disability, learning readiness (requests, accepts, or avoids information), and preferred learning style

In some health-care facilities, nurses are responsible for screening clients for nutritional problems. If the nurse finds a client at nutritional risk, she or he should make a referral to the dietitian.

Regulatory agencies of long-term care facilities require that clients have a nutritional assessment performed by a registered dietitian shortly after admission. The assessment identifies clients at nutritional risk. The care plan should reflect nutritional problems identified during the assessment.

Monitoring

All clients should be reassessed or monitored at appropriate intervals. Some clients in hospital intensive care units require continuous monitoring. Other clients require daily reassessment.

The **client care conference** (interdisciplinary conference) is a productive means of monitoring clients. It is most effective if all health-care workers come prepared. Before the conference, information on the nutritional care of the client should be gathered, including:

1. The client's initial nutritional assessment
2. The client's present body weight and weight history
3. A record of the client's recent food acceptances
4. Any changes in the client's medical condition
5. The client's diet order
6. Family support

With this information in hand, it is easy to determine most changes in the client's nutritional status. Weight loss is readily identified. A review of the client's **food acceptance record,** if available, can verify whether such a weight loss is likely a result of poor food intake.

Those clients whom health-care providers have determined to be at nutritional risk because of poor food intake should be treated; treatment may include a nutritional supplement, between-meal feedings, a change in the diet prescription, or a change in feeding status. If, for example, a client can no longer feed himself or herself, the client's feeding status would need to be changed from self-feed to assisted feeding. Monitoring the client's weight, laboratory values, and food intake is an important part of delivering high-quality nutritional care.

Counseling

All clients should be evaluated for nutritional counseling. The assumption that a client is not expected to be discharged and therefore is not entitled to education is unjustifiable. Educating the client about nutritional concerns helps the client assume responsibility for his or her own care, thus promoting self-esteem and a sense of worth.

Diet Manuals

Current accreditation standards (both long-term and acute-care) require all institutions that provide health care to have a diet manual available to all health-care workers. The diet manual defines and describes all diets used in the facility and includes information about the particular food service operation. What is included in a "soft diet" may vary slightly from one institution to another. For example, one soft diet may allow lettuce, whereas another may not. The diet manual is developed and approved jointly by all health-care professionals in a facility. Regional food preferences and the unique training of the facility's medical staff and other professionals influence the choice of food items allowed or avoided on special diets.

The administrative dietitian is usually responsible for initiating the selection of a diet manual or for writing the manual. Most aspects of the nutritional care given to clients are covered in such a manual, including nutritional supplements stocked by the pharmacy, purchasing, and dietary departments; dietary preparation for diagnostic procedures; kilocalorie count procedures; meal-service delivery schedules; client educational services; a listing of foods allowed, restricted, and avoided on the various diets; and nursing procedures to follow when transmitting a diet order.

When developing the manual, the dietitian usually consults with other department heads and members of the medical staff. After the manual is developed and written, it must be approved by the facility administrator and the medical staff. Physicians are usually requested to follow the manual when prescribing diets for clients. The medical staff, nursing department, and other professionals in the hospital can and do influence the nutritional care given to clients by participating in the diet manual approval process.

Diet Orders

The physician is responsible for prescribing a diet for the client. Just as you cannot administer a medication to a client without a medication order, you cannot serve a diet to a client without a written physician's diet order. One of the functions of the diet manual is to define a diet. The diet manual is the first place to look when clients request food items that are not being served to them. The diet manual may state, perhaps, that the food item is restricted or not allowed on the client's prescribed diet.

SPECIAL DIETS

The purpose of a special or modified diet is to restore or maintain a client's nutritional status by manipulating one or more of the following aspects of the diet:

1. Nutrients such as protein, calcium, iron, sodium, potassium, and vitamin K may be increased, decreased, or eliminated.
2. Kilocalories may be either restricted or increased.
3. Texture or consistency of foods may be an issue. For example, only clear liquids may be served.
4. Use of seasonings such as pepper may be restricted or eliminated.

All modified diets are variations of the general diet; the client nonetheless needs all the essential nutrients. For this reason, each modified diet must be carefully planned to provide each of the essential nutrients or a documented reason for not providing one or more essential nutrients.

Much confusion results when the terminology in the diet order is not the same as the terminology in the diet manual. For example, a low-salt diet may not be the same as a low-sodium diet as defined in the diet manual. Physicians may persist in ordering a low-salt or low-sodium diet, even though the diet manual requests that all sodium-restricted diets be ordered in units of sodium such as 2-gram sodium or 4-gram sodium.

Physicians may become confused because they have patients admitted at different facilities simultaneously. Many facilities have eliminated this confusion by defining a low-sodium and low-salt diet in the diet manual (the definitions for both low-salt and low-sodium diets differ markedly from one facility to another). Other vague diet orders are *salt-free, diabetic, regular diabetic, low-fat, fat-free,* and *as tolerated*. The nursing or dietetic staff should clarify all vague diet orders with the physician before the client is served. All health-care workers should become familiar with the terminology in the facility's diet manual.

Diet manuals are not usually designed to be used directly for client instruction. Much of the information in the diet manual is directed to physicians and other health-care workers to assist in the implementation of special diets. For example, many diet manuals describe indications and contraindications for use of a particular diet. An **indication** is the circumstance that indicates when the diet should be used. A **contraindication** describes a circum-

stance when the diet should not be used. The diet manual also lists nutrients deficient in a particular diet. This type of information may alarm and confuse some clients.

COMMON DIET ORDERS

Some common diet orders are for *clear liquid, full liquid, soft,* and *general* or *regular*. A clear-liquid diet is any transparent liquid that can be poured at room temperature. Gelatin, some juices, broth, tea, and coffee are clear liquids. A clear-liquid diet is nutritionally inadequate. Clear-liquid nutritional supplements, however, are available. A full-liquid diet is any liquid that can be poured at room temperature. Milk, custard, thinned hot cereals, all fruit juices, ice cream, and all items allowed on the clear-liquid diet are allowed on most full-liquid diets. The major difference between a clear-liquid and a full-liquid diet is that the latter contains milk and milk products (Table 15–1 and Boxes 15–1 and 15–2).

Soft diets vary greatly from one facility to another. For example, a mechanical soft diet is ordered when the client has only a few or no teeth (edentulous). A soft diet is ordered following surgery when easily digested foods are required. A facility that specializes in treating clients with eye, ear, nose, and throat disorders may have many types of soft diets. A pureed diet usually consists of foods that have been run through a blender or food processor to meet the consistency needs of the patient. Table 15–2 lists recommended foods on a pureed, mechanical soft, and soft diet.

A general or regular diet means that the client is on an unrestricted diet. Frequently, an *as tolerated* or *progressive* diet may be prescribed, which means that a clear-liquid diet is to be served initially and the diet advanced (full-liquid to soft to general) as the client is able to tolerate. The nurse is usually responsible for determining the client's tolerance for food just before tray delivery. This last-minute determination of client tolerance is necessary for many clients because of fluctuating medical status.

Diets for Diagnostic Procedures

Many **diagnostic** procedures that require dietary preparation are performed in hospitals. It is important to follow the facility's diet manual when preparing a client for a diagnostic procedure.

POOR CLIENT PREPARATION

Poor dietary preparation can force a client to have an expensive procedure repeated or postponed (Fig. 15–1). Figure 15–1A is an x-ray from a poorly prepared client.

| Table **15–1** | Composition of Liquid Diets |

DIET	PROTEIN (g)	FAT (g)	CARBOHYDRATE (g)	SODIUM (mEq)	POTASSIUM (mEq)	KILOCALORIES
Clear liquid	5	trace	70–95	65	20	375
Clear liquid with three 6-oz servings of Citrotein/Enlive	30	1	140–165	80	30	750
Full liquid	50	55	205	110	65	1500

Box 15–1 **Clear-Liquid Diet**

Description: The clear-liquid diet provides energy and fluid in a form that requires minimal digestive action.
Indications: The clear-liquid diet is prescribed when it is necessary to limit undigested food in the gastrointestinal tract, before bowel surgery, diagnostic imaging procedures, and colonoscopic examination. A clear-liquid diet is also used during acute stages of illness to assist with fluid and electrolyte replacement and as a first step in oral alimentation following intravenous feeding, surgery, and gastrointestinal disturbances.
Adequacy: This diet is inadequate in all nutrients and should be used only in the short term.

FOOD ALLOWED	FOODS TO AVOID
Coffee and tea	All other food and beverages
Carbonated beverages such as 7-Up and ginger ale	
Fruit-flavored gelatin and popsicles	
Apple, grape, or cranberry juice	
Clear fat-free broth and bouillon	
Sugar	

Recommended to Enhance Nutrition

Nutritional supplements such as Enlive (Ross) or Citrotein (Novartis)
High-protein broth and gelatin desserts are also available

Sample Breakfast, Lunch, and Dinner Menu

Clear apple, grape, or cranberry juice
Broth
Flavored gelatin
Coffee or tea
Sugar
Clear-liquid complete nutritional supplement if client is on this diet for longer than two meals

Box 15–2 **Full-Liquid Diet**

Description: The full-liquid diet provides foods and beverages that are liquid or may become liquid at body temperature.
Indications: This diet is used as a progression between clear liquids and a soft diet and following oral surgery. Acutely ill clients with a chewing or swallowing dysfunction and clients with oral, esophageal, or stomach disorder who are unable to tolerate solid foods because of strictures or other anatomical disorders find this diet useful.
Adequacy: This diet can be adequate in all nutrients according to the Recommended Dietary Allowances. Special care needs to be taken to meet folacin, iron, thiamin, niacin, vitamin A, fiber, and kcalorie allowances.

FOODS ALLOWED	FOODS NOT ALLOWED
BEVERAGES	
Any beverage that pours at room temperature	All others
Breads, cereals, and grains:	All others
Cooked refined cereals (thinned or strained) such as cream of wheat	
FRUITS	
All fruit juices	All others
VEGETABLES	
Any vegetable juice	All others
MEATS	
None	
MILK	
Any	
FATS	
Butter, margarine, cream, and oils	All others
OTHER	
Custard, ice cream, flavored gelatin, sherbet, sugar, and popsicles	All others and any made with coconut, nuts, or whole fruit

(Continued on the following page)

Special Notes

The use of a complete nutritional liquid supplement is often necessary to meet nutrient allowances for clients who follow this diet for longer than 3 days.

An oral supplement that contains fiber minimizes the potential for problems with constipation and abdominal cramping. However, liquid supplements with fiber are not indicated for all patients on full-liquid diets.

Sample Menu

BREAKFAST	LUNCH AND DINNER	SNACKS
1/2 cup fruit juice	1/2 cup fruit juice	A complete nutritional supplement as needed to meet protein and kilocalorie allowances
1/2 cup cream of wheat	1/2 cup vegetable juice	
1 cup pasteurized eggnog	1 cup strained cream soup	
Coffee, cream, and sugar	1/2 cup custard	
	8 oz Ensure or Sustacal or similar product	
	Coffee as desired	

Table 15–2   **Consistency Modifications—Recommended Foods**

FOOD GROUP	PUREED DIET	MECHANICAL SOFT DIET	SOFT DIET
Soups	Broth, bouillon, strained or blenderized cream soup	Broth, bouillon, strained or blenderized cream soup	Broth, bouillon, cream soup
Beverages	All	All	All
Meat	Strained or pureed meat or poultry, cheese used in cooking	Ground, moist meats, or poultry, flaked fish, eggs, cottage cheese, cheese, creamy peanut butter, soft casseroles	Moist, tender meat, fish, or poultry, eggs, cottage cheese, mild flavored cheese, creamy peanut butter, soft casseroles
Fat	Butter, margarine, cream, oil, gravy	Butter, margarine, cream, oil, gravy, salad dressing	Butter, margarine, cream, oil, gravy, crisp bacon, avocado, salad dressing
Milk	Milk, milk beverages, yogurt without fruit, nuts, or seeds, cocoa	Milk, milk beverages, yogurt without seeds or nuts, cocoa	Milk, milk beverages, yogurt without seeds or nuts, cocoa
Starch	Cooked, refined cereal, mashed potatoes	Cooked or refined ready-to-eat cereal, potatoes, rice, pasta, white, refined wheat, light rye bread or rolls, graham crackers as tolerated	Cooked or ready-to-eat cereal, potatoes, rice, pasta, white, refined wheat, light rye or graham bread, rolls, or crackers
Vegetables	Strained or pureed, juice	Soft, cooked, without hulls or tough skin as in peas and corn, juice	Soft, cooked, vegetables, limit strongly flavored vegetables and whole-kernel corn, lettuce and tomatoes
Fruit	Strained or pureed, juice	Cooked or canned fruit without seeds or skins, banana, juice	Cooked or canned fruit, banana, citrus fruit without membrane, melon, juice
Desserts	Gelatin, sherbet, ice cream without nuts or fruit, custard, pudding, fruit ice, popsicle	Gelatin, sherbet, ice cream without nuts or fruit, custard, pudding, fruit ice, popsicle	Gelatin, sherbet, ice cream without nuts, custard, pudding, cake, cookies without nuts or coconut, fruit ice, popsicle
Sweets	Sugar, honey, jelly, candy, flavorings	Sugar, honey, jelly, candy, flavorings	Sugar, honey, jelly, candy, flavorings
Miscellaneous	Seasonings, condiments	Seasonings, condiments	Seasonings, condiments

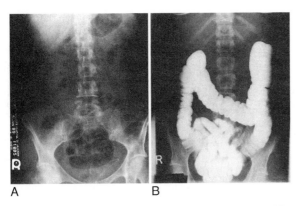

Figure **15–1** A, Image of a client who was poorly prepared for a barium enema. B, Image of a client who was adequately prepared for a barium enema. (Courtesy of Dr. Russell Tobe.)

Feces in the colon block the view of structures within the colon. Figure 15–1B shows the colon of a well-prepared client. In the absence of fecal material, the entire length of the colon can be visualized.

Some x-ray procedures are not only expensive but also uncomfortable. The client must have the procedure repeated if necessary bodily structures cannot be visualized. Although the specific dietary preparation for x-ray studies of the colon may vary from one facility to another, dietary preparation usually is somewhat similar. The client should be instructed not to eat or drink anything after midnight on the day of the imaging study. In addition, the client may need to follow a clear-liquid diet for 12 to 48 hours before the x-ray procedure.

Many clients undergo x-ray studies as outpatients. The nurse working in a physician's office is usually responsible for dietary instruction before these procedures. A reliable diet manual should be consulted before the scheduling of clients for such studies.

MISDIAGNOSIS

Poor dietary preparation can lead to a misdiagnosis. For example, a blood sample for a fasting blood glucose (FBS) test should be drawn on a **fasting** individual, that is, one who has not had any food (nor, sometimes, fluid) by mouth for at least 8 hours before the blood draw. If the client eats before the procedure, his or her blood glucose level may be elevated, and this elevation may cause a misdiagnosis of diabetes. A misdiagnosis may cause a client unnecessary anxiety and expense (Wellness Tip 15–1).

> *Wellness Tip* **15–1** • When a physician prescribes a diagnostic procedure for any outpatient, ask about the need for special dietary preparation. This question may prevent a misdiagnosis or the need to have a costly procedure repeated.

Importance of Nutritional Care

Malnutrition associated with acute and chronic disease is common in hospital settings. **Acute** means that the illness is characterized by a rapid onset, severe symptoms, and a short course. **Chronic** means that the illness has a long duration.

The presence and importance of malnutrition has been increasingly recognized over the past 30 years. It is one of the most common conditions affecting the care of hospitalized clients. Recent nutrition surveys in hospitals continue to suggest that upwards of 40% to 50% of patients, particularly those in intensive care units, have moderate to severe malnutrition (Pfau and Rombeau, 2004). Many patients come into hospitals malnourished, and their acute illnesses further worsens their malnutrition.

Malnutrition is associated with a 25 percent morbidity and a 5 percent mortality. **Morbidity** is defined as the rate of being diseased. **Mortality** is defined as the death rate. A malnourished client is thus more likely to be sicker and run a higher risk of death than a well-nourished client with the same diagnosis. Because malnutrition affects morbidity and mortality, it is also associated with a prolonged hospital stay.

Iatrogenic Malnutrition

The term **iatrogenic malnutrition** was first used in 1974 (Butterworth and Blackburn, 1975). *Iatrogenic malnutrition* is a less offensive phrase than *induced malnutrition,* that is, induced by a physician or an institution. Routine hospital practices such as extended periods of food or nutrient deprivation because of treatments, as well as diagnostic tests that interfere with the client's meal schedule or that cause a lack of appetite, are related to the high prevalence of malnutrition. Drug therapy may also affect a client's appetite. Some drugs cause drowsiness, lethargy, nausea, and anorexia. Problems related directly to an illness, such as pain, unconsciousness, paralysis, vomiting, and diarrhea, can also interfere with eating.

Today many institutions have written policies and procedures for nurses and dietitians to follow to minimize the likelihood of iatrogenic malnutrition. The tasks nurses should perform to combat institutional malnutrition are discussed in Clinical Application 15–1.

Methods of Nutrient Delivery

Nutrients can be delivered to the client orally in foods or supplements, by tube feeding, or parenterally through veins. An **enteral tube feeding** means the feeding of an appropriate formula or liquid via a tube to a client's gastrointestinal tract. A **parenteral feeding** designates any intravenous route.

Oral Delivery

Most institutionalized clients are fed orally. All of the factors mentioned throughout this text influence whether the food items served are actually consumed by the client. Whenever possible, the client should be encouraged to eat foods, not only as an optimal way to obtain nutrients but also because it is beneficial for the client to continue to experience the normal psychological and physical pleasure associated with eating.

The Menu

An institution's menu can be selective or nonselective. A selective menu is similar to a restaurant menu; clients can choose the specific menu items that appeal to them.

Methods for Nurses to Combat Iatrogenic Malnutrition

Nursing actions can affect the nutritional health of institutionalized clients. All of the following behaviors minimize the likelihood of malnutrition:

Recording height and weight

Regular communication among nurses, physicians, dietitians, and other health-care workers

Food tray viewing (monitoring) and documentation of client's food intake

Good food sanitation for oral and enteral feedings

Knowledge of the importance of good nutrition, nutritional supplements, and the composition of vitamin mixtures

Monitoring the length of time clients are NPO, on liquid diets, and on intravenous feedings of only glucose

Appreciation of the role of nutrition in the prevention and recovery from infection

Recognition of the increased nutritional needs due to injury or illness

Monitoring of stool frequency, urinary losses, losses by suction tubes, drainage, and so forth

Recording of weight at regular intervals

Monitoring of behavior patterns, vomiting, and any unusual comments clients make about food

Monitoring of client fluid intake and output

Everyone has food likes and dislikes; what appeals to one client may not appeal to another. Clients eat best when they fill out their own menus or a close significant other does so for them. Marking the menu is one way in which a client can participate daily in care planning.

Some institutions do not have a selective menu. Only one kind of meal is prepared and served to all clients. Food and labor required for institutions providing a selective menu is more expensive than for institutions providing a nonselective menu. However, many clients may fail to eat the food when the menu is nonselective.

Eating Environment

Health-care workers need to create as pleasant an environment as possible immediately before and during mealtime. The room should be checked for objectionable odors, sounds, and sights. Obviously, a full bedside commode or an emesis basin discourages eating. The client should be prepared to eat when the tray arrives. Cleaning the client's hands and face helps the client become more enthusiastic about eating. The client's bedside table should be cleared of all miscellaneous items so that the table can be used for the client's tray. Because all food loses and gains temperature quickly, unnecessary delays in serving the tray should be avoided. The client should be properly positioned to eat. This includes elevating the head of the bed (if condition permits) and positioning the bedside table to the correct height.

Some clients may find the odor of food offensive. For these clients, it is best for the nurse not to uncover the food items directly in front of them, so as to minimize the risk of nausea.

Assisted Feeding Versus Self-Feeding

Some clients must be fed. Food should be offered in bite-sized portions and in the order that the client prefers. Nurses should check the temperature of all hot liquids against the inside of their wrists before offering them to the client. Clients should not be rushed during feeding. Talking with the client while feeding makes mealtime more pleasant and signals to the client that he or she is not rushed. Sitting while feeding the client also indicates a willingness to spend time with the client and encourages relaxation.

Some nurses have found they can enhance a client's food intake by using the following technique:

- Sit behind the client.
- Place your right arm over the client's arm (if you and the client are right-handed).
- Place a fork or spoon with food in either the client's hand or your own hand (depending on the client's ability to do this maneuver).
- Guide the client's hand to his or her mouth.

This technique mimics normal eating behavior. In a long-term care facility, it is important that a client's ability to feed himself or herself be reevaluated at regular intervals. Any client's condition can change, and health-care workers need to constantly be aware of any changes in the client's condition.

Assisting the Disabled Client

A client with a disability may require either total or partial assistance with eating. Partial assistance may include opening milk cartons and plastic bags containing condiments and eating utensils, buttering the bread, and cutting the meat. Visually impaired clients may be able to feed themselves once they are told where the food is placed on the plate. The usual technique is to describe food placement in terms of hours on a clock face.

Some clients can feed themselves but may be very slow, clumsy, and messy. A large napkin under the chin may assist in cleanup. Offering hot beverages in small amounts may minimize the likelihood of an accident.

Sometimes a particular quality of a food offered to clients may influence whether they can feed themselves; the consistency of food is one example. A thin liquid may cause some clients to choke. A thicker substance such as yogurt may be better tolerated. Some disabled people are able to manage finger foods such as French fries or hard-cooked eggs. It is best to learn the food tolerances and preferences of disabled clients by observation and simply by asking them what they can tolerate.

Health-care workers should encourage clients to remain as independent as possible in all the activities of daily living, including eating. If a client cannot feed himself or herself, an evaluation should be made. Some clients' inability to feed themselves may be related to neuromuscular disabilities. Many special eating devices have been developed to assist such clients. The occupational therapist has had special training in the selection and fitting of such eating devices.

Supplemental Feedings

Many clients are unable to consume sufficient kilocalories or nutrients because of anorexia or an increased need for nutrients. The first step with this type of client is to offer additional foods at or between meals. Any between-meal feedings must adhere to the client's diet order. A kilocalorie count should be started for poor eaters; kilocalorie counts are one method to monitor the effectiveness of nutritional care. If the client will not accept the supplemental feedings, another treatment approach may be needed.

Liquid supplementation is often useful; many clients accept liquids better than solids. Many debilitated clients seem to feel less full after drinking a beverage than after eating a comparable number of kilocalories and nutrients in foods. Liquid supplements can include milk, milk shakes, and instant breakfast drinks. Many different commercially prepared liquid formulas are available. Four different types of supplements are used as oral feedings: modular supplements, intact or "polymeric" formulas, elemental or "predigested" formulas, and disease-specific formulas.

MODULAR SUPPLEMENTS

A **modular supplement** contains only one nutrient. Modular supplements are designed for clients who require the addition of only one nutrient. Moducal, Nutrisource CHO, Polycose, and Sumacal are supplements produced by different manufacturers that contain only carbohydrate. Medium-chain triglycerides supply only one form of lipid. Microlipid is another example of a of lipid supplement (see Appendix). Modular supplements for protein include Pro Mod, Propac, Pro-Mix, and Casec. Modular supplements are available in a liquid or powder form and can be added to foods, other types of oral supplements, or tube feedings.

INTACT OR "POLYMERIC" FORMULAS

An **intact** or **"polymeric" formula** is used when the gastrointestinal tract is functional and the client needs all of the essential nutrients in a specified volume. There are dozens of such products on the market. A complete supplement should always be used when the formula is the sole source of nutrition. Ensure, Sustacal, Resource, and Meritene are examples of complete nutritional supplements. Some complete nutritional supplements are also designed for tube feedings; the consistency and flavor of a feeding designed to be tube-fed will probably not be acceptable to the client when fed orally.

Intact formulas differ from one another. Some contain lactose and some do not. Some provide fiber. The product may be a powder for reconstitution, a liquid, or a pudding. It may be flavored or unflavored. The percentages of kilocalories derived from carbohydrates, fats, and proteins may be different.

The carbohydrate, fat, and protein may be derived from various sources. For example, the protein source in Meritene is concentrated skim milk, whereas the protein source in Ensure is sodium and calcium caseinates and a soy-protein isolate. For many reasons, the source of any of the three energy nutrients may be important. For example,

Meritene, Carnation Instant Breakfast, and Sustagen are not good supplements to use for a client with a lactose intolerance. Citrotein and Enlive are clear liquid polymeric formulas.

Commercial supplements should be used only after the client's requirements for nutrients have been assessed. Some health-care workers still think that if some is good, more is better, and they therefore encourage the client to consume greater amounts of oral supplement. Excess nutrients, however, are rarely beneficial. Not only do clients become frustrated because they cannot consume the entire supplement served to them, but to do so may be medically harmful. Many organs in the human body are in a stress situation in the poorly nourished client. Why subject the client's kidneys or liver to unnecessary work if the nutrients cannot be used efficiently? A suggested procedure to follow when determining the volume of an oral supplement to serve to a client is demonstrated in Clinical Calculation 15–1.

ELEMENTAL OR "PREDIGESTED" FORMULAS

Another group of oral supplements includes **elemental** or **"predigested" formulas**. Examples of elemental or predigested formulas include Flexical, Vital, and Vivonex. The nutrients in these formulas are easier to digest or already partially digested. For example, maltrodextrins, corn syrup solids, oligosaccharides, and glucose polymers are rapidly hydrolyzed by maltase and oligosaccharidases, which are apt to be present in the small intestine in higher concentrations than lactase.

Protein is either partially or totally predigested. Partially predigested protein (small peptides) offer an advantage over totally predigested protein (single amino acids). Peptides and free amino acids do not inhibit each other's transport across the gastrointestinal tract, and absorption of nitrogen is actually improved by the inclusion of small peptides. Easier-to-digest fats include medium-chain triglycerides. Partially digested fats include monoglycerides and diglycerides.

Predigested formulas contain little lactose and residue and may be given orally or through a tube. These formulas are very expensive and are designed only for use with clients with limited gastrointestinal function or metabolic disorders. Because they are less palatable than **intact feedings**, client acceptance is sometimes a problem when they are administered orally.

DISEASE-SPECIFIC FORMULAS

The last group of oral supplements includes those designed for clients with specific metabolic problems. For example, special formulas are available for clients with liver (Hepatic-Aid, Travasob Hepatic), pulmonary (Respalor, Pulmocare), and kidney disorders (Suplena, Amin-Aid, Travasob Renal). These special formulas are discussed in subsequent chapters.

Oral supplements are also used extensively to wean clients from both tube and parenteral feedings. Once a client ceases to consume foods orally, a transition period is always necessary to reacclimate the client back to oral feedings. This process can sometimes take a couple days

Clinical Calculation 15–1

How Much Oral Supplement Is Indicated?

1. Place client on a kilocalorie count.
2. Calculate client's kilocalorie allowance.
3. Select an appropriate oral supplement for the client. Some hospitals allow clients to taste several supplements and choose the one most palatable to them.
4. Determine the difference between the client's recorded food intake and kilocalorie allowance.
5. Determine the kilocalorie concentration of the formula. This can be done by referring to either the appropriate table in the diet manual or the supplement's label. Usually formulas are between 1.0 to 2.0 kcal/mL.
6. Determine how many milliliters of formula are needed to meet the client's kilocalorie allowance.
7. Divide the total milliliters needed by the number of feedings to be offered.
8. Calculate the client's protein allowance (0.8 g/kg).
9. Check to make sure that the client's protein allowance will be met by the combination of recorded protein intake and volume to be provided in the supplement. Also check to make sure that the client will not be receiving more than twice the RDA for protein.

Example:

1. Assume that the client ate 550 kcal.
2. Assume that the client is a woman who weighs 132 pounds and, is 55 years of age, and is 5 ft 2 in. tall and reports 30 minutes of daily physical activity ((See Table 6–2 overweight and moderately active)

Client's estimated need for kilocalories is 13 kcal/pound
13 X 132 = 1716 kilocalories
3. Assume that the client has tasted several supplements and prefers Nutren 1.0
4. The client's estimated need for kilocalories is 1716
The client ate 550 kcal
The difference is 1166 kcal
5. Nutren 1.0 contains 1.0 kcal/ml (information obtained from the product's label).
6. The client needs about 1166 ml to meet her estimated kilocalorie need.
7. The client stated she would prefer to drink this feeding five times per day, some on each tray, and at two between-meal feedings.
Round up to 1200 to simplify math 1200 divided by 5 = 240 ml
8. Assume from the client's recorded food intake that she is eating about 10 g of protein per day. A woman weighing 60 kg has a protein allowance of 0.8 g/kg.
60 kg × 0.8 g/kg = 48 g of protein
Subtract the 10 g eaten from trays
48 g – 10 g = 38 g
The supplement should provide at least 38 g of protein and no more than 86 g [(48 X 2) – 10 of protein.†
9. Nutren 1.0 contains 10 g of protein per 250 mL (one can).
10 g of protein X 5 cans (of 250 ml each) = 50 g 50 g of protein from oral supplement + 10 g of protein from food = 60 g
The client's protein allowance will more than be met by 1200 mL of Nutren 1.0 and food, but will not exceed the 200% guideline.

---

*This product is available in both quarts and 250-mL units. Some institutions stock only 250-mL units and may prefer to dispense this feeding in 250-mL units. In this situation, divide 250 mL into 1200 mL.
†It is important that the feeding and food not provide more than twice the client's protein allowance. In this case, 48 × 2 = 96 g. As the client is eating about 10 g of protein per day and will consume about 50 g more in the supplement, her total protein intake would be approximately 60 g/day. This amount does not exceed twice her RDA for protein and is therefore acceptable.

---

to months. An enteral formula comparison chart can be found in the Appendix K.

Enteral Tube Feeding

Tube feedings are the second way nutrients can be delivered to clients. With some medical conditions, oral feeding is impossible, insufficient, or impractical. Several common conditions in which a tube feeding is indicated are listed in Table 15–3.

Tube feedings, like oral supplements, can be made from table foods or purchased commercially prepared. If the client's finances are tight and the client has no impairment of digestion and absorption, he or she can be taught to prepare a tube feeding from table foods before discharge. Home-prepared tube feedings are less expensive than commercially prepared feedings but more prone to contamination. Many of the commercial products described in the previous section can be used by tube-fed clients.

Medical literature has addressed the subject of tube feedings for clients with dementia (Climent, 2000; Vollman, 2000). Both of these articles advocate ending the use of stomach tubes to feed people with advanced Alzheimer's disease and other types of dementia. Patients with these conditions frequently pull the tubes out, which leads nursing home and hospital staff to place the patients in restraints. An argument can be made that tube feedings deprive patients of the enjoyment that can be derived from eating and the social satisfaction that accompanies eating by hand. For this reason, most institutions have strict guidelines that all nurses must follow before inserting a tube feeding into any patient.

Gastrointestinal Function

The gastrointestinal tract should always be used to the extent possible. Oral supplements should be considered before tube feeding; tube feeding should always be

Table 15–3 Conditions Indicating a Tube Feeding*

CONDITION	EXAMPLES
Client has mechanical difficulties that make chewing and/or swallowing impossible or difficult	Obstruction of the esophagus, weakness or nausea, mouth sores, throat inflammation
Client has an intestinal disease and cannot digest or absorb food adequately	Malabsorption syndromes
Client refuses to eat or cannot eat	Anorexia nervosa
Client is unable to consume a sufficient amount of food because of clinical condition	Coma, serious infections, trauma victims, clients with large kilocalorie requirements

*Other conditions will be discussed in subsequent chapters.

considered before intravenous feeding. Tube feeding is safer, cheaper, and more physiological than intravenous feeding; in other words, it more nearly mimics normal feeding conditions. Nutrients should be supplied intact rather than predigested if the client has normal digestion. **Intact nutrients** are nutrients that are not predigested. With intact nutrients, the body must keep producing all the secretions and enzymes necessary for digestion, thereby forcing the gastrointestinal tract to function.

Tube Placement

Feeding tubes can enter the body through the nose or through a surgically made opening. A **nasogastric (NG) tube** runs from the nose to the stomach. A **nasoduodenal (ND) tube** runs from the nose to the duodenum. A **nasojejunal (NJ) tube** runs from the nose to the jejunum. These types of tubes are designed for short-term use only because of client discomfort and tissue irritation.

When long-term tube feeding is needed or a tube cannot be inserted through the nose, an **ostomy,** or surgically created opening, is created. An **esophagostomy** is a surgical opening into the esophagus through which a feeding tube is passed. A **gastrostomy** is a surgical opening in the stomach through which a feeding tube is passed; this is the most common tube insertion method.

Percutaneous endoscopic gastrostomy or PEG tube placement is used for clients who require a feeding tube long term. A PEG tube can be placed **percutaneously** with the aid of an **endoscope** or surgically if the patient is already undergoing abdominal surgery or has a condition that makes working with an endoscope difficult. Percutaneous endoscopic jejunostomy (PEJ) tube placement is generally reserved for clients who are not candidates for a PEG. A client who has had a gastrectomy (stomach removal) procedure requires a PEJ tube placement.

A critical responsibility of nurses is assessment of feeding tube placement. The most reliable method of determining tube placement is radiography. Tubes have been mispositioned in such dangerous locations as the lungs and even the brain (Metheny and Titler, 2001).

Unfortunately, feeding tubes migrate (after x-ray) and may move out of the stomach or jejunum. Tube migration places the client at risk for aspiration because the tube may move into the trachea. The client is also at risk if he or she regurgitates the feeding. **Regurgitation** means to cause to flow backward. If the feeding backs up into the client's lungs, a lung infection can develop.

When a client has inhaled fluids regurgitated from the stomach, he or she may develop aspiration pneumonia. **Aspiration** is the state whereby a substance has been drawn up into the nose, throat, or lungs. Pulmonary aspiration is a common occurrence in hospitalized patients. Enteral tube feeding increases the risk of aspiration and is associated with the development of nosocomial pneumonia, which significantly increases morbidity and mortality in critically ill patients.

In the past, many nurses were taught and institutions recommended the tinting of enteral feedings with blue dye to promote early detection of aspiration. Every time the patient was suctioned, the specimen was inspected against a white background for the presence of dye. The presence of blue color in suctioned specimens indicated aspiration of the feeding into the lungs. The blue dye was the favored color because blue is not a color found in secretions. It is now widely recognized that blue dye has toxic effects. These effects include lactic acidosis, altered mental status, hypotension, hyperthermia, and rapid death (Super, 2003). Other problems associated with the use of blue dye include bacterial contamination of the dye solution. Many professionals believe the use of blue dye in enteral feedings formulas should be abandoned. The FDA issued a health advisory in 2003 citing several reports of toxicity, including death with FD&C Blue No. 1 (www.fda accessed, 2003).

Many practitioners consider an analysis of the color and pH of fluid intentionally aspirated from a tube to be the second best method (after x-ray) to assess tube placement. A pH-paper reading of between 0 and 4 indicates the tube is likely in the stomach and helps rule out inadvertent respiratory placement. Gastric fluid is most often grassy green, tan to off-white, bloody, or brown (Metheny and Titler, 2001). Tracheobronchial fluid is usually off-white and heavily tinged with mucus. Although they are not infallible methods, pH and color analysis to assess tube placement can offer valuable clues.

Contamination

Unfortunately, tube feedings provide an excellent environment for the growth of microorganisms. When a tube feeding becomes contaminated with bacteria, the client receiving the feeding may become ill and may suffer from gastrointestinal problems such as nausea, vomiting, or diarrhea. For this reason, many hospitals and nursing homes use only commercially prepared tube feedings (as opposed to those prepared in-house from table foods). Commercial feedings are packaged under sterile conditions. Most hospitals do not have a sterile area in their dietary departments. Even commercially prepared formulas can become contaminated if they are not handled safely after opening.

To prevent contamination, first check the can for the correct product, flavor, expiration date, and any signs of contamination such as swelling. If the can is swollen, notify your supervisor. Do not administer a feeding from a damaged can. Other cans in the same shipment should be checked for contamination.

Good personal hygiene is important. The following recommendations help reduce the possibility of contamination:

* Always wash your hands before opening the can.
* Wash the top of the can carefully before opening the can.
* Shake the can well before opening it.
* If a can opener is needed, be sure it is clean.
* Transfer the formula into a clean container.
* Use sterile, bottled, or boiled water to dilute the formula (if indicated).
* Label any remaining formula carefully with the client's name, room number, the date the formula was opened, the amount in the container, the name of the product, and other pertinent information. Other information may include whether the formula is diluted or contains medications, vitamins, or other additives.
* Store the formula in the refrigerator in a covered container. When a new supply of formula is received, place it in the rear of the storage area so that the older formula is used first.
* Once opened, most formulas should be discarded after 24 hours.

Administration

Tube feedings can be administered continuously, intermittently, or by **bolus**. Clogging of the tube occurs significantly more often with continuous rather than intermittent feedings.

CONTINUOUS FEEDING

Many professionals feel that **continuous feeding** is preferable to other methods. A continuous feeding is always recommended for formulas delivered directly into the small intestine. One recommended rate is 30 to 50 milliliters per hour, increasing daily by 25 milliliters per hour to the rate necessary to meet energy needs. This gradual increase in the formula's volume gives the client's gastrointestinal tract a chance to adjust to the formula and helps prevent many complications that occur in tube-fed clients. Safety precautions for continuous feedings include (1) flushing the tube with water every 4 to 6 hours and (2) allowing no more than a 4-hour hang time for each bag of formula unless the formula is packaged in a sterilized delivery system. These procedures help prevent contamination and bacterial growth. An infusion pump is necessary for precise control of a continuous feeding.

INTERMITTENT FEEDING

An **intermittent feeding** means giving a 4- to 6-hour volume of feeding solution over 20 to 30 minutes. Clients tolerate intermittent feedings much better than bolus feedings because these feedings more closely approximate normal eating behavior. The tube needs to be flushed after each feeding to minimize bacterial growth and prevent contamination.

BOLUS FEEDING

Bolus feeding means giving a 4- to 6-hour volume of feeding solution within a few minutes. A client is thus fed only four to six times per day. Feedings given by this method are frequently poorly tolerated, with clients complaining of abdominal discomfort, nausea, fullness, and cramping. Some clients, however, can tolerate bolus feedings after they have had a period of adjustment to the tube feeding. Bolus feedings are usually poorly tolerated for feedings that enter the intestines.

The adjustment period should follow the procedure described above, that is, the volume of feeding is slowly increased. Clients on bolus feedings should be instructed not to recline for at least 2 hours following the feeding. Tubes should be irrigated (flushed with water) after each bolus feeding to prevent contamination. The patient with normal gastric function can usually tolerate 500 ml of formula at each feeding (Blouch and Mueller, 2004).

Potential Complications

Complications fall into three categories: mechanical, gastrointestinal, and metabolic. Table 15–4 reviews these complications of tube-fed clients and lists system-specific prevention strategies. Metabolic complications are discussed in later chapters.

Osmolality

The osmolality of a solution is based on the number of dissolved particles in the solution. The greater the number of particles, the higher the osmolality.

At a given concentration, the smaller the particle size, the greater the number of particles present. Oral supplements and tube feedings with a high osmolality draw body fluid into the bowel, resulting in a fluid imbalance. The symptoms are diarrhea, nausea, and flushing. The osmolality of normal body fluids is approximately 300 milliosmoles per kilogram. Predigested nutrients have a higher osmolality than intact nutrients. An **isotonic** feeding has an osmolality of 300 milliosmoles, the same osmotic pressure as body fluids. Table 15–5 lists the osmolality of selected formulas.

Sensitivity to the osmolality of oral supplements and tube feedings varies greatly from one individual to another. A high-osmolality feeding can provide a more concentrated source of nutrients than a feeding of lower osmolality. All clients need a period of adjustment to a high-osmolality formula. Most clients are able to eventually develop a tolerance to a high-osmolality formula; some clients, however, are more likely to develop symptoms of an intolerance. These include debilitated clients, clients with gastrointestinal disorders, preoperative and postoperative clients, gastrostomy and **jejunostomy** clients, and clients whose gastrointestinal tract has not been challenged by food for a significant period of time.

Table 15–4 **Common Mechanical, Gastrointestinal, and Metabolic Complications of Tube-Fed Clients and Prevention Strategies**

COMPLICATION	PREVENTION STRATEGY
MECHANICAL	
Tube irritation	Consider using a smaller or softer tube
	Lubricate the tube before insertion
Tube obstruction	Flush tube after use
	Do not mix medications with the formula
	Use liquid medications if available
	Crush other medications thoroughly
	Use an infusion pump to maintain a constant flow
	Feeding should not be started until tube placement is radiographically confirmed
Aspiration and regurgitation	Elevate head of client's bed greater than or equal to 30 degrees at all times
	Discontinue feedings at least 30 to 60 minutes before treatments where head must be lowered (e.g., chest percussion)
	If the client has an endotracheal tube in place, keep the cuff inflated during feedings
	Test pH of aspirate with pH paper or meter
	a. pH of tracheobronchial secretions is alkaline, >7.4
	b. pH of gastric secretions is acidic, <5.0
	c. As the tube moves from the acid stomach to the alkaline duodenum, pH will change from acid to alkaline
Tube displacement	Place a black mark at the point where the tube, once properly placed, exits the nostril
	Replace tube and obtain physician's order to confirm with x-ray imaging
GASTROINTESTINAL	
Cramping, distention, bloating, gas pains, nausea, vomiting, diarrhea*	Initiate and increase amount of formula gradually
	Bring formula to room temperature before feeding
	Change to a lactose-free formula
	Decrease fat context of formula
	Administer drug therapy as ordered, e.g., Lactinex, kaolin-pectin, Lomotil
	Change to formula with a lower osmolality
	Change to formula with a different fiber content
	Practice good personal hygiene when handling any feeding product
	Evaluate diarrhea-causing medications the client may be receiving (e.g., antibiotics, digitalis)
METABOLIC	
Dehydration	Assess client's fluid requirements before treatment
	Monitor hydration status
Overhydration	Assess client's fluid requirements before treatment
	Monitor hydration status
Hyperglycemia	Initiate feedings at a low rate
	Monitor blood glucose
	Use hyperglycemic medication if necessary
	Select low-carbohydrate formula
	Evaluate total kilocalories provided; overfeeding in a critically ill patient exacerbates hyperglycemia
Hypernatremia	Assess client's fluid and electrolyte status before treatment
	Provide adequate fluids
Hyponatremia	Assess client's fluid and electrolyte status before treatment
	Restrict fluids
	Supplement feeding with rehydration solution and saline
	Diuretic therapy may be beneficial
Hypophosphatemia	Monitor serum levels
	Replenish phosphorus levels before refeeding
Hypercapnia	Select low-carbohydrate high-fat formula
Hypokalemia	Monitor serum levels
	Supplement feeding with potassium if necessary
Hyperkalemia	Reduce potassium intake
	Monitor potassium levels

*The most commonly cited complication of tube feeding is diarrhea.

Table 15–5 Osmolality of Selected Formulas

FORMULA	mOm/kg H$_2$	DESCRIPTION
f.a.a. (Free Amino Acid Diet)	700	Elemental formula
Vivonex RTH*	700	Elemental formula
Ensure	590	Intact or polymeric
Isocal	270	Intact or polymeric

*Please note the wide range in osmolality of the various formulas.
*Ready to hang

Administration of Medications to a Tube-Fed Client

All health-care workers should be aware of potential drug-food interactions to minimize or prevent complications (see Chapter 17). Clinical Application 15–2 discusses suggested procedures for administering medications through feeding tubes. Medications can be physically incompatible with the tube feeding because of changes in the feeding's viscosity (thickness) or flow characteristics. Some medications may also cause the feeding to separate, granulate, or coagulate.

Monitoring the Tube-Fed Client

Nutritional status, fluid balance, and gastrointestinal tolerance all need to be monitored in tube-fed clients. Whether the client requires daily or weekly monitoring depends on client acuity, duration of feeding, and the practice in the individual facility.

Nutritional status monitoring begins with a comparison of the client's kilocalorie and protein allowances to the volume and composition of the nutritional product utilized. Initially the client's kilocalorie and protein allowances are not usually met because a tube feeding is usually started at a low volume to increase gastrointestinal tolerance. Changes in the client's medical status and treatment, physical activity, and tolerance to the tube feeding may continually alter the volume and kind of feeding the client requires. Thus, the kilocaloric and protein content of the tube feeding requires reassessment.

In stable clients, serum levels of sodium, blood urea nitrogen, hemoglobin, and albumin are indicators of fluid status. Urine osmolality can be used to monitor hydration status. Urine osmolality is normally in the range of 50 to 1400 mOsm, with a usual range 300 to 900 mOsm and an average of 850 mOsm. Decreased osmolality indicates overhydration, and increased osmolality indicates dehydration. Fluid intake and output need to be recorded daily. Fluid intake should be at least 500 mL greater than output in clients who are neither overhydrated nor underhydrated. This 500-mL surplus is needed to cover insensible losses in feces and from the skin and lungs. Clinical signs of hydration status include skin turgor, presence of axillary sweat, condition of the mucous membranes, and the presence or absence of edema. Constipation is another possible sign of dehydration. Critically ill clients are usually overhydrated, whereas stable clients are often dehydrated (Skipper, 1998).

Clinical Application 15–2

Procedures for Administering Medications Through Feeding Tubes

Procedures for the administration of medications through feeding tubes may vary slightly from one institution or facility to another. The following suggested procedures, however, are common in most facilities:

1. If possible, administer drugs in liquid form.
2. If the drug is not available in liquid form, consult with the pharmacist; he or she may be able to procure a liquid form or similar drug provided by the American Society of Hospital Pharmacists in Pediatric Extemporaneous Formulation List of the manufacturer's suggestions.
3. Exercise caution when calculating equivalent liquid doses. Many liquid dosage forms are intended for pediatric use, and the dose of the drug must be adjusted appropriately for adults.
4. Administer crushed tablets only when no other alternatives are available.
5. If crushed tablets are administered, crush the tablet to a fine powder and mix with water. Do not crush any tablet on the list of oral drugs that should not be crushed. Do not crush drugs with a sustained-release action or an enteric coating. If in doubt, consult with the pharmacist.
6. Administer each drug separately. Do not mix all the medications for one dosing time. Flush with at least 5 mL (1 tsp) of water between each medication.
7. Flush the tube with at least 30 mL of water before giving the medication and before restarting the tube feeding.
8. To avoid causing gastric irritation and diarrhea, drugs that are hypertonic or irritating to the cells that line the gastrointestinal tract, such as potassium chloride, should be diluted in at least 30 mL of water before administration.
9. If the medication is ordered to be added to the feeding, observe the feeding after the addition for any reaction or precipitation. Shake the solution thoroughly. Label the feedings with at least the name and amount of the drug added, the time, date, and your initials.
10. Drugs usually administered with meals to avoid gastric irritation, such as indomethacin, should also be diluted with water before administration.
11. Sustained- or slow-release formulations of drugs that are used for once-daily dosing may need to have divided dosing schedules when administered in liquid form.

Gastrointestinal tolerance can be assessed by the absence or presence of diarrhea, bowel sounds, nausea, distension, and vomiting. The type of feeding delivered, the volume given, or the delivery rate can cause diarrhea. Diarrhea is frequently caused by medications. Antibiotics, laxatives, H$_2$ receptor blockers, and antacids with magnesium can cause stools to become watery. Medications that contain sorbital can also have a laxative effect (Burnham, 2000).

Gastric residuals are usually measured several times daily or about every 4 hours. Because elevated residuals indicate delayed gastric emptying and a potentially increased risk for aspiration, feedings are advanced only when gastric residuals are within acceptable limits (150 to 200 ml) (Skippper, 1998). Measurement of gastric residuals in a stable alert client who has a well-established tolerance to the tube feeding is usually not necessary. Feedings continuously dripped into the intestines do not normally produce a gastric residue because there is no place for the fluid to collect. Gastric residue measurement is most relevant in critically ill patients and others at risk for gastroparesis (Blouch and Mueller, 2004).

Home Enteral Nutrition

Many clients on tube feedings are being discharged from hospitals and nursing homes. Most hospitals and nursing homes that discharge clients on home enteral nutrition (HEN) have a **nutrition support service**. The delivery of effective nutritional support requires a team effort. Team members usually include the physician, pharmacist, nurse clinician, dietitian, and social worker. Team functions vary from one facility to another. Members of nutrition support teams assess, monitor, and educate clients. Some nutrition support service team members also arrange for client follow-up in outpatient clinics or in the home.

Parenteral Nutrition

Parenteral nutrition in which nutrients are delivered to the client through the veins (intravenously) is the third means of feeding. **Peripheral parenteral nutrition (PPN)** means to feed the client via a vein away from the center of the body (Fig. 15–2). In **total parenteral nutrition (TPN),** the client is fed via a central vein. Clients are also fed via a central line that has been inserted peripherally and threaded into the subclavian or jugular veins. This is called a **PIC line**. The terminology is confusing. It is important to note if the line terminates peripherally or centrally. TPN, PIC lines, and PPN can be used to provide partial or total daily nutritional requirements. Clients who cannot or should not be fed through the gastrointestinal tract are some of the candidates for TPN, PIC lines, and PPN. See Box 15–3 for appropriate indications for the use of PPN and TPN.

Peripheral Parenteral Nutrition (PPN)

Intravenous (IV) feeding (peripheral parenteral nutrition [PPN]) is routine in most health-care institutions. IV solutions, usually containing water, dextrose, electrolytes, and occasionally other nutrients, are used to maintain fluid, electrolyte, and acid-base balance. Intravenous solutions do contain kilocalories. The calculation of the kilocalorie content of an intravenous solution is demonstrated in Clinical Calculation 15–2.

Amino acids and fat can be supplied peripherally. To prevent ketosis, intravenous lipid emulsions should contribute no more than 60 percent of the total kilocalories provided. Dextrose concentrations are limited to approximately 10 percent, because peripheral veins cannot withstand concentrations greater than 900 milliosmoles per kilogram. Thus, PPN has often failed to provide adequate kilocalories and other nutrients for repair and replacement of losses. PPN has been used to supplement a partially successful enteral nutrition program.

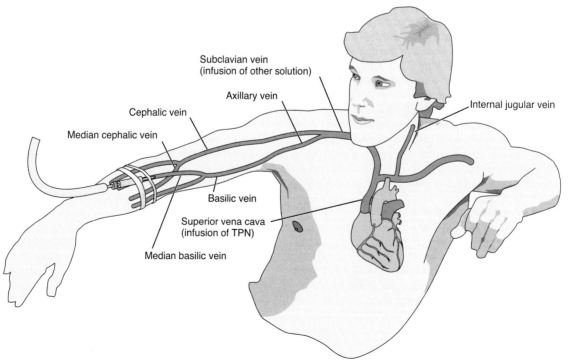

Figure **15–2** Correct placement of a peripherally placed central catheter (PICC).

Box 15–3 Indications for Peripheral Parenteral Nutrition (PPN) and Total Parenteral Nutrition (TPN)

PPN

PPN is an effective method of nutritional support for clients with mild to moderate nutritional deficiencies who are unable to receive enteral nutrition or for whom the central venous route is inaccessible or undesirable. Specifically, PPN is indicated for clients:

- Who are expected to be NPO for 5 days
- Who have inadequate GI function expected to last 5 to 7 days
- Who are making the transition to an oral diet or tube feeding
- In whom central venous access is contraindicated
- Who are malnourished and expected to be NPO for several days

- Who have energy and protein requirements that can be met with PPN (1800 kcalories per day or less)

TPN/PIC

Potential candidates for TPN/PIC include those clients who are anticipated to require nutritional support for longer than 10 days or who have an increased requirement for energy, such as clients:

- Who need preoperative preparation but are severely malnourished
- Who have postoperative surgical complications
- Who have inflammatory bowel disease
- Who have inadequate oral intake or malabsorption

A system for PPN (called all-in-one or three-in-one) has been developed that allows a higher osmotic load (1200 to 1350 milliosmoles per liter) to be delivered peripherally. Lipids, amino acids, dextrose, electrolytes, trace elements, and vitamins are all incorporated in one container. Tolerance of this higher osmotic mixture in peripheral veins might be attributed to the buffering and dilution effects of intravenous fats in combination with the higher pH of the amino acid solutions and the addition of heparin to the mixture.

The ratio of nonprotein to protein kilocalories, important in peripheral feedings, is discussed in Chapter 24.

Clinical Calculation 15–2

Calculation of Kilocalories in IV Solutions

D_5W means 5 percent dextrose in water. The subscript following the D tells you the percent of dextrose in the solution. Other common concentrations of sugar and water are $D_{10}W$ and $D_{50}W$.

A 5 percent concentration of dextrose means 100 mL of water contains 5 g of dextrose. A 10 percent concentration of dextrose means 100 mL of water contains 10 g of dextrose. A 50 percent concentration of dextrose means 100 mL of water contains 50 g of dextrose. A simple proportion should be used to calculate the number of kilocalories in any given volume of a solution.

The formula is:

$$\frac{\text{percent of concentration}}{100 \text{ mL}} = \frac{\times \text{ grams of dextrose}}{\substack{\text{volume of solution} \\ \text{client received}}}$$

For example, a client has received 1000 mL of D_5W:

$$\frac{5 \text{ gram of dextrose}}{100 \text{ mL}} = \frac{\times \text{ grams of dextrose}}{1000}$$

$$= 50 \text{ grams of dextrose}$$

Proportions are solved by cross-multiplication and division: (5 g × 1000 mL) divided by 100 mL = 50 g of dextrose. One gram of carbohydrate given intravenously provides 3.4 kcal; thus, 50 g multiplied by 3.4 kcal/g = 170 kcal.

Total Parenteral Nutrition (TPN) and PIC Lines

When nutrients are infused into a central vein, parenteral nutrition is often referred to as total parenteral nutrition (TPN) or **hyperalimentation**. Hyperalimentation is actually a misnomer because it implies that the solution exceeds nutritional requirements. The **superior vena cava,** one of the largest-diameter veins in the human body, is often used for TPN. Total parenteral nutrition can deliver greater nutrient loads, because the blood flow in the superior vena cava rapidly dilutes these solutions 1000-fold. Concentrations for both dextrose and amino acids are determined by the client's needs. See Clinical Calculation 15–3 for an explanation and demonstration of the calculation of a sample TPN solution. A line inserted peripherally but threaded into a central vein is hyperalimentation.

INSERTION AND CARE OF TPN LINE

The physician inserts the TPN line usually through the subclavian vein and into the superior vena cava. A highly trained nurse often inserts a PIC line. It can be inserted at the client's bedside using strict aseptic technique. TPN and PIC solutions are sterile mixtures of dextrose, amino acids, lipid emulsion, electrolytes, vitamins, trace elements, and other additives. The pharmacist usually prepares these solutions. Careful attention is required to provide vitamins and minerals to clients maintained on TPN/PIC solutions to prevent problems such as Wernicke-Korsakoff syndrome (Chapter 7).

Total parenteral nutrition has both advantages and disadvantages. Central TPN should not be carried out without experienced personnel and proper facilities. One disadvantage of solutions that terminate into central veins is that it takes a highly trained staff to provide safe administration and close monitoring, and the solution itself is

Clinical Calculation 15–3

Calculation of a Sample TPN Solution/TPN Energy Nutrient Content (or PIC line)

TPN/PIC solutions are usually packed in 500-mL bags. Pharmacists prefer to use dextrose and amino acids in 500-mL bags and vary the concentration of the nutrients to achieve the appropriate nutritional parameters. For example, a 500-mL bag of dextrose mixed with a 500-mL bag of amino acids equals 1000 mL. Lipids are usually provided as 250 mL of 20 percent lipid (1/2 bag) or 500 mL (one bag) of 10 percent lipid. The client's needs for kilocalories, protein, and fat can be amlommodated by individualizing the concentration of each energy nutrient. For example, dextrose can be ordered from 5 to 70 percent, noted as D_5, D_{40}, D_{50}, etc. Commonly used concentrations of amino acids are 5 percent, 8.5 percent, and 10 percent.

Nutritional Values Used in Computations of TPN Solutions

Dextrose = 3.4 kcal/g
20 percent lipid = 2.0 kcal/cc
10 percent lipid = 1.1 kcal/cc
Protein = 4.0 kcal/g
1 g of nitrogen = 6.25 g protein

Calculate the total kilocalories, nonprotein kilocalories, grams of nitrogen, calorie/nitrogen ratio, and percent kilocalories from fat in 500 mL D_{50}, 500 mL 10 percent amino acids, and 250 cc 10 percent lipid.

Dextrose	Percent concentration × volume = grams of dextrose	0.50 × 500 = 250 g dextrose
	Grams of dextrose × 3.4 kcal/g = kcal of solution	250 g dextrose × 3.4 kcal/g = 850 kcal
Amino acids	Percent concentration × volume = grams of protein	0.10 × 500 mL = 50 g protein
	Grams of protein × kcal/g = protein kcal	50 g protein × 4 kcal/g = 200 kcal
Lipids	Kcal/cc × volume in cc = fat kcal	1.1 × 250 mL = 275 kcal
Total kilocalories	Add kcal from dextrose, protein, and lipid	850 + 200 + 275 = 1325 kcal
Percent kilocalories from fat	Kcal from fat divided by total kcal = percent fat kcal	275 divided by 1325 = 21 percent fat

costly. This makes the therapy very costly. The nurse is usually responsible for assessing, monitoring, and educating the client destined for home parental nutrition. The clinical dietitian on the team usually has an advanced degree and special training. The dietitian is responsible for constant nutrition assessment, monitoring, interpretation of data, and calculating formula needs with the physician.

MONITORING

Careful administration of the central lines solutions is important. Most reputable institutions have a strict protocol that must be followed by all health-care professionals. (A **protocol** is a description of steps to be followed when performing a procedure.) Protocols vary widely from one institution to another. Most TPN protocols include a slow start, a strict schedule, close monitoring, instructions for increasing the volume, maintenance of a constant rate, and instructions for a slow withdrawal. The solution may require adjustment, which can be made by increasing or decreasing any or all of the nutrients. All long-term TPN/PIC line patients should receive ongoing monitoring by a home-care clinician, including an assessment of micronutrient status, to ensure adequacy of the nutrition support regimen (Falk, 2002). All long-term patients on this therapy also should receive ongoing monitoring by a home-care clinician, including an assessment of micronutrient status to ensure adequacy of the nutrition support regimen (Falk, 2002). Careful monitoring of the client's response to central line nutrition and taking corrective measures when needed are essential for safe administration of these solutions.

Many metabolic complications are possible with TPN. Rapid shifts of potassium, phosphorus, and magnesium intracellularly result in a lowering of their concentrations in the serum. The solution may need to be altered if there is a drop in the serum values of these electrolytes. Providing glucose in excess of kilocaloric needs can result in several problems, including carbon dioxide retention with respiratory difficulty. High glucose content of solutions also leads to hyperglycemia. Therefore, glucose levels should be assessed regularly. Liver function test results will become abnormal after an excess glucose load. Excess glucose may lead to hyperlipidemia and fatty deposits in the liver.

The avoidance of metabolic complications directly related to a glucose overload is one reason TPN clients need to be monitored closely. These complications can be avoided by providing only an appropriate and not an excessive amount of kilocalories. In addition, an initial slow infusion at low concentrations prevents complications. Box 15–4 lists general recommendations for TPN monitoring.

TRANSITION AND COMBINATION FEEDINGS

Clients need a transition period from TPN to oral feedings. Some physicians prefer to wean clients from TPN by using tube feeding. Other physicians prefer to avoid the tube and wean clients orally. In the latter case, as the client's oral intake increases, the TPN solution is gradually withdrawn. Expect clients who have been on TPN for a significant period of time to experience some difficulty with oral feedings. They may need much encouragement to eat.

One of the problems with TPN is that the gastrointestinal tract does not have to work during its administration. Consequently the gastrointestinal tract will have undergone some atrophy. Oral foods should be offered slowly during the weaning process. Some physicians avoid this problem by allowing some clients to consume a clear-liquid or light diet while on TPN, if their condition permits.

HOME PARENTERAL NUTRITION

Increasingly, clients are being discharged on TPN. These clients need adequate follow-up by either the hospital or a community home health agency. The pharmacist is responsible for the storage of TPN solutions in most institutions. Nurses involved in home parenteral nutrition need to be aware that vitamin degradation during the storage of total parenteral nutrition mixtures is significant and affects clinical outcome (Dupertuis, 2003). Factors affecting vitamin degradation include TPN bag material, temperature, and length of time between TPN compounding and end of infusion into the patient. The home-care nurse needs to work closely with the pharmacist and patient to minimize nutrient losses in TPN solutions.

Box 15–4 **Monitoring TPN**

Initial Assessment

- Vital signs (respiration, pulse, temperature)
- Body weight and height
- Serum electrolytes, glucose, creatinine, blood urea nitrogen levels
- Serum magnesium, calcium, phosphorus levels
- Serum triglycerides and cholesterol levels
- Liver function tests
- Serum albumin and prealbumin
- Complete blood count
- Energy (estimated or measured), protein, fluid, and micronutrient needs

Routine Every 4 to 8 Hours

- Vital signs

Every 24 Hours

- Weight
- Fluid intake and output
- Serum electrolytes, glucose, creatinine, blood urea nitrogen levels; daily for 5 days or until stable; then twice a week

Weekly

- Serum ammonia, SGOT*, serum calcium, phosphorus, magnesium, total protein, and albumin
- Complete blood count
- Reassessment of actual oral, enteral, and TPN intake

Other monitors may be indicated depending on the client's clinical condition.

*Serum glutamic oxaloacetic transaminase is a liver enzyme that reflects liver cellular damage when elevated (as opposed to liver obstructive disease)

SUMMARY

The nutritional care of clients is a joint responsibility of the dietary and nursing departments. All nurses who work in institutions need to know not only how meals are distributed to clients but also current meal-service schedules, which affect the administration of medications and the scheduling of clients for procedures. Nutritional care includes three areas: assessing the client's need for nutrients, monitoring nutrient intake, and counseling clients about nutritional needs.

Nutrients can be delivered to clients orally, via tube feeding, or parenterally. See Figure 15–3 for a nutritional support decision tree. One principle is followed when selecting a feeding route: if the gastrointestinal tract works, use it to maximum capability. Every means should be attempted to assist clients to eat orally and independently. Oral feedings should be considered before tube feeding. Tube feeding should be considered before intravenous feeding. Intravenous feeding can be delivered peripherally or centrally. Clients on either tube feedings or intravenous feedings need to be closely monitored.

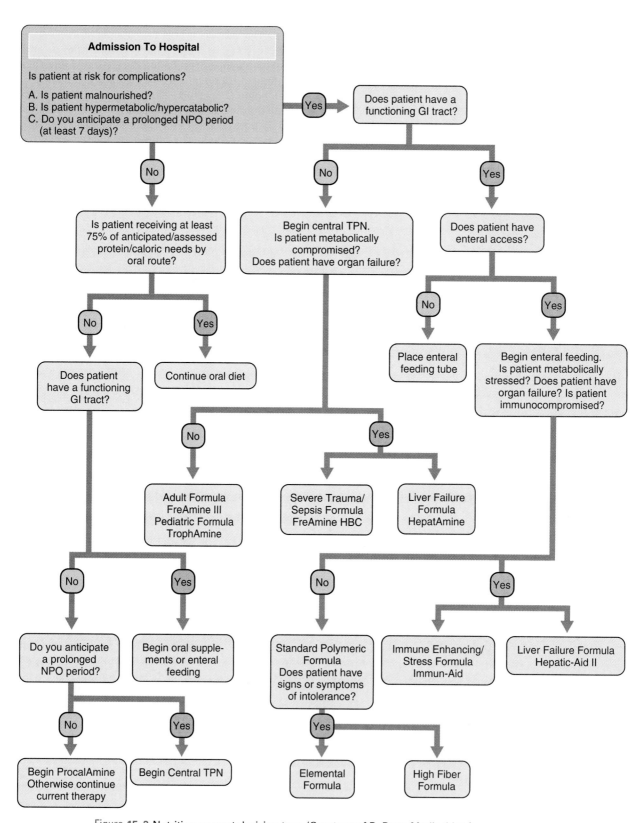

Figure **15–3** Nutrition support decision tree. (Courtesy of B. Baun Medical Inc.)

CASE STUDY 15-1

P was brought into the emergency room by ambulance with his mother. The mother stated her son was hit by a car while riding his bike. P is 11 years old, 4 ft 11 in tall, and weighs 89 lb. The client's mother stated her son was well before the accident. In the emergency room, it was observed that both his eyes were surrounded by contusions and his throat and the left side of his face were swollen. Communication with the client was at first minimal because it was painful for him to speak. An intravenous solution of D_5W was started in the emergency room. He was also shown to have a fractured femur. Surgery was required to reset the bone. The physician determined that **traction** would be necessary. P was expected to require traction, and thus hospitalization, for 3 to 5 weeks.

Five days later, P is still having problems swallowing. He has not progressed beyond sips of clear liquids. The kilocalorie count shows an average daily intake of 395 kcal, with only 8 g of protein for the past 3 days. P appears to be in pain when he swallows and has choked twice on larger sips of the clear liquids. The client speaks only in single words or short sentences. It is still painful for him to talk. The swelling in his esophagus has decreased enough to allow the insertion of a small silicone feeding tube. The physician has ordered a nasogastric feeding tube with Enrich. The order reads:

Day 1 Continuous drip 50 mL/h 1/2 strength
Day 2 Continuous drip 50 mL/h 3/4 strength
Day 3 Continuous drip 50 mL/h full strength
Day 4 Continuous drip 84 mL/h full strength

Enrich contains 1.1 kcal/mL and 39.7 g of protein per 1000 mL. P may have ice chips and small amounts of clear liquids in addition to the tube feeding as desired. The physician states, "The client will remain on a tube feeding until he can consume his kilocalorie requirement orally. This client requires adequate nutrition to enable the femur to heal properly." P is not expected to be discharged on a home enteral tube feeding. His prognosis is good, and he is expected to make a full recovery.

The physician inserts the nasogastric tube because of the swelling in the esophagus and the danger of a perforation. The nurse assists at the client's bedside. The client holds the nurse's hand tightly as the tube is inserted. He has a worried look on his face, increased facial perspiration, and increased pulse/respirations during the procedure.

NURSING CARE PLAN

SUBJECTIVE DATA Client held hand tightly during nasogastric tube insertion and appeared worried, apprehensive, and jittery.

OBJECTIVE DATA Client is a trauma victim who showed increased perspiration and increased pulse/respirations during the tube insertion procedure.

NURSING DIAGNOSIS NANDA, Fear (NANDA, 2003, with permission) related to enteral nutrition therapy and situational crisis as evidenced by tension during tube insertion and increased pulse/respirations and perspiration.

DESIRED OUTCOMES EVALUATION CRITERIA	NURSING ACTIONS/ INTERVENTIONS	RATIONALE
NOC: (Moorhead, Johnson, and Maas, 2004, with permission) The client will state he needs the food in the tube feeding to heal his leg until he is eating better.	NIC: Fear Control (Dochterman and Bulechek, 2004, with permission) Explain enteral nutrition therapy procedures as performed. As the client's condition permits, be available for listening and talking. Encourage the client to acknowledge and express feelings.	A tube feeding is unfamiliar to most clients. Knowledge about the procedure may relax the client. The client needs to vent his feelings about both the tube feeding and the situational crisis (the accident).

C T Q CRITICAL THINKING QUESTIONS

1. What would you do if the client pulled out the tube after insertion?
2. How would you reassess the client's continued need for a tube feeding?

3. How should this client be monitored while on the tube feeding?

⟩⟩⟩ CHAPTER REVIEW

1. Modular formula feedings:
   a. Always have a low osmolality
   b. Are designed for clients with malabsorption
   c. Contain a limited number of nutrients
   d. Are always predigested

2. A(n) _____ provides all of the essential nutrients in a specified volume.
   a. Intact or polymeric formula
   b. Modular feeding
   c. Intravenous feeding
   d. Clear-liquid diet

3. Careful administration of total parenteral nutrition includes all of the following except:
   a. A slow start
   b. Close monitoring
   c. Abrupt withdrawal
   d. A strict schedule

4. Among the following, diarrhea in a tube-fed client is most likely related to:
   a. A continuous-infusion feeding
   b. A contamination
   c. A fluid deficit
   d. Insufficient kilocalories

5. Which of the following is not a recommended procedure for administering medications through a tube feeding?
   a. Mix all of the medications together, crush thoroughly, mix with water, and add to the formula.
   b. If at all possible, use medications in the liquid form.
   c. Flush the tube with at least 30 milliliters of water before giving the medication and before resuming the tube-feeding formula.
   d. If a medication is ordered to be added to the formula, observe the feeding after the addition for any reaction or precipitation.

✚ CLINICAL ANALYSIS

1. Mr. J, 58 years old, visits his physician with a complaint of abdominal pain. He is scheduled for a diagnostic work-up, which will include a **barium enema** (x-ray study of his colon). Before this procedure, the nurse should instruct the client to:
   a. Eat a large breakfast on the day of the examination, such as orange juice, cereal, toast, scrambled eggs, and milk.
   b. Drink ample fluids on the morning of the examination, including at least 12 ounces of juice, 1 cup of gelatin, and broth.
   c. Take nothing orally after midnight on the day of the examination and consume only gelatin, clear broth, tea, coffee, and grape, apple, or cranberry juice on the day before the examination.
   d. Drink milk, juices, and coffee and eat only strained cream soups, ice cream, and gelatin on the day before the examination and take nothing orally after midnight.

2. Ms. L has a jejunostomy. She was discharged from the hospital last week after receiving instructions on home care from the nutrition support service. The local pharmacy is out of the Vivonex formula she has been instructed to use. As the nurse, you recommend that:
   a. She substitute Ensure
   b. She substitute Polycose
   c. She contact the Nutrition Support Service for instructions
   d. She substitute an intact or polymeric formula

3. Mr. W has been receiving a tube feeding of Ensure via nasogastric tube for 3 weeks via a bolus infusion. He has just started to have loose stools (300 milliliters each × 6 today). You should first suspect the following to be responsible for the diarrhea:
   a. A new medication added to his treatment plan
   b. Bacterial contamination
   c. Intolerance to the bolus delivery method
   d. Lactose intolerance

REFERENCES

American Dietetic Association: Manual of Clinical Dietetics, ed 6. Chicago, American Dietetic Association, 2000.

Blouch, AC, and Mueller, C: Enteral and Parenteral Nutrition Support in Food, Nutrition and Diet Therapy. Elsevier, Philadelphia, 2004.

Byrom, SE: Nutrition and Dietetics. Churchill Livingston & Wilkins, Edinburgh, UK, 2002.

Burnham, TH (ed): Drug Facts and Comparisons, ed 8. Lippincott, Williams & Wilkins, Philadelphia, 2004.

Butterworth, CE: The skeleton in the hospital closet. Nutrition Today 9:8, 1975.

Butterworth, CE, and Blackburn, GL: Hospital malnutrition and how to assess the nutritional status of a patient. Nutrition Today 10:8, 1975.

Climent, J: Tube feeding bad for patients with dementia. BMJ 320:335, 2000.

Dochterman, JM, and Bulechek, GM: Nursing Interventions Classification (NIC), ed 4. Mosby, Philadelphia, 2004.

Dupertuis, YM: Physical characteristics of total parenteral nutrition bags significantly affect the stability of vitamins C and B_1: A controlled prospective study. J Parenter Enteral Nutr 26:310, 2002.

Falk, A: Evaluating the effectiveness of a micronutrient assessment tool for long-term total parenteral nutrition patients. 17:240, 2002.

Food and Drug Administration: FDA Public Health Advisory. Reports of Blue Discoloration and Death in Patients Receiving Enteral Feedings Tinted with the Dye, FD&C No. 1. Accessed January 2004 at www.cfsan.fda.gov.

Gillick, M: Rethinking the role of tube feedings in patients. N Engl J Med 342:206, 2000.

Healthy People 2010. U.S. Department of Health and Human Services, Washington, DC, 2000.

Metheny, N, and Titler, MG: Assessing placement of feeding tubes. Am J Nurs 101:36, 2001.

Moorhead, S, Johnson, M, and Maas, M: Nursing Outcomes Classification (NOC), ed 3. Mosby, Philadelphia, 2004.

NANDA International: Nursing Diagnoses: Definitions and Classification, 2003–2004. NANDA International, Philadelphia, 2003.

Pfau, PR, and Rombeau, JL: Nutrition. Med Clin North Am 84:1209, 2000.

Phillips, LD: Manual of Intravenous Therapy. FA Davis, Philadelphia, 1994.

Skipper, A: A Dietitian's Handbook of Enteral and Parenteral Nutrition. Aspen Publications, Gaithersburg, Maryland, 1998.

Souba, W: Nutrition support correspondence. N Engl J Med. 336:41, 1997.

Super, J: Tube feedings making you blue. Drug Therapy Topics. University of Washington Medical Center 32:6, 2003.

Vollmann, J, et al: Rethinking the role of tube feeding in patients with advanced dementia [letter]. N Engl J Med 342:1755, 2000.

Wolfsen, HC, et al: Tube dysfunction following percutaneous gastrostomy and jejunostomy. Gastrointest Endosc 36:261, 1990.

CHAPTER 16

Complementary Medicine: Nutritional Aspects

Learning Objectives

After completing this chapter, the student should be able to:

1. Compare and contrast the regulatory processes for products sold in the United States as dietary supplements with those for products marketed as drugs.
2. List examples of adverse effects from five commonly used complementary medicines.
3. Identify interactions that can occur between botanical remedies and prescription and over-the-counter medications.
4. Compose neutral questions to assess a client's intake of supplements.
5. Discuss the use of special dietary supplements by athletes.

Although vitamin and mineral supplements are part of complementary medicine (Institute of Medicine, 2005), this chapter is chiefly concerned with two categories of complementary medicine, botanical remedies and ergogenic aids (substances supposed to enhance athletic performance). Both are sold in the United States as dietary supplements for reasons described in this chapter. In addition, over-the-counter substances that fit neither category, glucosamine and probiotics, merit consideration because of their frequent appearances in medical literature. Examples of the wide range of products being sold as dietary supplements are included here, but the sample does not begin to constitute a comprehensive review of the market. The fact that a particular item is mentioned does not imply endorsement. On the contrary, many of the cases are included to stimulate a strong sense of caution regarding these supplements. With these products, even more than with over-the-counter or prescription medications, the watchword is "let the buyer beware." Particular groups are at greater risk of adverse effects than others. An analysis of calls to 11 poison-control centers found increased severity of symptoms associated with the con-

sumption of several ingredients, long-term use, and older age (Palmer et al, 2003).

Botanical Remedies

Although the term *herbal medicine* is commonly used to describe the use of plant products sold as dietary supplements, some experts have objected to this phrase. Strictly speaking, an herb is a flowering plant whose stems above the ground are not woody (Stashower and Torres, 1995), and a shrub is a woody plant smaller than a tree, usually with permanent stems branching from or near the ground. Both herbs and shrubs are used as medicinal sources, including mainstream medicines. Here the term *botanical medicine* is used to mean the use of plant products that are not regulated as drugs in the United States but are sold as nutritional supplements.

Botanical products have been used to treat illnesses for centuries. Some of these products have been refined and synthesized to become drugs marketed by pharmaceutical companies. Digitalis originally was derived from purple foxglove. Morphine came from the opium poppy, quinine from cinchona bark, and aspirin from willow bark. The latter botanical caused anaphylaxis in a 25-year-old white woman who ingested two capsules of a dietary supplement promoted for weight loss that contained willow bark. She was known to have an allergy to aspirin and was successfully treated in an emergency room (Boullata, McDonnell, and Oliva, 2003). Reserpine from snakeroot, a centuries-old Hindu remedy for snake bite, mental illness, and anxiety, was not accepted into Western medicine until the 1940s, when it came to be used as a tranquilizer and an antihypertensive drug. Plants directly provide about 25 percent of currently used drugs; another 25 percent are chemically altered natural products (Sheehan, 1998).

All of these drugs can be used to treat illness, but they can also produce illness if misused or unwisely used. As detailed in Chapters 7 and 8, excessive ingestion of vitamins and minerals can produce disease just as insufficient amounts can. A basic premise of toxicology is that no chemical substance is absolutely safe; therefore, no chemical substance should be considered entirely harmless (Omaye, 1998). It follows, then, that believing any substance to be safe simply because it is "natural" is a major error of logic.

In the relatively recent past, ingredients of medicines were kept secret, the same medicine was sold to treat or cure multiple unrelated illnesses, and certain medicines were distributed by unlicensed peddlers. Even among medical practitioners, revealing the contents of the prescription and giving client educational information are relatively new developments. Forty or 50 years ago, nurses were expected not to divulge to a client the name of the medicine he or she was receiving.

With botanical products, nature keeps some of the ingredients secret. Not all the constituents of these products have been identified, and they may exert more than one physiological effect in the human body (Huang et al, 2004). Therefore, when ingesting one of them, a person takes not only the active ingredient that is purported to have the desired medicinal effect but also other substances in the plant tissue as well. Among these other substances may be defensive chemicals the plant has evolved to protect itself from predators (Sheehan, 1998).

Regulation of Pharmaceuticals and Dietary Supplements

Laws of various countries treat drugs and dietary supplements differently. Botanicals are regulated as drugs in most countries except the United States (Huang et al, 2004). In France and Germany, 30 to 40 percent of physicians use herbal remedies as their primary treatment options (Watkins, 2002a). Even within the United States, some states regulate certain substances more stringently than do others. To the extent permitted by law, the Food and Drug Administration (FDA) is responsible for regulating pharmaceuticals and dietary supplements. In Germany, a similar agency, Commission E, has that responsibility.

Food and Drug Administration

Although the FDA oversees the safety of dietary supplements, the rules governing their testing, processing, and labeling are vastly different from the rules governing prescription and over-the-counter drugs. Before receiving permission to market a new drug, the pharmaceutical company must conduct rigorous tests on animals and on people in randomized, double-blind clinical trials. Randomization requires that participants be assigned by coin toss or equivalent unbiased method to receive the investigative drug or not. **Double-blind** trials are experiments in which neither the subject nor the investigator knows whether a subject is receiving the treatment or a placebo.

Even after approval by the FDA, each company is granted the exclusive right or patent to manufacture the drug for a limited time only, after which other drug companies may copy, manufacture, and sell it. The patent application process is very long and expensive and is one reason sellers of botanical products give for not applying for a patent. Naturally occurring substances and laws of nature may not be patented. The process by which such a substance is purified or manufactured may be the subject of a process patent claim if it is new and not obvious.

In 1994, Congress removed dietary supplements from the labeling provisions of the Nutrition Labeling and Education Act of 1990. Under the provisions of the Dietary Supplement Health Education Act of 1994, referred to by the acronym DSHEA, dietary supplements can be sold unless shown by the FDA to be unsafe, adulterated, or labeled in a misleading manner. The burden of proof in this case rests with the FDA, not with the manufacturer, and no prior notice from the manufacturer of intent to sell is required. In contrast, in Canada, France, and Germany, dietary supplements are regulated as drugs requiring premarketing approval of safety and the burden of proof lies with the manufacturer (Institute of Medicine, 2005).

Despite a long history of use, little is known about toxicity of botanical medicines. Most such knowledge has been acquired from acute cases of toxicity sporadically reported, but recently scientific studies have been conducted. Manufacturers and distributors of dietary supplements are not required to record, investigate, or forward to the FDA any reports of illness or injury from their products (Huang et al, 2004).

Under DSHEA, a dietary supplement is defined as any product taken by mouth that contains a "so-called 'dietary ingredient'" (U.S. Food and Drug Administration, 1999) and

1. Contains one or more nutrients, herbs, botanicals, or a concentrate, metabolite, or constituent extract from the ingredients previously mentioned
2. Is in the form of a supplement (meaning pill, tablet, capsule, liquid, or powder)
3. Is not represented as a food or sole item of a meal or the human diet
4. Includes a similar new drug or biologic approved under previous legislation and not currently being investigated (Food Institute, undated)

DSHEA does not limit the serving size or the amount of nutrients in any form of dietary supplement, but its regulations spell out the nature of the claims made for a product on the label and its format.

The following types of statements are allowed:

1. Health claims that have substantial scientific support plus those allowed pursuant to a court decision, Pearson v. Shalala. The latter ruling disallowed the FDA's rejection of health claims for the benefits of fiber and antioxidants on cancer risk, of omega-3 fatty acids on coronary heart disease risk, and of the effective dose of folic acid in preventing neural tube defects. Most health claims apply only to foods (Institute of Medicine, 2005).
2. Nutrient content claims describe the level of the nutrient or dietary ingredient in a product compared with an established daily value. These claims can also state the contents of the product as a percentage of the product or compare the product's contents as a percentage of another product (Institute of Medicine, 2005).
3. Structure-function claims describe the product's effect on structure or function of the body or on general well-being. These claims must also include the following

information displayed prominently on the label: "**This statement has not been evaluated by the Food and Drug Administration. This product is not intended to diagnose, treat, cure or prevent any disease.**" In addition, the FDA must be notified within 30 days of placing a product with a structure-function claim on the market (Institute of Medicine, 2005).

A product is considered to be misbranded if it fails to list the name and quantity of each ingredient and to have the identity and strength represented (Green, Catlin, and Starcevic, 2001).

By contrast, the rules for labeling the nutrient content of foods in the United States are much more stringent than those applied to dietary supplements in that substantiation through research or scientific agreement is needed for information to be permitted on a food label. Most herbal products, because the evidence is inadequate to permit health or nutrient content claims, must use structure-function claims (Institute of Medicine, 2005). The standard for the structure-function claim for dietary supplements is simply that it be truthful and not misleading. Some manufacturers have been issued warnings for violating the rules. See Box 16–1.

German Commission E

Filling a role in Europe similar to that of the FDA in this country, German Commission E is a governmental regulatory agency that has evaluated the safety and **efficacy** of botanicals based on clinical trials, cases, and scientific literature. Although admitting that herbal remedies in Germany must meet purity standards not presently in force in the United States, critics of the German system point to a double standard regarding proof of efficacy or effectiveness.

The standard of proof accepted by German Commission E for herbal remedies is set lower than for conventional drugs (Angell and Kassirer, 1999). Hundreds of preparations have been licensed in Germany by Commission E and are regulated as over-the-counter or prescription medications (Barrett, Kiefer, and Rabago, 1999). Since 1978, German Commission E has published more than 320 monographs on botanical products. This information has been translated into English by the American Botanical Council (http://www.HerbalGram.org). Someone considering the use of botanical preparations should review the evidence presented by German Commission E and the American Botanical Council before deciding.

Box 16–1 FDA Actions Regarding Dietary Supplements

The Food and Drug Administration has seized dietary supplements that had been marketed using unsubstantiated claims about their effects on the structure and function of the body and has issued warning letters to marketers making such claims and to those promoting their products as treatments or preventives for disease. The agency has successfully pursued civil and criminal action against firms and individuals that did not comply with the regulations (U.S. Food and Drug Administration, 2002a). Unauthorized health claims or claims suggesting the food is intended to treat, cure, or mitigate disease subjects the food to regulation as a drug (U.S. Food and Drug Administration, 2001b).

The agency also has warned manufacturers regarding the addition of botanical and other novel ingredients to conventional foods (U.S. Food and Drug Administration, 2001a). Such ingredients must be preapproved by the FDA or appear on the GRAS (Generally Recognized as Safe) list. All other additions constitute adulteration of the food, making it illegal to import into or sell in the United States (U.S. Food and Drug Administration, 2001b). In just 6 months, the FDA inspected 180 domestic dietary supplement manufacturing plants, issued 119 warning letters to distributors, refused entry to 1171 foreign shipments, and seized or supervised the destruction of products reportedly valued at $18 million (Crawford, 2004). A warning to consumers to avoid a product purported to bolster infants' immunity was posted because the product was represented as an infant formula (U.S. Food and Drug Administration, 2004b).

In 2004, the FDA banned the sale of currently marketed dietary supplements containing a source of ephedrine alkaloids such as ephedra, Ma huang, Sida cordifolia, and pinellia (U.S. Food and Drug Administration, 2004e). When chemically synthesized, *ephedrine* and *pseudoephedrine* (that are metabolized in the body from ephedrine alkaloids) are regulated as drugs. Moreover, scientific evidence shows the risk to the circulatory system far outweighs any short-term benefits to dieters or athletes (U.S. Food and Drug Administration, 2004a). Ephedra had already been banned by the National Football League, the National Collegiate Athletic Association, and the International Olympic Committee. Soon after ephedra contributed to the death of one of its athletes at age 23 from multiple organ failure due to heat stroke, minor league baseball also banned ephedra (Meadows, 2003).

The FDA has issued a consumer advisory and solicited input from health-care professionals regarding adverse effects of another botanical product, kava (U.S. Food and Drug Administration, 2002b). Australia, Canada, France, Germany, and Switzerland have restricted the sale of kava-containing products because of potential liver toxicity, and two cases requiring liver transplantation have occurred in the United States (Centers for Disease Control, 2002). Shortly after Health Canada issued the advisory, however, 65 percent of stores surveyed in Toronto still recommended kava, of which only 41 percent mentioned safety concerns (Mills et al, 2004).

Enforcement after the fact is only one activity of the agency. It also provides information to educate marketers and consumers on the FDA Web site, http://www.fda.gov.

Botanicals are Big Business

Sales of dietary supplements, totaling 29,000 different products excluding vitamins and minerals, are estimated to have risen from $4.5 billion in 1994 to $7.2 billion in 1998 (American Dietetic Association, 2001). Based on sales, the most popular botanical products in the United States are ginkgo biloba, reaping $290 million in 2000, followed by St. John's wort, with $235 million, and echinacea, with $211 million (Challener, 2002).

In a national survey, 14 percent of the respondents had taken at least one herbal/nonvitamin-nonmineral supplement in the week preceding the interview (Kaufman et al, 2002) and an estimated 32.7 percent of health maintenance organization adult subscribers in northern California used nonvitamin-nonmineral dietary supplements (Schaffer et al, 2003). Nearly one-sixth (15.9 percent) of a nationally representative sample of U.S. women used at least one herbal supplement in 2000 compared with 13.2 percent of U.S. men. Women most likely to use the most common herbal supplements were non-Hispanic white, 35 to 64 years of age, more educated, not poor, current alcohol users, living in the South and West. They also were more likely than other women to have functional limitations and chronic conditions (Yu, Ghandour, and Huang, 2004).

Areas of Concern with Botanicals

Because the FDA's responsibility begins only after the products have been packaged and marketed, the maintenance of quality is the responsibility of the manufacturer. Four major areas of concern with botanicals involve the lack of standardization of the products, the potential for contamination with dangerous substances, interactions with other drugs, and the difficulty obtaining reliable information.

Lack of Standardization

The potency of botanical products can vary with the climate and soil conditions and with the life cycle of the plants from which they come. Great differences in the quantities of active ingredients have been found, depending on the source, the species and part of the plant used, storage conditions (Borins, 1998), inclusion of look-alike plants, time of harvest, method of processing, and country of origin. Without consistent products, research cannot be generalized as a basis for evidence-based practice (Institute of Medicine, 2005).

Furthermore, it is not safe to assume that naturally occurring plant constituents are maintained at equivalent levels of biological activity when extracted, dried, and compacted into tablets (American Dietetic Association, 1999). A "seed to shelf" standardization process would minimize batch-to-batch variations in botanical products but is not currently in place (Huang et al, 2004) .

Even worse, botanical products can come to market not containing the ingredients on the label. For example, analysis of echinacea preparations determined that labeled species content was correct in only 52 percent of the samples and 10 percent contained no echinacea at all (Gilroy et al, 2003). Analysis of 54 samples of St. John's wort determined that just 2 of them (3.7 percent) contained active

ingredients within 10 percent of the amounts stated on the label (Draves and Walker, 2003). A slightly better result was reported in an analysis of 25 commercial ginseng preparations that determined all the plant products were correctly identified by botanical species; however, concentrations of marker compounds differed significantly from labeled amounts (Harkey et al, 2001). Brand-name products with ingredients within 20 percent of the labeled amount are reported by brand name on a Web page, http://www.consumerlab.com.

A traditional Chinese botanical product, jin bu huan (JBH; *Lycopodium serratum*), is used as a sedative and analgesic. Three unrelated children in Colorado, 13 months to 30 months of age, accidentally ingested 7 to 60 tablets of this remedy. All of the children experienced central nervous system depression and recovered after treatment in emergency rooms. Analysis of the tablets in all three cases revealed substances from the plant genus *Stephania* but none from *Polygala* as the label indicated. In this case, because the package insert also stated various medical indications for the product, it fell under the drug regulating authority of the FDA (Centers for Disease Control, 1993b).

The same situation, tablets containing components of the genera *Stephania* and *Corydalis* but not *Polygala*, led to acute hepatitis in two women, ages 24 and 66 years, who ingested 4 to 16 tablets per week for 2 to 3 months. A third woman was treated for acute hepatitis, having purchased jin bu huan from the same store as the other two women had used, but the contents of the third woman's tablets were not reported (Centers for Disease Control, 1993a).

Discerning the species of a plant product by visual inspection is not possible in some cases. Chinese star anise (*Illicium verum*) when used as a spice is on the **GRAS List** but Japanese star anise (*Illicium anisatum*) causes neurologic and gastrointestinal toxicities. Seven infants, aged 2 to 12 weeks, were treated at Miami Children's Hospital for star anise poisoning. Symptoms included irritability, hyperexcitability, vomiting, abnormal eye movements, and seizures (Ize-Ludlow et al, 2004). After approximately 40 individuals, including about 15 infants, became ill following ingestion of star anise teas, the FDA issued an advisory to not drink such beverages because the particular variety of star anise involved in these illnesses could not be identified (U.S. Food and Drug, 2003).

Potential for Contamination with Dangerous Substances

The desired botanical product may be contaminated with toxic substances. For example, within four days in March, the California Department of Health Services screened Asian patent medicines collected from retail herbal stores for undeclared pharmaceuticals and heavy metal contaminants. Of 243 samples tested for pharmaceuticals, 7 percent contained undeclared pharmaceuticals, the most common being *ephedrine, chlorpheniramine, methyltestosterone,* and *phenacetin*. Of the 251 samples tested for heavy metals, 10 percent contained lead, 14 percent contained arsenic, and 14 percent contained mercury. These contaminants were not found in trace amounts. The United States Pharmacopoeia limits the presence of heavy metals in most oral pharmaceuticals to 30 parts per million (ppm),

The United States Pharmacopeia (USP), legally recognized since 1906, is a compendium of standards for drugs issued and revised periodically by a national committee of pharmacists, pharmacologists, physicians, chemists, biologists, and other allied personnel. Official drugs listed therein must meet standards of purity and strength as determined by chemical analysis or animal responses to specified doses.

The National Formulary (NF) is a list of drugs of established usefulness that are not listed in the U.S. Pharmacopeia. The NF was originally issued by the American Pharmaceutical Association but since 1980 has been published by the U.S. Pharmacopeial Convention.

with lower limits for lead, arsenic, and mercury (Box 16–2). These contaminated samples had means of 54.9 ppm of lead, 14,553 ppm of arsenic, and 1046 ppm of mercury (Ko, 1998).

CONTAMINATION WITH DRUGS

In 1994, the New York City Department of Health investigated seven cases of **anticholinergic** poisoning in members of three different families. (Anticholinergic drugs inhibit the transmission of parasympathetic nerve impulses, making them useful drugs to reduce smooth-muscle spasms, dilate the pupil of the eye, and decrease gastrointestinal and bronchial secretions.) Symptoms of toxicity appeared in these 10- to 40-year-old clients within 2 hours of drinking tea made from leaves labeled "Paraguay tea" purchased commercially. Laboratory tests confirmed the presence of the anticholinergic drugs *atropine, scopolamine,* and *hyoscyamine* in these particular leaves, which are not present in the holly tree supposedly used for Paraguay tea. The investigation pinpointed the one grocery store handling the tea from a distributor who purchased the leaves from a farmer, had it shipped in bulk to New York, and packaged it for sale (Centers for Disease Control, 1995).

In another case, mixtures of herbs for "internal cleansing" led to *digitalis* poisoning in two women. Each sought medical treatment for nausea, vomiting, and palpitations. The first client experienced nausea and severe vomiting within 24 hours of beginning the cleansing program but continued the regimen for 2 additional days. She discontinued the program but then restarted it at reduced dosage 2 days before seeking treatment in the emergency room for nausea, irregular heartbeat, and hot flashes. The second client began the cleansing program 5 days before admission, discontinued it after 3 days, and sought medical care for visual disturbances, shortness of breath, and chest pressure in addition to nausea, vomiting, and palpitations. An investigation by the FDA revealed the ingredient labeled plantain contained cardiac glycosides. The two women had consumed the same brand-name product with the same lot number. The raw material was traced to the supplier. Approximately 2700 kilograms (3 tons) of the plantain had been imported from Germany over a 2-year period. More that 150 manufacturers, distributors, and retailers received potentially contaminated plantain. Thirteen voluntary recalls were initiated by manufacturers and distributors. Eight firms received warning letters from the FDA, which issued two press releases and posted warnings for consumers on the FDA Web site (Slifman et al, 1998).

While studying natural anti-inflammatory substances in human placental blood, investigators detected an unknown substance. It was subsequently identified as the drug *colchicine* that is used to treat gout and was traced to five women who consumed ginkgo biloba during pregnancy and also was found in samples of ginkgo biloba distributed commercially in the area. This drug has the potential to be teratogenic or damaging to a fetus (Petty et al, 2001).

CONTAMINATION WITH HEAVY METALS

A 43-year-old man sought treatment for abdominal pain. He received an extensive medical work-up, including multiple blood tests, urine tests, abdominal and chest radiographs, abdominal ultrasounds, an upper gastrointestinal series with barium, gastroscopy, and colonoscopy. Finally the cause of his problem was determined to be lead poisoning. The source of the lead was tablets of "Indian plants," dispensed in an unlabeled plastic container by a person he consulted for his diabetes. Beginning with two tablets per day, the man had increased his intake to eight tablets per day. Each tablet was found to contain 10 milligrams of lead (Beigel, Ostfeld, and Schoenfeld, 1998).

An asymptomatic case of lead poisoning was discovered in a 33-year-old Cambodian woman, but not her husband or their two children, when they attended a lead-screening clinic sponsored by a nursing school. The investigators concluded that the source of the lead was the red dye in "Koo So Pills" or "Koo Sar Pills" (the label and the package insert did not agree) she had taken at the rate of six per day for 7 days per month for 3 to 4 years for menstrual cramps (Centers for Disease Control, 1999). A less-positive outcome occurred in a preterm infant with the highest blood lead level recorded in a surviving neonate due to its mother's long-term ingestion of lead-contaminated herbal tablets (Tait et al, 2002). Another incidental finding occurred when Chinese herbal balls were confiscated by the U.S. Fish and Wildlife Service in a case of alleged endangered-species violations. The herbal balls were subsequently tested for contaminants. These were factory-produced products manufactured in China that were supposed to contain herbs and honey to be consumed as a tea. Of the nine herbal balls tested, eight contained arsenic and mercury and one contained just arsenic (Espinoza, Mann, and Bleasdell, 1995).

During 2000 to 2003, 12 cases of lead poisoning associated with ayurvedic remedies were reported to the CDC. These occurred among adults in California, Massachusetts, New Hampshire, New York, and Texas. Eleven of the affected persons were natives of India or Nepal; the twelfth's birthplace is unknown. Some branches of ayurvedic medicine use heavy metals therapeutically, so technically the lead is not a contaminant. Remedies taken by nine of the clients were tested for lead content that ranged from 0 to 96,000 ppm. These cases illustrate the need for culturally appropriate assessment and teaching about potential ill effects of folk medicine. Young children and fetuses of pregnant women are at special risk for the toxic effects of lead, because these products are used to treat infertility in women (Centers for Disease Control, 2004).

Similarly, an investigation in 2003 identified lead, mercury, or arsenic in 14 of 70 ayurvedic herbal medicines purchased within 20 miles of Boston City Hall. Lead was found in 13 products, mercury and arsenic in 6 each. If taken as recommended by the manufacturers, each of these 14 herbal medicines could result in heavy metal intakes above standards published in the U.S. Pharmacopeia and by the U.S. Environmental Protection Agency (Saper et al, 2004).

Interactions with Other Drugs

Surveys have revealed significant proportions of clients combining botanical products with prescription medications. Of 458 outpatient veterans, 43 percent were taking at least one dietary supplement with prescription medications, of which 45 percent had a potential for a significant drug-dietary supplement interaction (Peng et al, 2004). Of 944 emergency department clients, 14.3 percent reported regular use of dietary supplements, of whom 79.3 percent were taking supplements with prescription medications, and yet 69 percent were unable to identify a specific reason for using the supplements (Rogers, Gough, and Brewer, 2001).

A literature review of 41 case reports or case series and 17 clinical trials reporting herb-drug interactions in humans indicated that many of the botanical products covered individually in the following pages can have serious clinical consequences (Izzo and Ernst, 2001). The interactions thus identified in this review (with garlic, ginkgo, ginseng, and St. John's wort) are incorporated into the following section.

As many as 70 percent of clients do not reveal their use of herbal medicines to their physicians and pharmacists, which places them at risk of drug-dietary supplement interactions (Pribitkin and Boger, 2001). Forty-five percent of children seen in the emergency department had been given an herbal product by their caregivers, of whom just 45 percent reported discussing the herbal therapy with the child's primary health-care provider (Lanski et al, 2003).

Over an 11-week period, 22 percent of presurgical patients at one large medical center reported the use of herbal remedies, a practice more frequent in women and clients aged 40 to 60 years of age and most often involving, in rank order, echinacea, ginkgo biloba, St. John's wort, garlic, and ginseng (Tsen et al, 2000), the last four of which

have the potential to increase bleeding times. So many people are taking botanical products that the American Society of Anesthesiologists (1999) issued a warning to consumers of herbal medicine to stop taking the products 2 to 3 weeks before scheduled surgery. Possible interactions cited were an unintended deepening of anesthesia and problems with bleeding and blood pressure.

Difficulty Obtaining Reliable Information

Often the source of information about a dietary supplement is the seller of the product. In a Canadian test of health food stores in which a case was presented of a child with Crohn's disease, an employee at 72 percent of the stores recommended a treatment. Only one of the 32 stores had an employee who advised consulting a physician without recommending a product, and three others advised medical consultation in addition to recommending a product (Calder, Issenman, and Cawdron, 2000).

The editors of the New England Journal of Medicine found it necessary to link a caution to a 1990 article on human growth hormone, because an Internet seller referenced the article inappropriately in promotional materials. The caution reiterated the view in the 1990 editorial that human growth hormone use in the elderly is not justified (Drazen, 2003).

Analysis of 443 Web sites identified 55 percent that contained claims to treat, prevent, diagnose, or cure specific diseases despite the prohibition of such statements (Morris and Avorn, 2003). A specific search of 208 Web sites for St. John's wort discovered that just 22 percent correctly listed depression as the only indication for the herb and only 22 percent listed at least one drug interaction with St. John's wort (Martin-Facklam et al, 2002).

An additional problem when searching for reliable information is a language barrier. There are few publications in the English language supporting the combinations of herbal products, yet they are widely distributed by nutrition and health food stores, pharmacies, and supermarkets (Haller, 2002).

An evaluation of 22 books on botanical dietary supplements written for health professionals found that editors of some books were highly qualified while others lacked the qualifications to summarize scientific information in a balanced, unbiased manner. Many books contained unsubstantiated statements. The books judged to be of the highest quality provided primary references to support all statements and also advised the reader that insufficient information is available to assess potential drug interactions and safety during pregnancy and lactation (Chambliss et al, 2002). Because of the wide variation among references, multiple sources should be consulted to obtain information about product safety and quality (Institute of Medicine, 2005). Suggestions for clients regarding the use of dietary supplements are given in the Appendix L.

Potentially Safe Botanical Products

Nine botanical products that have been judged to be relatively safe are reviewed next. Professors of pharmacy categorized seven herbal remedies as potentially safe: Asian ginseng, feverfew, garlic, ginkgo, saw palmetto, St. John's wort, and valerian (Klepser and Klepser, 1999). Echinacea and ginger are also included because of their popularity in the United States and appearances in medical literature. Four of these products, garlic, ginger, ginseng, and valerian, are on the FDA GRAS list (O'Hara et al, 1998).

Any substance, even pure water, can be unsafe in excessive amounts or for particular people in certain situations. Good clinical judgment is necessary for the practitioner seeking to help the client. Knowledge and caution are necessary for the client to weigh the risks and benefits of botanical therapy (Fig. 16–1).

Asian Ginseng (Panax ginseng)

Traditionally used short-term in Chinese medicine for 2000 years (Watkins, 2002a), Asian ginseng is used in Germany as a tonic to combat lassitude, debility, and lack of energy and concentration (Klepser and Klepser, 1999). The active ingredients, known as ginsenosides, are present in varying quantities in different parts of the plant, with highest concentration believed to be in the root. At least 28 ginsenosides have been isolated, each of which produces unique effects on the central nervous system, the cardiovascular system, and other body systems. Some ginsenosides' effects are direct opposites of other ginsenosides' effects (Klepser and Klepser, 1999), and a single ginsenoside initiates multiple actions in the same tissue (Attele, Wu, and Yuan, 1999). An 8-week prospective, double-blind, placebo-controlled, randomized clinical trial involving 43 men and 40 women with a mean age of 25.7 years found no support for claims that ginseng, at either its clinically recommended level or at twice that level, enhances affect or mood in healthy young adults (Cardinal and Engels, 2001).

Cautions: It is recommended that ginseng not be used by children, pregnant women, and persons with hypertension, psychological imbalances, headaches, heart palpitations, insomnia, asthma, inflammation, or infections with high fever. Severe hypotension upon withdrawal of the herb has been reported (Sheehan, 1998). Ginseng may decrease blood glucose levels and thus should be used with caution with antidiabetic agents (Nursing 2004 Herbal). *Adverse effects* include hypertension, euphoria, restlessness, nervousness, insomnia, skin eruptions, edema, and diarrhea. Ginseng may exert an estrogen-like effect in postmenopausal women, resulting in diffuse breast nodularity and vaginal bleeding. Vaginal bleeding was reported following the use of ginseng face cream for 1 month (Miller, 1998). *Drug Interactions:* Concomitant use with anticoagulants and nonsteroidal anti-inflammatory drugs (NSAIDs) should be avoided (Miller, 1998). Use with **monoamine oxidase inhibitors (MAOIs)** may cause headache, irritability, and visual hallucinations. Concomitant use should be avoided (Nursing 2004 Herbal). Some of the components of ginseng are structurally similar to *digoxin,* which with some assay techniques caused falsely elevated or falsely depressed serum test results (Dasgupta et al, 2003). Ginseng lowers blood concentrations of alcohol and *warfarin* and induces mania if used concomitantly with *phenelzine* (Izzo and Ernst, 2001).

Echinacea (Echinacea purpurea, Echinacea pallida)

Echinacea purpurea, also called purple coneflower, is native to America and was used to treat wounds by the American Indians (Mullins and Heddle, 2002). Its root and leaf extracts are used as therapeutic agents (see Fig. 16–2). Between 1919 and 1950, echinacea was listed in the National Formulary (Box 16–2). In Germany, echinacea is dispensed through 2 million physicians' prescriptions per year (Barrett, Kiefer, and Rabago, 1999).

Echinacea stimulates phagocytosis and lymphocyte activity (Watkins, 2002b) and is considered helpful for bolstering the immune system, especially for colds, flu, and chronic upper respiratory or urinary tract infections, but the opposite effect, immunosuppression, has been

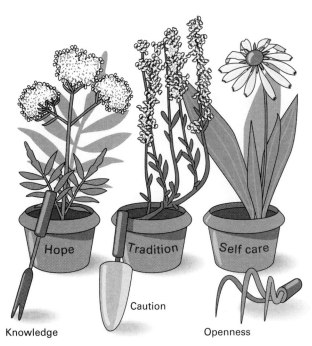

Figure **16–1** Many people use botanical products because of their cultural traditions, seeking a measure of self-care and hope. Those who use botanical products, however, need to cultivate knowledge and caution in their choices. They also should practice openness with their health-care providers.

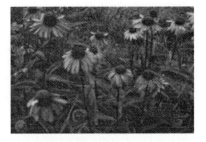

ECHINACEA PURPUREA

Figure **16–2** Echinacea purpurea (purple coneflower) is a member of the daisy family, as is apparent from the illustration. (Reprinted from Venes, 2001, p 633, with permission.)

reported with long-term use (Capriotti, 1999). Echinacea was judged to be effective in reducing symptoms of the common cold in a sample of 95 individuals (Lindenmuth and Lindenmuth, 2000) and in 282 subjects in a randomized, double-blind, placebo-controlled trial with a standardized formulation (Goel et al, 2004). It was not effective in preventing colds or decreasing their duration in 108 individuals (Grimm and Muller, 1999) or in 148 young adults given unrefined echinacea (Barrett et al, 2002). Neither was it effective in treating symptoms in 2- to 11-year-old children but was associated with an increased risk of rash (Taylor et al, 2003).

Cautions: Echinacea is not recommended for longer than 8 weeks of use orally or 3 weeks parenterally. The healthcare provider should be consulted before taking echinacea if the client is a child or a woman who is pregnant, planning to become pregnant, or lactating; however, in a prospective study, 206 women who took echinacea during pregnancy were no more likely to deliver infants with major or minor malformations than control group women (Gallo et al, 2000). A person with allergies, especially to members of the daisy family (aster, camomile, chrysanthemum, daisy, dandelion, goldenrod, marigold, ragweed, St. John's wort, sunflower, thistle, yarrow, and zinnia) should consult his or her health-care provider before taking this herb. *Adverse Effects:* Instances of adverse reactions to echinacea were reported in Australia, including seven individuals who reacted after their first known exposures. Of the 56 cases reported, 6 persons experienced anaphylasis, 10 urticaria/angioedema, and 13 acute asthma. More than half the clients were known to have allergies, and those who are atopic particularly should be cautioned about the possibility of cross-reactivity between echinacea and other environmental allergens (Mullins and Heddle, 2002). *Drug Interactions:* Echinacea may cause liver toxicity, especially when used with other hepatotoxic drugs. It decreases the effectiveness of immunosuppressants and protease inhibitors and should not be used with those classes of drugs (Nursing 2004 Herbal). Echinacea has been shown to inhibit intestinal enzymes of the cytochrome P450 metabolic pathway and to induce hepatic enzymes of the same system (see Chapter 17), so that caution is needed with drugs whose curative amount approaches its tolerated amount, such as *cyclosporine, phenytoin,* and *theophylline* (Huang et al, 2004). The most common complaint is of an unpleasant taste.

Feverfew (Tanacetum parthenium)

Encapsulated leaves of feverfew have been approved by the Canadian Health Protection Branch to prevent migraine headaches. Feverfew has 35 identified components, one of which is thought to produce the pharmacologic effects of inhibiting prostaglandin synthesis, platelet aggregation, and phagocytosis, among other actions (Nursing 2004 Herbal). Five randomized, placebo-controlled, double-blind trials assessing the efficacy of feverfew for preventing migraine were judged to provide insufficient evidence of an effect of feverfew over and above placebo, but no major safety problems were identified (Pittler and Ernst, 2004).

Cautions: Feverfew should be avoided in pregnancy, lactation, for children under 2 years of age, and persons allergic to plants in the daisy family (see examples under echinacea cautions). *Adverse Effects:* Gastrointestinal ulcers or canker sores occur in 5 to 15 percent of users, and abrupt cessation may cause postfeverfew syndrome, characterized by tension headaches, insomnia, joint pain and stiffness, and lethargy (Nursing 2004 Herbal). *Drug Interactions:* Feverfew may interact with anticoagulants and potentiate the antiplatelet effect of *aspirin.* NSAIDs interfere with feverfew's effects (Vickers and Zollman, 1999).

Garlic (Allium sativum)

Following a folk medicine practice that may have merit, Filipinos commonly consume garlic daily to combat hypertension (Purnell and Paulanka, 2003). Mentioned as a remedy in 5000-year-old East Indian records (Watkins, 2002b), garlic contains more than one compound, apparently wielding opposite biological effects. Also, the complex chemistry of garlic makes it plausible that variations in processing can yield quite different preparations (Amagase et al, 2001). In addition, homogenized raw garlic has been reported to exert antioxidant potential, whereas higher doses have been shown to be toxic to the heart, liver, and kidney (Banerjee, Mukherjee, and Maulik, 2003). Evidence from available studies suggests a preventive effect of garlic consumption in stomach and colorectal cancers (Fleischauer and Arab, 2001).

German Commission E indicates garlic for *the support of dietary measures* for treating hyperlipoproteinemia and to prevent arteriosclerosis. Over a 4-year period, high-dose garlic powder reduced the increase in arteriosclerotic plaque volume by 5 to 18 percent (Koscielny et al, 1999), and a **meta-analysis** of 13 randomized, double-blinded, placebo-controlled trials determined garlic produces a modest reduction in cholesterol compared to placebo (Stevinson, Pittler, and Ernst, 2000). Garlic apparently does not affect high-density cholesterol (Watkins, 2002b). Optimal effects are achieved by consuming raw cloves or enteric-coated tablets, because the purported active ingredient is degraded by crushing, heat, and acid (O'Hara et al, 1998). Garlic is known to inhibit platelet function and to increase levels of two antioxidant enzymes. A case of spontaneous spinal epidural hematoma was attributed to the 87-year-old man's consumption of four cloves of garlic daily for an unreported length of time to prevent heart disease (Rose et al, 1990). Although randomized trials have been reported, researchers admit the characteristic odor of garlic is difficult to hide for the purposes of double-blinded studies. Because the active ingredients are sulfur derivatives and pungent, odorless preparations of garlic are likely worthless (Watkins, 2002b).

Cautions: Any form of garlic should be stopped at least 7 days before surgery (Watkins, 2002a). Allergies have been reported (Perez-Pimiento et al, 1999), and topical application has produced second-degree burns (Baruchin et al, 2001; Rafaat and Leung, 2000). Clients who are pregnant or breast-feeding should limit intake to amounts used in cooking. *Adverse Effects:* Garlic has been reported to cause heartburn, flatulence, sweating, light-headedness, and excessive menstrual flow (Klepser and Klepser, 1999). The side effects of malodorous breath and skin can be moderated by consuming the garlic with protein or by taking **enteric-coated** tablets that dissolve in the intestine rather than the stomach (O'Hara et al, 1998). *Drug Interactions:* Garlic inhibits one of the cytochrome P450 metabolic pathway enzymes that may result in hepatotoxic levels of some anesthetics (Sorensen, 2002). Garlic decreases metabolism of *acetaminophen*, producing higher blood levels of the drug, decreases blood glucose levels if taken with antidiabetic agents, and may increase bleeding time if taken with anticoagulants (Nursing 2004 Herbal).

Ginger (Zingiber officinale)

The ancient Greeks and Romans used ginger as a digestive aid, as did people in East Indian and Chinese cultures. Sailors have used ginger for motion sickness. Western versions of the medicinal herb include ginger ale, ginger beer, and ginger tea. The root of this plant has been shown to reduce nausea and vertigo better than placebo. Ginger improves gastroduodenal motility (Micklefield et al, 1999) so that its mechanism of action is local rather than affecting the central nervous system (Miller, 1998).

Two of three randomized controlled trials testing ginger's effectiveness for postoperative nausea and vomiting suggested that ginger was superior to placebo and equally effective as *metoclopramide*. Three randomized controlled trials concerning seasickness, morning sickness, and chemotherapy-induced nausea collectively favored ginger over placebo (Ernst and Pittler, 2000). Another double-blinded trial involving 70 women with nausea and vomiting of pregnancy received either oral ginger or an identical placebo for 4 days. The number of vomiting episodes decreased significantly and nausea symptoms improved significantly in the ginger group compared with the placebo group, without detectable adverse effects on the pregnancy outcomes (Vutyavanich, Kraisarin, and Ruangsri, 2001). A randomized, controlled equivalence trial involving 291 pregnant women showed ginger to be equivalent to vitamin B_6 in reducing nausea, retching, and vomiting (Smith et al, 2004). *Adverse Effects:* Ginger prolongs bleeding times. Other side effects are heartburn and diarrhea. *Drug Interactions:* Avoid using ginger with anticoagulant drugs. A 76-year-old white European woman controlled on long-term anticoagulant therapy began using ginger products. Several weeks later, her laboratory test showed excessive anticoagulation and she developed nosebleeds (epistaxis). The laboratory test returned to therapeutic range after ginger was stopped and vitamin K_1 was given (Kruth et al, 2004).

Ginkgo (Ginkgo biloba)

This is the earth's oldest living tree species, the only tree to survive Hiroshima and Nagasaki, with individual trees reaching an age of 1000 years (Watkins, 2002a). In Germany, ginkgo is prescribed for treatment of cerebral circulatory disturbances and dementia and for peripheral arterial insufficiency. Its extract dilates arteries, inhibits arterial spasms, and decreases blood viscosity, but results may not be apparent for 6 to 8 weeks (Watkins, 2002a). Meta-

analysis of eight randomized, placebo-controlled, double-blind trials found a significant increase in pain-free walking distance in favor of ginkgo biloba (Pittler and Ernst, 2000). In seven of eight clinical studies, statistically and clinically significant effects of ginkgo on cerebral insufficiency were shown compared with placebo. An application to the treatment of dementia has been proposed (Le Bars et al, 1997). Trials in healthy individuals have shown mixed results. In a randomized, double-blind, placebo-controlled, 6-week trial, 230 healthy men and women showed no improvement in memory or cognitive function (Solomon et al, 2002), but another placebo-controlled, multidose, double-blind trial found that ginkgo biloba produced improvement in attention over a period of 6 hours in healthy young volunteers (Kennedy, Scholey, and Wesnes, 2000).

Adverse Effects: Individuals have experienced spontaneous bleeding while taking ginkgo. A 70-year-old man bled into the anterior chamber of the eye 1 week after adding ginkgo to his aspirin regimen following coronary artery bypass surgery. A 78-year-old woman, stabilized on *warfarin* for 5 years after coronary bypass surgery, sustained a left **parietal** hemorrhage after using ginkgo for 2 months. A 72-year-old woman developed a **subdural hematoma** after taking ginkgo for 6 to 7 months. A 33-year-old woman suffered bilateral subdural hematomas after taking it for 2 years (Cupp, 1999). Post-laparoscopic cholecystectomy bleeding occurred in a client taking ginkgo biloba (Fessenden, Wittenborn, and Clarke, 2001) and in a liver transplant client necessitating exploratory laparotomy. The latter client continued taking ginkgo without informing his physicians until he suffered an eye hemorrhage (Hauser, Gayowski, and Singh, 2002). *Drug Interactions:* Taking ginkgo with *aspirin* or any nonsteroidal anti-inflammatory drug (NSAID) or anticoagulants is ill-advised. Ginkgo may also diminish the effectiveness of anticonvulsant drugs and potentiate the risk of seizures with medications known to decrease the seizure threshold, such as tricyclic antidepressants (Miller, 1998). Two cases are reported of seizures after ingestion of 50 to 70 ginkgo seeds (Klepser and Klepser, 1999; Miwa et al, 2001). Other interactions are elevated blood pressure with a thiazide diuretic (Izzo and Ernst, 2001) and coma with the antidepressant *trazodone* following as few as four doses of ginkgo (Nursing 2004 Herbal). The most commonly reported adverse effects of ginkgo are gastric disturbances, headache, dizziness, and vertigo.

St. John's Wort (Hypericum perforatum)

References to this herb are found in the works of Hippocrates (460–375 BC), the Father of Medicine (Watkins, 2002a). In use as a treatment for psychiatric disorders since the 15th century, St. John's wort (Fig. 16–3) is indicated by German Commission E as supportive treatment for anxiety and mild to moderate depression, but its mechanism of action remains unknown, and 6 to 12 weeks may elapse before effects are seen (Watkins, 2002a). At least 13 active ingredients have been isolated (Klepser and Klepser, 1999). Meta-analysis of 22 randomized controlled trials showed St. John's wort to be significantly more effective than placebo but not significantly different in efficacy from active antidepressants; however, adverse effects occurred more frequently with standard antidepressants than with St. John's wort (Whiskey, Werneke, and Taylor, 2001). Theories suggest that St. John's wort may act as a monoamine oxidase inhibitor (MAOI) or a selective serotonin reuptake inhibitor (SSRI). One source recommends that clients should be advised to separate foods rich in tyramine from intake of St. John's wort (Nursing 2004 Herbal), although Ang-Lee, Moss, and Yuan (2001) describe the MAO inhibition as insignificant in vivo. The interaction of MAOIs with tyramine in foods is explained in Chapter 17.

Cautions: St. John's wort should be avoided in pregnancy because of its **abortifacient** action and because of its teratogenic potential. It has mutagenic effects on sperm and ova, so women *and men* planning a pregnancy should not use St. John's wort (Nursing 2004 Drug). It also may cause allergy. The section on echinacea concerning possible sources of cross-reactivity applies to St. John's wort as well. Because photosensitivity is common with the use of this botanical preparation, people taking it may need to protect themselves from exposure to the sun. A case report of subacute toxic neuropathy was attributed to demyelination of cutaneous axons due to singlet oxygen and free radicals produced from hypericins' exposure to light (Bove, 1998). *Adverse Reactions:* St. John's wort is reported to cause gastrointestinal irritation, tiredness, and restlessness. *Drug Interactions:* Use with other drugs causing photosensitivity should be avoided (Miller, 1998). Two cases of rejection of transplanted hearts (11 and 20 months after surgery) due to interference with the metabolism of *cyclosporin* were attributed to beginning the use of St. John's wort, self-prescribed and prescribed by a psychiatrist, 3 weeks before symptoms appeared (Ruschitzka et al, 2000). St. John's wort interferes with the metabolism of medications by inducing the cytochrome P450 metabolic pathway (see Chapter 17). Experimental evidence from healthy volunteers showed that a 14-day course of St. John's wort significantly induced of one of the cytochrome P450 enzymes, as measured by changes in *alprazolam* **pharmacokinetics**. This suggests that long-term administration of St. John's wort may result in diminished clinical effectiveness or increased dosage requirements for all CYP

3A4 substrates, which represent at least 50 percent of all marketed medications (Markowitz et al, 2003). An experiment with healthy premenopausal women showed concomitant use of St. John's wort with a combination oral contraceptive produced effects on the contraceptive's metabolism consistent with increased CYP3A activity. Therefore, women taking St. John's wort along with oral contraceptives should be counseled to expect breakthrough bleeding and should consider adding a barrier method of contraception to their precautions (Hall et al, 2003). St. John's wort has been shown to decrease blood concentrations of *amitriptyline, cyclosporin, digoxin, indinavir, nevirapine, theophylline,* and *warfarin* (Ioannides, 2002; Izzo and Ernst, 2001). In contrast, St. John's wort may prolong the effects of anesthesia (American Society of Anesthesiologists, 2000) and increase the effects of monoamine oxidase inhibitors and selective serotonin reuptake inhibitors, increasing the risk of toxicity.

Saw Palmetto (Serenoa repens)

Until 1950, saw palmetto tea was included in the U.S. Pharmacopeia and the National Formulary (Watkins, 2002b). The German Commission E has indicated saw palmetto to decrease difficulties with urination associated with benign prostatic hypertrophy (BPH). Its mechanism of action is unknown, but it may inhibit the binding of dihydrotestosterone to androgen receptors in prostate cells or inhibit the enzyme responsible for converting *testosterone* to dihydrotestosterone. Compared with *finasteride,* saw palmetto produces similar improvement in urinary tract symptoms and urinary flow but with fewer adverse effects (Wilt et al, 1998). Teas made with saw palmetto are probably ineffective, because the active components are insoluble in water (Klepser and Klepser, 1999).

Cautions: Pregnant women and children should not take saw palmetto. Adults and children with hormone-dependent illnesses other than benign prostatic hypertrophy or breast cancer should avoid this herb (Nursing 2004 Herbal). *Adverse effects* are headache, nausea, and upset stomach. A severe intraoperative hemorrhage that required 10 units of blood products to control during resection of a brain tumor was attributed to saw palmetto because the client's prolonged bleeding time returned to normal a few days after discontinuing saw palmetto (Cheema, El-Mefty, and Jazieh, 2001). *Drug Interactions:* None have been reported, but the prudent person would avoid concurrent use of other hormonal therapies (Miller, 1998).

Valerian (Valeriana officinalis)

The Greek physician Galan (130–299 AD) recommended valerian for insomnia (Watkins, 2002c). It has official pharmacopoeial status in Europe, but although it may correct numerous causes of insomnia, the variety and the instability of its components creates problems with standardization (Houghton, 1999). Valerian is recommended by German Commission E to manage restlessness and nervous disorders of sleep. Its mode of action affecting the central nervous system is incompletely understood. Some 44 constituents of valerian have been isolated. Compared with placebo, valerian significantly improved sleep quality

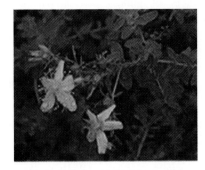

SAINT JOHN'S WORT

Figure **16–3** St. John's wort grows 1- to 3-feet tall in fields and beside roads in the United States, flowering from June through September. (Reprinted from Venes, 2001, p 1832, with permission.)

in habitually poor or irregular sleepers. It has not been observed to change sleep stages (Miller, 1998). Valerian may require 1 to 4 weeks of continuous use to show effect, and it has not been judged safe for children or pregnant or lactating women (Watkins, 2002c). *Adverse effects* are headaches, hangover, excitability, insomnia, uneasiness, cardiac disturbances, ataxia, decreased sensibility, hypothermia, hallucinations, and increased muscle relaxation (Klepser and Klepser, 1999). At higher than recommended doses taken for a long time, *benzodiazepine*-like withdrawal symptoms may occur when the herb is discontinued so that weaning over 2 weeks is advised (Watkins, 2002c). *Drug Interactions:* Since valerian prolongs *thiopental-* and *pentobarbital*-induced sleep, it should not be used with barbiturates (Miller, 1998).

A summary of the main uses of the nine botanical products mentioned above and some situations in which they should be avoided appear in Table 16–1. Use with anticoagulants and during pregnancy are the most frequent contraindications cited. The absence of such a warning should

Table 16–1 **Commonly Used Botanicals' Main Uses and Avoidance Situations**

PRODUCT	MAIN USE*	INTERACTS WITH	AVOID IN
Asian ginseng (Panax ginseng)	To combat lack of energy	Anticoagulants Digoxin Estrogen MAOIs NSAIDs	Asthma Children Hypertension Pregnancy Psychological imbalances
Echinacea (E. purpurea, E. pallida)	To bolster the immune system	Anabolic steroids Immunosuppressants Preotease inhibitors Other hepatotoxic drugs	Allergies to the daisy family Children Pregnancy Lactation
Feverfew (Tanacetum parthenium)	To prevent migraine headaches	Anticoagulants Aspirin NSAIDs	Allergies to the daisy family Children younger than 2 years Pregnancy Lactation
Garlic (Allium sativum)	To treat hyperlipoproteinemia	Acetaminophen Anticoagulants Antidiabetic drugs	Pregnancy and lactation in more than cooking amounts Allergies
Ginger (Zingiber officinale)	To aid digestion and treat motion sickness	Anticoagulants	
Ginkgo (Ginkgo biloba)	To improve cerebral circulation	Anticoagulants Anticonvulsants Aspirin Drugs that decrease seizure threshold NSAIDs Thiazide diuretics Trazodone Tricyclic antidepressants	Anticoagulants Seizures
Saw palmetto (Serenoa repens)	To decrease urination difficulty	Other hormonal therapies	Hormonal-dependent illnesses except BPH and breast cancer Children Pregnancy
St. John's wort (Hypericum perforatum)	To support treatment for anxiety and depression	Amitriptyline Anticoagulants Cyclosporin Digoxin Drugs causing photo-sensitivity Indinavir MAOIs Oral contraceptives Serotonin-reuptake inhibitors Theophylline Tyramine-rich foods (possible)	Allergies to the daisy family Pregnancy (abortifacient) Planning a pregnancy (women and men) Sun exposure
Valerian (Valeriana officinalis)	To manage restlessness and disorders of sleep	Barbiturates	Children Pregnancy Lactation

*As listed in Canada or Germany. U.S. labeling may be reworded.

not be construed as evidence of safety, however. Sufficient data may not have been gathered. As the use of herbal medicines increases, more adverse effects and interactions appear in the literature.

When Things Go Wrong

Sometimes the use of home remedies goes terribly wrong, often because of human error. As the following cases illustrate, poor choices of botanicals, lack of sufficient knowledge about plants, and failure to accept recommendations can lead to serious consequences.

Choosing Toxic Plants

Chaparral (*Larrea tridentata*) is an evergreen desert shrub found in the southwestern United States and Mexico that has been used to treat several diseases and to prevent conception (Sheehan, 1998). Federal investigation of 18 reported cases of liver toxicity confirmed that chaparral ingestion caused 13 of them. Twelve of the 13 clients had ingested tablets or capsules from various manufacturers; the other person consumed chaparral as a tea. Cessation of ingestion of chaparral resulted in resolution in 11 clients but the remaining two underwent liver transplantation. The pathophysiology of chaparral-associated liver toxicity is unclear, but the two clients requiring liver transplantation took chaparral capsules for longer than a year, compared with the other clients, who reported having ingested it for 2.8 to 24 weeks (Sheikh, Philen, and Love, 1997).

One of the individuals who received a liver transplant after being poisoned with chaparral went through extensive blood tests, an abdominal ultrasound, and CT scan. The latter reveal gallbladder pathology. An exploratory laparotomy was performed. Severe acute hepatitis was diagnosed by liver biopsy. At that point, the client's husband revealed that she had ingested two capsules of chaparral daily for 10 months, along with a pinch of garlic powder and a tea made from nettle and chickweed. Three weeks before admission, the client had developed symptoms of flu and *increased* her dose of chaparral to six capsules per day (Gordon et al, 1995). Two Canadian clients also developed acute hepatitis after ingesting chaparral leaf, one for 2 months and one for 3 months, but recovered after discontinuing use of the botanical product (Batchelor, Heathcote, and Wanless, 1995).

Herbal supplements accounted for the most cases of fulminant liver failure (onset of encephalopathy within 8 weeks of onset of jaundice in the absence of preexisting liver disease) referred to one liver transplant service in a 22-month period. That etiology exceeded liver failure cases due to *acetaminophen* toxicity and viral hepatitis (Estes et al, 2003).

Misidentifying Plants

A 72-year-old woman became ill after drinking a tea she thought to be made of borage leaves. She developed nausea, vomiting, diarrhea, flickering in her eyes, and palpitations. Her electrocardiogram showed intermittent atrioventricular blockage. Her blood levels of *digitoxin* and *digoxin/* were 133.5 and 3.93 ng/mL (toxic >25 ng/mL

and >2.4 ng/mL), respectively. Symptomatic treatment was all that was necessary. The cause was attributed to her gathering of foxglove leaves, mistaking them for borage (Brustbauer and Wenisch, 1997).

In a similar case, an 18-month-old boy developed liver disease after consuming a tea supposedly made with peppermint and coltsfoot (*Tussilago farfara*) since 3 months of age. Conservative treatment led to a complete recovery within 2 months. Analysis of the leaves indicated that the parents had gathered alpendost (*Adenostyles alliariae*), mistaking it for coltsfoot (Sperl et al, 1995). Even without the misidentification, however, the intended mixture is not harmless, because coltsfoot is a direct hepatotoxin (Haller et al, 2002).

Tragedy resulted from giving Hispanic infants tea from homegrown "mint" plants. The first infant's mother did not reveal the use of "mint" tea until the second hospital day. After the 8-week-old infant died, autopsy revealed liver necrosis, hemorrhagic kidneys, left adrenal hemorrhage, bilateral lung consolidation, and diffuse cerebral edema with ischemic necrosis. The second infant, 6 months old, had been given the tea three times a week since he was 3 months old. Laboratory testing of the leaves from the involved plants and the infants' sera confirmed the source of the poison to be pennyroyal oil, a highly toxic agent used by herbalists to induce menstruation or abortion. The second infant received some "mint" tea the evening before admission when he had vomited and had a fever. Although the second infant lived, he was left with liver and brain dysfunction. Medical opinion was that he tolerated the pennyroyal oil until he seemed to develop a viral infection, which precipitated the acute illness (Bakerink et al, 1996).

Increasing the Dose

A uterine stimulant, blue cohosh (*Caulophyllum thalictroides*), was prescribed by a midwife as follows. Beginning 1 month before her due date, the pregnant woman was to take one tablet daily to induce uterine contractions. The woman took three tablets per day for 3 weeks. Spontaneous onset of labor resulted in precipitous delivery 1 hour later. The amniotic fluid was slightly stained with meconium. Within 20 minutes of birth, the infant became cyanotic and required mechanical ventilation. An electrocardiogram revealed an acute myocardial infarction. He was extubated at 21 days of age and discharged from the hospital at 31 days of age. At 2 years of age, he displayed normal growth and development despite cardiomegaly and mildly reduced left ventricular function, for which he received *digoxin*. The long-term prognosis was guarded. Congenital anomalies were ruled out, and the cause for this newborn's heart attack was attributed to the blue cohosh, which contains an alkaloid known to produce toxic effects on the myocardium of laboratory animals (Jones and Lawson, 1998).

A client may increase the dose of a dangerous substance inadvertently, as happened to a 44-year-old man who sought medical assistance for worsening muscle cramps. He volunteered the fact that he had been drinking up to 4 liters of black tea daily for 25 years and recently switched to the Earl Grey brand because of gastric pain he attributed to his usual brand. One week after the change, he noticed repeated muscle cramps in his right foot that eventually affected his left foot, right calf, and hands. Additionally, he complained of pressure in his eyes, associated with blurred vision, particularly in darkness. He received an extensive diagnostic work-up with negative results. The client, assuming that there was a connection between his symptoms and his tea consumption, stopped drinking Earl Grey. Within 1 week, his symptoms had completely disappeared and did not recur if he limited his intake of Earl Grey to 1 liter per day. A simple explanation of his pathology is related to bergamot oil, an extract from the rind of the bergamot orange, which is added to black tea to give Earl Grey a pleasant, refreshing scent. Bergamot oil has a strong phototoxic effect, which led to it being widely banned as an ingredient in cosmetics and tanning products, but it is used therapeutically in several skin diseases. In this client, a chemical component of the oil selectively blocked potassium channels in the affected nerves (Finsterer, 2002). This situation could have been avoided if the client had adopted the advice underpinning a good diet: balance, moderation, and variety.

Another report of adverse effects of bergamot oil used in complementary medicine relates to aromatherapy. Two clients developed phototoxic skin reactions within 48 to 72 hours after exposure to bergamot aromatherapy oil and subsequent ultraviolet exposure. One client had no history of direct contact with the aromatherapy oil but developed blister-like skin lesions after exposure to aerosolized (evaporated) aromatherapy oil in a sauna and subsequent ultraviolet radiation in a tanning salon (Kaddu, Kerl, and Wolf, 2001).

Bergamot oil is also found in colognes called "Florida Water" or "Kananga Water," popular with Hispanic, African American, and Caribbean people who use them for spiritual blessing, treating headaches, and personal hygiene. These products may increase risk of phototoxic dermatitis as described above (Wang, Sterling, and Don, 2002).

A Prudent Course

Several issues arise when health-care providers assist clients who are attempting to maximize their health. The fact that many botanical products have been used for centuries does not negate the dangers cited in this chapter. Clearly in this market, "let the buyer beware" holds true. Aside from changing the law, what can be done to protect clients?

Thorough assessment is vital. In several of the worst cases cited, the fact that herbal remedies were used did not come to light until late in the treatment cycle. Did health-care providers ask the clients about use of botanical products? If so, was it done in a manner that permitted them to reveal their practices without feeling ridiculed or condemned? Written questionnaires are not as effective as personal interviews in eliciting information about the use of botanical products (Ang-Lee, Moss, and Yuan, 2001).

Education is essential. Without disparaging a client's background, the health-care provider must counter the ill-advised attitude that "Everything natural is safe." Substances strong enough to produce the effects attributed to botanical preparations are medicines, no matter what the law currently allows for distribution. Such substances should be treated with respect. Use of childproof containers should be encouraged.

All health-care providers must educate themselves about botanical products, because many of their clients will be using them. The *Physicians' Desk Reference for Herbal Medicines,* shown in Figure 16–4, first published in 1998, symbolizes the recognition of complementary and alternative medicine by mainstream medicine. Now in the 3rd edition, the reference offers credible information to healthcare providers. Staying alert to press releases and general news items about botanical medicine helps healthcare providers keep up to date as well.

Awareness of the dangers is essential. More than one source has recommended that the following botanicals

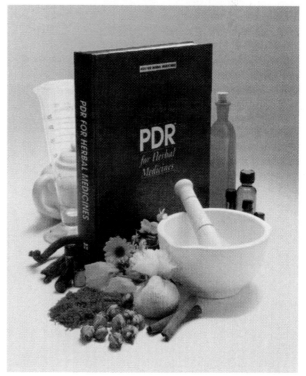

Physician's Desk Reference®
Introduces

PDR® for Herbal Medicines

The First Authoritative Herbal Guide
for Healthcare Professionals

Figure **16–4** The first edition of the Physician's Desk Reference for Herbal Medicines was published in 1998. (Gruenwald, J [ed]: Physicians Desk Reference for Herbal Medicines, 1998, courtesy of Medical Economics Company. Used with permission.)

The Nursing Process and Botanical Remedies

Ask clients these questions about botanical use:

Assessment

What kinds of herbal products, dietary supplements, or other natural remedies do you take?

Do you find the recommended dose satisfactory?

Are you taking any prescription or over-the-counter medications for the same purpose? Or for opposite purposes?

Have you used this product before? For how long?

Where do you obtain these products?

Is anyone else in your household taking botanical products?

Are you allergic to any plant products?

Are you pregnant, planning to become pregnant, or breast-feeding?

Analysis

Ask the pharmacist or look up botanical remedies in the PDR for Herbal Medicines, in a reference authored by registered pharmacists, or on the Internet at http://www.rxlist.com, if necessary. Additional internet sources are the Office of Dietary Supplements of the National Institutes of Health at http://ods.od.nih.gov/Health_Information/IBIDS.aspx and the American Association of Poison Control Centers at http://www. aapcc.org.

Identify problem areas.

Planning

Prioritize problems to be addressed as to seriousness:

Products with known toxic effects.

Products given to children.

Home-grown plant materials.

Products with interactions to drugs the client is receiving.

Implementation

Document findings in the record.

Encourage client to discuss use with primary health-care provider.

Offer educational advice to the client and document it.

Encourage use of single-herb formulations rather than conglomerates.

If long-term studies establishing the safety of a product are lacking, encourage client to limit use to several weeks.

Teach client that multiple products taken for the same effect can lead to trouble.

Discourage use of botanical products for infants, children, pregnant women, and the elderly without professional medical advice.

If the client wishes to use these products, reinforce the need to abide by recommended doses and to consistently use the same reputable supplier.

Encourage client to monitor for side effects and report them to health-care provider or the FDA's MEDWATCH at 1-800-FDA-1088 or on the Internet at http://www.fda.gov/medwatch/report/consumer/consumer.htm.

Evaluation

Follow up the actions of the client at each visit.

Are there new symptoms?

Have the products, brands, or doses been changed?

Have any products been stopped or new ones added?

Does the client think the products are effective? Wh or why not?

SOURCE: Adapted from Cirigliano and Sun, 1998; Cupp, 1999; Glisson, Crawford, and Street, 1999; Smolinske, 1999, and Yager, Siegfried, and DiMatteo, 1999.

be avoided: borage, chaparral, comfrey, ephedra, germander, kombucha, lobelia, pennyroyal, sassafras, and wormwood (Baker, 1999; Brody, 1999; Consumer Reports, 2004; Haller, et al, 2002; Klepser and Klepser, 1999; and Sheehan, 1998).

A general nursing process approach to botanical use is given in Clinical Application 16–1. The potential exists, as more knowledge accumulates, that botanicals might be used in conjunction with pharmaceuticals to take advantage of their synergistic effects, perhaps reducing dosages of each (Sorensen, 2002).

Ergogenic Aids

An ergogenic aid is a means to increase work output or the potential of work output. For athletes it is any means of enhancing energy utilization, including energy production, control, and efficiency. An estimated one to three million male and female athletes in the United States alone have used anabolic steroids (Silver, 2001), but in 2004, the Food and Drug Administration warned manufacturers to stop distributing androstenedione (see Box 16–3). Athletes in training, attempting to build a competitive edge, often alter their dietary intake and consume various supplements. This section summarizes some of these actions and cites scientific opinion as to the safety and effectiveness of the practices. Many athletic organizations prohibit the use of certain pharmacologic, physiologic, and nutritional aids, so before using any of these supplements, the athlete, with the advice of the health-care provider, parents, and coach, should evaluate the supplement carefully.

1. Is the link between the purported aid and known physiology and biochemistry logical?
2. Has the use been critiqued in peer-reviewed journals?

Box 16–3 FDA Stops Distribution of Androstenedione

In March 2004, the Food and Drug Administration warned 23 manufacturers to cease distributing the dietary supplement androstenedione that acts as a steroid once it is metabolized by the body. Such metabolized steroids are unavailable without a physician's prescription. The National Collegiate Athletics Association, the National Football League, and the International Olympic Committee had previously banned the use of androstenedione. Potential long-term effects of androstenedione are listed in the following table.

MEN	CHILDREN	WOMEN
Testicular atrophy	Early onset of puberty	Male pattern baldness
Impotence	Premature cessation of bone growth	Permanent clitoral enlargement
Breast enlargement	Boys: testicular atrophy	Increased facial hair
	Breast enlargement	Deepened voice
	Girls: Severe acne	Menstrual irregularities
	Excessive body and facial hair	Blood clots
	Deepened voice	
	Permanent clitoral enlargement	
	Disruption of menstrual cycle	

SOURCE: Adapted from U.S. Food and Drug Administration, 2004c and 2004d.

3. What are the safety, ethical, and legal consequences of using the aid, including the rules of athletic conferences and the International Olympic Committee?

The use of ergogenic aids for improved physical prowess has roots in ancient history. Athletes and soldiers in the past consumed selected animal parts to acquire some of the animal's strength, speed, or agility. Some ergogenic aids clearly fall into the classes of nutrients included in Unit I of this text, whereas others do not, although they may be substances with physiological functions. For the sake of uniformity, the ergogenic aids included here will be categorized either as nutrients corresponding to those in Unit I or as nonnutrients.

Nutrients

Various investigators have tested the effects on physical performance of altering ingestion of carbohydrate, protein, and antioxidant vitamins and minerals. Additionally, procedures to maximize water retention have been researched.

Carbohydrates

Carbohydrate loading has evidence-based support of being both ergogenic and safe (Juhn, 2002). Consuming carbohydrates immediately before or after exercise augments performance by increasing muscle glycogen stores, delaying fatigue, and enhancing recovery. An endurance athlete's carbohydrate consumption should be at least 60 percent of kilocaloric intake normally and 70 percent of energy intake for several days prior to competition. Ingesting carbohydrate 3 to 6 hours before exercise enhances performance (Applegate, 1999). Fatigue can be reduced by adding carbohydrate to the fluids consumed so that 30 to 60 grams of rapidly absorbed carbohydrate are ingested during each hour of an athletic

event (Coyle, 2004). If an athlete is glycogen-depleted after exercise, a carbohydrate intake of 1.5 grams per kilogram of body weight during the first 30 minutes and again every 2 hours for 4 to 6 hours will be adequate to replace glycogen stores (American College of Sports Medicine, 2000).

Protein and Amino Acids

Athletes involved in intense training may have greater protein needs than sedentary individuals. Protein recommendations for endurance athletes are 1.2 to 1.4 grams per kilogram of body weight per day, but resistance and strength-trained athletes may need 1.6 to 1.7 grams per kilogram of body weight per day (American College of Sports Medicine, 2000), an intake that is possible through a normal diet that maintains energy balance. Most protein supplements on the market contain relatively little protein compared with 3 ounces of chicken with 27 grams and the same amount of light tuna with 35 grams. The same advice holds here as in other areas of nutrition: read the labels. There is no scientific evidence that protein supplementation enhances metabolic efficiency and increases muscle mass (Lawrence and Kirby, 2002).

GLUTAMINE

Glutamine is an important fuel for some cells of the immune system and may have specific immunostimulatory effects. Oral glutamine, compared with placebo, appeared to have a beneficial effect on the incidence of infections reported by runners after a marathon (Castell and Newsholme, 1998). There is some evidence that this amino acid supplement promotes muscle growth and decreases exercise-induced immunosuppression, thus decreasing incidence of upper respiratory infections, but long-term studies have not been conducted (Kreider, 1999). Levels of plasma amino acids, mainly glutamine, were decreased in

Olympic athletes suffering from chronic fatigue and infection. Inadequate protein intake appeared to be a factor, because 7 of the 12 athletes in the chronic fatigue group had restricted dietary intake of dairy products and animal protein (Kingsbury, Kay, and Hjelm, 1998). The few scientific studies available suggest that glutamine is effective only for athletes with a true deficiency (Beduschi, 2003).

BRANCHED-CHAIN AMINO ACIDS (BCAA)

Leucine, isoleucine, and valine are branched-chain amino acids that make up about one-third of muscle protein (Mero, 1999). Significant decreases in levels of plasma leucine follow exercise sessions. Theoretically, supplementation with branched-chain amino acids (BCAA) during intense training could reduce exercise-induced muscle damage and consequently lead to greater gains in fat-free mass (Kreider, 1999). Leucine or its metabolite, beta-hydroxy beta-methylbutyrate (beta-HMB), has been reported to increase fat-free mass in college football players and in elderly men and women, but no significant difference was found between it and placebo in two other studies (Kreider, 1999). Most reviews suggest that supplementation with BCAA is not effective as an ergogenic aid (Beduschi, 2003).

Dietary Antioxidants and Minerals

The potential for antioxidants to enhance recovery from exercise is related to their ability to detoxify free radicals, which are produced during strenuous exercise. Some evidence supports the concept that supplemental dietary antioxidant intake protects against oxidative stress due to exercise and perhaps also enhances recovery and minimizes muscle soreness (Applegate, 1999). Antioxidants are essential components of the diet, but additional oral supplementation does not increase endurance or strength (Juhn, 2003).

Chromium is promoted as an ergogenic supplement, but there is no conclusive evidence supporting its effectiveness in enhancing athletic performance (Lawrence and Kirby, 2002). It appears to have no efficacy as a body-building supplement (Fillmore et al, 1999) or as a means to enhance body composition (Kobla and Volpe, 2000).

Water

Although proper hydration with fluids and electrolytes is necessary, hard evidence is lacking regarding the best strategies to prevent exercise-induced cramping (Fillmore et al, 1999). When possible, fluids should be ingested at rates that closely match the sweating rate. When that is not possible, some athletes exercising in a cold or temperate environment might tolerate loss of 2 percent of body weight without significant risk to performance or well-being. In a hot environment, however, that degree of dehydration impairs power and predisposes the athlete to heat injury (Coyle, 2004).

A different theory on etiology proposes that a spinal neural mechanism may induce cramping that is unrelated to biochemical changes in either blood or in the affected skeletal muscles (Noakes, 1998). This theory, supported by electromyographic (EMG) data obtained from runners during exercise-associated muscle cramps, suggests the cause is muscle fatigue that provokes abnormal spinal reflex activity. In this case, passive stretching relieves the cramp (Schwellnus, Derman, and Noakes, 1997).

Nonnutrients

Among the ergogenic aids promoted for athletes are several substances that occur in the human body as a result of metabolism and one commonly ingested foreign substance, caffeine. The United States Olympic Committee (USOC) has banned many drugs. The lists are accessible at its Web site, http://www.usoc.org.

Bicarbonate

Muscular activity generates lactic acid as a waste product with consequent lowering of blood pH. The drop in pH is thought to inhibit the resynthesis of ATP and to inhibit muscle contraction. One physiological buffer is bicarbonate. Sodium bicarbonate (baking soda) has been shown to be an effective ergogenic aid during exercise lasting approximately 1 to 7 minutes (Applegate, 1999). McNaughton, Dalton, and Palmer (1999) showed sodium bicarbonate to be significantly more effective than placebo or no intervention in decreasing fatigue during 60-minute cycling sessions.

Creatine

Creatine is a nonprotein substance synthesized in the body from the amino acids arginine, glycine, and methionine. When combined with phosphate, the resulting compound, phosphocreatine, serves as a storage form of energy that is released with anaerobic muscle contraction. Increasing the supply of creatine supposedly would increase muscle creatine and phosphocreatine concentration, leading to a higher rate of ATP resynthesis (Mujika and Padilla, 1997). **Endogenous** synthesis produces 1 to 2 grams of creatine per day, while dietary fish and meat provide another 1 to 2 grams. Creatine is eliminated by its irreversible conversion to creatinine at a rate of approximately 1 to 2 grams per day (Juhn and Tarnopolsky, 1998).

Oral creatine supplements have promoted gains in lean body mass in most individuals when used with resistance training and have enhanced power and strength (Racette, 2003). Creatine appears to have scientific support as enhancing exercise performance in high-intensity, short-term tasks with little recovery time between repetitions (Beduschi, 2003) and is ergogenic in repetitive anaerobic cycling sprints but not running or swimming (Juhn, 2003). Without large clinical trials, the safety of creatine is unknown; moreover, adverse kidney and liver effects have been reported (Lawrence and Kirby, 2002). Creatine supplementation does result in weight gain that initially is the result of water retention, which complicates the task of designing double-blind, placebo-controlled studies (Juhn and Tarnopolsky, 1998).

As many as 28 percent of college athletes admit taking creatine, and in a New York suburb, 5.6 percent of middle and high school athletes, aged 10 to 18, admitted to using it, most commonly those participating in football, wrestling, hockey, gymnastics, and lacrosse (Metzl et al, 2001). Young athletes, however, must be cautious about taking creatine, because its effects on growth and development are unknown and long-term safety has not been established (Racette, 2003).

Glycerol

Glycerol is an alcohol that is a component of fats. The pharmaceutical grade of glycerol is called glycerin(e). It is used to moisten chapped skin, as an ingredient in suppositories for constipation, and as a sweetening agent in medications. Taken orally, it acts as an osmotic diuretic to reduce intracranial pressure and intraocular pressure.

As an ergogenic aid, glycerol has been tested as a means of hyperhydration to prevent dehydration. Although oral glycerin does enhance fluid retention, its effectiveness in improving athletic performance is controversial and largely unsubstantiated (Wagner, 1999), and Coyle states that athletes do not benefit from glycerol (2004). Appropriate hydration without glycerol is recommended.

Caffeine

Caffeine dosing before exercise delays the onset of fatigue and may enhance performance of high-intensity exercise. Caffeine has also been shown to increase speed and/or power output in activities that last as little as 60 seconds or as long as 2 hours. Its ingestion before exercise does not lead to dehydration, and it is metabolized similarly in males and females. The mechanism(s) by which caffeine produces ergogenic effects are unknown, but the theory that it enhances fat oxidation and spares muscle glycogen has little support and would only partially explain the effect. Caffeine may work, in part, by creating a more favorable intracellular ionic environment in active muscle that could facilitate force production by each motor unit (Graham, 2001). Despite its ready availability, caffeine has side effects and causes some drug interactions, but it has evidence-based support of being both ergogenic and safe (Juhn, 2002).

Making Wise Decisions

Athletes often make tremendous sacrifices in the pursuit of excellence. Their drive and dedication is admirable, but rash judgments about the substances they take into their bodies are not. Clients need guidance in gathering and evaluating evidence about the safety and efficacy of nutritional supplements marketed for athletes. If an athlete chooses to take a nutritional supplement, the recommended dose should be used. More is not better. Physicians and dietitians specialize in sports medicine to help the athlete's decision making. One such physician cautions that nutritional supplements have not been tested in or approved for use by children or adolescents and that their use in this population should be approached with trepidation (Metzl, 1999).

Basic nutrition principles hold true for athletes as well as less-active people. Increased kilocalories because of the activity, consuming proportionate protein, and drinking adequate water are appropriate approaches to athletic training. Extra snacks of sports drinks, fruit juices, low-fat milk, yogurt, whole-grain cereal, fruit, and pretzels are good choices to increase kilocaloric intake in a healthful manner.

A particular problem occurs in sports for which body size or weight is crucial. The deaths of collegiate wrestlers trying to "cut weight" were reported in Chapter 9. Other activities with weight consideration that might lead to unwise dieting are gymnastics, cross-country track, crew (rowing), and dance.

Other Possibly Beneficial Products

Several additional products that do not fit into botanical or ergogenic categories show promise in certain situations. Glucosamine has been favorably evaluated in the medical literature regarding its impact on osteoarthritis. Probiotics have been found effective for various conditions, and an unusual use of a food ingredient evokes interest.

Glucosamine

Glucosamine, available as a dietary supplement, is a molecular building block found in joint cartilage (Morelli, Naquin, and Weaver, 2003) that has been evaluated by medical researchers. As with other dietary supplements, it may take 4 to 6 weeks to see an effect that is also maintained for about the same time after stopping the supplement (Hochberg and Dougados, 2001). In 12 of 13 randomized controlled trials, glucosamine was found to be superior to placebo. In four trials comparing glucosamine to an NSAID, glucosamine was superior in two and equivalent in two. Thus, glucosamine was judged to be effective and safe in osteoarthritis, but more research was recommended to confirm the long-term effectiveness and level of toxicity (Towheed et al, 2001). In contrast to simply controlling pain, two 3-year randomized, placebo-controlled studies showed glucosamine to have a disease-modifying effect on osteoarthritis of the knee as measured by radiographs (Bruyere et al, 2004; Reginster et al, 2001). A meta-analysis of randomized, placebo-controlled trials reported glucosamine to have a highly significant effect on all outcomes, including joint space narrowing (Richy et al, 2003).

In North America, glucosamine is an over-the-counter dietary supplement, and preparations made by different manufacturers may vary. An ongoing long-term clinical trial in the United States will possibly standardize this therapy and produce appropriate recommendations (Zerkak and Dougados, 2004). Meanwhile, some formulations are distributed by pharmaceutical companies, a feature that might give a consumer greater confidence in the sanitation and standardization of their production.

Probiotics

Probiotics emerged as a popular treatment in 1908 because fermented foods were associated with longevity (Teitelbaum, 2005). Certain beneficial microorganisms were described in Chapter 12, and products containing them are available in foods and as dietary supplements. **Probiotics** are live microbial food supplements that benefit the person when ingested by improving the microbial balance of the intestine. The main action of probiotics is reinforcement of the intestinal mucosal barrier against deleterious agents (Fioramonti, Theodorou, and Bueno, 2003). A second category of supplement encompasses **prebiotics,** nondigestible food ingredients that encourage favorable microorganisms. The most extensively studied and widely used probiotics are Lactobacillus and Bifidobacterium. Adverse effects include occasional reports of bacteremias and endocarditis associated with Lactobacillus usually occurring in severely immunocompromised persons (Kopp-Hoolihan, 2001). Clients who may benefit from probiotics include those with allergies, diarrhea, and impaired immune function.

In allergy, probiotics may improve the mucosal barrier of the intestine. In children they are thought to promote the development of the immune system (Kopp-Hoolihan, 2001). A relationship has been found between allergies and decreased exposure to multiple organisms that results from better sanitation in the Western world. To counter this dearth of bacteria in a child's environment, probiotics are suggested to stimulate the gut immune system, thus reducing atopic disease (Vanderhoof and Young, 2003). A double-blind, randomized, placebo-controlled trial that gave Lactobacillus GG to pregnant women who had at least one first-degree relative or partner with atopic disease and to their infants for 6 months reduced atopic eczema by half at age 2 years compared with the placebo group (Kalliomaki, 2001).

Prevention and treatment of diarrhea in children has been extensively studied. Very low birth weight infants given *Lactobacillus acidophilus* and *Bifidobacterium infantis* with breast milk had significantly lower incidences of death or necrotizing enterocolitis (see Clinical Application 12–5) than infants receiving only breast milk (Lin et al, 2005). Nevertheless, special caution is urged when introducing new and potentially infectious agents to immunologically immature infants (Kliegman and Willoughby, 2005).

A meta-analysis of randomized, blinded, controlled trials determined that Lactobacillus reduced diarrhea frequency and duration compared with placebo (Van Niel et al, 2002). Similarly, adding Lactobacillus GG to oral rehydration solutions significantly reduced the number of hours of diarrhea caused by rotavirus compared with placebo (Guandalini et al, 2000). In sum, probiotics show promise in the treatment of acute infectious diarrhea and the prevention of antibiotic-associated diarrhea such that they are becoming accepted pediatric therapies (Van Niel, 2005).

Studies of healthy aging individuals suggest that dietary supplementation with probiotics may reduce the impaired immunity associated with aging (Hebuterne, 2003). Supplementation of healthy elderly persons with

Bifidobacterium lactis showed increases in measures of leukocyte activity in their blood samples. As is often the case with supplements, the greatest changes in immunity occurred in the subjects with poor pretreatment immune responses (Gill et al, 2001). In a similar study, using Lactobacillus or Bifidobacterium supplements, lymphocytes from subjects older than 70 years showed significantly greater tumoricidal activity than those from younger subjects (Gill, Rutherford, and Cross, 2001).

Probiotics can be found in fermented or aged milk and milk products, other fermented products, breast milk, and supplements. Food sources of probiotics enhance the probiotic's stability by buffering stomach acid and also contain other nutrients. The most reliable food source is yogurt labeled "Live & Active Culture." In order for a this seal to appear on a container of yogurt, the product must contain at least 100 million bacteria per gram of yogurt at the time it is made and must not have been heat treated because that kills the bacteria. Additionally, to maximize desired effects, one should choose fresh yogurts since bacteria counts decrease as the expiration date approaches (Yale-New Haven, 2005).

Clients choosing to use supplements should use well-known species of bacteria and increase their intakes to the desired amount gradually over 2 or 3 weeks to minimize side effects. Many studies of diarrhea, lactose intolerance, and biomarkers for colon cancer indicate an effective dose of probiotics would be about 1 liter of acidophilus milk daily, but lesser amounts may be beneficial to some individuals, particularly if accompanied by prebiotics (Kopp-Hoolihan, 2001). Examples of prebiotics are wheat, barley, rye, asparagus, banana, onions, garlic, and tomatoes (Brown, 2005, Kennedy, Kirk, and Gardiner, 2000).

Peppermint Oil

A novel use of this food flavoring product is to apply it topically to relieve pain. A physician's personal experience obtaining headache relief after applying the remedy purchased at his local grocery store to his forehead and temples led to recommendations to friends who also obtained relief. Eventually he offered the therapy to a client who was more impressed with his personal testimony than the research he cited (Richard, 1998). The basis for Richard's venture into complementary medicine was a double-blind, placebo-controlled study that showed no significant difference between the efficacy of 1000 mg of acetaminophen and 10% peppermint oil in ethanol solution, both providing relief from tension headaches compared with their placebos (Gobel et al, 1996).

Another case report involves a 76-year-old woman with intractable pain following herpes zoster. Application of neat peppermint oil containing 10 percent menthol to her skin resulted in almost immediate improvement in her pain that persisted for 4 to 6 hours. She continued to use the remedy for 2 months without adverse effects (Davies, Harding, and Baranowski, 2002).

SUMMARY

Botanical remedies are plant products sold as dietary supplements. With few exceptions, under United States law as of this writing, they are exempt from many of the regulations governing prescription and over-the-counter medications. Although the FDA oversees the safety of botanicals, the responsibility for proving a product is *unsafe* is the *government's*. That power was exercised with the botanical ephedra and the ergogenic aid androstenedione. With prescription and nonprescription drugs, in contrast, the *manufacturer* must demonstrate the medicine is *safe*.

Botanical products are commonly used in other countries. In Germany, they are often prescribed based on evaluations by German Commission E. Those evaluations have been published and can be consulted in the search for reliable information.

Frequently, adults taking prescription medicines also use botanical products or high-dose vitamins or both, commonly without the knowledge of their health-care provider. Areas of concern with botanical products are the lack of standardization and quality control and the contamination of the products with dangerous substances. Even botanicals that are considered reasonably safe should sometimes be avoided. The drug interaction most often cited for the botanicals included in the chapter was with anticoagulants, sometimes causing severe illnesses.

Although not as systematically monitored as prescription and over-the-counter drugs, adverse effects from botanical products are investigated, usually when the client becomes acutely ill after consuming a product. If a person wishes to use botanical products, he or she should avoid products with known toxic effects, investigate suppliers' reputations, take only the recommended dose and only for several weeks, and be as alert for side effects as one would be with prescription or over-the-counter medications. The health-care provider should be consulted *before* infants, children, pregnant women, and the elderly are given botanical products (see Wellness Tip 16–1).

> **Wellness Tip 16–1** • If a person is interested in botanical or ergogenic products, several steps are necessary to minimize risks:
>
> 1. Accumulate as much information as possible. Investigate the credibility of the source of the information.
> 2. Be careful. Proceed slowly. Use single-ingredient supplements in preference to mixtures.
> 3. Avoid food items that have botanical products added.
> 4. Use for a short time only.
> 5. Discuss the program with the primary-care provider.
> 6. Do not use in infants, children, pregnant women, or the elderly.
> 7. Be a minimalist. These substances are taken with the expectation of medicinal results. They are not harmless because they are "natural."

Ergogenic aids are supplements intended to improve athletic performance. As with botanical products, the data supporting the use of many of the aids are sparse, and long-term studies have yet to be performed. The results of many laboratory studies have not been confirmed by athletes in competition. Just because an item is available over the counter does not mean it is safe. Although there is agreement that athletes require additional protein, it can be obtained through a balanced diet that includes sufficient energy for their needs.

Other dietary supplements such as glucosamine and probiotics are proving to be beneficial and may become incorporated into mainstream medical practice. Health-care providers should educate themselves about complementary medicine products, query clients about their use of these supplements, and assist clients in making wise decisions by discussing their risks and benefits. An open mind is an asset when confronted with novel treatments, but caution is the watchword.

CASE STUDY 16–1

Ms. P is a 25-year-old white woman who is attending a well-baby clinic. Her infant is 2 months old, in good health, and achieving satisfactory weight gain on breast milk. Ms. P, her husband, and two other children recently moved to this area, and her previous health-care providers are unavailable to her.

During her intake interview, she relates that, aside from relations with her mother-in-law, who now resides within a few miles of Mr. and Ms. P, the family is adjusting well. Ms. P becomes teary-eyed when describing the situation. The mother-in-law offers multiple suggestions that Ms. P is uncomfortable about implementing, but she is beginning to run out of excuses. Of greatest concern is the mother-in-law's insistence that the baby be given "mint tea" to settle its stomach when it regurgitates. Thus far, Ms. P has resisted the suggestion, but Mr. P is losing patience with her "stubbornness," since his mother successfully raised 11 children and "what's a little tea going to hurt?"

(Continued on the following page)

CASE STUDY *(Continued)*

NURSING CARE PLAN

SUBJECTIVE DATA   Verbalized uncertainty about choices
Verbalized feelings of distress about situation
Delayed decision making and implementation

OBJECTIVE DATA   Visibly upset and teary-eyed discussing her plight

NURSING DIAGNOSIS   NANDA: Decisional Conflict (NANDA, 2003, with permission) concerning infant care practices
Related to conflicting advice from tradition-based mother-in-law and health-care providers

DESIRED OUTCOMES EVALUATION CRITERIA	NURSING ACTIONS/ INTERVENTIONS	RATIONALE
NOC: Decision Making (Moorhead, Johnson, and Maas, 2004, with permission)	NIC: Decision Making Support (Dochterman and Bulechek, 2004, with permission)	
Identifies relevant information	Provide or reinforce information about infant feeding.	American Academy of Pediatrics recommends breast-feeding without supplements of any kind. Regurgitation is very common until 6 months of age and does not indicate pathology that needs treatment.
Recognizes contradiction with others' desires	Help client formulate her reasons to explain to husband and mother-in-law. Role-play the encounter if the client wishes.	Regular tea decreases iron absorption. "Mint" tea, especially from homegrown leaves, has been toxic to infants. Practice stating one's position and counterarguments can help a person maintain focus and composure in the actual situation.
Acknowledges social context of the situation	Assist client to identify persons whose opinions the mother-in-law would respect to encourage collaborative efforts to benefit the child. Support client as she tries to maintain her role as primary caregiver of the infant.	Expanding the context to acknowledge all the adults involved are attempting to provide the best care they can for the infant may transform the situation beyond a battle of wills. Reinforce the fact that she has made good decisions regarding her older children.

C T Q   CRITICAL THINKING QUESTIONS

1. Identify potential compromises that might be made in this situation.
2. How do you visualize the mother-in-law? Does that image affect how you would approach this situation?

3. Devise a Plan B for the possibility that the sample Nursing Care Plan is not successful.

≫ CHAPTER REVIEW

1. Which of the following statements is true of botanical remedies?
   a. One brand is as good as another, since manufacturing is regulated by the government.
   b. These naturally occurring substances are inherently safer than prescription medicines.
   c. Many people are willing to try them to improve their health status.
   d. The rules governing their production and marketing are the same as for over-the-counter medications.

2. For which of the following clients would the nurse follow-up immediately if the child's mother relates that she gives the child herbal tea?
   a. A 2-month-old
   b. An 18-month-old
   c. A 3-year-old
   d. A 4-year-old

3. If a person wishes to drink herbal tea, which of the following products would be the safest to consume?
   a. Tea from plants grown at home

b. Tea sold in a grocery store with a food nutrition label

c. Tea purchased in bulk from a health food store

d. Tea ordered over the Internet

4. Which class of medications is likely to interact with the most botanicals covered in the chapter?

a. Barbiturates

b. Anticoagulants

c. Hormones

d. Vitamins

5. For which of the following items is there most agreement that athletes require increased amounts compared with more sedentary individuals?

a. Protein

b. Creatine

c. Glucosamine

d. Glycerol

 ## CLINICAL ANALYSIS

1. Maria G. is pregnant with her third child. She tells the clinic nurse that she takes some herbal products "to keep my strength up and get me through the day." Which of the following products would raise the greatest concern for the nurse?

a. Natural vitamin C

b. Ginger

c. St. John's wort

d. Valerian

2. Which of the following responses by the nurse would be most helpful to maintaining a positive relationship with Maria?

a. "Who told you to take herbal medicines?"

b. "Let me write those herbs down on your chart. How do you spell them?"

c. "Does your doctor know you are taking these herbs?"

d. "It's not just herbs. Most medicines should be avoided in pregnancy to be on the safe side."

3. Theresa is a freshman member of a college golf team. After fainting on the 16th hole, she was taken to the health clinic for treatment. The admission assessment by the nurse should include height, weight, blood pressure, and

a. Food preferences

b. Theresa's knowledge of the Dietary Guidelines for Americans

c. History of recent travel

d. Use of botanical products and supplements

REFERENCES

Amagase, H, et al: Intake of garlic and its bioactive components. J Nutr 131:955S, 2001.

American College of Sports Medicine, American Dietetic Association, and Dietitians of Canada: Joint Position Statement: nutrition and athletic performance. Med Sci Sports Exerc 32:2130, 2000.

American Dietetic Association: Food fortification and dietary supplements. J Am Diet Assoc 101:115, 2001.

American Dietetic Association: Position on functional foods. J Am Diet Assoc 99:1278, 1999.

American Society of Anesthesiologists. Anesthesiologists warn: If you're taking herbal products, tell your doctor before surgery. Press release May 26, 1999. Accessed May 16, 2000 at http://www.asahq.org/PublicEducation/herbal.html.

American Society of Anesthesiologists: What you should know about your patients' use of herbal medicines. Professional Information dated March 21, 2000. Accessed May 16, 2000 at http://www.asahq.org/ProfInfo/herb/herbbro.html.

Angell, M, and Kassirer, JP: Drs. Angell and Kassirer reply [letter]. N Engl J Med 340:566, 1999.

Ang-Lee, MK, Moss, J, and Yuan, C-S: Herbal medicines and perioperative care. JAMA 286:208, 2001.

Applegate, E: Effective nutritional ergogenic aids. Int J Sport Nutr 9:229, 1999.

Attele, AS, Wu, JA, and Yuan, CS: Ginseng pharmacology: Multiple constituents and multiple actions. Biochem Pharmacol 58:1685, 1999.

Baker, J: Be smart, beware. AARP Bulletin, May 1999, 14.

Bakerink, JA, et al: Multiple organ failure after ingestion of pennyroyal oil from herbal tea in two infants. Pediatrics 98:944, 1996.

Banerjee, SK, Mukherjee, PK, and Maulik, SK: Garlic as an antioxidant: The good, the bad and the ugly. Phytother Res 17:97, 2003.

Barrett, B, Kiefer, D, and Rabago, D: Assessing the risks and benefits of herbal medicine: An overview of scientific evidence. Altern Ther Health Med 5:40, 1999.

Barrett, BP, et al: Treatment of the common cold with unrefined echinacea. Ann Intern Med 137:939, 2002.

Baruchin, AM, et al: Garlic burns. Burns 27:781, 2001.

Batchelor, WB, Heathcote, J, and Wanless, IR: Chaparral-induced hepatic injury. Am J Gastroenterol 90:831, 1995.

Beduschi, G: Current popular ergogenic aids used in sports: A critical review. Nutr Diet 60:104, 2003.

Beigel, Y, Ostfeld, I, and Schoenfeld, N: A leading question. N Engl J Med 339:827, 1998.

Borins, M: The dangers of using herbs. Postgrad Med 104:91, 1998.

Boullata, JI, McDonnell, PJ, and Oliva, CD: Anaphylactic reaction to a dietary supplement containing willow bark. Ann Pharmacother 37:832, 2003.

Bove, GM: Acute neuropathy after exposure to sun in a patient treated with St. John's wort. Lancet 352:1121, 1998.

Brody, JE: Americans gamble on herbs as medicine. NY Times, February 9, 1999.

Brown, JE: Nutrition Through the Life Cycle, ed 2. Thomson Wadsworth, Belmont, CA, 2005.

Brustbauer, R, and Wenisch, C: Bradycardiac atrial fibrillation after consuming herbal tea [in German]. English abstract. Dtsch Med Wochenschr 122:930, 1997.

Bruyere, O, et al: Glucosamine sulfate reduces osteoarthritis progression in postmenopausal women with knee osteoarthritis: Evidence from two 3-year studies. Menopause 11:138, 2004.

Calder, J, Issenman, R, and Cawdron, R: Health information provided by retail health food outlets. Can J Gastroenterol 14:767, 2000.

Capriotti, T: Exploring the "herbal jungle." Med Surg Nursing 8:53, 1999.

Cardinal, BJ, and Engels, HJ: Ginseng does not enhance psychological well-being in healthy, young adults: Results of a double-blind, placebo-controlled, randomized clinical trial. J Am Diet Assoc 101:655, 2001.

Castell, LM, and Newsholme, EA: Glutamine and the effects of exhaustive exercise on the immune response. Can J Physiol Pharmacol 76:524, 1998.

Centers for Disease Control: Adult lead poisoning from an Asian remedy for menstrual cramps—Connecticut, 1997. MMWR

48:27, 1999. Accessed August 11, 1999 at http://www.cdc.gov/epo/mmwr/preview/mmwrhtml/00056277.htm.

Centers for Disease Control: Anticholinergic poisoning associated with an herbal tea—New York City, 1994. MMWR 44:193, 1995. Accessed September 28, 1999 at http://www.cdc.gov/epo/mmwr/preview/mmwrhtml/00022295.htm.

Centers for Disease Control: Hepatic toxicity possibly associated with kava-containing products—United States, Germany, and Switzerland, 1999–2002. MMWR 51:1065, 2002. Accessed May 19, 2004 at http://www.cdc.gov/mmrw/PDF/wk/mm5147.pdg.

Centers for Disease Control: Jin Bu Huan toxicity in adults—Los Angeles, 1993. MMWR 42:920, 1993a. Accessed May 12, 2005 at http://www.cdc.gov/epo/mmwr/preview/mmwrhtml/00022295.htm

Centers for Disease Control: Jin Bu Huan toxicity in children—Colorado, 1993. MMWR 42:633, 1993b. Accessed October 21, 1999 at http://www.cdc.gov/epo/mmwr/preview/mmwrhtml/00021421.htm.

Centers for Disease Control: Lead poisoning associated with ayurvedic medications—Five states, 2000–2003. MMWR 53:582, 2004. Accessed August 4, 2004 at http://www.cdc.gov/mmwr/preview/mmwrhtml/mm5326a3.htm.

Challener, C: Changing fortunes for dietary supplements: sales of herbal supplements continue their slump, as a few rising stars emerge in non-specialty supplements. Chemical Market Reporter. 261:FR11, June 17, 2002.

Chambliss, WG, et al: Assessment of the quality of reference books on botanical dietary supplements. J Am Pharm Assoc 42:723, 2002.

Cheema, P, El-Mefty, O, and Jazieh, AR: Intraoperative haemorrhage associated with the use of extract of Saw Palmetto herb: A case report and review of literature. J Intern Med 250:167, 2001.

Cirigliano, M, and Sun, A: Advising patients about herbal therapies [letter]. JAMA 280, 1565, 1998.

Consumer Reports: Dangerous supplements still at large. 69: May 12, 2004.

Coyle, EF: Fluid and fuel intake during exercise. J Sports Sci 22:39, 2004.

Crawford, LM: Speech before American Society for Pharmacology and Experimental Therapeutics and American Society for Nutritional Sciences, April 19, 2004. Accessed May 27, 2004 at http://www.fda.gov/oc/speeches/2004/aspet0419.html.

Cupp, MJ: Herbal remedies: Adverse effects and drug interactions. Am Fam Physician 59:1239, 1999.

Dasgupta, A, et al: Effect of Asian and Siberian ginseng on serum digoxin measurement by five digoxin immunoassays: Significant variation in digoxin-like immunoreactivity among commercial ginsengs. Am J Clin Pathol 119:298, 2003.

Davies, SJ, Harding, LM, and Baranowski, AP: A novel treatment of postherpetic neuralgia using peppermint oil. Clin J Pain 18:200, 2002.

Dochterman, J, and Bulechek, G (eds): Nursing Interventions Classification (NIC), ed 4. Mosby, St. Louis, 2004.

Draves, AH, and Walker SE: Analysis of the hypericin and pseudo-hypericin content of commercially available St. John's wort preparations. Can J Clin Pharmacol 10:114, 2003.

Drazen, JM: Inappropriate advertising of dietary supplements. N Engl J Med 348:777, 2003.

Ernst, E, and Pittler, MH: Efficacy of ginger for nausea and vomiting: A systematic review of randomized clinical trials. Br J Anaesth 84:367, 2000.

Espinoza, EO, Mann, M-J, and Bleasdell, B: Arsenic and mercury in traditional Chinese herbal balls [letter]. N Engl J Med 333:803, 1995.

Estes, JD, et al: High prevalence of potentially hepatotoxic herbal supplement use in patients with fulminant hepatic failure. Arch Surg 138:852, 2003.

Fessenden, JM, Wittenborn, W, and Clarke, L: Ginkgo biloba: A case report of herbal medicine and bleeding postoperatively from a laparoscopic cholecystectomy. Am Surg 67:33, 2001.

Fillmore, CM, et al: Nutrition and dietary supplements. Phys Med Rehabil Clin N Am 10:673, 2000.

Finsterer, J: Earl Grey tea intoxication. Lancet 359: 1484, 2002.

Fioramonti, J, Theodorou, V, and Bueno, L: Probiotics: What are they? What are their effects on gut physiology? Best Pract Res Clin Gastroenterol 17:711, 2003.

Fleischauer, AT, and Arab, L: Garlic and cancer: A critical review of the epidemiologic literature. J Nutr 131:1032S, 2001.

Food Institute of Canada. Appendix II: Dietary Supplement and Health Education Act of 1994. Accessed October 10, 1999 at http://foodnet.fic.ca/industry/appii.html.

Gallo, M, et al: Pregnancy outcome following gestational exposure to echinacea: A prospective controlled study. Arch Intern Med 160:3141, 2000.

Gill, HS, et al: Enhancement of immunity in the elderly by dietary supplementation with the probiotic Bifidobacterium lactis HN019. Am J Clin Nutr 74:833, 2001.

Gill, HS, Rutherfurd, KJ, and Cross, ML: Dietary probiotic supplementation enhances natural killer cell activity in the elderly: An investigation of age-related immunological changes. J Clin Immunol 21:264, 2001.

Gilroy, CM, et al: Echinacea and truth in labelling. Arch Intern Med 163:699, 2003.

Glisson, J, Crawford, R, and Street, S: Review, critique, and guidelines for the use of herbs and homeopathy. Nurs Pract 23:44, 1999.

Goel, V, et al: Efficacy of a standardized echinacea preparation (Echinilin) for the treatment of the common cold: A randomized, double-blind, placebo-controlled trial. J Clin Pharm Ther 29:75, 2004.

Gobel, H, et al: Effektivität von Oleum menthae piperitae und von Paracetamol in der Therapie des Kopfschmerzes vom Spannungstyp: Effectiveness of Oleum menthae piperitae and paracetamol in therapy of headache of the tension type [English abstract]. Nervenarzt 67:672, 1996.

Gordon, DW, et al: Chaparral ingestion. JAMA 273:489, 1995.

Graham, TE: Caffeine and exercise: Metabolism, endurance and performance. Sports Med 31:785, 2001.

Green, GA, Catlin, DH, and Starcevic, B: Analysis of over-the-counter dietary supplements. Clin J Sport Med 11:254, 2001.

Grimm, W, and Muller, HH: A randomized controlled trial of the effect of fluid extract of Echinacea purpurea on the incidence and severity of colds and respiratory infections. Am J Med 106:138, 1999.

Gruenwald, J (ed): Physicians Desk Reference for Herbal Medicines. Medical Economics, Oradell, NJ, 1998.

Guandalini, S, et al: Lactobacillus GG administered in oral rehydration solution in children with acute diarrhea: A multicenter European trial. J Pediatr Gastroenterol Nutr 30:54, 2000.

Hall, SD, et al: The interaction between St. John's wort and an oral contraceptive. Clin Pharmacol Ther 74:525, 2003.

Haller, CA, et al: Making a diagnosis of herbal-related toxic hepatitis. West J Med 176:39, 2002.

Harkey, MR, et al: Variability in commercial ginseng products: An analysis of 25 preparations. Am J Clin Nutr 73:1101, 2001.

Hauser, D, Gayowski, T, and Singh, N: Bleeding complications precipitated by unrecognized Ginkgo biloba use after liver transplantation. Transpl Int 15:377, 2002.

Hebuterne, X: Gut changes attributed to ageing: Effects on intestinal microflora. Curr Opin Clin Nutr Metab Care 6:49, 2003.

Hochberg, MC, and Dougados, M: Pharmacological therapy of osteoarthritis. Best Pract Res Clin Rheumatol 15:583, 2001.

Houghton, PJ: The scientific basis for the reputed activity of valerian. J Pharm Pharmacol 51:505, 1999.

Huang, SM, et al: Drug interactions with herbal products and grapefruit juice: A conference report. Clin Pharmacol Ther 75:1, 2004.

Institute of Medicine Committee on the Use of Complementary and Alternative Medicine. Complementary and Alternative Medicine in the United States. National Academies Press, Washington, DC, 2005. Accessed May 13, 2005 at http://www.nap.edu/openbook/0309092701/html.

Ioannides, C: Pharmacokinetic interactions between herbal remedies and medicinal drugs. Xenobiotica 32:451, 2002.

Ize-Ludlow, D, et al: Neurotoxicities in infants seen with the consumption of star anise tea. Pediatrics 114:e653, 2004.

Izzo, AA, and Ernst, E: Interactions between herbal medicines and prescribed drugs: A systematic review. Drugs 61:2163, 2001.

Jones, TK, and Lawson, BM: Profound neonatal congestive heart failure caused by maternal consumption of blue cohosh herbal medication. J Pediatr 132:550, 1998.

Juhn, MS: Ergogenic aids in aerobic activity. Curr Sports Med Rep 1:233, 2002.

Juhn, M: Popular sports supplements and ergogenic aids. Sports Med 33:921, 2003.

Juhn, MS, and Tarnopolsky, M: Oral creatine supplementation and athletic performance: A critical review. Clin J Sport Med 8:286, 1998.

Kaddu, S, Kerl, H, and Wolf, P: Accidental bullous phototoxic reactions to bergamot aromatherapy oil. J Am Acad Dermatol 45:458, 2001.

Kalliomaki, M, et al: Probiotics in primary prevention of atopic disease: A randomised placebo-controlled trial. Lancet 357:1076, 2001.

Kaufman, DW, et al: Recent patterns of medication use in the ambulatory adult population of the United States. JAMA 287:337, 2002.

Kennedy, DO, Scholey, AB, and Wesnes, KA: The dose-dependent cognitive effects of acute administration of Ginkgo biloba to healthy young volunteers. Psychopharmacology 151:416, 2000.

Kennedy, RJ, Kirk, SJ, and Gardiner, KR: Promotion of a favorable gut flora in inflammatory bowel disease. JPEN 24:189, 2000.

Kingsbury, KJ, Kay, L, and Hjelm, M: Contrasting plasma free amino acid patterns in elite athletes: Association with fatigue and infection. Br J Sports Med 32:25, 1998.

Klepser, TB, and Klepser, ME: Unsafe and potentially safe herbal therapies. Am J Health Syst Pharm 56:125, 1999.

Kliegman, RM, and Willoughby, RE: Prevention of necrotizing enterocolitis with probiotics. Pediatrics 115:171, 2005.

Ko, RJ: Adulterants in Asian patent medicines. N Engl J Med 339:847, 1998.

Kobla, HV, and Volpe, SL: Chromium, exercise, and body composition. Crit Rev Food Sci Nutr 40:291, 2000.

Kopp-Hoolihan, L: Prophylactic and therapeutic use of probiotics: A review. J Am Diet Assoc 101:229, 2001.

Koscielny, J, et al: The antiatherosclerotic effect of Allium sativum. Atherosclerosis 144:237, 1999.

Kreider, RB: Dietary supplements and the promotion of muscle growth with resistance exercise. Sports Med 27:97, 1999.

Kruth, P, et al: Ginger-associated overanticoagulation by phenprocoumon. Ann Pharmacother 38:257, 2004.

Lanski, SL, et al: Herbal therapy use in a pediatric emergency department population: Expect the unexpected. Pediatrics 111:981, 2003.

Lawrence, ME, and Kirby, DF: Nutrition and sports supplements: Fact or fiction. J Clin Gastroenterol 35:299, 2002.

Le Bars, PL, et al: A placebo-controlled, double-blind, randomized trial of an extract of Ginkgo biloba for dementia. JAMA 278:1327, 1997.

Lin, HC, et al: Oral probiotics reduce the incidence and severity of necrotizing enterocolitis in very low birth weight infants. Pediatrics 115:1, 2005.

Lindenmuth, GF, and Lindenmuth, EB: The efficacy of echinacea compound herbal tea preparation on the severity and duration of upper respiratory and flu symptoms: A randomized, double-blind placebo-controlled study. J Altern Complement Med 6:327, 2000.

Markowitz, JS, et al: Effect of St. John's wort on drug metabolism by induction of cytochrome P450 3A4 enzyme. JAMA 290:1500, 2003.

Martin-Facklam, M, et al: Quality markers of drug information on the Internet: An evaluation of sites about St. John's wort. Am J Med 113:740, 2002.

McNaughton, L, Dalton, B, and Palmer, G: Sodium bicarbonate can be used as an ergogenic aid in high intensity, competitive cycle ergometry of 1 h duration. Eur J Appl Physiol 80:64, 1999.

Meadows, M. Public health officials caution against ephedra use. FDA Consumer 37:8, 2003.

Mero, A: Leucine supplementation and intensive training. Sports Med 27:347, 1999.

Metzl, JD: Strength training and nutritional supplement use in adolescents. Curr Opin Pediatr 11:292, 1999.

Metzl, JD, et al: Creatine use among young athletes. Pediatrics 108:421, 2001.

Micklefield, GH, et al: Effects of ginger on gastroduodenal motility. Int J Clin Pharmacol Ther 37:341, 1999.

Miller, LG: Herbal medicinals. Arch Intern Med 158:2200, 1998.

Mills, E, et al: Impact of federal safety advisories on health food store advice. J Gen Intern Med 19:269, 2004.

Miwa, H, et al: Generalized convulsions after consuming a large amount of ginkgo nuts. Epilepsia 42:280, 2001.

Moorhead, S, Johnson, M, and Maas, M (eds): Nursing Outcomes Classification (NOC), ed 3. Mosby, St. Louis, 2004.

Morelli, V, Naquin, C, and Weaver, V: Alternative therapies for traditional disease states: Osteoarthritis. Am Fam Physician 67:339, 2003.

Morris, CA, and Avorn, J: Internet marketing of herbal products. JAMA 290:1505, 2003.

Mujika, I, and Padilla, S: Creatine supplementation as an ergogenic aid for sports performance in highly trained athletes: A critical review. Int J Sports Med 18:491, 1997.

Mullins, RJ, and Heddle, R: Adverse reactions associated with echinacea: The Australian experience. Ann Allergy Asthma Immunol 88:42, 2002.

NANDA International: Nursing Diagnoses: Definitions and Classification, 2003–2004. NANDA International, Philadelphia, 2003.

Noakes, TD: Fluid and electrolyte disturbances in heat illness. Int J Sports Med 19:S146, 1998.

Nursing 2004 Drug Handbook, ed 24. Lippincott Williams & Wilkins, Philadelphia, 2004.

Nursing 2004 Herbal Medicine Handbook, ed 2. Lippincott Williams & Wilkins, Philadelphia, 2004.

O'Hara, MA, et al: A review of 12 commonly used medicinal herbs. Arch Fam Med 7:523, 1998.

Omaye, ST: Safety facets of antioxidant supplements. Top Clin Nutr 14:26, 1998.

Palmer, ME, et al: Adverse events associated with dietary supplements: An observational study. Lancet 361:101, 2003.

Peng, CC, et al: Incidence and severity of potential drug-dietary supplement interactions in primary care patients: An exploratory study of 2 outpatient practices. Arch Intern Med 164:630, 2004.

Perez-Pimiento, AJ, et al: Anaphylactic reaction to young garlic. Allergy 54:626, 1999.

Petty, HR, et al: Identification of colchicine in placental blood from patients using herbal medicines. Chem Res Toxicol 14:1254, 2001.

Pittler, MH, and Ernst, E: Feverfew for preventing migraine. Cochrane Database Syst Rev 1:CD003230, 2004.

Pittler, MH, and Ernst, E: Ginkgo biloba extract for the treatment of intermittent claudication: A meta-analysis of randomized trials. Am J Med 108:276, 2000.

Pribitkin, ED, and Boger, G: Herbal therapy: What every facial plastic surgeon must know. Arch Facial Plast Surg 3:127, 2001.

Purnell, LD, and Paulanka, BJ: Transcultural Health Care, ed 2. FA Davis, Philadelphia, 2003.

Racette, SB: Creatine supplementation and athletic performance. J Orthop Sports Phys Ther 33:615, 2003.

Rafaat, M, and Leung, AK: Garlic burns. Pediatr Dermatol 17:475, 2000.

Reginster, JY, et al: Long-term effects of glucosamine sulphate on osteoarthritis progression: A randomised, placebo-controlled clinical trial. Lancet 357:251, 2001.

Richard, D: What counts as evidence? Arch Fam Med 7:598, 1998.

Richy, F, et al: Structural and symptomatic efficacy of glucosamine and chondroitin in knee osteoarthritis. Arch Intern Med 163:1514, 2003.

Rogers, EA, Gough, JE, and Brewer, KL: Are emergency department patients at risk for herb-drug interactions? Acad Emerg Med 8:932, 2001.

Rose, KD, et al: Spontaneous spinal epidural hematoma with associated platelet dysfunction from excessive garlic ingestion: A case report. Neurosurgery 26:280, 1990.

Ruschitzka, F, et al: Acute heart transplant rejection due to Saint John's wort. Lancet 355:548, 2000.

Saper, RB, et al: Heavy metal content of ayurvedic herbal medicine products. JAMA 292:2868, 2004.

Schaffer, DM, et al: Nonvitamin, nonmineral supplement use over a 12-month period by adult members of a large health maintenance organization. J Am Diet Assoc 103:1500, 2003.

Schwellnus, MP, Derman, EW, and Noakes, TD: Aetiology of skeletal muscle "cramps" during exercise: A novel hypothesis. J Sports Sci 15:277, 1997.

Sheehan, DM: Herbal medicines, phytoestrogens and toxicity: Risk:benefit considerations. Proc Soc Exp Biol Med 217:379, 1998.

Sheikh, NM, Philen, RM, and Love, L: Chaparral-associated hepatotoxicity. Arch Intern Med 157:913, 1997.

Silver, MD: Use of ergogenic aids by athletes. J Am Acad Orthop Surg 9:61, 2001.

Slifman, NR, et al: Contamination of botanical dietary supplements by Digitalis lanata. N Engl J Med 339:806, 1998.

Smith, C, et al: A randomized controlled trial of ginger to treat nausea and vomiting in pregnancy. Obstet Gynecol 103:639, 2004.

Smolinske, SC: Dietary supplement-drug interactions. J Am Med Womens Assoc 54:191, 1999.

Solomon, PR, et al: Ginkgo for memory enhancement. JAMA 288:835, 2002.

Sperl, W, et al: Reversible hepatic veno-occlusive disease in an infant after consumption of pyrrolizidine-containing herbal tea. Eur J Pediatr 154:112, 1995.

Sorensen, JM: Herb-drug, food-drug, nutrient-drug, and drug-drug interactions. J Alter Complement Med 8:293, 2002.

Stashower, ME, and Torres, RZ: Chaparral and liver toxicity [letter]. JAMA 274:871, 1995.

Stevinson, C, Pittler, MH, and Ernst, E: Garlic for treating hypercholesterolemia. Ann Intern Med 133:420, 2000.

Tait, PA, et al: Severe congenital lead poisoning in a preterm infant due to a herbal remedy. Med J Aust 177:193, 2002.

Taylor, JA, et al: Efficacy and safety of echinacea in treating upper respiratory tract infections in children: a randomized controlled trial. JAMA 290:2824, 2003.

Teitelbaum, JE: Probiotics and the treatment of infectious diarrhea. Pediatr Infec Dis J 24:267, 2005.

Towheed, TE, et al: Glucosamine therapy for treating osteoarthritis. Cochrane Database Syst Rev 1:CD002946, 2001.

Tsen, LC, et al: Alternative medicine use in presurgical patients. Anesthesiology 93:148, 2000.

United States Food and Drug Administration: Dietary supplement enforcement report. December 18, 2002a. Accessed May 26, 2004 at http://www.fda.gov/oc/nutritioninitiative/report.html.

United States Food and Drug Administration: FDA issues advisory on star anise "teas." September 10, 2003. Accessed May 13, 2005 at http://www.fda.gov/bbs/topics/NEWS/2003/NEW00941.html.

United States Food and Drug Administration: FDA issues regulation prohibiting sale of dietary supplements containing ephedrine alkaloids and reiterates its advice that consumers stop using these products. February 6, 2004a. Accessed May 26, 2004 at http://www.cfsan.fda.gov/~lrd/fpephed6.html.

United States Food and Drug Administration: FDA warns consumers not to feed infants "Better than Formula Ultra Infant Immune Booster 117," January 23, 2004b. Accessed May 26, 2004 at http://www.cfsan.fda.gov/~lrd/fpinf2.html.

United States Food and Drug Administration: Health effects of androstenedione. March 11, 2004c. Accessed June 8, 2004 at http://www.fda.gov/oc/whitepapers/andro.html.

United States Food and Drug Administration: HHS launches crackdown on products containing andro. March 11, 2004d. Accessed June 8, 2004 at http://www.fda.gov/bbs/topics/news/2004/hhs_031104.html.

United States Food and Drug Administration: Questions and answers about FDA's actions on dietary supplements containing ephedrine alkaloids. February 6, 2004e. Accessed May 26, 2004 at http://www.fda.gov/oc/initiatives/ephedra/february2004/qa_020604.html.

United States Food and Drug Administration Center for Food Safety and Applied Nutrition. Kava-containing dietary supplements may be associated with severe liver injury, March 25, 2002b. Accessed May 27, 2004 at http://www.cfsan.fda.gov/~dms/addskava.html.

United States Food and Drug Administration Center for Food Safety and Applied Nutrition: Letter to manufacturers regarding botanicals and other novel ingredients in conventional foods. January 30, 2001a. Accessed May 26, 2004 at http://www.cfsan.fda.gov/?~dms/ds-ltr15.html.

United States Food and Drug Administration Center for Food Safety and Applied Nutrition. Overview of Dietary Supplements. January 2001b. Accessed May 27, 2004 at http://vm.cfsan.fda.gov/~dms/ds-oview.html.

United States Food and Drug Administration Center for Food Safety and Applied Nutrition. Overview of Dietary Supplements. May 1997, Updated April 1999. Accessed August 21, 1999 at http://vm.cfsan.fada.gov/~dms/ds-oview.html.

Vanderhoof, JA, and Young, RJ: Role of probiotics in the management of patients with food allergy. Ann Allergy Asthma Immunol 90(Suppl 3):99, 2003.

Van Niel, CW: Probiotics: Not just for treatment anymore. Pediatrics 115:174, 2005.

Van Niel, CW, et al: Lactobacillus therapy for acute infectious diarrhea in children: A meta-analysis. Pediatrics 109:678, 2002.

Vickers, A, and Zollman, C: Herbal medicine. BMJ 319:1050, 1999.

Vutyavanich, T, Kraisarin, T, and Ruangsri, R: Ginger for nausea and vomiting in pregnancy: Randomized, double-masked, placebo-controlled trial. Obstet Gynecol 97:577, 2001.

Wagner, DR: Hyperhydrating with glycerol: Implications for athletic performance. J Am Diet Assoc 99:207, 1999.

Wang, L, Sterling, B, and Don, P: Berloque dermatitis induced by "Florida water." Cutis. 70:29, 2002.

Watkins, RW: Herbal therapeutics: The top 12 remedies, first of three parts. Emerg Med 34:43, 2002a.

Watkins, RW: Herbal therapeutics: The top 12 remedies, second of three parts. Er... Ied 34:12, 2002b.

Watkins, RW: Herbal therapeutics: The top 12 remedies, third of three parts. Emerg Med 34:33, 2002c.

Whiskey, E, Werneke, U, and Taylor, D: A systematic review and meta-analysis of Hypericum perforatum in depression: A comprehensive clinical review. Int Clin Psychopharmacol 16:239, 2001.

Wilt, TJ, et al: Saw palmetto extracts for treatment of benign prostatic hyperplasia: A systematic review. JAMA 280:1604, 1998.

Yager, J, Siegfried, SL, and DiMatteo, TL: Use of alternative remedies by psychiatric patients: Illustrative vignettes and a discussion of the issues. Am J Psychiatry 156:1432, 1999.

Yale-New Haven Nutrition Advisor: Understanding yogurt. March 10, 2005. Accessed May 13, 2005 at http://www.ynhh.org/online/nutrition/advisor/yogurt.html

Yu, SM, Ghandour, RM, and Huang, ZJ: Herbal supplement use among US women, 2000. J Am Med Womens Assoc 59:17, 2004.

Zerkak, D, and Dougados, M: The use of glucosamine therapy in osteoarthritis. Curr Pain Headache Rep 8:507, 2004.

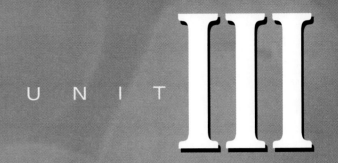

U N I T **III**

Clinical Nutrition

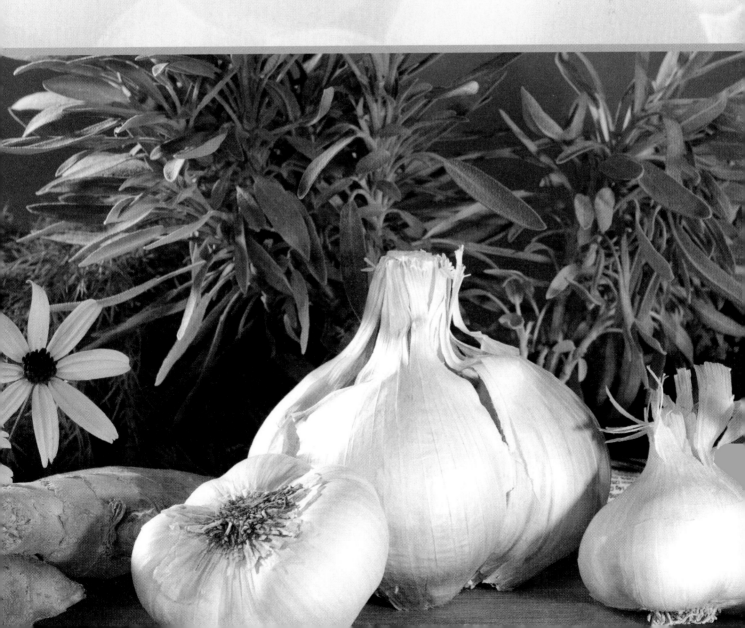

CHAPTER 17

Food, Nutrient, and Drug Interactions

Learning Objectives

After completing this chapter, the student should be able to:

1. Explain the importance of proper scheduling of medications in relation to food intake.
2. Identify two groups of clients likely to experience food-drug interactions.
3. Recognize certain food and drug interactions covered in the text.
4. Describe four ways in which nutrients and drugs can interact and give an example of each.
5. Discuss one potentially life-threatening food-drug interaction and design nursing interventions to avoid this possibility.
6. Name several drug-nutrient interactions that affect water balance in the body.

Medication or legal drug use is widespread in the United States. A population-based survey indicated that 81 percent of respondents used at least one medication the previous week, 50 percent took at least one prescription drug, and 7 percent took five or more prescription drugs. Sixteen percent of those taking prescription drugs also took herbal remedies or dietary supplements (Kaufman et al, 2002). Some drugs interact with other drugs, foods, and nutrients in ways that can be beneficial or detrimental. This chapter explains and gives examples of some of the ways in which drugs interact with foods (including beverages), nutrients (including nutrient formulas and, briefly, TPN), and the nonnutrient components of foods. An interaction is the process of one substance affecting another. The food or nutrient can enhance the action of a drug or inhibit it. Similarly, a drug can facilitate the body's use of nutrients or impede it. In no sense is the information in the chapter exhaustive. The drugs included here illustrate the broad range of interactions and do not necessarily reflect the preferred treatment for the conditions mentioned. In all cases, pharmaceutical resources should be consulted when administering medications.

A drug is a substance, other than a food, that is intended to affect a structure or function of the body. As used in this text, the term *drug* includes alcohol and both prescription and over-the-counter drugs. As is the usual practice in medical literature, the **generic names** of drugs are used here.

The Effects of Drugs on Nutritional Status

Any person who takes a drug risks potentially harmful effects from food and drug interactions. Nutritional status can be affected because these interactions might alter (1) food intake, (2) the absorption of nutrients or drugs, (3) the metabolism of nutrients or drugs, or (4) the excretion of nutrients or drugs. Some known interactions are considered clinically desirable because they help control a disease process. For example, by controlling a client's dietary vitamin K, the effect of *warfarin*, an anticoagulant, is maximized. Many effects that result from food and drug interactions are undesirable. These include nutritional deficiencies, growth retardation in children, loss of disease control, and acute toxic reactions. Some individuals, especially the elderly, are at higher risk than others for suffering unwanted effects.

Identifying Clients at High Risk

Persons at highest risk for food and drug interactions are those who (1) take many drugs, including alcohol; (2) require long-term drug therapy; or (3) have poor or marginal nutrition. These and other risk-increasing factors are listed in Clinical Application 17–1. The elderly are particularly vulnerable because they are more likely to have several of the risk factors mentioned. Forty-four percent of men and 57 percent of women over the age of 65 reported taking 5 or more medications the week preceding the survey, and 12 percent of each gender took 10 or more (see Fig. 17–1). Nineteen percent of these elderly men and 23 percent of the women took five or more prescription drugs (Kaufman et al, 2002). The elderly are likely to be on long-term regimens for chronic diseases, further increasing the

Factors Increasing the Risk of Drug-Nutrient Interactions

The risk of a drug-nutrient interaction is increased if a client:

- Is malnourished
- Consumes alcohol
- Takes a high-potency vitamin or mineral supplement
- Is receiving many drugs

or if the client's drugs:

- Are given with meals
- Are instilled into a feeding tube
- Are prescribed long-term to control chronic disease
- Are known to cause malabsorption or have antinutrient effects

In any of the above situations, the following are appropriate:

- A careful search of pharmacology literature
- A thorough assessment
- An ongoing effort to monitor the client's status

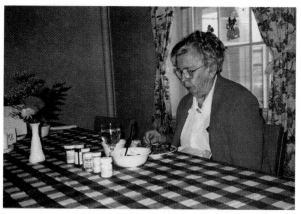

Figure **17–2** This woman has several risk factors for drug-nutrient interactions. She is elderly, is on a multiple-drug regimen, and takes some of her medications with a meal.

risk of adverse effects (Fig. 17–2). The elderly are also more prone to food-drug interactions as a result of self-medication, noncompliance with prescribed regimens, and changes in their needs associated with aging. Clinical Application 17–2 lists factors that should trigger investigation of the client's risk of drug-nutrient interactions. Other groups at risk of food and drug interactions are infants and adolescents because of higher nutrient needs and immature detoxification systems, the latter of particular concern with adolescents who also use alcohol (Alonzo-Aperta and Varela-Moreiras, 2000).

Minimizing Food and Drug Interactions

Known adverse outcomes of food and drug interactions can be offset by changes in drug dosage, diet, or both. Because drugs often increase or decrease the absorption of nutrients, it may be necessary to change (1) the route of administration, (2) the dose of a drug, (3) the time interval between doses, and/or (4) whether the drug is administered with food. For example, therapeutic drug levels may not be achieved or may take longer to build up in the body if less of the drug is absorbed because of an interaction with food. This could prolong a disease or prevent its cure. Dosage adjustments often minimize such effects.

Certain foods or nutrients (including supplements) may be (1) added to the diet, (2) deleted from the diet, or (3) required in increased or reduced amounts to counterbalance adverse nutrient-drug interactions. For example, protein inhibits the absorption of *phenytoin*, an anticonvulsant drug, whereas carbohydrate increases its absorption. Depending on the desired therapeutic effect, dietary intake

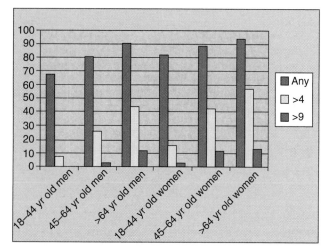

Figure **17–1** Percentages of adults who took at least 1, 5 or more, or 10 or more medications in the week surveyed. Medications included prescription, over-the-counter, vitamin/mineral, or herbal supplements. The most frequently used products were multivitamins (26 percent of adults) and acetaminophen (23 percent), ibuprofen and aspirin (17 percent each), and vitamin E (10 percent). All other medications were used by fewer than 10 percent of the respondents. (Adapted from Kaufman et al, 2002.)

Screening Clients at Risk of Drug-Nutrient Interactions

Further nutritional assessment may be in order if the client:

1. Reports a recent weight change
2. Abuses alcohol
3. Consumes a modified diet including one characterized by significant changes in protein content
4. Takes medication with meals
5. Has a worsening of signs and symptoms of the disease
6. Displays laboratory values indicating nutrient depletion
7. Receives medications known to interfere with nutrition

of protein and/or carbohydrate may be modified in amount or schedule. Food and drug interactions can be complex, especially if the client is on a multiple-drug regimen or is at high risk for other reasons. Health-care professionals need a sound knowledge of potential food and drug interactions and the ability to apply their knowledge in practice. Physicians, dietitians, pharmacists, and nurses share responsibility for being aware of and for preventing or controlling such interactions. The clinical pharmacist can be a valuable ally of the nurse when scheduling medications for optimal effect. Likewise, nurses may ask a clinical dietitian to assess a client's risk for food-drug interactions. Because of the multitude of medications available and the complexity of potential interactions, most health-care organizations use computer-generated client profiles that include all the medications the client is to receive and thereby can identify known interactions. A good reference library on the clinical unit also helps provide information.

The Effects of Drugs on Foods and Nutrients

Drugs can (1) affect food intake, (2) alter the absorption of nutrients through both luminal and mucosal effects, (3) modify the metabolism of nutrients, and (4) increase or decrease the excretion of certain nutrients.

The Effects of Drugs on Food Intake

Even before food is ingested, drugs can affect food intake. Several drugs increase or decrease appetite, interfere with the senses of taste and smell, or cause gastric irritation. Food is sometimes used to temper these and other side effects of drugs.

Decreased Appetite

Central nervous system stimulants, including *dextroamphetamine* and *methylphenidate*, both used in the treatment of narcolepsy or the management of attention deficit hyperactivity disorder (ADHD), have the effect of depressing the desire for food. One of the side effects of these stimulants in children is slowed growth so that height and weight should be regularly monitored. **Antineoplastic drugs** (agents that prevent the development, growth, or proliferation of malignant cells) are well known for causing a loss of appetite (anorexia). Other side effects, including severe nausea, vomiting, and **stomatitis,** exacerbate anorexia. Examples of such antineoplastic drugs are *bleomycin, plicamycin,* and *vincristine.* Poor appetite can also result from drugs that cause a dry mouth. Many antihistamines, including *brompheniramine* and *diphenhydramine,* decrease saliva output, thereby causing decreased appetite. Bulk-forming laxatives containing *psyllium* may reduce appetite because of a feeling of abdominal fullness.

When assessing a client with a weight-loss history or one taking drugs known to cause food and drug interactions, nurses should review the client's drug regimen. All intake, including physician-prescribed and self-prescribed drugs as well as nutritional supplements, is pertinent to include in such a nutritional assessment.

Increased Appetite

Some antidepressants, such as *doxepin,* may promote appetite and lead to marked weight gain. Another such drug, *bupropion,* can either increase or decrease appetite. *Medroxyprogesterone,* a female hormone used as an oral contraceptive and in cyclic hormone therapy after menopause, also increases appetite. This hormone occurs naturally in the second half of the menstrual cycle and in pregnancy (to support the growth requirements of the mother and fetus). To minimize the effect of increased appetite, if weight gain is not desired, several nursing interventions might be appropriate. Instructing the client to increase the fiber content of the diet, especially with fruits and vegetables, and encouraging the client to drink six to eight glasses of water daily, to eat slowly, and to chew food thoroughly are strategies that may prove helpful.

Changes in Taste or Smell

The senses of taste and smell influence how one responds to foods. Some drugs alter the perception of these senses, making foods and beverages taste bitter, metallic, or unpleasant. Although this usually leads to a decreased appetite, some individuals try to rid themselves of the sensation by eating constantly. *Acetylsalicylic acid (ASA),* more commonly known as *aspirin,* is a drug used to control pain or to reduce fever. It also is taken in small daily doses to decrease the risk of heart attacks. One gram of *aspirin,* about three adult-dose tablets, increases the taste perception of bitterness. An anti-infective reserved for tuberculosis and other serious infections, *streptomycin,* is partially excreted in the saliva. One result is a metallic or bitter taste, even when the drug is administered by intramuscular injection.

Lithium, an antimanic drug, causes a metallic taste sensation. Other common side effects of this drug related to nutritional intake are dry mouth, anorexia, nausea, vomiting, and diarrhea. *Lithium* also has serious interactions with a person's fluid and electrolyte balance (covered later in the chapter).

Penicillamine, a drug given for rheumatoid arthritis and for **Wilson's disease,** in which a genetic defect prevents excretion of copper (see Chapter 8), causes a loss of taste and smell. *Penicillamine* binds with copper so that it can be excreted by the kidney. The loss of taste and smell is caused by zinc deficiency because *penicillamine* also binds with zinc, causing its excretion. The angiotensin-converting enzyme (ACE) inhibitors, such as *captopril,* used to treat hypertension, cause a loss of taste perception that usually resolves within 8 to 12 weeks despite continued therapy (Deglin and Vallerand, 2005). A postulated mechanism of action is decreased salivary magnesium concentration (Utermohlen, 1999). Nursing interventions that may help a client with taste changes include providing good oral hygiene before meals and avoiding bitter foods in favor of the other taste sensations—sweet, sour, or salty.

Gastric Irritation

Drugs that cause gastric irritation are often taken with food to reduce this side effect. *Aspirin* can cause gastric bleeding and over time can lead to anemia. Taking *aspirin* with food, milk, crackers, or a full glass of water reduces the likelihood of stomach irritation. Other NSAIDs (nonsteroidal anti-inflammatory drugs) and certain potassium supplements are also associated with gastric irritation.

The Effects of Drugs on Nutrient Absorption

Drugs can affect the absorption of nutrients in several ways. Drug-induced alterations in absorption are categorized according to two general mechanisms of action: luminal effects or mucosal effects.

Luminal Effects

Drug-induced changes within the intestine that affect the absorption of nutrients or drugs without altering the intestine itself are called **luminal effects.** These drug-induced changes may affect peristalsis, pH, or the formation of complexes.

PERISTALSIS

Laxatives may interfere with the absorption of nutrients and other drugs because they stimulate peristalsis and thus cause rapid transit of intestinal contents. Long-term use may result in physical dependence and electrolyte imbalances. An over-the-counter laxatives ingredient, *bisacodyl*, interferes with the uptake of glucose, water, calcium, sodium, and potassium by the cells.

A relatively short period of malabsorption with diarrhea may interfere with the absorption of vitamin K. This interference in turn enhances the activity of *warfarin*, especially if the person's intake of green vegetables has been sparse. Clients taking *warfarin* who experience diarrhea or decreased food intake should have their prothrombin times or INRs (International Normalized Ratios) monitored more frequently than usual and *warfarin* dosages adjusted accordingly (Smith, Aljazairi, and Fuller, 1999).

Other drugs may slow peristalsis and thus cause a longer transit time. The long-term use of either *docusate*, a stool softener, or *chlorpromazine*, an antipsychotic drug, results in the increased absorption of cholesterol, an undesirable side effect in most clients.

CHANGES IN pH

The absorption of weakly acidic drugs takes place in the stomach, whereas the absorption of neutral and alkaline drugs takes place in the small intestine. Drug-induced changes in the pH of these sites influence the absorption of both nutrients and drugs. For example, an acid pH is necessary for folic acid absorption. It is also required for intrinsic factor to combine with vitamin B_{12} and protect it until it reaches the ileum. Because long-term *antacid* or *potassium* therapy neutralizes gastric acidity, the result is a decrease in the absorption of thiamin, folic acid, and vitamin B_{12}. The histamine H_2 antagonists, such as *cimetidine*, and the gastric acid-pump inhibitor *omeprazole* also decrease vitamin B_{12} absorption because of altered gastric pH (Utermohlen, 1999). *Antacids* and *potassium* also decrease the absorption of iron because an acid medium is necessary to convert ferric iron (Fe^{3+}) to ferrous iron ($2+$), the more absorbable form.

FORMATION OF COMPLEXES

Sometimes foods or nutrients bind with or form complexes with drugs. This combining can increase, decrease, or prevent the absorption of one or the other.

Cholestyramine, a lipid-lowering agent, binds with bile salts, which increases the excretion of cholesterol. Unfortunately, it may also bind with the fat-soluble vitamins A, D, E, and K. These vitamins are then excreted along with the cholesterol. Because vitamin K is not stored in the body in significant amounts, *cholestyramine* therapy can lead to a deficiency of clotting factors and result in hemorrhage. Fortunately, water-soluble forms of these vitamins are available for clients who need them. *Cholestyramine* also interferes with the absorption of folic acid, vitamin B_{12}, calcium, and iron, necessitating vigilant monitoring of the client's nutritional status. *Mineral oil*, a lubricant, is sometimes used as a laxative. The fat-soluble vitamins dissolve in the indigestible oil and are excreted, as are calcium and phosphorus. Therefore, taking mineral oil on a long-term, daily basis is undesirable. In addition, children and elderly adults with relaxed cardiac sphincters are at risk for aspiration pneumonia if they regurgitate the mineral oil. These untoward side effects as well as recommended dietary interventions (see Chapter 22) should be taught to clients seeking advice regarding self-treatment of constipation.

Mucosal Effects

The luminal effects do not affect the tissues or organs. In contrast, **mucosal effects** are drug-induced changes that affect the absorption of nutrients or drugs by damaging or altering tissue structures. Mucosal effects include decreased digestive enzymes, damaged intestinal mucosa, and inhibited transport mechanisms.

DECREASED DIGESTIVE ENZYMES

Hundreds of enzymes are involved in digestion. Many drugs, including alcohol, can destroy the structural integrity of digestive organs by damaging tissues. This usually causes decreased enzyme production, resulting in poor nutrient absorption. Long-term *alcohol* consumption damages the pancreas, decreasing enzyme production. Thus, the breakdown of amino acids and fats, chiefly accomplished by the action of pancreatic enzymes, is slowed or insufficiently completed. The result is reduced or poor absorption of amino acids and fats.

DAMAGED INTESTINAL MUCOSA

Several drugs contribute to the malabsorption of other drugs by their damaging effect on the intestinal mucosa. Some drugs produce general malabsorption, and other drugs are more specific and decrease the absorption of only certain nutrients. *Alcohol* abuse causes several changes in the intestinal mucosa that lead to the malabsorption of many nutrients. Most commonly affected are thiamin and magnesium, but folic acid, niacin, and pyridoxine also may be malabsorbed.

Because *neomycin*, an anti-infective agent, inhibits protein synthesis in bacteria and is poorly absorbed at usual doses but remains in the bowel, it is sometimes used to reduce the bacterial count in the bowel before intestinal surgery. Changes produced in the intestinal mucosa by *neomycin* lead to the decreased absorption of fat, vitamins A, D, and K, folic acid, and vitamin B$_{12}$. This malabsorption is not likely to cause problems when the drug is used short-term.

Gastrointestinal tract cells, because of their short life and rapid turnover, are killed by many antineoplastic drugs, such as *methotrexate*. Among other side effects, *methotrexate* therapy results in the malabsorption of vitamin B$_{12}$, folic acid, and calcium.

Colchicine, an antigout drug, may cause generalized malabsorption because it damages the intestinal mucosa. The consequences are inhibited absorption of vitamin B$_{12}$, folic acid, and calcium. In addition, *colchicine* reduces the absorption of fat, lactose, and carotene.

INHIBITED TRANSPORT MECHANISMS

Several nutrients have to be helped across the intestinal membrane to the bloodstream. A number of drugs impair the absorption of nutrients through their effects on the transport mechanism. For example, the sedative/hypnotic drug *glutethimide* impairs the transport of calcium.

Phenytoin, a drug used to control epileptic seizures or heart rhythm irregularities, is a folic acid antagonist that competes with the vitamin for binding sites. Among women with epilepsy, major malformations were detected in 3.8 percent of fetuses exposed to antiepileptic drugs compared with 0.8 percent in fetuses not exposed. Varying degrees of risk were associated with individual drugs, with low serum folate at the end of the first trimester, and with lower educational attainment of the mother (Kaaja, Kaaja, and Hiilesmaa, 2003). Spacing of doses of the antiepileptic drug throughout the day is recommended to control blood levels (Morrell, 1998), as is treatment with just one anticonvulsant drug whenever possible and folate supplementation before and during pregnancy (Pennell, 2003). Reduced folic acid absorption also occurs with *sulfasalazine*, an anti-inflammatory agent used to treat ulcerative colitis. The decrease in absorption is caused by the inhibited transport of folic acid.

An additional interaction of *phenytoin* and other anticonvulsants with vitamins involves an unknown mechanism, possibly an alteration in absorption of vitamins or interference with synthesis of niacin from tryptophan. Nevertheless, a case of pellagra in a client with cerebral palsy receiving *phenytoin, valproic acid,* and *diazepam* for years was treated with multiple therapies from numerous physicians before the correct diagnosis was reached. Symptoms resolved in 2 months with niacin and multivitamin supplementation, and the cause was attributed to the anticonvulsants (Lyon and Fairley, 2002). Three weeks of *phenytoin* therapy was credited with causing a pellagrous dermatitis in a 3-year-old child that resolved within 3 weeks of niacin supplementation and 2 weeks of replacing *phenytoin* with *carbamazepine* (Kaur et al, 2002).

The Effects of Drugs on Nutrient Metabolism

Many drugs alter the metabolism of nutrients. Drugs can affect the metabolism of energy nutrients and also can disrupt vitamin metabolism through a variety of mechanisms.

Alteration of Energy Nutrient Metabolism

Corticosteroids are hormones that are produced by the adrenal gland. Pharmaceutical doses of these drugs are given for their anti-inflammatory effects. The side effects of the drug are signs and symptoms like those of Cushing's syndrome, a disease that results from oversecretion of *corticosteroids*. The metabolism of all the energy nutrients is affected. *Corticosteroids* stimulate the conversion of fat and protein to glucose resulting in hyperglycemia or a worsening of preexisting diabetes. *Corticosteroids* increase the catabolism of the matrix of the bone, inhibit the osteoblasts from building new bone, and prevent the liver from processing vitamin D. When this lack of vitamin D results in insufficient calcium absorption by the intestine, parathyroid hormone causes withdrawal of calcium from the bones and osteoporosis results. Similar protein wasting affects the skin and skeletal muscle, producing easy bruising and weakness. *Corticosteroids* also cause a redistribution of fat deposits to the trunk, the back of the neck, and the face so that the person eventually develops a "moon face" and/or a "buffalo hump."

Interference with Vitamin Metabolism

Although vitamins have specific and singular functions in the body, several mechanisms can interfere with their proper metabolism. The same vitamin may be affected by different drugs at various phases of its metabolism.

VITAMIN K

Anti-infective drugs, besides fighting pathogens, destroy beneficial intestinal bacteria that synthesize vitamin K. Cerebral hemorrhage in a 4-month-old infant was attributed to *isoniazid* and *rifampin* therapy for congenital tuberculosis (Kobayashi et al, 2002). A practice of instituting vitamin K prophylaxis in severely ill clients, those on extended courses of antibiotics, and those consuming inadequate diets has been proposed (Bhat and Deshukh, 2003). In some clients, consuming buttermilk or yogurt with active bacterial cultures helps to replace the intestinal bacteria (see Chapter 16).

The anticoagulant *warfarin* is given to inhibit the synthesis of vitamin K dependent clotting Factors II, VII, IX and X and thus prolong clotting time and "thin the blood." Eating large amounts of foods high in vitamin K during anticoagulant therapy with *warfarin* decreases or may even negate the desired effect of the drug. Clients should not stop eating foods containing vitamin K, but they should avoid large variations in the amounts eaten. A problem might arise if they eat mounds of green leafy vegetables one day and then none for the following several days. Even beverages such as green tea can be a significant source of vitamin K. A case of interaction with *warfarin* was reported in a 44-year-old client who had been stabilized on the drug but who later drank one-half to one gallon of green tea per day (Taylor and Wilt, 1999).

An additional side effect of *warfarin* therapy involves the function of vitamin K in bone metabolism. Both in bone and kidney, vitamin K-dependent calcium-binding proteins have been identified (Gropper, Smith, and Groff, 2005). Clients receiving long-term *warfarin* therapy have been shown to have decreased bone mineral density (Sato et al, 1997); however, *warfarin* was not associated with increased risk of hip fracture in 52,701 elderly clients (Mamdani et al, 2003). An experiment using diets that decreased vitamin K intake by 80 percent or increased it by 500 percent during a 4-day in-hospital stay demonstrated significant changes in their INRs thus supporting the relevance of diet to therapeutic anticoagulation (Franco et al, 2004). Table 17–1 summarizes instructions for clients taking *warfarin* products. The explanation for including cranberry juice in the table appears in the section Interference with Cytochrome P450 Pathways later in this chapter.

THE B VITAMINS

Methotrexate, an antineoplastic agent, is an antagonist of folic acid. It successfully destroys cancer cells because they too require folic acid for DNA replication. In the process, the efforts of normal body cells to divide are also impaired.

Both the antituberculosis drug *isoniazid* and the anti-Parkinson agent *levodopa* form a complex with vitamin B_6. The kidney then excretes this complex in the urine rather than returning it to the bloodstream. Individuals most at risk for peripheral neuritis from vitamin B_6 deficiency are clients who are pregnant or elderly or who have diabetes, alcoholism, or uremia (Utermohlen, 1999). Supplemental *pyridoxine* may be added to a *levodopa* regimen to correct a vitamin B_6 deficiency, but this will decrease the effectiveness of *levodopa*. An additional consequence of vitamin B_6 deficiency is an inability to convert tryptophan to nicotinic acid, resulting in a niacin deficiency (Kelly et al, 1998). Because isoniazid is structurally similar to niacin, the body recognizes it as niacin and reduces its production of the vitamin; thus, pellagra is a complication of isoniazid therapy (Ozturk et al, 2001).

An exceptional case of a client's dietary pattern predisposing to adverse effects from anesthesia relates to vegetarianism and nitrous oxide. The woman so affected had been a vegetarian for 10 years and for 5 years had restricted her intake to apples, nuts, and raw vegetables while avoiding legumes. (See Chapters 7 and 12 regarding vegetarianism and vitamin B_{12} deficiency.) Nitrous oxide was one component of the anesthesia this client received to repair a traumatic hip fracture. Six weeks later, she was unable to walk and was diagnosed with degeneration of the spinal cord. The deficiency in this case was caused by the known action of nitrous oxide to oxidize the cobalt atom in cobal-

amin to an inactive state, thus reducing the effectiveness of cobalamin-dependent enzymes. The client improved with cobalamin injections but still had some residual effects 1 year after anesthesia (Rosener and Dichgans, 1996).

Low serum levels of vitamins B_6 and B_{12} were found in women taking oral contraceptives. Since low vitamin B_6 levels are independently associated with increased risk for arterial and venous thromboembolism, this finding could partly account for the increased risk of thromboembolism in oral contraceptive users (Lussana et al, 2003). Low-dose contraceptives were associated with significantly lower vitamin B_{12} levels, with frank cobalamin deficiency discovered in 13 percent of 71 treated subjects versus none of the 170 control subjects (Sutterlin et al, 2003). Neither study found an association between oral contraceptive use and folate status.

VITAMIN D

Phenytoin, an anticonvulsant, interferes with the liver's processing of vitamin D. Clients receiving long-term therapy need an estimated 15 to 25 micrograms of vitamin D daily to prevent rickets or osteomalacia. Other medications that increase the metabolism of vitamin D, possibly resulting in low serum levels of the vitamin, include *carbamazepine, phenobarbital,* and *rifampin* (Linus Pauling Institute, 2004).

Effects of Drugs on Nutrient Excretion

Drugs usually cause excessive excretion, rather than retention, of nutrients. Drugs can act on the excretion of nutrients in four ways: they can (1) compete with nutrients for binding sites, (2) form chemical bonds with the nutrient, (3) deplete the nutrient supply in the body's tissues, and (4) interfere with the kidneys' reabsorption of the nutrient into the bloodstream.

Competition for Binding Sites

Many drugs circulate in the bloodstream attached to plasma proteins. These proteins serve a similar function in relation to some nutrients. The plasma protein and its hitchhiker drug or nutrient form a large particle. Sometimes there are too few binding sites on the plasma proteins for all of the drug or nutrient. When that happens, excess drug or nutrient accumulates as free, small particles in the bloodstream. The kidney is likely to excrete these small particles rather than to restore them to the

---

Table 17–1 **Dietary Restrictions for Oral Anticoagulant Therapy**

AVOID	ONE SERVING PER DAY, 1 CUP RAW OR 1/2 CUP COOKED	CHECK WITH PRESCRIBER IF LARGE INCREASES OR DECREASES
Kale (except garnish)	Broccoli	Green vegetables
Parsley (except garnish)	Brussels sprouts	Garbanzo beans
Natto (Japanese)	Spinach	Lentils
	Turnip or other greens	Soybeans or soybean oil
		Liver
		Green tea
		Cranberry juice

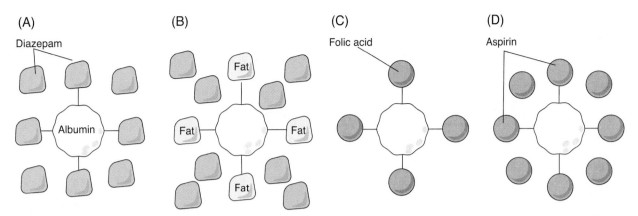

Figure 17–3 a, Four molecules of diazepam are bound to the albumin molecule, leaving the other four molecules of diazepam free to leave the bloodstream for the central nervous system. b, Fat displaces the diazepam from the albumin molecule so that all eight molecules of diazepam are immediately free to exert sedative effects on the central nervous system. c, Four molecules of folic acid are attached to the albumin molecule and able to circulate through the kidney intact. d, Aspirin displaces the folic acid from the albumin molecule, and the separate molecules of folic acid are likely to be excreted in the urine.

bloodstream. One common drug that interferes in this manner with a nutrient is *acetylsalicylic acid*, or *aspirin*. It displaces folic acid from its plasma protein. The kidney then excretes the folic acid in the urine.

A client with low levels of serum albumin as a result of malnutrition is at risk for drug toxicity with drugs that are usually highly bound to albumin. The drug that is bound to protein is inactive, whereas the unbound drug circulating in the blood is active and able to exert its intended therapeutic effect. Examples of drugs with an affinity to bind to protein are *salicylates, warfarin*, and *thiopental* (Yaffe and Sonawane, 1997). Figure 17–3 sketches two consequences of the competition between drugs and foods or nutrients for protein binding sites. Management of the client receiving enteral nutrition and warfarin may involve separation of the drug from the feeding and certainly will require careful monitoring of INRs (Fitzgerald, 2005; Society of Hospital Pharmacists, 2005).

Formation of Chemical Bonds

To combat heavy-metal poisoning, an antidote drug is administered that combines chemically with the metal. The drug plus the metal then is excreted harmlessly. As with many treatments, the drug is not specific and will combine with nutrients as well as the noxious heavy metal, such as lead or mercury. An example of this type of interaction involves *penicillamine* that is used for adjunct treatment of heavy metal poisoning but also for rheumatoid arthritis resistant to conventional therapy (Deglin and Vallerand, 2005). It forms a stable bond with zinc, copper, iron, and other metals, causing excessive excretion and thus possibly leading to deficiencies. Therefore, penicillamine should be taken without food or milk to avoid a high risk of treatment failure (Schmidt and Dalhoff, 2002).

Depletion of Nutrients in Tissues

As part of its overall catabolic effect, the anti-inflammatory glucocorticoid *prednisone* depletes tissues of ascorbic acid. The ascorbic acid accumulates in the blood and is excreted. Because ascorbic acid is necessary for the healing of wounds, one side effect of prednisone and other corticosteroids is poor wound healing. When *alcohol* is present, folic acid "leaks" from the liver into the bloodstream, allowing for excessive excretion in the urine. This interaction can lead to folic acid deficiency.

Interference with Reabsorption by the Kidney

Many diuretic agents prevent normal reabsorption of sodium into the bloodstream within the kidney. This increases the amount of sodium excreted by the kidney into the urine. Along with the sodium, water is excreted. Often the drug's action is not specific enough to dispose of sodium alone. Many diuretics also cause loss of potassium. Sometimes the client must take pharmacologic doses of potassium to prevent hypokalemia. One diuretic, *furosemide*, produces calcium loss in addition to potassium loss by the same mechanism. In contrast, other diuretics, for example, *amiloride, spironolactone*, and *triamterene*, are potassium sparing, eliminating the need for supplementation.

Diuretics lead to increased excretion not only of electrolytes but also of water-soluble vitamins. Diuretic administration to individuals older than 50 years was significantly related to worsening thiamin status (Suter et al, 2000). Table 17–2 summarizes the effects of drugs on foods and nutrients. Figure 17–4 shows some of the nutritional effects related to changes in the gastrointestinal tract caused by medications.

The Effects of Foods and Nutrients on Drugs

Foods and nutrients can decrease, delay, or increase the absorption of drugs. They can also cause alterations in drug metabolism.

The Effects of Foods on Drug Absorption

The interaction of food with a drug can be used to therapeutic advantage in some cases. In other situations,

Table 17–2 The Effects of Drugs on Nutrients

DRUG GROUP	DRUG	EFFECTS/ACTION ON NUTRIENT	MECHANISM OF ACTION
ALTERATION IN FOOD INTAKE			
Analgesic	Acetylsalicylic acid	Decreases appetite	Altered taste; gastric irritation
Antidepressants	Bupropion	Increases/decreases appetite	Side effects
	Doxepin	Increases appetite	Side effect
Antihistamine	Brompheneramine, diphenhydramine	Decrease appetite	Side effect: dry mouth
Antihypertensive	Captopril	Decreases appetite	Loss of taste sensation
Anti-infective	Streptomycin	Decreases appetite/overeating	Altered taste
Antimanic	Lithium	Decreases appetite	Altered taste; side effects: dry mouth, anorexia, nausea, vomiting
Antineoplastic	Bleomycin, plicamycin, vincristine	Decrease appetite	Side effects: anorexia, nausea, vomiting, stomatitis
Chelating agent	Penicillamine	Decreases appetite/overeating	Altered taste and smell
CNS stimulant	Dextroamphetamine, methylphenidate	Decrease appetite	Depressed desire for food
Hormone	Medroxyprogesterone	Increases appetite	Natural effect of hormone
Laxative	Psyllium	Decreases appetite	Gives feeling of fullness
ALTERATION IN NUTRIENT ABSORPTION			
Alcohol	Ethanol	Decreases absorption of amino acids, fat, thiamin, folic acid, niacin, pyridoxine, and magnesium	Decreased enzyme production, damaged intestinal mucosa
Antacids	Aluminum hydroxide, calcium carbonate, magnesium hydroxide	Decrease absorption of folic acid, vitamin B_{12}, and iron	Reduced gastric acidity
Anticonvulsant	Phenytoin	Reduces absorption of folic acid	Competition for binding sites
		Pellagra	Possible interference with absorption or with tryptophan metabolism
Antigout agent	Colchicine	Malabsorption of vitamin B_{12}, folic acid, calcium; reduces absorption of fat, lactose, and carotene	Damaged intestinal mucosa
Anti-infective	Neomycin	Decreases absorption of fat, fat-soluble vitamins, vitamin B_{12}, lactose, iron, sucrose, sodium, potassium, and calcium	Damaged intestinal mucosa
Anti-inflammatory agent	Sulfasalazine	Reduces absorption of folic acid, iron	Inhibited transport mechanism
Antineoplastic	Methotrexate	Decreases absorption of vitamin B_{12}, folic acid, and calcium	Damaged intestinal mucosa
Antipsychotic	Chlorpromazine	Increases absorption of cholesterol	Altered peristalsis
Electrolyte therapy	Potassium	Decreases absorption of folic acid, vitamin B_{12}, and iron	Reduced gastric acidity
Gastric acid-pump inhibitor	Omeprazole	Decreases vitamin B_{12} absorption	Reduced gastric acidity
Histamine H_2 receptor antagonist	Cimetidine	Decreases vitamin B_{12} absorption	Reduced gastric acidity
Laxatives	Bisacodyl	Interferes with uptake of glucose, potassium, calcium, sodium, and water	Increased peristalsis
	Docusate	Increases absorption of cholesterol	Altered peristalsis
	Mineral oil	Decreases absorption of vitamins A, D, E, and K, calcium, and phosphorus	Formation of complexes
Lipid-lowering agent	Cholestyramine	Interferes with absorption of vitamins A, D, K, B_{12}, folic acid, and the mineral calcium	Formation of complexes
Sedative/hypnotic	Glutethimide	Leads to calcium deficiency	Impaired transport mechanism

DRUG GROUP	DRUG	EFFECTS/ACTION ON NUTRIENT	MECHANISM OF ACTION
ALTERATION IN NUTRIENT METABOLISM			
Alcohol	Ethanol	Amino acids and fats poorly utilized	Damaged intestinal mucosa
Anticoagulant	Warfarin	Counteracting vitamin K is desired effect	Inhibits synthesis of vitamin K dependent clotting Factors II, VII, IX and X
Anticonvulsant	Phenytoin, carbamazepine, phenobarbital	Vitamin D deficiency	Impeded conversion of vitamin D to intermediate form
Anti-infective	Broad spectrum antibiotics	Decrease vitamin K synthesis	Destruction of intestinal bacteria
Antineoplastic	Methotrexate	Folic acid deficiency	Folic acid antagonist
Anti-Parkinson agent	Levodopa	Vitamin B_6 deficiency leading to niacin deficiency	Formation of complexes leading to increased urinary excretion of the vitamin
Antitubercular agents	Isoniazid	Vitamin B_6 deficiency leading to niacin deficiency; pellagra	Formation of complexes leading to increased urinary excretion; similar structure to niacin suppresses endogenous production of the vitamin
	Isoniazid, rifampin	Vitamin K deficiency, hemorrhage in newborn	Destruction of intestinal bacteria
	Rifampin	Vitamin D deficiency	Impeded conversion of vitamin D to intermediate form
Glucocorticoids	Cortisone, hydrocortisone, methylprednisolone, prednisone	Decrease glucose tolerance; alter fat deposition, producing "moon face" and/or "buffalo hump"; increase catabolism of bone, resulting in osteoporosis	Protein catabolism; mobilization of fats; conversion of fat and protein to glucose
Hormones/oral contraceptives	Estrogen/progesterone	Decreased serum levels of vitamin B_6 and vitamin B_{12}; low levels of vitamin B_6 associated with thromboembolus; frank cobalamin deficiencies reported	Multiple mechanisms
ALTERATION IN NUTRIENT EXCRETION			
Alcohol	Ethanol	Increases excretion of folic acid	Nutrient not retained in liver
Analgesic/anesthetic	Acetylsalicylic acid, thiopental	Increases excretion of folic acid	Competition for binding sites
Anticoagulant	Warfarin	Increased excretion if low serum albumin	Competition for binding sites
Chelating agent	Penicillamine	Increases excretion of metals: zinc, copper, and iron	Formation of chemical bonds
Diuretic	Furosemide	Increases excretion of sodium, potassium, calcium, and water-soluble vitamins	Interference with reabsorption by kidneys
Glucocorticoid	Prednisone	Increases excretion of vitamin C	Catabolism of tissues

knowledge of interactions helps the health-care team schedule meals and medication doses to the best advantage of the client.

Decreased or Delayed Absorption

Food, nonnutrient components of foods, or nutrients in food may decrease or delay the absorption of drugs. A strict protocol is used for *alendronate*, a bone resorption inhibitor given for osteoporosis. It must be taken first thing in the morning with plain water 30 minutes before any other medications, food, or beverages. Any intake other than water significantly decreases absorption. Moreover, the person must remain upright for 30 minutes to facilitate passage through the pylorus and minimize risk of esophageal irritation.

Melphalan, an antineoplastic drug, should be given without food because it competes with amino acids for absorption. Another antineoplastic drug given for leukemia,

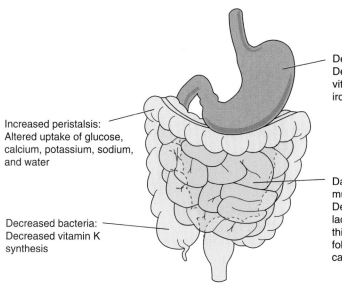

Decreased acidity:
Decreased folic acid,
vitamin B$_{12}$, and
iron absorption

Increased peristalsis:
Altered uptake of glucose,
calcium, potassium, sodium,
and water

Damaged intestinal
mucosa:
Decreased absorption of
lactose, fat, amino acid,
thiamin, niacin, vitamin B$_6$,
folic acid, vitamin B$_{12}$,
calcium, iron, and magnesium

Decreased bacteria:
Decreased vitamin K
synthesis

Figure **17–4** Both therapeutic effects (decreased gastric acidity and increased peristalsis) and side effects (damaged intestinal mucosa and decreased colon bacteria) can adversely affect nutrient utilization.

mercaptopurine, should be taken without food, because food causes oxidation of the drug into inactive metabolites. Taking either of these antineoplastic drugs with food risks treatment failure (Schmidt and Dalhoff, 2002).

Food delays the absorption of *cortisone*, a *glucocorticoid* used as an anti-inflammatory drug. Taking *cortisone* with food produces a more consistent blood level of the drug than taking it without food. Other factors, such as a drug's susceptibility to acid degradation or its ability to form insoluble complexes, also influence whether a drug is administered with food or between meals.

GASTROINTESTINAL pH

Food in the stomach, acidic fruit or vegetable juices, and carbonated beverages increase gastric acidity. Anti-infective drugs particularly susceptible to acid degradation are *penicillin V, cloxacillin,* and *ampicillin.* A risk of treatment failure occurs if *azithromycin* or *isoniazid* is taken with food (Schmidt and Dalhoff, 2002). An acid medium breaks down these drugs, resulting in a less-effective blood level. To diminish such acid degradation, these anti-infective drugs are administered with a full glass of water 1 hour before or 2 hours after meals. Conversely, individuals with less gastric acid, such as young infants and the elderly, may achieve higher blood levels of these drugs than intended. Achlorhydria that often affects clients with AIDS severely impairs the absorption of the antifungal agents *itraconazole* and *ketoconazole.* Giving the medications with cola increases their **bioavailability** sufficiently to permit oral dosing (Schmidt and Dalhuff, 2002).

Drugs formulated to dissolve in the intestine rather than in the stomach are **enteric-coated;** an acid-resistant shell covers the active ingredient (Fig. 17–5). The stomach's environment normally is acid, and the duodenum's is alkaline. Milk raises the pH of the stomach, making it more alkaline. Taking enteric-coated drugs with milk allows the coating to dissolve early and thereby decreases the action of the drug. Some formulations of *erythromycin*, an anti-infective drug, are enteric-coated and should not be taken

with milk. Alcohol and hot beverages can also cause premature erosion of the enteric-coating on drugs.

FOODS CONTAINING IRON OR CALCIUM

Tetracycline, an anti-infective agent, combines with the salts of iron, calcium, magnesium, or aluminum to form insoluble compounds. The drug and the nutrient thus bound are both unavailable for absorption. For this reason, *tetracycline* should not be administered within 1 to 3 hours of taking iron supplements or eating iron-containing foods (red meat, egg yolks), milk or other dairy products, or antacids containing magnesium, aluminum, and/or calcium. Tetracycline should be taken without food or milk to avoid a high risk of treatment failure due to chelation. Bioavailability of tetracycline is reduced up to 57 percent when taken with food, 65 percent with dairy products, and 81 percent with iron supplements. Even a small amount of milk in coffee or tea can reduce the drug's bioavailability by 49 percent (Schmidt and Dalhoff, 2002). Another class of anti-infective drugs, the *fluoroquinolones*, including

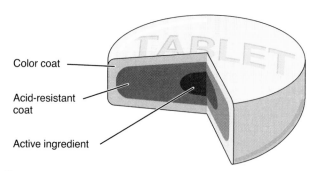

Color coat

Acid-resistant
coat

Active ingredient

Figure **17–5** Enteric-coated tablet. Substances that penetrate the acid-resistant coating defeat the purpose of this type of tablet. (Reprinted from Clayton, BD, and Stock, YN: Basic Pharmacology for Nurses, ed 9. Mosby, St. Louis, 1989, p 56, with permission.)

ciprofloxacin, combine with calcium, iron, and zinc, resulting in decreased absorption of the anti-infective drugs to such an extent as to produce treatment failures (Gregg, 1999). *Ciprofloxacin* should not be taken with dairy products or calcium-fortified juices alone but may be taken with a meal containing those items (Huang and Lesko, 2004). The bioavailability of ciprofloxacin was decreased by 28 percent when administered orally to normal subjects with Ensure (Society of Hospital Pharmacists, 2005) and reduced by 27 to 72 percent when administered with enteral feeding so that withholding tube feedings for one hour before and after the dose of medication is delivered is suggested (Finch, 2001).

ENERGY NUTRIENTS

A rich protein diet impairs the clinical effect of *levodopa*, a drug used in the management of Parkinson's disease, thought to be the result of competition for carriers at the blood-brain barrier between levodopa and large neutral amino acids such as phenylalanine, tyrosine, and tryptophan (Brown, 2005). A separation of 3 hours between administration of *levodopa* and ingestion of high-protein food improves absorption. Clients with Parkinson's disease may find that daytime restriction of protein intake gives them a higher level of functioning. Consuming their required protein at bedtime is a compensatory strategy (Utermohlen, 1999). Protein inhibits the absorption of *methyldopa* (an antihypertensive) and of *theophylline,* a bronchodilator used to treat asthma and chronic obstructive pulmonary disease, and delays the action of *phenytoin* (an anticonvulsant). Serum phenytoin levels decreased 72 percent when the drug was administered with continuous enteral nutrition so that withholding the tube feeding for two hours before and after the dose of phenytoin is recommended (Finch, 2001). In contrast, toxicity can occur if an enteral feeding is discontinued without adjusting the *phenytoin* dosage (Schmidt and Dalhoff, 2002).

A high-fiber meal decreases the absorption of *digoxin,* a drug used to treat congestive heart failure and certain cardiac arrhythmias by slowing and strengthening cardiac contractions. A high-fiber diet may lead to treatment failure with *lovastatin,* the cholesterol-lowering agent, but taking the drug with fat increases its solubility and effect (Schmidt and Dalhoff, 2002). The pectin in apples and jelly reduces the absorption of *acetaminophen,* an analgesic.

Fatty meals inhibit the absorption of *zidovudine,* an antiretroviral drug used in the management of human immunodeficiency virus (HIV) infections (Gregg, 1999). Another antiretroviral drug, *indinavir,* has a high risk of treatment failure if taken with food that may precipitate the drug (Schmidt and Dalhoff, 2002).

Increased Absorption

Foods and nutrients may also increase or facilitate the absorption of drugs. Some drugs are affected in one or more ways by one or more nutrients. *Levodopa* has a second interaction with food. Although protein impairs the absorption of *levodopa,* carbohydrate facilitates it. Giving *levodopa* with carbohydrate-rich snacks improves the absorption of the drug. Similarly, protein delays the anti-

convulsant action of *phenytoin,* but the presence of carbohydrate increases the absorption. An unusual situation, using a diet in cases of poor control of a seizures with medication, is detailed in Clinical Application 17–3.

In general, protein inhibits the absorption of *theophylline,* a bronchodilator given for asthma or chronic obstructive pulmonary disease, but carbohydrate accelerates its absorption. Various preparations of controlled-release *theophylline,* however, responded differently in relation to food intake (Utermohlen, 1999), so administration information for the specific product should be sought.

The antiprotozoal drug *atovaquone,* given for *Pneumocystis carinii* pneumonia, should be taken with a fatty meal to increase the drug's solubility. Absorption of *griseofulvin,* an antifungal drug, is promoted by bile secretion so that administration with a fatty meal is required to avoid treatment failure, especially in children. Increased effectiveness of *nifedipine* sustained-release is achieved through a consistent relationship with meals, because bile secretion promotes the drug's absorption. Similarly, *tacrolimus,* an immunosuppressant, and *isotretinoin,* the vitamin A metabolite given for severe acne (see Chapter 11), have increased solubility with fat intake and should be taken with a consistent relationship to meals to avoid fluctuations in drug effects (Schmidt and Dalhoff, 2002).

Clinical Application 17–3

The Ketogenic Diet for Seizure Control in Children

Some children with epilepsy who are poorly controlled with medication benefit from a high-fat, low-carbohydrate, ketogenic diet. Although no reliable evidence from randomized controlled trials support its use, large observational studies, some prospective, suggest it results in decreased seizure activity (Levy and Cooper, 2003) as well as decreased medication use (DiMario and Holland, 2002; Hemingway et al, 2001). The mechanism of action is unknown, but animal studies suggest that acetone has an anticonvulsant effect. Whether the diet generates a sufficient concentration to confirm this theory awaits further research (Likhodii and Burnham, 2002).

The ketogenic diet is not easy to follow, sometimes requiring inpatient stays to initiate the diet (Mandel et al, 2002), and it has a high rate of discontinuance, 41 percent within 6 months (Lightstone et al, 2001). In addition, the diet has several known complications. Kidney stones have been reported in 10 percent of clients (Kielb et al, 2000), and a small study revealed cardiac abnormalities in 15 percent of clients (Best et al, 2000). The ketogenic diet can provide sufficient nutrition to maintain normal growth, but very young children grow poorly on the diet and require careful monitoring (Vining et al, 2002).

Nevertheless, the ketogenic diet provides an option for families with a child suffering from difficult-to-control seizures. It requires specialty dietary and medical care and an extremely motivated family.

The Effects of Foods on Drug Metabolism

Foods can alter the metabolism of drugs. One metabolic food-drug interaction, described in the following section, can be life-threatening, and another can affect many drugs.

Monoamine Oxidase Inhibitors

The usual abbreviation for this group of drugs is **MAOI (monoamine oxidase inhibitor).** Several antidepressants are monoamine oxidase inhibitors, and some other drugs produce similar reactions (see the drugs listed in Table 17–3).

MECHANISM OF DRUG ACTION

These drugs prevent the breakdown of tyramine and **dopamine,** chemicals necessary for proper functioning of the nervous system. The drugs' therapeutic effect is to increase the concentration of epinephrine, norepinephrine, serotonin, and dopamine in the central nervous system, thus counteracting depression.

In the peripheral nervous system, MAO inhibitors also prevent the release of the norepinephrine that builds up in the nerves. The stores of norepinephrine become especially high in the nerves that regulate the size of blood vessels. The result is a decreased ability to constrict peripheral blood vessels. The vasodilation thus produced leads to hypotension. To compound the situation, the drugs also inhibit the body's normal response to a low blood pressure, an increased heart rate. Thus, the individual displays the unusual combination of hypotension and bradycardia.

EFFECT OF FOODS ON MAO INHIBITORS

Some foods contain **tyramine,** a metabolic intermediate product in the conversion of the amino acid tyrosine to epinephrine. Foods that contain degraded protein, such as aged cheese, are high in tyramine. When a client taking MAOIs consumes foods or beverages high in tyramine, the drugs prevent the normal breakdown of tyramine. As a consequence, the tyramine oversupply leads to excessive epinephrine, producing hypertension. Sometimes the blood pressure is severely elevated, which can cause intracranial hemorrhage.

As with many substances, individuals' responses to tyramine vary. Several factors interact to determine the severity of reaction: (1) the amount of tyramine ingested, (2) the dose of the MAOI, (3) client susceptibility, and (4) the time between the drug dose and a tyramine-containing meal.

TYRAMINE-RICH FOODS

Many foods contain enough tyramine to create problems for clients receiving MAOIs. These include foods and beverages such as cheese, beer, and Chianti wine, in which

Table 17–3 **Tyramine-Restricted Diet**

DESCRIPTION	INDICATION	ADEQUACY
Restricts food with naturally high levels of tyramine.	Used when clients receive drugs classified as monoamine oxidase (MAO) inhibitors and those with MAO inhibitor activity. Antidepressants: *Isocarboxazid, Phenelzine; Tranylcypromine* Anti-infectives: *Furazolidone; Isoniazid, Linezolid* Antineoplastics: *Procarbazine* Antiparkinson: *Selegiline*	Adequate in all nutrients according to the current Recommended Dietary Allowances if the individual makes appropriate food choices.

FOOD GROUP	TO AVOID	TO USE MODERATELY
Breads and cereals	None	None
Fruit and vegetables	Avocados Bananas Figs Broad (fava) beans Chinese pea pods Eggplant Italian flat beans Mixed Chinese vegetables	None
Dairy	Aged cheese (brick, blue, brie, cheddar, Camembert, Swiss, Romano, Roquefort, mozzarella, Parmesan, provolone) Yogurt	Gouda cheese Processed American cheese
Meat and fish	Any canned meat Beef or chicken liver Sausage (bologna, salami, pepperoni, summer) Fish (caviar, dried fish, salt herring)	
Beverages	Ale, beer, sherry, red and white wines	Coffee, colas, hot chocolate (1–3 cups per day)
Other	Chocolate, bouillon and other protein extracts, meat tenderizer, soy sauce, yeast concentrates	

aging is used to enhance flavor. The amount of tyramine varies even in different samples of a particular food. Table 17–3 describes the tyramine-restricted diet. Because this interaction can be life-threatening, the best advice to give a client is to avoid all foods capable of causing problems, even though a small amount of the food, or a given batch of a product, might be safe. New formulations of antidepressant MAO inhibitors, such as *moclobemide* and *brofaromin,* with limited tyramine potentiation are more selective in targeting the central nervous system and do not require severe dietary restrictions (Utermohlen, 1999; Youdim and Weinstock, 2004). Even so, experts advise that those treated with *moclobemide,* until further research is available, avoid the consumption of excessive amounts of aged or overripe cheese and yeast extracts (Youdim and Weinstock, 2004).

Interference with Cytochrome P450 Pathways

Cytochrome P450 (CYP450) is a superfamily of enzymes found mainly in the liver but also in the gastrointestinal tract, lungs, and kidneys. The three major families of isoenzymes are CPY1, CPY2, and CPY3 (Anderson, 2002). The isoenzyme CYP3A4, the main form in the small intestine, is estimated to participate in the metabolism of more than 50 percent of all pharmaceutical agents, a function that may have evolved to protect the body from toxins. After uptake by the intestinal epithelial cells (enterocytes), many substances are metabolized by CYP3A4 or returned to the intestinal lumen by a transporter protein (Kane and Lipsky, 2000), thus limiting the amount of the substance available for absorption. This process, along with similar enzymatic actions in the liver, is called the **first-pass effect.** Individuals show a wide variation in the amount of CYP3A4 in the liver and the intestine due to genetic, physiological, and environmental effects so that persons with more of the isoenzyme show greater effects to its inhibition than those with lesser amounts of intestinal CYP3A4 (Anderson, 2002; Kane and Lipsky, 2000).

GRAPEFRUIT JUICE

An accidental discovery in 1989 that grapefruit juice, used to mask the taste of alcohol in a study, enhanced the absorption of *felodipine* has spurred research into the underlying mechanism. It appears that grapefruit juice's major effect is through the inhibition of intestinal CYP3A4 so that the oral bioavailability of affected drugs is increased dramatically, in some cases sufficient to cause drug toxicity or treatment failure, whereas the same drugs administered intravenously accompanied by oral grapefruit juice are unaffected. A single glass (250 milliliters) of grapefruit juice is enough to produce measurable effects for 24 hours, presumably until the body manufactures more of the enzyme. Although less quantification is documented, consumption of grapefruit sections also impacts drug absorption, as does intake of juice from Seville oranges (Harris, Jung, and Tsunoda, 2003). Applying this knowledge to clinical practice is complicated by the fact that even within a given class of drugs, not all agents are metabolized by CYP3A4, so some medications in the class are affected by grapefruit juice and others are not. Some

examples follow, but they are by no means all-inclusive and undoubtedly more research will be conducted.

The calcium channel blockers, given to manage hypertension and angina pectoris, include *felodipine,* the prototype interactor with grapefruit juice, *nisoldipine,* and *nicardipine,* which interact similarly. With two other calcium channel blockers, *nifedipine* and *amlodipine,* little or no interaction with grapefruit juice is seen, presumably because they have a higher bioavailability compared with the first three. Similarly, grapefruit juice increases the bioavailability of the benzodiazepines *diazepam, midazolam,* and *triazolam* but not *alprazolam.* Two statin drugs, given to lower cholesterol and prevent ischemic heart disease, *simvastatin* and *lovastatin,* had greatly increased blood levels when given with grapefruit juice, but *atorvastatin* showed a lesser effect and *pravastatin* no effect (Dahan and Altman, 2004) because *pravastatin* is not exclusively metabolized by CYP3A4 (Schmidt and Dalhuff, 2002).

Cyclosporine, an immunosuppressive agent used to prevent transplant rejection, is metabolized by intestinal CYP3A4, and elevated blood levels have occurred when administered with grapefruit juice. Because *cyclosporine* has a narrow **therapeutic index** and serious side effects, avoidance of grapefruit juice during therapy is well advised (Dahan and Altman, 2004). The antifungal agent *ketoconazole* is a CYP3A4 inhibitor that, when administered with *cyclosporine,* permits a lower dose of *cyclosporine* to achieve the desired therapeutic effect at a savings in cost. Suggestion that grapefruit juice be substituted for *ketoconazole* for this purpose is ill advised due to inconsistencies in the concentration of the active metabolites in the juice (Kane and Lipsky, 2000).

CRANBERRY JUICE

A similar mechanism but a different isoenzyme is proposed to explain an interaction between *warfarin* and cranberry juice. Following a chest infection, a client subsisted almost solely on cranberry juice for 2 weeks while taking his prescribed medications, *digoxin, phenytoin,* and *warfarin.* He died of gastrointestinal and pericardial hemorrhage. Warfarin is mainly metabolized by the cytochrome P450 isoenzyme CYP2C9, and cranberry juice contains flavonoids known to inhibit P450 enzymes (Suvarna, Pirmohamed, and Henderson, 2003). Another case of a persistently elevated INR occurred in a client with a prosthetic mitral valve 2 weeks after the client began drinking cranberry juice. Subsequent symptoms included postoperative bleeding problems (Grant, 2004).

Effects of Other Nutrients

Certain nutrients increase the amount of a drug in the bloodstream, thus increasing or decreasing the risk of toxicity. For example, fat displaces the antianxiety drug *diazepam* from **protein binding sites,** thus increasing the amount of unbound drug circulating in the bloodstream. This increased serum concentration leads to increased activity of the drug.

Normal potassium and calcium levels are necessary for adequate muscle function, including that of the heart. Hypokalemia or hypercalcemia increases the risk of toxicity from digitalis. Clients receiving digitalis and loop diuretics, a common combination, require careful monitoring.

Table 17–4 summarizes the effects of foods and nutrients on drugs. Thus far, the chapter has been concerned with oral administration of medications and oral or enteral feeding. The use of TPN requires even more sophisticated knowledge of interactions, as briefly outlined in Clinical Application 17–4.

Occasionally, a food or beverage contains a drug that produces untoward effects. For example, a woman was seen in a dermatology clinic for a persistent rash, worsened by sunlight. She habitually drank 500 milliliters of tonic water daily. Tonic water is a carbonated mixer that contains lemon, lime, sweeteners, and *quinine*, a drug used to treat malaria. The amount of *quinine* in the water, 40 milligrams in 500 milliliters, was much less than that given pharmacologically to adults. Among *quinine's* side effects, however, is a skin rash. Once the woman stopped drinking tonic water, her skin problem was cured (Wagner, Diffey, and Ive, 1994). Although the United States Food and Drug Administration banned its use for nocturnal leg cramps due to lack of safety and efficacy, *quinine* is widely available in beverages. Anecdotal reports suggest that products containing *quinine* may produce neurological signs and symptoms, confusion, altered mental status, seizures, and coma (Brasic, 2003).

Effects of Nonnutrient Intakes

Although it is not a nutrient and has been on the GRAS list since 1958, caffeine should be included in a dietary assessment. The most common sources of caffeine for Americans are coffee, tea, soft drinks, and chocolate.

Table 17–4　The Effects of Foods and Nutrients on Drugs

EFFECT	TYPE OF FOOD/NUTRIENT	ACTION ON DRUG
Decreased or delayed absorption	Any food	Significantly decreases absorption of *alendronate*
		Oxidizes *mercaptopurine** into inactive metabolites
		Gastric acid breaks down *azithromycin** and *isoniazid**
		Precipitates *indinavir**
		Delays absorption of *cortisone*
	Amino acids in proteins	Inhibit transfer of *levodopa* across blood-brain barrier
		Impair absorption of *methyldopa* and *theophylline*
		Delay action of *phenytoin*
		Compete for absorption with *melphalan**
	Acidic juices, carbonated beverages	Degrade *penicillin V, cloxacillin*, and *amphicillin*
	Milk	Increases pH of stomach, causing premature erosion of enteric coatings
	Calcium in dairy products Iron supplements	Combine with *tetracycline** to impair absorption
	Foods high in calcium, iron, or zinc (dairy products, red meat)	Combine with *fluoroquinolones* such as *ciprofloxacin** to decrease absorption
	High-fiber meal	Decreases absorption of *digoxin* and *lovastatin**
	Alcohol, hot beverages	Cause premature erosion of enteric coatings
	Pectin in jelly, apples	Reduces absorption of *acetaminophen*
	Carbohydrate	Decreases absorption of *isoniazid*
	Fatty foods	Inhibit absorption of *zidovudine*
Increased absorption	Carbohydrate	Enhances absorption of *levodopa, phenytoin,* and *theophylline*
	Fatty foods	Enhance absorption of *griseofulvin,** *lovastatin*
		Increase solubility of *atovaquone, isotretinoin,* and *tacrolimus*
	Cola	Increases gastric acidity to aid absorption of *itraconazole* and *ketoconazole*
Altered metabolism	Fat	Enhances activity of *diazepam* by displacing it from protein binding sites
	Tyramine-containing foods	May cause hypertensive crisis when combined with *MAO inhibitors*†
	Grapefruit juice	Inhibits CYP3A4 to increase the bioavailability of *cyclosporine, diazepam, felodipine, lovastatin, midazolam, nicardipine, nisoldipine, simvastatin, triasolam,* and many others
	Cranberry juice	Presumably inhibits CYP2C9 to increase the bioavailability of *warfarin*†
	Caffeine	Inhibits CYP1A2 to potentially increase the bioavailability of *clozapine, enoxacin, fluvoxamine, imipramine, mexiletine,* and *theophylline*

*Risk of treatment failure.
†May be life-threatening.

Clinical Application 17-4

Preventing Drug Interactions with TPN

TPN is a complex formulation of dextrose, amino acids, fat emulsion, electrolytes, vitamins, and trace elements. Up to 38 additives may be included, each having individual characteristics that might contribute to interactions. TPN is not recommended as a drug delivery vehicle because of limited or unreliable compatibility information. The preferred mode of medication administration is to separate the drugs from the TPN. This can be accomplished by using multiple lumen catheters, alternating the TPN infusion with medication infusion, or, if possible, oral administration of medications. Compatible medications may be coinfused with TPN through auxiliary units.

Only the histamine H2 antagonists, *famotidine* and *ranitidine*, and *insulin* can be admixed with both dextrose-amino acid (2-in-1) and dextrose-amino acid-fat emulsion (3-in-1) formulations. Information is available on Y-site compatibility that for individual drugs varies with the formulation. For instance, *erythromycin* and *magnesium sulfate* are compatible with 2-in-1 solutions but not 3-in-1, whereas *cefazolin* and *sodium bicarbonate* are compatible with 3-in-1 solutions but not 2-in-1.

Multivitamins should be admixed immediately before infusion. Thiamin and vitamin A are known to have a short stability in TPN. Night-blindness developed in a client whose TPN was admixed in the pharmacy and later delivered to the home. Even more serious, calcium phosphate precipitates in TPN caused two deaths. Interactions may become apparent as in these cases or if the catheter becomes plugged, but loss of effectiveness of the drug or the TPN can also occur. Administration of drugs in TPN or by coinfusion should be avoided if at all possible.

SOURCE: Summarized from Mirtallo, 2004.

Another isoenzyme in the cytochrome P450 family is involved in the metabolism of caffeine as well as several pharmaceutical preparations. CYP1A2, primarily found in the liver, participates in the metabolism of the selective serotonin reuptake inhibitor (SSRI) *fluvoxamine* given for obsessive-compulsive disorder, the antiarrhythmic *mexiletine*, the antipsychotic *clozapine*, the tricyclic antidepressant *imipramine*, the bronchodilator *theophylline*, and anti-infective *enoxacin*. All of these drugs reportedly are potent inhibitors of the isoenzyme. Thus, pharmacokinetic interactions at the CYP1A2 enzyme level may cause toxic effects if caffeine is consumed with these drugs (Carrillo and Benitz, 2000; Harris, Jang, and Tsunoda, 2003).

The Body's Homeostatic Mechanisms Affect Drug Levels

In addition to nutritional status, the status of the person's acid-base balance and fluid and electrolyte balance affects the excretion of drugs. To consider either acid-base balance or fluid and electrolyte balance in isolation risks oversimplifying the body's functions. The functions of these two regulatory systems are interwoven.

Acid-Base Balance

The kidneys play a major role in maintaining the normal composition of the blood and tissue fluid. The contents of urine, therefore, reflect the metabolic state of the body. The end products of the foods that are consumed and the drugs that are taken make the urine either more acid or more alkaline. Freshly voided urine usually has an acid pH, averaging about 6.0.

Alkaline Urine

Large amounts of citrus juices, greater than 1 liter per day (Smith, 1995), or a vegetarian diet causes the urine to become alkaline. When the body is producing alkaline urine, the kidneys take longer to excrete alkaline drugs. Higher levels of the drugs remain in the bloodstream for a longer period. Examples of alkaline drugs are the cardiac antidysrhythmic *quinidine*, the tricyclic antidepressant *imipramine*, and *amphetamine* stimulants. If the client's metabolism leads to alkaline urine, these drugs have more pronounced and prolonged effects. Clients treated with these drugs should neither change the amounts of citrus juice they consume nor become vegetarians without consulting the physician.

The opposite effect occurs when a person's metabolism produces alkaline urine and the drugs are acidic. The kidney excretes acidic drugs faster than usual if the urine is alkaline. One acidic drug that should spring to mind immediately is *acetylsalicylic acid*, or *aspirin*. Another acidic drug is the barbiturate *phenobarbital*, commonly used as an anticonvulsant. The kidney excretes both of these drugs faster than normal if the client is producing alkaline urine.

Acid Urine

Large doses of *ascorbic acid* (vitamin C) make the urine more acidic. Vitamin C is sometimes given specifically for the purpose of acidifying the urine. For example, a urinary pH of 5.5 or less is necessary for the urinary anti-infective drug *methenamine* to be effective. In an acid urine, the drug becomes ammonia and formaldehyde, both bactericidal chemicals.

Sulfonamides are antimicrobial drugs that are often given for urinary tract infections. One of the possible side effects of sulfonamides is **crystalluria,** crystallization of the drug in the urinary tract. Although some drugs crystallize more readily than others, these drugs are more likely to crystallize in concentrated or acid urine. For this reason, clients should be instructed to drink ample fluid. It may also be necessary to deliberately alkalinize the urine with another drug or diet modification to prevent crystallization. Table 17–5 summarizes the effects of urinary pH on the excretion of drugs.

Fluid and Electrolyte Balance

A person's fluid and electrolyte status also interacts with drugs. Potassium intake, sodium and water intake, and licorice can cause serious imbalances in fluid and electrolyte status in certain situations.

Salt Substitutes and ACE Inhibitors

The angiotensin-converting enzyme (ACE) inhibitors lower blood pressure by preventing conversion of angiotensin I to

Table **17–5** **Effects of Urinary pH on Drugs**

	ALKALINE URINE	ACID URINE
Increased excretion	Acetylsalicylic acid Phenobarbital	Amphetamines Imipramine Quinidine
Decreased excretion	Amphetamines Imipramine Quinidine	Acetylsalicylic acid Phenobarbital
Necessary for adequate effect	Sulfonamides	Methenamine

angiotensin II, thereby decreasing aldosterone secretion and increasing excretion of sodium and water (see Fig. 9–5.) Clients receiving ACE inhibitors such as *captopril, enalapril,* and *lisinopril* should be monitored for hyperkalemia. The excessive serum potassium may be related to potassium-sparing diuretics or potassium-containing salt substitutes. One client had to be resuscitated following cardiac arrest before the contribution of a salt substitute to his hyperkalemia became apparent (Ray, Dorman, and Watson, 1999).

Sodium, Fluids, and Lithium

Both sodium intake and increased fluid intake affect the antimanic drug *lithium*. This drug is absorbed, distributed, and excreted with sodium. Therefore, decreased sodium intake with decreased fluid intake may lead to *lithium* retention. Signs and symptoms of lithium toxicity include drowsiness, confusion, hand tremor, blurred vision, vertigo, and seizures (Ament, Bertolino, and Liszewski, 2000). Conversely, increased sodium intake and increased fluid intake increase the excretion of *lithium* and decrease its antimanic effect, thus worsening signs and symptoms of mania. Because of this important interaction, clients who take *lithium* are taught to monitor the concentration or **specific gravity** of their urine.

Licorice

Licorice, a flavoring agent, contains glycyrrhizic acid, which, when metabolized, inhibits an enzyme that controls the conversion of cortisol to cortisone in the kidney. As little as "a couple of twists" per day can counteract the effects of diuretics and increase the mineralocorticoid effects of corticosteroids (Utermohlen, 1999). When eaten in excess, licorice can cause sodium and water retention, hypertension, hypokalemia, and alkalosis. Control of hypertension took 8 months for a 49-year-old woman who, unbeknownst to her physician, consumed large quantities of a licorice-flavored sweet (Dellow, Unwin, and Honour, 1999). Another client suffered life-threatening hypokalemic paralysis caused by consumption of licorice as a tea sweetener (a common custom among the Arab population) superimposed on long-term consumption of licorice candy (Elinav and Chajek-Shaul, 2003). A third case involved an elderly Asian man whose muscle weakness progressed to paralysis. He was hypertensive, hypokalemic, and in metabolic alkalosis, attributed to a 3-year daily ingestion of tea flavored with natural licorice root (Lin et al, 2003). Obviously these clients did not realize the risks of their habits. Besides these deliberate ingestions, however, a person may consume it unknowingly because licorice is used to flavor many foods, some chewing tobacco, chewing gum, alcoholic beverages, and some laxatives.

Responsibilities of Health-Care Professionals

The task of administering medications correctly in relation to food and nutrient intake might seem overwhelming. The clinical pharmacist can provide valuable assistance in planning appropriate scheduling. Identifying the interactions with higher risks of toxicity or treatment failure and preventing those adverse effects should take priority, especially with clients receiving many medications. The Joint Commission on the Accreditation of Healthcare Organizations mandates that clients be given information on the medications they receive, including potential dietary interactions. Although the dietitian is charged with this responsibility, the successful completion of the task requires cooperation from the health-care team. Box 17–1 lists some principles for charting client teaching.

As more information becomes available, particularly in the area of genetic variations in capability to metabolize drugs, individualized treatment with medications may become possible (Haga and Burke, 2004). Identification of genetic variations in the capacity to metabolize phenytoin (van der Weide et al, 2001) and pravastatin (Chasman et al, 2004) with resulting consequences for dosing have been reported. Meanwhile, managing a medication regimen with general rules is a challenging but worthwhile effort. The consequences of improper scheduling of drugs and foods or nutrients can be treatment failure, toxicity, and/or increased expense.

Box **17–1** **Charting Tips**

- Record the client's knowledge at the start of your teaching.
- Identify information discussed.
- Indicate evidence, such as verbalization or recitation, that indicates client understood your teaching.
- Whenever possible, give the client a choice. If the client makes a choice, chart the decision as the client's.
- Document educational materials given to the client.

SUMMARY

This chapter has only touched the surface of the subject of food and drug interactions. For every drug included in the chapter, many others had to be omitted. Commonly prescribed drugs and those that have significant interactions with foods are included, as are various modes of food and drug interactions.

Persons at highest risk for food-drug interactions are those who (1) take many drugs, including alcohol; (2) require long-term drug therapy; (3) have poor or marginal nutrition; or (4) have immature or impaired metabolic systems. All clients should be instructed about how to prevent or manage possible interactions (Wellness Tips 17–1). Food-drug interactions can affect (1) food intake, (2) absorption of nutrients or drugs, (3) metabolism of nutrients or drugs, and (4) excretion of nutrients or drugs.

 17–1 • Learn as much as possible about proper administration of medications in relation to food intake.
- Be especially cautious about combining medications with alcohol intake.
- If a medication with known nutrient interactions is necessary long-term, discuss appropriate proactive nutritional interventions with the health-care provider.

- Follow the package directions regarding the maximum use of over-the-counter medications.
- If several health-care providers are prescribing medications, be sure each knows the entire regimen being followed, including dietary intake.
- Maintain a balanced, varied, and moderate diet.

Medications influence food intake by decreasing or increasing appetite, causing taste changes, or provoking gastric irritation. Drugs affect nutrient absorption through luminal or mucosal effects and impact nutrient metabolism through many mechanisms. Medications affect the excretion of nutrients by competing for binding sites, forming chemical bonds, depleting nutrients in tissues, and interfering with kidney reabsorption. In addition, foods and nutrients can affect drug levels and actions by increasing or decreasing absorption and altering the medication's metabolism. Four particularly important nutrient-drug interactions are those of (1) tyramine-containing foods with MAO inhibitors, (2) sodium and water with lithium, (3) vitamin K with warfarin, and (4) grapefruit juice with many medications. Also at risk are clients in unstable acid-base or fluid and electrolyte balance and those with alterations in serum proteins.

CASE STUDY 17-1

Mrs. S, a 72-year-old client, is being seen by the home health nurse to reaffirm her suitability for independent living. She has a history of congestive heart failure for which she has been successfully treated with digoxin 0.125 mg daily for the past 6 months. Mrs. S takes the tablet with her usual breakfast of orange juice, raisin toast, and tea.

Recently she has had difficulty with constipation. Obtaining information on bowel hygiene on her own, she decided to improve her nutritional intake by adding a high-fiber cereal to her breakfast.

After 1 week, her constipation has been relieved, but she now is becoming fatigued easily. When climbing a flight of stairs she finds it necessary to rest twice en route. The nurse asked Mrs. S to weigh herself. Mrs. S reported she had gained 5 lb in 2 weeks. Based on the above data and her observations, the home health nurse prepared a nursing care plan. The portion of it pertinent to food and drug interactions appears below.

NURSING CARE PLAN

SUBJECTIVE DATA Easily fatigued
Short of breath <1 flight of stairs
History of constipation, relieved by addition of high-fiber cereal to diet
Medications: digoxin, 0.125 mg daily in morning with breakfast

OBJECTIVE DATA Alert, oriented, cooperative. Vital signs normal except pulse 90 beats per minute. Weight gain: 5 lb over 2 weeks.

NURSING DIAGNOSIS NANDA: Deficient Knowledge (NANDA, 2003, with permission) related to food-drug interaction as evidenced by beginning signs of heart failure

(Continued on the following page)

CASE STUDY (Continued)

DESIRED OUTCOMES EVALUATION CRITERIA	NURSING ACTIONS/INTERVENTIONS	RATIONALE
NOC: Knowledge: Diet (Moorhead, Johnson, and Maas, 2004, with permission) Client will revise medication or meal schedule immediately to maximize effectiveness of digoxin.	NIC: Teaching: Prescribed Medication (Dochterman and Bulechek, 2004, with permission) Teach client to separate digoxin from high-fiber foods.	High-fiber foods decrease the absorption of digitalis preparations.

C T Q CRITICAL THINKING QUESTIONS

1. What additional assessment data could impact the resolution of this situation?
2. In what way might this scenario develop such that the nurse should contact the client's physician during the home visit?

3. How would you approach the follow-up care of this client?

>>> CHAPTER REVIEW

1. Which of the following clients is at greatest risk for food-drug interaction?
   a. A 50-year-old man with no current disease who takes one baby aspirin daily to prevent heart disease
   b. A 75-year-old woman taking medication for several chronic diseases
   c. A 39-year-old man who usually consumes two cocktails before dinner
   d. A 25-year-old pregnant woman who is taking a prenatal vitamin supplement and calcium tablets

2. How do food and drugs interact?
   a. Drugs may affect food intake.
   b. Either may affect the absorption of the other.
   c. Certain foods and drugs specifically interfere with the metabolism of the other.
   d. Nutrients and drugs can increase or decrease the rate of excretion of one another.
   e. All of the above are true.

3. Which of the following statements by a client prescribed simvastatin would indicate he understood the instructions?

   a. "One glass of grapefruit juice a day is as much as I can have."
   b. "I can have grapefruit juice for breakfast since I take the pill at bedtime."
   c. "I won't drink grapefruit juice while I am taking this drug."
   d. "I won't drink grapefruit juice but eating grapefruit sections is okay."

4. A client taking lithium is most likely to experience increased mania with:
   a. Decreased fluid intake and decreased sodium intake
   b. Decreased fluid intake and increased potassium intake
   c. Increased sodium intake and decreased potassium intake
   d. Increased sodium intake and increased fluid intake

5. Individuals taking the anticoagulant warfarin must be counseled to consume no more than one serving per day of:
   a. Broccoli or spinach
   b. Vegetable oils
   c. Kale and parsley
   d. Dried apricots and dates

CLINICAL ANALYSIS

Mr. A is being admitted to a long-term care facility. He is a 45-year-old post-trauma client. The motor vehicle accident in which he became paralyzed below the waist also killed his wife and daughter. The accident occurred 6 months ago. In the meantime, he has been treated at a rehabilitation center. He is depressed and freely sharing his feelings of guilt and loss. The depression has interfered with his progress toward rehabilitation and also contributed to a 20-pound weight loss since the accident. After many trials of various antidepressants, he is now receiving phenelzine. The following questions relate to his care.

1. To ensure that everyone caring for Mr. A is alerted to potential complications related to his drug therapy, the nurse

begins a nursing care plan. The nursing diagnosis that best states this problem as described by the data is:
   a. Ineffective coping related to deaths of family members as evidenced by expressions of grief and guilt.
   b. Imbalanced nutrition, less than body requirements, related to inappropriate scheduling of medications in relation to meals.
   c. Deficient knowledge related to potential food-drug interaction between tyramine-containing foods and monoamine oxidase inhibitor.
   d. Noncompliance with dietary plan related to low motivation to return to the home he had shared with his wife and daughter.

2. Close attention to Mr. A's diet is essential. Which of the following foods will he have to avoid completely?
   a. Baked beans, dates, and roast beef
   b. Sugar, molasses, and maple syrup
   c. Bologna, cheddar cheese, and wine
   d. Green beans, whole-wheat bread, and oranges

3. When teaching nursing assistants about the dietary restrictions needed by Mr. A, the nurse should be sure the nursing assistants understand that:

a. The potential complication can be life-threatening.
b. Mr. A is to be kept unaware of the seriousness of his condition.
c. As time goes on, the forbidden foods can be added to the diet slowly, one at a time.
d. If Mr. A does not cooperate in his dietary care, his paralysis is likely to worsen.

REFERENCES

Alonzo-Aperte, E, and Varela-Moreiras, G: Drugs-nutrient interactions: A potential problem during adolescence. Eur J Clin Nutr 54:S69, 2000.

Ament, PW, Bertolino, JG, and Liszewski, JL: Clinically significant drug interactions. Am Fam Physician 61:1745, 2000. Accessed May 15, 2005 at http://www.aafp.org/afp/20000315/1745.html.

Anderson, GD: Sex differences in drug metabolism: Cytochrome P-450 and uridine diphosphate glucoronosyltransferase. J Gender Specific Med 5:25, 2002.

Best, TH, et al: Cardiac complications in pediatric patients on the ketogenic diet. Neurology 54:2328, 2000.

Bhat, RV, and Deshmukh, CT: A study of vitamin K status in children on prolonged antibiotic therapy. Indian Pediatr 40:36, 2003.

Brasic, JR: Risks of the consumption of beverages containing quinine. Psychol Rep 93:1022, 2003.

Brown, JE: Nutrition Through the Life Cycle, ed 2. Thomson Wadsworth, Belmont, CA, 2005.

Carrillo, JA, and Benitez, J: Clinically significant pharmacokinetic interactions between dietary caffeine and medications. Clin Pharmacokinet 39:127, 2000.

Chasman, DT, et al: Pharmacogenetic study of statin therapy and cholesterol reduction. JAMA 291:2821, 2004.

Dahan, A, and Altman, H: Food-drug interaction: Grapefruit juice augments drug bioavailability—mechanism, extent and relevance. Eur J Clin Nutr 58:1, 2004.

Deglin, JH, and Vallerand, AH: Davis's Drug Guide for Nurses, ed 9. FA Davis, Philadelphia, 2005.

Dellow, EL, Unwin, RH, and Honour, JW: Pontefract cakes can be bad for you: Refractory hypertension and liquorice excess. Nephrol Dial Transplant 14:218, 1999.

DiMario, FJ, and Holland, J: The ketogenic diet: A review of the experience at Connecticut Children's Medical Center. Pediatr Neurol 26:288, 2002.

Dochterman, J, and Bulechek, G (eds): Nursing Interventions Classification (NIC), ed 4. Mosby, St. Louis, 2004.

Elinav, E, and Chajek-Shaul, T: Licorice consumption causing severe hypokalemic paralysis. Mayo Clin Proc 78:767, 2003.

Finch, C: Medication and enteral tube feedings: Clinically significant interactions. J Crit Illn 16:20, 2001.

Fitzgerald, MA: What do I need to know about drug interactions with enteral feedings? Medscape Nurses. Accessed March 9, 2005 at http://www.medscape.com/viewarticle/498270.

Franco, V, et al: Role of vitamin K intake in chronic oral anticoagulation: Prospective evidence from observational and randomized protocols. Am J Med 116:651, 2004.

Grant, P: Warfarin and cranberry juice: An interaction? J Heart Valve Dis 13:25, 2004.

Gregg, CR: Drug interactions and anti-infective therapies. Am J Med 106:227, 1999.

Gropper, SS, Smith, JL, and Groff, JL: Advanced Nutrition and Human Metabolism, ed 4. Wadsworth, Belmont, CA, 2005.

Haga, SB, and Burke, W: Using pharmacogenetics to improve drug safety and efficacy. JAMA 291:2869, 2004.

Harris, RZ, Jang, GR, and Tsunoda, S: Dietary effects on drug metabolism and transport. Clin Pharmacokinet 42:1071, 2003.

Hemingway, C, et al: The ketogenic diet: A 3- to 6-year follow-up of 150 children enrolled prospectively. Pediatrics 108:898, 2001.

Huang, SM, and Lesko, LJ: Drug-drug, drug-dietary supplement, and drug-citrus fruit and other food interactions: What have we learned? J Clin Pharmacol 44:559, 2004.

Kaaja, E, Kaaja, R, and Hiilesmaa, V: Major malformations in offspring of women with epilepsy. Neurology 60:575, 2003.

Kane, GC, and Lipsky, JJ: Drug-grapefruit juice interactions. Mayo Clin Proc 75:933, 2000.

Kaufman, DW, et al: Recent patterns of medication use in the ambulatory adult population of the United States. JAMA 287:337, 2002.

Kaur, S, et al: Pellagrous dermatitis induced by phenytoin [letter]. Pediatr Dermatol 19:93, 2002.

Kelly, MP, et al: A diagnostically reasoned case study with particular emphasis on B_6 and zinc imbalance directed by clinical history and nutrition physical examination findings. Nutr Clin Pract 13:32, 1998.

Kielb, S, et al: Nephrolithiasis associated with the ketogenic diet. J Urol 164:464, 2000.

Kobayashi, K, et al: Cerebral hemorrhage associated with vitamin K deficiency in congenital tuberculosis treated with isoniazid and rifampin. Pediatr Infect Dis J 21:1088, 2002.

Levy, R, and Cooper, P: Ketogenic diet for epilepsy. Cochrane Database Syst Rev 3:CD001903, 2003.

Lightstone, L, et al: Reasons for failure of the ketogenic diet. J Neurosci Nurs 33:292, 2001.

Likhodii, SS, and Bernham, WM: Ketogenic diet: Does acetone stop seizures? Med Sci Monit 8:HY 19, 2002.

Lin, SH, et al: An unusual cause of hypokalemic paralysis: Chronic licorice ingestion. Am J Med Sci 325:153, 2003.

Linus Pauling Institute: Vitamin D. Oregon State University. Accessed April 15, 2004 at http://lpi.oregonstate.edu/infocenter/vitamins/vitaminD.

Lussana, F, et al: Blood levels of homocysteine, folate, vitamin B_6 and B_{12} in women using oral contraceptives compared to nonusers. Thromb Res 112:37, 2003.

Lyon, VB, and Fairley, JA: Anticonvulsant-induced pellagra. J Am Acad Dermatol 46:597, 2002.

Mamdani, M, et al: Warfarin therapy and risk of hip fracture among elderly patients. Pharmacotherapy 23:1, 2003.

Mandel, A, et al: Medical costs are reduced when children with intractable epilepsy are successfully treated with the ketogenic diet. J Am Diet Assoc 102:396, 2002.

Mirtallo, JM: Complications associated with drug and nutrient interactions. J Infus Nurs 27:19, 2004.

Moorhead, S, Johnson, M, and Maas, M (eds): Nursing Outcomes Classification (NOC), ed 3. Mosby, St. Louis, 2004.

Morrell, MJ: Guidelines for the care of women with epilepsy. Neurology 51(Suppl 14):S21, 1998.

NANDA International: Nursing Diagnoses: Definitions and Classification, 2003–2004. NANDA International, Philadelphia, 2003.

Ozturk, F, et al: Pellagra: A sporadic pediatric case with a full triad of symptoms. Cutis 68:31, 2001.

Pennell, PB: The importance of monotherapy in pregnancy. Neurology 60(Suppl 4):S31, 2003.

Ray, KK, Dorman, S, and Watson, RDS: Severe hyperkalemia due to the concomitant use of salt substitutes and ACE inhibitors in hypertension: A potentially life threatening interaction. J Hum Hypertens 13:717, 1999.

Rosener, M, and Dichgans, J: Severe combined degeneration of the spinal cord after nitrous oxide anesthesia in a vegetarian [letter]. J Neurol Neurosurg Psychiatry 60:354, 1996.

Sato, Y, et al: Long-term oral anticoagulation reduces bone mass in patients with previous hemispheric infarction and nonrheumatic atrial fibrillation. Stroke 28:2390, 1997.

Schmidt, LE, and Dalhoff, K: Food-drug interactions. Drugs 62:1481, 2002.

Smith, CH: Drug-food/food-drug interactions. In Morley, JE, Glick, Z, and Rubenstein, LZ (eds): Geriatric Nutrition, ed 2. Raven Press, New York, 1995.

Smith, JK, Aljazairi, A, and Fuller, SH: INR elevation associated with diarrhea in a patient receiving warfarin. Ann Pharmacother 33:301, 1999.

Society of Hospital Pharmacists of Hong Kong: Drug-enteral tube feeding interaction. Accessed May 15, 2005 at http://www.shphk.org.hk/index.php?option=com_content&task=view&id=200&Itemid=38

Suter, PM, et al: Diuretic use: a risk for subclinical thiamine deficiency in elderly patients. N Nutr Health Aging 4:69, 2000.

Sutterlin, MW, et al: Serum folate and vitamin B_{12} levels in women using modern oral contraceptives containing 20 microg ethinyl estradiol. Eur J Obstet Gynecol Reprod Biol 107:57, 2003.

Suvarna, R, Pirmohamed, M, and Henderson, L: Possible interaction between warfarin and cranberry juice. BMJ 327: 1454, 2003.

Taylor, JR, and Wilt, VM: Probable antagonism of warfarin by green tea. Ann Pharmacother 33:426, 1999.

Utermohlen, V: Diet, nutrition, and drug interactions. In Shils, ME, et al (eds): Modern Nutrition in Health and Disease, ed 9. Lippincott Williams & Wilkins, Philadelphia, 1999.

van der Weide, J, et al: The effect of genetic polymorphism of cytochrome P450 CYP2C9 on phenytoin dose requirement. Pharmacogenetics 11:287, 2001.

Vining, EP, et al: Growth of children on the ketogenic diet. Dev Med Child Neurol 44:796, 2002.

Wagner, GH, Diffey, BL, and Ive, FA: "I'll have mine with a twist of lemon": Quinine photosensitivity from excessive intake of tonic water [letter]. Br J Dermatol 131:734, 1994.

Yaffe, SJ, and Sonawane, BR: Drug therapy and the role of nutrition. In Walker, WA, and Watkins, JB: Nutrition in Pediatrics, ed 2. BC Decker, Hamilton, Ontario, 1997.

Youdim, MB, and Weinstock, M: Therapeutic applications of selective and non-selective inhibitors of monoamine oxidase A and B that do not cause significant tyramine potentiation. Neurotoxicology 25:243, 2004.

CHAPTER 18

Weight Control

Learning Objectives

After completing this chapter, the student should be able to:

1. List basic principles of energy imbalance.
2. Discuss the effects of weight loss on the body.
3. Identify the medical, psychological, and social problems associated with too much and too little body fat.
4. Discuss the federal guidelines for the identification, evaluation, and treatment of overweight and obesity in adults.
5. Describe the symptoms commonly exhibited by a client with anorexia nervosa and/or bulimia.
6. Evaluate at least three fad diets used for weight reduction.

Weight management and control are issues for many people. Obesity accounts for more than $93 billion in direct health-care expenses each year (Manson and Bassuk, 2003). It has been estimated that 280,000 people each year die from complications related to excess weight (Gendreau, 2003). Forty-four percent of women and 29 percent of men reported trying to lose weight at any given time (Serdula et al, 1999). Approximately 85 percent of those who lose weight will regain their original weight within 5 years (Saltzman, 2004). Although this sounds dismal, 15 percent of all people who lose weight are successful over the long term. Weight control, although difficult, is not impossible, and the financial and health benefits of weight control both to the individual and society are enormous. The federal government published guidelines on the identification, evaluation, and treatment of overweight and obesity in the United States. The information in this chapter is consistent with these guidelines.

This chapter discusses (1) terminology and classification, (2) the prevalence of energy imbalance, (3) basic scientific principles of energy metabolism and body composition, (4) consequences of obesity, (5) theories about obesity, (6) screening clients for treatment (7) Federal Guidelines on the Identification, Evaluation, and Treatment of Overweight and Obesity, and (8) reduced body mass.

The goal of this chapter is to provide a foundation to enable the evaluation of further research and treatment options. On a more personal level, the hope is that the reader who wants to control body weight may find the motivation and gain practical information on how to do this safely.

Terminology and Classification

The classification of an individual as underweight, normal weight, overweight, mildly obese, moderately obese, or severely or extremely obese historically has been difficult for the scientific community. How a person is classified often determines whether treatment is indicated and the kind of treatment that is appropriate. **Obesity** and, to a lesser extent, overweight are characterized by an excess accumulation of body fat. Height-weight tables, for lack of a better method, have been widely used historically to assist the health-care community in the classification of overly fat clients. Athletes and athletic clubs frequently use percent body fat for individual evaluation. The National Institutes of Health recommends the use of body mass index (BMI) by health-care professionals. Height-weight tables, percent body fat, and body mass index are discussed separately in the following sections, along with the merits and limitations of each method.

Height and Weight

Percent body weight is computed from height-weight tables. The Metropolitan Life Insurance Company produced the first height-weight table in 1942. The original purpose of this table was to determine life insurance rates based on life expectancy studies. People who weighed more than the amounts recommended on the tables either paid higher premiums or were rejected when they applied for life insurance. The medical community adopted these tables for health purposes.

The term ***ideal body weight*** means a person's weight as compared to the weight in the Ideal Height-Weight Table. The Metropolitan Life Insurance Company released the Ideal Height-Weight Table in 1943. The term ***desirable*** *body weight* means a person's weight as compared to the weight shown on the Desirable Height-Weight Table, which the Metropolitan Life Insurance Company released in 1959. The data used to compile these tables were based on extensive mortality studies of insured lives conducted by the Association of Life Insurance Medical Directors of America and Society of Actuaries.

In 1983, the Metropolitan Life Insurance Company issued a new table. This table is based on mortality data collected from the 1979 Build Study. Data collected showed that a modest increase in weight (2 to 13 pounds) did not result in a decreased life expectancy. Thus, the weights in the 1983 table are about 2 to 13 pounds heavier than those in the 1959 table in each gender, frame size, and height category. The weights on this table are not necessarily based on a healthy body weight but on death rates. In this text, the 1983 Height-Weight Table is used.

Much controversy exists concerning which height-weight table best meets the health needs of the population. In fact, many other organizations and researchers have developed their own height-weight tables because of a dissatisfaction with the Metropolitan Life Insurance Company's tables. It is important to realize that height-weight tables of the Metropolitan Life Insurance Company are based on mortality (death rates), which are not necessarily the weights at which people are healthy, perform their jobs optimally, or even look their best. Height-weight tables cannot replace a thorough body audit, an accurate diet history, information about exercise patterns, or measurement of a client's body fat content.

Percent Reasonable Body Weight

Mild, moderate, and extreme obesity are often expressed in terms of percent reasonable body weight (RBW). *Overweight* is often used to mean 10 to 20 percent above RBW. *Obese* is often used to mean more than 20 percent above RBW. The obese client may be classified further as:

- **mildly obese:** 20 to 40 percent overweight, or 120 to 140 percent RBW
- **moderately obese:** 41 to 100 percent overweight, or 141 to 200 percent RBW
- **severely (extremely) obese:** greater than 100 percent overweight, or 200 percent RBW

All researchers and the medical community do not universally accept the classification of the degree of obesity by this method. However, some members of the medical community use this method in medical record documentation.

Percent Body Fat

The terms *overweight* and *obesity* are used to describe excessive accumulations of body fat that are detrimental to health and well-being. Although an RBW expressed as a percent over 120 or a body mass index in excess of 30 kg/m^2 may alert the health-care worker that the client may be overly fat, this is not always foolproof. Two examples are discussed next to illustrate this concept.

First, consider a 5-foot 4-inch female (without shoes) with a medium frame weighed with indoor clothing. According

to the 1983 Metropolitan Height and Weight Table for Adults, she should weigh 127 to 141 pounds. Let's review the calculation of RBW. Subtract 127 pounds from 141 pounds for a difference of 14 pounds. Divide 14 pounds by 2 for an answer of 7 pounds. Add 7 pounds to 127 pounds for a sum of 134 pounds. A weight of 134 pounds is this client's RBW. Let's say this client weighs 134 pounds. Her RBW would be 100 percent. Can we automatically conclude that this client is not obese? The answer is no. The optimal fat content for females is 18 to 22 percent. A more accurate definition of *obesity for females* is a fat content greater than 33 percent. A person at her reasonable body weight is metabolically obese if her body fat content exceeds 33 percent. The female in this example may have all the health risks of obesity even at 100 percent RBW if her body fat content exceeds 33 percent. Some researchers believe that a percent body fat of 30 classifies a person as obese. The medical and scientific communities do not universally accept the definitions of obesity.

Second, consider a 5-foot 9-inch male (without shoes) with a medium frame size weighed with indoor clothing. According to the Metropolitan Height and Weight Table for Adults, this individual should weigh 158 to 180 pounds. The same process can be used to derive his reasonable body weight. First, subtract 158 pounds from 180 pounds for an answer of 22 pounds. Next, divide 22 pounds by 2 for an answer of 11 pounds. Add 11 pounds to 158 pounds to calculate his RBW, which is 169 pounds. Let's say this client weights 225 pounds. That weight, 225 pounds, divided by 169 pounds equals 133 percent. Can we automatically classify this client as moderately obese? The answer is again no. This client may have a body fat content of only 15 percent. The optimal fat content for males is 15 to 19 percent. This individual may be a trained athlete and the excess weight the result of increased muscle mass. A fat content in excess of 25 percent is considered *obese for males*. Some researchers dispute this numerical value and believe it should be lower.

At least half of body fat is located subcutaneously (just beneath the skin). Therefore, the measurement of skinfold thickness is commonly used to estimate a person's body fat content. In this chapter, the four-site measurement technique to determine percent body fat is discussed. This technique requires minimal calculations. Figure 18–1 (A, B, C, D) illustrates how to perform these measurements.

The worksheet in Clinical Calculation 18–1 can be used to calculate a client's percent body fat using skin calipers. A total of 12 measurements should be taken at four different sites. The three numbers obtained at each site are added together and averaged to give a value of one number per site. All of these numbers are added together and compared with the number on a standard table to determine the client's percent body fat. A standard table is provided in Appendix E. This procedure takes time and requires accurate measurements.

Other techniques to estimate body fat involve underwater weighing, tissue x-rays, ultrasound, electrical conductivity, electrical impedance, computed tomographic scans, and magnetic resonance imaging scans. Electrical impedance is widely used in athletic clubs and gyms (Fig. 18–2). The other procedures are expensive and not

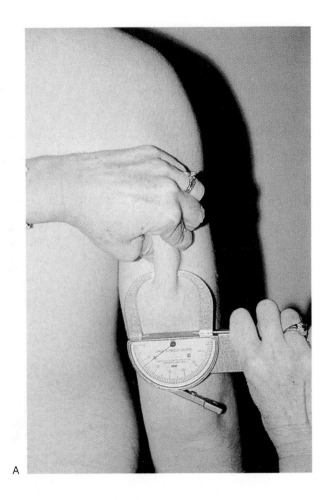

A

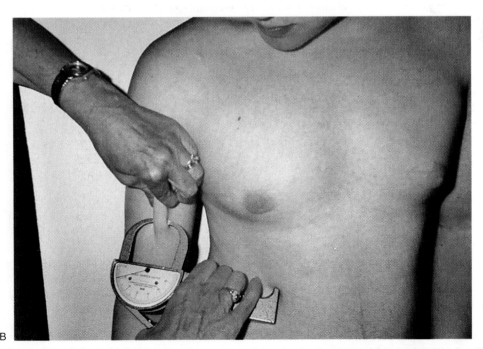

B

Figure 18–1 Directions for skin calipers. A, Triceps: Between the tip of the olecranon process of the ulna (elbow) and the scapula (shoulder). B, Biceps-midpoint muscle belly: This will generally be a point on the arm just opposite the nipple. C, Subscapular: Below tip inferior angle scapula 45 degrees to vertical (back, just under shoulder blade). D, Suprailiac: Above the iliac crest in mid-axillary line (approximately 2.5 cm above the hip bone).

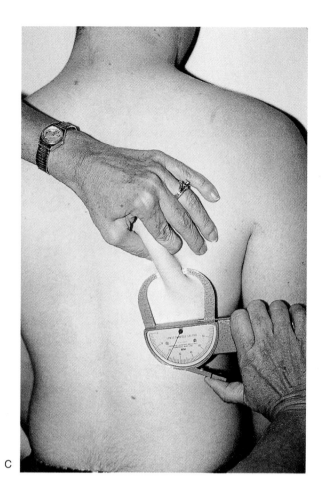

C

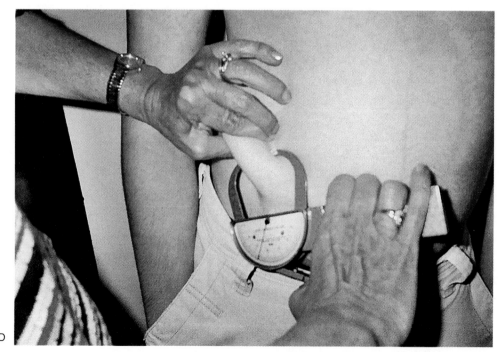

D

Figure **18-1** *(Continued)*

Clinical Calculation 18–1

Calculating Body Fat Content Using the Four-Site Technique

Worksheet for Calculating Percent Body Fat Using Skin Calipers

SKINFOLD MEASUREMENTS	1	2	3	=	TOTAL ÷ 3 = AVERAGE
Biceps		+	+	=	
Triceps		+	+	=	
Subscapular		+	+	=	
Suprailiac		+	+	=	

Total value of the average of four sites: _____

Procedure to Calculate Percent Body Fat Using Skin Calipers in Adults

1. Take skinfold measurements directly on the skin, not through clothing.
2. Pick up and hold the skinfold with one hand while measuring it with calipers held by the other hand.
3. Take three measurements at each of the four sites. Then average the three measurements of each skinfold to arrive at a final figure.

   - Biceps: measure the muscle belly of the biceps. This will generally be a point on the straightened arm just opposite the nipple.
   - Triceps
   - Subscapular: measure on the back just under the shoulder blade.
   - Suprailiac: measure approximately 1 inch above the hip bone.

4. Add the averages of all skinfold sites to arrive at a total skinfold measurement.
5. To determine the percent body fat, compare the total measurement with the values in the appropriate Body Fat and Skinfolds table located in Appendix E.

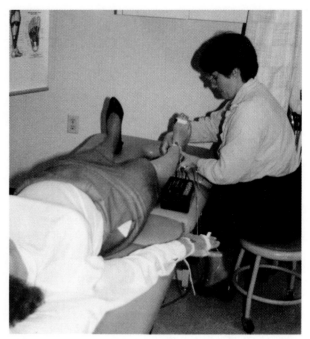

Figure **18–2** The measurement of a client's percent body fat using bioelectrical impedance. This method is widely used by athletes to measure changes in body composition as a result of training. For example, a decrease in percent body fat and a stable body weight indicate an increase in muscle mass.

available in clinical settings. Limitations include less accuracy in extremely obese persons, states of overhydration and underhydration, hormone abnormalities, and the need for a qualified technician; these are of limited usefulness for persons trying to lose weight.

Body Mass Index

A client's **body mass index (BMI)** is his or her body weight in kilograms divided by height in meters squared. BMI can be determined without doing any calculations by using a body mass index chart (Table 18–1). The BMI is an indicator of optimal weight for health and is different from lean body mass or percent body fat calculations because it considers only height and weight. A BMI of 20 to 25 kilograms per meter squared is normal. Overweight clients have a BMI of 25 to 30. Obese clients have a BMI above 30 (National Institutes of Health, 1998). Severe or extreme obesity is characterized by a BMI above 40. The BMI can also be used to estimate relative risk for disease compared

to people of normal weight. Table 18–2 classifies overweight and obesity by BMI. The National Institutes of Health (NIH) recommends and encourages all health-care professionals to use BMI to classify clients as underweight, normal weight, overweight, and so on in clinical settings.

Waist Circumference

Although BMI and waist circumference are frequently correlated, this is not always the case. For example, a person with thin arms and legs may have a low BMI and a high waist circumference. Because an individual with abdominal obesity is at a greater health risk than an individual with gluteal-femoral obesity, the panel recommends that the waist circumference be used to assess abdominal fat content. Men with a waist circumference greater than 40 inches, or 102 cm, and women with a waist circumference greater than 35 inches, or 88 cm, are at a high risk. A high waist circumference with a high BMI increases disease risk. In some populations, waist circumference is a better indicator of relative disease risk than is BMI; examples include Asian-Americans and persons of Asian descent living elsewhere. Waist circumference also assumes greater value at older ages. Individuals with a BMI greater than 35 kg/m² do not usually need to have their waist circumference measured because it usually is greater than the 40 and 35 inches.

Prevalence and Incidence of Overweight and Obesity

Prevalence means the total number of cases of a specific disease divided by the number of individuals in

Table 18–1   Body Mass Index Chart

BMI	19	20	21	22	23	24	25	26	27	28	29	30	31	32	33	34	35	36
HEIGHT (INCHES)								**BODY WEIGHT (POUNDS)**										
58	91	96	100	105	110	115	119	124	129	134	138	143	148	153	158	162	167	172
59	94	99	104	109	114	119	124	128	133	138	143	148	153	158	163	168	173	178
60	97	102	107	119	118	123	128	133	138	143	148	153	158	163	168	174	179	184
61	100	106	111	116	122	127	132	137	143	148	153	158	164	169	174	180	185	190
62	104	109	115	120	126	131	136	142	147	153	158	164	169	175	180	186	191	196
63	107	113	118	124	130	135	141	146	152	158	163	169	175	180	186	191	197	203
64	110	116	122	128	134	140	145	151	157	163	169	174	180	186	192	197	204	209
65	114	120	126	132	138	144	150	156	162	168	174	180	186	199	198	204	210	216
66	118	124	130	136	142	148	155	161	167	173	179	186	192	198	204	210	216	223
67	121	127	134	140	146	153	159	166	172	178	185	191	198	204	211	217	223	230
68	125	131	138	144	151	158	164	171	177	184	190	197	203	210	216	223	230	236
69	128	135	142	149	155	162	169	176	182	189	196	203	209	216	223	230	236	243
70	132	139	146	153	160	167	174	181	188	195	202	209	216	222	229	236	243	250
71	136	143	150	157	165	172	179	186	193	200	208	215	222	229	236	243	250	257
72	140	147	154	162	169	177	184	191	199	206	213	221	228	235	242	250	258	265
73	144	151	159	166	174	182	189	197	204	212	219	227	235	242	250	257	265	272
74	148	155	163	171	179	186	194	202	210	218	225	233	241	249	256	264	272	280
75	152	160	168	176	184	192	200	208	216	224	232	240	248	256	264	272	279	287
76	156	164	172	180	189	197	205	213	221	230	238	246	254	263	271	279	287	295

BMI	37	38	39	40	41	42	43	44	45	46	47	48	49	50	51	52	53	54
HEIGHT (INCHES)								**BODY WEIGHT (POUNDS)**										
58	177	181	186	191	196	201	205	210	215	220	224	229	234	239	244	248	353	258
59	183	188	193	198	203	208	212	217	222	227	232	237	242	247	252	257	262	267
60	189	194	199	204	209	215	220	225	230	235	240	245	250	255	261	266	271	276
61	195	201	206	211	217	222	227	232	238	243	248	254	259	264	269	275	280	285
62	202	207	213	218	224	229	235	240	246	251	256	262	267	273	778	284	289	295
63	208	214	220	225	231	237	242	248	254	259	265	270	278	282	287	293	299	304
64	215	221	227	239	238	244	250	256	262	267	273	279	285	291	296	302	308	314
65	292	228	234	240	246	252	258	264	270	276	282	288	294	300	306	312	318	324
66	229	235	241	247	253	260	266	272	278	284	291	297	303	309	315	322	398	334
67	336	242	249	255	261	268	274	280	287	293	299	306	312	319	399	331	338	344
68	243	249	256	262	269	276	282	289	295	302	308	315	329	328	335	341	348	354
69	250	257	263	270	277	284	291	297	304	311	318	324	331	338	349	351	358	365
70	257	264	271	278	285	292	299	306	313	320	327	334	341	348	355	362	369	376
71	265	272	279	286	293	301	308	315	322	329	338	343	351	358	365	379	379	386
72	272	279	287	294	302	309	316	324	331	338	346	353	361	368	375	383	390	397
73	280	288	295	302	310	318	325	333	340	348	355	363	371	378	386	393	401	408
74	287	295	303	311	319	326	334	342	350	358	365	373	381	389	396	404	419	420
75	295	303	311	319	397	335	343	351	359	367	375	383	391	399	407	415	423	431
76	304	312	320	328	336	344	353	361	369	377	385	394	402	410	418	496	435	443

To use the table, find the appropriate height in the left-hand column. Move across to a given weight. The number at the top of the column is the BMI at that height and weight. Pounds have been rounded off.

Table 18–2   Classification of Overweight and Obesity by Body Mass Index (BMI)

	OBESITY CLASS	BMI (kg/m^2)
Underweight		<18.5
Normal		18.5 to 24.9
Overweight		25.0 to 29.9
Obesity	I	30.0 to 34.9
	II	35.0 to 39.9
Severe or Extreme Obesity	III	≥40

SOURCE: National Institutes of Health: Clinical Guidelines on the Identification, Evaluation, and Treatment of Overweight and Obesity, 1998.

the population at a certain time. Currently, about 66 percent of U.S. adults are classified as overweight or obese, compared with 25 percent in the 1960s (Manson and Bassuk, 2003). Thirty-four percent of the adult population is overweight (BMI 25 to 29.9). Twenty-seven percent is obese (BMI 30 to 39.9) (Yanovski and Yanovski, 2002). The prevalence of clinically extreme (severe) obesity (≥100 pounds overweight or BMI >40) is increasing much faster than obesity (Sturm, 2003).

Many experts are concerned about the incidence and prevalence of obesity in the nation's children. **Incidence** is defined as the frequency of occurrence of any event or condition over time and in relation to the population in which it occurs. Asian children have the lowest incidence of obesity. Native Americans have the highest incidence of obesity. Several studies suggest that one-third or more infants in the Western industrialized world are too heavy. The prevalence of overweight children and adolescence (defined as BMI in the 95th percentile or higher for age and sex) has more than doubled since 1976 (Manson and Bassuk, 2003). Current statistics from the National Center for Health Statistics estimate obesity prevalence to be 20 percent among young adults (National Center for Health Statistics, 2003).

Basic Science of Energy Imbalance

Nutrition is a science supported by a research base. The scientific method to understanding anything involves recognizing a problem, formulating a hypothesis (or question), accumulating data that answer the question, and analyzing the findings, as distinguished from an intuitive approach. As health-care providers, we have a responsibility to understand the basic science behind the information we disseminate. The federal government's guidelines are based on science. The recommendations are based on evidence that has been replicated or a joint consensus of expert judgment. Nursing students are encouraged to take a course in scientific methodology to learn how to evaluate scientific research. The science of nutrition is based on peer-reviewed research that can be replicated. Yet all scientific information should be critically read and evaluated.

Energy Imbalance

Energy imbalance results when the number of **kilocalories** eaten does not equal the number used for energy. An individual can determine whether food intake is meeting energy needs by monitoring his or her weight. If more kilocalories are eaten than are used by the body, weight gain will occur. If fewer kilocalories are eaten than are used by the body (and protein intake is adequate), weight loss will occur. (A low-protein intake over an extended period will eventually lead to fluid retention and a subsequent weight gain from the fluid retained. In this situation, energy imbalance is difficult to ascertain by body weight alone.) In cases in which a single health-care provider or a group with access to the medical record follows the progress of a client for an extended time, energy balance can be assessed by monitoring the normally hydrated client's weight history.

There are two basic principles of energy imbalance. First, it takes a specific number of kilocalories to gain or lose a pound of body fat. Second, the body stores energy and uses stored energy in a highly specific manner.

The Five-Hundred Rule

To lose 1 pound of body fat per week, an individual must eat 500 kilocalories fewer per day than his or her body *expends* for 7 days. To gain 1 pound of body fat per week, the individual must eat 500 kilocalories more per day for 7 days than his or her body expends. The gain or loss of body fat need not occur during the course of a week; the kilocalorie surplus or deficit may occur over a month or year. The principle is the same. The total number of kilocalories required to gain or lose a pound of body fat is 3500. Wellness Tip 18–1 discusses one implication of the five-hundred rule.

 18–1 • Too many kilocalories from any source of carbohydrates, fat, and/or protein promote weight gain.

The five-hundred rule means that weight loss is independent of diet composition. It does not matter whether the kcalories are from fat, carbohydrate, or protein—eating more kcalories than the body expends will result in weight gain.

Body Fat Stores

Excess kilocalories from any source (fat, carbohydrate, or protein) are stored as body fat in adipose tissue. The human body is able to store adipose fat tissue in unlimited amounts. This can lead to overweight and, eventually, obesity. During a kilocalorie deficit, the body first seeks the energy necessary to sustain body functions in glycogen stores, which are limited. When a kilocalorie deficit occurs for longer than about 1 day, the body seeks the energy necessary to sustain its functions in both body fat stores (adipose tissue) and body protein stores (organ and muscle mass).

Energy Imbalance and Body Composition

Weight loss affects body composition, and body composition affects health. The human body's two largest components are fat and lean body mass that includes protein. Protein is stored primarily in muscle tissue, organs, and certain body chemicals. Preservation of lean body mass and optimal health goes hand in hand. A loss of structural body content (e.g., heart and respiratory muscles, kidney, liver, body chemicals) is undesirable. Exercise can preserve and somewhat increase lean body mass. Weight gain increases body fat content. Weight loss decreases both body fat and lean body mass. An understanding of the difference between body fat content and lean body mass content is crucial to understanding the science of energy imbalance. The health benefits of weight loss are all related to a loss of body fat and not a loss of lean body mass.

Loss of Fat Versus Loss of Water and Protein

Most people, especially the overweight, can lose only about 2 pounds of body fat a week by eating less. Any weight loss beyond that is probably due to loss of water and/or lean muscle tissue. There is always some loss of body protein along with body fat during weight loss. This is because lean body mass is more metabolically active and therefore burns more kilocalories than fat tissue. The loss of body protein from reduced food intake is greater than the loss of body protein from a combination of reduced food intake and regular exercise. Also, the greater the rate of weight loss, the more organ and muscle mass is lost.

Variation With the Severity of Obesity

Weight loss affects body composition of lean and obese people differently. The amount of lean body mass an individual loses during weight reduction depends on the degree of severity of his or her obesity. Obese animals tolerate starvation better than thin ones, and the same is true of humans (Forbes, 1999). *Tolerate* means that they conserve body protein during weight loss. This means overweight and mildly obese individuals are at a higher risk of becoming protein-depleted during rapid weight loss. Rapid weight loss (0.5 to 1.0 pounds per day), if sustained for many weeks, is associated with an excessive loss of lean body mass and protein depletion of the heart (Van Itallie, 1988). Malnutrition of the heart muscle can lead to sudden death. As individuals lose more and more fat during rapid weight loss, their ability to conserve lean body mass decreases. Thus, the length of time an individual diets as well as his or her beginning total body fat content has an impact on the amount of lean body mass lost.

Consequences of Obesity

The problems of obesity can lead to many adverse consequences. The distribution of body fat affects a person's susceptibility to medical problems, and the **psychological** ramifications of obesity are significant. Clients are often enmeshed in a tangle of cultural, religious, emotional, societal, and perceptual issues. Many clients find great difficulty in breaking the cycle of behaviors that contribute to obesity. A greater understanding of each issue equips the health-care provider with the tools necessary to educate and encourage overweight and obese clients.

Social

The social consequences of obesity are connected to cultural expectations and the documented prejudice many obese people experience.

Cultural Expectations

Culture, in this context, refers to the convictions of a given people during a given period. Currently, many Americans are preoccupied with leanness. Leanness is perceived as being attractive and desirable. Fatness is perceived as being unattractive and undesirable. Yet what is and has been considered attractive has changed over time. Leanness has not

always been the preferred body build. For example, during the 1800s, the overly fat body was considered the most attractive. Carrying excess weight meant that the person was well-to-do, that he or she could afford to overeat. Many experts think that our society is slowly changing perceptions of what is attractive. For example, women with well-developed muscles are perceived as being more attractive to many than her lean, not-so-muscular counterparts. The increased numbers of female bodybuilders demonstrate this attitudinal change.

In the United States, obese people have been under intense pressure to lose weight. This is evidenced by billions of dollars being spent on weight-reduction programs and special foods each year. In an effort to be more attractive, many obese clients try to lose weight. Over time, however, most people regain the weight they have lost and often regain an additional few pounds over and above their original weight. Thus, a self-defeating cycle begins.

Prejudice Documented

Several classic studies show that obese persons are the objects of prejudice and unfair discrimination. In a 7-year follow-up study of women 16 to 24 years old, obese women were less likely to have been married and had less schooling, lower incomes, and higher rates of household poverty than those with other chronic medical conditions (Gortmaker et al, 1993; Canning and Mayer, 1966). Health-care workers should try to understand their own feelings about fatness, obesity, and obese persons. All too often, health-care workers insult obese clients without being aware of it. For example, comments made in front of clients, such as "It will take three of us to move this client," are hurtful. Clients benefit when health-care workers are sensitive to their psychological needs. Above all else, nurses should treat obese clients with respect, kindness, and patience.

Psychological

Obesity can be associated with a range of psychological problems, which may also result from food restriction (Box 18–1). One important psychological consequence of obesity is body image disturbances.

Box 18–1 **Psychological Consequences of Food Restriction**

Food restriction either voluntary or involuntary has consequences. Xenophon in ancient Greece described a "ravenous hunger" in soldiers who had been deprived of food during a military campaign (Stunkard, 1993). During World War II, Keyes et al studied the effects of semistarvation on subjects (Keyes et al, 1950). Cocina and Dixon studied the effects of food deprivation on rats (Cocina and Dixon, 1983). In all of these studies, the subjects responded to food deprivation with extraordinarily similar behaviors. First, restrained eaters did not necessarily have much, if any, long-term weight loss. Second, restraining one's eating made one highly susceptible to bouts of excessive eating even after restrictions are

lifted. Third, study subjects exhibited **cognitive** and emotional changes when food was restricted, including heightened emotional responsiveness; cognitive disruptions, including distractibility; and a focus on food and eating (Polivy, 1996).

Health-care providers need to caution clients about the consequences of restrained eating. Overweight clients need to be helped to give up their crash diets and to be advised to eat balanced healthful diets that include whole grains, fruits, vegetables, and nonfat dairy products. Abandonment of the short term "diet mentality" and adoption of long-term lifestyle changes will enhance physical and psychological well-being.

Body Image Disturbances

Body image is the mental picture a person has of himself or herself. A disturbed body image can manifest itself in two ways. First, people with distorted body images are usually dissatisfied with their bodies. Chronic complaints, demands for extra attention, and frequent negative statements made by clients about the way they look may be signs of an underlying body image disturbance. Second, persons with distorted body images frequently do not view their bodies realistically. For example, people may view themselves as having certain body parts larger than they actually are. A later section in this chapter discusses clients with anorexia nervosa, a mental health disorder, who frequently have body image disturbances. Very thin clients who have this condition frequently view themselves as overweight despite valid evidence to the contrary.

A classic study showed that body image disturbances are not found in emotionally healthy obese individuals (Stunkard and Mendelson, 1961). Body image disturbances are most common in young women of the middle and upper-middle classes who have been obese since childhood. Many of them have a generalized neurotic disturbance, and their parents and peers have criticized them for their obesity (Stunkard and Burt, 1967; Stunkard and Mendelson, 1961).

Medical

Obesity is considered a major health problem in the United States and is also considered a chronic medical condition. Excessive body weight has been associated with nonfatal disease risks and chronic disease.

Life Expectancy

One method to evaluate life expectancy for individuals is in terms of the number of years of life lost (YLL) because of a medical condition. The YLL is defined as the difference between the number of years a person would be expected to live if he/she did not have a condition and the number of years he/she could be expected to live with a medical condition. There are differences in YLL for obese people between whites and blacks, men and women, and young and old. For any given degree of overweight, young adults generally had more years of life lost then did older adults. Adult white men between 20 to 30 years with a severe degree of obesity (BMI >45) lost 13 years of life. Blacks at younger ages with severe levels of obesity had a YLL of 20 for men and 5 for women (Fontaine et al, 2003). Among black men and women older than 60 years, overweight and moderate obesity were generally not associated with YLL. Obesity lessens life expectancy for the young.

Disease Risk

Obesity is associated with many chronic diseases. Obesity is strongly linked to heart disease as well as high blood pressure, high cholesterol levels, and non-insulin-dependent diabetes mellitus. Even a moderately elevated BMI is a significant predictor of hypertension and of diabetes in both whites and blacks, and the incidence of these conditions increases similarly in both ethnic groups as BMI increases (Stevens et al, 2002). Obesity is also associated with sleep apnea, gallbladder disease, fatty liver, lung function impairment, endocrine abnormalities, childbearing and childbirth complications, trauma to the weight-bearing joints, excessive protein in the urine, **dysphoria,** and increased hemoglobin concentration. Overweight is a risk factor for dementia (Gustafson et al, 2003). Overweight men have higher rates for colorectal and prostate cancer, and overweight women have higher rates for cancer of the ovary and of the breast.

Metabolic syndrome, also called **dysmetabolic syndrome X,** is associated with excess body weight. This condition is characterized by abdominal obesity, elevated triglyceride levels, elevated small-density lipoprotein particles, elevated low high-density lipoprotein cholesterol, raised blood pressure, insulin resistance, and prothrombic proinflammatory states (Blackburn and Bevins, 2003). The complications of the syndrome can develop in fewer than 15 years. All components of the metabolic syndrome are positively affected by weight loss. Healthy weight loss-producing behaviors over a lifetime are associated with decreased insulin resistance, improved blood lipid levels, and reduced blood pressure levels.

Many nonfatal risks are also associated with obesity. A nonfatal risk is a hazard that does not decrease life expectancy but does decrease the quality of life for an individual. Back and joint pain is one example of a nonfatal health risk. Much research is underway to determine whether weight loss can prevent chronic diseases; however, once **comorbidity** factors are present, lifestyle strategies should be directed toward the improvement of metabolic parameters associated with the comorbidity (Franz, 1998). Poor blood glucose levels were more closely associated with heart disease among clients with diabetes than was body weight. Therefore, health-care providers may need to carefully consider whom they treat for obesity and why. Most experts recommend weight reduction counseling for the prevention of weight gain. On the other hand, treatment efforts for obese clients with a comorbidity such as diabetes should be directed at normalization of blood glucose and lipid levels first and weight reduction second.

The distribution of body fat affects risks. Abdominal obesity is more dangerous than gluteal-femoral obesity (Blackburn and Bevins, 2003). In **abdominal obesity** the excess weight is between the client's chest and pelvis. Clients with abdominal obesity are said to be shaped like an apple. Clients with abdominal obesity are especially vulnerable to chronic disease risks associated with excessive body weight. In **gluteal-femoral obesity** the excess weight is around the client's buttocks, hips, and thighs. Clients with gluteal-femoral obesity are said to be pear-shaped. Clients with gluteal-femoral obesity are not as susceptible to chronic disease risks associated with excessive body fat.

The treatment of obesity is an important means of controlling some major chronic and degenerative diseases. For example, blood pressure levels can be reduced by a diet high in fruits and vegetables and low in fat. Up to 2 1/2 cups of fruits and 4 cups of vegetables are recommended for a very active 18-year old male. Up to 1 1/2 cups of fruits and 2 cups of vegetables are recommended for a sedentary 65-year old female.

Factors That Influence Food Intake

Lifestyle behaviors, human physiology, and, questionably, macronutrient energy distribution influence food intake.

Lifestyle Behaviors

Behaviors affect how much is eaten. It has been known for over 20 years that the greater the variety of food served, the more kcalories will be spontaneously consumed. Buffets that offer dozens of food items are not a good idea for someone trying to lose weight. The effect of weekend days on kcaloric intake is substantial. One study found that people over the age of 2 consume more kcalories, fat, and alcohol Friday through Sunday compared with the rest of the week, with an average increase of 82 kcalories per day (Haines et al, 2003). This 82 kcalories equals 3.6 pounds of body fat per year. Eating at regular times and planning non-food-related activities for weekends may assist in weight control. People who regularly skip breakfast were 450 percent more likely to be obese. Those eating four or more times daily were 45 percent less likely to be obese (YunSheng et al, 2003). The fourth meal was a small snack. Skipping meals is not a good weight-control strategy. Eating meals away from home is associated with increased energy intake (CDC, 2004). The length of time spent chewing food is associated with food intake. The more foods need to be chewed, the less kilocalories are eaten. The intake of sweetened soda is associated with a positive energy balance (CDC, 2004). Soda, although not as concentrated a source of kilocalories as fat, may still contribute a significant source of kilocalories to the diet because of the amount often consumed. The faster food is eaten, the more is consumed. Serving hot soup at the beginning of a meal will slow down eating. Most people will wait for the soup to cool before consumption. This will slow down eating and can be a practical weight-control strategy. Eating patterns and behaviors influence food intake.

Lifestyle behaviors that are responsible for decreased energy expenditure also increase body weight. The more hours spent watching television, the less time is spent being physically active. The same can be said for computer and video games. The enjoyment of physical activity should start young. Examples of appropriate activities for young children include ballet lessons, tricycle or bike riding, walking daily with a family member, swimming lessons, and sledding (see Fig. 18–3). Small daily decreases in energy expenditure may be significant over the course of a year. Lifestyle behaviors such as the use of television remote controls, telephone extensions, and garage door openers all decrease energy expenditure. Communities need to develop safe areas for children to play. Local school districts should be encouraged to offer more opportunities for our young to be active in a noncompetitive environment. The totally sedentary child has the most health benefit to gain from physical activity and is more uncomfortable in a competitive situation.

Human Physiology

Numerous hormones and neuropeptides that stimulate or inhibit food intake through central or peripheral mecha-

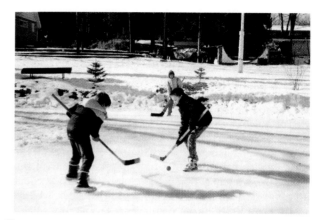

Figure **18–3** Youngsters who engage in year-round sports activities are better able to maintain their weight than others.

nisms have been identified and investigated in experimental models, as have molecules that affect metabolic rates and energy expenditure (Lowell and Spiegelman, 2000). Figure 18–4 illustrates multiple molecules and pathways involved in internal food intake regulation. In general, there is redundancy and counterbalance among these pathways so that, for instance, the inhibitory effect of one molecule is dampened by another. This complex redundancy and counterbalance makes the effective treatment of obesity complex. Perhaps in the future, as researchers learn more about the human energy balance system, more effective and safe treatments for energy imbalances may be available.

Macronutrient Energy Composition

Is it possible that a particular macronutrient composition (fat, CHO, and protein) might result in lower spontaneous energy intake, reduced hunger, and greater satiety? After a single meal, for example, the satiating power of protein is superior to carbohydrate, which in turn is superior to fat (Eisenstein et al, 2002). In one study after 6 months, subjects eating a diet with 25% protein, 45% CHO, and 30% fat consumed fewer kilocalories and lost more weight compared with those consuming a diet with 12% protein and a commensurate increase in CHO (Skov et al, 1999). In anther study published in 2003, subjects lost more weight initially on a 20-gram per day CHO diet than on a low-fat 1200- to 1500-kcal diet (Foster, Wyatt, and Hill, 2003). However, at the 12-month end of the study, the difference in weight between the lower and higher CHO diet group was no longer significant. It appears that reducing dietary CHO to very low levels may confer an advantage over several months. If hunger is suppressed and intake is reduced, this micronutrient mix might be an effective strategy for some (Saltzman, 2004). Critics of the very-low-carbohydrate diet cite potential effects on bone health and cardiovascular risk factors from a high-fat, high-protein diet. Consumption of high levels of saturated fats without adverse effects on cardiovascular disease is inconsistent with a large body of epidemiological and intervention data (Bonow and Eckel, 2003).

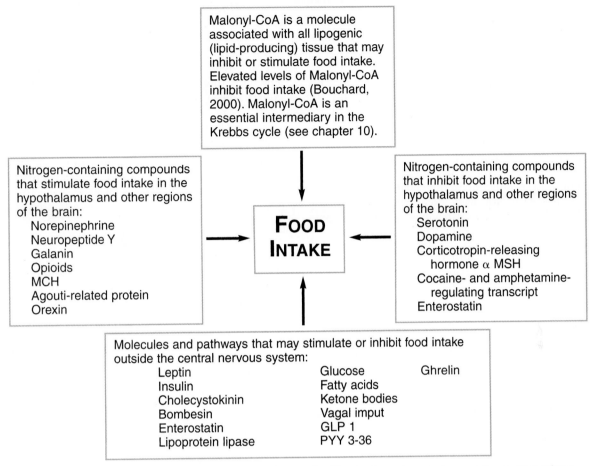

Figure 18–4 The hormones, molecules, and pathways that influence food intake through central or peripheral mechanisms. (Adapted from Bouchard, C: Inhibition of food intake by inhibitors of fatty acid synthase. N Engl J Med 343:25, 1889, 2000.)

Glycemic Index

Some people believe that eating carbohydrates that have a low glycemic index (GI) may result in a spontaneous reduction in food intake. GI is a measure of how much the blood glucose level increases following consumption of a particular food that contains a given amount of CHO. A slice of white bread or glucose is the reference food. All other foods' GIs are set in comparison to white bread or glucose and are ranked according to their potential to raise blood glucose as compared with the reference white bread or glucose. Foods with a low GI are thought to promote satiety and decrease food intake. The glycemic index of mixed meals is not known. Following are some examples of the glycemic index of selected foods. Note the reference food is white bread:

- White Bread 100
- Glucose 138
- Fructose 26
- Honey 126
- Whole-Wheat Bread 100
- Rye, (whole grain), pumpernickel 88
- Cornflakes 121
- Banana 84
- Baked Potato 116
- Kidney Beans, canned 74
- Ice Cream 69
- Sucrose 83
- White Rice, polished (boiled 10–25 minutes) 81
- Oatmeal 85
- All-Bran 74
- Plum 34
- Sweet Potato 70
- Lentils, (green canned) 74
- Skim Milk 46
- Orange 59
- Orange juice 71
- Yogurt 52
- Soybeans, (canned) 22

Many factors influence a food's glycemic index. The rate of consumption and the time of day a food is eaten may increase or decrease a particular food's GI. Other components in a food besides carbohydrate influence a food's GI, including fat, fiber, and protein content and starch characteristics. How the food is cooked and processed influences GI. Physiologic effects, including pregastric hydrolysis, gastric emptying rate, intestinal response, hydrolysis and absorption, pancreatic and gut hormone response, and colonic effects, influence a food's GI. Nondietary factors that influence a food's GI include medications taken, stress, physical activity, and overall health status.

Clinical use of glycemic index as a guide to food selection may provide a health benefit and appears to be without adverse effects. Hints to incorporate the GI into the diet follow:

- Keep it simple—substitute whole grains and fresh fruits and beans for lower-GI foods.
- Focus on foods that contribute the most CHO, such as bread, breakfast foods, and potatoes.
- Do not worry about foods that contribute 5 or less grams of CHO in a serving. Some nutritionally dense foods, such as carrots, have a higher GI but low amount of total CHO in a serving.

Obesity and Poor Metabolism

Some obese individuals actually require fewer kilocalories for normal body functions than do lean individuals. Some obese individuals use kilocalories very efficiently and may have poor metabolism.

THE FUNCTION OF BROWN FAT

Brown fat, a special type of fat cell, accounts for less than 1 percent of total body weight. The function of brown fat is to burn kilocalories and release the energy as heat. Energy released as heat is not stored as body fat. Some obese people may have defective brown fat or less brown fat than lean people.

THE SET POINT THEORY

The set point theory argues that each individual has a unique, relatively stable, adult body weight that is the result of several biologic factors. The obese person may have a higher set point than his or her lean counterpart.

THE NUMBER OF FAT CELLS

Obese individuals have many more fat cells than do their lean counterparts. A kilocalorie deficit can reduce the fat in each cell but cannot break down the entire cell. Once manufactured, a fat cell exists until death. Empty fat cells pressure the reduced obese person to fill the depleted cells. The reduced obese person must learn to constantly ignore internal hunger signals. Although obese individuals are able to do this for a short period, long-term adaptation to hunger pains is difficult.

ENZYMES IN THE METABOLIC CHAIN

Lipoprotein lipase is an enzyme that is involved in the uptake of fatty acids for the manufacture of fat in individual fat cells. Research has shown that the activity of this enzyme increases during weight reduction. This action makes the fat cell even more efficient in synthesizing fats.

Theories About Obesity

Theories about obesity are plentiful (Box 18–2). The truth may be that any one of these theories is accurate for a specific client but that none is true for everyone. For example, research has shown that obese mice have a deficiency of the hormone leptin. Some researchers have referred to an obesity gene called ob gene. The ob gene produces leptin, a hormone that, if all is working correctly, helps to prevent obesity. Leptin is produced by the adipocytes and travels through the blood presumably to the hypothalamus. Leptin appears to act as an adipostat by signaling the brain regarding adipose tissue stores. Administration of exogenous leptin to deficient rodents leads to decreased food intake, increased metabolic activity, and weight loss (Shils et al, 1999). Many experts think leptin acts as an **afferent** satiety signal. There is a strong correlation among serum leptin concentrations, percentage body fat, and body mass index. However, some obese mice have elevated levels of leptin in their serum. For this group of mice, the pathology is not a deficiency of leptin but perhaps a receptor or a postreceptor defect in the hypothalamus. After leptin was discovered, scientists were hopeful that it could be used to effectively treat obesity. The therapeutic promise of leptin as an appetite and weight-restraining agent to be used in obese humans has been considerably dampened by the

---

Box 18–2 **Frequently Asked Questions About Theories of Obesity**

Can a Malfunctioning Hypothalamus Cause Weight Gain?

The brain partially controls hunger and satiety. The hypothalamus in the brain appears to be the center for weight control. Satiety is the feeling of satisfaction after eating. Appetite refers to the pleasant sensation based on previous experience that causes a person to seek food to eat. **Hunger** is the physical sensation caused by a lack of food, characterized by a dull or acute pain at or around the lower portion of the chest. A malfunctioning hypothalamus could cause an individual to receive incorrect hunger signals, thus stimulating continued eating and signaling weight gain. Appetite, satiety, and hunger may be incorrectly processed by a malfunctioning hypothalamus.

Various areas of the hypothalamus are sensitive to at least 13 neurochemicals, and these areas are involved in the regulation of hunger, eating, and satiety. The ventromedial nucleus and the lateral lobe in the hypothalamus are the two most significant areas. The ventromedial nucleus, which is activated by **serotonin** and antagonized by norepinephrine, mediates satiety. The lateral lobe, which is activated by norepinephrine and/or dopamine and antagonized by serotonin, mediates hunger and thirst. Selective hypothalamic neurotransmitters are now being considered as medications to alter the brain sensation of hunger, appetite, and satiety. However, more research is necessary to better understand long-term and short-term effects of these medications.

discovery that most such persons are resistant to its actions (Balasubramanyam, 2003).

Several other hormones and brain chemicals besides leptin are involved in appetite and the feeling of satiety. Researchers believe that there are probably others that have not been discovered yet. Two hormones made in the gut called PYY3-36 and ghrelin have been identified. PYY3-36 is secreted by cells lining the intestines after eating. The amount of the hormone that is secreted is proportional to kcaloric meal content. PYY3-36 signals the brain that the body is no longer hungry after a meal. Ghrelin is a hormone that increases food intake in rodents and humans (Cummings et al, 2002). Ghrelin blood levels increase after weight loss. One hormone increases food intake, and one hormone decreases food intake. The human body's energy balance system is complex and not fully understood and has redundant controls. However, each year researchers learn more about appetite and hunger control. The system evolved to help the human body survive famine by helping people to gain weight, not lose weight.

Biology alone is not fully responsible for excess body weight. Identical twins raised in different environments (adopted and nonadopted) have been studied extensively. From these studies, many experts believe obesity is about 33 percent genetic and 66 percent environmental (food and exercise behaviors) (Romsos, 1996). Keep the theories about obesity in mind when counseling a client who is overweight, obese, or underweight. There is more than one cause for the development and maintenance of obesity. However, body weight can be decreased by a modification of food and exercise behaviors. Health-care professionals should not give up treating these clients. Overweight and obese clients in well-designed programs can achieve a weight loss of as much as 10 percent of baseline weight, a weight loss than can be maintained for a sustained period of time (1 year or longer) (National Institutes of Health, 1998).

Fad Diets

Many kinds of fad diets have come and gone. Typically, such diets limit the person to a few specific foods or food combinations. Among the most popular diets are programs that limit dietary carbohydrate, the so-called "low-carbohydrate

diets." One recent study found weight loss was indeed greater on a low-carbohydrate diet at the end of 6 months; however, at the end of 12 months, the difference in weight loss between those on a low-carbohydrate diet and a higher-carbohydrate diet was no longer significant (Saltzman, 2004). By default, these diets are higher in protein and fat. This diet does not meet the recommendations of the American Heart Association, the American Cancer Society, and the American Dietetic Association and may be harmful over the long term. High fat intake has been associated with many chronic and degenerative diseases. Consumption of high levels of saturated fat without adverse effects on cardiovascular disease is inconsistent with a large body of epidemiologic and intervention data (Bonow and Eckel, 2003).

These diets are low in vitamins A and C and fiber. The National Cancer Institute believes the elimination of fruits, vegetables, whole grains, and beans may increase the risk of cancer. Athletic performance is reduced on a low-carbohydrate diet because a high-carbohydrate diet enhances performance during strenuous athletic events. Rising blood pressure and elevated uric acid levels from too much protein may cause gout. Uric acid and calcium oxalate stones are more likely to form on a high-protein diet. Over time, excess protein intake, especially from animal sources, increases the loss of calcium in the urine, which may contribute to osteoporosis (www. foodandhealth.com, accessed 2003). The most important factors contributing to weight loss in several studies were the degree of energy restriction and the duration of the study (Saltzman, 2004), not the macronutrient partitioning of the diet. The lower the kcalorie intake and the longer someone follows the diet, the more weight is lost.

Another example of a fad diet is the grapefruit diet. On this diet, the individual is allowed only grapefruit. Such a diet cannot possibly lead to a lifelong change in eating behaviors and is not nutritionally balanced. Table 18–3 lists three popular diets along with the rationale for the diet (according to each diet's author) and a brief description. These diets are not widely endorsed by the health-care community; however, it is important for health-care professionals to know what their clients are eating and thinking.

Table 18–3 **Common Diets Discussed in the Popular Media for Weight Control**

NAME OF DIET	RATIONALE OF DIET'S AUTHOR	DESCRIPTION
Atkins	Claims processed CHO and insulin rather than excess kcalories are responsible for weight gain and obesity.	Restricts CHO and encourages protein with the use of vitamin and mineral supplements
South Beach	The faster sugars and starches are absorbed, the more weight is gained. Low glycemic index meals suppress appetite and reduce food intake later in the same day in comparison to higher glycemic index meals (see below).	Three phases: • Severe CHO restriction for first 2 weeks • Reintroduction of "good CHO" (those with a low glycemic index, such as whole grains, fruits, vegetables) during phases 2 and 3 • Consistent meal times and water
Zone	Only through eating in the "Zone" can the body reach its physical peak. The author claims most people gain weight because they have an imbalance of energy nutrients. The kilocalorie intake of the meal plans are between 1000 and 1700 calories.	The zone is 40 percent CHO, 30 percent protein, and 30 percent fat. All food is measured and only precise portions sizes are eaten. CHO serving sizes are small (1/8 cup of pasta)

Screening

How do health professionals decide whom to treat or not treat? Not all clients should be encouraged to lose weight. Repeating gaining and losing weight is harmful. Inappropriate weight-loss methods, including repeated crash diets, can have damaging effects on physical health and psychological well-being.

Responsible weight-loss programs screen clients for the following.

1. Is weight loss indicated for this client? Is the client internally motivated to lose weight? The basic motivation to undergo treatment must originate from the client.
2. What level of health supervision is necessary? Are clients screened for psychosocial conditions that would make weight loss inappropriate? Are clients at medical risk, requiring a physician's care?
3. What factors in the client's history and lifestyle are relevant to the weight-loss program? For example, a weight-loss program that costs a significant amount of money may not be affordable for low-income clients.
4. Does the diet attempt to adapt weight-reduction approaches to the needs of diverse client groups?

The best candidates for weight reduction are those who express the desire to change their total lifestyle. The client must be motivated enough to agree to participate in routine exercise program, follow a low-kilocalorie diet, and change lifelong food behaviors. A significant time investment on the client's part is necessary. Capacity to succeed is best demonstrated by deeds rather than words. For example, will the client attend all program sessions and self-monitor his or her food intake?

In addition, the best candidates for weight reduction are not under stress currently. Stressful life events such as a recent divorce, death of a significant other, or change in living situation or job status decrease the chances of success.

Most individuals associate weight loss with being more attractive. The association between weight loss and wellness is a secondary consideration. The health benefits of weight loss are related to a loss of body fat, not a loss of lean body mass. The individual who loses a high amount of lean body mass rather than fat derives minimal health benefits from weight loss.

Setting Realistic Goals

Nurses can assist clients in setting realistic goals for weight reduction and encourage loss of modest amounts of weight. Often clients have an unrealistic weight-loss goal. Despite considerable professional agreement that modest weight losses of 5 to 10 percent are successful for reducing comorbid conditions associated with obesity, obese patients often desire weight losses two to three times greater than this (Foster et al, 2001). For example, the weight-reduction diet may be planned to allow for a 1 pound per week weight loss. The client may expect to lose 5 pounds per week. A female client may expect to be able eventually to wear a size 5 dress as a result of dieting. This is not a realistic expectation for some clients with large bones.

All overweight clients should be educated to stop gaining weight. Health-care workers provide a valuable service when they teach clients how to prevent weight gain.

Federal Guidelines on the Identification of Overweight and Obesity in Adults

There are clearly advantages to weight loss by overweight and obese clients. Chief among the reasons to avoid weight gain is to decrease the risk of disease and treat some persons who already have an obesity-related disorder. The treatment of energy imbalances depends on an understanding of the degree of overweight and obesity.

Advantages of Weight Loss

The panel that developed the federal clinical guidelines for the identification of overweight and obesity in adults focused on the medical benefits to be derived from weight loss. This panel recommended:

- Weight loss to lower blood pressure in overweight and obese persons with high blood pressure.
- Weight loss to lower elevated levels of cholesterol, low-density lipoprotein cholesterol, and triglycerides and to raise low levels of high-density lipoprotein cholesterol in overweight and obese persons with dyslipidemia (see Chapter 20).
- Some weight loss to lower elevated blood glucose levels in overweight and obese persons with type 2 diabetes.

Measurement of Degree of Overweight and Obesity

According to the federal guidelines, practitioners should use the body mass index and waist circumference to classify the degree of energy imbalance in clients. Body weight alone can be used to follow weight loss and to determine efficacy of treatment (National Institutes of Health, 1998). The reason the use of BMI is advocated in clinical practice is ease of measurement and cost.

Other Risk Factors

Persons with cardiovascular disease or diabetes mellitus with evident obesity should be evaluated for weight loss. The panel recognized that the decision to quit smoking should be given priority over weight loss.

Federal Guidelines on the Evaluation and Treatment of Overweight and Obesity

The federal guidelines address goals for weight loss, how to achieve weight loss, goals for weight maintenance, how to maintain weight loss, and special treatment groups.

Goals for Weight Loss

The initial goal of weight loss should be to reduce body weight by 10 percent from the baseline. With success, further weight loss can be attempted, if indicated. Safe weight loss occurs at about 1 to 2 pounds per week for a period of 6 months, with the subsequent strategy based on the amount of weight lost (National Institutes of Health, 1998).

How to Achieve Weight Loss

The panel explores a variety of weight-loss options to achieve weight loss, including dietary therapy, physical activity, behavior therapy, combined therapy, pharmacotherapy, and weight-loss surgery. The approach taken should depend on professional evaluation and the client's BMI, waist circumference, and other risk factors (National Institutes of Health, 1998).

Diet Therapy

A diet for weight loss would be reduced in total kilocalories but adequate in all nutrients. The diet should contain adequate protein, all essential vitamins and minerals, a small amount of fat, dietary fiber, and enough carbohydrate to prevent ketosis. More specifically, the diet should provide at least 130 grams of carbohydrate, 25 to 35 grams of fiber, and contain all the essential nutrients. The meal plan should be one the client can and will follow. When clients are given a standardized meal plan on paper, weight loss is not usually successful. However, when behavior modification, nutritional counseling, and exercise recommendations support the meal plan, weight loss can be more successful.

Different clients need different types of meal plans or dietary directions. A few clients just want to be told what to eat and will follow through with appropriate behaviors. Some clients want and require simplified instructions. They do not want to invest the time in learning a complicated diet. A Food Pyramid Guide dietary plan may work well for this type of client (provided behavior modifications and the need for exercise are also discussed). Portion control needs to be emphasized with this approach. Reasonable portion sizes are indicated on the MyPyramid guide (www.MyPyramid.gov, accessed 2005) and Exchange Lists.

A common tool used for teaching clients how to eat to lose weight is the American Diabetic and Dietetic Association's Exchange Lists. This approach has been successful for clients who want detailed information and are willing to invest the time required to learn food exchanges. This approach clearly spells out portion sizes. Patients often request a diet such as this when admitted to an institution, and health-care employees need a guide to go by when they serve and monitor weight-reduction diets. The ADA Exchange Lists are located in Appendix A.

Sometimes clients (outpatients) are unable to change their food intake so drastically. In this situation, nutritional counselors should encourage clients to make major behavioral changes in their eating habits slowly. The goal in weight-reduction counseling is to help the client make permanent lifestyle changes. The current recommendation is that clients should be encouraged to change only one or two negative food behaviors at a time. For example, if the nutrition counselor recommends that the client substitute skim milk for whole milk, it is not wise to simultaneously discourage the use of sweets. The goal is to encourage permanent changes in eating behavior, so the client needs time to make the necessary adjustments. With this in mind, perhaps it is best to review one food item or group at a time with some clients. After the client has changed negative behaviors associated with one food item or group, recommendations can be suggested to change negative behaviors associated with another food item or group.

Changing a negative behavior usually take several weeks. Priority should be given to eliminating foods in the fat, milk, and meat lists that are high in fat and in which the client overindulges. An average woman will lose weight on a 1200-kilocalorie diet. Larger women and most men will lose weight on a 1500-kilocalorie diet.

Physical Activity

Population studies conducted in the United States, Great Britain, and France have suggested that the rapidly increasing prevalence of obesity in recent decades may be largely due to increasing sedentary behaviors, perhaps to a greater extent than dietary excesses (Weinser et al, 1998). The propensity to be physically inactive seems to be at least partly determined by genetics. Individuals with certain body builds may be genetically predisposed to engage in less spontaneous physical activity and to have relatively low energy requirements. However, physical activity behaviors also influence whether we stay lean or become obese. One study showed that within twin pairs, the twin who reported being more physically active was generally less obese than the more sedentary sibling (Samaras et al, 1999). Another study showed that physical activity in previously sedentary adults led to weight loss even when they were not dieting and had not been encouraged to lose weight (Stentz et al, 2004). Some dietitians, in their role as nutrition counselors, advocate a nondieting approach to weight control. Exercise and healthy eating is encouraged instead of adherence to a rigid diet plan.

The panel recommends that physical activity be part of a comprehensive weight-loss therapy and weight maintenance program because it (1) modestly contributes to weight loss in overweight and obese adults, (2) may decrease abdominal fat, (3) increases cardiopulmonary fitness, and (4) may help with weight loss. The combination of a reduced-kilocalorie diet and increased physical activity is recommended because it produces weight loss, decreases abdominal fat, and increases cardiopulmonary fitness. Initially, moderate levels of exercise for 30 to 45 minutes 3 to 5 days per week should be encouraged. All adults should set a long-term goal to accumulate at least 30 minutes or more of moderate-intensity physical activity on most, and preferably all, days of the week. (National Institutes of Health, 1998). Wellness Tip 18–2 encourages exercise.

Wellness *Tip* **18–2** • Everyone should set a long-term goal to accumulate 30 minutes or more of moderate-intensity physical activity on most days of the week.

To identify those individuals at a major heart disease risk, a physician should screen all clients before exercise recommendations are made. Clients with known heart, lung, or metabolic disease should have a physician-supervised stress test before beginning an exercise program.

When following an exercise program, fluid intake should be adequate. Individuals should drink water before, during, and after exercise. Close attention should be paid to thirst to prevent dehydration. Four ounces of water every 15 minutes is usually sufficient, but at very high temperatures this may not be adequate. The thirst mechanism may not be adequate to prevent dehydration in many elderly persons and in individuals involved in heavy exercise during hot weather. Such persons need to be taught to drink water even if they are not thirsty.

Behavior Modification

Behavior modification is a useful adjunct when incorporated into treatment for weight loss and weight maintenance. A client's motivation to enter weight-loss therapy and his or her readiness to implement the weight-control plan require evaluation. Permanent weight loss can result only from a permanent change in eating and exercise behaviors. The behavioral strategies most commonly applied in weight-reduction programs include self-monitoring, stimulus control, slowed-down eating, a reward system, and cognitive behavior modification. Box 18–3 lists specific techniques used to help clients modify their behaviors. See Wellness Tip 18–3.

 18–3 • To lose weight, keep a food diary. Behavior modification in combination with exercise helps prevent weight gain and promote weight loss.

SELF-MONITORING

Clients keep their own food records, track their body weights, and record exercise completed during self-monitoring. Many clients come to regard self-monitoring of their food intake as the single most helpful strategy in a weight-reduction program. Recording of food intake seems to work best when clients know they must turn in the records to their nutritional counselor.

Requiring clients to monitor their weight once a week is also a helpful behavioral strategy. When clients are gaining weight, they tend to avoid scales and mirrors (Foreyt, 2004). Requiring clients to weigh themselves helps to keep them on their eating plan. Clients should also be asked to record their exercise in a notebook. Again, the notebook should be reviewed regularly in the training program.

STIMULUS CONTROL

Stimulus-control strategies are designed to help clients rearrange their lifestyle to reduce the chances of inappropriate eating habits. Clients are taught to examine their behaviors to determine which ones may trigger them to eat inappropriately. For example, a truck driver may eat two doughnuts every morning for breakfast because he or she drives past the bakery on the way to work. The nutritional counselor may recommend that this client take a different route to work to reduce the probability of his or her buying doughnuts.

SLOWED-DOWN EATING

Some overweight and obese people eat very rapidly. It takes approximately 20 minutes from the time food has been eaten for the brain to receive the message that food has been consumed. An individual can consume many extra kilocalories in 20 minutes. These clients are frequently taught several behavioral techniques to slow down their eating.

REWARD SYSTEM

Many clients respond better to any type of suggested behavioral change when they are working for specific rewards. In one program, for example, a client earns tokens whenever he or she performs a desirable behavior. The tokens are redeemable at the hospital's gift shop for merchandise.

Box 18–3 **Weight Control: Behavior Modification Techniques**

Self-Monitoring

- Keep a food diary and record all food intake.
- Keep a weekly graph of weight change.
- Keep an exercise diary.

Stimulus Control

- At home, limit all food intake to one specific place.
- Plan food intake for each day.
- Rearrange your schedule to avoid inappropriate eating.
- Sit down at a table while eating.
- At a party, sit a distance from snack foods, eat before you go, and substitute lower kilocalorie drinks for alcohol.
- Decide beforehand what you will order at a restaurant.
- Save or reschedule everyday activities for times when you are hungry.
- Avoid boredom; keep a list of activities on the refrigerator.

Slowed-Down Eating

- Drink a glass of water before each meal. Drink sips of water between bites of food.

- Swallow food before putting more food on the utensil.
- Try to be the last one to finish eating.
- Pause for a minute during your meal and attempt to increase the number of pauses.

Reward Yourself

- Chart your progress.
- Make an agreement with yourself or a significant other for a meaningful reward.
- Do not reward yourself with food.

Cognitive Strategies

- View exercise as a means of controlling hunger.
- Practice relaxation techniques.
- Imagine yourself ordering a side salad, diet dressing, low-fat milk, and a small hamburger at a fast-food restaurant.
- Visualize yourself enjoying a fresh apple in preference to apple pie.

COGNITIVE STRATEGIES

Many weight-reduction programs include cognitive strategies. The goal of cognitive strategies is to increase the client's knowledge of his or her eating behaviors so that he or she can develop skills to cope with inappropriate behaviors. Teaching the client to relax is one type of cognitive strategy. The use of imagery is another, for example, asking clients to imagine themselves coping successfully with anxiety-arousing events.

Pharmacotherapy

Weight-loss drugs approved by the FDA may be used as part of a comprehensive weight-loss program including diet and physical activity for clients with a BMI greater than or equal to 30 with no concomitant obesity-related risk factors or diseases according to the new federal guidelines. For clients with a BMI greater than or equal to 27 with concomitant obesity-related risk factors or diseases, medications may also be indicated. Drugs should never be used without lifestyle modification (National Institutes of Health, 1998). Drug therapy for obesity should be continually monitored for efficacy and safety and discontinued if the client does not lose weight. Table 18–4 lists weight-loss medications, actions, and adverse effects. Many researchers have come to the conclusion that long-term treatment, including pharmacotherapy, may be necessary for many obese clients (Poston, 1998). However, few medications approved by the FDA are available for long-term treatment of obesity, they do not work for all individuals, and on average they induce only modest weight loss (Yanorski and Yanorski, 2002). However, new medications are currently in clinical trials including Rimonabant. Some promising future developments involve PYY, ghrelin, and other neuropeptides. Pharmaceutical companies will make enormous profits when a safe medication for weight control is developed and profits will be enormous.

Weight-Loss Surgery

Weight-loss surgery is an option in carefully selected clients with clinically extreme or severe obesity (BMI ≥40, or ≥35 with comorbid conditions) when less-invasive methods of weight loss have failed and the client is at high risk for obesity-associated morbidity or mortality (National Institutes of Health, 1998).

Many different surgical procedures have been and are being used to treat obesity. The removal of fat tissue through a vacuum hose is called **liposuction. Lipectomy** is surgical removal of adipose tissue. Both of these procedures are done more for cosmetic reasons than for weight control. A **jejunoileal bypass** involves the removal of a part of the small intestine. Clients lose weight after this procedure because they cannot absorb all the food they eat, although this places these clients at a nutritional risk. The jejunoileal bypass procedure is rarely performed currently; however, health-care providers are likely to encounter patients who have had this procedure. All gastric (stomach) procedures either route food around (bypass) or through only part of the stomach (reduction). Diagrams of **gastric stapling** and **gastric bypass (roux-en-Y),** two common procedures, are shown in Figure 18–5. When the stomach is smaller or reduced, only a limited amount of food can be consumed at one feeding. This induces weight loss from reduced kilocalorie intake. Clinical Application 18–1 discusses problems that clients often encounter after gastric surgery for weight reduction and suggests general guidelines for these clients to follow. Clients should be followed carefully postoperatively due to risks for deficiencies such as iron, folacin, and vitamin B_{12}. Clients are also at risk for maladaptive eating behavior.

The results that can be expected from gastric surgery procedures should always be spelled out to clients. No permanent effects can be promised, and having the surgery does not mean that afterward the client can overeat indefinitely without weight gain. Ninety percent of weight loss occurs in the first year, and clients often begin to gain again in the second and third years. Only a minority achieve a weight as low as 125 percent of healthy body weight. The procedure should be viewed as a tool to be used in conjunction with behavioral training—the small pouch helps clients learn to reduce the amount of food consumed and slows down their intake. After the first year, due to stretching of the pouch or intestinal adaptation, much of the effect of the surgery can be negated and the lost weight may be regained.

Goals for Weight-Loss Maintenance

Weight regain often occurs after weight loss. A program of dietary therapy, physical activity, and behavior therapy enhances the likelihood of weight-loss maintenance. Drug therapy can also be used according to the guidelines published by the National Institutes of Health; however, drug safety and efficacy beyond 1 year of total treatment have not been established.

How Weight Loss Is Maintained

The literature suggests using weight-loss and weight-maintenance therapies that provide a greater frequency

---

Table 18–4 Weight-Loss Drugs

DRUG	ACTION	ADVERSE EFFECTS
Sibutramine (Meridia)	Norepinephrine, dopamine, and serotonin reuptake inhibitor	Increase in heart rate and blood pressure, heart palpitations and vasodilation Reports worldwide of deaths
Orlistat	Inhibits pancreatic lipase, decreases fat absorption	Decrease in absorption of fat-soluble vitamins Soft stools and anal leakage Possible link to breast cancer

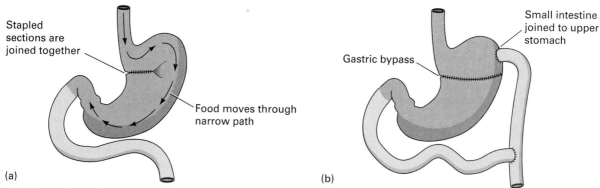

Figure **18–5** Illustrations of two common surgical procedures used to treat obesity: A, Gastric stapling; B, Gastric bypass.

of contacts between clients and practitioners over the long term. This can lead to more successful weight loss and weight maintenance (National Institutes of Health, 1998).

Obese clients who successfully lost weight and kept the lost weight off report the following (Foreyt, 2004):

- Clients who have kept off excess body weight report they have at least 30 minutes of moderate exercise each day, have a strong social support network, lost the weight gradually over a 6-month period, changed their attitudes toward their body weight, and made realistic lifestyle changes.
- They eat smaller portion sizes.
- They avoid food high in fat.
- Seventy-seven percent of clients who kept food records kept off previously lost weight versus 29 percent who did not keep food records.

- They eat a minimum of 35 servings of fruits and vegetables per week.
- They undereat 2 days per week.
- Nutritional portioned foods (Weight Watchers or Healthy Choice TV dinners and diet beverages) as meal replacements were widely used by successful dieters.
- The most frequently reported exercise was walking.
- The more structured the weight-loss program was, the more successful the participants were.

The Role of Nutrition Educators

All health-care workers become confused about their role as nutrition educators. Appropriate roles for nutrition educators include:

- Provide accurate information.
- Warn against dangerous practices such as self-imposed

Clinical Application 18–1

Complications of Gastroplasty and Gastric Bypass

There are many potential acute complications of gastric surgery for weight reduction. These include:

1. Nausea, vomiting, bloating, and/or heartburn: These signs and symptoms can be caused by overeating, not chewing food well, eating too quickly, drinking cold or carbonated beverages, using drinking straws, or eating gassy foods.
2. Staple disruption (for gastric stapling procedures): The result of loosened staples is that a larger intake of food is necessary before satiety can be achieved. Excessive food intake or vomiting can cause the staples to become disrupted.
3. Obstruction: An obstruction is the blockage of a structure. In this case, a blockage can occur close to the area stapled. A frequent cause of obstruction is poorly chewed food. The result is stomach pain, nausea, and vomiting.
4. Dumping syndrome: Intake of concentrated sweets and large quantities of fluids causes quick dumping of food into the small intestine. Abdominal fullness, nausea,

diarrhea 15 minutes after eating, warmth, weakness, fainting, racing pulse, and cold sweats are symptoms of this syndrome.
5. Among the long-term risks is osteoporosis, due to decreased calcium absorption.

Guidelines for the Client Following Gastric Surgery for Weight Reduction

The client who has had gastric surgery for weight reduction may find the following general guidelines helpful:

1. Eat three to six small meals per day.
2. Eat slowly.
3. Chew food thoroughly.
4. Eat very small quantities.
5. Stop eating when full.
6. Drink most fluids between meals.
7. Select a balanced diet.
8. Take a multivitamin-multimineral supplement.
9. Exercise regularly.

starvation diets that eliminate one or more of the major food groups and encourage the intake of only one food group.

- Guide clients to understand the risks and benefits of weight loss and weight-loss programs, products, medicines, procedures.
- Teach clients to evaluate the risks and benefits for themselves.
- When appropriate, refer clients to health-care professionals, including physicians and dietitians.
- In states where there are regulations, assist in efforts to enforce these standards for safe weight loss.

Special Treatment Groups

The federal panel discussed three groups of people that merit special consideration: smokers, older adults, and culturally diverse groups. All smokers, regardless of their weight status, should first quit smoking. Prevention of further weight gain should be encouraged. If weight gain occurs, it should be treated through diet, physical activity, and behavior therapy, maintaining the primary emphasis on abstinence from smoking (National Institutes of Health, 1998). Weight reduction in older adults should be guided by an evaluation of the potential benefits of weight loss for day-to-day functioning and reduction of the risk of future cardiovascular events, as well as the client's motivation to lose weight. Care should be taken in this group to ensure that any weight-loss program minimizes the likelihood of adverse effects on bone health or other aspects of nutritional status. A standard approach to weight loss may work differently in different cultural groups, a factor that must be considered when setting expectations about treatment outcomes. For example, female subjects who participated in one study indicated that weight-control methods and socioenvironmental context in which they conduct their lives merits attention (Tyler, Allan, and Alcozer, 1997).

Prevention of Overweight and Obesity

The current epidemic of obesity is partially caused by an environment that promotes excessive food intake and discourages physical activity. Prevention of excess body fat is the key to a healthy body weight. Clinical Application 18–2 offers some ways to prevent and control excess body fat. Figure 18–6 illustrates the crucial need to provide opportunities for children to engage in enjoyable physical activity.

The Client With Reduced Body Mass

Clients with a reduced body mass are as difficult, if not more difficult, to treat as overly fat clients. Body fat has important roles in insulation and protection of body organs. A client with a low body fat content usually has a

---

Clinical Application 18–2

Prevention and Control of Excess Body Fat

Weight maintenance is the key to weight control. How can we as health-care workers help clients achieve and maintain a healthy body weight?

We know it takes more kilocalories to support body protein content than body fat content. Health-care workers should first encourage patients to exercise more to increase their body protein content. Many experts believe that our society's increasingly sedentary lifestyle may be responsible for the increasing prevalence of obesity.

Second, eating fat is fattening. Here are some reasons to avoid dietary fat:

1. Teaspoon for teaspoon, fat contains more kilocalories than either carbohydrate or protein.
2. There is very little energy cost to convert fat in food to body fat. Carbohydrates in food must be converted to fat before carbohydrate can be stored in fat cells. This conversion requires an expenditure of kilocalories. Kilocalories used to convert carbohydrate in food to body fat are not stored as body fat.
3. Once a fat cell has been manufactured, there is no evidence that it can ever be broken down; it exists until death. When dieting, a person can reduce the amount of fat in each fat cell but not break down the cell completely. Some researchers believe that an empty fat cell sends a message to the reduced-obese person's brain to eat. The reduced-obese/overweight person

must learn to cope with a message constantly coming from the brain to eat. This is another reason why it is very difficult for a client to keep weight off permanently. Prevention of weight gain is the easiest way to maintain a reasonable body weight.

Third, a low-fiber intake may predispose a client to obesity. Fiber has a high satiety value. Obesity is uncommon among the populations of countries where a high proportion of dietary kilocalories is consumed as starchy vegetables. Educating clients to eat at least the recommended six servings of starch (preferably whole grain) and five to nine servings of fruits and vegetables may help clients achieve satiety. Many starches, fruits, and vegetables contain appreciable amounts of fiber. There is some evidence that fiber consumption may predict weight gain more strongly than total or saturated fat consumption (Ludwig et al, 1999).

Adherence to a low-fat and low-fiber diet will not always result in a permanent weight loss. An individual can still gain weight on a low-fat diet if he or she overeats foods high in carbohydrates (especially sugary drinks). Portion control is important. For some people, the most valuable information on the food label is the serving size.

To summarize, the health-care worker can educate clients to (1) exercise more, (2) eat less fat, (3) eat more fiber, (4) use portion control, and (5) avoid sweetened soda.

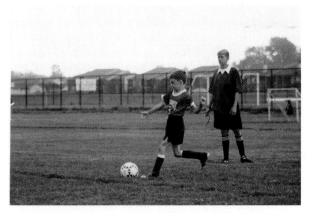

Figure **18–6** The parents who provide their child with the opportunity to engage in physical activity have given that child a special gift with life-long benefits.

loss of lean body mass as well, and loss of this functioning tissue concerns clinicians. Women cease to ovulate and menstruate when the percent of body fat falls below a certain level. The client may experience cardiac abnormalities and become more prone to infections. These clients are at risk for osteoporosis in the long term.

Classification

Methods similar to those used to diagnose overly fat clients can be used to diagnose clients with reduced body mass. A person whose weight is more than 15 percent below a reasonable body weight (RBW) may be classified as underweight. A man with a body fat content less than 15 percent and a woman with a body fat content less than 18 percent may be classified as having a reduced body mass. A BMI less than 20 percent may indicate that the client has a reduced body mass.

Consequences

Long-term follow-up of studies indicates that excessive leanness is associated with increased mortality and decreased life expectancy. However, the causes of mortality are different from those associated with excess weight. An excessively lean person is almost twice as likely to succumb to respiratory diseases such as tuberculosis. In addition, these clients have greater difficulty maintaining body temperature during cold weather. Infections and disturbances of the gastrointestinal tract are more likely in an underweight person, as is fragile bone structure and osteoporotic changes.

Causes

A person may be underweight because of genetic factors or because of a long-term or recent weight loss. As part of the nutrition screening process, the health-care worker should ask the client about any change in body weight. A good question is, "Have you experienced any undesired weight loss?" If the client responds yes, it is important to determine the time frame of the weight loss. However, a

response such as "I have always been lean" indicates a life-time pattern and may reveal that the client's leanness is genetic. A response of, "No, I intentionally lost weight" may reveal an anorexic client.

Rapid Loss Increases Risk

The greater the rate of weight loss, the more the client is at a nutritional risk. **Rate** means loss per unit of time. For example, a 20-pound weight loss in 2 weeks is an excessive weight loss. Such a client has lost a large amount of lean body mass. However, a 20-pound weight loss during a 20-week period could be attributed mostly to a loss of body fat with a minimal loss of lean body mass. If the client began with surplus body fat stores, a loss of 20 pounds may not place this client at a high nutritional risk. If the client had a reduced body mass, even a slow weight loss may place him or her at a nutritional risk.

Not all changes in body weight are caused by insufficient kilocalorie intake. For example, a client may lose several pounds of body weight over the course of a single day as a result of diuretic therapy. The weight loss in this instance would be due to water loss and not to body fat or protein loss.

One method to determine whether a client is eating enough food is to monitor his or her food intake. Kilocalorie intake is monitored by recording actual food consumption and calculating the kilocalories eaten. This can be done using several software programs, such as Food Processor or Diet Analysis.

Eating Disorders

Eating disorders may be caused by psychological factors and may result in nutritional problems. Many experts are concerned about the prevalence of anorexia nervosa and bulimia.

Anorexia Nervosa

Anorexia nervosa is a medical condition that results from self-imposed starvation. An estimated 0.5 to 3.7 percent of females suffer from anorexia nervosa (American Psychiatric Association Work Group on Eating Disorders, 2000). Symptoms include:

1. Loss of 20 to 40 percent of usual body weight (UBW); refer to Clinical Calculation 18–2 to calculate UBW
2. Decreased resting energy expenditure (REE)
3. **Amenorrhea** (cessation of menstruation)
4. Constipation
5. Excessive hair loss
6. Abnormal sleeping patterns
7. Preoccupation with food
8. Body image disturbance
9. Misconception about physical status
10. Intake of only 500 to 800 kilocalories per day
11. Slow eating
12. Increased physical activity
13. Social isolation
14. Intense fear of becoming obese
15. Poor muscle tone

This disorder may be life threatening. Among females, the disorder begins before age 20 in one-half and before age 21 in three-fourths. This disorder occurs 8 to 12 times more frequently in females than males (Huse and Lucas, 1999). The client may resort to a variety of devices to lose weight, including starvation, vomiting, and laxative use.

Bulimia

Bulimia is much more common than anorexia nervosa, especially during adolescence and young adulthood. The mean age for females at diagnosis was 23 years. An estimated 1.1 to 4.2 percent of females have bulimia nervosa in their lifetime (American Psychiatric Association Work Group on Eating Disorders, 2000). The condition is rare in males. Bulimics binge and purge. **Binging** involves the consumption of as much as 5000 to 20,000 kilocalories per day. **Purging** is the intentional clearing of food out of the system by vomiting and/or using enemas, laxatives, and diuretics. Athletes such as ballerinas and gymnasts sometimes are bulimic. The female triad is a serious syndrome comprising three interrelated components: (1) disordered eating, (2) amenorrhea, and (3) osteoporosis (Wast, 1998).

Treatment of Eating Disorders

There are many approaches to treatment of eating disorders, including nutritional counseling, behavioral therapy, family therapy, and group therapy. It is important to help the client discover the reason he or she chooses to eat, not

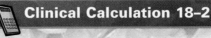

Clinical Calculation 18–2

Percent Usual Body Weight

The health-care worker can calculate the client's percent usual body weight (UBW). The formula is:

Present weight divided by usual reported
body weight × 100 = Usual weight

A 5-percent weight loss in 1 month may not be significant. However, a 5-percent weight loss over a week may be significant. The kcal deficit may be related to a recent change in medication, an underlying but as yet undiagnosed condition, a recent change in living situation, or not taking the time to eat.

eat, binge, or purge. Some of these clients have symptoms including a fixation on food, weight, physique, or exercise (Zerbe, 1999). Some clients are admitted to the hospital for treatment. Careful recording of kilocalories consumed is indicated. Sometimes nurses are asked to sit with these clients and watch them eat. These clients may attempt to hide food in their clothes, mouth, bedding, or anywhere else. It is sometimes necessary for the nurse to accompany these clients to the bathroom. Clients with eating disorders have been known to flush their food down the toilet. For these reasons, the physicians of such clients often order daily weighing.

SUMMARY

Energy imbalance results from an inequality of energy intake and expenditure. The reason an individual eats more or fewer kilocalories than needed to maintain a stable body weight is now only partially understood. Weight loss decreases *both* body fat and lean body mass. Care needs to be taken to minimize the loss of lean body mass during weight reduction. Exercise should be encouraged because it helps minimize the loss of lean body mass. The federal government has guidelines on the identification, evaluation, and treatment of overweight and obesity in adults. Exercise, a well-balanced diet, and behavior modification are all essential components of a sound weight-reduction program. Medications and surgical interventions may be indicated for individuals who meet the criteria set by the guidelines. Treating the client who has a reduced body mass is a concern for health-care workers.

CASE STUDY 18–1

The client arrives at the physician's office for a routine blood pressure check. Her blood pressure is 150/95. Her medications are 100 mg Lopressor bid and 10 mg atace qd. The client works nights as a cashier at a service station and days at a dry cleaner. Her BMI is 28. She recently had a stress test that was considered normal. The doctor would like the client to lose weight to help lower her blood pressure.

(Continued on the following page)

CASE STUDY *(Continued)*

NURSING CARE PLAN

SUBJECTIVE DATA Client stated, "I can barely afford my blood pressure medication, and the doctor has encouraged me to lose about 14 pounds. I know I need to eat less and exercise more. I need to spend less money on medications. I completed the sixth grade in school." A food frequency record showed that this client usually eats four times each day. Her usual pattern includes 3 cups of low-fat milk, 8 starches (mostly refined), 1/2 cup of vegetables, 1 piece of fruit, 6 to 8 ounces of meat, 5 fats, 1 dessert, and an occasional beer. She eats fast food two nights each week and has pizza weekly for lunch.

OBJECTIVE DATA Blood pressure 150/95; Height 5 ft 6 in; BMI 28; waist circumference 36; stress test was normal

NURSING DIAGNOSIS NANDA: Imbalanced Nutrition: more than body requirements (NANDA, 2003, with permission) as evidenced by client's statements and a BMI of 28 and a waist circumference of 36

DESIRED OUTCOMES EVALUATION CRITERIA	NURSING ACTIONS/INTERVENTIONS	RATIONALE
NOC: Knowledge: Diet (Moorhead, Johnson, and Maas, 2004, with permission)	NIC: Teaching: Diet (Dochterman and Bulechek, 2004, with permission)	
Increase physical activity.	Recommend Mrs. R monitor her exercise behaviors and try to walk at least 30 minutes three times per week and increase to 7 days per week as able.	Self-monitoring of lifestyle behaviors promotes behavioral change. The most sedentary individuals receive the most health benefit from even small amounts of exercise.
Consume foods in appropriate portions following the MyPyramid Guide.	Review food pyramid model with Mrs. R with emphasis on whole grains and fruits and vegetables and the avoidance of fats. Review portion sizes indicated on this teaching tool.	The MyPyramid Guide is a good tool to use for clients with a lower reading level and promotes a high-fiber, low-fat diet.
Will enlist a supportive person to walk with her or talk to when tempted to eat.	Assist client to identify such a person among her relatives and friends.	A strong social support system fosters success.
Client will state why a weight loss of 1 to 2 pounds a week may reduce her blood pressure.	Explain to client that the rate of weight loss is important and why.	A 1- to 2-pound per week weight loss will minimize the loss of lean body mass. Self-starvation rarely results in long-term weight loss for overweight clients.

C T Q CRITICAL THINKING QUESTIONS

1. What foods does this client need to eat less and what foods does she need to eat more?
2. What would you tell the client if after 1 week she gained a pound even though she had given up her daily dessert and had increased her vegetable intake to 5 servings each day?
3. What other dietary modifications would you recommend?

⟫⟫ CHAPTER REVIEW

1. To lose 2 pounds of body fat per week, an individual must eat _____ fewer kilocalories each day for 7 days without a change in energy expenditure.
   a. 1000
   b. 1500
   c. 2000
   d. 2500

2. A very rapid rate of weight loss (1 pound per day) in an adult who is slightly overweight:
   a. Usually encourages permanent changes in behavior
   b. May lead to sudden death in some clients
   c. Will preserve lean body mass
   d. Fosters long-term weight maintenance

3. An obese client should be enrolled in a weight-management program and meet the following criteria before medications are tried:
   a. BMI of 20 and a waist circumference of 30 inches

b. Waist circumference in a male of at least 35 inches and a BMI of 27

c. A BMI of 27 and no concomitant obesity-related risk factors

d. BMI of 30 or greater and a waist circumference of at least 35 inches in a female

4. A client with anorexia nervosa:
   a. Has an increased resting energy expenditure
   b. Frequently complains of constipation

c. Is not likely to have a body image disturbance

d. Typically seeks the company of others

5. An elderly overweight smoker should first be encouraged to:
   a. Lose weight
   b. Quit smoking
   c. Lose weight and quit smoking using any means possible
   d. Be evaluated to determine if weight loss is indicated and bone health is adequate

CLINICAL ANALYSIS

1. Mrs. R is a 40-year-old mother of three. She has arthritis in both knees. She weighs 180 pounds, has a medium frame, and is 5 feet, 3 inches tall. Her BMI is 32. Her physician has told her to lose weight to help reduce her knee pain. According to Mrs. R, she never thought she was overweight until she was 24 years old. At this time, her weight started increasing. When she weighed 140 pounds, she started to diet. One time she lost a total of 25 pounds, which she promptly regained plus an additional 5 pounds. The client described four additional **weight cycles.** Mrs. R claims she cannot exercise because "it is too painful on my knees." She has tried every conceivable type of diet, including a comprehensive medically supervised weight-control program. Mrs. R states that for the past year, no matter how little she eats, she cannot lose weight even on a 1200-kilocalorie diet. Mrs. R:
   a. Apparently knows a great deal about low-kilocalorie foods, because she has successfully lost weight before
   b. Knows very little about foods, because she always regained the weight she lost
   c. Lacks motivation, because she has an inability to follow through with the appropriate behavior

d. Should be discouraged from further attempts to control her weight

2. Mrs. M had a slow weight gain for about 10 years. She asks for advice concerning how to best manage her weight. Mrs. M lives a sedentary lifestyle, eats three well-balanced meals each day, and enjoys going out to dinner with her husband one night each week. Her BMI is 27. Mrs. M would most likely benefit from:
   a. Decreasing her meal frequency
   b. Increasing her physical activity
   c. Taking a medication to lose weight
   d. Not going out to dinner with her husband each week

3. Mr. P wants to lose weight and has a BMI of 30 and a waist circumference of 41. Initially, the nurse should advise Mr. P to:
   a. Follow a 1200-calorie diet
   b. Ask his doctor for a medication to assist in weight reduction
   c. Self-monitor and write down his food intake and physical activity
   d. Refer client to a surgeon for an evaluation

REFERENCES

American Dietetic and Diabetic Associations: Exchange lists for Meal Planning. American Dietetic Association. Chicago, 2003.

American Psychiatric Association Work Group on Eating Disorders: Practice guidelines for the treatment of patients and eating disorders (revision). Am J Psych 157(Suppl 1):1, 2000.

Balasubramanyam, A: Adipocyte-brain communications in the regulation of energy balance. Accessed February 2004 at www.medscape.com/px.

Batterham, RL: Inhibition of food intake in obese subjects by peptide YY$_{3-36}$. N Engl J Med 349:941, 2003.

Blackburn, GL, and Bevins, LC: The obesity epidemic: Prevention and treatment of metabolic syndrome. Accessed August 2003 at www.medscape.com/viewprogram/2015-pnt.

Bonow, RO, and Eckel, RH: Diet, obesity, and cardiovascular risk. N Engl J Med 348:2057, 2003.

Bouchard, C: Inhibition of food intake by inhibitors of fatty acid synthase. N Engl J Med 343:1888, 2000.

Canning, H, and Mayer, J: Obesity: Its possible effect on college acceptance. N Engl J Med 275:1172, 1966.

CDC: Trends in Intake of Energy and Macronutrients—United States, 1971–2000. Accessed February 2004 at www.cdc.gov/mmwr/preview.

Coscina, DV, and Dixon, LM: Body weight regulation in anorexia nervosa: Insights from an animal model. In Darby, PL, Garfield, PE, Garner, DM, et al (eds): Anorexia Nervosa: Recent Developments. Allan R. Liss, New York, 1983.

Cummings, DE, et al: Plasma ghrelin levels after diet-induced weight loss or gastric bypass surgery. N Engl J Med 346:1623, 2002.

Dochterman, JC, and Bulechek, GM: Nursing Interventions Classification (NIC), ed 4. Mosby, Philadelphia, 2004.

Eisenstein, J, et al: High-protein weight-loss diets: Are they safe and do they work? A review of experimental and epidemiologic data. Nutr Rev 60:189, 2002.

Fontaine, KR, et al: Years of life lost due to obesity. JAMA 289:187, 2003.

Forbes, GB: Body composition. In Shils, ME, et al (eds): Body Composition. Modern Nutrition in Health and Disease, ed 9. Williams & Wilkins, Baltimore, 1999.

Foreyt, JP: Lifestyle approaches to the IRS. Accessed February 2004 at www.medscape.com/viewarticle/467200-3.

Foster, GD, et al: Obese patients perceptions of treatment outcomes and the factors that influence them. Arch Intern Med 161:2133, 2001.

Foster, GD, Wyatt, HR, and Hill, JO: A randomized trial of low-carbohydrate diet for obesity. N Engl J Med 348:2082, 2003.

Frantz, MJ: Managing obesity in patients with comorbidities: The Obesity Epidemic. J Am Diet Assoc 98(Suppl 2):s39, 1998.

Gabbay, RA and Flier, JS: Transmembrane Signaling: A Tutorial. In Shils, ME, et al (eds): Modern Nutrition in Health and Disease, ed 9. Williams & Wilkins, Baltimore, p. 594. 1999.

Gendreau, GD: The supersizing of America, MSU Today. East Lansing, Fall, 2003.

Gortmaker, SL, et al: Social and economic consequences of overweight in adolescence and young adulthood. N Engl J Med 329:1008, 1993.

Gustafson, D, et al: An 18-year follow-up of overweight and risk of Alzheimer disease. Arch Intern Med 163:1524, 2003.

Haines, PS, et al: Weekend eating in the United States is linked to greater energy, fat, and alcohol intake. Obesity Res 11:945, 2003.

Huse, P, and Lucas, AR: Behavioral disorders affecting food intake: Anorexia nervosa, bulimia nervosa, and other psychiatric conditions. In Shils, ME, et al (eds): Modern Nutrition in Health and Disease. Williams & Wilkins, Baltimore, 1999.

Keyes, A, Brozek, J, Mickelson, O, et al: The Biology of Human Starvation. 2 vols. University of Minnesota Press, Minneapolis, 1950.

Lowell, BB, and Spiegelman, BM: Toward a molecular understanding of adaptive thermogenesis. Nature 404:652, 2000.

Ludwig, DS, et al: Dietary fiber, weight gain, and cardiovascular disease risk factors in young adults. JAMA 282:1539, 1999.

Manson, JE, and Bassuk, SS: Obesity in the United States. JAMA 289:2, 2003.

Moorhead, S, Johnson, M, and Maas, M: Nursing Outcomes Classification (NOC), ed 3. Mosby, Philadelphia, 2004.

NANDA International: Definitions and Classification, 2003–2004. NANDA International, Philadelphia, 2003.

National Center for Health Statistics: Report on the 2001 National Interview Survey. Accessed February 2004 at www.cdc.gov/about/major/nhis/released.

National Institutes of Health and National Heart, Lung, and Blood Institute: Clinical Guidelines on the Identification, Evaluation, and Treatment of Overweight and Obesity in Adults. Bethesda, MD, June 1998.

Polivy, J: Psychological consequences of food restriction. J Am Diet Assoc 96:589, 1996.

Poston, WS II, et al: Challenges in obesity management. South Med J 8:710, 1998.

Pyle, RL, Mitchell, JE, and Eckert, ED: Bulimia: A report of 34 cases. J Clin Psychiatry 42:60, 1981.

Romsos, D: "Gene-Whiz": The Obesity/Gene Connection (unpublished lecture). 23rd Annual Nutrition Conference. Michigan State University, East Lansing, MI, March 6, 1996.

Saltzman, E: Low carbohydrate and high-protein diets for treatment of obesity. Accessed February 2004 at www.cyberrounds.com/conf/nutrition/2004-02-05.

Samaras, K, et al: Genetic and environmental influences on total-body and central abdominal fat: The effect of physical activity in twin females. Ann Intern Med 130:873, 1999.

Serdula, MK, et al: Prevalence of attempting weight loss and strategies for controlling weight. JAMA 282:1353, 1999.

Skov, A, et al: Randomized trial on a protein vs. carbohydrate in ad libitum fat reduced diet for the treatment of obesity. Int J Obes 23:528, 1999.

Stentz, CA, et al: Effects of the amount of exercise on body weight, body composition, and measures of central obesity. Arch Intern Med 164:1, 2004.

Stevens, J, et al: The effect of decision rules on the choice of body mass index cutoff for obesity: Examples from African American and white women. Am J Clin Nutr 75:986, 2002.

Stunkard, AJ: A history of binge eating. In Fairbanks, CG, and Wilson, GT (eds): Binge Eating, Assessment, and Treatment. Guilford Press, New York, 1993.

Stunkard, AJ, and Burt, V: Obesity and body image II: Age of onset of disturbances in the body image. Am J Psychiatry 123:1443, 1967.

Stunkard, AJ, and Mendelson, M: Disturbances in body image of some obese persons. J Am Diet Assoc 38:328, 1961.

Sturm, R: Increases in severe obesity in the US, 1986–2000. Arch Intern Med 163:2146, 2003.

Tyler, DO, Allan, JD, and Alcozer, FR: Weight loss methods used by African American and Euro-American women. Res Nurs Health 20:413, 1997.

Van Itallie, TB: Obesity. In Jeejeebhoy, KN (ed): Current Therapy in Nutrition. BC Decker, Toronto, Canada, 1988.

Wast, RV: The female athlete: The triad of disordered eating, amenorrhea, and osteoporosis. Sports Med 2:63, 1998.

Weinsier, RL, et al: The etiology of obesity: Relative contribution of metabolic factors, diet, and physical activity. Am J Med 105:145, 1998. www.foodandhealth.com, accessed May 2000.

Yanovski, JA, and Yanovski, SZ: Obesity. N Engl J Med 346:8, 2002.

Yunsheng, MA, et al: Association between eating patterns and obesity in a free-living US adult population. Epidemiology 158:85, 2003.

Venes, D (eds): Tabers Cyclopedic Medical Dictionary. 19th ed. FA Davis Publishing Co., Philadelphia, 2001.

Zerbe, KJ: Anorexia nervosa: When the pursuit of bodily perfection becomes a killer. Postgrad Med 1:161, 1999.

Diet in Diabetes Mellitus and Hypoglycemia

After completing this chapter, the student should be able to:

1. Define and classify diabetes mellitus and describe the treatment for each type.
2. Discuss the goals of nutritional care for persons with diabetes mellitus.
3. List nutritional guidelines for illness, exercise, delayed meals, alcohol, hypoglycemic episodes, vitamin/mineral supplementation, and eating out for people with diabetes.
4. Describe dietary treatment for reactive hypoglycemia as compared to diabetes mellitus.

This chapter introduces the importance of nutrition in diabetes and hypoglycemia. These two diseases are associated with insulin secretion and/or resistance to insulin accompanied by characteristic long-term complications. Diabetes mellitus is caused by the low secretion and/or utilization of insulin. Hypoglycemia is caused by excessive secretion of insulin. Diabetes mellitus has been diagnosed in approximately 18.2 million people, or 6.3 percent of the population in the United States. An additional 5.2 million individuals are believed to have undiagnosed diabetes. Each year more than one million new cases are diagnosed in people over 20 years of age (www.cdc.gov, accessed March, 2004). Wellness Tip 19–1 discusses the importance of early diagnosis of diabetes. Nationally, diabetes is the seventh leading cause of death. Hypoglycemia is much rarer than diabetes mellitus. Nutrition is integral to the management of diabetes.

Wellness Tip **19–1** • Approximately half of all individuals with diabetes are undiagnosed. Do you or any of your family members have any of the signs or symptoms of this disease? Early detection and treatment of diabetes reduces morbidity and mortality.

Definition and Classification

Diabetes mellitus is characterized by the passage of sweet urine, excessive urine production, thirst, excessive hunger, and, in some cases, weight loss. Records from the ancient Greeks described this condition as early as the first century A.D. Diabetes mellitus can be defined as a group of disorders with measurable persistent hyperglycemia. **Hyperglycemia** means an elevated level of glucose in the blood. Definitions and classifications for the various subclasses of diabetes mellitus have been standardized. The following sections define and classify the major types of diabetes.

Definition

Diabetes is diagnosed and defined by laboratory analysis. Fasting glucose levels of at least 126 milligrams per **deciliter** (mg/dL) are required for a diagnosis of diabetes in nonpregnant adults. Fasting is defined as no kilocalorie intake for at least 8 hours. A fasting blood glucose level ≥100 to 126 is diagnosed as prediabetes or **impaired fasting glucose** (www.diabetes.org, accessed June, 2004). This must be confirmed as described below. Casual or random blood glucose (RBG) greater than 200 mg/dL plus classic symptoms (increased urination, increased thirst, weight loss) is also an established method to diagnose diabetes in adults and children. A random or casual blood glucose between 140 and 199 mg/dL is diagnostic of pre-diabetes. Random means the blood sample is tested without regard to time of day, prior diet, and physical activity. Refer to Clinical Application 19–1 for an explanation of other tests used for diabetes.

Classification

There are two major forms of diabetes: **type 1 and type 2** (note the use of Arabic numerals). The American Diabetes Association recommends the use of three additional categories to classify diabetes: secondary diabetes, prediabetes, and gestational diabetes.

Type 1

Type 1 diabetes has also been called **insulin-dependent diabetes mellitus (IDDM),** juvenile-onset diabetes, and type I diabetes. All of these terms are still used in medical

Clinical Application 19–1

Laboratory Tests for Diabetes

Several types of biochemical tests are discussed below: fasting blood sugar, glucose tolerance test, urine tests, and glycolated hemoglobin.

FASTING BLOOD SUGAR

A measurement of a **fasting blood sugar (FBS)** is performed routinely on most diabetic clients. In preparation, the client should be instructed not to eat or drink for 8 hours before the test. Water is the exception, as it will not interfere with test results. The test ideally should be done after at least 3 days of unrestricted diet ($\geq$150 g carbohydrate per day) and unlimited physical activity. The individual should remain seated and not smoke throughout the test. If the client usually takes insulin or a hypoglycemic agent, the medication should not be taken or given until the blood test is done. Normal FBS should be less than 100 mg/dL. A finding of 126 mg/dL is diagnostic of diabetes mellitus.

GLUCOSE TOLERANCE TEST

In the **glucose tolerance test,** 75 grams of anhydrous glucose dissolved in water is given orally or intravenously after a fasting blood sugar sample has been drawn. Blood samples are then drawn at specified intervals. The client's ability to process glucose can be evaluated by this means. A blood glucose value above or equal to 200 mg/dL at 2 hours and at least one other sample at less than 2 hours are required for the diagnosis in nonpregnant adults. A normal 2-hour blood sample would have an upper level of 140 mg/dL. Values between 140 and 199 mg/dL are indicative of impaired glucose tolerance or pre-diabetes. In the absence of unequivocal hyperglycemia, these criteria should be confirmed by reat testing on a different day (American Diabetes Association, 2005).

Clients may need to discontinue certain drugs for 3 days before the test. Also, a high-carbohydrate diet of 300 g of carbohydrate per day should be followed for the same period. The client should be given written instructions explaining the pretest dietary requirements. An inadequate diet before the glucose tolerance test may diminish carbohydrate tolerance and cause high glucose levels, creating a false-positive result. During the test, the client should be instructed not to have anything by mouth except water. Tobacco, coffee, and tea can alter the test results.

URINE TESTS

For most people, when blood glucose reaches 180 to 200 mg/100 mL, the kidneys begin to spill glucose into the urine. This point of spillage is called the **renal threshold.**

At one time, this test was assumed to reflect the glucose content of the blood, but the renal threshold varies from individual to individual. The renal threshold may also change in a given individual with decreasing kidney function. Although urine tests are used as screening tests, they are less reliable than the blood glucose tests available for home use.

URINE ACETONE

As a consequence of the body's inability to metabolize glucose, fat is partially broken down for energy. The intermediate products of fat breakdown are ketone bodies. These ketone bodies build up in the blood because the quantity of fat being catabolized exceeds the body's capacity to process these intermediate products effectively. As this occurs, ketone bodies begin to spill into the urine. One of the ketone bodies is acetone, which can be measured in the urine. The presence of acetone in the urine is called **ketonuria.** Ketonuria is a sign that the diabetes is out of control. Clients are often taught to test for urinary ketones if their blood glucose level exceeds 240 mg/dL. When a client exhibits ketonuria, the physician and diabetes educator should be consulted for changes in the diet prescription or insulin dosage.

GLYCOSYLATED HEMOGLOBIN (A1C)

Glucose attaches to the hemoglobin molecule in a one-way reaction throughout the 120-day life of the red blood cell. In a high-glucose environment, a greater percentage of the hemoglobin is glycosylated. This blood test is performed on a random blood sample; the client does not have to fast. The result is not influenced by exercise or diabetic drugs. For good glycemic control, the AIC should be <7 (referenced to a nondiabetic range of 4.0 to 6.0 percent using a DCCT-based assay).

Because the **glycosylated hemoglobin** value reflects the average blood glucose level for the preceding 2 to 3 months, it is a good test of the effectiveness of long-term therapy. A client cannot follow the prescribed regimen for just a few days before a doctor's visit and claim otherwise. Glycosylated hemoglobin will be 4 to 8 percent of the total hemoglobin in adults without diabetes. In clients with diabetes, a value of 7 percent indicates good control of the disease, and greater than 8 percent is considered high.

An A1C is recommended at least two times a year for those in good control and more often if the HbAic is greater than 8 percent or when there is a change in the treatment plan.

---

records. Patients with this disorder cannot survive without daily doses of insulin because the pancreas does not produce sufficient insulin for glucose uptake. This results in elevation of blood glucose. These variations in blood glucose levels make these patients prone to two conditions. The first condition is **ketoacidosis.** The signs of ketoacidosis are hyperglycemia and excessive ketones.

Ketoacidosis is discussed further later in this chapter. The second condition is **hypoglycemia,** or a low blood glucose level. Type 1 diabetes can occur at any age, although its usual onset is during childhood. Five to 10 percent of people with diabetes have type 1. The onset of this disorder is usually abrupt, and the condition is difficult to control.

Type 2

Type 2 diabetes has also been called **non-insulin-dependent diabetes mellitus (NIDDM),** adult-onset diabetes, and type II diabetes. Persons with type 2 are not insulin dependent or prone to ketoacidosis. However, some of them do use insulin because of persistent hyperglycemia. Also, insulin is the preferred medication to treat persons with type 2 diabetes with a critical illness. Clients with this condition can manufacture some insulin but do not make a sufficient amount or cannot use insulin efficiently. Typically, the non-insulin-dependent diabetic client develops his or her condition after age 45. Most of these clients are obese, and weight reduction usually improves their ability to process glucose. Excess body fat seems to be related to a decrease in the number of cell receptor sites. About 90 to 95 percent of all people with diabetes in the United States have type 2. The prevalence of type 2 diabetes is markedly increased among Native Americans, African Americans, Hispanic Americans, and Pacific Islanders. The cultural implications of these statistics were discussed in the Chapter 2. The onset of this disorder is gradual. The condition is usually easier to control than type 1. Table 19–1 summarizes the differences between types 1 and 2.

Maturity-onset diabetes in the young (MODY) is a term used to describe a diabetes disorder that is found in clients younger than 25 years old. This condition is genetic. A parent with MODY has a 50 percent chance of passing on MODY to his or her children (The Diabetes Monitor, www.diabetesmonitor, accessed June, 2004). Clients with MODY do not always need insulin treatment and often can be treated with oral agents and a weight-reduction diet.

Other Specific Types

Most diabetes results from a primary failure of insulin production and/or use, but diabetes can occur as a result of a variety of disorders, including pancreatitis, cystic fibrosis, surgical removal of the pancreas, Cushing's disease, or pharmacological doses of glucocorticoids (e.g., prednisone) or other hormones or drugs. The term **secondary diabetes** is sometimes used when one of these disorders is responsible for the hyperglycemia. The diabetes may be resolved if the cause is alleviated. If the cause is not cor-rectable, secondary diabetes is treated similarly to other forms of diabetes.

IMPAIRED GLUCOSE TOLERANCE (IGT)/IMPAIRED FASTING GLUCOSE (IFG)/PRE-DIABETES

Impaired glucose tolerance (IGT) and impaired fasting glucose (IFG) are terms that refer to a metabolic state intermediate between normal and glucose homeostasis and diabetes. The American Diabetes Association encourages the use of the term pre-diabetes. Individuals who have a fasting glucose level of greater than 110 mg/dL but less than 126 mg/dL on more than two occasions meet the criteria for IGT or IFG. IGT may represent a step in the development of types 1 and 2 diabetes. In fact, 25 percent of clients with IGT later develop diabetes mellitus.

GESTATIONAL DIABETES

Gestational diabetes (GDM) is the term for glucose intolerance in pregnancy. Women who are diagnosed as diabetic before pregnancy are not classified as having gestational diabetes. Clinical Application 19–2 discusses diabetes mellitus in pregnancy. A fasting plasma glucose level of >126 mg/dL or a casual plasma glucose >200 mg/dL meets the criteria for the diagnosis of diabetes (American Diabetes Association, 2004). The condition usually disappears after childbirth. However, women who have had gestational diabetes are at an increased risk for developing type 2 diabetes as they age.

Normal Nutrient Metabolism

An understanding of diabetes mellitus is based on knowledge of the pancreas, the organ that produces insulin. It is also important to understand the cellular sources of glucose, the normal blood glucose curve, and the functions of insulin and other hormones. All of these are discussed in the following sections of this chapter.

Anatomy of the Pancreas

The pancreas is a gland that lies behind the stomach. It has both exocrine and endocrine secretions. The exocrine functions of the pancreas include the flow of enzymes into

Table 19–1 **Insulin-Dependent and Non-Insulin-Dependent Diabetes Mellitus**

	TYPE 1	TYPE 2
Cause	Beta cells damaged	Tissues resist insulin
Most common age at onset	Under 20 years	Over 45 years
Medication	1. Insulin injections OR 2. Insulin injections and oral agents	1. None OR 2. Oral agents OR 3. Some individuals may require insulin injections to attain optimal blood glucose levels
	3. Insulin drip during critical illness	4. Insulin drip during critical illness
Usual body build	Thin, underweight	Obese
Nutrition therapy	Integration of insulin therapy, activity, and food intake Consistent timing of food intake	Achievement of near-normal glucose, lipid, and blood pressure goals Weight loss is desirable and possible with some clients

Diabetes in Pregnancy

Pregnancy raises blood insulin levels in all women. It is an adaptive mechanism. Early in pregnancy, the woman's body cells store energy. Later, the woman's tissues become insulin resistant so that the fetus can draw on energy stores when the woman is fasting.

When the pregnant woman has or develops hyperglycemia, the mother's blood glucose crosses the placenta but her insulin does not. Then the fetus produces more insulin, which increases his/her fat deposition. Women with diabetes have large babies for this reason.

Perinatal mortality of infants born to women with diabetes is higher than that of infants of women who do not have diabetes. Ketosis in early pregnancy can produce congenital malformations, central nervous system disorders, and low intelligence. With strict control of the diabetes, however, 97 percent of the fetuses survive, compared with 98 to 99 percent born to women without diabetes.

Insulin resistance is greater in the morning in pregnant women. For this reason, usually only 39 grams of CHO are planned into the breakfast meal plan. There is a heightened tendency for maternal ketosis during fasting, and the possible adverse effects of ketones on the fetus suggest that periods of fasting during pregnancy should be avoided. Small, frequent feedings throughout the day are recommended. A bedtime snack that contains between 15 and 45 grams of CHO is recommended to minimize an accelerated production of ketones, which has been known to occur during sleeping. Clients should be reminded not to skip meals. Following is a summary of these recommendations:

- Breakfast: 30 grams of CHO
- Lunch and dinner: 60 grams of CHO
- Snacks: between 15 and 45 grams of CHO (dependent on the client's energy allowance based on individual assessment)
- Recommend bedtime snack for all clients
- Include protein and fat at each meal (amount dependent on client's energy allowance based on individual assessment)

Nutritional regulation is central to management of diabetes in pregnant women. During pregnancy, the most commonly recommended kilocalorie distribution is 40 to 45 percent carbohydrate, 20 to 25 percent protein, and 30 to 40 percent fat. The treatment goal is to prevent hypoglycemia, defined as fasting plasma concentrations of 70 to 90 mg/dL and 2-hour postprandial plasma glucose levels of less than 140 mg/dL. Some medical experts believe that this goal is too rigid because hypoglycemia during early pregnancy may be **teratogenic** (causing abnormal development of the embryo). Hypoglycemic agents have been shown to cause significant risk to the fetus. In most instances, women are advised to discontinue use of hypoglycemic agents before conception. If medication is necessary to control hyperglycemia, insulin is safer for the fetus.

Early pregnancy loss and congenital malformations can be minimized by optimal medical care and client education before conception in women with diabetes. Contraception, timing of conception, control of metabolic state, self-management techniques, assessment of diabetic complications, and other medical complications should be discussed with the female client of child-bearing age. The desired outcome of glycemia control in the preconception phase of care is to lower glycohemoglobin so as to achieve maximum fertility and optimal embryo and fetal development (American Diabetes Association, 1996a). Preconception counseling is best accomplished by a multidisciplinary team approach including a endocrinolgoist; internist or family practice physician; obstetrician; and diabetes educators, including nurses, registered dietitians, social workers, and other specialists as necessary. Self-management skills essential for control during pregnancy include (Position Paper of the American Dietetic Association, 1996a):

- Using an appropriate meal plan
- Timing of meals and snacks
- Planning physical activity
- Choosing time and site of insulin injections
- Using carbohydrate and glucagon for hypoglycemia
- Reducing stress, coping with denial
- Testing capillary blood glucose
- Self-adjusting insulin doses

---

the intestine through **ducts.** Endocrine secretions (hormones) flow directly into the bloodstream.

Clusters of cells in the pancreas called the **islets of Langerhans** produce three hormones. These islets contain three types of cells: alpha, beta, and delta. The alpha cells produce **glucagon,** the beta cells produce insulin, and the delta cells produce **somatostatin** (Fig. 19–1). Special sensors at junctions of the three types of cells monitor levels of blood glucose and stimulate the release of the appropriate hormone.

Functions of Insulin

Insulin is the only hormone that lowers blood glucose. A person normally secretes insulin in response to an elevated blood glucose level. Insulin decreases blood glucose by accelerating its movement from the blood into the cells. As glucose enters the cells, it may be metabolized to yield energy, may be stored as glycogen, or may be converted to fat (Table 19–2). The ultimate fate of glucose once it is inside the cell depends on body need and the amount of glucose that enters the cell. The cells' energy needs will be met first. If cells have available glucose over and above immediate energy needs, the excess glucose is stored as glycogen. Insulin stimulates the storage of glucose as glycogen. Once the glycogen stores are filled to capacity, any remaining glucose is converted to fat. The body can store about 0.4 pound of glycogen, which is equal to 800 kilocalories.

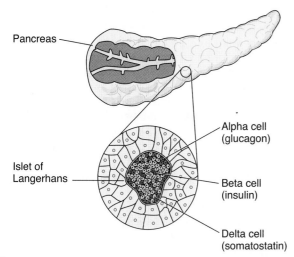

Figure **19–1** View of the pancreas and an enlarged islet of Langerhans. Alpha cells secrete glucagon, beta cells secrete insulin, and delta cells secrete somatostatin.

Insulin influences the metabolism of protein and fat. Insulin stimulates entry of amino acids into cells and enhances protein formation. It also enhances fat storage in adipose tissue and indirectly inhibits the breakdown of fat for energy. If the body has ample glucose available for energy, protein and fat need not be broken down to meet energy needs. If the body does not have glucose available for energy, it will use dietary protein or break down internal body protein stores to meet its immediate need for energy.

Insulin levels fluctuate in the blood. Normally, blood insulin levels increase as the blood glucose level increases. A high level of insulin in the blood signals the cells not to break down stores for energy (Table 19–3). An anabolic, or building, state exists when metabolism is normal and glucose and insulin levels are high. Normally insulin levels decrease as the blood sugar level decreases. A low level of insulin in the blood indirectly signals the body to begin to break down body stores for glucose. A catabolic, or breaking-down, state exists when metabolism is normal and glucose and insulin levels are low. Figure 19–2 illustrates glucose use by the cells.

Other Hormones

Glucagon and somatostatin assist in coordinating the storage and mobilization of the energy nutrients (carbohy-

Table **19–2** Metabolic Activities Promoted by Insulin

ACTIVITY	NAME OF METABOLIC PATHWAY
Movement of glucose into cells	None
Energy production from glucose	Glycolysis
Manufacture of glycogen	Glycogenesis
Fat formation from carbohydrate and protein	Lipogenesis

Note: "Genesis" means building up.

Table **19–3** Metabolic Activities Inhibited by a High Level of Insulin

ACTIVITY	NAME OF METABOLIC PATHWAY
Movement of glucose from noncarbohydrate sources, e.g., glycerol and amino acids	Gluconeogenesis
Release of glucose from glycogen	Glycogenolysis
Breakdown of fat from adipose tissue	Lipolysis

Note: "Genesis" means building up.

drate, fat, and protein). Glucagon increases blood glucose levels and stimulates the breakdown of body protein and fat stores. Somatostatin acts locally within the islets of Langerhans to depress the secretion of both insulin and glucagon. Evidence has shown that these hormones may not be at optimal levels in some clients with diabetes.

Cellular Sources of Glucose

The cells obtain glucose from both the food that is eaten and internal glucose stores. Almost all of the carbohydrate eaten (except fiber), about 50 percent of the protein eaten, and about 10 percent of the fat eaten will enter the blood as glucose. The internal body stores that can be converted to glucose are glycogen, some protein, and the glycerol portion of triglycerides. Body fat is stored as triglycerides in adipose tissue. To understand diabetes, it is necessary

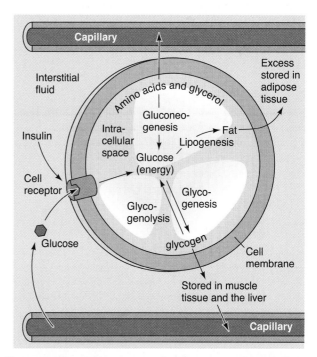

Figure **19–2** Insulin is necessary for glucose to gain entry into a cell. Once inside the cell, glucose can meet several fates: it can be burned as energy or stored as glycogen, or the glycerol portion of a fat molecule or some amino acids can be broken down into glucose. Some amino acids will be converted to glucose if the cell requires glucose.

to know how the body coordinates all internal and external sources of glucose to maintain a normal blood glucose range.

Blood Glucose Curve

Given the vital need for every cell to have an uninterrupted supply of energy, the human body has evolved to allow an uninterrupted energy supply to reach cells without continuous eating. A normal blood glucose range is usually about 70 to 100 mg/dL. (Some laboratories assign a normal blood glucose range of 80 to 110 mg/dL. The difference is the result of the type of equipment the laboratory uses and not the glucose content of the blood.) The blood glucose level increases after eating and decreases in the fasting state. Figure 19–3 illustrates the normal blood glucose curve.

Causes of Diabetes

The causes of diabetes include genetic factors, lifestyle, and viral infections. Although these causes are explained separately for the sake of clarity, in reality they are often interconnected.

Genetic Factors

Some of the susceptibility to diabetes is genetic. Researchers have discovered that people with type 1 diabetes have certain genes associated with their immune response. These particular genes are often found in children with type 1 diabetes. However, not everyone with these genes develops clinical diabetes. Before diabetes becomes apparent, this genetic susceptibility is often triggered by the individual's lifestyle or other environmental factors. These factors cause a series of events that results in damage to or destruction of the pancreatic beta cells. Inheritance is even more prominent in the development of type 2 than in type 1 diabetes, as the next section describes.

Insulin Resistance

A person may be genetically susceptible to **insulin resistance.** Insulin resistance occurs when both an individual's glucose and blood insulin levels are elevated. Insulin may not be released at the right times and/or be unable to assist the movement of glucose into the cells because of a lack of receptor sites. Before glucose can enter the cells, the insulin must first attach itself to specific receptor sites on the cells' outer surfaces. Persons with type 2 diabetes may lack enough receptor sites, have faulty receptor sites, or have postreceptor defects. Excess body fat seems to be related to a decrease in the number of receptor sites. Type 2 diabetes is often associated with insulin resistance.

Lifestyle

A healthy lifestyle is particularly important for the *prevention* of diabetes in genetically susceptible clients. Excessive body fat, inactivity, and stress are risk factors for diabetes, as highlighted in Wellness Tip 19–2. Up to 90 percent of clients with type 2 diabetes have a higher than recommended percent of body fat. A loss of body fat alone is sometimes sufficient to balance the insulin produced with a modified food intake. At least a dozen studies have demonstrated that weight loss reduces insulin resistance and increases peripheral glucose uptake (Maggio and Pi-Sunyer, 1997). Inactivity is a lifestyle risk factor that predisposes one to diabetes. Sometimes emotional or physical stress is the stimulus that causes hyperglycemia. The body's stress response involves the release of epinephrine from the adrenal glands. One action of epinephrine is to raise the blood sugar level so the person has energy for the "fight or flight" response.

Wellness*Tip* **19–2** • Excess body fat, inactivity, and stress are lifestyle choices that can increase the risk of diabetes. Type 2 diabetes can sometimes be prevented with good lifestyle choices.

Viral Infections

Links have been noted between viral epidemics and the onset of diabetes. During the late fall and winter months, a disproportionate number of cases of type 1 diabetes are diagnosed. Because these seasons are also associated with peak occurrence of childhood viral diseases, it is possible that a causal connection exists between viral epidemics and the onset of type 1 diabetes.

Antibodies to pancreatic islet cells have been found in some people with diabetes. Type 1 diabetes is usually an autoimmune disease that is characterized by the presence of a variety of autoantibodies on the surface of or within the beta cells of the pancreas. Individuals with more than one autoantibody (i.e., ICA, IAA, GAD, IA-2) are at a high risk for type 1 diabetes (www.medscape.com/, accessed May 2000). In **autoimmune diseases,** the body cannot recognize its own cells but rather treats them as foreign invaders. The event that provokes this process usually is a viral infection. These elevated antibodies may be detected in about 90 percent of clients before the diagnosis of diabetes. Physicians order laboratory tests to check the levels of these antibodies in clients' blood. If the levels are elevated, the physician can inform the client of his or her situation. It is inappropriate to inform a client of a highly probable prognosis unless treatment options are presented and offered at the same time. However, after speaking to a client, physicians frequently will request other

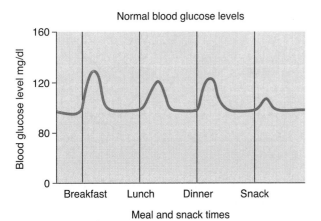

Normal blood glucose levels

Figure **19–3** A person's blood glucose level normally goes up after food consumption and then down between feedings.

health-care professionals to explain in detail to the client the treatment options.

Signs and Symptoms of Diabetes

The classic triad of signs and symptoms includes **polyuria,** increased urination; **polydipsia,** increased thirst; and **polyphagia,** increased appetite and weight loss. The triad is most commonly seen in type 1 diabetes. The following section describes these and other signs and symptoms commonly seen in persons with diabetes.

Classic Triad

In diabetes, glucose cannot optimally move from the intravascular space across a cell membrane into the intracellular space. This is why the diabetic person's blood glucose level remains elevated after eating. Under normal circumstances, the blood glucose level does not increase excessively because excess glucose undergoes glycolysis and is readily converted to adipose tissue or stored as glycogen inside the cell. As the glucose-rich blood circulates through the kidneys, these organs reabsorb all the glucose of which they are capable. After this point is reached, glucose enters the urine. **Glycosuria** means an abnormally high amount of glucose in the urine. As the glucose exits the body in the urine, water is pulled out, also as a result of the osmotic effect of glucose. This results in polyuria, or a large urine output. The large loss of water causes excessive thirst and polydipsia and prompts the person to drink fluids.

When glucose is not available for energy inside the cells, the body begins to break down protein and fat for energy. In untreated type 1 diabetes, the body's cells are starving. These starving cells send a message to the brain to turn on the person's appetite. The person responds by eating to satisfy the craving for food. The third symptom or sign of diabetes is polyphagia, an abnormal increase in appetite. Polyphagia, polyuria, and polydipsia are the three classic signs or symptoms reported or seen in clients with diabetes.

Other Signs and Symptoms

The abnormal carbohydrate metabolism of diabetes and its effects on the body's tissues cause other problems. Weight loss is more commonly seen in clients with type 1 diabetes than in clients with type 2. Blurred vision is common in both types. The need for good eye care is discussed in Wellness Tip 19–3. Fatigue is frequently seen in these clients. High glucose levels impair white blood cell functioning, thus increasing the client's susceptibility to infection. Commonly involved agents are *Staphylococcus aureus* and *Candida albicans* involving the skin and mucous membranes. Recurrent furuncle (boil, caused by localized infection), **vaginitis** (inflammation of the vagina), or bladder infections in a client may stimulate testing for diabetes. Poor wound healing is related to decreased circulation. Circulatory problems in men may manifest as impotence.

under control. Diabetes is the leading cause of adult blindness in the United States. Often no symptoms appear before damage occurs.

Complications

Both acute and chronic complications occur with diabetes mellitus. Acute complications require immediate care. Chronic complications include diseases of the eye, kidneys, heart, and nervous system. Chronic complications are responsible for the increased death rate among individuals with diabetes and the diminished quality of life that many of these clients experience.

Acute Clinical Situations

Three acute complications are seen in clients with diabetes: **diabetic ketoacidosis (DKA),** hyperglycemic hyperosmolar nonketotic syndrome, and **hypoglycemia.**

Ketoacidosis

Individuals with type 1 diabetes who experience a profound insulin deficiency may progress to the condition of ketoacidosis. The three main precipitating factors in ketoacidosis are a decreased or missed dose of insulin, an illness or infection, or uncontrolled disease in a previously undiagnosed person. Ketoacidosis is a complex, life-threatening condition that demands emergency treatment. The predominant clinical manifestations of dehydration, acidosis, and electrolyte imbalances and general principles of treatment are discussed next.

DEHYDRATION

Without insulin, glucose cannot be transferred across the cell membranes into the cells. A greatly increased number of glucose molecules (300 to 800 mg/dL) in the blood exert an osmotic effect, causing water to move from within the cells to the intravascular space and producing cellular dehydration. The body excretes the excess water, glucose, and electrolytes in the urine.

ACIDOSIS

Unaware that the problem is not lack of glucose but lack of insulin, the body proceeds to increase blood glucose by mobilizing protein and fat from the tissues to be converted to glucose by the liver. Because the human body can use only the glycerol portion of the triglyceride molecule for glucose, the fatty acid portion is processed into ketones. Normally the ketones are metabolized and excreted as carbon dioxide and water. Under conditions of ketoacidosis, however, the body cannot metabolize this overload of ketones rapidly enough to maintain homeostasis, and thus the client has excessive ketones in the blood (ketonemia) and spills ketones in the urine (ketonuria). Acetone is one of the ketone bodies for which urine is tested. The ketone bodies are acid, and thus the term ketoacidosis.

The body can initiate several homeostatic mechanisms as it attempts to correct the acidosis. It decreases the level of carbonic acid in the blood by increasing the excretion of carbon dioxide through involuntary deep, gasping rapid breaths called **Kussmaul respirations.** The client's breath

 19–3 • Keep your eyes working by keeping your blood pressure and blood glucose

has a fruity odor from the ketonemia. The kidney increases the hydrogen ion content or acidity of the urine it excretes. Buffering of hydrogen can occur in the cells also, where it displaces potassium to the extracellular fluid.

ELECTROLYTE IMBALANCES

Clients with severe ketoacidosis may excrete 6.5 liters of fluid and 400 to 500 milliequivalents of sodium, potassium, and chloride in 24 hours. A fluid loss of 15 percent of body weight is not unusual. Most critical in the treatment of electrolyte imbalances in diabetic ketoacidosis is the body's level of potassium. As the cells are being catabolized for fuel, the intracellular potassium is transferred to the intravascular space. Serum potassium levels can be low, normal, or elevated in the person with ketoacidosis, depending on the body's current coping mechanism. Regardless of the serum concentrations of potassium and sodium, the pathological process of diabetic ketoacidosis depletes these electrolytes. Either hypokalemia or hyperkalemia can lead to cardiac arrhythmias and must be carefully managed in clients with ketoacidosis.

TREATMENT

Clients with severe diabetic ketoacidosis are critically ill. Treatment includes supplemental insulin, fluid and electrolyte replacement, and medical monitoring. Serum electrolyte levels change dramatically once treatment commences. Intensive care is necessary to provide the careful monitoring and frequent adjustments in therapy required as the fluids and electrolytes are being replaced. Intravenous regular insulin will permit the use of carbohydrate for energy and will halt the body's excessive use of fat, which has produced the ketone bodies. Insulin drives glucose back into the cells. Potassium, too, moves from the intravascular space to the intracellular space, necessitating frequent measurement of the serum levels of both glucose and potassium. When the client recovers, identification of the precipitating factor for the ketoacidosis and education focused on preventing additional occurrences are essential.

Hyperglycemic Hyperosmolar Nonketotic Syndrome

The four signs of **hyperglycemic hyperosmolar nonketotic syndrome (HHNS)** are blood glucose level greater than 600 mg/dL, absence of or slight ketosis, plasma hyperosmolality, and profound dehydration. This life-threatening emergency is usually seen in the elderly or people with undiagnosed type 2 diabetes. HHNS is like DKA except that the insulin deficiency is not as severe, so increased **lipolysis** (the breakdown of body lipid stores) does not occur. Because these clients do not have symptoms of vomiting, nausea, and acidosis brought on by severe ketosis, as do clients with type 1 diabetes, they often do not seek prompt medical help. Their blood sugar levels are higher and their dehydration more severe than is seen in ketoacidosis.

In these clients, prolonged osmotic diuresis and dehydration secondary to hyperglycemia lead to decreased renal blood flow and allow the blood glucose to reach very high levels. Medications that cause an increase in blood glucose levels, chronic disease, and infection may con-

tribute to this condition. Examples of medications that cause hyperglycemia with diabetes include corticosteroids, such as hydrocortisone and prednisone; thiazide diuretics, such as lasix, hydrodiuril, and naturetin; dilantin; and estrogens. Treatment includes correction of the electrolyte imbalance, hyperglycemia, and dehydration.

Hypoglycemia

In both type 1 and type 2 diabetes (treated with medications), an individual can develop hypoglycemia. Hypoglycemia may be caused by too much insulin (accidental or deliberate), too little food intake, a delayed meal, excessive exercise, alcohol (especially in the fasting state), and/or medications such as oral hypoglycemic agents. Symptoms may include confusion, headache, double vision, rapid heartbeat, sweating, hunger, seizure, and coma. The treatment of hypoglycemia is discussed later in this chapter.

Chronic Complications

Clients with both type 1 and type 2 diabetes of sufficient duration are vulnerable to serious complications involving the eyes, kidneys, and nervous system. Diabetic **retinopathy** is a disorder that involves the retina. Diabetes is a leading cause of blindness and of visual loss in the adult U.S. population. The blurred vision reported by these clients is related to retinopathy. These clients are also at a higher risk for cataracts.

Diabetic neuropathy is a chronic complication of diabetes mellitus. Clients may complain of a lack of sensation in their extremities. They may puncture, cut, or burn their feet and not feel any pain. A wound may become infected and heal poorly. Gangrene, or tissue death, may follow. The treatment for gangrene is amputation. **Neuropathy** can affect gastric or intestinal motility, erectile function, bladder function, cardiac function, and vascular tone. **Gastroparesis** (paralysis of the stomach with delayed gastric emptying) may occur and alter the absorption of meals, which makes glycemic control problematic. Cardiovascular disease is more common in these clients. Diabetic **nephropathy,** or kidney disease, is another common complication in diabetic clients. Tragically, some clients with diabetes do not take the threat of chronic complications seriously until much damage has occurred.

Treatment

The current medical goal is to *normalize* the blood glucose throughout the day and control blood pressure and blood lipids. A normal fasting blood glucose level is less 100 mg/dL before a meal and less than 140 mg/dL 2 hours after a meal. Realistic target levels for individuals with diabetes treated intensively are 70 to 140 mg/dL before meals, less than 180 mg/dL 2 hours after meals, and glycosylated hemoglobin within 1 percent of normal. A landmark study known as the Diabetes Control and Complications Trial (DCCT) in individuals with IDDM demonstrated that intensive control of blood glucose levels delays the onset and slows the progression of diabetic retinopathy, nephropathy, and neuropathy (Diabetes Control and Complications Trial Research Group, 1993). According to this study's results, people with type 1 diabetes who followed a tightly controlled regimen, compared with those who followed a standard regimen, showed reductions of approximately:

- 76 percent in progression of diabetic retinopathy
- 54 percent in albuminuria (albumin in the urine, which may be a sign of renal impairment)
- 36 percent in **microalbuminuria** (a more sensitive indicator of protein in the urine, which may be an early warning of renal impairment)
- 60 percent in rates of neuropathy

A tightly controlled regimen is not without problems, however. Among these is an increased incidence of insulin-induced hypoglycemic episodes (Allen, 2001). Clients undergoing intensive diabetes treatment do not face deterioration in the quality of their lives, even while the rigor of their diabetes care is increased (Diabetes Control and Complication Trial Research Group, 1996). This evidence has been further strengthened by a recent report from the United Kingdom Prospective Diabetes Study (UKPDS), which demonstrated that intensive therapy for type 2 diabetes significantly lowered the rate of diabetes-related events (UK Prospective Diabetes Study Group, 1998).

Blood pressure and blood lipids should also be controlled and monitored for clients with diabetes. Systolic blood pressure for nonpregnant adults is ideally below 130 mmHg and diastolic blood pressure below 80 mmHg. Lipid management includes (American Diabetes Association, 2005):

In individuals with diabetes aged >40 years with total cholesterol greater than or equal to 135 mg/dl, without overt cardiovascular disease, statin therapy to achieve an LDL reduction of 30–40% regardless of baseline LDL levels is recommended. The primary goal is an LDL <100 mg/dl.

For persons with diabetes aged <40 years without overt cardiovascular disease, but at increased risk (due to other cardiovascular risk factors or long duration of diabetes), who do not achieve lipid goals with lifestyle modifications alone, the addition of pharmacological therapy is appropriate and primary goal is an LDL <100 mg/dl.

People with diabetes and overt cardiovascular disease are at very high risk for further events and should be treated with a statin. A lower LDL cholesterol goal of <70 mg/dl using a high dose statin, is an option in these high-risk patients with diabetes and overt cardiovascular disease.

All health-care workers should assist the general population in the early detection of diabetes and prevention of complications. As Figure 19–4 emphasizes, the three cornerstones of the management of diabetes after diagnosis are physical activity, medication, and nutritional management. Self-monitoring of blood glucose levels enables the client to assess how each of these factors interacts. Blood glucose monitoring, physical activity, medication, and diet are discussed next.

Self-Monitoring of Blood Glucose

Many individuals monitor their own blood glucose levels with a device called a blood glucose meter. This procedure is called **self-monitoring of blood glucose (SMBG).** Individual response to medication, diet, and exercise can be determined with this advanced technology. SMBG can be performed using a single drop of blood. The client obtains the drop of blood from a finger with either a lancet

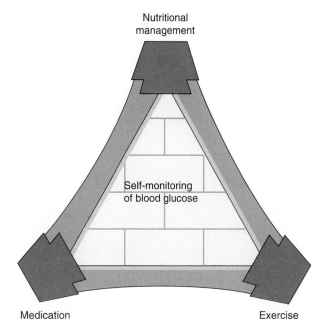

Figure **19–4** Nutritional management, medication, and exercise are the three components of treatment for diabetes. Each of these cornerstones has an influence on blood glucose levels. An individual can identify how each of these cornerstones impacts his or her blood glucose level by self-monitoring blood glucose.

or a spring-loaded device. The blood sample is placed in the meter, and the test results are available in less than 1 minute. The client can then adjust insulin dose and food and exercise behaviors accordingly. Many experts consider SMBG to be the most important development in diabetes management since the discovery of insulin. SMBG can also be done with a newer device that is easier to use because it does not require a skin poke and a drop of blood. The device is held next to the skin and the blood glucose is noted on the display.

SMBG has allowed clients to try to normalize their blood glucose levels throughout the day. Health-care workers need to carefully teach clients how to interpret the results of SMBG (Fig. 19–5). Continual reassessment of

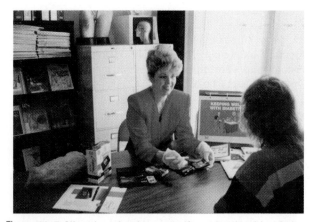

Figure **19–5** Client learning how to self-monitor her blood glucose levels. Note that the nurse is wearing personal protective equipment: gloves.

the client's technique and blood glucose records is necessary to guide treatment decisions. To evaluate the need for changes in diet or medications, monitoring should be done at least twice a day; four times a day for 3 days each week is preferable for clients who are stable. If near-normalization of blood glucose is the treatment goal, SMBG must be done four to eight times daily (before and 2 hours after each meal and/or snack). During acute illness, more frequent self-monitoring is indicated. Once the blood glucose is stabilized, SMBG can be done less frequently.

Physical Activity

Exercise plays a key role in the management of diabetes. All individuals with diabetes who exercise should be encouraged to follow these guidelines:

1. Wear proper footwear, and use other protective equipment if necessary.
2. Avoid exercise in extremely hot and cold environments.
3. Inspect feet daily and after exercise for open areas, blisters, punctures, swelling, and redness; report any of these signs to the physician immediately.
4. Avoid exercise during periods of poor metabolic control (blood glucose levels that are <60 or >240 mg/dL levels).
5. Wear a diabetes ID badge or bracelet.
6. Carry a source of glucose in case of a decrease in blood glucose, as exercise decreases blood glucose levels.

Exercise and Type 2 Diabetes

Physical activity is widely endorsed for persons with type 2 diabetes. Physical activity increases the number and binding capacity of insulin receptors, assists in lowering blood glucose levels, and reduces insulin requirements in persons who use insulin. Improved blood lipid levels occur in some clients who engage in regular exercise. This helps delay or prevent the cardiovascular disease complications often seen in these clients. Exercise also assists in weight control and improves muscle strength and flexibility.

Aerobic exercise should be encouraged at 50 to 70 percent maximum heart rate and of at least 40 minutes duration to promote breakdown of body fat. Daily exercise is recommended, but three times a week is considered the minimum required to aid blood glucose management. Current research suggests that three 10-minute exercise sessions provide a substantial health benefit, especially for the sedentary individual. The strategy to break down activity sessions into shorter, more frequent increments may be helpful to clients who have difficulty being physically active.

Exercise and Type 1 Diabetes

The American Diabetes Association strongly endorses an exercise program for people with type 1 diabetes because of the potential to improve cardiovascular fitness and psychological well-being. Exercise involves some risk for individuals with type 1 diabetes because it changes insulin requirements in sometimes unpredictable ways more than 24 hours after the exercise. Retinopathy, neuropathy, and renal disease may worsen in some clients with type 1 diabetes who exercise. Blood pressure may also become elevated. For this type of client, self-monitoring of blood glucose should be incorporated into a modified exercise program tailored to individual client needs and limitations. The client should demonstrate the ability to self-treat a hypoglycemic episode.

Exercise, SMBG, and Food Intake

Type 1 clients with diabetes who do exercise and all type 2 clients who engage in nonroutine exercise should monitor their blood glucose levels before, during, and after exercise. If the blood glucose level is greater than 100 mg/dL before exercise, there is usually no need for additional food if the planned exercise is of short duration and low intensity. Exercise of long duration and high intensity generally requires more kilocalories. Snacks that contain an additional 15 to 30 grams of carbohydrate-containing food should be ingested for every 30 to 60 minutes of exercise. Good choices for snack foods include fruit, starch, and milk exchanges. To prevent wide swings in blood glucose levels, care should be taken not to overeat. Too much food will cause the blood glucose level to go up too high and subsequently to drop too low. Exercise is best done 60 to 90 minutes after meals, when the blood glucose level is highest.

Medications

Two types of medications are used with diabetic clients: insulin and oral hypoglycemic agents. Clients with type 1 diabetes require insulin. Clients with type 2 diabetes may not require any medication or may need to have an oral hypoglycemic agent or insulin prescribed. Frequently, clients with type 2 diabetes are able to discontinue the medication after a loss of body fat.

Insulin

Almost all the insulin used in the United States is human. Human insulin is manufactured by recombinant-DNA technology (biosynthetic). Human insulin (**Humulin**) produces few allergic reactions. Insulin cannot be taken orally because the gastrointestinal tract enzymes would digest it before absorption. Insulin must be administered by needle either **subcutaneously** (beneath the skin) or intravenously (IV). Only regular insulin is given IV. The substances used to delay absorption of intermediate- and long-acting insulins are not designed for IV administration. Regular insulin is usually administered IV only for the severely hyperglycemic or hospitalized client.

Insulin can also be administered with an insulin pump. These pumps are designed to provide a small inflow of insulin continuously and large inflows before eating, thus mimicking normal insulin secretion. Continuous subcutaneous insulin infusion (CSII) or insulin pumps have been available for nearly 20 years, but only recently have they been widely used.

Medications are described according to the onset, peak, and duration of action. A bolus dose of insulin is short acting and designed to cover needs for one meal. A basal dose of insulin is longer acting and usually injected once or twice a day. Table 19–4 lists the times of onset, peak, and duration of insulin. Variation in duration makes it possible

Table 19–4 Times of Onset, Peak, and Duration of Action for Rapid-Acting, Intermediate-Acting, and Long-Acting Insulin

	TIMES IN HOURS		
	ONSET	**PEAK**	**DURATION**
INSULIN BOLUS (SHORT ACTING)			
Humalog	5–15 min	1–2 hour	3 1/2–5 hour
NovoLog	10–20 min	1–3 hour	3–5 hour
Regular	30–60 min	2–4 hour	6–8 hour
BASAL (QD) NOT TX INTENSIVELY (2 × QD)			
Lantus*	1 hour	None	24 hour
NPH	1–1 1/2 hour	4–10 hour	14–18 hour
70/30†	1/2 hour	2–3 hour and 4–10 hour	14–18 hour
Lente	1 1/4 hour	7–15 hour	24 hour
Ultralente	4–6 hour	10–16 hour	>36 hour

*Lantus is a long-acting insulin that is designed to be given at HS. Lantus has no pronounced peaks with a relatively constant level over 24 hours. The FDA approved Lantus in early 2000.
†Mixture is 70% NPH and 30% regular.
A typical meal is a combination of CHO, fiber, fat, and protein. CHO is digested and absorbed in about 1 to 2 hours. Meals containing moderate or high fat or protein may require additional bolus insulin to overcome insulin resistance. In addition, fat takes longer to digest than CHO. For this reason, after a moderate or high-fat meal, the bolus dose of insulin may need to be split (some taken with the meal and some taken after the meal) to achieve optimal blood glucose control. A high-fiber meal (>5 grams/serving) also delays the digestion and absorption of CHO. The best control is achieved when the bolus dose of insulin is split. Clients should be taught to do this by a Certified Diabetes Educator.
SOURCES: Killion, KH: Facts and Comparison. Wolters Kluwer, St. Louis, 2003; Ryan-Turek, T: Latest Therapies and Technology in Diabetes Treatment. Michigan Dietetic Association Spring Conference, Midland, MI, 2003.

to inject insulin in a pattern that is as close as possible to normal insulin activity. Ideally, the medication is planned around the diet, not vice versa. Most experts know that it is far easier to change a medication than a food behavior.

Oral Hypoglycemic Agents

Oral hypoglycemic agents lower blood glucose levels in type 2 diabetes. These drugs stimulate insulin release from the pancreatic beta cells, reduce glucose output from the liver, and increase the uptake of glucose in tissues. Many new oral agents are being prescribed in the United States, and many more are in development (Table 19–5). Recently, oral agents and insulin administered simultaneously have been used successfully to treat type 1 diabetes. Commonly prescribed oral hypoglycemic agents include glipizide, glyburide, glimiperide, metformin, acarbose, and tolazamide. Oral agents are increasingly being used in combinations. Many of the new oral agents work on different cell receptor

Table 19–5 Diabetes Oral Medications and Major Actions

CLASSIFICATION	MAJOR ACTIONS	GENERIC NAME (TRADE NAME)	COMMENTS
Sulfonylureas	Stimulate insulin release by the pancreas and may help decrease liver glucose production.	Glipizides (Glucotrol) Glyburide (Glynase, Micronase, and Diabeta)	Glipizide must be taken on an empty stomach. Glyburide can be taken with food or on an empty stomach. Low toxicity. Use caution with elderly.
Biguanides	Decrease liver production of glucose. Increase glucose uptake into tissues.	Metformin (Glucophage)	Given in 2–3 doses per day with meals. Not metabolized. Often used in combination with sulfonylureas.
Meglitinide	Stimulates immediate insulin release from pancreas as needed for meals.	Repaglinide (Pradin)	Given in 2–4 doses per day 15–30 minutes before meals.
Alpha-Glucosidase Inhibitors	Slow the rate of digestion of starches and complex sugars.	Acarbose (Precose)	Given in 3 doses per day with meals. 98 percent not absorbed. Rest excreted by kidneys.

SOURCE: Adapted from Quick Reference Guide to Diabetes for Health Care Providers by Michigan Diabetes Outreach Network. www.Diabetes-midon.org and Sodon Sentinel, Vol. 4, Issue 4 by Michigan Diabetes Outreach Network.

sites. For example, metformin and acarbose can be added to sulfonylurea (e.g., glimiperide, glyburide) with an additional 0.5 to 2 percent reduction in HbA1C level (Zimmerman and Hagan, 1998).

Medical Nutritional Management

Diabetes is directly related to how the body uses food. Nutrition is thus an essential component of management for all persons with diabetes. Studies have shown that clients report improved health, better control of body weight, improved control of blood glucose blood pressure and lipid levels, and improved use of insulin when they adhere to dietary recommendations. The goals of nutritional care for persons with diabetes are the control and prevention of complications. This involves the promotion of normal nutrition and dietary modification to control blood glucose and lipid levels. Clients' nutritional goals need to be determined individually. There is **no** "diabetic diet" or "ADA diet," but several meal-planning approaches are widely endorsed by the American Diabetes Association and the American Dietetic Association.

The next sections describe the overall goals of nutritional care, the need to individualize nutritional care to meet each client's goals, assessment of client readiness to change negative eating behaviors, survival skills needed by all clients with diabetes, and various meal-planning approaches that are widely used for these clients.

Nutritional Goals

The goal of medical nutritional therapy is to educate the person with diabetes to make changes in food and exercise habits that lead to improved metabolic control. Specifically, the client needs assistance with:

1. The attainment and maintenance of near-normal blood glucose levels as feasible by the coordination of food intake, **endogenous** and **exogenous** insulin and/or hypoglycemic agents, and physical activity. This is a challenge in some clients who have fluctuating endogenous insulin production.
2. The attainment and maintenance of optimal serum lipid levels and blood pressure
3. Provision of adequate kilocalories to
   - attain and maintain a healthy body weight for adults and normal growth and development for children
   - recover from illnesses
   - meet the metabolic needs of pregnancy and lactation
4. The prevention and treatment of the acute and chronic complications of diabetes, such as renal disease, autonomic neuropathy, hypertension, and cardiovascular disease
5. Improvement of overall health through good nutrition. *MyPyramid and Dietary Guidelines for Americans* illustrate and summarize nutritional guidelines for all Americans, including people with diabetes.

Goal Priority

The medications prescribed, the type of diabetes the individual has, and the client's desire to change behavior determine goal priority. A high priority for the person tak-

ing insulin is to facilitate consistency in the timing of meals and snacks to prevent wide swings in blood glucose. This requires coordination among exercise, insulin, and food intake. A high priority for the individual with type 2 diabetes is achieving glucose, blood pressure, and lipid goals. To achieve these goals, diet is a cornerstone of treatment. Weight reduction for these clients usually improves short-term glycemic levels and long-term metabolic control. The client's motivation to lose weight needs to be carefully assessed by the health-care educator.

Meal Frequency

Meal spacing is more crucial in type 1 than in type 2 diabetes. Consistent timing and meal size assist in stabilization of blood glucose levels in type 1 diabetes. In general, people with diabetes benefit from eating on a regular basis (every 4 to 5 hours) while awake.

Client Readiness to Change Behavior

Food behaviors are difficult to change. Although some clients with diabetes do successfully change or alter food behaviors to enhance their outcomes, many clients do not, will not, or cannot change harmful food behaviors. Modification of harmful behaviors involves progression through five stages: precontemplation, contemplation, preparation, action, and maintenance. Individuals typically recycle through these stages several times before terminating negative behaviors. Following is a brief description of each of these stages:

1. *Precontemplation:* individuals exhibit no intention to change behavior in the foreseeable future.
2. *Contemplation:* individuals know they have a problem and they are seriously thinking about overcoming the harmful behavior but are not ready to take action.
3. *Preparation:* individuals plan to take action in the near future, may have taken action unsuccessfully in the past, and may report small behavioral changes.
4. *Action:* individuals modify their behavior, experiences, and/or environment to overcome the harmful behavior. This stage requires considerable commitment of time and energy.
5. *Maintenance:* individuals continue to work to prevent relapse and to consolidate gains.

Health-care workers can assist clients in the precontemplation and contemplation stages by attempting to raise patients' consciousness about the benefits of behavioral change. Stimulus control and reinforcement also help patients become more aware of the need to alter behaviors (see Chapter 18, Weight Control). The most difficult problems posed by clients for the health educator are at the precontemplation phase (Jacobson, 1993).

The health-care educator needs to carefully consider how much information the client desires and how ready he or she is to change food behaviors. An educational tool that takes 3 to 4 hours to review with a client is inappropriate for someone who is willing to devote just a few minutes to learning about his or her diet. In contrast, the client who wants to learn everything he or she can about self-care will not be satisfied with an elementary meal plan.

Survival Skills

The American Diabetes and Dietetic associations recommend that the newly diagnosed client initially learn basic "survival skills." See Box 19–1 for information the client needs to know immediately. Appendix L has handouts on survival skills for clients on medication and treated by diet alone. Once the client has demonstrated an understanding of this basic knowledge, a firm foundation has been set for the acquisition of additional, more individualized information. Individualized food/meal plans and insulin regimens provide flexibility to accommodate lifestyle, age, and overall health status (American Diabetes Association, 2003).

Meal-Planning Approaches

There are about a dozen appropriate meal-planning approaches. The most elementary approaches include *MyPyramid, Dietary Guidelines for Americans,* and *The First Step in Diabetes Meal Planning.* Any one of these meal-planning approaches is considered survival-skill level information. After the client has demonstrated an understanding of the meal-planning approach initially used by the health educator, the use of a more advanced approach should be considered. The client will achieve optimal blood glucose and lipid control with a more sophisticated meal-planning approach. Two of the more widely used, more advanced

---

Box 19–1 **Survival Information for the Client With Diabetes**

Initial education for the client with diabetes should include basic knowledge that will facilitate the maintenance of acceptable (safe) blood glucose levels. Individuals with diabetes must come to accept responsibility for self-management and the need for ongoing education. Survival skills are typically reviewed with these clients during the first educational session.

1. Diabetes is caused by a lack of insulin and/or an inability to use the insulin the body produces. There is no cure for diabetes, but it can be controlled through diet, exercise, and medications.
2. An acceptable blood glucose is <100 mg/dL **preprandial plasma glucose** (before meals and fasting) and less than 180 mg/dL **peak postprandial plasma glucose** (about 2 hours after meals). The client is said to be adequately controlled if the blood glucose level is between these numbers relative to the time meals are eaten. Better control can be possible with more finely controlled blood glucose levels.
3. Monitoring and recording blood glucose levels can be done with a blood glucose monitor. All individuals with diabetes are encouraged to monitor their blood glucose levels. Hospital nurses and dietitians, home health-care agencies, and health-care workers in physicians' offices can teach the client how to monitor blood glucose levels.
4. Nutrition is an important part of blood glucose control. The MyPyramid provides an initial acceptable dietary guide of what foods should be eaten. Foods chosen from the MyPyramid guide should be divided into three or more equal feedings. Carbohydrate-containing foods are especially important to distribute evenly throughout the day. It is important to eat at regular times each day, to avoid skipping meals, and to eat about the same amount each day. Try to limit fat, salt, sugar, and alcohol intake. Portion control is important. Alcohol consumption on an empty stomach may cause a low blood glucose reaction. Try to increase intake of fruits, vegetables, and whole grains.
5. Exercise is beneficial for most people with diabetes; however, before beginning any exercise program, consult the doctor. Exercise is the most beneficial when the blood glucose is below 200 mg/dL. Regular exercise is more beneficial than sporadic exercise and best done 60 to 90 minutes after eating.
6. An understanding of the peak, onset, and duration of any medication used to treat a high blood glucose is important. Good insulin injection technique (if applicable) is essential.
7. A high blood glucose (greater than 240 mg/dL) is potentially dangerous, especially if untreated. Always check the urine for ketones if the blood glucose is more than 240 mg/dL. Contact the physician if the blood glucose is greater than 240 mg/dL and the urine is positive for ketones.
8. A blood glucose of less than 60 mg/dL is dangerous and may lead to confusion, disorientation, and coma. Signs of a low blood glucose include sweating, slurred speech, headache, weakness, tremors, hunger, nervousness, tingling of the lips, and rapid heart beat. In the event these signs are noted, immediately:
   a. Ingest 15 to 20 grams of glucose (sucrose can be substituted as a second choice).
   b. Glucose tablets or $\frac{1}{2}$ cup of orange juice or 6 hard candies is equal to this amount of CHO.
   c. Initial response to treatment should be seen in 10 to 20 minutes.
   d. Evaluate blood glucose in about 60 minutes, as additional treatment may be necessary.
   e. Repeat the process if blood glucose is less than 100 mg/dL.
9. Over the long term, diabetes can lead to foot problems, including infection and amputation. Check the feet (and legs) daily. Look for sores, redness, infection, drainage, swelling, or bruises. Report problems to the doctor early. Keep the feet clean and dry. Never go barefoot. Protect any area where sensation is lost.
10. Have an annual examination with a board-certified ophthalmologist (a doctor specializing in eye care). Diabetes is the leading cause of adult blindness in the United States. Often there are no symptoms before damage occurs.
11. The person with diabetes should wear a personal identification bracelet or necklace.

meal-planning systems are discussed next. Various meal-planning approaches are discussed in Table 19–6.

THE EXCHANGE LISTS OF THE AMERICAN DIETETIC AND THE AMERICAN DIABETES ASSOCIATIONS

This approach to meal planning, introduced in Chapter 2, Individualized Nutritional Care, teaches the learner about food composition and portion sizes. For example, many clients do not know that sugars are carbohydrates and oil is fat. Many clients think that however much they eat of a food item is a portion size. Exchange Lists are one method to learn about food; however, it is not the only method. Many clients find this method of menu planning too complex. Unfortunately, many health educators in the past have insisted clients learn this approach to meal planning. It is important to individualize lesson plans for each client. Usually the registered dietitian reviews this approach with the client and then the nurse reinforces the dietitian's teaching. The educator needs to anticipate spending a total of 1 to 2 hours to thoroughly explain this approach to a client (Fig. 19–6). This can best be accomplished in two or more sessions. *The Exchange Lists of the American Dietetic and American Diabetes Associations* is used to calculate energy nutrient distribution.

ENERGY NUTRIENT DISTRIBUTION

Total energy requirements for the individual with diabetes do not differ from those for individuals without diabetes. Therefore, please refer to Chapter 6, Energy Balance, to determine the total kilocalorie requirement for a person. The distribution of energy nutrients refers to the percentage of total kilocalories that should be derived from carbohydrate, fat, and protein. Distribution also refers to the division of carbohydrate, fat, and protein among the day's

Table 19–6 **Meal-Planning Approaches**

APPROACH	COMMENTS	AVAILABILITY
MyPyramid	Initial phase of teaching.	A colorful version is available from the National Dairy Council, 10255 West Higgins Road, Suite 900, Rosemont, IL 60018-4233; 1-708-803-2000.
	Provides a basic foundation in normal nutrition.	www.MyPyramid.gov accessed May, 2005
	Does not emphasize meal consistency.	
Dietary Guidelines	Initial phase of teaching.	United States Department of Agriculture Home & Garden Bulletin #232, Local Cooperative Extension Office.
	Provides a basic foundation in normal nutrition, 40 pages in length.	
	Does not emphasize meal consistency.	
The First Step in Diabetes	Initial phase in teaching.	The American Dietetic Association, 216 West Jackson Boulevard, Suite 800, Chicago, IL 60606-6995; 1-800-366-1655.
Meal Planning	Combines MyPyramid and Dietary Guidelines and provides information on meal consistency in a simplified format.	
CHO Counting	Progressive teaching tool that leads to maximum control of blood glucose and lipid levels.	The American Dietetic Association, 216 West Jackson Boulevard, Suite 800, Chicago, IL 60606-6995; 1-800-366-1655.
Level I Level II Level III		
	Decreased emphasis on balance and variety.	
Month-O-Meals	Each book contains 28 complete and interchangeable menus for breakfast, lunch, dinner, and snacks.	The American Dietetic Association, 216 West Jackson Boulevard, Suite 800, Chicago, IL 60606-6995; 1-800-366-1655.
	Excellent approach for the client who "just wants to be told what and when to eat."	
Exchange Lists of the American Dietetic and the American Diabetes Associations	Allows the health-care educator to distribute all of the energy nutrients.	The American Dietetic Association, 216 West Jackson Boulevard, Suite 800, Chicago, IL 60606-6995; 1-800-366-1655.
	More emphasis on the importance of eating a balanced diet than the CHO-counting approach.	
	Time consuming to learn and teach.	

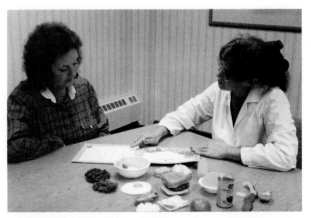

Figure **19–6** A diabetes educator providing nutritional counseling. The use of food models facilitates the learning process and teaches portion control.

meals/feedings. Another term in use is macronutrient partitioning. Clinical Calculation 19–1 shows how the percentage of energy nutrients is converted to grams of carbohydrate, fat, and protein and distributed throughout the day's meals/feedings. The next three sections elaborate on energy nutrient distribution.

CARBOHYDRATE AND MONOUNSATURATED FAT

These two macronutrients are discussed together because they can to some extent be substituted for each other to supply energy. Carbohydrate and monounsaturated fat should ideally provide 60 to 70 percent of the total kilocalories. Dietary Guidelines for Americans recommends all people choose a variety of fiber-containing food, such as whole grains, fruits, and vegetables, because they provide vitamins, minerals, fiber, and other substances that optimize health (Franz, 2003). Considerations for a more definitive partitioning between carbohydrate and monounsaturated fat include:

- In weight-maintaining diets for type 2 clients with diabetes, replacing carbohydrate with monounsaturated fat reduces postprandial glycemia and triglyceridemia (Garg et al, 1994).
- Increased fat intake in ad libitum diets may promote weight gain and contribute to insulin resistance (Marshall, Bessesen, and Hamman, 1997).

The contribution of carbohydrate and monounsaturated fat to kilocalorie intake should be individualized based on nutrition assessment, laboratory results, and weight and treatment goals.

Clinical Calculation 19–1

How to Distribute the Energy Nutrients and Calculate a Diet Using the Exchange System

In the following example, an 1800-kcal diet is being converted to 55 percent carbohydrate, 20 percent protein, and 25 percent fat.

$$1800 \text{ kcal} \times 0.55 = \frac{990 \text{ kcal}}{4 \text{ kcal/g}} = 248 \text{ g carbohydrate}$$

$$1800 \text{ kcal} \times 0.20 = \frac{360 \text{ kcal}}{4 \text{ kcal/g}} = 90 \text{ g protein}$$

$$1800 \text{ kcal} \times 0.25 = \frac{450 \text{ kcal}}{9 \text{ kcal/g}} = 50 \text{ g fat}$$

In the following example, 248 g of carbohydrate, 90 g of protein, and 50 g of fat are converted to a 1/5, 2/5, 1/5, and 1/5 distribution. Each fraction represents one meal; thus, 1/5 of the energy nutrients are to be provided each at breakfast, supper, and the evening snack; 2/5 of the energy nutrients are to be provided at the noon meal. Please note: 1/5 equals 20 percent, and 2/5 equals 40 percent.

$$248 \text{ g of carbohydrate} \times 0.20 = 50 \text{ g} \times 3 \text{ meals} = 150$$

$$248 \text{ g of carbohydrate} \times 0.20 = 99 \text{ g} \times 1 \text{ meals} = \frac{99}{249}$$

$$90 \text{ g of protein} \times 0.20 = 18 \text{ g} \times 3 \text{ meals} = 54$$

$$90 \text{ g of carbohydrate} \times 0.40 = 36 \text{ g} \times 1 \text{ meal} = \frac{36}{90}$$

Because only a small percentage of dietary fat enters the bloodstream as glucose, normally fat is not calculated into the distribution. Lunch (2/5 distribution) would contain about 99 g of carbohydrate and 36 g of protein. Each of the other meals (1/5 distribution) would contain about 50 g of carbohydrate and 18 g of protein.

The next step is to determine the number of exchanges to be provided from each of the six exchange groups. There is no exact method used to determine this step. Usually the client is consulted to determine the amount of nonfat milk, fruits, vegetables, and so forth that he or she would be willing to consume. An effort should be made to calculate the diet with at least the recommended amount of food in the MyPyramid guide. Many health-care workers determine the amount of nonfat milk, fruits, and vegetables to be provided first. This is followed by the grams of carbohydrate to be contributed by these groups. The remaining carbohydrate is then allocated to the starch group.

The protein is determined by first calculating the amount previously provided by nonfat milk, vegetables, and starches; the remaining protein is then allocated to meat exchanges. The fat is determined by first calculating the amount previously provided by the meat exchanges; the remaining fat is then allocated to fat exchanges. The calculations and meal plan for our sample 1800 kcal with 55 percent carbohydrate, 20 percent protein, and 25 percent fat with a 1/5, 2/5, 1/5, and 1/5 distribution appear in Table 19–7.

Table 19–7 Sample 1800-Kilocalorie Diabetic Diet*

Division of Energy Nutrients and Exchanges

EXCHANGE LIST	NUMBER OF DAILY EXCHANGES	PROTEIN (90 g)	FAT (50 g)	CARBOHYDRATE (218 g)	BREAKFAST	LUNCH	DINNER	HS
Skim milk	2	16	0	24	1/2	1		1/2
Starch	11	33	0	165	2	4	3	2
Fruit	3	0	0	45	1	1	0	1
Vegetable	3	6	0	15	0	2	1	0
Meat	5	35	25	0	1	2	1	1
Fat	5	0	25	0	1	1	2	1

Meal Plan and Sample Menus

MEAL PAN	SAMPLE MENU 1	SAMPLE MENU 2
BREAKFAST		
1/2 cup skim milk	1/2 cup skim milk	1/2 cup skim milk
2 starch	2 slices of toast	1 cup of oatmeal
1 fruit	1/2 cup orange juice	1/2 banana
1 meat	1/4 cup low-cholesterol egg substitute	1 low-fat sausage link
1 fat	1 tsp margarine	2 pecans
LUNCH		
1 skim milk	1 cup skim milk	1 cup skim milk
4 starch	1 cup brown rice	2 slices of bread†
		1 cup broth-type vegetable soup and 3 ginger snaps
1 fruit	1 apple	1/2 cup pineapple juice
2 vegetables	1 cup green beans	1/2 cup asparagus and 1 cup raw carrots
2 meat	2 oz stir-fried chicken	2 slices low-fat cheese†
1 fat	1 tsp oil	1 tsp margarine†
DINNER		
3 starch	1 large baked potato	1/4 10-in pizza, thin crust, and 2 bread sticks (4 × 1/2 in)
1 vegetable	1/2 cup broccoli‡	Sliced tomato
Free vegetable	Lettuce salad	Lettuce salad
1 meat	1 oz ground beef	(on pizza)
2 fat	2 tbsp sour cream‡	(on pizza)
	1 tbsp French dressing	1 tbsp Italian dressing
Free	Coffee	Diet soft drink
HS		
1/2 skim milk	1/2 cup skim milk	1/2 cup skim milk
2 starch	1 1/2 oz pretzels	6 cups hot-air-popped popcorn
1 fruit	15 grapes	1 peach
1 meat	1 oz low-fat cheese stick	1 tbsp Parmesan cheese
1 fat	2 walnuts	1 tbsp diet margarine

*The calculations and meal plan based on 55 percent carbohydrate, 20 percent protein, and 25 percent fat with a 1/5, 2/5, 1/5, and 1/5 distribution.
†Cheese sandwich.
‡Potato toppings.

The American Diabetes Association published these general guidelines that pertain to carbohydrates (American Diabetes Association, 2003):

- The total amount of CHO in a feeding is more important than the source or type.
- CHO and monounsaturated fat should provide 60 to 70 percent of energy intake. Consider the metabolic profile and need for weight loss when determining the monounsaturated fat content of the diet.
- Sucrose and sucrose-containing foods do not need to be restricted.
- Nonnutritive sweeteners are safe when consumed within the acceptable daily intake levels established by the FDA.
- There is no reason to recommend that people with diabetes consume a greater amount of fiber than other Americans.
- The use of low-glycemic-index foods may reduce postprandial hyperglycemia; insufficient evidence of any long-term benefits of using low-glycemic-index diets precludes them as a primary strategy in food/meal planning.

Clinical Application 19–3 discusses the glycemic index of

foods. Note that glucose has a high glycemic index, honey has a low glycemic index, and sucrose falls somewhere between them. White bread, potatoes, and cornflakes all have a higher glycemic index than sucrose. Thus, it is incorrect to tell a client that sucrose and honey cause the blood glucose level to increase faster or higher than an equal amount of carbohydrate from some starches. A client may ask why a particular food that contains starch

Clinical Application 19–3

Glycemic Index (GI)

The use of glycemic index in clinical practice is contro- versial and widely discussed in the popular media. Clients have many questions about glycemic index. Different food sources that contain equal amounts of carbohydrate have been found not to have an equal impact on blood glucose levels. The **glycemia index** of food attempts to classify foods according to their impact on blood glucose. The higher the glycemic index value, the higher the blood glu- cose would be expected to rise after ingestion of the food.

Foods high in water-soluble fiber, in the raw state, high in binders, and eaten as part of a mixed meal reduce the glycemia response. Dairy products, pasta, dried peas, and legumes are examples of foods with a low glycemic index. Potatoes, some cereals, and bread are examples of foods with a high glycemic index.

Food is usually eaten as mixed nutrient sources. For example, spaghetti is usually eaten with tomato sauce or as part of a meal. Because a mixed meal tends to dilute the glycemia index of any one of the meal's constituents, the glycemia index is rarely taught in clinical practice. However, some highly motivated and well-educated people with diabetes are beginning to use information about the glycemic index of foods to assist in meal planning. Thus it is important to understand this concept. Glycemic index should not be the primary strategy for food/meal planning but an adjunct approach with another meal-planning system. The following table compares effects of foods based on equal amounts of carbohydrate, not serving sizes or energy content. By convention, white bread is assigned a value of 100. Some researchers use glucose as the reference food. Therefore, glucose would have a GI of 100 and the GI of other foods would be adjusted accordingly.

FOOD	GLYCEMIC INDEX
Glucose	138
Potato, russet, baked	135
Cornflakes	119
White bread	100
White table sugar (sucrose)	86
Rice	83
Banana	79
All-bran cereal	73
Spaghetti	66
Dried peas	56
Apple	53
Ice cream	52
Milk	49
Honey (fructose)	30

causes the blood glucose level to increase rapidly, and knowledge of the glycemic index of that particular food may help answer the client's question. Clients who monitor their blood glucose levels have many such questions and look to all health-care professionals for information.

PROTEIN

The need for protein in the diabetic population is the same as for the general population if renal function is normal. Excessive amounts of dietary protein should be avoided in people with diabetes, just as members of the general pop- ulation should avoid it. The concept that excessive dietary protein may have a health risk is discussed in the Chapter 5 on protein. The American Diabetic Association has made these recommendations concerning protein (American Diabetic Association, 2003):

- Although protein is just as potent a stimulant of insulin secretion as CHO, ingested protein does not increase plasma glucose concentration in those with controlled type 2 diabetes.
- There is no evidence to suggest that usual protein intake (15 to 20 percent of total energy) should be modified if renal function is normal.
- In individuals with microalbuminuria, reduction of pro- tein to 0.8 to 1.0 g/kg/body weight per day, and in indi- viduals with overt nephropathy reduction to 0.8 g/kg/body weight per day, may slow the progression of nephropathy.
- The long-term effects of diets low in CHO and high in protein and fat are unknown and may have specific renal and CVD risks.

FAT

The primary goal regarding dietary fat in clients with dia- betes is to decrease saturated fat and cholesterol intake (Franz, 2003). The American Diabetes Association pub- lished these guidelines that pertain to fat (American Diabetes Association, 2003):

- <10% of energy intake should be derived from saturated fats. Those with LDL ≥100 mg/dL may benefit from low- ering dietary saturated fat intake to <7% of energy intake.
- Dietary cholesterol should be <300 mg/day. Those with LDL cholesterol ≥100 mg/dL may benefit from lowering cholesterol to <200 mg per day.
- Minimize intake of *trans*-unsaturated fatty acids.
- About 10% of energy intake should be derived from polyunsaturated fats.

Some people with diabetes have better glucose control on high-monounsaturated-fat diets (40 to 45 percent of the kcalories). If a diet is 40 to 45 percent fat, the carbohydrate content of the diet drops to 35 to 45 percent. Diabetes is a complicated disease, and clients with diabetes benefit from a highly individualized approach to diet manipula- tion. Some patients with hypertriglyceridemia and ele- vated LDL cholesterol levels respond better to a 40 to 45 percent high-monounsaturated-fat diet (Nuttall and Chasuk, 1998). This is why the percent of kilocalories from fat and the kind of fat consumed by persons with diabetes merit consideration. This concept requires rigid compliance. Individual evaluation by a registered dietitian is necessary to assess feasibility.

Not all clients with diabetes have these lipid abnormalities. In epidemiological studies, an increased plasma triglyceride and low HDL cholesterol have been associated with an increased risk for clinically apparent cardiovascular disease in people with diabetes. Overall, cardiovascular disease is at least two to three times more common in patients with type 2 diabetes (Nuttall and Chasuk, 1998).

CARBOHYDRATE COUNTING

In 1995, the American Diabetes and Dietetic Associations introduced carbohydrate counting, a new menu-planning concept. Carbohydrate counting refers to a teaching tool that includes three progressive levels of difficulty, achievement, and self-care to be mastered by the client. These three progressive levels are designated Level I, Level II, and Level III. They are summarized in Table 19–8. Because carbohydrate is assumed to be the main factor affecting postprandial blood glucose elevation, priority is given to counting the total amount of carbohydrate consumed at one meal and/or snack as opposed to the source of the carbohydrate. Diabetes educators use Level I, then Level II,

and possibly Level III as a client masters the previously taught level. The advantages of the carbohydrate-counting meal plan concept include single-nutrient focused, more precise matching of food and insulin, flexible food choices, a potential for improved blood glucose, and client-controlled treatment. Challenges for the client who uses this system may include the need to weigh and measure food, maintenance of extensive food records, monitoring of the blood glucose before and after eating, the need to calculate grams of carbohydrate consumed, the need to maintain healthful eating, and weight management.

Knowledge of carbohydrate counting is often a prerequisite before consideration for insulin pump therapy. It is also a prerequisite for clients who want to learn how to calculate insulin:carbohydrate ratios. This type of teaching is usually done by a certified diabetes educator (CDE) and is considered Level III teaching.

The rationale for carbohydrate counting is a carbohydrate = a carbohydrate = a carbohydrate or one starch exchange = one fruit exchange = one milk exchange. One carbohydrate unit (or exchange) is about 15 grams of carbohydrate with an acceptable range of 8 to 22 grams per carbohydrate choice. Food labels, tables of food composition, and *Exchange Lists for Meal Planning* are some of the tools clients can use to determine the carbohydrate

Table 19–8 **Carbohydrate Counting**

TITLE	LEVEL I	LEVEL II	LEVEL III
MyPyramid	Getting Started	Moving On	Intensive Diabetes Management Using Carbohydrate/Insulin Ratios
Educational concepts	Foods that should be eaten Importance of eating on time Use of foods to counteract hypoglycemia	Rationale for meal plan Expands on the selection of healthy foods	Sets the stage for self-management skills that provide flexibility and best control of diabetes
		Provides additional tips for meal planning	The nutrient content of food
			Interpretation of food labels Use of dietetic foods and sweeteners Advice for dealing with fast food, eating out, and parties
Client goals	Carbohydrate dietary consistency Flexible food choices	Adjust food, medication, and activities based on patterns from client daily records	Adjust insulin dose using ratio of carbohydrate/insulin dosage
Intended audiences	Type 1 Type 2 GDM	Person on diet only, oral agents, or insulin who has mastered basics of carbohydrate counting	People on intensive therapy People who have mastered insulin adjustment and supplementation
Primary distribution channels	Physician's offices Hospitals HMOs Clinics with registered dietitians on staff	Settings with a registered dietitian or certified diabetes educator who has diabetes training and experience	Settings with health-care team trained in intensive insulin therapy

content of a particular food. Following is a typical meal plan for a client who has been taught to count carbohydrates:

Breakfast: 3 carbohydrates (range, 38 to 52 grams)
Example: 1 whole bagel and 8 ounces (oz) skim milk
Lunch: 3 carbohydrates (range, 38 to 52 grams)
Example: 8 oz regular cola, 1 fresh orange, and 1 slice whole-wheat bread
Dinner: 3 carbohydrates (range, 38 to 52 grams)
Example: 1 1/2 cups pasta
Snack: 1 carbohydrate (range, 8 to 22 grams)
Example: 8 oz skim milk

Most health-care workers (including students) underestimate the amount of time a client must be willing to spend to learn the carbohydrate counting. The American Diabetes Association and the American Dietetic Association estimate that clients need between 90 and 180 minutes to master one level of this menu-planning system (The American Diabetes Association and the American Dietetic Association, 1995). Client visits (usually three) should be spread over several months. One study documented that patients who received three sessions with a registered dietitian experienced significant improvements in glucose control (FBG and HbA1c), serum cholesterol, and weight (Franz et al, 1995). However, clients learn new information and change eating behaviors at different rates. Each client benefits from an individualized teaching plan. The need for lifelong learning should be emphasized.

Protein and fat intake are not counted with this meal-planning system but should be given some consideration. Clients are usually counseled to eat about the same amount of protein each day and choose foods that are low in fat. For example, based on an individualized assessment, a client may be counseled to choose a food that provides approximately 3 grams of fat or less for each carbohydrate (15 grams). Thus, if a client is considering a canned entrée containing 30 grams of carbohydrate, he or she knows the food is not a good choice if it contains more than 6 grams of fat (Zeman and Ney, 1996).

Special Considerations

Persons with diabetes frequently ask questions about nutritional problems related to vitamin and mineral supplementation, alcohol, acute illness, eating out, and delayed meals. The following sections discuss these nutrition-related problems.

Vitamin and Mineral Supplementation

There is no evidence that people with diabetes benefit from vitamin or mineral supplementation solely because they have diabetes. Exceptions include folate for prevention of birth defects and calcium for prevention of bone disease (American Diabetes Association, 2003). Two minerals commonly mentioned in relation to diabetes are chromium and magnesium. Chromium deficiency has been related, hypothetically, to development of diabetes in humans for years, but persuasive studies in Western people are not available that recommend chromium supplementation for diabetic individuals. Most people with diabetes are not chromium deficient, and thus chromium supplementation cannot be

routinely recommended (Anderson, 1999). Similarly, magnesium should be used as a dietary supplement only if hypomagnesemia (low levels of magnesium in the blood) is demonstrated (Anderson, 1999).

Individuals on very-low-calorie diets (less than 800 kilocalories) or pregnant women may need a vitamin and mineral supplement. Any disease condition that normally affects the ingestion, digestion, absorption, metabolism, and excretion of nutrients may require a supplement as it would for the person without diabetes.

Alcohol

The moderate use of alcohol does not adversely affect diabetes in the well-controlled client. Recommendations follow (American Diabetes Association, 2003):

For insulin users:

- Limit to one drink for women and two drinks for men per day. One drink is defined as 12 oz beer, 5 oz wine, or 1.5 oz distilled spirits.
- Drink only with food to minimize hypoglycemia.
- Do not cut back on food.
- If history of alcohol abuse, abstain.
- Abstain during pregnancy.

For noninsulin users:

- Substitute for fat kilocalories.
- Limit to promote weight loss or maintenance.
- Limit with elevated triglycerides.
- If there is a history of alcohol abuse, abstain.
- Abstain during pregnancy.

Nutrition During Acute Illness Episodes

Acute illness affects everyone, including the person with diabetes. Colds and flu-like symptoms can be fatal for some people with diabetes unless precautions are taken. Secretion of both glucagon and epinephrine increases during illness and contributes to an increase in blood glucose levels. This may lead to a loss of glucose, fluid, and electrolytes. Dehydration, electrolyte depletion, and a loss of nutrients may follow. Acute illnesses can lead to DKA in IDDM and to HHNS in NIDDM.

Dehydration is more rapid when electrolytes and fluids are not replaced. Vomiting, diarrhea, and fever all result in fluid loss. During acute illness, the individual should be instructed to monitor his or her blood glucose level every 2 to 4 hours until the symptoms subside. Urine ketone levels should be checked. The following guidelines are recommended (www.diabetes-midon.org, accessed March 2004):

- If the blood glucose is over 250 mg/dL: drink kilocalorie-free, caffeine-free liquids in place of a meal. Also, consume additional liquids from kilocalorie- and caffeine-free sources.
- If the blood glucose is between 180 and 250 mg/dL: drink or eat 15 grams of CHO in place of a meal (one carbohydrate). Also, consume additional liquid from kilocalorie- and caffeine-free sources.
- If the blood glucose is under 180 mg/dL: drink or eat usual mealtime CHO amount. If vomiting occurs after insulin administration, the client may need to sip sugar

water every 20 to 30 minutes to maintain blood glucose of 100 to 180 mg/dL.

- When the glucose drops to less than 100 mg/dL and vomiting persists, immediate attention is required. Hospitalization may be necessary.

Increased fluids reduce the risk of dehydration. Clients who are vomiting or nauseated and are unable to tolerate regular food should drink liquids that contain carbohydrate and/or electrolytes (Table 19–9). A general guideline is that approximately 15 grams of carbohydrate should be consumed every 1 to 2 hours. Some clients have an individually calculated sick-day menu based on the carbohydrate content of their regular diet.

Other meal-planning tips that may prove helpful during periods of acute illness include (1) increasing water intake, even for clients who can eat regular food; (2) eating smaller, more frequent feedings; and (3) eating soft, easily digested foods.

Table 19–9 Easily Consumed Carbohydrate-Containing Foods for "Sick Days"

FOOD	AMOUNT	GRAMS OF CARBOHYDRATE
Regular cola	1/2 cup	13
Ginger ale	3/4 cup	16
Milk	1 cup	12
Apple juice	1/2 cup	15
Grape juice	1/2 cup	15
Orange juice	1/2 cup	15
Pineapple juice	1/2 cup	15
Prune juice	1/3 cup	15
Regular gelatin	1/2 cup	20
Sherbet	1/2 cup	30
Tomato juice*	1/2 cup	5

*High in sodium.

Clinical Application 19–4

Children with Diabetes

Kilocalorie allowances are based on a person's weight. As a rough estimate, a 1-year-old child needs 1000 kcal per day. For older children, 100 kcal per year of age are added to the daily intake. For a 9-year-old child, this would equal 1900 kcal. Typically, 55 percent of the total kilocalories should be consumed as carbohydrate. 1900 kcal multiplied by 55 percent equals 1045 kcal. To convert kilocalories from carbohydrate to grams of carbohydrate, divide by 4. 1045 kcal divided by 4 kcal/g equals 260 g of carbohydrate.

How these grams of carbohydrate are divided among the day depends on the child's prescribed medications and lifestyle. Let's assume the child eats three meals and two snacks (at mid-afternoon and bedtime) and takes one dose of basal insulin in the morning and three doses of regular insulin, one before each meal.

The diet could be planned to provide 20 percent of the carbohydrate at each feeding. Twenty percent of 260 g of carbohydrate equals 52 g or 3 1/2 carbohydrate choices. The child and the child's parents would be instructed to provide about 52 g of carbohydrate at each feeding.

As long as the child eats balanced meals that provide all the essential nutrients, the source of the carbohydrate is not important. Scientific evidence has shown that the use of sucrose as part of the meal plan does not impair blood glucose control in individuals with type I and type II diabetes (American Dietetic Association, 2000). A typical menu for the child follows:

Grams of Carbohydrate

BREAKFAST	ACCEPTABLE RANGE, 46 TO 60
1/2 cup Honey Nut Cheerios	12 (package label)
3/4 cup skim milk	9 (exchange value)
1/2 cup orange juice	15 (exchange value)
1 slice toast	15 (exchange value)
1 tsp peanut butter	0
Total carbohydrates	51

LUNCH	
Ham and cheese sandwich with 2 slices of bread	30 (exchange value)
1 apple	15 (exchange value)
3/4 cup skim milk	9 (exchange value)
Carrot sticks	0 (free with this system)
Total carbohydrates	54

MID-AFTERNOON SNACK	
3/4 cup apple juice	23 (exchange value)
13 animal crackers	25 (exchange value)
Total carbohydrates	48

DINNER	
15-in cheese pizza	39 (table of food composition)
6 oz regular cola	20 (table of food composition)
Total carbohydrates	59

BEDTIME SNACK	
1/2 cup skim milk	6 (exchange value)
Raw broccoli with dip	0 (free with this system)
10 (1 1/2 oz) whole-wheat crackers (no added fat)	30 (exchange value)
1/2 oz jelly beans	14 (table of food composition)
Total carbohydrates	50
Total carbohydrates for the day	262

Eating Out and Fast Foods

The best advice for persons with diabetes who enjoy eating out is that they know their meal-planning system and order small. For example, an individual counting carbohydrates and eating a small hamburger at McDonald's with a side salad, diet dressing, and a glass of skim milk would count:

3 carbohydrates	Grams of CHO
2 starches (hamburger bun)	30
1 milk	12
Total	42

The individual can always mix 4 ounces of orange juice with diet soft drinks for a fruit punch beverage if he or she needs an additional 15 grams of carbohydrate. Some fast-food restaurants offer fresh fruit.

Hypoglycemia in Diabetes Mellitus (The 15-15 Rule)

The immediate treatment goal for a glucose level of less than 60 mg/dL is to increase blood glucose to within a normal level as rapidly as possible. Take care not to overtreat hypoglycemia. If the client is monitoring his or her blood glucose level, at the first sign or symptom of hypoglycemia, he or she should measure the blood glucose level. If the blood glucose level is less than 60 mg/dL, 15 grams of carbohydrate should be consumed. Fifteen grams of carbohydrate are equal to 2 to 3 glucose tablets, 6 to 10 Lifesavers candies, or 4 to 6 ounces of juice. Fifteen minutes later, he or she should measure the blood glucose a second time. This is called the 15-15 rule. The process may need to be repeated a second time to achieve a blood glucose level between 70 and 110 mg/dL; check laboratory's normal range. Treat with 15 grams of carbohydrate, wait 15 minutes, and retest. If the reaction is not resolved, treat again. Overtreatment can be avoided by adherence to the 15-15 rule. Clients who do not test their blood glucose levels should be taught to do so.

Clients should be advised to carry a source of carbohydrate with them at all times. A snack should be consumed if a meal or snack is delayed (preplanned or not preplanned) by a half hour or more. At least one significant other should be instructed about hypoglycemia and the 15-15 rule.

Teaching Self-Care

Persons with diabetes ultimately treat themselves. The better educated the individual is about diabetes, the greater the likelihood of his or her avoiding the acute and chronic complications of this disease. Many public health departments, hospitals, and clinics hold classes for clients with diabetes. Newly diagnosed clients with diabetes need to learn survival skills. Health-care workers often have to repeat instructions several times before the client understands the survival skills being taught. Because of the genetic predisposition toward diabetes, many newly diagnosed clients have relatives who have suffered from the acute and chronic complications of diabetes. Hearing about such complications first hand often creates fear in newly diagnosed clients. They need time to accept their condition. Occasionally, it may take as long as a full year before clients can grasp the principles of self-care. This is especially difficult for children (see Clinical Application 19-4). During hospitalization, it is extremely difficult to effectively educate clients. Follow-up with a certified diabetes educator (CDE) and a registered dietitian (RD) is crucial.

Hypoglycemia

Hypoglycemia, caused by increased endogenous insulin production (hyperinsulinism), is rarer than diabetes mellitus. Hyperinsulinism is most likely caused by islet cell tumors or, less often, by reactive hypoglycemia. Hypoglycemia that occurs 1 to 3 hours after a meal and resolves spontaneously with the ingestion of carbohydrate is often termed reactive hypoglycemia.

The dietary management of reactive hypoglycemia consists of avoiding simple carbohydrates and sometimes taking small, frequent feedings. The meal plans for diabetes offer a reasonable guide to meal planning. Table 19–10 is a 1-day meal plan for this type of diet.

Table 19–10   **Sample Meal Plan for Hypoglycemic Diet**

EXCHANGE GROUP	SAMPLE MENU
MORNING	
1 fruit	1/2 cup unsweetened orange juice
1 starch	3/4 cup whole-grain cereal
1 meat	1 low-fat cheese or
1/2 skim milk	1/2 cup skim milk
Free	Decaffeinated coffee
MID-MORNING	
1 meat	1 tbsp peanut butter
1 starch	4 whole-grain crackers
NOON	
Chef salad	
2–4 meat	2–4 oz lean meat
1 vegetable	Lettuce, tomatoes, and
1 fat	Dressing
1 fruit	1 small piece fresh fruit
1 skim milk	1 cup skim milk
1 starch	2 breadsticks (4 × 1/2 in)
MID-AFTERNOON	
1 meat	1 oz low-fat cheese
1 starch	4 whole-grain crackers
EVENING	
2–4 meat	2–4 oz lean meat
1 starch	1/2 cup potato or pasta
1 vegetable	1/2 cup vegetable
1 fat	Lettuce salad with dressing
1 fruit	1 piece fresh fruit
Free	Decaffeinated coffee or tea
BEDTIME	
1 starch and	1/2 sandwich (1 slice whole-grain
1 meat	bread and 1 oz lean meat)
1 vegetable	Fresh vegetables
Free	Decaffeinated beverage

SUMMARY

Diabetes mellitus is caused by an undersecretion or underutilization of insulin and/or receptor or postreceptor defects. Diabetes is actually a group of disorders with a common sign of hyperglycemia. The two major types of diabetes are type 1 and type 2. Impaired glucose tolerance or impaired fasting glucose, secondary diabetes, and gestational diabetes are other categories of this disease. Persons with diabetes suffer from acute and chronic complications. Treatment involves medication, nutrition management, and exercise. Nutrition is a fundamental part of treatment. Hypoglycemia, a rarer condition than diabetes, is caused by oversecretion of insulin and is also treated with dietary manipulation.

CASE STUDY 19-1

Mrs. S, a 45-year-old black woman, was admitted to the hospital with medical diagnoses of type 2 diabetes and cellulitis of the left leg. Her admitting height was 5 ft 5 in, and weight 200 lb (BMI = 33.5). Wrist measurement shows Mrs. S has a large frame. Vital signs were temperature 98.6°F, pulse 70 beats per minute, respirations 16 per minute, and blood pressure 160/95.

Mrs. S reported a gradual increase in her weight since her third child was born 20 years ago. That baby weighed 12 lb. Two previous pregnancies produced infants weighing 10 and 11 lb. She has no known allergies.

None of the children live at home. Mrs. S lives with her husband, who works as a construction laborer. She has been seasonally employed as a hotel maid at a nearby resort. Health insurance coverage is sporadic. They have a new insurance policy now.

Mrs. S is the oldest of six children. Her father died of a heart attack at age 60. Her mother died of a stroke at age 62 following 15 years of treatment for diabetes mellitus. The sister who is closest to Mrs. S in age developed diabetes mellitus 3 years ago and is being treated with oral medication. Their youngest sister was diagnosed as an insulin-dependent diabetic at age 18 following an episode of mumps.

Mrs. S reports a good appetite and a fluid intake of about 3 quarts per day. Her favorite beverage is iced tea with sugar and lemon. She does most of the grocery shopping and cooking.

Mrs. S hit her left ankle with the screen door about 2 months ago. The resulting sore has not healed but has gotten worse. Mrs. S knows that a sore that does not heal is a sign of cancer, which is why she sought medical attention. The ankle now has an open lesion 5 cm in diameter over the lateral ankle bone. The entire foot is swollen to twice the size of the right foot. The bandage over the sore had greenish-yellow drainage on it.

A random blood glucose test in the doctor's office 3 hours after her last meal was 400 mg/dL. Her urine glucose was negative for ketones. Before she left the office, the physician told Mrs. S she has type 2 diabetes mellitus.

The physician prescribed the following care for Mrs. S:

- Bed rest with left leg elevated
- Bedside commode
- Diet assessment and teaching
- Multivitamin, 1 capsule, daily
- Culture and sensitivity of drainage from left leg
- Cefuroxime, 250 mg, orally every 12 hours
- Warm, moist dressing to left leg ulcer four times per day
- Fasting blood sugar (FBS), electrolytes in AM

The admitting nurse constructed the following Nursing Care Plan for Mrs. S.

NURSING CARE PLAN

SUBJECTIVE DATA Family history of diabetes mellitus
Large appetite
Large fluid intake
Delay in seeking medical attention

OBJECTIVE DATA Obesity (BMI = 33.5)
Newly diagnosed type 2 diabetes
Possible hypertension (only one reading given)
Open lesion 5 cm diameter over left lateral ankle; purulent discharge

NURSING DIAGNOSIS NANDA: Ineffective Health Maintenance, related to inappropriate self-care (NANDA, 2003, with permission) as evidenced by delay in seeking medical attention

DESIRED OUTCOMES EVALUATION CRITERIA	NURSING ACTIONS/ INTERVENTIONS	RATIONALE
NOC: Knowledge: Treatment Regimen (Moorhead, Johnson, and Maas, 2004, with permission) Client will verbalize self-care measures related to type 2 by hospital discharge.	NIC: Teaching: Disease Process (Dochterman and Bulechek, 2004, with permission) Refer to dietitian for nutritional assessment and education.	The cornerstone of treatment of type 2 is weight loss. Although any weight loss will help, to reach a healthy weight, Mrs. S needs to lose 51 lb. A dietitian's expertise is needed.
	Review survival skills with client (see Appendix for client teaching tool).	The American Diabetes Association recommends all patients with diabetes learn survival skills if they do not know this core information.
Client will verbalize willingness to continue nursing/medical regimen after discharge.	Refer to social worker for sources of medical attention when uninsured.	Social workers are most familiar with community resources.
	Teach principles of wound care, including effect of high blood sugar on infection.	If Mrs. S understands that high blood sugar feeds the bacteria causing the infection, she may be more willing to work hard to control the diabetes.
	Reinforce dietitian's instruction. Have Mrs. S state the Dietary Guidelines and the reason why they are important.	Knowledge usually precedes behavior change.
	Have Mrs. S describe the meal plan she follows.	Short periods of instruction are most effective; frequent review of the material will help the client master it.
	Ask physician to discuss exercise regimen when the blood sugar is under control.	Mrs. S needs a prescribed exercise program suited to her level of conditioning.

CTQ CRITICAL THINKING QUESTIONS

1. The client would like to learn how to monitor her own blood glucose levels (as the nurses do) before discharge. How would the nurse, in the role of client advocate, arrange for this to be done? Why is a physician's written order important?
2. The client's fasting blood glucose level has decreased steadily during her 3-day hospitalization. On the morning of discharge, the FBS was 150 mg/dL. The client stated, "It has come down enough. Now I don't need to worry about the diabetes any longer." How would you respond?
3. Why is a referral to a certified diabetes educator crucial for this client?

≫ CHAPTER REVIEW

1. If a client has a history of ketoacidosis, he or she most likely has which type of diabetes:
   a. Type 1
   b. Type 2
   c. Pituitary
   d. Gestational

2. The following statement is true:
   a. Acute illness lowers blood glucose levels.
   b. Fluid and electrolyte replacement is essential during episodes of acute illness in all persons with diabetes.
   c. Persons with diabetes who have an acute illness require a vitamin and mineral supplement.
   d. Persons with diabetes should never eat forms of simple sugar.

3. Dietary guidelines for people with diabetes include:
   a. One serving of alcohol daily
   b. Consume no more than 2000 milligrams of sodium each day
   c. Restrict fat intake to less than 10 percent of total kilocalories
   d. Consume at least 20 to 35 grams of fiber each day

4. For most clients, the cornerstone of treatment of type 2 diabetes is:
   a. Stress management
   b. Meal planning
   c. Strict adherence to five planned meals per day
   d. Hypoglycemic drugs

5. The diet for reactive hypoglycemia includes the following features:
   a. Small, frequent meals with restricted simple sugars
   b. Three meals with ample simple sugars and high complex carbohydrate
   c. Four to six small meals that are high in fat
   d. Three high-carbohydrate meals that are moderate in fat

CLINICAL ANALYSIS

Ms. N, a 14-year-old, was diagnosed 1 year ago with type 1 diabetes mellitus. Her blood sugar levels have been stable on an intermediate-acting insulin and a 370-gram CHO diet. The teenager is now being seen in the doctor's office for routine follow-up. The nurse is reviewing Ms. N's knowledge of self-care.

1. To assess knowledge, the nurse asks how the client would handle a day when the client could not eat solid foods. Which of the following answers would show understanding of the usual procedure?
   a. Skip insulin that day.
   b. Call the doctor after missing one meal.
   c. Replace the carbohydrates in the meal plan with liquids containing equal amounts of carbohydrate.
   d. Take half her usual insulin dose and double the usual fluid intake.

2. The client plays volleyball for the high-school team and is moderately active during practices and games. SMBG records indicate a daily glucose level of between 120 and 140 mg/dL prior to the time she usually plays volleyball. Which of the following behaviors are appropriate for her before playing?
   a. No additional food is indicated.
   b. Increase intake by 15 grams of carbohydrate.
   c. Decrease intake by 15 grams of carbohydrate.
   d. Increase intake by one vegetable exchange and one fat exchange.

3. The client states, "I am getting tired of pricking my finger several times a day. Why can't I manage my diabetes with urine testing like my grandmother?" Which of the following responses by the nurse would be most appropriate?
   a. "The urine test is more accurate in older people."
   b. "The point at which sugar is spilled in the urine varies even for one individual. Therefore, the blood test is more accurate."
   c. "Urine tests are more costly."
   d. "The blood test is the newest thing. Your grandmother's doctor must be old-fashioned."

REFERENCES

Allen, A, et al: Risk factors for frequent and severe hypoglycemia in type 1 diabetes. Diabetes Care 24:1878, 2001.

American Diabetes Association: Summary for the 2005 clinical practice recommendations. Diabetes Care. 28:53, 2005.

American Diabetes Association: Diagnosis and classification of diabetes mellitus. Diabetes Care. 28:237-S42, 2005.

American Diabetes Association: Preconception care of women with diabetes [position paper]. Diabetes Care 19(Suppl):525, 1996.

American Diabetes Association: 2003 Nutrition recommendations for diabetes. Order code 59111-02, 2003.

American Diabetes Association: Summary of 2004 clinical practice recommendations. Diabetes Care 27:S3, 2004

American Diabetes Association: www.diabetes.org/home. Accessed January 2005.

American Diabetes Association: Maximizing the Role of Nutrition in Diabetes Management. American Diabetes Association, Alexandria, VA, 1994.

American Diabetes and Dietetic Association: Exchange Lists for Weight Reduction. Daley, Chicago, 2003.

American Dietetic Association: Basic Carbohydrate Counting. American Dietetic Association, Chicago, 2003.

American Dietetic Association: Advanced Carbohydrate Counting. American Dietetic Association, Chicago, 2003.

American Diabetes Association and National Institutes of Diabetes: Digestive and Kidney Diseases: Position statement. The prevention or delay of type 2 diabetes. Diabetes Care 25:742, 2002.

American Dietetic Association: Nutrition recommendations and principles for people with diabetes mellitus [position paper]. J Am Diet Assoc 94:504, 1994.

American Dietetic Association: Manual of Clinical Dietetics, ed 6. American Dietetic Association, Chicago, 2000.

Anderson, JW: Nutritional management of diabetes mellitus. In Shils, ME, et al (eds): Modern Nutrition in Health and Disease, ed 9. Williams & Wilkins, Baltimore, 1999.

Centers for Disease Control: www.cdc.gov/health/diabetes. Accessed January 2005.

Diabetes Control and Complication Trial Group: Influence of intensive treatment on quality-of-life outcomes in the diabetes control and complications trial. Diabetes Care 19:195, 1996.

Diabetes Control and Complication Trial Group: The effect of intensive treatment of diabetes on the development and progression of long-term complications in insulin-dependent diabetes mellitus. N Engl J Med 329:977, 1993.

Dochterman, JC, and Bulechek, GM: Nursing Interventions Classification (NIC), ed 4. Mosby, Philadelphia, 2004.

Franz, MJ, et al: Effectiveness of medical nutrition therapy provided by dietitians in the management of noninsulin-dependent diabetes: A randomized, controlled clinical trail. J Am Diet Assoc 95:1009, 1995.

Franz, MJ, et al: Evidence-based nutrition principles and recommendations for the treatment and prevention of diabetes and related complications. Diabetes Care 25:148, 2003.

Guyton, AC, and Hall, JE: Textbook of Medical Physiology, ed 10. Saunders, Philadelphia, 2000.

Garg, A, et al: Effect of varying carbohydrate content of diet for patients with non-insulin dependent diabetes mellitus. JAMA 271:1421, 1994.

Holcomb, CA, Heim, DL, and Loughin, TM: Physical activity minimizes the association of body fatness with abdominal obesity in white, premenopausal women: Results from the third national health and nutrition examination survey. J Am Diet Assoc 104:1854, 2004.

Jacobson, AM: Commentary. Diabetes Spectrum 6:36, 1993.

Killion, KH: Facts and Comparisons. Kluwer, St. Louis, 2003.

Maggio, C, and Pi-Sunyer, X: The prevention and treatment of obesity: Application to type-2 diabetes. Diabetes Care 20:1744, 1997.

Marshall, JA, Bessesen, DH, and Hamman, RF: High monounsaturated fat and low starch and fiber are associated with hyperinsulinemia. JAMA 40:430, 1997.

Michigan Diabetes Outreach Network: Quick Reference Guide to Diabetes for Health Care Providers. SODON (Southern Michigan Outreach Diabetes Network): Southern Michigan Diabetes Outreach Network Newsletter. Vol. 4, Issue 4. Coldwater, MI, November 1999.

Moorhead, S, Johnson, M, and Maas, M: Nursing Outcomes Classification (NOC), ed 3. Mosby, Philadelphia, 2004.

NANDA International: Nursing Diagnoses: Definitions and Classification, 2003–2004. NANDA International, Philadelphia, 2003.

Nuttall, FQ, and Chasuk, RM: Nutrition and the management of type 2 diabetes. J Fam Pract 47(5 suppl), 1998.

Ryan-Turek, T: Latest therapies and technology in diabetes treatment. Michigan Dietetic Association Conference. Midland, MI, 2003.

The Diabetes Monitor: http://www.diabetesmonitor.com/. Accessed January 2005.

UK Prospective Diabetes Study Group: Intensive blood-glucose control with sulphonylurea or insulin compared with conventional treatment and the risk of complications in patients with type 2 diabetes (UKPDS 33). Lancet 352:837, 1998.

www.diabetes-midon.org. Accessed November 16, 1999.

www.medscape.com/ADA/DC/2000.v23no01s.01/pnt-dc23s01.01.html.

Zeman, FJ, and Ney, DM: Applications in Medical Nutritional Therapy. Merril, Columbus, 1996.

Zimmerman, BR, and Hagen, MD: An evaluation of new agents in the treatment of type 2 diabetes. J Fam Pract 47(Suppl 5):S37, 1998.

CHAPTER 20

Diet in Cardiovascular Disease

After completing this chapter, the student should be able to:

1. Discuss the relationship of diet to the development of cardiovascular disease.
2. Distinguish between type II and type IV hyperlipoproteinemias as to aggravating factors and dietary modifications.
3. Identify strategies that are likely to reduce the risk of cardiovascular disease.
4. Describe the 2-gram sodium diet.
5. List several flavorings and seasonings that can be substituted for salt on a sodium-restricted diet.

The cardiovascular system includes not only the heart and blood vessels but the blood-forming organs as well. This chapter covers common diseases of the heart and blood vessels that can be influenced by diet modification. Conditions resulting from faulty blood forming are included in other chapters. Iron-deficiency anemia is found in Chapter 8 on minerals, and pernicious anemia is found in Chapter 7 on vitamins and in Chapter 11 on pregnancy. Nutritional care of leukemia clients is included in Chapter 23, Diet in Cancer.

Occurrence of Cardiovascular Disease

Despite declines in recent years, heart disease and stroke remain the first and third leading causes of death in the United States, respectively. Of all U.S. deaths in 2001, heart disease accounted for 29.0 percent and stroke for 6.8 percent (Centers for Disease Control, 2004a). These findings pertain to all groups except men and Hispanics, for whom cerebrovascular disease is the fourth leading cause of death (Anderson and Smith, 2003).

Heart disease has been the leading cause of death in the United States since 1921. The death rate began declining in the 1950s, even before the advances in coronary care and current medications were available. As is evident in Figure 20–1, death rates from coronary heart disease are declining more rapidly than those from stroke. Moreover, the decreases in death rates for heart disease are not evenly distributed throughout the country or the population. Interactive maps of heart disease death rates by state, region, gender, and ethnicity are available (see Fig. 20–2).

Ethnicity also influences morbidity, and genetic differences are being discovered that help explain the differences. Myocardial infarction (MI) risk-associated genotypes have been identified that occurred at a significantly higher rate in African Americans than in European Americans. Whereas 9.1 percent of African Americans had all three of the high-risk genotypes studied, none of the European Americans did (Lanfear et al, 2004). Additionally, two adrenergic receptor genotypes have been found to increase the risk of heart failure in blacks, one of which in homozygous persons increases risk more than five times (Small et al, 2002).

Stroke has been the third leading cause of death since 1938. The southeastern United States is known as the "Stroke Belt." Age-adjusted death rates for cerebrovascular diseases for North and South Carolina, Georgia, Arkansas, Louisiana, Mississippi, Tennessee, and the District of Columbia are the highest reported except for American Samoa, Guam, and the Virgin Islands (Centers for Disease Control, 1999). The Carolinas and Georgia, the stroke belt's "buckle" have mortality rates twice as high as the rest of the nation (Steefel, 2004).

Throughout the United States, non-Hispanic blacks had approximately four times the risk of stroke mortality as non-Hispanic whites at ages 35 to 54 and three times the risk at ages 55 to 64. Suggested reasons for the ethnic differences include greater prevalence of risk factors for stroke, such as obesity, uncontrolled hypertension, physical inactivity, poor nutrition, diabetes, and smoking, as well as barriers to health care, such as lack of health insurance, inadequate transportation, and unfamiliarity with early warning signs of stroke (Centers for Disease Control, 2000). Figure 20–3 is an example of the data available on stroke death rates from the Centers for Disease Control.

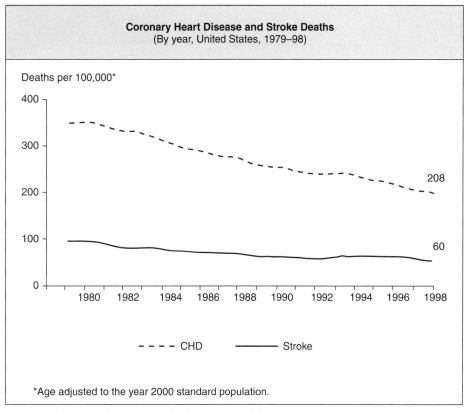

Coronary Heart Disease and Stroke Deaths
(By year, United States, 1979–98)

Deaths per 100,000*

208

60

- - - - CHD   ——— Stroke

*Age adjusted to the year 2000 standard population.

Source: CDC, NCHS, National Vital Statistics System (NVSS), 1979–98

Figure **20–1** Age-adjusted death rates per 100,000 population for coronary heart disease and stroke, United States, 1979–1998. (Centers for Disease Control, 2004.)

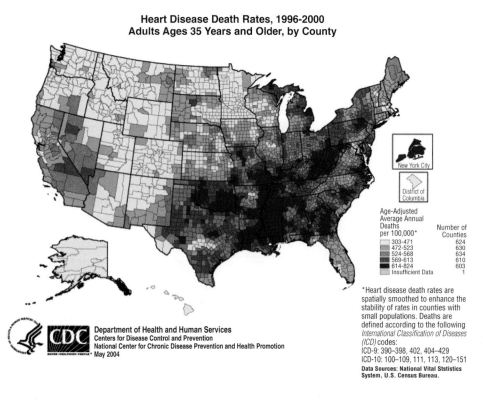

Heart Disease Death Rates, 1996-2000
Adults Ages 35 Years and Older, by County

New York City

District of Columbia

Age-Adjusted
Average Annual
Deaths
per 100,000*   Number of
                             Counties

	303-471	624
	472-523	630
	524-568	634
	569-613	610
	614-824	603
	Insufficient Data	1

*Heart disease death rates are spatially smoothed to enhance the stability of rates in counties with small populations. Deaths are defined according to the following *International Classification of Diseases (ICD)* codes:
ICD-9: 390–398, 402, 404–429
ICD-10: 100–109, 111, 113, 120–151
Data Sources: National Vital Ststistics System, U.S. Census Bureau.

Department of Health and Human Services
Centers for Disease Control and Prevention
National Center for Chronic Disease Prevention and Health Promotion
May 2004

Figure **20–2** Heart disease death rates, 1996–2000, by county. Available as an interactive file at http://www.cdc.gov/cvh/maps/ heart_disease_map_all.htm (accessed September 14, 2004).

**Smoothed County Stroke Death Rates
1991–1998**

**Total Population
Ages 35 Years and Older**

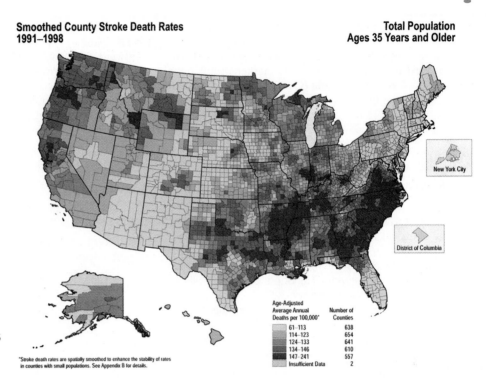

Figure **20–3** Stroke death rates, 1991–1998, by county. Available as an interactive file at http://apps. nccd.cdc.gov/giscvh/(jfwduj45ven5 44zb0hgsss55)/maps.aspx (accessed September 14, 2004).

Underlying Pathology

Two major pathological conditions contribute to cardiovascular disease. One is atherosclerosis, the most common form of **arteriosclerosis.** The second is hypertension, which is included here as contributing to pathology and later in the chapter as a risk factor for cardiovascular disease.

Atherosclerosis

In **atherosclerosis,** fatty deposits of cholesterol, fat, or other substances accumulate inside the artery. Initially, the deposited material, or plaque, is soft, but later it becomes fibrosed or hard. This disease process interferes with the pumping of blood through the artery in two ways: (1) the deposits gradually make the lumen smaller and smaller, and (2) the fibrosis makes it progressively harder

for the artery to constrict or dilate in response to the tissues' needs for oxygenated blood (Fig. 20–4). When the lumen, or opening through the artery, is 70 percent blocked by atherosclerotic plaque, the person is likely to show symptoms of impaired circulation distal to the obstruction. The atherosclerotic process begins early in life. People 15 to 34 years old with normal lipoprotein levels, autopsied after trauma or accidents, had evidence of atherosclerosis that was associated with smoking, hypertension, obesity, and impaired glucose tolerance (McGill et al, 2001).

Because half of myocardial infarction clients do not have abnormal blood lipids (both explained later), other factors that might affect a person's risk profile are being explored. One of these is serum homocysteine, because homocysteinemia has been reported to be an independent

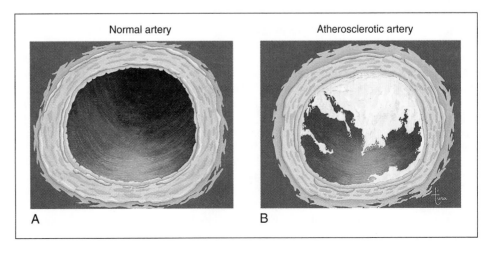

Figure **20–4** Cross-section of a normal coronary artery (left) and an atherosclerotic artery (right). Note both the narrowed diameter and the roughness within the lumen in the diseased artery. (Reprinted from Scanlon and Sanders, 2003, p 265, with permission.)

risk factor for atherosclerosis (see Clinical Application 20–1).

Another factor that has recently been associated with atherosclerosis is inflammation. One marker of inflammation, plasma **C-reactive protein (CRP),** an abnormal protein produced by the liver in response to acute inflammation,

has been extensively investigated in relation to atherosclerosis. Numerous studies have shown a strong association between CRP levels and future vascular events, whether coronary, cerebrovascular, or peripheral vascular disease, with minimal correlation to low-density lipoprotein cholesterol, expanded upon later (Backes, Howard, and Moriarty,

---

Clinical Application 20–1

Homocysteine and Atherosclerosis

HISTORY
Thirty years ago, extensive atherosclerosis was found on autopsy of individuals with elevated plasma homocysteine levels due to errors of metabolism. This autosomal recessive genetic disease, homocystinuria, occurs in about 1 of 300,000 live births with a higher prevalence in Ireland and New South Wales (Refsum et al, 2004). When untreated, homocystinuria results in thromboembolic events in 50 percent of the clients and a 20 percent mortality rate before the age of 30 (Nygard et al, 1997).

CORRELATIONAL STUDIES
Even among individuals without homocysteinuria, a link has been found between plasma homocysteine levels and atherosclerosis. In adults without prior myocardial infarction, a plasma homocysteine level higher than the median for age and gender predicted the risk of the development of congestive heart failure (Vasan et al, 2003). Among clients with coronary heart disease, those with the highest levels of homocysteine had four times the risk of stroke as those with the lowest levels (Tanne et al, 2003). Whether the association between high plasma concentrations of homocysteine and vascular disease is causal is unclear (Schwammenthal and Tanne, 2004). In addition, a Norwegian study found homocysteine levels not only related to cardiovascular mortality but also to cancer mortality and all-cause mortality (Vollset et al, 2001).

PATHOPHYSIOLOGY
Homocysteine is an amino acid produced as the sulfur-containing essential amino acid methionine is metabolized in the body. Homocysteine is not ingested and normally not detectable in the plasma or urine because it is processed intracellularly (Klor et al, 1997). High levels of homocysteine are thought to damage the lining of the arteries.

Hyperhomocysteinemia, in the absence of kidney disease, indicates faulty metabolism due to vitamin deficiency (folate, B_{12}, B_6) or a genetic defect (Selhub and D'Angelo, 1997). Evidence of dietary deficiency was shown in a study of vegans, 28 percent of whom had inadequate cobalamin status and 38 percent of whom had elevated homocysteine levels, with the length of vegetarianism significantly correlating to homocysteine concentration (Waldman et al, 2004). Mutation of a gene that encodes an enzyme that regulates homocysteine metabolism has been found in some individuals with elevated serum homocysteine. An analysis of many studies, however, showed significantly elevated homocysteine levels in clients with and without the mutation who had ischemic

heart disease, deep vein thrombosis, or stroke (Wald, Law, and Morris, 2002).

DIETARY/SUPPLEMENTARY ASSOCIATIONS
Clients given folic acid, cobalamin, and pyridoxine for 6 months following coronary angioplasty were significantly less likely to require revascularization than those given placebo (Schnyder et al, 2002). Adding low or high doses of folic acid, cobalamin, and pyridoxine to a multivitamin regimen for clients following nondisabling cerebral infarctions produced moderate reduction of total homocysteine but had no effect on vascular outcomes during 2 years of follow-up (Toole et al, 2004).

RECOMMENDATIONS
Hyperhomocysteinemia as an independent risk factor for cardiovascular disease is thought to be responsible for about 10 percent of total risk. The Homocysteine Studies Collaboration (2002) concluded that homocysteine is at most a modest independent predictor of ischemic heart disease and stroke risk in healthy populations but that more studies are needed on genetic variants and on the effects of vitamin supplementation. Some experts, however, recommend vitamin supplements to reduce homocysteine in clients at particular risk of cardiovascular events, because such interventions are inexpensive and well-tolerated (Schwammenthal and Tanne, 2004; Stanger et al, 2004).

Recent fortification of grain with folic acid, although initiated to prevent neural tube defects during pregnancy, may coincidentally reduce hyperhomocysteinemia. A comparison of blood samples from groups of middle-aged and older adults showed that the prevalence of high homocysteine levels was 48 percent less in those tested after fortification was implemented than in those tested before fortification (Jacques et al, 1999).

The dearth of definitive answers to the significance of homocysteine levels in the blood illustrates the difficulty of researching biological events in a changing environment. For individuals who elect to monitor their homocysteine levels, clear and cautious interpretation by the health-care provider is essential. A group of experts recommended standardization of collection and processing protocols but was unable to reach consensus about the use of homocysteine to assess risk of cardiovascular risk (Refsum et al, 2004). Meanwhile, avoiding smoking, maintaining desirable cholesterol levels, and controlling weight and blood pressure are definitely recommended to reduce the risks of cardiovascular disease.

2004). Confirmation of an inflammatory process in athero-sclerosis expands the rationale for the use of aspirin to prevent cardiovascular disease. In addition to its anticoag-ulant properties, it is an anti-inflammatory agent. Infectious agents may play a role in the pathogenesis of atheroscle-rosis through a number of mechanisms so that chronic, persistent infection may favor proinflammatory changes in the vascular wall (Kol and Santini, 2004).

Hypertension

Blood pressure is the force exerted against the walls of the arteries by the pumping action of the heart. It is recorded in two numbers, such as 120/80. The top number, **systolic pressure,** is the pressure when the heart beats. The bot-tom number, **diastolic pressure,** is the pressure between beats. Both pressures are reported in millimeters of mer-cury (mmHg). Except in persons younger than 50 years, systolic pressure is a more important risk factor than dias-tolic pressure (U.S. Department of Health and Human Services, 2003).

Diagnosis of Hypertension

Hypertension, which affects about 40 million people in the United States, is defined as blood pressure of 140/90 or higher on at least three occasions on different dates. The category also includes persons taking antihypertensive medication. Several readings are taken on various days to eliminate the possibility of excitement or nervousness causing a transient elevation. Hypertension is classified as Stage 1 or 2 (Table 20–1). Blood pressure measurement should be part of a child's health assessment beginning at the age of 3 years. For children, prehypertension is blood pressure at or above the 90th percentile and hypertension is blood pressure at or above the 95th percentile according to height, gender, and age (National High Blood Pressure Education Program, 2004).

A person with hypertension may not feel sick, so blood pressure screening is often offered as a community service (Fig. 20–5). Along with temperature, pulse, and respira-tions, blood pressure is a vital sign. The National Stroke Association recommends blood pressure checks for all clients at every health-care visit and the use of home blood pressure monitoring for hypertensive clients (Gorelick et al, 1999).

Types of Hypertension

Depending on the cause of the hypertension, it is labeled primary or secondary. About 90 percent of hypertensive

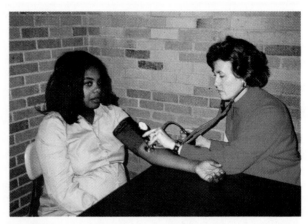

Figure **20–5** Hypertension is a silent killer. Blood pressure mon-itoring is a part of most health system visits. Even children are occasionally hypertensive and should have blood pressure checked beginning at age 3.

clients have primary or **essential hypertension.** There is no single, clear-cut cause for this high blood pressure.

Secondary hypertension occurs in response to another event or disease process in the body. One such event is pregnancy, during which hypertension may occur (see Chapter 11). Medications also can cause secondary hyper-tension. Birth control pills that contain progesterone stim-ulate the production of renin (recall Fig. 9–5), which may result in an elevation in blood pressure. As detailed in Chapter 17, the combined intake of monoamine oxidase (MAO) inhibitors and tyramine-rich foods or beverages can cause hypertension. Secondary hypertension also can result from diseases of the kidney, adrenal glands, or nerv-ous system.

Positive Feedback Cycle

Many cardiovascular conditions have interlocking causative factors. The interaction between atherosclerosis and hypertension is an example of a **positive feedback cycle.** In this situation, the presence of the second condi-tion worsens the first. Atherosclerosis narrows the lumen of the arteries, and the smaller opening increases the blood pressure. Then the higher blood pressure forces more lipids into the arterial wall, worsening the atherosclerosis, and the cycle is repeated.

End Result of Pathology

Most people do not have either atherosclerosis or hyper-tension. More commonly, they have both conditions.

Table **20–1** Classification of Blood Pressure for Adults and Children

CLASSIFICATION	mmHg SYSTOLIC	mmHg DIASTOLIC	PERCENTILE DENOTING CLASSIFICATION IN CHILDREN AND ADOLESCENTS
Normal	<120	and <80	<90th
Prehypertension	120–139	or 80–89	90th to 95th (Children) >120/80 (Adolescents)
Stage 1 hypertension	140–159	or 90–99	95th to (99th + 5 mmHg)
Stage 2 hypertension	>159	or >99	>99th + 5 mmHg

SOURCE: Adapted from National High Blood Pressure Education Working Group, 2004 and U.S. Department of Health and Human Services, 2003.

Although many organs are likely to be damaged by atherosclerosis and hypertension, the major concern is the effect on the heart and brain, as described in the following sections on coronary heart disease and cerebrovascular disease.

Coronary Heart Disease

When the coronary arteries that supply the heart muscle with blood become blocked, the result is **coronary heart disease (CHD)** or coronary artery disease (CAD), which affects 12.2 million people in the United States. If the blockage is temporary, due to increased activity and the body's increased demand for oxygen, the person may experience **angina pectoris**, or severe pain and a sense of constriction about the heart. Rest and the administration of vasodilating medications commonly produce relief, but changes in diet and lifestyle are necessary to stave off heart damage. But if the vessel is blocked by atherosclerotic plaque, by a **thrombus** (blood clot), or by an **embolus** (a circulating mass of undissolved matter), the heart tissues beyond the point of obstruction receive no oxygen or nutrients. When this happens, the person exhibits signs and symptoms of a **coronary occlusion,** or a heart attack. When the blood supply cannot be restored quickly, myocardial cells in the affected area die. The medical diagnosis then becomes **myocardial infarction** (MI), which occurs in about 1.5 million people in the United States annually.

Congestive Heart Failure

When the heart cannot keep up with the demands on it, in other words, when **cardiac output** is not adequate to meet the circulatory demands of the body, a sequence of events sets up another positive feedback cycle. **Congestive heart failure (CHF)** occurs when the heart is unable to maintain adequate circulation of the blood. Causes may include atherosclerosis, hypertension, myocardial infarction, rheumatic fever, or a birth defect. The right side of the heart normally collects the blood returning from the body and pumps it to the lungs to excrete carbon dioxide and absorb oxygen. If the right ventricle is failing, usually due to lung disease, the blood backs up into the veins that empty into the right atrium, and the client has the signs of peripheral edema. As a result of fluid volume excess and edema of the small bowel, the client suffers from anorexia and nausea.

The left side of the heart normally receives the oxygenated blood from the lungs and pumps it out to the body. If the left ventricle is failing, usually following a myocardial infarction, the blood that cannot be pumped effectively to the body backs up in the blood vessels of the lungs. Next the fluid from the blood is forced into the lung tissue. The client will display shortness of breath and moist lung sounds and will expectorate frothy pink sputum.

In addition, if the heart cannot pump enough to maintain blood pressure, the body implements the renin response. Angiotensin II constricts the blood vessels, raising blood pressure. Aldosterone causes the kidney to conserve sodium, and with it, water (Fig. 9–5). More fluid fills the blood vessels. The higher blood pressure pushes this fluid out into the interstitial spaces, causing edema.

Obviously, one side of the heart cannot function for long if the other side is failing. Nevertheless, the health-care worker learns to look for early signs of heart failure in the extremities in right-sided failure or in the lungs in left-sided failure. Nearly 0.5 million persons are diagnosed with heart failure for the first time each year (American College of Cardiology, 2002), and almost 75 percent of the nearly 5 million clients with heart failure in the United States are older than 65 years (Centers for Disease Control, 2004b). The prognosis after development of CHF is grim, with a median survival of 1.7 years in men and 3.2 years in women (Lloyd-Jones, 2001), but treatment of hypertension reduces the incidence of heart failure by approximately 50 percent, even among very elderly clients (Baker, 2002).

Clients often see CHF as an acute disease that is resolved once they return home rather than the chronic disease it is. Therefore they do not manage it well between acute episodes. Self-management at home includes daily weights so that a gain of 3 to 5 pounds triggers follow-up with the primary healthcare provider for adjustment of therapy (Horowitz, Rein, and Leventhal, 2004).

Cerebrovascular Accident

When a blood vessel in the brain becomes blocked by atherosclerosis (ischemic stroke), the tissue supplied by that artery dies. This is the most common cause of **cerebrovascular accidents (CVAs),** or strokes, in the United States. Strokes also can be caused by an embolus or by a ruptured blood vessel. Cerebrovascular accidents, affecting 4.4 million people in the United States, are usually secondary to atherosclerosis, hypertension, or a combination of both. Each year, 600,000 strokes occur in the United States, resulting in about 158,000 deaths (Centers for Disease Control, 2004b). Hemorrhagic and ischemic strokes are common complications of acute myocardial infarction (Angeja et al, 2001), with about one in 40 clients suffering an ischemic stroke within 6 months of discharge following myocardial infarction. Among Medicare clients with myocardial infarction, independent predictors of ischemic stroke were age 75 or older, black race, no aspirin at discharge, frailty, prior stroke, atrial fibrillation, diabetes, hypertension, and history of peripheral vascular disease (Lichtman et al, 2002).

Stroke is called a "brain attack" and early treatment can minimize its long term effects but people often ignore initial signs and symptoms. In 2002, at one stroke center in North Carolina only 50 percent of clients displaying stroke symptoms arrived by ambulance and 75 percent arrived some 26 hours after the appearance of symptoms (Steefel, 2004).

Diets have been linked to the occurrence of strokes. Fish consumption one to three times per month reduced the risk of ischemic stroke by 43 percent compared with men who ate fish less than once per month (He et al, 2002). Increased risk for stroke was associated with low serum potassium levels among diuretic users and with low dietary potassium intake among persons not taking diuretics (Green et al, 2002).

Peripheral Vascular Disease (PVD)

This is a broad classification of diseases affecting arteries and veins distal to the heart. Atherosclerosis is a major causative factor of peripheral vascular disease (PVD), affecting about 3 percent of clients younger than 55 years of age, 11 percent of those 65 to 74 years of age, and 20 percent of those age 75 years and older. Cerebrovascular/carotid disease, abdominal aortic aneurysms, and peripheral arterial occlusive disease are the most common peripheral vascular conditions seen in primary care (Dillavou and Kahn, 2003). Signs and symptoms vary depending on the vessels affected, the extent of the damage, and the duration of the problem. The effects of peripheral vascular disease range from limitation of activities to amputation of digits or extremities due to gangrene to sudden death in the case of aortic aneurysm.

Risk Factors in Cardiovascular Disease

The occurrence of cardiovascular disease in a person cannot be predicted with certainty. Many attributes and behaviors interact to produce the illness.

Unchangeable Risk Factors

Age, gender, race, family history, and personal medical history can be predictive of atherosclerosis and hypertension in some people. None of these risk factors can be modified to prevent disease.

Age, Gender, and Race

Age-related changes account for many cardiovascular events. For example, hypertension usually develops at about age 50 to 60, and coronary atherosclerosis becomes problematic more frequently in individuals over the age of 40.

Gender-related occurrence of coronary heart disease is readily apparent, as risk increases in males after age 45 and females after age 55. Until menopause, women have less atherosclerosis and coronary heart disease than men, but women past menopause and younger diabetic women are stricken with coronary heart disease just as often as men are. Women have a higher prevalence of hypertension than men and also are less likely to be under current treatment and to have the condition under control (Centers for Disease Control, 2005).

Ethnicity as a risk factor is evident: the prevalence of hypertension is 27 percent in non-Hispanic whites compared with 41 percent in non-Hispanic blacks, who have 1.5 times the heart disease mortality and 1.8 times the stroke mortality as whites (Bassett et al, 2002; Centers for Disease Control, 2005).

Family and Prior Medical Histories

A few cardiovascular diseases can be traced to particular genes, but for the most part, it is likely that many genes interact to affect response to nutrients that result in disease (Krauss, 2000). Whatever the pathophysiology, a family history of premature coronary heart disease in a parent or sibling increases a person's risk of the disease. Premature coronary heart disease occurs before age 55 in males and 65 in females (Expert Panel, 2001).

Of special concern are the inherited **hyperlipoproteinemias,** or increased lipoproteins and lipids in the bloodstream (Table 20–2). One of these hyperlipoproteinemias, type IV, is very common and is often associated with **non-insulin-dependent diabetes mellitus (NIDDM).** Some of the other types are seen less often. All six types have a connection to food intake of fats, carbohydrates, or both. Blood plasma values vary in each condition. For example, type I hyperlipoproteinemia is aggravated by fat, and the chylomicrons (see Table 20–3) are elevated because they carry exogenous triglycerides that cannot be broken down. Thus, plasma triglyceride levels are elevated as well.

Type II hyperlipoproteinemia results from a single gene defect in the cell receptor that binds circulating low-density lipoproteins. It is an autosomal dominant characteristic. Individuals with this defect have a rate of coronary heart disease 25 times that of the normal population. In addition, clients with the subgroup type IIA hyperlipoproteinemia generally develop heart disease 15 years earlier than the rest of the population. Some even suffer heart attacks in infancy and childhood.

Besides the inherited disorders of lipid metabolism, hyperlipoproteinemia can develop secondary to other conditions and environmental factors such as diet. Diabetes mellitus, alcohol consumption, oral contraceptives, kidney

Table 20–2   Inherited Hyperlipoproteinemias

				Increased Plasma Values				
				Lipoprotein			Lipid	
TYPE	FREQUENCY	INHERITANCE PATTERN	AGGRAVATED BY	CHYLOMICRONS	VLDL	LDL	CHOLESTEROL	TRIGLYCERIDES
I	Very rare	Autosomal recessive	Fat	X				X
IIA	Common	Autosomal dominant	Fat			X	X	
IIB	Common	Autosomal dominant	Fat		X	X	X	X
III	Uncommon	Multifactorial	CHO	Remnants			X	X
IV	Very common	Autosomal dominant	CHO		X			X
V	Rare	Autosomal recessive	Fat and CHO	X	X		X	X

SOURCE: Adapted from Dietary Management, 1980, and Fauci et al, 1998.

disease, liver disease, and hypothyroidism can either cause or aggravate existing lipid disorders.

A person's medical history is pertinent when evaluating risks of cardiovascular disease. The risk of heart attack rises more sharply after surgical menopause (removal of the ovaries) than after natural menopause. A person who has already suffered a stroke has an increased risk of a subsequent stroke.

Changeable Risk Factors

Unlike age, gender, race, and family or personal history, some risk factors for cardiovascular disease can be modified. The major changeable risk factors are hypertension, serum cholesterol, obesity, diabetes mellitus, physical inactivity, alcohol intake, and cigarette smoking. These are detailed in the following sections.

Hypertension

Hypertension is the major risk factor for stroke. Approximately 29 percent of the adults in the United States have high blood pressure. Unfortunately, only about 63 percent of people with pressures greater than 140/90 are aware of it, about 55 percent of them are being treated, and about 30 percent are adequately controlled (Centers for Disease Control, 2005). Older age, higher BMI, and non-Hispanic black race/ethnicity are associated with increased rates of hypertension, whereas female gender, Hispanic ethnicity, and age greater than 59 years are associated with lower rates of control compared with men, younger individuals, and non-Hispanic whites (Hajjar and Kotchen, 2003). Antihypertensive therapy has been related to decreased incidences of stroke of 35 to 40 percent, of myocardial infarction of 20 to 25 percent, and of heart failure of more than 50 percent (U.S. Department of Health and Human Services, 2003).

Two dietary influences have been related to hypertension: high salt intake and low intakes of potassium, calcium, and magnesium.

HIGH SALT INTAKE

Age-related increases in blood pressure are related to salt intake. Blood pressure values increase with age everywhere but in extremely remote areas of the world and are significantly related to salt intake. Although sodium has been identified as the major influence on blood pressure, it does not increase blood pressure when administered with anions other than chloride (Kotchen and Kotchen, 1999). Moreover, not everyone is equally responsive to salt intake. Individuals most likely to benefit from salt restriction include African Americans, older people, and clients with hypertension or diabetes. It is generally accepted that the differences in response to sodium has a genetic basis (Gropper, Smith, and Groff, 2005).

LOW CALCIUM, POTASSIUM, AND MAGNESIUM INTAKES

Low intakes of these three minerals have been associated with hypertension. The results of 33 clinical trials showed that potassium supplementation reduced mean blood pressure by 4.4 mmHg systolic and 2.45 mmHg diastolic (Whelton and He, 1999). In addition, high potassium intake produces a greater reduction in blood pressure in African Americans than in whites and in individuals with a high salt intake (Kotchen and Kotchen, 1999).

After noting in the 1970s that communities with hard water had lower death rates from cardiovascular disease than those with soft water, many researchers studied the effects of calcium on hypertension (Brown, 2005). In general, benefits are seen in individuals with low calcium intakes. Diets containing less than 600 milligrams of calcium daily are most clearly associated with hypertension. Dietary calcium is also inversely related to systolic blood pressure in young children (Kotchen and Kotchen, 1999) and to age-related increases of systolic blood pressure and pulse pressure (Hajjar, Grim, and Kotchen, 2003).

In regulating vascular tone, calcium interacts with cellular magnesium. A deficiency of magnesium results in decreased functioning of enzymes, membrane pumps, and ion pumps, leading to exaggerated effects of calcium and vasoconstriction (Dakshinamurti and Dakshinamurti, 2001). Epidemiological and experimental studies demonstrate an inverse association between magnesium levels and blood pressure, supporting a role for magnesium in the pathogenesis of hypertension; however, clinical studies have been less convincing so that the value of magnesium in the prevention and management of essential hypertension is unclear. The clinical use of magnesium with the greatest potential in hypertension management is in the treatment of preeclampsia and eclampsia (Touyz, 2003). See Chapter 11.

As is commonly is seen in nutrition studies, an intake of certain foods can be correlated with an increase or reduction of disease, but individual nutrients when tested are not. It may be that the individual nutrient selected to be tested has a small effect alone but works in conjunction with other nutrients or that the substance in the food causing the effect has not been identified. Obtaining adequate dietary intake from food, not supplements, is recommended.

Elevated Blood Cholesterol

Despite its categorization as a risk factor for cardiovascular disease, **cholesterol** serves vital functions in the body. It is a component of the nerve tissue of the brain and spinal cord, of the tissues of the liver, the adrenal glands, and the kidneys, and of bile. Cholesterol is a precursor of adrenal hormones and the sex hormones. Blood cholesterol levels, however, are frequently measured to monitor risk, to promote health, and to prevent disease. The recommended frequency is every 5 years in adults aged 20 and older.

Universal screening of children's cholesterol is not recommended, but rather the need for screening is determined by family history. Children of parents or grandparents with documented cardiovascular disease occurring before the age of 55 years and children whose family histories are unavailable should be screened at the discretion of the physician (Hyperlipidemia, 2004). Children who do have elevated serum cholesterol levels have to be managed carefully so that sufficient food is provided to support growth.

RELATIONSHIP TO DIET

About 1000 milligrams of cholesterol is processed in the body per day, but less than one-third of the body's store of cholesterol comes from diet, and that is exclusively derived from foods of animal origin. Nearly all of the body's tissues can synthesize cholesterol, with the liver and the intestine producing the most. Most people can produce less cholesterol or increase its excretion in response to high levels of dietary cholesterol, but others respond weakly, a phenomenon that may be genetically based and seems to affect just synthesis by the liver and not by other tissues (Gropper, Smith, and Groff, 2005).

Consumption of substances other than dietary cholesterol can also influence serum cholesterol levels. *Trans* unsaturated fatty acids in vegetable oil products have been identified as a risk factor for cardiovascular disease because they raise LDL-C levels and lower HDL-C levels (see next section). About 63 to 75 percent of the intake of *trans*-fatty acids is derived from baked goods, fried fast foods, and other prepared foods, rather than from margarines (Ascherio, Katan, and Stampfer, 1999). *Trans*-fatty acids are not specified on food labels, but a proposal by the FDA would include *trans*-fatty acids on labels by the year 2006 (U.S. Food and Drug Administration, 2003). The heart-healthiest margarines have less than 3 grams per tablespoon of saturated and *trans* fats combined (compared to 7.5 grams in butter). Those would include tub and squeeze margarines (Mayo Clinic staff, 2004), but new *trans*-free products are likely to be marketed.

Coffee intake has shown mixed effects on cholesterol. Boiled or unfiltered coffee (common in Scandinavia and Turkey) contains cafestol and kahweol that promote increased plasma concentration of cholesterol in humans (Ranheim and Halvorsen, 2005). Analysis of multiple studies identified a dose-response relation between coffee consumption and both total cholesterol and LDL cholesterol, with greater increases in hyperlipidemic clients and with caffeinated or boiled coffee. Trials using filtered coffee demonstrated very little increase in serum cholesterol (Jee et al, 2001). Instant coffee has been filtered in the manufacturing process, and many coffeemakers require filters.

LIPOPROTEINS AS RISK FACTORS

Lipids such as triglycerides (the major form of dietary fat and of stored body fat) and cholesterol (a sterol with fat-like properties) cannot dissolve in water or the blood but are bound to proteins for transportation in the bloodstream. These fat-carrying complex molecules consisting of triglycerides, cholesterol, phospholipids, and proteins are called lipoproteins. There are four main classes of lipoproteins: **chylomicrons, very low-density lipoproteins (VLDL), low-density lipoproteins (LDL),** and **high-density lipoproteins (HDL).** Table 20–3 summarizes the functions, significance, and normal laboratory values of these four classes of lipoproteins. Intermediate density lipoproteins (between VLDL and LDL) also exist in the bloodstream for short periods of time but have little nutritional or physiological significance (Gropper, Smith, and Groff, 2005).

A laboratory test of **apolipoproteins,** the protein components of lipoproteins, is now used to determine LDL:HDL ratios more reliably than simply measuring cholesterol levels. For instance, **apolipoprotein A,** (apo A) is the primary HDL apoprotein and apolipoprotein B (apo B) the major LDL apoprotein (Gropper, Smith, and Groff, 2005), The apolipoproteins help keep lipids in solution, direct the lipids toward the correct organs and tissues, and assist in regulating lipid metabolism by activating and inactivating enzymes required for the process. Apo A levels are inversely related to the risk for developing coronary artery disease (Schnell, Leeuwen, and Kranpitz, 2003).

SERUM CHOLESTEROL AS A RISK FACTOR

Blood tests for serum cholesterol are reported as total cholesterol, LDL cholesterol (LDL-C) or HDL cholesterol (HDL-C) based upon cholesterol's association with the two major transport lipoproteins. Serum cholesterol itself is neither good nor bad, but the lipoproteins are associated with greater or lesser risk of coronary heart disease.

LDL cholesterol is deposited into macrophages in the endothelial wall on its way to becoming part of atherosclerotic plaque. Two types of LDL receptors have been identified in the macrophages. One type recognizes unoxidized

Table 20–3   Functions and Significance of Various Lipoproteins

LIPOPROTEIN	NORMAL VALUE IN 12- TO 14-HOUR FASTING SPECIMEN	FUNCTION	CLINICAL SIGNIFICANCE
Chylomicrons	0	Transport exogenous triglycerides from intestines to blood stream	Formed in small intestine; present in blood only after a meal
VLDL	3–32 mg/dL	Main transporter of endogenous triglyceride	Synthesized by liver from free fatty acids, glycerol, and carbohydrate
LDL	38–40 mg/dL	Transports cholesterol to body cells	Evolves from VLDLs as body's cells remove triglyceride from them and attach cholesterol; carrier of about 60 percent of total serum cholesterol; the higher the LDL level, the greater the risk of CHD.
HDL	20–48 mg/dL	Transports cholesterol from body cells to liver to be excreted	Synthesized by liver and intestines; the higher the HDL level, the lower the risk of CHD; aerobic exercise increases HDL level in men but only slightly in women.

LDL and limits the amount taken into the cell once a sufficient amount has been accumulated. The other type recognizes oxidized LDL but does not stop its entry into the cell (Spencer, Carson, and Crouch, 1999). Because it is thought that oxidized LDL is more atherogenic than unoxidized LDL, much current research involves antioxidants. Box 20–1 summarizes some of these conflicting findings.

The higher the serum LDL cholesterol, the greater is the risk of CHD. Based on a 10-year risk of CHD, recommendations have been made to guide clinical judgment in the treatment of hyperlipoproteinemia. The primary target of cholesterol-lowering regimens is LDL-C. The goals of therapy are to lower the LDL-C value to

1. below 160 mg/dL if fewer than two other risk factors for cardiovascular disease are present
2. below 130 mg/dL if two or more other risk factors are present
3. below 100 mg/dL if coronary heart disease exists or if the person has *CHD risk equivalents* (i.e., diabetes or other atherosclerotic disease) that equate the risk to established CHD (Expert Panel, 2001).

A tool to calculate risk and other materials are available at http://nhlbi.nih.gov/guidelines/cholesterol/profmats.htm.

Conversely, the higher a person's HDL–C level, the lower is the risk of coronary heart disease. A person with a high HDL-C level (60 mg/dL or more) can subtract one other risk factor when tallying risk (Expert Panel, 2001). Genetic factors account for about half the variation in the serum HDL levels in the population (Grundy, 1999). As an example, individuals in rural Italy with very low HDL levels have been found to have a mutated version of apo A that is particularly effective in clearing plaque from arteries. Five weekly infusions of a recombinant version of that effective Italian apo A produced significant regression of coronary atherosclerosis in a small multicenter study in the United States (Nissen et al, 2003).

Obesity

Obesity has been recognized as a major modifiable risk factor for cardiovascular disease, second only to cigarette smoking (Sharma, 2003). Weight reduction can raise HDL-C levels by 5 to 10 percent (Denke, 2002). People who are overweight have two to six times the risk of developing hypertension as people with a healthy body weight, and an estimated 50 percent of hypertension could be prevented by weight control. Even a 22-pound weight loss is estimated to lower systolic blood pressure by 5 to 20 mmHg (U.S. Department of Health and Human Services, 2003).

Obesity is also related to heart failure. Compared to persons with normal BMIs, obese women had 2.1 times the risk of heart failure and obese men had 1.9 times the risk. For each increment of 1.0 on the BMI scale, heart failure risk increased by 5 percent for men and 7 percent for women (Kenchaiah et al, 2002).

The location of the body fat is significant: abdominal obesity is related to cardiovascular disease and diabetes mellitus more than is **gluteal-femoral obesity.** Waist circumferences of more than 40 inches in men and 35 inches

in women are related to increased risk of cardiovascular disease (Krauss et al, 2000).

Diabetes Mellitus

At any given cholesterol level, diabetic persons have a two to three times higher risk of atherosclerosis than other people. Diabetic women lose the preventive advantages usually associated with premenopausal women regarding cardiovascular risk.

Insulin is required to maintain adequate levels of **lipoprotein lipase,** an enzyme that breaks down chylomicrons. When lipoprotein lipase is inadequate, chylomicrons and VLDL particles accumulate in the blood. After the diabetes is controlled, serum lipid levels decrease. Lipoprotein lipase is more active in physically active subjects and increases with exercise. This factor is very important in the management of type 2 (NIDDM) diabetes. Another example of altered physiology is described in Box 20–2, relating undernutrition in utero to increased risk for diabetes mellitus and cardiovascular disease in adulthood.

Physical Inactivity

Lack of exercise contributes to many other risk factors for cardiovascular disease. For instance, activity is inversely related to blood pressure independent of being overweight in both sexes and across all ages. As well, increased physical activity has been accompanied by increased HDL-C levels with its attendant lessening of risk (Denke, 2002).

EFFECT WELL DOCUMENTED

The more active a person is, the less likely is the development of cardiovascular disease. Forty-six percent of Mexican American women, 40 percent of non-Hispanic black women, and 33 percent of Mexican American men report no leisure time activity that likely accounts for some of the variation in hypertension prevalence (Bassett et al, 2002). Men who ran 1 hour or more per week had 42 percent lower risk of coronary heart disease than men who did not run (Tanasescu et al, 2002). Even walking less than 2 hours per week reduced the risk of stroke in women by 25 percent, with greater activity reducing risk further (Costa, 2002).

Thus, moderately intense physical activity, such as brisk walking for 30 to 45 minutes on most days of the week, is recommended. Irregular bouts of heavy physical activity such as occur in weight lifting and rowing are not recommended for clients with hypertension because they raise blood pressure (Russell and Suter, 2001).

METABOLIC SYNDROME

A particular constellation of signs and symptoms labeled **metabolic syndrome** increases the risk of cardiovascular disease. Metabolic syndrome was identified in 4.6, 22.4, and 59.6 percent of normal-weight, overweight, and obese men, respectively, and correspondingly in 6.2, 28.1, and 50.0 percent of women (Park et al, 2003). Clients with this condition display three or more of the following signs: glucose intolerance, hypertriglyceridemia, low HDL cholesterol,

Box 20-1 **Research on Antioxidants in Cardiovascular Disease**

Vitamins

Based on the theory that oxidation of LDL initiates atherosclerosis, antioxidant vitamins have been extensively studied in relation to cardiovascular disease. Observational studies of antioxidant-rich foods have found some associations with reduced cardiovascular disease, but randomized controlled trials of supplements, the gold-standard of medical research, have failed to provide sufficient evidence to support taking supplements. For example, observational studies have linked vitamin E and beta-carotene to decreases in cardiovascular events, but clinical trials have failed to confirm any benefit. A meta-analysis of those two antioxidants involving 81,788 persons in a randomized trial of vitamin E and 138,113 people in beta-carotene trials found no less cardiovascular disease with vitamin E and a small but significant *increase* in all-cause mortality with beta-carotene (Vivekananthan et al, 2003).

Specifying death as an end point creates a demanding research project. Vitamin A supplementation did not reduce the incidence of coronary death, and no trials of its effect on atherosclerotic CVD have been reported. Studies of vitamin C showed mixed results, with one good-quality study showing reduced cardiovascular and all-cause mortality. No randomized clinical trial of primary prevention has measured the effect of vitamin C alone on cardiovascular outcomes (Morris and Carson, 2003). A possible reason for mixed results in randomized trials is genetic. Postmenopausal women given vitamin E and vitamin C for 2.8 years showed more or less coronary atherosclerosis depending on their type of haptoglobin, a protein that transports hemoglobin from lysed red blood cells to the liver, with increased effects, for better or worse, in women with diabetes (Levy et al, 2004).

Extrapolating to humans from animal studies is open to error. For instance, the subtypes of haptoglobin occur only in humans. In addition, an animal's diet can be completely controlled but that of free-living humans not only is uncontrolled but also may be subject to reporting error depending on the method and frequency of data collection. Numerous studies have reported that compared with those who do not take supplements, people who do take them are thinner, more physically active, nonsmoking, nondrinking, better educated, of higher socioeconomic status, and have less early coronary disease in their families (Morris and Carson, 2003). These are just the people who would need supplementation least.

While antioxidants eventually may be deemed useful in preventing diseases and there is solid evidence linking oxidative processes to human disease, thus far a beneficial effect on cardiovascular disease has not been proved (Brown and Crowley, 2005). In fact, antioxidants (vitamins E and C, beta-carotene, and selenium) blunted the increases in HDL-C normally associated with simvastatin and niacin therapy in persons with CAD due to a striking selective effect on apo A (Cheung et al, 2001).

Although recent RDAs specify supplements or fortified food for subgroups of the population (see Chapter 7), the best advice for healthy people is still variety, balance, and moderation in food and limiting supplements to a multivitamin-multimineral product at RDA levels. Oxidation is a necessary physiological process in which some oxidative products act against invading bacteria so that consuming large doses of antioxidants could upset the body's defenses. The declining heart disease rate has been correlated with increased fruit and vegetable consumption in the United States, a safe means of achieving optimal blood concentrations of antioxidants.

The U.S. Preventive Services Task Force (2003) could not recommend for or against the use of antioxidant vitamin supplements to prevent cardiovascular disease or cancer because of insufficient evidence either way. It did recommend against using beta-carotene supplements because of lack of benefit to middle-aged and older adults as well as demonstrated associations with higher incidence of lung cancer and higher all-cause mortality in heavy smokers.

Flavonoids

Vitamins are not the only antioxidant-functioning elements of the diet. **Flavonoids** are chemicals found in most plants that reportedly have many actions in the body including that of antioxidant. Tea is the major source of flavonoids in Western populations, and a daily intake of more than 375 mL was associated with a 43 percent less risk of myocardial infarction compared with non-tea drinkers (Geleijnse et al, 2002). A meta-analysis involving more than 100,000 people found a 20 percent lower risk of CHD mortality in those in the top third of flavonol (a subclass of flavonoids) intake compared with the bottom third. The richest sources of flavonols were tea (mostly black), onions, apples, and broccoli (Huxley and Neil, 2003). Notice, too, that broccoli contains vitamins A and C besides flavonoids, attesting to the difficulty of teasing out the cause of a particular health benefit attributed to foods.

Moderate wine consumption has been touted to prevent cardiovascular disease. (See the section on alcohol later in this chapter.) Purple grape juice decreased platelet aggregation in humans, suggesting the flavonoids in grape juice, not the alcohol in wine, might be the active ingredient protecting the heart (Freedman et al, 2001). Similar studies on individual food products have been reported; however, caution is necessary. Adding the supposedly beneficial food without subtracting equal kilocalories is likely to lead to unwanted weight gain. Moreover, until knowledge about flavonoids' bioavailability and metabolism is accrued, prudence dictates avoidance of supplements or fortified products (Duthie, Duthie, and Kyle, 2000).

Box 20–2 **Fetal Nutrition and Cardiovascular Disease in Adulthood**

Environmental influences before and shortly after birth are generally accepted as important determinants of the risk of cardiovascular disease and diabetes mellitus in adulthood (Hofman, Jackson, and Knight, 2004). Prenatal nutrition may be a factor determining cardiovascular disease risk in that retrospective cohort studies indicate that low birth weight and disproportion at birth are powerful predictors of later disease risk (Langley-Evans, 2001). Programming of the fetus may result from adaptations invoked when the materno-placental nutrient supply fails to match the fetal nutrient demand (Godfrey and Barker, 2001) such as shunting of fuels to the developing brain at the expense of the muscles and pancreas (Sperling, 2004). Studies have connected low birth weight, thinness, and short body length at birth with high death rates from cardiovascular disease and high prevalence of type 2 diabetes mellitus (Barker, 1999). The associations are seen in small-for-gestational-age (SGA) babies, rather than premature infants, and are independent of social class or lifestyle. Babies who are thin at birth tend to be insulin resistant as adults and have a high prevalence of diabetes mellitus, hypertension, and hyperlipidemia as adults. It is suggested that undernutrition during gestation alters the relationships between glucose and insulin and between growth hormone and insulin-like growth factors. In this way, the fetus adapts to its environment to permit survival, but its changed physiology makes the individual susceptible to cardiovascular disease in later life.

hypertension, and abdominal obesity (Expert Panel, 2001). Specific criteria are:

- Fasting blood glucose $>/=$ 100 mg/dL
- Triglycerides $>/=$ 150 mg/dL
- HDL-C <40 mg/dL in men; <50 mg/dL in women
- Blood pressure $>/=$ 130 mmHg systolic; $>/=$ 85 mmHg diastolic
- Waist circumference > 40 inches in men; > 35 inches in women

Insulin resistance and resulting hyperinsulinemia probably are responsible for the impairment in glucose homeostasis, dyslipidemia, and hypertension (Natali and Ferrannini, 2004). The estimated 47 million people in the United States with metabolic syndrome require immediate treatment, because these clients quickly develop diabetes, CAD, and stroke. Treatment is a multifaceted, including diet, exercise, and pharmacologic therapy (Scott, 2003).

Alcohol Consumption

Moderate alcohol intake has been linked to lower occurrence of cardiovascular events. In small amounts, alcohol seems to cause vasodilation, whereas at high doses it acts as a vasoconstrictor. Compared with men who consumed alcohol less than weekly, men who consumed any type of alcoholic beverage 3 to 4 days per week had a 32 percent less risk of myocardial infarction (Mukamal et al, 2003). Similarly, in survivors of acute myocardial infarctions, the risk of complications was reduced by 59 percent in those consuming about two **drinks** per day, mostly wine, compared with abstainers (de Lorgeril, Martin, and Paillard, 2002).

Modest doses of alcohol are thought to benefit the cardiovascular system by increasing HDL cholesterol or by altering blood clotting mechanisms. Large quantities of alcohol imbibed over years, however, may produce alcoholic cardiomyopathy with dilation and impaired contractility of the left or both ventricles (Schoppet and Maisch, 2001). Heavy doses of alcohol affect the brain long term as well as short term. Compared to occasional drinkers, those who consumed more than four drinks per day had a 68-percent increase in risk of stroke, primarily confined to hemorrhagic stroke (Iso et al, 2004).

Many studies have found wine drinkers to be significantly different from consumers of other alcoholic beverages. Typical of the conclusions drawn is the following. Wine drinkers had a lower mortality risk than beer or liquor drinkers in an investigation of over 128,000 California adults, but whether that risk was due to nonalcoholic wine ingredients, drinking patterns, or other traits was not clear (Klatsky et al, 2003). That uncertainty, coupled with other major health consequences of alcohol consumption, has led the American Heart Association to recommend against alcohol as a cardioprotective substance (Krauss et al, 2000).

Cigarette Smoking

Among the major coronary risk factors, cigarette smoking has been shown to be harmful to the heart and blood vessels whether from active smoking or second-hand smoking. An independent relationship exists between cigarette smoking and cardiovascular disease, but smoking also greatly increases the risk of cardiovascular diseases in individuals with other coronary risk factors (Leone, 2003). The exact toxic components among the thousands of pharmacologically active substances present in tobacco smoke and their mechanisms affecting cardiovascular dysfunction are largely unknown, but smoking does increase inflammation, thrombosis, and oxidation of low-density lipoprotein cholesterol (Ambrose and Barua, 2004).

Smoking cessation increases HDL-C levels by 5 to 10 percent (Denke, 2002). Risks are not reduced by smoking cigarettes with lower tar and nicotine, but persons who have smoked only pipes or cigars seem to have a lower risk for cardiovascular diseases (Burns, 2003). After 6 weeks compared with a control group, postmenopausal women who stopped smoking had lower daytime systolic pressures and heart rates partly due to reduced sympathetic nervous system activity (Oncken et al, 2001). Smoking cessation after myocardial infarction reduces subsequent cardiovascular mortality by nearly 50 percent, leading to a recommendation to implement smoking cessation strategies, including behavioral counseling and medications, for smokers with CVD (Thomson and Rigotti, 2003).

Several of the major risk factors for cardiovascular disease not only exert individual effects but also contribute to

Table 20–4 Risk Factors for Cardiovascular Disease

UNCHANGEABLE	CHANGEABLE
Age	Hypertension
Gender	High blood cholesterol
Race	Obesity
Heredity	Diabetes mellitus
Family history	Physical inactivity
Prior medical history	Cigarette smoking
	Alcohol intake

a cascade effect. For instance, race and physical inactivity affect obesity, and all three factors impact blood pressure. Major risk factors for cardiovascular disease are listed in Table 20–4.

Dietary Prevention and Treatment of Cardiovascular Disease

The American Heart Association revised its dietary guidelines and broadened the approach to encompass lifestyle rather than only food. The major focus is concerned with a healthy eating pattern, a healthy body weight, a desirable lipoprotein profile, and a normal blood pressure (Krauss et al, 2000). Guidelines for the general population are quite detailed and replace the AHA Step I Diet. The Therapeutic Lifestyle Changes (TLC) Diet is indicated for those for individuals with or at greater risk of cardiovascular disease and replaces the Step II Diet. It assumes an individualized program will be supervised by an appropriate health-care provider. Planning strategies is especially important if the client is unwilling to adapt all the recommended lifestyle changes. A registered dietitian can help prioritize those actions likely to have the greatest impact on risk. The major components of the dietary guidelines are elaborated upon below.

Healthy Diet Pattern

The preferred dietary pattern is listed in Table 20–5. A balance should be attained over several days. Emphasis is placed on five or more daily servings of fruits and vegetables, six or more daily servings of grains, particularly whole grains, and two weekly servings of fish. Low-fat or

Table 20–5 Outline of Treatments to Prevent and Treat Cardiovascular Disease

GROUP	OVERALL DIET PATTERN (TO BE BALANCED OVER SEVERAL DAYS)	TO ACHIEVE APPROPRIATE BODY WEIGHT	TO ACHIEVE DESIRABLE BLOOD CHOLESTEROL	TO ACHIEVE DESIRABLE BLOOD PRESSURE	ADJUNCTIVE TREATMENTS
General population (Replaces Step I Diet)	5 or more daily servings of whole fruits and vegetables* 6 or more daily servings grains, especially whole* 2 servings/ week of fish Low-fat or nonfat dairy products Legumes Poultry Lean meat	Match energy intake to needs	Limit saturated and *trans* fats to 10 percent of kilocalories Limit dietary cholesterol to 300 mg/day Substitute unsaturated fat from fish, nuts, legumes, and vegetables for saturated and *trans* fats	Limit salt to 6 grams/day (2400 mg sodium) Limit alcohol to 1 standard drink (women) or 2 standard drinks (men)/day Maintain healthy body weight	
Therapeutic lifestyle changes (TLC)† For individuals with increased blood lipids, CV disease, insulin resistance, diabetes, CHF, renal disease (Replaces Step II Diet)	As above	As above plus moderate physical activity to use about 200 kilocalories/day	Limit saturated and *trans* fats to 7 percent of kilocalories Limit dietary cholesterol to 200 mg/day Up to 20% of total kilocalories from monounsaturated and 10% from polyunsaturated fats may be prescribed for clients with diabetes or metabolic syndrome	As above	After 6 weeks on TLC program, soluble fiber and plant sterols may be added. After another 6 weeks, cholesterol-lowering medications may be prescribed.

*These amounts could total 25 grams of fiber daily.
†Progress of clients requiring this therapy should be regularly monitored.
SOURCE: Adapted from American Heart Association, Undated; Expert Panel, 2001; and Krauss et al, 2000.

nonfat dairy products, legumes, poultry, and lean meat complete the pattern.

Fruits and Vegetables

A high intake of fruits and vegetables is linked to lower risk of heart disease, hypertension, and stroke (Krauss, 2000). Recent large, prospective studies also show a direct inverse association between fruit and vegetable intake and the occurrence of CVD incidents such as coronary heart disease and stroke, but the mechanisms whereby fruits and vegetables exert their effects are unclear and are likely to be multiple. Many nutrients and phytochemicals in fruits and vegetables could work alone or together to reduce CVD risk. Although it is important to continue the search for causation, it is equally important to apply current knowledge to encourage increased fruit and vegetable intake (Bazzano, Serdula, and Liu, 2003). Whole fruits and vegetables, rather than juices, should be consumed to maintain consumption of adequate fiber. Individuals consuming diets very high in vegetables, fruit, and nuts (55 grams of fiber per 1000 kilocalories) obtained a 33 percent reduction in LDL cholesterol compared with starch-based or low-fat diets, with maximum lipid reductions occurring within 1 week (Jenkins et al, 2001).

Grain Products

Diets high in grain products and fiber have been associated with lower risk of cardiovascular disease (Krauss et al, 2000). In women, higher intake of whole grains, but not total grains, was associated with a lower risk of ischemic stroke (Liu et al, 2000). Likewise, men who consumed one or more servings per day of whole-grain cereal had a 17 percent lower risk of total mortality and a 20 percent lower risk of CVD mortality than men who rarely or never consumed it (Liu et al, 2003).

Foods containing psyllium seed husk (e.g. Kellogg's Bran Buds) may make a health claim that the food, as part of a diet low in saturated fat and cholesterol, may reduce the risk of coronary heart disease. To qualify, the food must provide at least 1.7 grams of soluble fiber in an amount customarily consumed. To obtain the result achieved in the controlled studies on which the FDA approval was based, a person would have to consume 4 servings per day (U.S. Food and Drug Administration, 1998). Indeed, consumption of 10.2 grams of psyllium per day for six months lowered serum LDL cholesterol by 7% in persons already consuming a low-fat diet (Anderson et al, 2000).

Healthy Body Weight

The general population is encouraged to balance kilocalorie intake with energy output to meet this goal. The TLC Diet specifies adopting an exercise program requiring the expenditure of 200 kilocalories per day. The health-care professional monitoring individuals requiring the TLC Diet will help the client design an effective and safe exercise program. Principles of weight control are covered in Chapter 18.

Desirable Lipoprotein Profile

Saturated fat is the chief dietary determinant of serum LDL cholesterol (Krauss, 2000). Reducing intakes of saturated fat and *trans* fat are priority dietary interventions in the prevention and treatment of **hypercholesterolemia.** Two particular foods, fish and soy products, have demonstrated cholesterol-lowering effects.

Saturated and Trans Fats

For the general population, saturated plus *trans* fats should be limited to 10 percent of kilocalories and dietary cholesterol limited to 300 milligrams per day. Unsaturated fat from fish, nuts, legumes, and vegetables can substitute for saturated and *trans* fats. Meats, fish, and poultry should be baked, broiled, or grilled, not fried. Legumes also contribute soluble fiber to the diet.

The TLC Diet limits saturated plus *trans* fats to 7 percent of kilocalories and cholesterol to 200 milligrams per day. For clients with diabetes or metabolic syndrome, up to 20 percent of kilocalories may come from monounsaturated fats and 10 percent from polyunsaturated fats to reduce carbohydrate intake. Since foods are blends of fats of different saturation levels (Fig. 4–3), diet choices are based on selection of those that supply the most of a desired degree of saturation. Figure 20–6 delineates various foods providing significant amounts of the various fats. Monounsaturated fats may significantly lower LDL cholesterol as well as protect against blood clots, but any oil contributes substantial kilocalories that may be important to body weight. See Figure 20–7 for information on a popular source of monounsaturated fatty acids.

Reducing saturated fat intake decreases serum cholesterol more than reducing dietary cholesterol does. Using nonfat or low-fat dairy products rather than higher fat ones can reduce fat intake by as much as 90 percent. This is an especially important strategy, because milk fat contains more cholesterol-raising fatty acids than meat fat does (Grundy, 1999). Cooking methods also affect the fat in meat. For instance, warm water rinsing of cooked, crumbled ground beef containing 30 percent fat reduced its fat content by 33 to 52 percent (Love and Prusa, 1992). Other techniques to reduce fat in meat are shown in Figure 20–8.

Fish Intake

Not all animal fat is equally threatening to one's heart and blood vessels. Eskimos following their traditional diet eat a lot of animal fat; they also have a low rate of CHD. Many researchers attribute this to the high omega-3 fatty acid content of the fish Eskimos eat.

MODERATION

The type and amount of fish affects health outcomes. Compared with women who ate fish less than once per month, those who ate fish one to three times per month had a 21 percent lower risk of CHD and those who ate it once per week had a 29 percent lower risk. More frequent fish meals produced smaller gains: 31 percent lower risk with two to four times per week and 34 percent lower risk with five or more times per week (Hu et al, 2002). Regarding stroke risk, one weekly portion of fish was inversely related to ischemic stroke, but "Eskimo" intakes may increase risk of hemorrhagic stroke possibly because omega-3 fatty

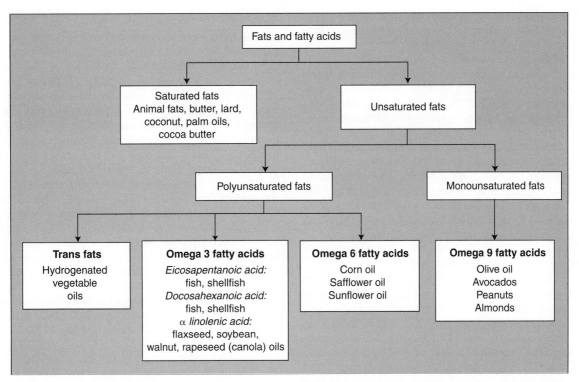

Figure **20–6** Fatty acids and their common food sources. Omega-3 fatty acids are particularly desirable in a heart healthy diet. (Adapted from Din, Newby, and Flapan, 2004.)

acids are known to decrease platelet aggregation (Kris-Etherton, Harris, and Appel, 2002).

MARINE OMEGA-3 FATTY ACIDS

Foods rich in marine omega-3 fatty acids, **eicosapentaenoic acid (EPA)** and docosahexaenoic acid (DHA), result in decreased occurrences of arrhythmia and sudden death, lower plasma triglycerides, and reduced blood clotting tendencies. Furthermore, alpha-linolenic acid from plant sources has been associated with reduced risk of myocardial infarction and of fatal ischemic heart disease in women (Krauss, 2000). Docosahexanoic acid (DHA) in adi-pose tissue is useful as a long-term marker of fatty fish intake, whereas alpha-linolenic acid is mostly metabolized, and when it is stored it is converted to DHA so that blood levels of alpha-linolenic acid would reflect recent food intake (Albert et al, 2002). Persons consuming diets enriched with omega-3 fatty acids had a 20 percent lower

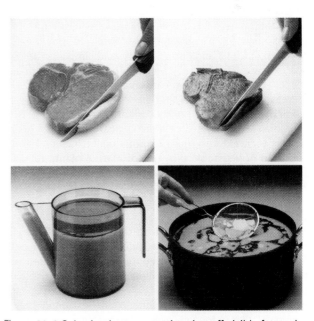

Figure **20–8** Selecting lean meat, trimming off visible fat, and skimming fat from meat juices reduce the amount of fat consumed. (From the National Live Stock and Meat Board, 444 North Michigan Avenue, Chicago, IL 60611, with permission.)

Figure **20–7** CA-NO-LA (Canadian oil) is derived from a variation of rapeseed developed by traditional plant breeding. It is high in monounsaturated fatty acids. (Photograph compliments of Canada's Canola Industry, used with permission.)

risk of nonfatal myocardial infarction and a 30 percent lower risk of fatal myocardial infarction than those taking control diets or placebo (Bucher et al, 2002).

One proposed mechanism for these beneficial effects was tested with people scheduled for carotid endarterectomy who received placebo, omega-6 fatty acids as sunflower oil, or omega-3 fatty acids as fish oil. Those receiving the fish oil had more stable plaque that incorporated omega-3 fatty acids, whereas the other two groups did not (Thies et al, 2003). Fish that contain omega-3 fatty acids include herring, mackerel, rainbow trout, salmon, sardines, swordfish, and tuna, but commercially prepared fried fish are low in omega-3 fatty acids and high in *trans* fats. Up to 3 grams per day of marine omega-3 fatty acids are considered Generally Recognized As Safe (GRAS) by the FDA, but individuals taking larger amounts should be monitored by a physician because of the risk of bleeding (Kris-Etherton, Harris, and Appel, 2002).

Based upon supportive but not conclusive research that they may reduce the risk of coronary heart disease, in 2000 the FDA approved a qualified health claim for DHA- and EPA-containing supplements and in 2004 for foods that contain significant amounts of those omega-3 fatty acids. Foods specifically mentioned were salmon, lake trout, tuna and herring. The FDA further recommends that consumers not exceed a total intake of 3 grams per day of EPA and DHA omega-3 fatty acids, with no more than 2 grams per day coming from a dietary supplement (U.S. Food and Drug Administration, 2004).

Clinical studies suggest that tissue levels of long-chain omega-3 fatty acids are depressed in vegetarians, particularly in vegans. Both of those diets, especially the vegan, are relatively low in α-linolenic acid (ALA) and provide little, if any, eicosapentaenoic acid (EPA) and docosahexaenoic acid (DHA). Conversion of ALA by the body to the more active longer-chain metabolites is less than 5 to 10 percent efficient for EPA and 2 to 5 percent for DHA. Thus, total omega-3 requirements may be higher for vegetarians than for nonvegetarians. Moreover, the balance between omega-3 and omega-6 fatty acids impacts the conversion rate. Thus, it may be wise to consult a dietitian if the client is at risk for cardiovascular disease or has increased need for EPA and DHA (pregnant or lactating women) or is likely to poorly convert ALA to EPA and DHA (persons with diabetes or neurological disorders, premature infants, elderly). Interventions might include careful selection of vegetable oils, use of marine plants or DHA-rich eggs, as well as supplements (Davis and Kris-Etherton, 2003).

MERCURY CAUTION

An additional concern has been raised about mercury in fish as a health risk, because, unlike the case with polychlorinated biphenyl (PCB) contamination, skinning and trimming the fish does not significantly reduce the mercury in contaminated fish (Kris-Etherton, Harris, and Appel, 2002). One study in nine countries found higher mercury levels in toenails associated with increased risk of MI and also with decreased DHA in adipose tissue, suggesting mercury may diminish the cardioprotective effect of eating fish (Guallar et al, 2002).

Soy Protein

Clinical trials have shown that consumption of soy protein compared with other proteins such as those from milk or meat can lower total and LDL cholesterol levels. The key is to replace some of the animal protein with soy protein. In 1999 the FDA approved a health claim for soy-containing foods stating that including soy protein in a diet low in saturated fat and cholesterol may reduce the risk of CHD by lowering blood cholesterol levels. Because 25 grams of soy protein daily in the diet is needed to show a significant cholesterol-lowering effect, in order to qualify for this health claim, a food must contain at least 6.25 grams of soy protein per serving (U.S. Food and Drug Administration, 1999).

The hypocholesterolemic effect of soy protein is greatest in moderate to severe rather than mild elevations in plasma lipids (Hecker, 2001). Soy protein seems to directly activate LDL receptors in the human liver that is normally not very effective in removing LDL from circulation, thus providing a different mechanism to reduce plasma cholesterol reduction than pathways taken by other dietary and pharmacologic interventions (Brown, 2005; Sirtori and Lovati, 2001). Figure 20–9 shows the many choices available utilizing soy.

Not all research is easily or quickly interpreted. Clinical Application 20–2 describes apparent paradoxes in diet and diseases in different countries.

Diets Tailored to Types of Hyperlipoproteinemia

Because of altered physiology, clients with the different types of hyperlipoproteinemia may need modified cholesterol-lowering diets (Table 20–6). The dietitian works with clients to maximize compliance. Although some of the clients may need cholesterol-lowering drug therapy, adjunct dietary therapy is likely to reduce the amount of medication required. Cholesterol-lowering drugs are recommended in addition to, not instead of, dietary modification.

Beyond the general recommendations to lower saturated fat consumption, clients with hyperlipoproteinemia need more stringent diets. All of these clients who are overweight are urged to lose the excess weight. Alcohol is the energy nutrient with the strongest linear association to serum triglycerides, and limiting intake to one standard drink per day can reduce triglyceride levels by 50 percent. Also, in persons with elevated serum triglycerides, a high-sucrose intake further increases triglyceride levels. Almost any recipe can be satisfactorily made with two-thirds to three-fourths the usual sugar while increasing the amounts of vanilla extract and cinnamon to give the impression of sweetness. Clients who have followed a very-low-fat diet may have a carbohydrate-induced hypertriglyceridemia (Denke, 2002). Refer again to Table 20–2 in relation to the following diet modifications for the different types of hyperlipoproteinemias.

TYPE I

This person is deficient in the enzyme triglyceride lipase. The serum chylomicrons are elevated because they carry the exogenous triglyceride in the bloodstream after meals. To treat this condition, food sources of triglyceride are restricted. Usually a 20- to 30-gram fat diet is prescribed,

Daily Soyfood Guide Pyramid

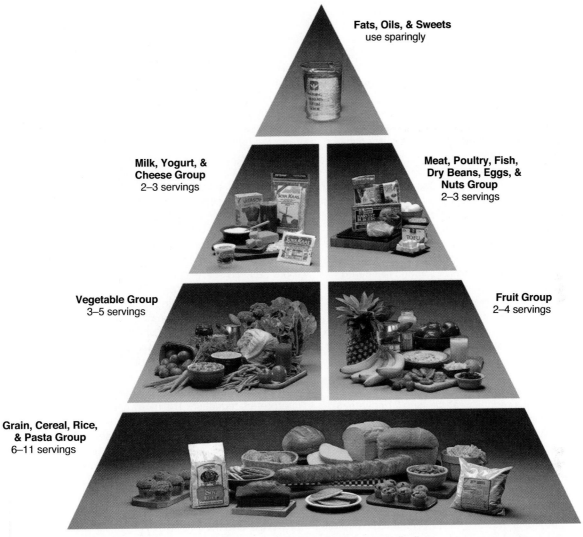

It's easy to include soyfoods in your daily diet.

Figure **20–9** Daily Soyfood Guide Pyramid. Soy products include oil, milk, cheese, yogurt, beans, burgers, tofu, grits, and flour. (From Indiana Soybean Development Council, with permission.)

which generally limits the person to 3 to 4 ounces of lean meat per day and results in a diet deriving less than 10 percent of energy from fat (Grundy, 1999).

TYPE IIA

This diet contains less than 200 milligrams of cholesterol per day. LDL and cholesterol elevations characterize Type IIA hyperlipoproteinemia. Polyunsaturated and monounsaturated fats should outnumber saturated fats by a factor of 1.5 or 2 to 1.

TYPE IIB

This diet is the same as for Type IIA, plus limitation in alcohol and high-carbohydrate foods, especially simple sugars. In Type IIB hyperlipoproteinemia, triglyceride levels are elevated, whereas in Type IIA they are not. Alcohol and car-

bohydrate stimulate triglyceride production and therefore are to be restricted. Usually the diet is calculated to provide only 40 percent of the kilocalories from carbohydrate.

TYPE III

Carbohydrate aggravates Type III hyperlipoproteinemia. Here dietary carbohydrate is limited to 35 to 40 percent of kilocalories. Because triglycerides are elevated, alcohol and sugar should be restricted. If cholesterol levels continue to be high after weight loss, dietary cholesterol should be moderately reduced.

TYPE IV

This very common hyperlipoproteinemia also is aggravated by carbohydrate. Therefore, only 35 to 40 percent of kilocalories should come from carbohydrate. Triglycerides

The Limits of Population Studies: An Historical Perspective

In the 1960s, the lowest rates of heart disease reported among seven countries were in Japan and Greece. People in those two countries were poles apart in fat consumption: 10 percent of kilocalories in Japan and 40 percent on the island of Crete. But the Greeks derived less than 10 percent of kilocalories from animal protein and 33 percent of their kilocalories from olive oil, which is 82 percent monounsaturated. Diets high in monounsaturates enhance the resistance of LDL cholesterol to oxidation, whereas polyunsaturates are more susceptible to oxidation (Kratz et al, 2002).

Since 1976, a decrease in cardiovascular mortality in men and women was experienced in Spain, despite increased intakes of dairy products and meat, particularly pork and poultry. If attention focused only on those foods, the rationale for the decreased mortality would be missed. Most of the decrease in cardiovascular mortality was due to a decline in stroke mortality. Improved hypertension control, including decreased intake of salt and salt-cured foods, is thought to have influenced this trend. Other contributing factors were increased consumption of fruit and fish, reduction in cigarette smoking, and expanded access to clinical care, including a major increase in the use of aspirin as a platelet inhibitor (Serra-Majem et al, 1995).

Consumption of red wine is credited with conferring some protection against coronary heart disease. The "French Paradox" refers to that country's second lowest coronary heart disease mortality rate among 21 countries, in the face of its rank as having the highest alcohol intake and the highest wine intake. Other studies have shown a maximum protective effect of alcohol against CHD at one to two drinks per day. Higher alcohol intake is progressively associated with higher risks of cardiovascular disease and other causes of mortality. A 12-year study of French men indeed found a decrease in cardiovascular mortality of 30 percent associated with a daily intake of 48 grams of alcohol, mostly wine. In contrast, mortality by cancer and violent death was increased compared with that of abstainers (Renaud and Gueguen, 1998).

Men in eastern Finland have one of the highest recorded incidences of mortality from CHD. An association was reported between high levels of stored iron (as assessed by serum ferritin levels or ratio of serum transferrin receptor to serum ferritin) and increased risk for acute myocardial infarction (Salonen et al, 1992; Tuomainen et al, 1998). Iron overload thus was hypothesized to cause the higher occurrence of CHD in men compared with women. A study in Greece also correlated high dietary iron intake with increased risk of coronary artery disease in men and women 60 years of age or older (Tzonou et al, 1998). A more detailed study found no association between total iron intake and risk of myocardial infarction after adjustment for age and gender but did find high dietary intake of heme iron associated with occurrence of and mortality from myocardial infarction (Klipstein-Grosbusch et al, 1999), and a reanalysis of Salonen's data associated increased iron intake with increased consumption of red meat (American Heart Association, 2000).

Thus, evidence accumulates slowly and must be interpreted cautiously. The many correlations found in large studies are often statistically significant but do not prove causation and may not be clinically useful. Advice to clients should be based, as much as possible, on randomized clinical trials, the "gold standard" of medical practice.

---

are elevated, so sugar intake should be limited. Alcohol should be consumed at a rate of not more than 1 to 2 ounces per week, if at all.

TYPE V

This hyperlipoproteinemia is characterized by high serum levels of both chylomicrons and VLDL. Most clients with type V hyperlipoproteinemia display insulin resistance in the liver that apparently contributes to the production of VLDL. To control the chylomicronemia, a very-low-fat diet is prescribed. Obese clients are urged to lose weight and increase activity to decrease production of VLDL by the liver. Despite compliance with the dietary restrictions, some clients require triglyceride-lowering medications (Grundy, 1999).

Because all hyperlipoproteinemias are not the same, neither are the dietary treatments. Nurses should be informed about the differences and not assume that all clients with hyperlipoproteinemia receive the same diet prescription. For best results, the clinical dietitian should individualize the diet with the client.

Normal Blood Pressure

Specific guidelines centered on blood pressure concern salt intake, a healthy body weight, alcohol intake, and the DASH Diet. Strategies on weight control appear in Chapter 18. Information on the other three components of the program to control blood pressure are detailed below.

Maintain a Healthy Body Weight

Almost every trial of the effect of weight loss on blood pressure has shown a significant effect on blood pressure even without attaining a desirable body weight (Krauss et al, 2000). A 17.6-pound weight loss is associated with about an 8.5-mmHg decrease in systolic and 6.5-mmHg decrease in diastolic pressure in overweight hypertensive clients. Similarly, a combined exercise and weight-loss intervention has been shown to decrease systolic and diastolic pressures by 12.5 and 7.9 mmHg, respectively (Bacon et al, 2004).

Weight loss benefits multiple manifestations of metabolic syndrome. Individuals receiving a very low calorie

Table 20–6 **Cholesterol-Lowering Diets**

DESCRIPTION	INDICATION	ADEQUACY
These diets limit lipids and, for some clients, sugars.	These diets are prescribed when clients have elevated serum cholesterol. Consultation with a Registered Dietitian is encouraged to individualize a dietary plan.	The diets are adequate in all nutrients with the possible exception of iron because of the restriction on red meat. If the client is also on a sodium-restricted diet, imitation cheese, bacon, and eggs may exceed the prescription. Clients must be encouraged to consume enough energy to maintain a healthy body weight.

FOOD GROUP	RECOMMENDED FOODS
Milk	Skim milk, 1 percent milk, cultured buttermilk, evaporated skim or nonfat milk Nonfat or low-fat yogurt and frozen yogurt 1 or 2 percent fat cottage cheese Low-fat soft cheese: Farmer and pot cheese labeled no more than 2 to 6 g of fat/oz
Breads, cereals, and starches	Breads (made without whole milk, eggs, or butter): whole wheat, rye, pumpernickel, pita, white, bagels, English muffins, sandwich buns, dinner rolls, rice cakes Low-fat crackers: sticks, rye crisp, saltines, zwieback Hot cereals, most dry cold cereals Pasta: noodles, macaroni, spaghetti Rice Dried peas and beans, split peas, black-eyed peas, chick peas, kidney beans, navy beans, lentils, soybeans, low-fat tofu
Fruits and vegetables	Fresh, frozen, canned, or dried prepared without butter, cream, or cheese sauce

Meat, poultry, fish, shellfish	Lean meat with fat trimmed:
	    Beef—round, sirloin, chuck, loin
	    Lamb—leg, arm, loin, rib
	    Pork—tenderloin, leg, shoulder
	    Veal—all except ground
	Poultry without skin
	Fish: Fresh or frozen cod, flounder, haddock, halibut, trout; fresh or canned-in-water tuna
	Shellfish: Clams, crab, lobster, scallops, shrimp

Eggs	Egg whites, egg substitute
Fats and oils	Monounsaturated preferred (canola, olive, peanut oils) Low-fat dressings
Desserts and snacks	Low-fat frozen desserts: sorbet, sherbet, Italian ice, frozen yogurt, popsicles Angel food cake Low-fat cookies: fig bars, gingersnaps Low-fat candy: hard candy, jelly beans Low-fat snacks: pretzels, plain popcorn
Beverages	Nonfat beverages: carbonated drinks, juices, tea, coffee

diet achieved a 6.5-percent reduction in weight after 4 weeks along with decreases of 11.1 mmHg in systolic and 5.8 mmHg in diastolic pressure. Their blood glucose, triglycerides, and total cholesterol also declined 17 mg/dL, 94 mg/dL, and 37 mg/dL respectively. The decreases in glucose and cholesterol were maintained and further reductions in blood pressure and triglycerides were noted at 16.7 weeks, when a total weight loss of 15.1 percent was recorded (Case et al, 2002).

Limit Alcohol Intake

Individuals who choose to consume alcohol should limit intake to two standard-sized drinks per day for men and one drink for women and lighter-weight men. A standard drink contains 1/2 ounce of **ethanol,** an amount found in 12 ounces of beer or 5 ounces of wine or 1 ounce of 100-proof whiskey. High alcohol intake of more than three drinks per day has been linked to elevated blood pressure, and reduction of intake can lower blood pressure in hypertensive and normotensive men (Krauss et al, 2000) but a biologic mechanism for this link remains unclear (Klatsky, 2003). The pattern of drinking is also related to hypertension risk in that daily drinkers and those consuming alcohol without food had a significantly higher risk of hypertension compared with those drinking less than weekly and those drinking mostly with food (Stranges et al, 2004)

In one study, alcohol-dependent men received alcohol proportionate to body weight for 24 hours and then no alcohol for 24 hours. Eighty percent of the hypertensive subjects and 51 percent of the normotensive ones had significant decreases in blood pressure during the withdrawal period and were considered sensitive to alcohol (Estruch et al, 2003). Combined analysis of 15 trials found alcohol reduction to be associated with a significant lowering of systolic pressure by 3.31 mmHg and of diastolic pressure by 2.04 mmHg with greater decreases in blood pressure associated with larger percentage reductions in alcohol intake (Xin et al, 2001).

The DASH Diet

An 11-week clinical feeding trial of individuals with systolic blood pressure of less than 160 mmHg and diastolic pressures from 80 to 95 mmHg showed that dietary modification is effective in reducing blood pressure. The trial was named *Dietary Approaches to Stop Hypertension*, thus the resulting intervention is called the "DASH Diet." After 3 weeks on a *Control Diet*, low in fruits, vegetables, and dairy products with fat content typical of the United States, the participants were randomly assigned to continue on the *Control Diet* or to receive a *Fruits and Vegetables Diet* or a *Combination Diet* for 8 weeks. The *Fruits and Vegetables Diet* was similar to the *Control Diet* except that it provided more fruits and vegetables and fewer snacks and sweets. The *Combination Diet* was rich in fruits, vegetables, and low-fat dairy foods and had reduced amounts of total fat, saturated fat, and cholesterol than either of the other two diets. The potassium, magnesium, and calcium levels of the *Control Diet* were at about the 25th percentile of U.S. consumption, whereas those minerals in the *Fruits and Vegetables Diet* and the *Combination Diet* were close to the 75th percentile.

Weight reduction did not confound the results, because kilocalories were adjusted to maintain weight. Likewise, the three types of diets each contained about 3 grams of sodium, and individuals were permitted no more than three caffeinated beverages and no more than two standard alcoholic beverages per day. Reported intakes of alcohol were similar across all the diets. After 8 weeks on the experimental diets, the reductions in blood pressure shown in Table 20–7 were attained.

An outstanding feature of this trial was its emphasis, not on limiting or restricting foods but on increasing intake of certain foods. Commonly available foods, not specialty foods containing fat substitutes, were used throughout the trial. The features of the DASH diet are shown in Table 20–8 and Figure 20–10. The example is based on a 2000-kilocalorie diet. Individuals requiring more or less energy intake would need to make proportionate adjustments.

Limit Salt Intake

Analysis of randomized trials have shown that reducing sodium intake by 1800 milligrams per day produced an

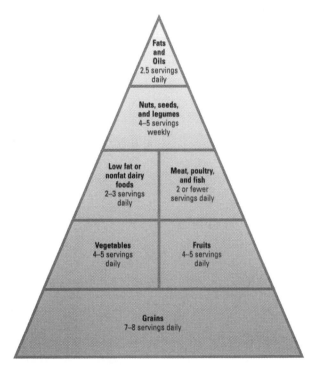

Figure 20–10 The Dash Diet, featuring fruits, vegetables, lowfat dairy products, and specifying servings of nuts, seeds, and beans, has been shown to reduce hypertension. The numbers of servings are based on a 2000-kilocalorie diet. (Adapted from National Institutes of Health, 1997.)

average of 4- and 2-mmHg reductions in systolic and diastolic pressures in people with hypertension. Those with normal pressure had smaller reductions (Krauss et al, 2000). A target of 6 grams of salt (2400 milligrams of sodium) has been set. To reach this goal, consumers should choose foods low in salt and limit the amount of salt added to food.

Depending on their clinical status, clients on a TLC Diet may have further restrictions on their sodium intake. Reductions beyond the population target are difficult to achieve without professional guidance and monitoring. In one case personally observed, a client who claimed to be following a low-sodium diet as an outpatient experienced electrolyte imbalances when hospitalized on a "real" dietitian-calculated, sodium-restricted diet.

Projected achievable decreases in systolic pressures from lifestyle changes appear in Table 20–9. Adapting all of the behaviors could have a significant effect on blood pressure, with the possibility of eliminating the need for medication or reducing the amount required to maintain a desirable pressure.

Table 20–7 **Reduction in Blood Pressure Compared to Control Diet**

| | Fruit and Vegetable Diet | | Combination (DASH) Diet | |
	SYSTOLIC	DIASTOLIC	SYSTOLIC	DIASTOLIC
Normotensive	2.8 mmHg	1.1 mmHg	5.5 mmHg	3.0 mmHg
Hypertensive	7.2 mmHg	2.8 mmHg	11.4 mmHg	5.5 mmHg

SOURCE: Adapted from Appel et al, 1997.

Table 20–8 The DASH Diet

FOOD GROUP	DAILY SERVINGS	SERVING SIZES	EXAMPLES AND NOTES	SIGNIFICANCE OF FOOD GROUP TO DASH DIET
Grains and grain products	7–8	1 slice bread 1/2 cup dry cereal 1/2 cup cooked cereal, rice, or pasta	Whole-wheat bread, English muffin, pita bread, bagel, cereals, grits, oatmeal	Major sources of energy and fiber
Vegetables	4–5	1 cup raw leafy 1/2 cup cooked 6 oz juice	Tomatoes, potatoes, carrots, peas, squash, broccoli, turnip greens, collards, kale, spinach, artichokes, sweet potatoes, beans	Rich sources of potassium, magnesium, and fiber
Fruits	4–5	6 oz juice 1 medium fruit 1/4 cup dried fruit 1/2 cup fresh, frozen, or canned fruit	Apricots, bananas, dates, oranges, grapefruit, mangoes, melons, peaches, pineapples, prunes, raisins, strawberries, tangerines	Important sources of potassium, magnesium, and fiber
Low-fat or non-fat dairy foods	2–3	8 oz milk 1 cup yogurt 1.5 oz cheese	Skim or 1 percent milk, skim or low-fat buttermilk, nonfat or low-fat yogurt, part-skim mozzarella cheese, nonfat cheese	Major sources of calcium and protein
Meats, poultry, and fish	2 or fewer	3 oz cooked meat, poultry, or fish	Select only lean; trim away visible fat, broil, roast, or boil instead of frying; remove skin from poultry	Rich sources of protein and magnesium
Nuts, seeds, and legumes	4–5 per week	1.5 oz. or 1/3 cup nuts 1/2 oz or 2 tbsp seeds 1/2 cup cooked legumes	Almonds, filberts, mixed nuts, peanuts, walnuts, sunflower seeds, kidney beans, lentils	Rich sources of energy, magnesium, potassium, protein, and fiber
Fats and oils	2.5	1 tsp	Canola, olive, peanut oils	Contain mainly monounsaturated fatty acids

SOURCE: Adapted from National Institutes of Health, 1997 and the ADA Exchange Lists, Appendix A.

Specialty Foods

More and more foods are packaged bearing health claims. Whole-grain foods high in soluble fiber may claim to reduce the risk of heart disease *in a low-fat diet*. Many popular foods are marketed in light or fat-free versions that nevertheless may contain significant kilocalories.

If a person's cholesterol is still in the undesirable range after 6 weeks on a TLC Diet, specialty foods containing plant sterols may be recommended *in prescribed amounts*, not as much as desired. These are marketed as table spreads (butter substitutes) and salad dressings. **Plant sterols** are compounds, which structurally resemble cholesterol but are not absorbed in the human body to any extent and actually inhibit the absorption of cholesterol. A dose of 2 grams per day can produce a 10-percent decrease in LDL-C levels (Denke, 2002). Monitoring for side effects of plant sterols is recommended. Decreases in bioavailability of beta-carotene and alpha-tocopherol have been reported

Table 20–9 Possible Effects of Lifestyle Changes on Blood Pressure

LIFESTYLE CHANGE	GOAL	APPROXIMATE ACHIEVABLE DECREASES IN SYSTOLIC PRESSURE
Weight reduction	BMI between 18.5 and 24.9	5 to 20 mmHg/10 Kg (22 lb) weight loss
DASH Diet	Low in total and saturated fat High in fruits, vegetables, and nonfat dairy foods	8 to 14 mmHg
Reduced salt intake	Maximum of 2.4 g sodium (6 g salt)	2 to 8 mmHg
Physical activity	Minimum 30 min/day most days	4 to 9 mmHg
Moderate alcohol intake	Maximum of 2 drinks/day for most men; 1/day for women and lighter weight men	2 to 4 mmHg
Total reduction possible	With 22 lb weight loss plus 4 other lifestyle changes	21 to 55 mmHg

SOURCE: Adapted from U.S. Department of Health and Human Services, 2003.

Table 20–10 **Labeling Regulations for Sodium Content Descriptions**

TERM	LEGAL DEFINITION
Free	Less than 5 mg of sodium per serving.
Salt Free	Must meet the criteria for free.
Very Low* Sodium	Less than 35 mg of sodium per serving. For meals and main dishes: 35 mg or less per 100 g.
Low* Sodium	Less than 140 mg of sodium per serving. Meals and main dishes: 140 mg or less per 100 g.
Reduced or Less	This term means that a nutritionally altered product contains 25 percent less sodium than the regular, or reference, product. However, a reduced claim cannot be made on a product if its reference food already meets the requirement for a "low" claim.
Light in Sodium or Lightly Salted	May be used on food in which the sodium content has been reduced by at least 50 percent compared with an appropriate reference food.
Unsalted or No Added Salt	Must declare "This is not a sodium-free food" on information panel if the food is not sodium free.

*Synonyms for low include "little," "few," and "low source oil."

(Richelle et al, 2004). There is one absolute contraindication to the use of plant sterols. In a rare autosomal recessive disorder called sitosterolemia, both cholesterol and plant sterols are absorbed at a high rate and are not removed effectively by the liver, resulting in accelerated atherosclerosis and premature coronary artery disease (Lee, Lu, and Patel, 2001).

Sodium-Controlled Diets

As many as one-third of mild hypertensive cases can be controlled with sodium restriction, usually a 2-gram sodium diet. Results may not be apparent for up to 8 weeks. The preference for salty foods is learned and culturally transmitted, even when heavy salting is no longer necessary for preservation of food. After 3 months on a sodium-restricted diet, most individuals lose their appetite for salt. Table 20–10 lists the legal definitions for sodium and salt descriptions on labels.

Unseen contributions to sodium intake may come from other beverages, over-the-counter medications, and drinking water. Table 20–11 lists sodium content of beverages.

Many toothpastes and mouthwashes contain significant amounts of sodium and should not be swallowed. Over-the-counter medications that may contain significant amounts of sodium include analgesics, antacids, antibiotics, antitussives, laxatives, and sedatives.

The American Heart Association recommends a limit of 20 milligrams of sodium per liter of water as a standard for persons who require a restricted sodium diet. As much as 42 percent of the nation's water supply exceeds this amount (Korch, 1986). Many municipal water supplies are softened, which can increase the water's sodium content excessively. Sodium in city water supplies has varied from 1.2 milligrams per liter in Seattle to 100 milligrams per liter in Phoenix. Many households have water softeners in their homes that increase the water's sodium content. Consideration should also be given to the sodium content of specialty bottled waters. "Mineral waters" contain from 8 to 172 milligrams of sodium per liter. "Read the label" is appropriate advice here. Clients who require a diet containing less than 2 grams of sodium may elect to use bottled, distilled, deionized, or demineralized water for drinking and cooking in order to

Table 20–11 **Examples of Varying Sodium Content of Beverages***

BEVERAGE†	Regular		Diet	
	SODIUM (mg)	KILOCALORIES	SODIUM (mg)	KILOCALORIES
Club soda			75	0
Coffee	4	0		
Cola	15	151		
With aspartame			21	2
With saccharin			75	2
Gatorade	39	123		
Ginger ale	25	125	130	4
Kool-Aid	0	150		
With aspartame			0	6
Lemonade	12	150		
Lemon-lime soda	41	149	70	4
Pepper-type	38	151	70	0
Root beer	49	152	170	4
Tea	2	0		

*Serving size is 12 fluid ounces.
†Sodium content may vary depending on the source of water.

consume preferred sodium-containing foods. Many dietitians work with clients to develop individualized diet plans. Some clients prefer a daily allotment of salt in a shaker to be used as desired. If this strategy is adopted, the foods high in sodium must be limited to a greater extent than for a standardized sodium-controlled diet.

Several salt substitutes are available. Many of them substitute potassium for sodium. These may be unsuitable for clients with kidney disease or those taking potassium-sparing diuretics or ACE inhibitors. Clients should consult their health-care providers about using salt substitutes. These products are for table use only. Salt substitutes are not appropriate for cooking because they turn bitter.

In clinical practice, diet orders such as "no-added-salt diet" or "low-sodium diet" require clarification. Usually, a facility's diet manual defines the terms. A "no-added-salt diet" may be calculated as 4 grams of sodium and a "low-sodium diet" as 2 grams in one facility but at different levels in another. Diet prescriptions should be written in milligrams of sodium to achieve the desired result. Table 20–12 describes diets with sodium controlled from 2 grams to 2000 milligrams per day. Figure 20–11 shows some of the seasonings permitted on a sodium-controlled diet.

As was indicated in Table 8–3, processed foods are heavily laden with sodium. Therefore, to affect the population's risk of cardiovascular disease, food manufacturers will have to be persuaded to decrease the amount of salt in the foods they produce. Likewise, the same action will be needed to decrease the amounts of saturated and *trans* fats in the food supply.

Table 20–12 **Sodium-Controlled Diets**

DESCRIPTION	INDICATION	ADEQUACY		
These diets control sodium intake to prescribed levels.	Clients with hypertension, congestive heart failure, fluid-retaining kidney or endocrine disease, or other edematous conditions.	The 500-mg and 250-mg diets may be deficient in some nutrients.		

FOOD ITEM OR GROUP	2 GRAMS SODIUM	1 GRAM SODIUM	500 mg SODIUM	200 mg SODIUM
Soups	LS*	LS	LS	LS
Milk	2 cups	2 cups	1 cup	LS
Bread	3 slices	3 slices	LS	LS
Cereal	1 serving	LS	LS	LS
Fruits	Free	Free	Free	Free
Egg	1	1	1	1
Meat/substitutes	6 oz	5 oz	4 oz	4 oz
Vegetables	LS	LS	LS	LS
Desserts	1 serving	LS	LS	LS
Margarine	5 tsp	3 tsp	3 tsp	LS
Condiments	LS	LS	LS	LS

*Any food in the following LS list.

FOOD GROUP	LOWER IN SODIUM (LS)	HIGHER IN SODIUM
Milk	Commercially made low-sodium milk Low-sodium cheese	All milk from animals Yogurt Regular cheese Commercial milk products
Breads and cereals	Bread and crackers prepared without salt Rice, barley, and pasta without added salt Baked goods made without salt, baking soda, or baking powder Unsalted cooked cereal Puffed rice, puffed wheat, shredded wheat Cornmeal, cornstarch	Commercial mixes Frozen bread dough Regular crackers Instant rice and pasta mixes Instant and quick-cooking cereals Commercial stuffing and casserole mixes Self-rising flour and cornmeal Baked goods and quick breads made with salt, baking soda, baking powder, or egg white
Fruits	Fresh, frozen, dried, or canned fruit without added sodium All fruit juices	Crystallized or glazed fruit Maraschino cherries Dried fruit with sodium preservatives
Vegetables	Fresh, frozen without salt, low-sodium canned vegetables except those listed at right	Canned and frozen vegetables and juices Sauerkraut

(Continued on the following page)

Table 20–12 **Sodium-Controlled Diets** *(Continued)*

FOOD GROUP	LOWER IN SODIUM (LS)	HIGHER IN SODIUM
Meat, poultry, fish, shellfish	Fresh, frozen, or canned low-sodium meat and poultry Low-sodium luncheon meats Eggs Low-sodium peanut butter Fresh fish Canned low-sodium tuna and salmon	Real and imitation bacon Luncheon meat Chipped or corned beef Smoked or salted meat or fish Kosher meat Frozen and powdered egg substitutes Regular peanut butter Brains, kidney, clams, lobster, crab, oysters, scallops, shrimp, and other shellfish
Fats and oils	Cooking oil Unsalted butter, margarine, salad dressings, and shortening	Salted butter and margarine Commercial salad dressings
Desserts and miscellaneous	Alcohol Coffee, coffee substitutes Lemonade Tea Low-sodium candy Unflavored gelatin Jam, jelly, maple syrup, honey Unsalted nuts and popcorn	Regular canned or frozen soups Soup mixes Salted popcorn, nuts, potato chips, snacks Instant cocoa or powdered drink mixes Canned fruit drinks Commercial pastry, candy, cakes, cookies, gelatin desserts
Condiments and seasonings	Sweet: allspice, almond extract, anise seed, apricot nectar, baking chocolate, cardamom, cinnamon, coriander, ginger, lemon extract, lemon juice, mace, maple extract, mint, nutmeg, orange extract, orange juice, peppermint extract, pineapple, pineapple juice, unsalted pecans, vanilla extract, unsalted walnuts, walnut extract Tangy: basil, bay leaves, caraway seeds, cayenne pepper, chili powder, chives, cloves, curry powder, dill weed, garlic, garlic powder (not salt), green pepper, horseradish without salt, marjoram, mustard powder (not prepared), mustard seed, onion powder (not salt) onions, oregano, paprika, parsley, pepper, poppy seed, rosemary, sage, savory, sesame seeds, tarragon, thyme, turmeric	Any salt Barbecue sauce Bouillon cubes or granules Catsup Chili sauce Tartar sauce Horseradish sauce Meat extracts, sauces, and tenderizers Kitchen Bouquet Gravy and sauce mixes Monosodium glutamate Prepared mustard Olives Pickles Saccharin, other sugar substitutes containing sodium Soy sauce Teriyaki sauce Worcestershire sauce

SAMPLE MENUS FOR 2 g SODIUM DIET

BREAKFAST	LUNCH AND DINNER
1/2 cup orange juice 1/2 cup shredded wheat 2 slices toast 2 tsp margarine 1 tbsp strawberry jam 1 cup 1 percent milk Sugar Coffee	3 oz chicken breast, turkey, or fish baked in lemon juice Baked potato 2 tsp margarine 1/2 cup broccoli Tossed salad with homemade oil and vinegar dressing 1 dinner roll 1/2 cup sherbet 1 cup 1 percent milk (day's total = 2 cups) Tea

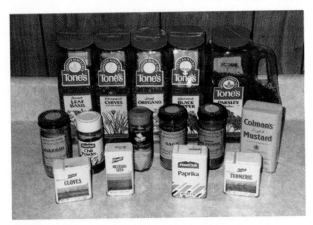

Figure 20–11 These are just a few of the many condiments and seasonings that are available to the client who needs to restrict sodium intake.

Other Modifications

Dietary intake may be adapted to the client's diagnosis and condition. Particular therapy may need regular monitoring and use of stimulants found in beverages may be restricted.

Due to Diagnosis or Condition

An acutely ill person may be in shock and a chronically ill person may have congestive heart failure. Both situations require modifications in diet.

SHOCK

After a heart attack, the client may be in shock. One adaptive response of the body is to slow gastrointestinal function. Thus the client should receive nothing by mouth while shock persists. Fluid is given intravenously to maintain fluid balance and to keep an access site open for intravenous medications. As the client recovers, the diet usually progresses from a 1000- to 1200-kilocalorie liquid diet to a soft diet of small, frequent meals. Large meals can increase the workload of the heart. Food is served at a moderate temperature. Very hot or very cold foods are thought to produce irregular heart rhythms.

CONGESTIVE HEART FAILURE

For clients in congestive heart failure, the diet order may read "as tolerated." Successfully nourishing them presents a challenge. Based on body weight, anthropometric measures, and plasma protein status, 50 to 68 percent of clients with congestive heart failure are malnourished. These clients frequently are anorectic due to unwelcome dietary changes, visceral congestion, and depression, but the loss of lean body mass exceeds that expected from anorexia alone (Hughes and Kostka, 1999). High-protein kilocalorie feeds do not reverse the abnormalities, signifying that the wasting that occurs in congestive heart failure is metabolic.

Food for the client with congestive heart failure should be nutrient-dense, easily eaten, and easily digested. An hour's rest before meals conserves energy. Large meals, which would exert upward pressure on the chest, are undesirable. Liquid formulas can be used to provide nutrients while moderating the feeling of fullness. It may be necessary to provide supplements of water-soluble vitamins and minerals that may be lost as fluid is excreted through treatment.

STROKE

Clients who have had a stroke may have chewing or swallowing problems. Often, thicker rather than thinner liquids are easier for a person with swallowing difficulty to manage. Nurses feeding clients with hemiplegia should place the food on the unaffected side of the tongue. Turning the client's head toward the weak side while he is sitting upright may help with swallowing. In addition, stroke clients may be aphasic and unable to communicate their needs or desires. A speech therapist is skilled in adaptive devices and restorative therapy for clients with dysphagia and aphasia.

Due To Particular Therapies or Habits

Both outpatients and hospitalized or institutionalized clients with cardiovascular diseases of all levels of acuity are treated with diuretics and will require knowledgeable caregiver and teachers. Similarly, the use of common stimulants found in beverages will have to be addressed by healthcare providers.

DIURETICS

Clients taking potassium-wasting diuretics may require dietary or supplemental potassium. The choices become more complex when the client is also on a sodium-controlled diet. In general, fruits are high in potassium and low in sodium. Another source of supplemental potassium to be assessed is a salt substitute.

ORAL ANTICOAGULANTS

The interaction between warfarin and vitamin K is included in Chapter 17. Table 17–1 summarizes dietary modifications for clients receiving oral anticoagulants.

CAFFEINE

The restrictions regarding the use of caffeine by clients with cardiovascular disease have been relaxed in some regions. Nevertheless, normal people have been observed to have serious **arrhythmias** after 9 or more cups of coffee or tea, whereas persons with histories of abnormal rhythms showed the same effects after 2 cups. Drinking more than 10 cups of caffeinated coffee per day was found to be a risk factor for sudden cardiac arrest in persons with coronary artery disease (de Vreede-Swagemakers et al, 1999). A comprehensive review indicated that, contrary to popular belief in habituation, blood pressure remains reactive to the pressor effects of caffeine in the diet. Although the impact of dietary caffeine on population blood pressure levels is likely to be only about 4/2 mmHg, caffeine use still could contribute to 14 percent of premature deaths from coronary heart disease and 20 percent from stroke

(James, 2004). Clinical judgment on the issue of caffeine varies so the protocol of the physician or the institution should be ascertained before providing caffeinated beverages to clients with cardiovascular diseases.

SUMMARY

Cardiovascular diseases are responsible for more deaths in the United States than are diseases of any other body system. Some of the risk factors, such as age, gender, race, and family and medical history, are beyond a person's control, but the major changeable risk factors can be modified. Those are hypertension, hypercholesterolemia, obesity, diabetes mellitus, physical inactivity, cigarette smoking, and excessive alcohol intake (Wellness Tips 20–1). Additional risk factors that affect hypertension are excessive salt intake and low intakes of potassium, calcium, and magnesium. Specific elevations of blood lipids and lipoproteins that are related to fat intake are closely linked to cardiovascular diseases.

Dietary modifications in cardiovascular disease most often involve cholesterol-lowering or sodium-controlling measures. The most common hyperlipoproteinemia is type IV, which requires restricted carbohydrate intake as well as controlled fat intake. Other qualities of the diet may require adjustment, such as potassium intake and the amount, timing, and texture of meals.

 20–1 • Know your risk for cardiovascular disease.

- To begin, select one risk factor to change that has the potential to significantly influence your risk profile.
- Make a commitment to modifying that risk factor. Solicit assistance from family and friends.
- Implement one strategy at a time.
- Visualize enjoying the action you are taking.
- Stay alert to reports of effective strategies. Wise and satisfying selections are facilitated when so many products are available.
- Lengthen your time frame to encompass the rest of your (healthy) life.

CASE STUDY 20–1

Mr. Z is a 59-year-old white man who was admitted to the acute-care hospital with a diagnosis of possible myocardial infarction. Subsequent testing proved Mr. Z did not have an infarction. His medical diagnoses are myocardial ischemia and type IV hyperlipoproteinemia. He is being readied for discharge to home.

Mr. Z is vice president for sales of a large manufacturing company. His business activities involve luncheon and dinner meetings at which alcohol consumption is common. He stated he has "at least one cocktail, usually two" with lunch and with dinner.

The clinical dietitian visited Mr. Z to instruct him on the diet prescribed by the physician. After the dietitian left, Mr. Z said to the nurse, "That diet is impossible for my situation. She just doesn't understand the business world. I don't believe there's anything wrong with my heart, anyway. It was just indigestion."

Providing client care is a dynamic process. Based on the above information, the nurse added the following modifications to Mr. Z's nursing care plan.

NURSING CARE PLAN

SUBJECTIVE DATA Reported alcohol intake of 2 to 4 oz per day
Perceived incompatibility of prescribed diet with lifestyle
Stated disbelief in medical diagnosis

OBJECTIVE DATA Elevated blood VLDL and triglyceride

NURSING DIAGNOSIS NANDA: Noncompliance (NANDA, 2003, with permission) related to denial of illness and negative perception of treatment regimen as evidenced by statements to nurse.

DESIRED OUTCOMES EVALUATION CRITERIA	NURSING ACTIONS/ INTERVENTIONS	RATIONALE
NOC: Health beliefs (Moorhead, Johnson, and Maas, 2004, with permission) Client will acknowledge consequences of noncompliant behavior by time of hospital discharge.	NIC: Decision Making Support (Dochterman and Bulechek, 2004, with permission) Review pathophysiology of hyper-lipoproteinemia and atherosclerosis with client. Analyze with the client the possibility of partial compliance. Obtain client's permission to discuss discharge instructions with significant other. Inform physician of extent of intended noncompliance.	Mr. Z is a competent adult. He is able to make his own choices. Repeating the information on atherosclerosis is an attempt to be sure his choice to reject the treatment regimen is informed. Perhaps the many changes required are overwhelming Mr. Z. One or two alter-ations might be acceptable as a starting point. Enlisting a support person might, over time, give Mr. Z reason to reconsider his decision. This is a change in the client's mental condition. It is appropriate to notify the physician and record it on the client's medical record.

CTQ CRITICAL THINKING QUESTIONS

1. How could additional assessment data regarding family history be helpful in interpreting this client's reaction? Would you expect his reaction to be different if the diagnosis of myocardial infarction had been confirmed?

2. What additional interventions have the potential to achieve the stated outcome before hospital discharge?

3. How would you plan for the follow-up care for this client?

⟫⟫ CHAPTER REVIEW

1. The DASH Diet to reduce hypertension emphasizes:
   a. Increased amounts of fruits, vegetables, nuts, seeds, and legumes
   b. Specialty formulas as meal replacements
   c. Carbohydrate control and counting similar to that used in diabetes mellitus treatment
   d. Increased amounts of protein through low-fat dairy prod-ucts and large servings of meats

2. The first action a hypertensive client should take to lower blood pressure is to:
   a. Restrict fluid to 1500 milliliters per day
   b. Eliminate saturated fat from the diet
   c. Lose weight if necessary
   d. Limit sodium intake to 1 gram per day

3. The Therapeutic Lifestyle Changes (TLC) Diet limits saturated and *trans* fat intake to _____ percent of daily kilocalories and cholesterol to _____ milligrams per day.

   a. 25, 500
   b. 20, 400
   c. 10, 300
   d. 7, 200

4. Which of the following seasonings are permitted on a sodium-controlled diet?
   a. Catsup, horseradish mustard, and tartar sauce
   b. Chili powder, green pepper, and caraway seeds
   c. Celery seeds, seasoned meat tenderizer, and teriyaki sauce
   d. Dry mustard, garlic, and Worcestershire sauce

5. A high-sucrose intake is related to cardiovascular disease because:
   a. Many cardiac clients have a genetic deficiency of sucrase.
   b. A high-sugar diet causes hyperactivity and hypertension.
   c. Excess sugar has to be excreted, causing premature aging of the kidney.
   d. Sucrose is positively related to triglyceride levels in the body.

CLINICAL ANALYSIS

Mr. T is a 55-year-old black man being seen in a health clinic for hypertension. His blood pressure was 150/102 3 months ago when he was first diagnosed. It has remained below that level but has not returned to normal. Today his blood pressure is 146/100.

Mr. T is 5 feet 9 inches tall and weighs 173 pounds. He has a medium frame. When first diagnosed, he weighed 178 pounds. A weight-loss diet with no added salt was prescribed, but progress has been slow.

Now the physician is prescribing a 2-gram sodium diet and starting Mr. T on a mild potassium-wasting diuretic. The clinic nurse is responsible for instructing the client.

1. Before he or she instructs Mr. T, which of the following actions by the nurse would best ensure his compliance with the diet?
   a. Doing a financial analysis to see if Mr. T can afford the special foods on his new diet
   b. Finding out which favorite foods Mr. T would have most difficulty giving up
   c. Listing the possible consequences of hypertension if it is not controlled
   d. Asking to see Mrs. T to instruct her on the preparation of foods for the new diet

2. Which of the following breakfasts would be best for Mr. T?
   a. Applesauce, raisin bran, 1 percent milk, and a bagel with cream cheese
   b. Canned pears, cornflakes, whole milk, and a cholesterol-free plain doughnut
   c. Cooked prunes, instant oatmeal, 2 percent milk, and raisin toast with margarine
   d. Orange juice, shredded wheat, skim milk, and whole-wheat toast with jelly

3. Mr. T has agreed to limit his alcohol intake to two drinks per week. He asks the nurse to recommend beverages compatible with his diet. Which of the following is the best choice?
   a. Tomato juice and bouillon
   b. Buttermilk and club soda
   c. Plain tea and fruit juice
   d. Gatorade and lemonade

REFERENCES

Albert, CM, et al: Blood levels of long-chain n-3 fatty acids and the risk of sudden death. N Engl J Med 346:1113, 2002.

Ambrose, JA, and Barua, RS: The pathophysiology of cigarette smoking and cardiovascular disease: An update. J Am Coll Cardiol 43:1731, 2004.

American College of Cardiology/American Heart Association Task Force on Practice Guidelines: ACC/AHA Guidelines for the Evaluation and Management of Chronic Heart Failure in the Adult, 2002. Accessed August 11, 2004 at http://www.acc.org/clinical/guidelines/failure/hf_index.htm.

American Heart Association: Iron and heart disease. 2000. Accessed June 5, 2000 at http://www.americanheart.org/Heart_and_Stroke_A_Z_Guide/iron.html.

American Heart Association: Step I, Step II, and TLC diets. Accessed September 1, 2004 at http://www.americanheart.org/presenter.jhtml?identifier=4764.

Anderson, JW, et al: Long-term cholesterol-lowering effects of psyllium as an adjunct to diet therapy in the treatment of hypercholesterolemia. Am J Clin Nutr 71:1433, 2000.

Anderson, RN, and Smith, BL: Deaths: Leading causes for 2001. Natl Vital Stat Rep 52:1, 2003. Accessed August 10, 2004 at http://www.cdc.gov/nchs/data/nvsr/nvsr52_09.pdf.

Angeja, BG, et al: Hormone therapy and the risk of stroke after acute myocardial infarction in postmenopausal women. J Am Coll Cardiol 38:1297, 2001.

Appel, LJ, et al: A clinical trial of the effects of dietary patterns on blood pressure. N Engl J Med 336:1117, 1997.

Ascherio, A, Katan, MB, and Stampfer, MJ: Trans fatty acids and coronary heart disease. N Engl J Med 340:1994, 1999.

Backes, JM, Howard, PA, and Moriarty, PM: Role of C-reactive protein in cardiovascular disease. Ann Pharmacother 38:110, 2004.

Bacon, SL, et al: Effects of exercise, diet and weight loss on high blood pressure. Sports Med 34:307, 2004.

Baker, DW: Prevention of heart failure. J Card Fail 8:333, 2002.

Barker, DJP: Fetal origins of cardiovascular disease. Ann Med 31(Suppl 1):3, 1999.

Bassett, DR, Jr, et al: Physical activity and ethnic differences in hypertension prevalence in the United States. Prev Med 34:179, 2002.

Bazzano, LA, Serdula, MK, and Liu, S: Dietary intake of fruits and vegetables and risk of cardiovascular disease. Curr Atheroscler Rep 5:492, 2003.

Brown, BG, and Crowley, J: Is there any hope for vitamin E? JAMA 293:1387, 2005.

Brown, JE: Nutrition Through the Life Cycle, ed 2. Thomson Wadsworth, Belmont, CA, 2005.

Bucher, HC, et al: N-3 polyunsaturated fatty acids in coronary heart disease: A meta-analysis of randomized controlled trials. Am J Med 112:298, 2002.

Burns, DM: Epidemiology of smoking-induced cardiovascular disease. Prog Cardiovasc Dis 46:11, 2003.

Case, CC, et al: Impact of weight loss on the metabolic syndrome. Diabetes Obes Metab 4:407, 2002.

Centers for Disease Control: Declining prevalence of no known major risk factors for heart disease and stroke among adults—United States, 1991–2001. MMWR 53:4, 2004a. Accessed August 10, 2004 at http://www.cdc.gov/mmwr/preview/mmwrhtml/mm5301a2.htm.

Centers for Disease Control: Age-specific excess deaths associated with stroke among racial/ethnic minority populations—United States, 1997. MMWR 49:94, 2000. Accessed March 1, 2000 at http://www.cdc.gov/epo/mmwr/preview/mmwrhtml/mm4905a2.htm.

Centers for Disease Control: Number of deaths, death rates, and age-adjusted death rates for major causes of death for the United States, each division, each state, Puerto Rico, Virgin Islands, Guam, and American Samoa, 1997. Natl Vital Stat Rep 47:82, 1999. Accessed December 9, 1999 at http://www.cdc.gov/nchs/fastats/pdf/47_19t24.pdf.

Centers for Disease Control: Racial/Ethnic Disparities in Prevalence, Treatment, and Control of Hypertension—United States, 1999–2002. MMWR 54:7, 2005.

Centers for Disease Control and National Institutes of Health: Healthy People 2010: Focus Area 12 Heart Disease and Stroke, August 06, 2004b. Accessed August 12, 2004 at http://www.cdc.gov/cvh/hp2010/objectives.htm#issues.

Cheung, MC, et al: Antioxidant supplements block the response of HDL to simvastatin-niacin therapy in patients with coronary artery disease and low HDL. Arterioscler Thromb Vasc Biol 21:1320, 2001.

Costa, FV: Non-pharmacological treatment of hypertension in women. J Hypertens 20:S57, 2002.

Dakshinamurti, K, and Dakshinamurti, S: Blood pressure regulation and micronutrients. Nutr Res Rev 14:3, 2001.

Davis, BC, and Kris-Etherton, PM: Achieving optimal essential fatty acid status in vegetarians: Current knowledge and practical implications. Am J Clin Nutr 78:640S, 2003.

Denke, MA: Dietary prescriptions to control dyslipidemias. Circulation 105:132, 2002.

de Lorgeril, M, et al: Wine drinking and risks of cardiovascular complications after recent acute myocardial infarction. Circulation 106:1465, 2002.

de Vreede-Swagemakers, JJ, et al: Risk indicators for out-of-hospital cardiac arrest in patients with coronary artery disease. J Clin Epidemiol 52:601, 1999.

Dietary Management of Hyperlipoproteinemias. A Handbook for Physicians and Dietitians. U.S. Department of Health, Education, and Welfare, Bethesda, MD, 1980.

Dillavou, E, and Kahn, MB: Peripheral vascular disease: Diagnosing and treating the 3 most common peripheral vasculopathies. Geriatrics 58:37, 2003.

Din, JN, Newby, DE, and Flapan, AD: Omega 3 fatty acids and cardiovascular disease—fishing for a natural treatment. BMJ 328:30, 2004.

Dochterman, J, and Bulechek, G (eds): Nursing Interventions Classification (NIC), ed 4. Mosby, St. Louis, 2004.

Duthie, GG, Duthie, SJ, and Kyle, JAM: Plant polyphenols in cancer and heart disease: Implications as nutritional antioxidants. Nutr Res Rev 13:79, 2000.

Estruch, R, et al: Effects of alcohol withdrawal on 24 hour ambulatory blood pressure among alcohol-dependent patients. Alcohol Clin Exp Res 27:2002, 2003.

Expert Panel on Detection, Evaluation and Treatment of High Blood Cholesterol in Adults: Executive summary of the third report of the Expert Panel on Detection, Evaluation and Treatment of High Blood Cholesterol in Adults (Adult Treatment Panel III). JAMA 285:2486, 2001.

Fauci, AS, et al: Harrison's Principles of Internal Medicine Companion Handbook. McGraw-Hill, New York, 1998.

Freedman, JE, et al: Select flavonoids and whole juice from purple grapes inhibit platelet function and enhance nitric oxide release. Circulation 103:2792, 2001.

Geleijnse, JM, et al: Inverse association of tea and flavonoid intakes with incident myocardial infarction: The Rotterdam Study. Am J Clin Nutr 75:880, 2002.

Godfrey, KM, and Barker, DJ: Fetal programming and adult health. Public Health Nutr 4:611, 2001.

Gorelick, PB, et al: Prevention of a first stroke: A review of guidelines and a multidisciplinary consensus statement from the National Stroke Association, 1999. Accessed August 10, 2004 at http://199.239.30.192/NationalStroke/ProfessionalResource/Prevention+Guidelines.htm.

Green, DM, et al: Serum potassium level and dietary potassium intake as risk factors for stroke. Neurology 59:314, 2002.

Gropper, SS, Smith, JL, and Groff, JL: Advanced Nutrition and Human Metabolism, ed 4. Wadsworth, Belmont, CA, 2005.

Grundy, SM: Nutrition and diet in the management of hyperlipidemia and atherosclerosis. In Shils, ME, et al (eds): Modern Nutrition in Health and Disease, ed 9. Lippincott Williams & Wilkins, Philadelphia, 1999.

Guallar, E, et al: Mercury, fish oils, and the risk of myocardial infarction. N Engl J Med 347:1747, 2002.

Hajjar, IM, Grim, CE, and Kotchen, TA: Dietary calcium lowers the age-related rise in blood pressure in the United States: the NHANES III survey. J Clin Hypertens 5:122, 2003.

Hajjar, I, and Kotchen, TA: Trends in prevalence, awareness, treatment, and control of hypertension in the United States, 1988–2000. JAMA 290:199, 2003.

He, K, et al: Fish consumption and the risk of stroke in men. JAMA 288:3230, 2002.

Hecker, KD: Effects of dietary animal and soy protein on cardiovascular disease risk factors. Curr Atheroscler Rep 3:471, 2001.

Hofman, PL, Jackson, WE, and Knight, DB: Premature birth and later insulin resistance. N Engl J Med 351:2179, 2004.

Horowitz, CR, Rein, SB, and Leventhal, H: A story of maladies, misconceptions and mishaps: effective management of heart failure. Soc Sci Med 58:631, 2004.

Hu, FB, et al: Fish and omega-3 fatty acid intake and risk of coronary heart disease in women. JAMA 287:1815, 2002.

Homocysteine Studies Collaboration: Homocysteine and risk of ischemic heart disease and stroke. JAMA 288:2015, 2002.

Hughes, C, and Kostka, P: Chronic congestive heart failure. In Shils, ME, et al (eds): Modern Nutrition in Health and Disease, ed 9. Lippincott Williams & Wilkins, Philadelphia, 1999.

Huxley, RR, and Neil, HA: The relation between dietary flavonol intake and coronary heart disease mortality: A meta-analysis of prospective cohort studies. Eur J Clin Nutr 57:904, 2003.

Hyperlipidemia. Kleinman, RE (ed): Pediatric Nutrition Handbook, ed 5. American Academy of Pediatrics, Elk Grove Village, IL, 2004.

Iso, H, et al: Alcohol consumption and risk of stroke among middle-aged men: The JPHC Study Cohort I. Stroke 35:1124, 2004.

Jacques, PF, et al: The effect of folic acid fortification on plasma folate and total homocysteine concentrations. N Engl J Med 340:1449, 1999.

James, JE: Critical review of dietary caffeine and blood pressure: A relationship that should be taken more seriously. Psychosom Med 66:63, 2004.

Jee, SH, et al: Coffee consumption and serum lipids: A meta-analysis of randomized controlled clinical trials. Am J Epidemiol 153:353, 2001.

Jenkins, DJ, et al: Effect of a very-high-fiber vegetable, fruit, and nut diet on serum lipids and colonic function. Metabolism 50:494, 2001.

Kenchaiah, S, et al: Obesity and the risk of heart failure. N Engl J Med 347:305, 2002.

Klatsky, AL: Alcohol and cardiovascular disease—more than one paradox to consider. Alcohol and hypertension: does it matter? Yes. J Cardiovasc Risk 10:21, 2003.

Klatsky, AL, et al: Wine, liquor, beer, and mortality. Am J Epidemiol 158:585, 2003.

Klipstein-Grosbusch, K, et al: Dietary iron and risk of myocardial infarction in the Rotterdam Study. Am J Epidemiol 149:421, 1999.

Klor, HU, et al: Nutrition and cardiovascular disease. Eur J Med Res 2:243, 1997.

Kol, A, and Santini, M: Infectious agents and atherosclerosis: current perspectives and unsolved issues. Ital Heart J 5:350, 2004.

Korch, GC: Sodium content of potable water: Dietary significance. J Am Diet Assoc 86:80, 1986.

Kotchen, TA, and Kotchen, JM: Nutrition, diet, and hypertension. In Shils, ME, et al (eds): Modern Nutrition in Health and Disease, ed 9. Lippincott Williams & Wilkins, Philadelphia, 1999.

Kratz, M, et al: Effects of dietary fatty acids on the composition and oxidizability of low-density lipoprotein. Eur J Clin Nutr 56:72, 2002.

Krauss, RM, et al: AHA dietary guidelines. Circulation 102:2284, 2000.

Kris-Etherton, PM, Harris, WS, and Appel, LJ: Fish consumption, fish oil, omega-3 fatty acids, and cardiovascular disease. Circulation 106:2747, 2002.

Lanfear, DE, et al: Genotypes associated with myocardial infarction risk are more common in African Americans than in European Americans. J Am Coll Cardiol 44:165, 2004.

Langley-Evans, SC: Fetal programming of cardiovascular function through exposure to maternal undernutrition. Proc Nutr Soc 60:505, 2001.

Lee, MH, Lu, K, and Patel, SB: Genetic basis of sitosterolemia. Curr Opin Lipidol 12:141, 2001.

Leone, A: Relationship between cigarette smoking and other coronary risk factors in atherosclerosis: Risk of cardiovascular disease and preventive measures. Curr Pharm Des 9:2417, 2003.

Levy, AP, et al: The effect of vitamin therapy on the progression of coronary artery atherosclerosis varies by haptoglobin type in postmenopausal women. Diabetes Care 27:925, 2004.

Lichtman, JH, et al: Risk and predictors of stroke after myocardial infarction among the elderly: Results from the Cooperative Cardiovascular Project. Circulation 105:1082, 2002.

Liu, S, et al: Is intake of breakfast cereals related to total and cause-specific mortality in men? Am J Clin Nutr 77:594, 2003.

Liu, S, et al: Whole grain consumption and risk of ischemic stroke in women: A prospective study. JAMA 284:1534, 2000.

Lloyd-Jones, DM: The risk of congestive heart failure: sobering lessons from the Framingham Heart Study. Curr Cardiol Rep 3:184, 2001.

Love, JA, and Prusa, KJ: Nutrient composition and sensory attributes of cooked ground beef: Effects of fat content, cooking method, and water rinsing. J Am Diet Assoc 92:1367, 1992.

Mayo Clinic Staff: Margarine vs. butter: Which is better for your heart? Accessed September 16, 2004 at http://www.mayoclinic.com/invoke.cfm?objectid=657E562B-7D04-4708-AAA6CAE9EB2CB068.

McGill, HC, et al: Effects of nonlipid risk factors on atherosclerosis in youth with a favorable lipoprotein level. Circulation 103:1546, 2001.

Moorhead, S, Johnson, M, and Maas, M (eds): Nursing Outcomes Classification (NOC), ed 3. Mosby, St. Louis, 2004.

Morris, CD, and Carson, S: Routine vitamin supplementation to prevent cardiovascular disease: A summary of the evidence for the U.S. Preventive Services Task Force. Ann Intern Med 139:56, 2003.

Mukamal, KJ, et al: Roles of drinking pattern and type of alcohol consumed in coronary heart disease in men. N Engl J Med 348:109, 2003.

NANDA International: Nursing Diagnoses: Definitions and Classification, 2003–2004. NANDA International, Philadelphia, 2003.

Natali, A, and Ferrannini, E: Hypertension, insulin resistance, and the metabolic syndrome. Endocrinol Metab Clin North Am 33:417, 2004.

National High Blood Pressure Education Program Working Group on High Blood Pressure in Children and Adolescents. Fourth report on the diagnosis, evaluation, and treatment of high blood pressure in children and adolescents. Pediatrics 114: 555, 2004. Accessed September 8, 2004 at http://pediatrics.appublications.org/cgi/content/full/114/2/S2/555.

National Institutes of Health. The DASH diet. Press Release, April 3, 1997. Accessed May 30, 2000 at http://www.nih.gov/news/pr/apr97/Dash.htm.

Nissen, SE, et al: Effect of recombinant ApoA-I Milano on coronary atherosclerosis in patients with acute coronary syndromes: a randomized controlled trial. JAMA 290:2292, 2003.

Nygard, O, et al: Plasma homocysteine levels and mortality in patients with coronary artery disease. N Engl J Med 337:230, 1997.

Oncken, CA, et al: Impact of smoking cessation on ambulatory blood pressure and heart rate in postmenopausal women. Am J Hypertens 14:942, 2001.

Park, YW, et al: The metabolic syndrome: prevalence and associated risk factor findings in the U.S. population from the Third National Health and Nutrition Examination Survey, 1988–1994. Arch Intern Med 163:427, 2003.

Ranheim, T, and Halvorsen, B: Coffee consumption and human health—beneficial or detrimental?—Mechanisms for effects of coffee consumption on different risk factors for cardiovascular disease and type 2 diabetes mellitus. Mol Nutr Food Res 49:274, 2005.

Refsum, H, et al: Facts and recommendations about total homocysteine determinations: An expert opinion. Clin Chem 50:3, 2004.

Renaud, S, and Gueguen, R: The French paradox and wine drinking. Novartis Found Symp 216:208, 1998.

Richelle, M, et al: Both free and esterified plant sterols reduce cholesterol absorption and the bioavailability of beta-carotene and alpha-tocopherol in normocholesterolemic humans. Am J Clin Nutr 80:171, 2004.

Russell, RM, and Suter, PM: Nutrition and blood pressure. Cyberounds Continuing Medical Education, 2001. Accessed August 10, 2004 at http://www.cyberounds.com/conferences/nutrition/conferences/current/conference.html.

Salonen, JT, et al: High stored iron levels are associated with excess risk of myocardial infarction in Eastern Finnish men. Circulation 86:803, 1992.

Scanlon, VC, and Sanders T: Essentials of Anatomy and Physiology, ed 4. FA Davis, Philadelphia, 2003.

Schnell, ZB, Van Leeuwen, AM, and Kranpitz, TR: Davis's Comprehensive Handbook of Laboratory and Diagnostic Tests with Nursing Implications. Philadelphia, FA Davis, 2003.

Schnyder, G, et al: Effect of homocysteine-lowering therapy with folic acid, vitamin B_{12}, and vitamin B_6 on clinical outcome after percutaneous coronary intervention. JAMA 288:973, 2002.

Schoppet, M, and Maisch, B: Alcohol and the heart. Herz 26:345, 2001.

Scott, CL: Diagnosis, prevention, and intervention for the metabolic syndrome. Am J Cardiol 92:35i, 2003.

Schwammenthal, Y, and Tanne, D: Homocysteine, B-vitamin supplementation, and stroke prevention: From observational to interventional trials. Lancet Neurol 3:493, 2004.

Selhub, J, and D'Angelo, A: Hyperhomocysteinemia and thrombosis: Acquired conditions. Thromb Haemost 78:527, 1997.

Serra-Majem, L, et al: How could changes in diet explain changes in coronary heart disease mortality in Spain? The Spanish paradox. Am J Clin Nutr 61(Suppl):1351S, 1995.

Sharma, AM: Obesity and cardiovascular risk. Growth Horm IGF Res 13:S10, 2003.

Sirtori, CR, and Lovati, MR: Soy proteins and cardiovascular disease. Curr Atheroscler Rep 3:47, 2001.

Small, KM, et al: Synergistic polymorphisms of B_1- and α_{2C}-adrenergic receptors and the risk of congestive heart failure. N Engl J Med 347:1135, 2002.

Spencer, AP, Carson, DS, and Crouch, MA: Vitamin E and coronary artery disease. Arch Intern Med 159:1313, 1999.

Sperling, MA: Prematurity—a window of opportunity? N Engl J Med 351:2229, 2004.

Stanger, O, et al: Clinical use and rational management of homocysteine, folic acid, and B vitamins in cardiovascular and thrombotic diseases. Z Kardiol 93:439, 2004.

Steefel, L: Race against time. Nurs Spectrum (Midwest) 5(1):8, 2004.

Stranges, S, et al: Relationship of alcohol drinking pattern to risk of hypertension: a population-based study. Hypertension 44:813, 2004.

Suter, PM, Sierro, C, and Vetter, W: Nutritional factors in the control of blood pressure and hypertension. Nutr Clin Care 5:9, 2002.

Tanasescu, M, et al: Exercise type and intensity in relation to coronary heart disease in men. JAMA 288:1994, 2002.

Tanne, et al: Elevated homocysteine in heart patients linked with higher stroke risk. Stroke 34 February 21. Rapid access issue, 2003. Accessed August 16, 2004 at http://www.americanheart.org/presenter.jhtml?identifier=3008854.

Thies, F, et al: Association of n-3 polyunsaturated fatty acids with stability of atherosclerotic plaques: A randomized controlled trial. Lancet 361:477, 2003.

Thomson, CC, and Rigotti, NA: Hospital- and clinic-based smoking cessation interventions for smokers with cardiovascular disease. Prog Cardiovasc Dis 45:459, 2003.

Toole, JF, et al: Lowering homocysteine in patients with ischemic stroke to prevent recurrent stroke, myocardial infarction, and death. JAMA 291:565, 2004.

Touyz, RM: Role of magnesium in the pathogenesis of hypertension. Mol Aspects Med 24:107, 2003.

Tuomainen, TP, et al: Association between body iron stores and the risk of acute myocardial infarction in men. Circulation 97:1461, 1998.

Tzonou, A, et al: Dietary iron and coronary heart disease risk: A study from Greece. Am J Epidemiol 147:161, 1998.

United States Department of Health and Human Services: The Seventh Report of the Joint National Committee on Prevention, Detection, Evaluation, and Treatment of High Blood Pressure. National Institutes of Health. Washington, DC, 2003. Accessed August 10, 2004 at http://www.nhlbi.nih.gov/guidelines/hypertension/express.pdf.

United States Food and Drug Administration: FDA allows foods containing psyllium to make health claim on reducing risk of heart disease. United States Department of Health and Human Services, Rockville, MD, February 17, 1998. Accessed May 18, 2005 at http://www.fda.gov/bbs/topics/ANSWERS/ ANS00850.html.

United States Food and Drug Administration: FDA announces qualified health claims for omega-3 fatty acids. United States Department of Health and Human Services, Rockville, MD, September 8, 2004. Accessed May 17, 2005 at http://www.fda.gov/bbs/topics/news/2004/NEW01115.html.

United States Food and Drug Administration: FDA approves new health claim for soy protein and coronary heart disease. United States Department of Health and Human Services, Rockville, MD, October 20, 1999. Accessed September 14, 2004 at http://www.fda.gov/bbs/topics/ANSWERS/ANS00980.html.

United States Food and Drug Administration: Food labeling; *trans* fatty acids in nutrition labeling. Federal Register 68:41433, 2003. Accessed May 16, 2005 at http://www.cfsan.fda.gov/~lrd/fr03711a.html.

United States Preventive Services Task Force: Vitamin supplementation to prevent cancer and cardiovascular disease. United States Department of Health and Human Services, Rockville, MD, 2003. Accessed September 2, 2004 at http://www.ahrq.gov/clinic/uspstf/uspsvita.htm.

Vasan, RS, et al: Plasma homocysteine and risk for congestive heart failure in adults without prior myocardial infarction. JAMA 289:1251, 2003.

Vivekananthan, DP, et al: Use of antioxidant vitamins for the prevention of cardiovascular disease: Meta-analysis of randomized trials. Lancet 361:2017, 2003.

Vollset, SE, et al: Plasma total homocysteine and cardiovascular and noncardiovascular mortality: The Hordaland Homocysteine Study. Am J Clin Nutr 74:130, 2001.

Wald, DS, Law, M, and Morris, JK: Homocysteine and cardiovascular disease: Evidence on causality from a meta-analysis. BMJ 325:1202, 2002.

Waldman, A, et al: Homocysteine and cobalamin status in German vegans. Public Health Nutr 7:467, 2004.

Whelton, PK, and He, J: Potassium in preventing and treating high blood pressure. Semin Nephrol 19:494, 1999.

Xin, X, et al: Effects of alcohol reduction on blood pressure: a meta-analysis of randomized controlled trials. Hypertension 38:1112, 2001.

Diet in Renal Disease

After completing this chapter, the student should be able to:

1. Identify the major causes of acute and chronic kidney failure.
2. List the goals of nutritional care for a client with kidney disease.
3. List the nutrients commonly modified in the dietary treatment of kidney disease.
4. Discuss the relationship among kilocaloric intake, dietary protein utilization, and uremia.
5. Discuss the nutritional care of clients with kidney disease in relation to their medical treatment.

Diet therapy for clients with kidney disease depends on an understanding of the normal function of the kidneys and basic concepts of pathophysiology of renal diseases. (**Renal** means pertaining to the kidneys.) The nutritional care of clients with renal disease is complex. These clients frequently must learn not just one diet in which one to seven nutrients are controlled but several different diets as their medical condition and the treatment approach change. The failure to adhere to necessary diet changes can result in death. One aspect of working with clients with renal disease is that inattentiveness to dietary restrictions can be measured objectively in weight changes or changes in blood chemistry.

This first part of this chapter discusses the internal structure and functions of the kidneys. Common kidney diseases, major forms of treatment available for clients, and the dietary treatment for renal disease are then presented. A brief discussion of urinary calculi and urinary tract infections concludes the chapter.

Anatomy and Physiology of the Kidneys

Internal Structure

The functioning unit of the kidney is the **nephron.** Each kidney contains about a million nephrons. Figure 21–1 shows an individual nephron. Each nephron has two main parts. The first part, **Bowman's capsule,** is the cup-shaped top of the nephron. Inside Bowman's capsule is a network of blood capillaries called the **glomerulus** (plural, *glomeruli*). The second part of the nephron is the **renal tubule.** (A **tubule** is a small tube or canal.) The renal tubule is the rope-like portion of the nephron. This rope-like structure ends at the collecting tubule. Several nephrons usually share a single **collecting tubule.**

Functions

The kidneys assist in the internal regulation of the body by performing the following functions:

1. *Filtration:* The kidneys remove the end products of metabolism and substances that have accumulated in the blood in undesirable amounts during the **filtration** process. Substances removed from the blood include urea, creatinine, uric acid, and urates. Undesirable amounts of chloride, potassium, sodium, and hydrogen ions are also filtered from the blood. The **glomerular filtration rate (GFR)** is the amount of fluid filtered each minute by all the glomeruli of both kidneys and is one index of kidney function. This is normally about 125 milliliters per minute (Fig. 21–2).
2. *Reabsorption:* Previously filtered substances (e.g., water and sodium) needed by the body are reabsorbed into the blood in the tubules.
3. *Secretion of Ions to Maintain Acid-Base Balance:* Secretion is the process of moving ions from the blood into the urine. Secretion allows for the amount of a particular substance to be excreted in the urine in concentrations greater than the concentration filtered from the plasma in the glomeruli. The kidneys regulate the balance between bicarbonate and carbonic acid by the secretion and exchange of hydrogen ions for sodium ions, which are used to form the base.
4. *Excretion:* The kidneys eliminate unwanted substances from the body as urine.
5. *Renal Control of Cardiac Output and Systemic Blood Pressure:* The kidneys adapt to changing cardiac output

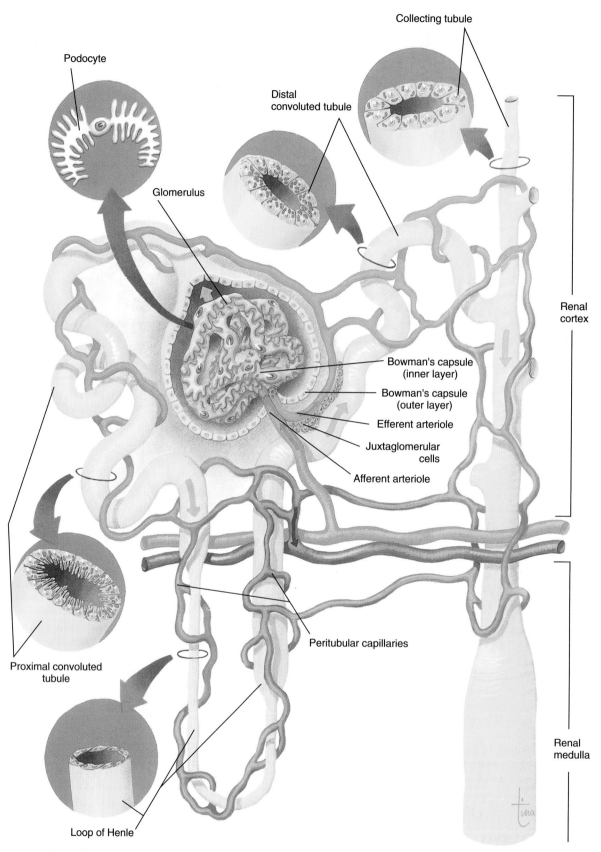

Podocyte

Glomerulus

Distal
convoluted tubule

Collecting tubule

Bowman's capsule
(inner layer)

Bowman's capsule
(outer layer)

Efferent arteriole

Juxtaglomerular
cells

Afferent arteriole

Renal
cortex

Peritubular capillaries

Proximal convoluted
tubule

Loop of Henle

Renal
medulla

Figure 21–1   A nephron with its associated blood vessels. The arrows indicate the direction of blood flow. (Reprinted from Scanlon, VC, and Sanders, T: Essentials of Anatomy and Physiology, ed 4. FA Davis, Philadelphia, 2003, with permission.)

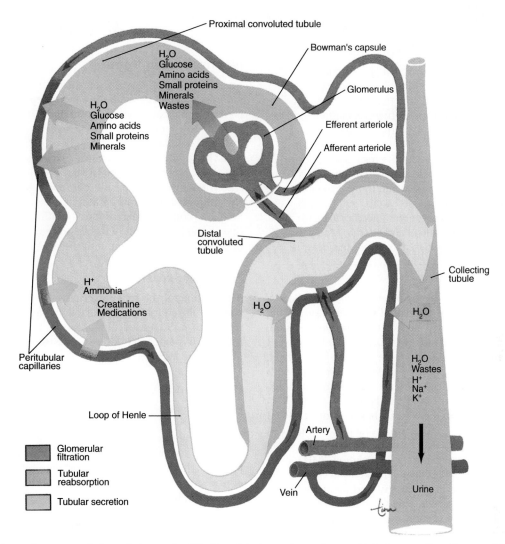

Figure **21–2** Schematic representation of glomerular filtration, tubular reabsorption, and tubular secretion. The renal tubule has been uncoiled, and the peritubular capillaries are shown adjacent to the tubule. (Reprinted from Scanlon, VC, and Sanders, T: Essentials of Anatomy and Physiology, ed 4. FA Davis, Philadelphia, 2003, with permission.)

by altering resistance to blood flow both at the beginning of the glomerulus and at the end.

6. *Calcium, Phosphorus, and Vitamin D:* The kidneys produce the active form of vitamin D, **calcitriol.** Activated vitamin D regulates the absorption of calcium and phosphorus from the intestinal tract and assists in the regulation of calcium and phosphorus levels in the blood.

7. *Erythropoietin:* The kidneys produce a hormone called **erythropoietin,** which stimulates maturation of red blood cells in bone marrow.

Kidney Disease

Because the kidneys perform so many different metabolic functions, kidney disease has serious consequences. This section of the text discusses the causes of kidney disease and describes several common kidney disorders.

Causes

Renal disease can be caused by many factors, including trauma, infections, birth defects, medications, chronic disease (e.g., atherosclerosis, diabetes, hypertension), and toxic metal consumption. Diabetic nephropathy is the most common cause of renal failure. A physiological stress such as a myocardial infarction or an extensive burn can precipitate renal disease by decreasing the perfusion of the kidney or markedly increasing catabolism. Clinical Application 21–1, which describes the renal response after myocardial infarction, describes the effect of reduced renal blood flow. Catabolism causes an increase in nitrogenous products and potassium; these must be excreted, thus overworking the kidneys. Renal disease is a feared complication of many pathologies and treatments, including radiocontrast materials used in diagnostic procedures, some antibiotics, and some pain medications.

Renal Response After a Myocardial Infarction

Immediately after a heart attack or MI, blood flow through the systemic circulation is diminished. Systemic circulation refers to the blood flow from the left part of the heart through the aorta and all branches (arteries) to the capillaries of the tissues. Systemic circulation also includes the blood's return to the heart through the veins. After a heart attack, blood flow to the myocardium, or heart muscle, is decreased and myocardial function is impaired. Less blood is thus delivered to the tissues. The kidneys sense the decreased cardiac output and try to compensate by reabsorption of additional water. This may lead to a fluid overload and edema. Most clients after a MI are on fluid restriction for this reason.

Obesity, poorly controlled diabetes, hypertension, and a high-protein diet increase the risk of renal disease. Losing weight reduces the severity of diabetes and hypertension, the two leading causes of kidney failure, and helps prevent those conditions in people who have not developed them. Normalization of blood glucose and lipid levels along with blood pressure control also decrease the risk of renal disease. The Diabetes Control and Complications Trail (DCCT) and United Kingdom Prospective Diabetes Study (UKPDS) have definitively shown that intensive diabetes therapy can significantly reduce the risk of overt nephropathy in people with diabetes (American Diabetes Association, 2004). Both systolic and diastolic hypertension markedly accelerate the progression of diabetic nephropathy, and aggressive anti-hypertension management is able to greatly decrease the rate of fall of GFR. There is some evidence that a habitually high intake of dietary protein (greater than 1.6 g/kg body weight) can cause kidney damage. These are among the reasons that all clients should be encouraged to follow the diets prescribed for them and faithfully take prescribed medications.

Glomerulonephritis

A general term for an inflammation of the kidneys is **nephritis.** This is the most common type of kidney disease. Inflammation of the glomeruli is called **glomerulonephritis,** which can be either acute or chronic. This condition often follows scarlet fever or a streptococcal infection of the respiratory tract. Young children and young adults are often victims. Symptoms include nausea, vomiting, fever, hypertension, blood in the urine (**hematuria**), a decreased output of urine (**oliguria**), protein in the urine (**proteinuria**), and edema. Recovery is usually complete. However, in some clients the disease progresses and becomes chronic. This leads to a progressive loss of kidney function. Some clients develop **anuria,** which is a total lack of urine output. Without treatment, this condition is fatal.

Specific Tubular Abnormalities

A structural problem in the renal tubules may result in abnormal reabsorption or lack of reabsorption of certain substances by the tubules. The effect of a tubular abnormality is that the blood is not effectively cleansed.

Nephrotic Syndrome

The result of a variety of diseases that damage the glomeruli capillary walls is called **nephrotic syndrome.** Signs of nephrotic syndrome include proteinuria, severe edema, low serum protein levels, anemia, and hyperlipoproteinemia. Usually the higher the hyperlipoproteinemia, the greater the proteinuria. The disease is caused by the degenerative changes in the kidneys' capillary walls, which consequently permit the passage of albumin into the **glomerular filtrate.** Water and sodium are retained. Edema is sometimes so severe that it masks tissue wasting due to the breakdown of tissue protein stores. The degree of malnutrition is hidden until the excess fluid is removed.

Nephrosclerosis

A hardening of the renal arteries is known as **nephrosclerosis.** This condition is caused by arteriosclerosis and results in a decreased blood supply to the kidneys. This leads to **hypertensive kidney disease** and can eventually destroy the kidney.

Progressive Nature of Kidney Failure

Kidney disease can be acute or chronic. The earliest clinical evidence of nephropathy is the appearance of low but abnormal levels (≥ 30 mg/day or 20 µg/min) of albumin in the urine, referred to as **microalbuminuria.** In **acute renal failure,** the kidneys stop working entirely or almost entirely. Acute renal failure occurs suddenly and is usually temporary. It can last for a few days or weeks.

Chronic renal failure occurs when progressively more nephrons are destroyed until the kidneys simply cannot perform vital functions. Chronic renal failure occurs over time and is usually irreversible.

As individual nephrons are damaged, the remaining nephrons work harder to maintain metabolic homeostasis. As each functional nephron's workload is increased, the nephron becomes more susceptible to work overload and damage. The normal composition of the blood is altered when the remaining functional nephrons cannot assume any additional workload. Serum levels of **blood urea nitrogen (BUN), creatinine,** and uric acid become elevated. In some clients, even though the underlying condition (e.g., diabetes mellitus, hypertension) is treated, chronic renal disease may lead to **end-stage renal failure.** During end-stage renal failure, most or all of the kidneys' ability to produce urine and regulate blood chemistries is severely compromised.

Often, the first sign of chronic renal failure is sodium depletion. This occurs when the kidneys lose their ability to reabsorb sodium in the tubule. Symptoms associated with sodium depletion include a reduction of renal blood flow, dehydration, lethargy, decreased glomerular filtration rate (GFR), uremia (see next section), and client deterioration. The client's blood pressure and body weight drop. Urine volume may be increased initially in chronic renal failure. A loss of body fat and protein content is responsible for the weight loss. The client's serum albumin level may fall as protein is lost in the urine.

As kidney function further deteriorates, some of these symptoms reverse. The kidneys lose the ability to excrete sodium. When this occurs, symptoms include sodium retention, overhydration, edema, hypertension, and CHF. The body can excrete little or no urine.

The GFR gradually declines in chronic renal failure. Chronic kidney disease has been formally classified into five stages based on the GFR. Stage 1 has been described as kidney damage with normal or increased GFR of ≥90. Stage 2 is kidney damage with mild decreased GFR of 60 to 89. Stage 3 is a moderate decreased GFR of 30 to 59, and Stage 4 is a severe decreased GFR of 15 to 29. Stage 5 is kidney failure with a GFR <15 (National Kidney Foundation, 2002). Most clients with a GFR below 25 milliliters per minute will eventually require either dialysis or transplantation, regardless of the original cause of failure. Stages 1 through 4 represent kidney damage categories where medical and nutritional management can impact and potentially delay progression to Stage 5 (Beto and Bansal, 2004).

If these measures were not implemented, **uremia** would develop. Uremia is the name given to the toxic condition associated with renal insufficiency. Uremia is produced by the retention in the blood of nitrogenous substances normally excreted by the kidneys. The uremic client manifests many symptoms in virtually every body system as toxic waste products build up in the blood. The client may complain of fatigue, weakness, and decreased mental ability. The client's muscles may twitch and cramp. Anorexia, nausea, vomiting, and **stomatitis,** an inflammation of the mouth, may be present. Sometimes clients complain of an unpleasant taste in the mouth. To further complicate matters, gastrointestinal ulcers and bleeding are common. All of these symptoms have a direct effect on the client's willingness to eat.

Health-care professionals have known for many decades that clients with chronic renal disease who have sustained a loss of GFR often continue to lose renal function until they develop terminal renal failure. Much research is ongoing to find a way to halt the progression of chronic renal failure. A high-protein diet, a high-phosphorus diet, a high-fat or high-cholesterol diet, a high vitamin C intake, glycemic control, and a vitamin D overdose are among the nutrition-related causes of progressive renal failure. Protein restriction and phosphate lowering may have benefits in selected patients (American Diabetes Association, 2004). For this reason, dietary intervention is now instituted simultaneously with the initial diagnosis. Aggressive antihypertensive treatment and the use of ACE inhibitors will slow the rate of progression of nephropathy (American Diabetes Association, 2004).

Treatment of Renal Disease

Renal functions cannot be assumed by another organ. There is no cure for chronic renal failure. However, many clients can be treated with dialysis (an artificial kidney) and/or a kidney transplant. Artificial kidneys have been used for about 45 years to treat clients with severe kidney failure.

Dialysis

Dialysis means the passage of solutes through a membrane. Two functions of the kidneys are (1) the removal of waste products and (2) the regulation of fluid and electrolyte balance. By removing waste products from the blood and assisting in the maintenance of fluid balance, dialysis reduces the symptoms of uremia, hypertension, and edema and the risk of CHF. Dialysis is usually started when the client develops symptoms of severe fluid overload, high potassium levels, acidosis, or symptoms of uremia. Dialysis cannot restore the lost hormonal functions of the kidney. In addition, dialysis cannot correct the anemia that occurs because of a lack of erythropoietin. Some dialysis clients still need treatment for hypertension.

Hemodialysis

During **hemodialysis,** blood is removed from the client's artery through a tube, is forced to flow over a semipermeable membrane where waste is removed, and then is rerouted back into the client's body through a vein. Before dialysis can be initiated, an access site that allows blood to be removed from the body and replaced back into the body at the time of dialysis must be surgically created. Figure 21–3 illustrates a client undergoing a hemodialysis treatment. A solution called the **dialysate** is placed on one side of the semipermeable membrane, and the client's blood flows on the other side. The dialysate is similar in composition to normal blood plasma. The client's blood has a higher concentration of urea and electrolytes than the dialysate has, so these substances diffuse from the blood into the dialysate. The dialysate also contains glucose, and the more glucose the dialysate contains, the more fluid will move from the blood into the dialysate by osmosis. This process pulls extra fluid from the blood. The composition of the dialysate varies according to the requirements of each client.

Hemodialysis treatments usually last 3 to 5 hours and are administered three times per week. Some clients are taught to perform their own dialysis treatments at home. Dialysis is not as effective as normal kidney function because blood cleansing occurs only when clients are attached to artificial kidneys. Normal kidneys clear the blood 24 hours a day, 7 days a week.

Peritoneal Dialysis

The **peritoneum** is the lining of the abdominal cavity. During **peritoneal dialysis,** the dialysate is placed directly into the client's abdomen. The dialysate enters the body through a permanent catheter placed in the abdominal cavity. The peritoneum thus functions as the semipermeable membrane.

INTERMITTENT PERITONEAL DIALYSIS

Between 1 and 2 liters of fluid are introduced into the abdominal cavity during **intermittent peritoneal dialysis.** The fluid is allowed to remain in the abdomen for about 30 minutes and then is drained from the body by gravity. One complete exchange takes about an hour. This process is repeated until the blood urea nitrogen level drops.

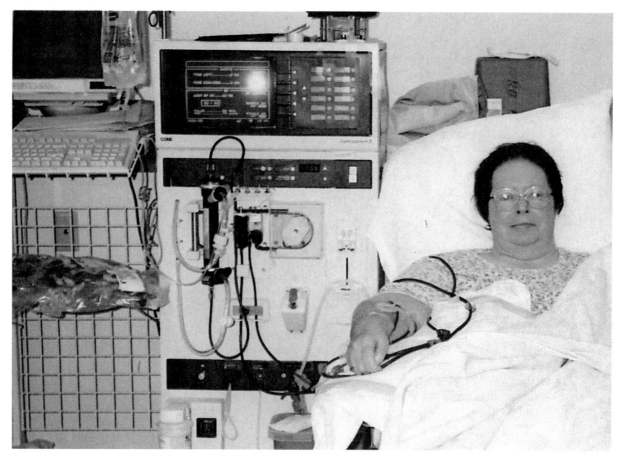

Figure **21–3** Client undergoing hemodialysis at dialysis center.

CONTINUOUS AMBULATORY PERITONEAL DIALYSIS

Continuous ambulatory peritoneal dialysis (CAPD) is one dialysis method chosen by many clients. One study showed that patients receiving peritoneal dialysis rate care higher than those receiving hemodialysis (Rubin et al, 2004). This is a form of self-dialysis. About 1 liter of dialysate is introduced into the abdominal cavity. The fluid remains in the cavity for 4 to 6 hours while the waste products diffuse into the dialysate. The dialysate is then replaced with a new solution. Clients can move about and pursue their activities of daily living during CAPD. The term *continuous* means that the client is dialyzing constantly. The advantage of CAPD is that the client's blood levels of sodium, potassium, creatinine, and nitrogen are kept within a much more stable range. Large shifts in fluid balance are also avoided. The decision about which treatment approach is best for an individual is based on medical condition, lifestyle behaviors, and personal preference. For example, a client with poor personal hygiene would not be a good candidate for CAPD because of a high risk for infection with this approach.

Kidney Transplant

A kidney transplant can restore full renal function. Immunosuppressants to prevent rejection of the trans-planted kidney are necessary. Some commonly used immunosuppressants are azathioprine, corticosteroids, and/or cyclosporine. These medications have many side effects, including diarrhea, nausea, and vomiting, which influence nutrient intake and absorption.

Nutritional Care of the Renal Client

The nutritional needs of clients with renal diseases are changing constantly. The reason for the change is that the disease state and treatment approach are not static. Clients with kidney disease require constant assessment, monitoring, and counseling. In addition, it is an ongoing challenge to provide quality nutritional care to these clients, who frequently must be coaxed to eat. Anorexia, nausea, and vomiting are frequent complaints. It is common for the dietitian to see these clients more than once each day for nutritional problems during hospitalization. Client-nurse interactions are important because nurses can influence and hopefully enhance patient adherence to prescribed diets. One study showed that 81.4% of hemodialysis patients have difficulty following diet modifications and 74.6% fluid restrictions (Kugler, Vlaminck, and Haverich, 2005). Close communication among all members of the health care team is vital to meeting the dynamic nutritional needs of these clients.

Malnutrition

Malnutrition in hemodialysis clients is associated with increased morality and morbidity. One study cited moderate to severe malnutrition in 34 percent of study participants (Kuhlmann et al, 1997). Among the reasons for the malnutrition are increased catabolism, metabolic derangement, decreased food intake, and low economic status. Oral supplements, tube feedings, intravenous feedings, and intra-dialytic parenteral nutrition have all been used to treat the protein-energy malnutrition seen in these clients. **Intra-dialytic** parenteral nutrition involves the administration of lipids, glucose, and amino acids into the peritoneal cavity.

Goals of Nutrition Therapy

Well-planned nutritional management is a fundamental part of any treatment plan for renal disease. Every client with renal disease requires an individualized diet based on the following goals:

1. Attain and maintain optimal nutritional status
2. Prevent net protein catabolism
3. Minimize uremic toxicity
4. Maintain adequate hydration status
5. Maintain normal serum potassium levels
6. Control the progression of renal osteodystrophy (discussed later)
7. Modify diet to meet other nutrition-related concern, such as diabetes, heart disease, gastrointestinal tract ulcers, and constipation
8. Retard the progression of renal failure and postpone the initiation of dialysis

No single diet is appropriate for all renal clients. Every client requires an individual assessment.

Dietary Components

Several basic components need to be monitored and, if possible, controlled in renal diets. These components are:

- Kilocalories
- Protein
- Sodium
- Potassium
- Phosphorus and calcium
- Fluid
- Saturated fat and cholesterol
- Iron, vitamins, and minerals

The need to restrict or encourage the consumption of any of these nutrients changes according to the client's medical status and treatment approach. For example, it may not be necessary for a client to control his or her phosphorus intake at one time, but it may be vital at another time.

Kilocalories

The intake of kilocalories is often increases for clients with renal disease. Clients on high-kilocalorie diets are usually given all the simple carbohydrates and monounsaturated and polyunsaturated fats they will eat. *Trans*-fats are minimized. The end products of fat and carbohydrate catabolism are carbon dioxide and water. Neither of these dietary constituents imposes a burden on the client's compromised excretory ability. Inadequate nonprotein kilocalories, however, will encourage tissue breakdown and aggravate the uremia. Clients with renal insufficiency need 35 to 40 kcal/kg per day. The use of a specialized oral supplement such as *ReNeph LP/HC* (LP = low protein; HC = high kilocalorie) by Ross Laboratories is one example of an appropriate oral supplement for clients who are unwilling to eat enough food. An adequate intake of kilocalories is crucial to the success of the dietary treatment.

Some individuals with diabetes mellitus and renal diseases still need to have their blood sugar levels controlled. For these clients, it may or may not be advisable to increase simple carbohydrates. The need to control their blood sugar is sometimes a secondary concern. In some cases, the primary nutritional goal is to decrease the uremia. Uremic diabetic clients may have relatively high amounts of sugar planned in their diets.

Some renal clients require an alternate feeding route to attain and maintain optimal nutritional status. Accordingly, some physicians order a peripheral intravenous infusion of lipids to supplement oral feedings. Total parenteral nutrition solutions for renal clients are commercially available.

Protein

A primary goal of nutritional therapy in renal clients is control of nitrogen intake. Control may mean an increase or decrease of dietary protein as the client's medical condition and treatment approach change. In addition, the kind of protein fed to the client may be important. Some physicians prescribe a diet of high-biological-value protein when the client has an extremely high BUN level. Eggs, meat, and dairy products are examples of foods that contain protein of high biologic value because animal products contain all the essential amino acids.

The benefits of a vegetarian diet for patients with renal failure have proven useful. Studies using human and animal models suggest that some plant proteins may increase survival rates and decrease proteinuria, glomerular filtration rate, renal blood flow, and histologic renal damage compared with nonvegetarian diets (American Dietetic Association, 1997). Vegetarian diets by nature are higher in potassium and phosphorus because of all the vegetables, whole grains, and fruits they contain. The goal is to eat the right combination of plant proteins while keeping potassium and phosphorus under control. A referral to a renal dietitian is indicated for these patients. Protein restrictions are effective only if the client also consumes adequate kilocalories. Beginning renal insufficiency is usually referred to as a predialysis situation and requires a restriction or modification of protein intake. Some physicians believe it is more difficult to clinically raise a depressed albumin than to clear the blood of the toxic end products of protein metabolism through dialysis. Because of the danger of tissue catabolism, a diet that provides less than 40 grams of protein per day is rarely indicated.

The treatment approach selected by the client and the physician influences protein requirements. Hemodialysis clients sometimes need increased protein because hemodialysis results in a loss of 1 to 2 grams of amino acids per hour of dialysis. A client on CAPD has an even higher protein need because he or she dialyzes continuously. During dialysis, protein passes out of the blood with the waste products and into the dialysate fluid. When the dialysate fluid is discarded, a significant amount of protein is lost from the body. A high-protein diet is necessary to replenish these losses.

Sodium

The desirable sodium intake for renal clients depends on individual circumstances and is usually determined by repeated measurements of sodium in the serum and in the urine (if any). Most clients require between 1 and 3 grams of sodium per day. The sodium intake of many clients with renal failure must be restricted to prevent sodium retention in the body with consequent generalized edema.

The disease that precipitated the renal failure plays a role in determining the need for a sodium restriction. Because glomerulonephritis, for example, is more likely to produce hypertension and fluid retention, sodium restriction is often necessary. Low levels of sodium, absence of edema, and normal or low blood pressure often characterize other renal diseases, such as pyelonephritis. **Pyelonephritis** is an inflammation of the central portion of the kidney. In this situation, sodium intake can be higher than in the other groups of diseases but is individualized to the client's needs.

Potassium

Dietary potassium, like sodium, needs to be evaluated on an individual basis. **Hypokalemia** (low blood potassium level) needs to be avoided because it introduces the danger of cardiac arrhythmias and eventually cardiac arrest. Boxes 21–1 and 21–2, respectively, list foods that are high and low in potassium. Salt substitutes are very high in potassium and should be avoided by most renal clients. It is important to recognize that a water softener may be a source of dietary potassium. The need to restrict potassium generally increases in clients with decreased urinary output.

ACE inhibitors have been shown to reduce the level of albuminuria and the rate of progression of renal disease to a greater degree than other hypertensive agents that lower blood pressure by an equal amount (American Diabetes Association, 2004). Use of ACE inhibitors may exacerbate hyperkalemia in clients with advanced renal insufficiency. If an ACE inhibitor is used, serum potassium levels should be monitored for the development of hyperkalemia. If the client's potassium level is elevated, a dietary potassium intake should be minimized. The recommended intake is 1.5 to 3.0 grams per day for most patients. In cases of anuria or when serum potassium exceeds 6.5 mEq/L, a diet intake of 20 to 25 mEq/L (about 780 to 975 mg K) is suggested. This suggestion is for the acute, critical-care patient because of its poor palpability (Inman, 1999). When urinary output is 500 to 100 cc and serum potassium is 5.5 to 6.5, a 40- to 60-mEq (about 1563 to 2345 mg K) intake is suggested. Fundamental to understanding medical nutritional therapy for clients with renal disease is that it is never appropriate to over-restrict the client's diet because of the danger of tissue catabolism and malnutrition.

The potassium content of fruits and vegetables varies according to the form in which they are eaten and the method of food preparation. For example, ½ cup of canned pears in heavy syrup has a potassium content of about 80

Box 21–1 High-Potassium Foods to Avoid

Dairy products	In excess of 2 cups per day
Meats	In excess of 6 oz per day
Starches	Bran cereals and bran products
Fruits	Avocado
	Bananas
	Orange, fresh
	Mango, fresh
	Nectarines
	Papayas
	Dried prunes
	All others if eaten in excess of allowance
Vegetables	Bamboo shoots
	Beet greens
	Baked potato, with skin
	Sweet potato fresh
	Spinach, cooked
	All others if eaten in excess of allowance
Others	Chocolate, cocoa
	Molasses
	Salt substitute
	Low-sodium broth
	Low-sodium baking powder
	Low-sodium baking soda
	Nuts

Box 21–2 Low-Potassium Foods and Beverages*

Gum drops
Hard, clear candy
Nondairy topping
Honey
Jams and jellies
Jelly beans
Lollipops
Marshmallows
Suckers
Sugar
Lifesavers
Chewing gum
Poly-Rich (nondairy creamer)
Cornstarch

Low-Potassium Beverages

Carbonated beverages
Lemonade
Limeade
Cranberry juice
Popsicles (1 stick—60 mL of fluid)
Hawaiian punch
Kool-Aid

Low-Potassium Unsweetened Beverages

Diet carbonated beverages
Diet lemonade
Diet Kool-Aid

*Note: Foods with sugar should not be eaten freely by diabetics.

milligrams, and one fresh pear has a potassium content of about 210 milligrams. Potassium is water soluble. For this reason, some renal clients on very low potassium diets are taught to use large amounts of water when preparing vegetables and to discard the water after cooking. This decreases the potassium content of the vegetables. Unfortunately, it also decreases the water-soluble vitamins in the food. This is one reason that most renal clients need vitamin supplements. Clients should be taught to eat the fruits or vegetables in the form given on the list.

Phosphorus, Vitamin D, and Calcium

Phosphorus, vitamin D, and calcium are all normally balanced in the body. In clients with kidney disease, vitamin D cannot be activated. This leads to a low serum calcium level. At the same time, the kidneys cannot excrete phosphorus. This leads to an elevated serum phosphorus level. When the serum calcium level drops, calcium is released from the bones because of the increased secretion of **parathyroid hormone (PTH).** PTH is secreted in an effort to correct the calcium imbalance. This chain of events may lead to renal **osteodystrophy,** which is a complication of chronic renal disease. **Renal osteodystrophy** leads to faulty bone formation.

Control of the blood levels of calcium and phosphorus involves three treatment approaches. First, clients with hypocalcemia and hyperphosphatemia are currently given calcitriol, the activated form of vitamin D. The second treatment approach is a dietary phosphorus restriction. Third, calcium supplements, a high-calcium diet, or both are frequently prescribed if the serum phosphorus is under control.

Phosphorus is found mainly in:

- Dairy products
- Dried beans and peas, such as kidney beans, split peas, and lentils
- Nuts and peanut butter
- Beverages such as cocoa, beer, and cola soft drinks

Clients on protein-restricted diets generally do not eat enough phosphorus to cause hyperphosphatemia. Clients on chronic renal dialysis with a more liberal protein intake may need to limit the intake of foods high in phosphorus.

Fluid

Predialysis (renal insufficiency) and dialysis clients generally must restrict fluid intake because their kidneys can no longer excrete excess fluid. Fluids need to be allocated between meals and medications. Table 21–1 lists guidelines to follow for distributing fluids between meals and medications. Clients on hemodialysis are restricted to 500 to 1000 milliliters plus 24-hour urinary output. This allows for some fluid gain between dialysis treatments. For predialysis clients, fluids are usually restricted to 500 milliliters plus output. For clients on CAPD, fluid restriction is "as tolerated" according to their daily weight fluctuations and blood pressure.

Saturated Fat and Cholesterol

Clients with renal disease frequently have hyperlipoproteinemia. High serum lipid levels increase the progression of renal disease, which contributes to an increased risk of cardiovascular disease. Total cholesterol levels may be increased up to tenfold. This is believed to be especially a problem in clients with nephrotic syndrome, diabetes, and/or an **LCAT deficiency.** LCAT is an enzyme that transports cholesterol from tissues to the liver for removal from the body. Most clients with an LCAT deficiency develop progressive glomerular injury.

Significant hypertriglyceridemia is often present in clients with a history of renal disease. The nutritional care of clients with elevated triglycerides (type 4 hyperlipoproteinemia) includes a modified fat diet and a modification of carbohydrate intake. Clients are usually counseled to avoid saturated fat and to increase their intake of polyunsaturated and monounsaturated fat. Thirty to 35 percent of the total kilocalories are provided as fat because excessive carbohydrate could worsen the hypertriglyceridemia (Moore, 1996). Simple sugars and alcohol are usually limited for the same reason.

Iron

The anemias seen in clients with renal disease may be due to a lack of erythropoietin; a decreased oral iron intake, which often occurs as a result of dietary restriction; or

---

Table 21–1 **Guidelines for Fluid-Restricted Clients**

IF THE FLUID RESTRICTION IS	USE THIS AMOUNT OF FLUIDS WITH MEALS	USE THIS AMOUNT OF FLUIDS WITH MEDICATIONS
1000 mL (4 cups)*	600 mL (2 1/2 cups)	400 mL (1 1/2 cups)
1200 mL (5 cups)	700 mL (3 cups)	500 mL (2 cups)
1500 mL (6 cups)	1000 mL (4 cups)	500 mL (2 cups)
2000 mL (8 cups)	1000 mL (4 cups)	1000 mL (4 cups)

All foods contain some fluids, but it is especially important to count the following as part of the fluid allowance:

Milliliters of Fluid Per 1/2 Cup					
Water	120	All juices	120	Watermelon	100
Coffee	120	Soda-pop	120	Sherbet	65
Tea	120	Ice	60	Ice cream	40
Sanka	120	Gelatin	100	Ice milk	40
Milk	120	Soup	120	Popsicle	80

*Approximate.

blood loss. *Epoetin alfa*, a pharmaceutical form of erythropoietin, may be used to increase red blood cell production and thereby correct the anemia. The treatment for iron-deficiency anemia is oral or parenteral iron products and an increase in dietary sources of iron. A diagnosis of iron-deficiency anemia can be made by a laboratory measure of ferritin. **Ferritin** is the storage form of iron found primarily in the liver. A small amount of ferritin circulates in the blood and reflects the amount of iron in body stores. A laboratory value of less than 12 micrograms per liter suggests iron deficiency.

Nutritional therapy with iron supplements consists of 210 milligrams of ferrous iron salts per day divided among three to four doses. Absorption is enhanced when iron supplements are taken on an empty stomach or with vitamin C.

Vitamin and Mineral Supplementation

Chronically uremic patients are prone to deficiencies of water-soluble vitamins unless supplements are given (Kopple, 1999). Losses are most notable with pyridoxine, ascorbic acid, and folic acid. Supplementation of these nutrients is recommended for clients on dialysis. Fat-soluble vitamins are not lost in the dialysate, and supplementation is not indicated except with vitamin D for another reason (see previous discussion). Because the body's ability to excrete excess fat-soluble vitamins is compromised, toxicity is a potential problem.

National Renal Diet

The American Dietetic Association and the National Kidney Foundation introduced the National Renal Diet in the fall of 1993. Because the dietary management of renal disease is tailored to the stage of disease and treatment approach, six meal-planning systems were developed. They are renal insufficiency without diabetes, renal insufficiency with diabetes, hemodialysis without diabetes, hemodialysis with diabetes, peritoneal dialysis without diabetes, and peritoneal dialysis with diabetes. These national meal-planning systems offer standardized guidelines for nutrition intervention and client education.

Each system provides food lists and calculation figures (derived from the average nutrient content of foods included in each list). Although the food lists developed for the client booklets were patterned after the *ADA Exchange Lists*, the varied nutritional requirements of clients with renal disease at different stages of treatment necessitated creation of specific food lists for each treatment modality. Table 21–2 shows the General Dietary Recommendations for Renal Patients by treatment approach. In addition, separate calculation figures and food lists were devised for clients with diabetes receiving each treatment modality, because foods high in sugars were excluded from the food lists for clients with diabetes.

Box 21–3 is an example of the calculation of a diet for a client receiving hemodialysis without diabetes (one of the six meal-planning systems). A case study and sample meal

Table 21–2 **Selected Nutritional Parameters for Varying Levels of Kidney Failure**

NUTRITIONAL PARAMETER	NORMAL KIDNEY FUNCTION	STAGES 1–4 CHRONIC KIDNEY DISEASE	STAGE 5 HEMODIALYSIS	STAGE 5 PERITONEAL DIALYSIS	TRANSPLANT
Calories (kcal/kg/day)	30–37	<60 years: 35 ≥60 years: 30–35	<60 years: 35 ≥60 years: 30–35	<60 years: 35 ≥60 years: 30–35, including calories from dialysis	Initial: 30–35 Maintenance: 25–30
Protein (gm/kg/d)	0.8	0.6–0.75 50 percent HBV	1.2 50 percent HBV	1.2–1.3 50 percent HBV	Initial: 1.3–1.5
Fat (percent total kcal)	30–35 percent Patients considered at highest risk for cardiovascular disease: emphasis on <10 percent saturated fat, PUFA, MUSA, 250–300 mg cholesterol/day				
Sodium (mg/d)	Unrestricted	2000	2000	2000	Unrestricted; monitor medication effect
Potassium (mg/d)	Unrestricted	Correlated to laboratory values	2000–3000 (8–17 mg/kg/d)	3000–4000 (8–17 mg/kg/d)	Unrestricted; monitor medication effect
Calcium (mg/d)	Unrestricted	1200	≤2000 from diet and medications	≤2000 from diet and medications	1200
Phosphorus (mg/d)	Unrestricted	Correlated to laboratory values	800–1000	800–1000	Unrestricted unless indicated
Fluid (ml/d)	Unrestricted	Unrestricted with normal urine output	1000 + urine output	Monitored; 1500–2000	Unrestricted unless indicated

Meant as guidelines only for initial assessment; individualization to patient's own metabolic status and coexisting metabolic conditions is essential for optimal care.

Abbreviations: HBV = high biological value; PUFA = polyunsaturated fatty acids; MUFA = monounsaturated fatty acids.

SOURCE: Reprinted from Beto, JA, and Bansal, VK: Medical Nutrition Therapy in Chronic Kidney Failure: Integrating Clinical Practice Guidelines. V104(3), 407. Copyright 2004, with permission from the American Dietetic Association.

Box 21–3 Calculating the Renal Diet: Hemodialysis Case Study

Average Calculation Figures for Renal Diets (No Diabetes)*

FOOD CHOICES	ENERGY KCAL	PRO g	CHO g	FAT g	Na mg	K mg	P mg
Milk	120	4	8	5	80	185	110
Nondairy milk substitute	140	0.5	12	10	40	80	30
Meat	65	7	…	4	25	100	65
Starch	90	2	18	1	80	35	35
Vegetable							
Low potassium	25	1	5	tr	15	70	20
Medium potassium	25	1	5	tr	15	150	20
High potassium	25	1	5	tr	15	270	20
Fruit							
Low potassium	70	0.5	17	…	tr	70	15
Medium potassium	70	0.5	17	…	tr	150	15
High potassium	70	0.5	17	…	tr	270	15
Fat	45	…	…	5	55	10	5
High-calorie	100	tr	25	…	15	20	5
Salt	…	…	…	…	250	…	…

Case Example

The client is a 55-year-old man who works full-time and has a sedentary lifestyle. He is 5 ft 10 in tall, has a medium frame, and weighs 68 kg. His ideal and usual weight is 76 kg. During the past 6 to 9 months, he has been anorectic and has had intermittent nausea and episodes of vomiting. He receives 4 hours of hemodialysis 3 times per week. His predialysis blood chemistry values were blood urea nitrogen, 22.50 mmol/L (63 mg/dL); sodium, 135 mmol/L (135 mEq/L); potassium, 4.0 mmol/L (4.0 mEq/L); phosphorus, 2.0 mmol/L (6.2 mg/dL); calcium, 2.25 mmoVL (9.0 mg/dL); and albumin, 33 g/L (3.3 g/dL). His urine output ranges between 800 and 1000 mL per day.

Daily Renal Diet Plan Goals

NUTRIENT	LEVEL	RATIONALE
Energy (kcal)	3000	40 kcal/kg HBW
Protein (g)	91	1.2 g/kg HBW
Sodium (mg)	2000	Control fluid weight gain
Potassium (mg)	3000 (75 mEq)	≤40 mg/kg HBW
Phosphorus (mg)	300	≤17 mg/kg HBW
Fluid (mL)	1500–1750	750 mL plus urine output

Sample Calculation of Renal Diet Plan for Hemodialysis

FOOD CHOICES	CHOICES NO.	ENERGY KCAL	PRO g	Na mg	K mg	P mg
Milk	1	120	4	80	185	110
Nondairy milk substitute	1	140	0.5	40	80	30
Meat	9	585	63	225	900	585
Starch	10	900	20	800	350	350
Vegetable	2	50	2	30	…	40
Low potassium		…	…	…	…	…
Medium potassium	(1)	…	…	…	150	…
High potassium	(1)	…	…	…	270	…
Fruit	3	210	1.5	…	…	45
Low potassium		…	…	…	…	…
Medium potassium	(1)	…	…	…	150	…
High potassium	(2)	…	…	…	540	…
Fat	10	450	…	550	100	50
High-calorie	5	500	…	75	100	25
Salt	1	…	…	250	…	…
Totals		2955	91	2050	2825	1235

*Because control of fat and carbohydrate intake is not a priority for all patients, practitioners may include their calculation in the meal plan on a case-by-case basis.

Abbreviations: PRO = protein; CHO = carbohydrate; Na = sodium; K = potassium; P = phosphorus; tr = trace; HBW = healthy body weight.

SOURCE: Monsen, ER: Meeting the challenge of the renal diet. Copyright American Dietetic Association. Reprinted by permission from Journal of the American Dietetic Association 93:638, 1993.

Box 21–4 **Condensed Renal Food Lists for Chronic Renal Failure, Hemodialysis**

Milk List

Approximate Nutrient Content: 4 g protein, 120 kcal, 80 mg sodium (Na), 185 mg potassium (K), 110 mg phosphorus (P)

Item	Amount
Milk	1/2 cup
Alterna (low-sodium milk substitute)	1 cup
Cream cheese	3 tbsp

Nondairy Milk Substitutes

Approximate Nutrient Content: 0.5 g protein, 140 kcal, 40 mg Na, 80 mg K, 30 mg P

Liquid nondairy creamer, polyunsaturated	1/2 cup
Dessert topping, nondairy, frozen	1/2 cup

Meat List

Approximate Nutrient Content: 7 g protein, 65 kcal, 25 mg Na, 100 mg K, 65 mg P

Low-cholesterol egg substitute	1/4 cup
Lean beef, pork, poultry	1 oz
Unsalted canned tuna	1/4 cup

Starch List

Approximate Nutrient Content: 2 g protein, 90 kcal, 80 mg Na, 35 mg K, 35 mg P

Bread (white, light rye, sourdough)	1 slice
Saltines, unsalted	4
Puffed wheat	1 cup
Rice, cooked	1/2 cup
Angel food cake	1 oz

Vegetable List

Approximate Nutrient Content: 1 g protein, 25 kcal, 15 mg Na, 20 mg P; serving size is 1 1/2 cup unless otherwise noted; prepared or canned without salt

Low Potassium (0–100 mg K)

Lettuce, all varieties	1 cup
Cucumber, peeled	

Medium Potassium (101 to 200 mg K)

Carrots	1 small, raw
Corn	1/2 ear
Broccoli	1/2 cup

High Potassium (201–350 mg K)

Tomato	1 medium
Potato, baked	1/2 medium
Spinach, cooked	

Fruit List

Approximate Nutrient Content: 0.5 g protein, 70 kcal, 15 mg P; serving size is 1/2 cup, unless otherwise noted

Low Potassium (0–100 mg K)

Applesauce	
Pears, canned	

Medium Potassium (101–200 mg K)

Apple, fresh	1 small
Watermelon	1 cup

High Potassium (201–350 mg K)

Orange juice	
Pear, fresh	1 medium

Fat List

Approximate Nutrient Content: trace protein, 45 kcal, 55 mg Na, 10 mg K, 5 mg P

Unsaturated Fats

Margarine	1 tsp
Mayo	1 tsp

Saturated Fats

Coconut	2 tbsp
Powdered coffee whitener	1 tbsp

High-Kilocalorie Choices

Approximate Nutrient Content: 100 kcal, 15 mg Na, 20 mg K, 5 mg P

Carbonated beverages, fruit flavors, root beer	1 cup
Kool-Aid	1 cup
Lemonade	1 cup
Tang	1 cup
Gum drops	15

plan are shown. Box 21–4 is a condensed food list for the client with chronic renal failure who is receiving hemodialysis treatments. A sample menu derived from the condensed renal food list and the sample daily meal plan are shown in Table 21–3.

Nutrient Guidelines for Adults With Renal Disease

As you can see, the nutritional care of renal clients is complex. Table 21–4 summarizes clinical situations, dietary interventions, and the rationale for nutrient control.

Renal Disease in Children

Growth failure is commonly seen in children with chronic renal failure treated with dialysis, but it is not an inevitable complication. Inadequate kilocaloric consumption and/or metabolic acidosis are reasons for the poor growth. These children often need to have their sodium, potassium, and protein intake rigidly controlled, and this may contribute to poor food intake. Anorexia and emotional disturbances are also contributing factors. Suggestions for improving children's intake include involving the children in selecting and preparing foods (insofar as possible); serving meals in an appealing, attractive manner (e.g., serving contrasting colors and textures of foods, using decorative tableware and dishes); serving small, frequent meals; ensuring that the child has someone with him or her at mealtime; and planning special mealtime events such as picnics (even if they have to be held in the hospital playroom).

Kidney Stones

Kidney stones may be found in the bladder, kidney, ureter, or urethra. During urine formation, the urine moves from the collecting tubules into the renal pelvis. From the **renal pelvis,** the urine moves down the **ureter** and into the urinary bladder. Finally, urine passes from the bladder down the urethra and exits the body. A stone, also called a **urinary calculus,** is a deposit of mineral salts held together by a thick, syrupy substance. A urinary calculus can block the movement of urine out of the body. Symptoms of a blockage include sudden severe pain with chills, fever, **hematuria** (blood in the urine), and an increased desire to urinate. A kidney stone can also pass out of the body with the urine.

MEAL PLAN	SAMPLE MENU	MEAL PLAN	SAMPLE MENU
Breakfast		*Afternoon Snack*	
1 nondairy milk substitute	1/2 cup liquid nondairy creamer, polyunsaturated	1 high-kilocalorie	1 cup Kool-Aid
		Supper	
1 high-potassium fruit	1/2 cup orange juice	1 high-potassium vegetable	1/2 cup cooked drained spinach
2 starches	1 cup puffed wheat and 1 slice light rye toast		
		1 high-potassium fruit	1 fresh pear
1 meat	1/4 cup low-cholesterol egg substitute	2 starches	1/2 cup rice and 1 oz angel food cake
2 fats	2 tsp margarine	4 meat	4 oz broiled chicken breast
Morning Snack		2 fats	2 tsp margarine (used on chicken)
1 high-kilocalorie	1 cup Tang	1 high-kilocalorie	1 cup root beer
Lunch		*Bedtime snack*	
1 medium-potassium vegetable	1 small raw carrot	1 milk	1/2 cup low-fat milk
1 medium-potassium fruit	1 small apple	2 starches	8 unsalted saltine crackers
		1 meat	1/4 cup unsalted canned tuna
2 starches	2 slices of sourdough white bread	2 fats	2 tsp mayo (for tuna salad)
4 meats	4 oz unsalted lean beef	1 high-kilocalorie	1 cup limeade
2 fats	2 tsp mayo		
1 high-kilocalorie	1 cup lemonade		

CLINICAL SITUATION	RATIONALE	INTERVENTION
Proteinuria	Protein lost in urine	Increase dietary protein
CAPD	Protein lost in dialysate	Increase dietary protein
Elevated BUN and creatinine (Uremia)	Body unable to excrete waste generated from protein metabolism in the amounts eaten and/or catabolized	Decrease dietary protein
		Increase nonprotein kilocalories
		Emphasis on proteins with high biologic value (animal origin)
Edema (Anuria)	Body unable to reabsorb and excrete sodium and fluid in the amounts consumed	Fluid restrictions
		Sodium restriction
Hyperkalemia	Body unable to excrete potassium	Potassium restriction
Hyperphosphatemia	May be related to an inability to activate vitamin D	Phosphorus restriction
	Body unable to excrete the amounts of phosphorus consumed and absorbed	Phosphate binders
Low ferritin levels	Iron deficiency; may be caused by blood loss and/or poor food intake	Increase kilocalories
		Increase nutrient density
		Iron supplements
		Vitamin C enhances iron absorption and should be consumed with meals
Poor growth, especially in children	Insufficient energy	Increase kilocalories to spare protein
Low number of red blood cells with normal ferritin level	Inability to manufacture erythropoietin	Epoetin alfa supplement
Elevated triglyceride levels	Common in renal patients	Type 4 hyperlipoproteinemia diet with modifications in fat and carbohydrate intake

Causes

The cause of most kidney stones is unknown. Some possible causes include an abnormal function of the parathyroid gland, disordered uric acid metabolism (as in gout), an excessive intake of animal protein, and immobility. At higher risk for kidney stones are men, people with a sedentary lifestyle, Asians, and whites. Typically, kidney stones occur in clients who are between ages 30 and 50. A determination of the stone's composition may lead to a restriction of dietary substrates (the substance acted on). Frequent dietary substrates of kidney stones are oxalic acid and purines.

Treatment

All clients with kidney stones should be advised to drink sufficient water to keep the urine volume above 2 liters per day. About 3000 milliliters or 13 cups of water per day are necessary to produce this amount of urine. The primary reason for increasing fluid intake is to prevent formation of concentrated urine, in which crystals are more likely to combine and precipitate.

Oxalates

Calcium oxalate is the most common constituent of kidney stones (Massey, 2003). Some individuals are genetically susceptible to stone formation. A diet that excludes foods high in oxalates (see Box 21–5) is frequently prescribed for clients with kidney stones if laboratory analysis shows a surgically removed or passed stone to be high in oxalates. It is likely that all stone formers will benefit from reduction of dietary oxalates but especially hyperoxaluric stone formers (Massey, 2003).

Calcium

Historically, if laboratory analysis of a surgically removed or passed stone was found to be high in calcium, a low-calcium diet was prescribed (600 milligrams per day). Today it is known that kidney stones are not usually caused by dietary calcium. In most individuals, kidney stones are usually less of a problem with an increased calcium intake than with a decreased calcium intake. A high-calcium diet binds the oxalate of dietary origin in the gastrointestinal tract and prevents its absorption, thereby reducing urinary oxalate formation (Weaver and Heanly, 1999).

Uric Acid Stones

Stones composed of uric acid are sometimes a complication of gout. **Gout** is a hereditary metabolic disease that is a form of arthritis. One symptom of gout is inflammation of the joints. The metabolism of uric acid is related to dietary purines. **Purines** are an end product of protein digestion. Thus, a purine-restricted diet is often prescribed for gout. Box 21–6 shows foods that are high, moderate, and low in purines. Many physicians do not prescribe a low-purine diet for the treatment of gout because the condition can be more effectively controlled by medications.

Box 21–5 **Foods High in Oxalic Acid**

	mg/100 g
Beverages	
Coffee, instant dry	143.0
Tea, brewed	12.5
Fruits	
Blackberries, raw	12.4
Gooseberries, raw	19.3
Plums, raw	11.9
Grains	
Bread, whole-wheat	20.9
Vegetables	
Beets, raw	72.2
Beets, boiled	109.0
Carrots, boiled	14.5
Green beans, raw	43.7
Green beans, boiled	29.7
Rhubarb, raw	537.0
Rhubarb, stewed	447.0
Spinach, boiled	571.0
Miscellaneous	
Cocoa, dry	623.0
Ovaltine, powder	45.9

SOURCE: Values taken from Pennington, JA, and Douglass, JA: Bowes and Church Food Values of Portions Commonly Used, ed 18. Lippincott Williams & Wilkins, 2004.

Box 21–6 **Purines in Food**

Group A: High Concentration (150–1000 mg/100 g)	
Liver	Sardines (in oil)
Kidney	Meat extracts
Sweetbreads	Consommé
Brain	Gravies
Heart	Fish roes
Anchovies	Herring

Group B: Moderate Amounts (50–150 mg/100 g)	
Meat, game, and fish other than those mentioned in Group A	
Fowl	Asparagus
Lentils	Cauliflower
Whole-grain cereals	Mushrooms
Beans	Spinach
Peas	

Group C: Very Small Amounts Need not be Restricted in Diet of Persons with Gout	
Vegetables other than those mentioned above	
Fruits of all kinds	Coffee
Milk	Tea
Cheese	Chocolate
Eggs	Carbonated beverages
Refined cereals, spaghetti, macaroni	Tapioca
Butter, fats, nuts, peanut butter*	Yeast
Sugars and sweets	
Vegetable soups	

*Fats interfere with the urinary excretion of urates and thus should be limited when attempting to promote excretion of uric acid.
SOURCE: From Venes, D (ed): Taber's Cyclopedic Medical Dictionary, ed 19. FA Davis, Philadelphia, 2001, with permission.

Surgery

Surgery is sometimes necessary to remove large kidney stones. Surgical removal of the stones prevents infection, reduces pain, and prevents a loss of kidney function.

Urinary Tract Infections

One form of **urinary tract infection (UTIs)** is **cystitis,** an inflammation of the bladder. This condition is prevalent in young women. Recurrent UTI means that the individual has three or more bouts of infection per year. A general nutrition measure includes acidifying the urine by taking large doses of vitamin C. Several studies have found that the regular intake of a cranberry juice beverage reduced the frequency of urinary tract infections (Kontiokari et al, 2001). Cranberry juice contains a substance with biologic activity that inhibits the growth of *E. coli* in the urinary tract. Clients with UTIs should be encouraged to drink ample fluids.

SUMMARY

The basic functional unit of the kidney is the nephron. Millions of nephrons work together to form urine and remove unnecessary substances from the blood. Glomerular filtration rate (GFR) is a measure of kidney function. The kidneys also are the site where vitamin D_3 (calcitriol) and erythropoietin are activated. Kidney failure can be acute or chronic. Chronic renal disease is progressive. Much research is aimed at finding a way to stop the downward spiral of GFR in clients who are diagnosed with chronic renal failure. Current research is focused on the role of dietary protein and phosphorus in the progression of kidney failure. Treatment for kidney failure is dialysis or a kidney transplant.

Nutritional management of clients with renal disease is a fundamental part of treatment. Clients with kidney disease require constant assessment, monitoring, and counseling. The dietary components that may need modification are kilocalories, protein, sodium, potassium, phosphorus, fluid, cholesterol, and saturated fat. Vitamin and mineral supplements are often prescribed. Frequently, the diet these clients follow must be further modified as their medical condition and treatment approach changes. A National Renal Diet has been developed for these clients.

Some nutritional intervention is necessary for clients with kidney stones and UTIs. The fluid intake of these clients should be high. Usually, clients with kidney stones need to avoid foods that contain substances likely to form stones.

CASE STUDY 21-1

Mr. U, a 25-year-old man, was admitted to the hospital from his doctor's office for a shunt implantation with subsequent hemodialysis planned. A college graduate, he is employed as an engineer. His medical record indicates that he had an episode of acute glomerulonephritis about 10 years ago. He contracted the disease after a streptococcal throat infection. At that time his symptoms were hematuria, oligalria, proteinuria, hypertension, and edema. He was discharged on a 4-g sodium diet.

Mr. U now complains of swollen ankles, headaches, and fatigue. He reports to have had a 10-lb weight gain over the past 6 weeks. His usual body weight is 170 lb; he is 5 ft 10 in tall and has a large frame. He now weighs 181 lb. His blood pressure is 155/99. Laboratory test results follow:

TEST	RESULTS	NORMAL RANGE
BUN	75 mg/dL	9–25 mg/dL
Creatinine	2 mg/dL	0.6–1.5 mg/dL
Serum phosphorus	4.4 mg/dL	3.0–4.5 mg/dL
Serum calcium	3.5 mg/dL	3.5–5.0 mg/dL
Hemoglobin	6 mg/dL	14–18 g/dL
Hematocrit	19 percent	42–52 percent
Potassium	4.0 mEq/L	3.5–5.0 mEq/L
Albumin	3.5 g/dL	3.5–5.5 g/dL
Urine volume	900 mL/day	1000–1500 mL
Proteinuria	1 +	None
GFR	10 mL/min	125 mL/min
Cholesterol	280 mg/dL	<200 mg/dL
Triglycerides	140 mg/dL	40–150 mg/dL

The doctor has prescribed a 60-g protein, 2000-kcal, 2-g sodium, low-saturated-fat, low-cholesterol diet and a fluid restriction of output plus 500 mL. Hemodialysis is ordered for three times a week. His medications include docusate sodium, furosemide, a multivitamin, vitamin B_6, and folic acid. Mr. U stated that the protein, fluid, saturated fat, and cholesterol restrictions are new to him.

(Continued on the following page)

NURSING CARE PLAN

SUBJECTIVE DATA Client complains of headaches, swollen ankles, and fatigue.

OBJECTIVE DATA Client has an elevated BUN, phosphorus, blood pressure, and **creatinine**. The client also has edema, a decreased GFR, hemoglobin, and hematocrit, and a decreased urinary output.

NURSING DIAGNOSIS NANDA: Excess Fluid Volume (NANDA, 2003, with permission) related to renal insufficiency as evidenced by client complaints of headaches, swollen ankles, fatigue, and decreased urinary output, edema formation, and hypertension.

NANDA: Deficient Knowledge (NANDA, 2003, with permission) related to disease progression as evidenced by statement that restrictions are new to him.

DESIRED OUTCOMES EVALUATION CRITERIA	NURSING ACTIONS/INTERVENTIONS	RATIONALE
NOC: Excess Fluid Volume (Moorhead, Johnson, and Maas, 2004, with permission)	NIC: Fluid Management (Dochterman and Bulechek, 2004, with permission)	
The client will demonstrate a stabilized fluid balance with a calculated fluid intake and a measured fluid output. Vital signs will progress toward the normal range.	Measure urinary output every shift and fluid intake.	Client's urinary output may vary, and fluid intake must be adjusted accordingly.
	Plan fluid intake with client; monitor fluid intake and body weight.	Fluid intake must be controlled to prevent excessive edema and control blood pressure. Daily weight is the best measure of fluid balance.
	Monitor BUN/creatinine results, as needed.	The client is currently unable to excrete waste generated from protein metabolism in amounts eaten and/or catabolized. As the client begins dialysis treatments, the BUN/creatinine levels should decrease, and the protein content of the diet will need to be adjusted accordingly.
	Monitor blood pressure, pulses, and lung sounds every 4 hours.	The client's fluid volume excess and decreased GFR may increase secretion of renin and raise blood pressure.
NOC: Deficient Knowledge: Treatment Regimen (Moorhead, Johnson, and Maas, 2004)	NIC: Teaching: Disease Process (Dochterman and Bulechek, 2004)	
The client will verbalize knowledge of condition and therapy regimen.	Encourage adequate kilocalorie intake.	The diet will not be effective in controlling BUN/creatinine levels unless adequate kilocalories are consumed.
	Discuss necessary changes in lifestyle and assist client to incorporate disease management into activities of daily living.	Because the client has a chronic disease, long-term compliance with the treatment approach will be necessary.
	Teach client to measure urinary output.	The client will need to learn to measure his own urinary output.
	Teach client to measure fluid intake daily; fluid intake should be 500 mL plus urinary output in milliliters.	The client will need to learn how to calculate his daily fluid intake based on his urinary output and insensible losses of fluid.
	Discuss with client the relationships of his symptoms (headaches, swollen ankles, fatigue) and signs (edema; decreased GFR, hemoglobin, hematocrit, urinary output; and elevated BUN/creatinine) to treatment approaches (hemodialysis and dietary restrictions).	Relating signs and symptoms to the client's treatment approach will assist him in understanding his treatment regimen.

DESIRED OUTCOMES EVALUATION CRITERIA	NURSING ACTIONS/INTERVENTIONS	RATIONALE
	Refer to the dietitian for dietary teaching.	The client's needs will best be met if referral to the dietitian is made as soon as possible. A diet as complicated as this client's will require several hours of instruction. Information is usually better retained if small amounts of information are given at frequent intervals.
The client will demonstrate behaviors consistent with dietary program.	Discuss with the client the importance of regular hemodialysis treatments.	Failure to receive regular hemodialysis treatments will result in an excessive fluid gain and abnormal laboratory values between treatments. Subsequent efforts to remove this excess fluid may result in a dangerous drop in blood pressure during the dialysis treatment.
	Monitor client's food intake.	The best method to evaluate whether the client has learned his dietary restrictions is to monitor food intake.

C T Q CRITICAL THINKING QUESTIONS

1. Explain the relationship of each dietary modification to the signs and symptoms Mr. U is experiencing.
2. Mr. U eats only about half his needed kilocalories. What should you do?
3. Mr. U develops a stomach ulcer. What should you recommend?
4. Mr. U decides he would like to try CAPD. How would his diet probably change?

⟩⟩⟩ CHAPTER REVIEW

1. Which of the following is a nutritional goal for a child with renal failure?
   a. Maintain current hydration status
   b. Promote normal growth and development
   c. Maximize uremia
   d. Stimulate client well-being

2. Kidney disease cannot be caused by:
   a. Consumption of toxic metals
   b. Consumption of 1 to 3 liters a day of water
   c. Average daily intake of 150 grams of protein a day
   d. Trauma

3. Kilocalories usually need to be increased in protein-restricted diets because an adequate kilocalorie intake:
   a. Assists in the control of serum potassium

   b. Is necessary to prevent renal anemia
   c. Controls and prevents osteodystrophy
   d. Spares protein

4. The _____ intake from food is not monitored in renal clients.
   a. Vitamin D
   b. Fluid
   c. Protein
   d. Sodium

5. The most important nutritional consideration in treating clients with kidney stones is to:
   a. Limit calcium intake
   b. Restrict all end products of protein metabolism
   c. Restrict all food sources of calcium, oxalic acid, and purines
   d. Increase fluid intake

✚ CLINICAL ANALYSIS

1. Bill, age 10, has acute glomerulonephritis. His mother explains that Bill had a streptococcal infection 1 week before the illness. When planning Bill's care, the nurse recognizes that he needs help in understanding his diet. Bill's restrictions will include:
   a. A low-fat diet
   b. A calcium restriction
   c. Measuring urine output (if any) daily and planning his fluid intake
   d. A high-protein diet

2. Mr. Jones, a 49-year-old mechanic, has been admitted to the hospital with diagnosis of renal failure. Mr. Jones has been following a 40-gram protein, 2-gram sodium, 2-gram potassium, 1000-milliliter fluid restriction for the past 5 years. Mr. Jones is scheduled for surgery tomorrow to have a permanent fistula

   implanted for hemodialysis. Mr. Jones's nutritional needs will change after he is maintained on hemodialysis to:
   a. More oranges, bananas, and baked potatoes
   b. More lean meat, eggs, low-fat milk, low-fat cheeses, soymilk, tofu, and peanut butter
   c. Less starches, breads, and cereals
   d. Less margarine, oil, and salad dressings

3. Mr. Jones is found to have an elevated serum phosphorus level after 6 months on hemodialysis. He should:
   a. Restrict his intake of dairy products
   b. Restrict his intake of red meats
   c. Increase his intake of sugar, honey, jam, jelly, and other simple sugars
   d. Discontinue his phosphate binders

REFERENCES

American Diabetes Association: Nephropathy in diabetes: Position statement. Diabetes Care 27:S79, 2004.

American Dietetic Association: Position of the American Dietetic Association: Vegetarian diets. J Am Diet Assoc 97:1317, 1997.

Beto, JA, and Bansal, VK: Medical nutrition therapy in chronic kidney failure: Integrating clinical practice guidelines. J Am Diet Assoc 104:404, 2004

Dochterman, J, and Bulechek, GM: Nursing Interventions Classification (NIC), ed 4. Mosby, St. Louis, 2004.

Inman, JI: A Clinical Guide to the Nutritional Care of the Renal Patient. New England Center for Nutrition Education, Inc, Stoughton, MA, 1999.

Kontiokari, T, et al: Randomised trial of cranberry lingoberry juice and lactobacillus GG drink for prevention of urinary tract infections in women. BMJ 322:1571, 2001.

Kopple, JD: Renal disorders and nutrition. In Shils, ME, Olson, JA, Shike, M, and Ross, CA (eds): Modern Nutrition in Health and Disease, ed 9. Williams & Wilkins, Baltimore, 1999.

Kugler, C, Vlaminck, H and Maes, AH: Nonadherence with diet and fluid restrictions among adults having hemodialysis. Journal of Nursing Scholarship. 37:25–29, 2005.

Kuhlmann, MK, et al: Malnutrition in hemodialysis patients: Self-assessment, medical evaluations, and "verifiable" parameters. Med Klin 1:13, 1997.

Massey, LK: Dietary influences on urinary oxalate and risk of kidney stones. Front Biosci 8:S584, 2003.

Moorhead, S, Johnson, M, and Maas, M (eds): Nursing Outcomes Classification (NOC), ed 3. Mosby, St. Louis, 2004.

Monsen, ER: Meeting the challenge of the renal diet. J Am Diet Assoc 93:6, 1993.

Moore, MC: Pocket Guide to Nutrition and Diet Therapy, ed 5. Mosby Year Book, St. Louis, 1996.

NANDA International: Nursing Diagnosis: Definitions and Classifications, 2003–2004. NANDA International, Philadelphia, 2003.

National Kidney Foundation: K/DOQI clinical practice guidelines for chronic kidney disease: Evaluation, classification and stratification. Am J Kidney Dis 39(suppl 1):S1, 2002.

Pennington, JA, and Souglass, JA: Bowers and Churches Food Values of Portions Commonly Used, ed 18. Lippincott Williams & Wilkins, Baltimore, 2004.

Rubin, HR, et al: Patient ratings of dialysis care with peritoneal dialysis vs. hemodialysis. JAMA 291:697, 2004.

Scanlon, VD, and Sanders, T: Essentials of Anatomy and Physiology, ed 4. FA Davis, Philadelphia, 2003.

Venes, D (eds): Taber's Cyclopedic Medical Dictionary, ed 19. FA Davis, Philadelphia, 2001.

Weaver, CM, and Heaney, RP: Calcium. In Shils, ME, Olson, JA, Shike, M, and Ross, CA (eds): Modern Nutrition in Health and Disease, ed 9. Williams & Wilkins, Baltimore, 1999.

Diet in Gastrointestinal Disease

After completing this chapter, the student should be able to:

1. Distinguish the dietary preparation for gastrointestinal surgery from dietary preparation for surgery on other body systems.
2. Identify nutritional deficiencies that may accompany diseases or treatment of the gastrointestinal tract.
3. Relate the pathophysiology of cirrhosis of the liver to the associated signs and symptoms.
4. List several nutritional consequences of alcoholism.
5. Discuss dietary modifications for common gastrointestinal diseases treated medically and surgically.

The gastrointestinal tract functions both as a barrier to substances from the environment and as an entry point for nutrients and other substances. Many disorders that affect the gastrointestinal tract and its accessory organs (liver, gallbladder, and pancreas) influence the nutritional status of clients. Most surgical procedures impact gastrointestinal tract function and require special dietary measures, both preoperatively and postoperatively. This chapter covers diet modifications for surgical clients and for clients with common gastrointestinal disorders and diseases.

Dietary Considerations With Surgical Clients

Because of its role in tissue building and healing, protein is particularly crucial in surgical clients. Protein depletion causes increased risk of infection and shock. Protein is essential for the manufacture of antibodies and white blood cells, which help the body to fight infection. Hypoalbuminemia (low serum albumin) prevents the return of interstitial fluid to the venous system, decreasing intravascular fluid, resulting in increased risk of shock because of low intravascular volume. A low serum albumin level increases the time needed to reduce edema that accompanies any trauma, including surgery, thus hampering circulation and healing. The serum albumin level, then, becomes a useful and readily available measure of protein status, and preoperative levels in individuals undergoing elective gastrointestinal surgery were inversely correlated with complications, time in the intensive care unit, resumption of oral intake, and mortality despite the inadequacy of preoperative nutritional assessment (Kudsk et al, 2003). Clinical Application 22–1 elaborates the possible consequences of malnutrition in surgical clients.

Persons with gastrointestinal disease are at special risk when facing surgery because such diseases interfere with

Surgical Clients With Rampant Dental Caries

Within a period of weeks, three clients on a gynecological surgical unit suffered postoperative wound disruptions. Each disruption was a **dehiscence,** a separation of the wound edges. Dehiscence occurs most frequently between the fifth and twelfth postoperative days. Risk factors for dehiscence include obesity, malnutrition, dehydration, abdominal distention, increased abdominal pressure from improper deep breathing and coughing, and infection.

All three clients had at least one of the risk factors. One client ran a postoperative fever, which could have been caused by infection or dehydration. The other two clients had such severely carious teeth it would have been difficult for them to chew in the months before surgery. They probably were malnourished.

It is suggested that nurses refer preoperative clients with marked dental caries to the dietitian for nutritional assessment. Carious teeth can cause and be caused by poor eating habits.

Table 22–1 Examples of Liver Functions

RELATED TO	PRODUCES/PROCESSES	STORES	BREAKS DOWN
Carbohydrate	Glucose from galactose and fructose Glucose from glycogen Glucose from glycerol and protein	Glycogen	
Fat	Fat from glucose Cholesterol Fatty acids and glycerol from cholesterol, phospholipids, and lipoproteins Lipoproteins Water-soluble bilirubin (from fat-soluble) Bile	Fat	
Protein	Albumin Some globulins Prothrombin Fibrinogen Transferrin Enzymes to convert ammonia to urea		
Vitamins	Retinol-binding protein Other transport proteins Activates thiamine Activates vitamin B_6 Processes vitamin D	A, D, E, K Thiamin Riboflavin B_6 Folic acid B_{12} Biotin	
Minerals		Iron	Worn-out red blood cells
Other			Acetaminophen Alcohol Aldosterone Bacteria Barbiturates Estrogen Glucocorticoids Morphine Progesterone Some anesthetics

nutrition. In cases involving gastrointestinal surgery, the gastrointestinal tract is incised and sutured, so postoperative feeding is postponed to allow healing. Special notice should be given to surgical clients with liver disease. The liver has many functions, some of which are listed in Table 22–1. Because of the liver's role in metabolizing and detoxifying drugs, clients with liver disease must be carefully managed when surgery is necessary. Drugs may accumulate in the bloodstream because the liver cannot metabolize them. Moreover, some anesthetics, analgesics, and anti-infectives are toxic to the liver.

Mild to severe malnutrition affected 39 percent of clients undergoing gastrointestinal or orthopedic surgical procedures, about two-thirds of whom received nutritional support, but nutritional assessment was sparse, with just 59 percent of those charts even containing an entry on the client's body weight (Bruun et al, 1999). Surprisingly little evidence is available to support a significant impact of early nutritional support on postoperative clinical outcomes, however, with the exception of severely malnourished clients who receive nutritional support for at least 7 days preoperatively (Huckleberry, 2004).

Preoperative Nutrition

Before elective surgery is undertaken, nutritional deficiencies should be identified and corrected. Many obese clients are instructed to lose weight to reduce the risks of surgery. If the client is anemic, an iron preparation may be prescribed. Other nutrients can be provided as needed. At least 2 to 3 weeks are required for objective evidence of the effectiveness of nutritional therapy. All surgical clients should receive instruction in the weeks before surgery.

Preoperative fasting protocols have been liberalized based on research showing slight risk of pulmonary aspiration with modern anesthetics. Guidelines for anesthesia administration to healthy individuals scheduled for elective procedures permit greater oral intake than in the past (see Table 22–2). The guidelines do not supplant the need for individual assessment. Nor do they apply to individuals with gastrointestinal motility or metabolic disorders, individuals with potential airway problems, or women in labor. In a study conducted shortly after publication of the guidelines, the average fast was 12 hours for liquids and 14

Table 22–2   Fasting Recommendations to Minimize Aspiration Risk

ORAL INTAKE	MINIMUM FASTING TIME	COMMENT
Clear liquids	2 hours	No alcohol
Breast milk	4 hours	
Infant formula and nonhuman milk	6 hours	
Light meal	6 hours	Example: toast and clear liquids
Regular meal including fat or meat	8 hours	Fat and meat delay gastric emptying

SOURCE: Adapted from American Society of Anesthesiologists, 1999.

hours for solids. Ninety-one percent of these nonobstetric, nongastrointestinal surgical clients had been instructed to remain NPO (nothing by mouth) after midnight, including 79 percent of those scheduled for surgery at noon or later (Crenshaw and Winslow, 2002).

Surgery of the gastrointestinal tract demands additional bowel preparation. Anti-infectives such as neomycin that remain mainly in the bowel may be given to kill intestinal bacteria. A low-residue diet for 2 to 3 days will minimize the feces left in the bowel. A low-residue diet reduces the fecal bulk by reducing food residue. **Residue** is the total solid material in the large intestine after digestion. A low-residue diet usually consists of foods that are easily digested and absorbed. Table 22–3 details a low-residue diet.

Table 22–3   Low-Residue Diet

DESCRIPTION	INDICATIONS	ADEQUACY
The low-residue diet limits milk and milk products and excludes any food made with seeds, nuts, and raw or dried fruits and vegetables. The purpose of the diet is to decrease colonic contents.	The diet can be used for severe diarrhea, partial bowel obstruction, and acute phases of inflammatory bowel diseases. Preoperatively the diet is used to minimize fecal volume and residue. Postoperatively the diet is used in the progression to a general diet. Long-term use of the diet is not recommended since it may aggravate symptoms during nonacute phases of disease.	Strict reduction in milk and milk products, vegetables, and fruits may necessitate supplementation of calcium, vitamin C, folate, and other nutrients.

FOOD GROUP	CHOOSE	DECREASE
Milk	2 cups/day Mild cheese	Strong cheese
Breads and cereals	White bread Refined cereals: cream of wheat, cream of rice, puffed rice, Rice Krispies, corn flakes Crackers without whole grains or seeds Rice, noodles, macaroni, spaghetti	Whole-grain breads Bread made with seeds, nuts, or bran Cracked-wheat bread Whole-grain rice or pasta
Fruits	Juice without pulp Ripe banana Cooked or canned apples, apricots, Royal Anne cherries, peaches, pears Strained fruit	Prunes and prune juice Fruits not on "allowed" list Dried fruit
Vegetables	Juice without pulp Lettuce Cooked or canned asparagus, green and wax beans, beets, carrots, eggplant, pumpkin, spinach, acorn squash, seedless tomatoes, tomato sauce or puree, white or sweet potatoes without skin Strained vegetables	Vegetables not on "allowed" list Dried peas and beans Potato skins or chips Fried potatoes
Meat, poultry, fish, shellfish, eggs	Lean tender meat without grease: ground or well-cooked (roasted, baked, or broiled) beef, lamb, ham, veal, pork, poultry, organ meats, fish Eggs except fried	Tough, fried, or spiced meats Fried eggs
Fats and oils	Smooth peanut butter Butter, oils Cream (deduct from milk allowance) Margarine	All other nuts Coconut Olives
Desserts and miscellaneous	Plain dessert made with allowed foods: fruit, ices, sherbet, ice cream, gelatin	Popcorn Seeds of any kind

(Continued on the following page)

Table 22–3 **Low-Residue Diet** *(Continued)*

FOOD GROUP	CHOOSE	DECREASE
Desserts and miscellaneous *(continued)*	Candy: gum drops, hard candy, jelly beans, plain chocolate, marshmallows, butterscotch	Whole spices
	Honey, sugar, molasses	Chili sauce
	Salt, pepper, ground seasonings	Rich gravy
	Plain gravy	Vinegar
	Milk sauces (deduct from milk allowance)	Alcohol
	Mayonnaise	
	Coffee, decaffeinated coffee	
	Jelly	
	Tea	
	Soda	Jam, marmalade

SAMPLE MENU	
Breakfast	Lunch/Dinner
Strained grapefruit juice	Baked halibut with clear lemon juice
Cream of wheat	Twice-baked potato (no onions)
Poached egg	Candied sweet potato (no nuts or whole spices)
White bagel with butter and honey	Canned pear and banana on lettuce
1/2 cup milk	French bread and margarine
Coffee	Rice pudding (no raisins; deduct milk from allowance)

Postoperative Nutrition

Postoperatively, the healing process requires increased amounts of protein, vitamins C and K, and zinc, along with adequate amounts of other nutrients. Vitamin C is necessary for collagen formation; vitamin K for blood clotting; and zinc for tissue growth, bone formation, skin integrity, cell-mediated immunity, and generalized host defense. Two antioxidants, vitamins E and C, given to critically ill surgical clients (91 percent of them trauma victims who are classified as surgical clients) resulted in 19 percent fewer lung complications and 57 percent less multiple organ failure than occurred in individuals receiving standard care. Those receiving vitamins also had shorter periods of mechanical ventilation and time in the intensive care unit (Nathens et al, 2002).

Intravenous fluids are continued after surgery. The usual minimum replacement is 2 liters of 5-percent glucose in water in 24 hours. This amount contains 100 grams of glucose and delivers 340 kilocalories. Although this will not meet a person's resting energy expenditure, it will prevent ketosis. Previously well-nourished adults generally have nutrient reserves for 3 to 4 days of semistarvation. To prevent excessive muscle protein from being used for energy, adequate nourishment should be delivered to the client within 3 days. In general, 25 kilocalories/kilogram of body weight per day is an acceptable and achievable intake, but clients with sepsis or trauma may need almost twice as much energy (Reid, 2004).

To avoid abdominal distention, oral feedings traditionally have been delayed until peristalsis returns and is detected with a stethoscope. Another sign of peristalsis is the passage via the rectum of **flatus** (gas). Ambulation as permitted helps clients pass the flatus and avoid uncomfortable distention. **Paralytic ileus** is a complication of abdominal surgery and other traumatic events or diseases. Peristalsis ceases and secretions and gas accumulate in the bowel, leading to distention and vomiting. Removal of secretions by suction is the usual treatment. To test the traditional practice of delaying oral intake until peristalsis returns, major radical oncologic or urogynecologic abdominal surgery clients received clear liquids on the first postoperative day and were started on a regular diet once they tolerated 500 mL of clear fluid on a given day. They were discharged 2 days earlier than individuals receiving the traditional treatment, with no differences in postoperative complications noted between the two groups (Steed et al, 2002). Another approach comparing women given low-residue diets 6 hours postoperatively after major gynecologic surgery with those given traditional dietary management reported no significant differences in postoperative complications, including paralytic ileus (MacMillan et al, 2000).

Clients are usually progressed from clear liquids to full liquids, a soft diet, and then a regular diet as soon as possible (see Chapter 15). The progression time varies with the client and surgical procedure. It may be hours or days. If "diet as tolerated" is ordered, the client should be asked what foods sound appealing. Sometimes, a full dinner tray when the client does not feel well "turns off" the small appetite he or she has. After gastrointestinal surgery, oral food and fluids are deferred longer than with other surgeries to allow healing. Giving the exact amount of food or fluid prescribed is important. More is not better if the client's stomach or intestine has been sutured. It is not advisable to give red liquids, such as gelatin or cranberry juice, after surgery on the mouth and throat so that vomitus is not mistaken for blood or vice versa.

Surgical removal of a part of the gastrointestinal tract, such as the stomach, duodenum, jejunum, or ileum, may result in malabsorption of specific nutrients, as illustrated in

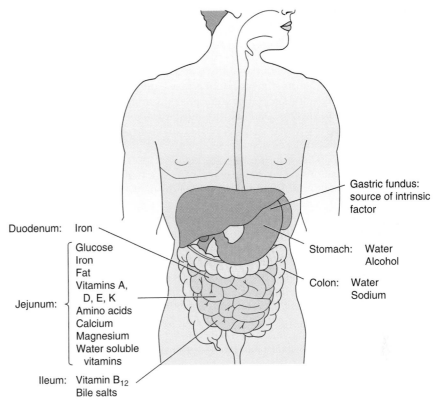

Figure **22–1** The chief sites of absorption for various nutrients. Disease or resection of an area will increase the risk of deficiency of specific nutrients. (Adapted from Scanlon, VC, and Sanders, T: Student Workbook for Essentials of Anatomy and Physiology, ed 4. FA Davis, Philadelphia, 2003, p 283, with permission.)

Figure 22–1. For example, intrinsic factor, which is secreted by the stomach, carries vitamin B_{12} to the ileum for absorption. Iron absorbed from the duodenum and the jejunum is necessary for hemoglobin synthesis. Glucose, amino acids, fat- and water-soluble vitamins, calcium, and magnesium, all absorbed in the jejunum, are necessary for metabolism. Bile salts are absorbed in the ileum. Although the loss of bile salts in the feces may seem harmless, the body ordinarily recycles these salts over and over in the management of fats. Prolonged impaired absorption of bile salts can result in failure to absorb fat and fat-soluble vitamins.

Disorders of the Mouth and Throat

Varied conditions such as dental caries, oral surgery, surgery of the head and neck, fractured jaw, cancer chemotherapy or radiation therapy can cause difficulty with chewing and swallowing. Special feeding techniques and scrupulous oral hygiene may be required. Often the client requires a feeding tube, as detailed in Chapter 15. Suggestions to manage dysphagia are described in Chapter 10, and interventions for anorexia appear in Chapter 23. Box 26–2 summarizes the dietary management of many symptoms.

Disorders of the Esophagus

The sole purpose of the **esophagus** is to conduct food to the stomach, but it sometimes malfunctions. Achalasia, gastroesophageal reflux, and hiatal hernia are types of esophageal disorders.

Achalasia

Failure of the gastrointestinal muscle fibers to relax where one part joins another is called **achalasia.** When it occurs in the **cardiac sphincter,** which separates the stomach from the esophagus, the condition is termed *cardiospasm.* The cause of achalasia is unknown, although autoimmunity has been suggested by several studies (Moses et al, 2003). Very hot or cold foods may trigger esophageal spasm, and anxiety seems to aggravate the condition. Symptoms are described as "something sticking in my throat" and a feeling of fullness behind the sternum (breastbone). Vomiting may occur with achalasia, and aspiration of vomitus can cause pneumonia.

In mild cases, avoiding spicy foods and minimizing dietary bulk may be effective. Diets for these clients require much individual attention. Rarely does one achalasia client have intolerances for the same foods as another client. Plenty of liquids with small, frequent meals may help. Treatment of more severe cases involves stretching the cardiac sphincter or surgically incising it to enlarge the passage.

Gastroesophageal Reflux Disease (GERD)

Some regurgitation of stomach contents into the esophagus occurs in normal individuals. Usually the presence of stomach contents in the esophagus stimulates esophageal contractions that return the refluxed material to the stomach. If excessive reflux occurs, either in frequency or volume, or if the esophagus fails to contract in response to stomach contents, the individual has **gastroesophageal reflux disease (GERD)** (also called *acid-reflux disorder*).

Gastroesophageal reflux disease, affecting 19 million people in the United States (Sandler et al, 2002), can usually be managed without surgery. This regurgitation is common in infancy and disappears with age, often to reappear in old age due to poor muscle tone of the cardiac sphincter. In infants, usually no treatment is undertaken unless there is evidence of aspiration of food into the respiratory tract or of failure to thrive. In adults, the most common underlying cause of gastroesophageal reflux is hiatal hernia, which is covered in the next section. Other conditions associated with GERD due to increased abdominal pressure are obesity and pregnancy. Some experts believe that gastroesophageal reflux may be caused by failure of the cardiac sphincter to operate properly. The stomach is normally protected from hydrochloric acid by a thick layer of mucus. Because the esophagus is not so protected, repeated bouts of gastroesophageal reflux can lead to esophagitis and ulcer formation that, when healed, may cause a stricture at the site of the scar tissue. The prominent symptom of gastroesophageal reflux is heartburn with pain occurring behind the sternum. Sometimes the pain radiates to the neck and the back of the throat. Lying down or bending over may increase reflux and aggravate the pain. If the passage becomes narrowed, dysphagia may become bothersome.

Treatment involves several conservative measures. Small, frequent meals often help. Protein is associated with tightening of the cardiac sphincter and is used in normal amounts in the diet. Foods often avoided because they relax the sphincter are fat, caffeine, peppermint, spearmint, and chocolate. Regardless of the type and amount of beverage consumed, alcohol facilitates the development of gastroesophageal reflux disease by reducing the pressure of the lower esophageal sphincter and esophageal motility (Bujanda, 2000). Smoking also relaxes the sphincter. Decaffeinated coffee and pepper are frequently avoided because they stimulate gastric secretion and acidic juices, such as citrus juices and tomato juice, also may be irritating.

A change in eating behaviors and lifestyle may assist in the control of gastroesophageal reflux. Chewing food thoroughly, not eating within 3 hours of bedtime, and sitting upright for 2 hours after meals may increase food tolerance. Liquids may accompany meals unless the client with GERD reports early satiety or distention. Raising the head of the bed 6 to 8 inches enables gravity to help keep stomach contents contained. Symptoms of overweight clients have decreased with weight loss (Fraser-Moodie et al, 1999). Table 22–4 details a diet for gastroesophageal reflux.

Table 22–4   **Diet for Gastroesophageal Reflux and Hiatal Hernia**

DESCRIPTION	INDICATIONS	ADEQUACY
The diet is designed to minimize reflux through timing of intake, texture control, limiting fat, and exclusion of sphincter relaxants and gas-forming foods. Adjunctive treatment involves positioning.	Esophageal reflux, hiatal hernia, esophageal ulcers, esophagitis, esophageal strictures, heartburn.	The diet may not meet the RDAs for vitamin C and iron in the premenopausal woman.

LIFESTYLE CHANGES	CHOOSE	DECREASE
Meal pattern	Six small meals 1/2 cup liquid with meals Other liquids >1 1/2 hours after meals >1/2 hour before meals	Eating within 3 hours of bedtime
Adjunction therapy	Elevate head of bed 6 inches Relax at mealtime Consider weight loss if needed	Lying down in the hour after eating
FOOD GROUP		
Milk	Skim milk, buttermilk, evaporated skim milk Skim milk cheese Cottage cheese Low-fat yogurt	Other milk Hot chocolate
Breads and cereals	White and whole-grain breads Plain rolls, biscuits, and muffins Plain crackers Any cereals except those on "decrease" list Rice Pasta	Pancakes, waffles, French toast Doughnuts, sweet rolls, nut breads Granola-type cereals with nuts and/or coconut
Fruits	Mild juices Any fruits except those on "decrease" list	Avocado Raw apples and melons Orange, grapefruit, and tomato juices

LIFESTYLE CHANGES	CHOOSE	DECREASE
Vegetables	Any vegetables except those on "decrease" list	Creamed or fried vegetables Hashed brown potatoes Broccoli, Brussels sprouts, cabbage, cauliflower, cucumber, dried peas or beans, onions, green pepper, rutabagas, sauerkraut, turnips
Meat, poultry, fish, shellfish eggs	6 oz/day: lean beef, pork, ham, lamb, liver, veal, fish, skinless poultry Eggs	Sausage, bacon, frankfurters, luncheon meats, canned meats and fish, duck, goose
Fats and oils	3 tsp/day: oil, butter, margarine, mild salad dressing 2 tbsp of the following may substitute for 1 tsp of fat: light cream, sour cream, nondairy cream Vegetable pan sprays as desired Low-fat salad dressings	Fried foods Gravies and sauces Cream Salad dressing Shortening, lard, or oils in excess of allowance Nuts, peanut butter
Desserts and miscellaneous	Plain cakes and cookies Gelatin, popsicles Sherbet and pudding made with skim milk Caffeine-free carbonated beverages Decaffeinated tea Fat-free broth, bouillon, consommé Soup made from allowed foods Cream soup made with skim milk Sugar, honey, syrup, molasses Jam, jelly, preserves Plain candy Salt Condiments and spices in small amounts Vanilla Vinegar	Ice cream, ice milk Pie, pastry Butter cake and icings Chocolate, coconut, cream, cream cheese, whipped cream, nuts, peppermint, spearmint Caffeinated beverages Decaffeinated coffee Tea Alcohol Potato chips Candy containing chocolate, nuts, coconut, or peppermint Popcorn Snack chips Pickles, relish Catsup, chili sauce Mustard Steak sauce

SAMPLE MENU

35 Minutes Before Breakfast
2 glasses of water

Breakfast
1/2 banana
1/2 cup oatmeal
1/2 cup skim milk
1 slice toast with Jam

Midmorning Snack
1/2 cup pineapple Juice
3 graham crackers

35 Minutes Before Meal
2 glasses of water

Lunch/Dinner
3 oz skinless chicken breast baked in lemon juice
1/2 baked potato with 1 tbsp sour cream
1/2 cup whole-kernel corn
3 small celery sticks
Hard roll with 1 tsp margarine
1/2 cup decaffeinated tea

35 Minutes Before Snack
2 glasses of water

Midafternoon/Evening Snack
1 cup low-fat yogurt

Hiatal Hernia

The *esophageal hiatus* is the opening in the diaphragm through which the esophagus is attached to the stomach. A **hiatal hernia** is a protrusion of the stomach through the esophageal hiatus into the chest cavity (Fig. 22–2). The symptoms of hiatal hernia are similar to those of gastroesophageal reflux, and its medical treatment is the same.

Persistent symptoms despite conservative treatment might lead the client to elect surgical repair of the hernia.

Disorders of the Stomach

Disorders of the stomach often require diet modification and, in some cases, surgery. The following sections concern two common disorders, gastritis and peptic ulcers,

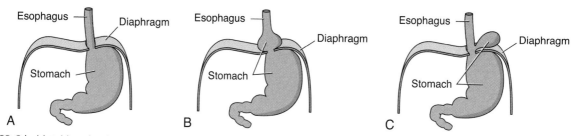

Figure 22–2 In hiatal hernia, the upper part of the stomach squeezes into the chest cavity through the esophageal opening in the diaphragm. A, Normal anatomy; B, Sliding hiatal hernia; C, Paraesophageal or rolling hiatal hernia. (Reprinted from Williams, LS, and Hopper, PD: Understanding Medical-Surgical Nursing, ed 2. FA Davis, Philadelphia, 2003, p 495, with permission.)

and one disorder mainly associated with diabetes mellitus, delayed gastric emptying. Also included is an exaggerated physiological response that can cause problems for older adults, postprandial hypotension.

Gastritis

Inflammation of the stomach is *gastritis.* Common causes of gastritis are the chronic use of aspirin and alcohol abuse. Other conditions that result in gastritis are food allergies, food poisoning, infections, radiation exposure, and stress. Symptoms of gastritis are anorexia, nausea, a feeling of fullness, and epigastric pain. Figure 22–3 illustrates the abdominal quadrants and regions used to record signs and symptoms revealed during the assessment process. Signs of gastritis are vomiting and eructating (belching).

The dietary treatment plan for gastritis includes having the client:

1. Eat at regular intervals.
2. Chew food, especially fibrous food, slowly and thoroughly.
3. Avoid foods that cause pain.

4. Avoid foods that cause gas, especially vegetables in the cabbage family, including broccoli, cauliflower, and Brussels sprouts.
5. Avoid the following:
   * gastric irritants such as caffeine and alcohol
   * nonsteroidal anti-inflammatory drugs (NSAIDs) such as aspirin
   * strong spices, including nutmeg, pepper, garlic, and chili powder
6. Eat in a relaxed manner.

More often than not, discovering which foods are responsible for the pain and discomfort of gastritis is a trial-and-error process. Tolerances vary from person to person. Prolonged or recurrent gastritis deserves medical attention.

Delayed Gastric Emptying

This condition can be associated with certain prescription drugs as well as the use of alcohol, tobacco, and marijuana. Low doses of alcohol accelerate gastric emptying, whereas high doses delay emptying and slow bowel motility

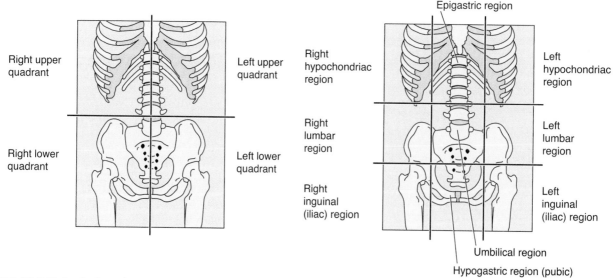

Figure 22–3 Abdominal quadrants and regions of the abdomen are used to describe locations of signs and symptoms. (Reprinted from Venes, D [ed]: Taber's Cyclopedic Medical Dictionary, ed 19. FA Davis, Philadelphia, 2001, p 4, by Beth Anne Willert, Dictionary Illustrator, with permission.)

(Bujanda, 2000). Delayed gastric emptying can occur in anorexia nervosa and in malnutrition, but up to 50 percent of clients with diabetes may be affected, with no clear association between length of disease and symptoms such as **postprandial** (after eating) abdominal pain, nausea, vomiting, and bloating. When it occurs with diabetes, delayed gastric emptying is termed *diabetic gastroparesis*, and it can accompany both insulin-dependent and non-insulin-dependent diabetes (Smith and Ferris, 2003). Treatment of delayed gastric emptying focuses on the cause of the disorder: removing offending drugs, intervening appropriately in malnutrition, and controlling hyperglycemia in clients with diabetes. Dietary interventions include eating small, frequent meals, replacing solids with liquids such as soups (which leave the stomach sooner than solids), reducing the fat ingested (which remains in the stomach longer than carbohydrate or protein) and decreasing fiber intake (Parkman, Hasler, and Fisher, 2004),

Peptic Ulcers

Both gastric (stomach) and duodenal ulcers are called *peptic ulcers*. Although treatments have improved, peptic ulcer disease was the primary diagnosis for 189,000 inpatient hospital stays and caused 4695 deaths in 1998 (Sandler et al, 2002).

Pathophysiology

An ulcer client's mucosa is not sufficiently resistant to the acids secreted by the stomach. If just the superficial cells are involved, the lesion is called an **erosion.** If the muscular layer of the stomach or duodenum is involved, the person has an **ulcer.** Infection with *Helicobacter pylori* is related to the occurrence of duodenal ulcers. The organism occurs worldwide and is found in about 20 to 30 percent of adults in developed countries; however, only a minority of these people develop duodenal ulcers (Heymann, 2004). In both Eastern and Western countries, peptic ulcer occurs most frequently during the winter months. Multiple other variations in geographical distribution, time trends, and gender differences indicate that while *H. pylori* is a major cause of peptic ulceration, other environmental and genetic factors contribute to ulcer formation (Lam, 2000).

Both *H. pylori* infection and nonsteroidal anti-inflammatory drug (NSAID) use independently and significantly increase the risk of peptic ulcer and ulcer bleeding. One-fourth of the cases of perforated peptic ulcer (see later) are attributed to the use of NSAIDs (Svanes, 2000), but peptic-ulcer disease is rare in *H. pylori*-negative, non-NSAID users (Huang, Sridhar, and Hunt, 2002). Long-term use of other medications such as potassium chloride and corticosteroids is also associated with ulcer formation. In addition, smoking predisposes a person to ulcer formation and complicates treatment.

Signs and Symptoms

A burning, cramping epigastric pain when the stomach is empty characterizes duodenal ulcer. This occurs 2 to 4 hours after eating or at night and is relieved by antacids or food. With gastric ulcer, the burning, gnawing epigastric pain occurs 1 to 2 hours after meals and is made worse by ingesting food (Williams and Hopper, 2003). One-fourth of ulcer clients experience bleeding, which occurs more often with duodenal than with gastric ulcers. If the blood is vomited immediately after bleeding begins, it is bright red. If it stays in contact with digestive juices for a while, the vomitus is brown-black and granular, resembling coffee grounds. The medical term for this is *coffee-ground emesis.* Other symptoms of peptic ulcer are nausea, anorexia, and sometimes weight loss.

Complications of Peptic Ulcers

Hemorrhage is a complication of peptic ulcers. Scar tissue from a healed ulcer can restrict the gastric outlet, causing pyloric obstruction. If the ulcer continues to erode through the entire stomach or intestinal wall, the result is a **perforated ulcer.** Leakage of gastrointestinal contents into the sterile abdominal cavity causes **peritonitis,** an inflammation of the peritoneum (the lining of the abdominal cavity). Most perforated ulcers in clients younger than 75 years of age are attributed to smoking (Svanes, 2000).

Treatment of Peptic Ulcers

Usually a course of medical treatment is prescribed first. If *H. pylori* infection is the cause, combinations of antibiotics and other drugs are recommended. Only if such treatment proves ineffective is surgery considered. A dietary approach has also been investigated. In asymptomatic clients with *H. pylori* infections, bifidobacterium- and lactobacillus-containing yogurt twice daily for 6 weeks effectively suppressed the infection (Wang et al, 2004).

MEDICAL TREATMENT

Before the advent of anti-ulcer medications, clients with peptic ulcers were usually advised to take antacids every 2 hours, alternating with milk and cream. One adverse effect of this treatment was milk alkali syndrome (see Chapter 8). New medications have revolutionized the treatment and are almost always effective without a drastic change in diet. In addition to antibiotics, commonly prescribed medications are *cimetidine, ranitidine*, and *famotidine*, which block histamine-stimulated gastric acid secretion, and *omeprazole*, which suppresses gastric acid production.

Diet does require some modification, however. Some experts recommend only three regular meals with no snacking between because food, including milk, stimulates gastric secretion. Other authorities recommend midmorning and midafternoon snacks. In both regimens, substances that cause gastric irritation are avoided. These include the same gastric irritants included in the section on gastritis. Clients should be encouraged to avoid or limit spices or foods that are not well tolerated. Changes in an ulcer client's lifestyle improve the chances of successful treatment. Since smoking stimulates secretion of gastric acid, ulcer clients should be advised not to smoke.

SURGICAL TREATMENT

When surgery is necessary, the ulcer is removed and the remaining gastrointestinal tract is sutured together. Surgical procedures designed to eliminate the diseased area include gastroduodenostomy (stomach and duodenum anastomosed) and gastrojejunostomy (stomach and jejunum anastomosed). **Anastomosis** is the surgical connection between tubular structures. Figure 22–4 illustrates these two procedures.

Following gastric surgery, parenteral and tube feeding are used singly or in combination. If tube feeding is used, the tube must be inserted beyond the area that was resected (removed). Once a client is advanced to an oral diet, he or she may experience the **dumping syndrome,** a complication of a surgical procedure that removes, disrupts, or bypasses the pyloric sphincter. Clinical Application 22–2 describes the dumping syndrome in more detail. Table 22–5 depicts a diet to prevent or treat the dumping syndrome. Long-term nutritional consequences of reconstructive surgery for peptic ulcer include iron deficiency anemia and osteomalacia. The deficiency of iron is related to decreased gastric acidity and decreased absorptive capacity of the duodenum. The mechanism for developing osteomalacia is incompletely described, although the duodenum is a major site for calcium absorption (Stenson, 1999).

Postprandial Hypotension

This refers to a drop in systolic blood pressure of 20 mmHg or more within 75 to 120 minutes after the beginning of a meal, most often resulting in dizziness and fatigue but also weakness, light-headedness, disturbed speech, and vision changes. The most severe hypotension occurs in individuals with neurological, cardiovascular, or renal diseases. Complications include higher incidence of coronary events, stroke, and total mortality (Malozemoff and Gentlemen, 2004). Normally the body compensates for the increased blood flow to the digestive tract following meals, but in the elderly the mechanisms maintaining adequate circulation to the rest of the body become less effective.

To prevent postprandial hypotension, a person should limit carbohydrate intake and take frequent small meals.

Clinical Application 22–2

Dumping Syndrome

The pyloric sphincter normally allows only small amounts of gastric contents into the duodenum at a time. After the pyloric sphincter is surgically removed, a concentrated liquid is suddenly "dumped" into the intestine. The concentrated contents then pull water from the bowel wall just as in osmotic diarrhea. Local effects are hyperperistalsis, diarrhea, abdominal pain, and vomiting 30 to 60 minutes after a meal. Systemic effects relate to deficient fluid volume: weakness, dizziness, sweating, decreased blood pressure, tachycardia, and palpitations. The dumping syndrome is most often associated with a total gastrectomy or a partial gastrectomy involving resection of two-thirds of the stomach. The same signs and symptoms can occur in a client receiving a tube feeding if the nasogastric tube is accidentally carried down into the duodenum.

Dietary treatment of the dumping syndrome attempts to delay gastric emptying and to distribute the increased osmolality in the bowel over time. This can be achieved by limiting the intake of simple sugars, consuming frequent meals, and limiting fluids with meals. Simple sugars increase the osmolality of the gastric contents and enhance the movement of food out of the stomach. Small, frequent meals will reduce the load on the intestine. Liquids should be taken between, rather than with, meals. Beverages should be low in simple carbohydrate. Very hot or cold foods will stimulate peristalsis and should be avoided. A nondietary intervention also helps to control the symptoms of the dumping syndrome. Lying down for 30 to 60 minutes after eating retains the meal in the stomach longer.

Special additives to delay gastric emptying are sometimes prescribed. Lying in a semirecumbent position for 90 minutes after eating and avoiding excessive exercise for 2 hours after meals can help to manage the condition. Scheduling of antihypertensive medications between rather than just before meals can be helpful as well (Malozemoff and Gentlemen, 2004).

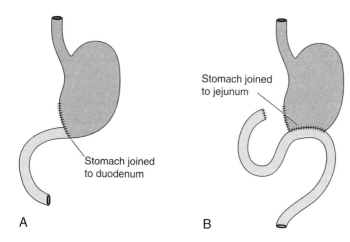

A Stomach joined to duodenum

Stomach joined to jejunum

B

Figure **22–4** Common gastric resection procedures. A, Gastroduodenostomy or Billroth I procedure; B, Gastrojejunostomy or Billroth II procedure. (Reprinted from Williams, LS, and Hopper, PD: Understanding Medical-Surgical Nursing, ed 2. FA Davis, Philadelphia, 2003, p 502, with permission.)

Table 22–5 **Diet for Dumping Syndrome**

DESCRIPTION	INDICATIONS	ADEQUACY
This diet consists of six small feedings, high in protein and low in simple sugars.	This diet and adjunct therapy, used after surgical removal of the pyloric sphincter or other treatments that speed gastric emptying, is designed to prevent rapid emptying of hypertonic gastric contents into the small intestine. Examples of such operative procedures include vagotomy, pyloroplasty, hemigastrectomy, total gastrectomy, esophagogastrectomy, Whipple's procedure, gastroenterostomy, and gastrojejunostomy. As the body adapts to its new condition, specific foods may be tolerated later in convalescence.	Deficiencies secondary to surgery or malabsorption may require supplementation. Among the nutrients likely to be needed are the vitamins B_{12}, D, and folic acid and the minerals calcium and iron.

LIFESTYLE CHANGES	CHOOSE	DECREASE
Meal pattern	Six small servings Eat slowly and chew thoroughly Lie down for 1/2 hour after meals	Fluids with meals
Adjunct therapy Food Group		
Milk	LactAid Aged cheese (>90 days)	Milk if lactose intolerant*
Breads and cereals	White, whole-wheat, rye, Jewish, Italian, and Vienna breads* Rolls, crackers, biscuits, and muffins (milk-free)* Any cooked or dry cereal, milk-free* Rice, noodles, spaghetti, macaroni	Frosted breads Sweet rolls, doughnuts, coffeecake Bread made with milk (unless tolerated)* Sugar-sweetened cereal Cereal containing milk*
Fruits	Fresh, frozen, or unsweetened canned fruits, banana Juices, fresh, frozen, canned, unsweetened, between meals only	Sweetened canned or frozen juices and fruits, dried fruit Raw fruits unless tolerated Juices with meals Those causing discomfort
Vegetables	Any as tolerated Juices between meals only	Juices with meals
Meat group	Any as tolerated	None
Fats and oils	Milk-free margarine if lactose intolerant* Oils Vegetable shortening	Any containing milk unless tolerated*
Desserts and miscellaneous	Artificially sweetened gelatin Angel food and sponge cakes Salt, pepper, spices as tolerated Mustard, catsup, pickles, relishes as tolerated Artificially sweetened beverages Decaffeinated tea and coffee, herbal tea Dietetic jam and jelly	Sugar-containing cakes, pies, cookies, ice cream,* sherbet* Seasonings that cause discomfort Caffeine-containing beverages Sugar, honey, syrup, molasses Jam, jelly Candy

SAMPLE MENU

30 Minutes Before Breakfast
Decaffeinated beverage
Artificial sweetener

Breakfast
1/2 banana
1 egg, poached
1 tsp milk-free margarine
Dietetic jelly

1 1/2 Hours After Breakfast
Orange juice
Midmorning Snack
1 slice whole-wheat toast
Dietetic jam

30 Minutes Before Lunch
1 cup LactAid

Lunch/Dinner
3 oz roast pork
Barley with butter
1/2 cup squash
1/2 cup fruit cocktail, drained

1 1/2 Hours After Meal
Decaffeinated beverage
Artificial sweetener

*If lactose restriction is necessary.

Disorders of the Intestines

Successful diagnostic studies of the bowel depend on proper preparation. It is imperative to empty the bowel for clear radiographic or endoscopic visualization. This is accomplished by laxatives and enemas. Often the client is advised to follow a low-residue diet for several days before diagnostic studies. Explaining the procedures and the necessity for them helps to gain the client's cooperation. The radiography department or the institution's diet manual lists the necessary protocols. The nurse should ensure that the client receives maximum nourishment when tests are completed for the day. Frequently, another series of tests is scheduled for the next day.

Problems With Elimination

Several problems with frequency and consistency of bowel movements are common. These include irritable bowel syndrome, diarrhea, and constipation.

Irritable Bowel Syndrome (IBS)

This condition is the most common disorder diagnosed by gastroenterologists and one of the more common ones encountered in general practice, with an overall prevalence of approximately 10 percent in most industrialized countries (Camilleri, 2001), affecting 15 million people in the United States (Sandler et al, 2002). Signs and symptoms of **irritable bowel syndrome** are diarrhea, constipation, or alternating diarrhea and constipation; abdominal pain; and flatulence. It is thought that altered gastrointestinal motility and increased sensitivity of the intestine may interact in irritable bowel syndrome, but other features, such as psychosocial factors, food intake, and prior infection, may contribute to its development (Camilleri, Heading, and Thompson, 2002). It is strongly recommended that lactose intolerance (Chapter 10), which was found and successfully treated in 24 percent of clients with irritable bowel syndrome, be excluded before diagnosing irritable bowel syndrome (Bohmer and Tuynman, 2001).

Treatment for irritable bowel syndrome is symptomatic. Offending foods should be identified and avoided. The most common foods identified are lactose and gluten, each accounting for about 40 percent of the identified causes of symptoms. In one study, more than half of clients could identify between two and five foods as creating problems (Carlson, 1998), and such identification makes the condition more manageable. Exclusion diets are time-consuming and not completely effective in identifying triggers, but an approach based on the client's immune response has had some success. Compared to clients consuming a sham diet, one excluding all foods to which the client had elevated IgG antibodies consumed for 12 weeks resulted in a 10 percent greater reduction in symptom score but a 26 percent reduction in fully compliant clients. In addition, relaxing the diet led to a 24 percent greater deterioration in symptoms in those on the true diet compared with the sham diet (Atkinson et al, 2004). For all clients, stress management techniques and bowel hygiene principles should be part of the teaching plan. A high-fiber diet, designed to avoid both constipation and increased pressure on the walls of the intestine, often provides symptomatic relief. Clients should be reassured that IBS does not harm the intestines, is unrelated to inflammatory bowel diseases (see below), and does not lead to cancer (National Digestive Diseases, 2003).

Diarrhea

Diarrhea is an important cause of morbidity and mortality in the elderly and in children (see Chapter 12). If an adult is in little jeopardy from an electrolyte imbalance, self-treatment for diarrhea following the conservative regimen listed in Table 22–6 is appropriate. Most instances of diarrhea in adults are self-limiting and resolve without treatment or the need for extensive medical work-up. On the other hand, large volumes of stool, severe abdominal pain, bloody stools, systemic symptoms such as fever, and prostration deserve investigation (Aranda-Michel and Giannella, 1999). In addition to these concerns, if the diarrhea is protracted or if a client has medical conditions for which fasting, dehydration, or infectious disease is a hazard, a physician should be consulted. In cases requiring a definite microbial cause for effective treatment, a

Table 22–6 Self-Treatment for Diarrhea*

TIME	ORAL INTAKE	COMMENTS
1st 12 h	Water or oral hydration solutions at room temperature	Easily absorbed fluids to maintain hydration
2nd 12 h	Clear liquids, no caffeine or extremes of temperature	If up to 5 percent body weight lost; if more than 5 percent lost, seek medical attention
		Very hot, very cold, or caffeinated beverages stimulate peristalsis
3rd 12 h	Full liquids	Experiment with milk in case lactose intolerance has developed
4th 12 h	Soft diet	Include applesauce or banana for **pectin;** rice, pasta, and bread without fat (digested by enzymes usually unaffected by gastroenteritis)
By 48th h	Regular diet	If diarrhea has not resolved and regular diet is not tolerated, seek medical treatment

*Appropriate for healthy adults.

new, faster method of identifying the microorganism causing infectious diarrhea involves analyzing the gases emitted from a stool specimen (Probert, Jones, and Ratcliffe, 2004).

Traveler's diarrhea, usually lasting less than 1 week, develops while a person is visiting in or just after returning from other countries. It affects 20 to 50 percent of travelers to Latin America, parts of the Caribbean, southern Asia, and Africa. To minimize risk, people should avoid drinking tap water, foods washed in water and served raw, ice, unpasteurized milk, sauces and salsas, uncooked seafood, and raw or poorly cooked meats. Foods obtained from street vendors are especially risky. Safe foods and beverages include carbonated bottled beverages, food cooked and served piping hot, and dry foods such as bread and cereal. Travelers should discuss prophylactic measures such as antibiotic prescriptions and probiotics with their health-care providers. Lactobacillus GG resists gastric acid and bile, adheres to and colonizes the bowel, and is considered a promising prophylactic agent for traveler's diarrhea (Connor and Landzberg, 2004).

Other causes of diarrhea may be iatrogenic (produced by treatment) such as tube feeding or antibiotic therapy. Total enteral nutrition supplemented with soluble fiber was shown to reduce the incidence of diarrhea in tube-fed mechanically ventilated septic patients (Spapen et al, 2001). Often yogurt or fermented milk products alleviate diarrhea accompanying antibiotic therapy by restoring microorganisms to the gut, by providing bacterial lactase to improve lactose absorption, and by increasing intestinal transit time (Heyman, 2000). In all cases, good handwashing for 30 seconds is likely to remove 95 percent of transient organisms and decrease the likelihood of transferring them to another (Musher and Musher, 2004).

Constipation

This condition is responsible for an estimated 2.5 million physician visits annually, with 100,000 referrals to gastroenterologists. The outcome of about 85 percent of these physician visits is a laxative prescription, contributing to the annual American laxative market of approximately $800 million. The average cost of diagnostic evaluation is approximately $3000, chiefly owing to colonoscopy expense (Faigel, 2002).

Each person develops a usual bowel pattern, so that a bowel movement every day or every second or third day may be perfectly normal for a given individual. **Constipation** refers to a decrease in a person's normal frequency of defecation, especially if the stool is hard, dry, or difficult to expel. It is essential that changes in bowel habits be investigated thoroughly to discover or rule out disease. Some medications, especially the taking of multiple medications, are risk factors for constipation. Opioids, diuretics, antidepressants, antihistamines, antispasmodics, anticonvulsants, and aluminum antacids were linked to the highest risk (Talley et al, 2003).

Once disease conditions have been ruled out, lifestyle changes can normalize elimination. Gradually increasing the fiber in the diet with adequate amounts of water and exercising regularly are the keys to overcoming constipa-

tion. Even laxative habits established for years can be reversed this way. A food-based remedy is highly effective in nursing home residents. The mixture is 2 cups of applesauce, 2 cups of unprocessed bran (All Bran), and 1 cup of 100 percent prune juice. The portion is 1 to 2 ounces with the evening meal. The mixture should be refrigerated and any unused amount discarded after 5 days (Gallagher-Allred, 1989). In some cases of fecal impaction, the client may experience diarrhea. Clinical Application 22–3 explains this paradox.

Problems With Absorption

Fat malabsorption may follow many diseases that damage the intestine. Celiac disease, or nontropical **sprue,** is a specific response to gluten-containing foods.

Fat Malabsorption

Several conditions hinder fat absorption. Many of the resulting symptoms are similar, despite the differences in the underlying pathology.

When fat is not well absorbed, the fat-soluble vitamins also are poorly absorbed and the fat content of the feces is increased. These extra fatty acids bind with calcium and magnesium to form soaps in the bowel. (A chemical soap results from the union of fatty acid and alkali.) The calcium bound in the soap is thus unavailable to bind with oxalate. An increased amount of oxalate is excreted through the kidney. This is not a harmless rerouting, however, because oxalate kidney stones can form as a result.

Treatment centers on careful selection of fats in the diet and appropriate supplementation of unavailable nutrients. Table 22–10 compares some food choices that are low in fat to similar items that are high in fat. Because pancreatic lipase or bile is unnecessary for their absorption, medium-chain triglycerides (MCTs) are often given to increase kilocalories. MCTs as well as amino acids and monosaccharides are absorbed into the portal vein, rather than into the lymphatic system as are other lipids. Usually MCTs are added to salad dressings, skim milk, or desserts. Because linoleic acid, an essential fatty acid, is missing from MCT, some regular fat is still needed in the diet. Supplements of the fat-soluble vitamins should be given in water-soluble form. To overcome malabsorption, the commonly used dose of supplements is twice the RDA.

Celiac Disease

An illness resembling this one was described in the first century AD. **Celiac disease** is also called **gluten-sensitive enteropathy** or nontropical sprue. It affects 1 in 133 people not at particular risk for the disease (Fasano et al, 2003) and is significantly underdiagnosed in the United States. Usually diagnosed in a child who becomes ill when cereals are added to the diet, the disease is sometimes discovered later without the classic signs and symptoms. Older children may present with short stature and adults commonly present with anemia (Israel et al, 2005). Celiac disease occurs in 10 percent of **first-degree relatives** (parent, sibling, child) of those with the disease and also in 70 percent of the identical twins of clients with the disease (Young and Thomas, 2004).

The disease is rare in blacks, Chinese, and Japanese and varies significantly by country (Connon, 1999). Because only a few genetically susceptible individuals develop celiac disease, its etiology is considered to be multifactorial involving a combination of (1) genetic predisposition, (2) ingestion of gluten, a protein in wheat, rye, and barley, and (3) an autoimmune response that produces chronic inflammation of the small intestine leading to atrophy of the intestinal villi in the jejunum (Young and Thomas, 2004). The consequence is malabsorption of all classes of nutrients except water.

The outstanding sign of celiac disease is **steatorrhea,** or excessive fat in the stools, which are foul-smelling, frothy, and bulky. Clients complain of bloating, diarrhea, and cramping abdominal pain. Some of this may be temporary as the result of lactase insufficiency. Untreated, the client's anorexia leads to weight loss and malnutrition marked by anemia, muscle wasting, edema from hypoalbuminemia, bleeding due to vitamin K deficiency, and bone pain and tetany from hypocalcemia. Clients with celiac disease, especially those who are untreated or whose disease is poorly controlled, may be at increased risk of developing osteoporosis (Kemppainen et al, 1999). The disease is not outgrown, and damage to the villi continues even without symptoms. Screening tests for specific antibodies are available and recommended for individuals at risk of the disease. Diagnosis is confirmed by small intestinal biopsy and by response to gluten-free diet (Israel et al, 2005) but the diet should not be changed until the diagnostic testing is completed (Allen, 2004).

Gluten sensitivity also has a skin manifestation, *dermatitis herpetiformis*, affecting approximately 25 percent clients with celiac disease (Collin and Reunala, 2003). Both diseases have a strong association with chromosome 6, but studies of identical twins indicate environmental factors determine the expression of this multifactorial disease (Hervonen et al, 2000).

The treatment is to remove gluten permanently from the diet. Although pure oats do not contain gluten, the grain is frequently contaminated during processing with wheat, rye, or barley. In fact, in a test of 3 brands of oats, only 25 percent of the samples would fit the definition of naturally gluten-free foods. Even oats processed in an "oats only" facility in Ireland had gluten 36 times that of gluten-free foods in one sample. Consequently, contamination of oats with wheat, barley and rye is a legitimate concern (Thompson, 2004). Removing gluten from the diet is easier said than done. It involves analyzing the label of every food the client ingests but assistance is available from the Celiac Disease Foundation at http://www.celiac.org. See Chapter 10 for an outline of a gluten-restricted diet. Fortunately, this treatment reverses the pathology almost completely, although it might take 3 to 6 months. Sometimes, secondary lactose intolerance results from mucosal damage and requires long-term management. Also, vitamin supplementation may be needed because most gluten-free products are not enriched (Thompson, 1999).

Inflammatory Bowel Diseases (IBD)

These diseases that affect approximately one million Americans (Lichtenstein, 2001) share similar characteristics but have some major differences. The two most common inflammatory bowel diseases are **Crohn's disease,** also known as *ileitis* or *regional enteritis*, and **ulcerative colitis.** Although the cause of both of these conditions is unknown, autoimmunity and genetic susceptibility may interact with the individual's environment to produce the illness. The stimulus for the abnormal immune response is likely common, nonpathogenic microorganisms in the intestine of which there are many. The digestive tract contains over 500 species of microorganisms and 100 trillion bacteria (Brown, 2005). More than 15 percent of clients with IBD have a first-degree relative with the disease (Lichtenstein and MacDermott, 2001). In addition, there is a strong and consistent association between smoking and Crohn's disease and between nonsmoking and ulcerative colitis, but the exact pathophysiological mechanisms for these associations remain unclear (Andus and Gross, 2000). Research is proceeding to identify genetic factors affecting intestinal flora and immunity to tailor individualized therapy with probiotics (Famularo et al, 2003) and to assess the anti-inflammatory effects of omega-3 fatty acids as treatments for IBD (Simopoulos, 2002).

The most common signs and symptoms of both Crohn's disease and ulcerative colitis are diarrhea, abdominal pain, and fever. Differences between the two diseases, in addition to the connection to smoking, include their locations in the gastrointestinal tract, the type of lesions involved, and complications (Table 22–7). Inflammatory bowel disease is systemic and can affect with many organs other than the bowel: liver, skin, joints, lungs, heart, kidneys, brain, and eye (Ghanchi, and Rembacken, 2003). In addition, whether due to the disease or medications such as corticosteroids prescribed for it, persons with IBD commonly have decreased bone mineral density (Lichtenstein, 2003). Clients with IBD had a 40 percent increase in fractures of the spine, hip, wrist, or rib, with a 74 percent increased risk for spinal fractures and a 59 percent increase for hip fractures (Bernstein et al, 2000). The nutritional care of clients with IBD is variable and depends on the nutritional status of the individual, the location and extent of the disease, and the nature of the surgical and medical management. In general, clients with Crohn's disease are more affected by the foods they consume than are clients with ulcerative colitis, but both groups reported

Table 22–7 **Differences Between Crohn's Disease and Ulcerative Colitis**

	CROHN'S DISEASE	ULCERATIVE COLITIS
Location	Anywhere in bowel Diseased areas alternate with healthy tissue	Large intestine Usually starts in rectum and spreads upward in continuous pattern
Lesions	Involves all layers of intestinal wall	Confined to mucosal and submucosal layers
Dietary intake	Many foods worsen symptoms	Fewer foods worsen symptoms
Environmental factors	Associated with smoking	Associated with nonsmoking
Complications	Fistula, obstruction, stricture	Toxic megacolon, fistula Increased risk of colon cancer

that bananas, carrots, potatoes, rice, roast chicken, and water did not worsen their symptoms and made them feel good (Joachim, 2000). Particularly for children with Crohn's disease, long-term enteral supplementation has extended remissions and supported growth (Griffiths, 1999).

Nutritional Therapy in Crohn's Disease

Crohn's disease may involve the small or the large intestine or both, as well as the stomach and esophagus in some cases. The emphasis of treatment is (1) to support the healing of tissue, (2) to avoid and/or prevent nutritional deficiencies, and (3) to prevent local trauma to inflamed areas. Bowel rest and TPN are as effective as corticosteroids at inducing remission for clients with active Crohn's disease, although the benefits are short-lived (Graham and Kandil, 2002). Parenteral and tube feedings may be used together or separately to meet nutritional goals. Increased frequency of Crohn's disease in Japan has been correlated with higher dietary fat intake (Hunter, 1998), leading to experiments with the amount of fat in a therapeutic diet An elemental diet promotes remission in active Crohn's disease; however, adding increasing amounts of fat as long-chain triglycerides decreases the effectiveness of the treatment (Bamba et al, 2003). When taking regular food, the client's diet is usually geared toward high-kilocaloric, high-protein, low-fat, and sometimes low-fiber or low-residue intake. Small, frequent feedings may assist in promoting comfort and adequate nutrition. Seasonings and chilled foods often aggravate symptoms. Restricting lactose is appropriate only in documented cases of intolerance.

Nutritional Therapy in Ulcerative Colitis

During an acute exacerbation of ulcerative colitis, tube feedings or total parenteral nutrition (TPN) may be given. A 4- to 6-week course of TPN achieves complete bowel rest. This choice may be necessary when the client has a fistula, obstruction, or abscess. Overall, ulcerative colitis has not been treated effectively with either elemental diets or TPN (Graham and Kandil, 2002). Dietary modification is usually based on client tolerance and avoidance of irritating foods. Despite clients' beliefs that food affected their disease course, no reported dietary behavior reduced the incidence of relapse of the illness (Jowett et al, 2004a). Parenteral supplements of iron and vitamin B_{12} may also be prescribed for these clients.

To maintain nutritional status, foods should not be eliminated from the diet without a fair trial. Restrictions should be limited to foods that produce gas or loose stools. Suspected foods should be tried in small amounts to determine tolerance levels. Early research has linked relapse from remission in ulcerative colitis to intakes of meat, particularly red and processed meat, protein, and alcohol. Compared to the lowest third, individuals in the highest third of meat consumption had three times the risk of relapse, of red and processed meats five times, of protein three times, and of alcohol 2.7 times. High sulphur or sulphate intakes were also associated with 2.8 and 2.6 times the risk of relapse (Jowett et al, 2004b). A suggested mechanism relates to colonic bacteria producing hydrogen sulfide from sulfur-containing amino acids, but further research is warranted (Magee et al, 2000; Tilg and Kaser, 2004). Work on testing the effectiveness of modifying the intestinal flora with probiotics and prebiotics is ongoing (Furrie et al, 2005; Kanauchi et al, 2005).

Surgical Treatment of Inflammatory Bowel Disease

Surgery may be recommended when inflammatory bowel disease becomes medically unmanageable. It may be curative in ulcerative colitis but is palliative in Crohn's disease. The portion of the bowel that is inflamed can be surgically resected. This results in a shorter gut. Resection of the small intestine may create additional nutritional hazards for the client (Clinical Application 22–4). A **colectomy** is the surgical removal of part or all of the colon. Other surgical procedures include ileostomy and colostomy, which may be either permanent or temporary.

In an **ileostomy,** the end of the remaining portion of the small intestine (the **ileum**) is attached to a surgically established opening in the abdominal wall called a **stoma,** from which the intestinal contents are discharged. In a **colostomy,** a part of the large intestine is resected and a stoma is created in the abdominal wall. Clients who have surgery to divert intestinal contents through the abdominal wall often suffer psychological trauma in addition to the physical change.

ILEOSTOMY

An ileostomy produces liquid drainage containing active enzymes, which irritate the skin. In addition, nutrient losses are great. A loss of as much as 2 liters of fluid per day immediately following surgery is possible. Clinical

Short Bowel Syndrome

Because the small intestine is 16 to 20 feet long in the adult, up to 50 percent can be removed, if necessary. Depending on the site of resection, the remaining bowel adjusts by becoming longer, thicker, and wider to increase its absorptive capacity. This process may take up to 6 months, however, and occurs only if the client receives food or tube feedings that stimulate gastrointestinal function. In cases in which the ileocecal valve and/or 80 percent of the small bowel is removed, the body cannot completely compensate for the loss.

Signs and symptoms of short bowel syndrome are diarrhea, weight loss, and muscle wasting. These are related to protein and fat malabsorption. Poor absorption of iron, calcium, or magnesium leads to anemia, hypocalcemia, or hypomagnesemia, respectively.

Treatment of short bowel syndrome can be intensive and requires consultation with a dietitian. Early nourishment is provided by TPN. When enteral feeding begins, elemental formulas may be chosen because they are completely absorbed in the proximal small intestine. When food is taken, it should be eaten as small low-fat meals, with medium-chain triglycerides replacing regular fats. Liquids should be taken between meals, and juices and regular soda may need to be diluted to half-strength to prevent osmotic diarrhea (Lykins and Stockwell, 1998).

In clients with intestinal failure who become intolerant to parenteral nutrition, small bowel transplantation can be a lifesaving procedure. Lengthening the small intestine by transplanting sections of a donor's small intestine is sometimes an option, but rejection rates are 50 percent or more despite the use of immunosuppressant drugs. Sepsis rates are also higher for clients who have had small bowel transplantation than for those who have received other organs because of bacterial translocation from the gut (Ghanekar and Grant, 2001).

Application 22–5 describes innovations for controlling ileostomy drainage. Over time the bowel adapts to some extent, and drainage decreases to 300 to 500 milliliters. This amount, however, is more than the 100 to 200 milliliters of water lost in the normal stool. Additional nutrient losses in ileostomy clients include sodium, potassium, and vitamin B$_{12}$.

COLOSTOMY

In contrast to an ileostomy, a colostomy after the convalescent period may be so continent that a dry dressing is all that is necessary to cover the stoma. The client may do daily irrigations or not, as the surgeon suggests. Sometimes, after the initial learning process, the client knows best.

DIETARY GUIDELINES FOR OSTOMY CLIENTS

A soft or general diet is usually served to ostomy clients after recovery from surgery. Stringy, high-fiber foods are

Continent Ileostomies

Ordinarily if an ileostomy is performed, the client must wear an appliance to contain the drainage. Other procedures afford a measure of control of the drainage. Continent ileostomies sometimes can be constructed from the remaining intestine, creating an intestinal reservoir just inside the abdominal wall. The reservoir is emptied by inserting a catheter into the stoma several times a day. Sometimes an ileoanal anastomosis is done so that the anal sphincter can be used to control elimination. Even after the bowel adapts to its shorter length, the client has 7 to 10 bowel movements per day.

It is important for the nurse to know which procedure has been performed so that the surgeon's and client's expectations can be reinforced when teaching the client.

---

initially avoided until a definite tolerance has been demonstrated. Stringy, high-fiber foods include celery, coconut, corn, cabbage, coleslaw, membranes on citrus fruits, peas, popcorn, spinach, dried fruit, nuts, sauerkraut, pineapple, seeds, and fruit and vegetable skins. Some clients avoid fish, eggs, beer, and carbonated beverages because they produce excessive odor.

Clients with ostomies should be encouraged to (1) eat at regular intervals; (2) chew food well to avoid blockage at the stoma site; (3) drink adequate amounts of fluid; (4) avoid foods that produce excessive gas, loose stools, offensive odors, and/or undesirable bulk; and (5) avoid excessive weight gain. Dietary restrictions are usually based on individual tolerance.

Diverticular Disease

A **diverticulum** (plural: diverticula) is an outpouching of intestinal membrane through a weakness in the intestine's muscular layer (Fig. 22–5). Diverticula are present in 10 percent of the U.S. population, in about 33 to 50 percent of the elderly, and in 60 percent of those older than 80. In 1998, diverticular disease was the primary diagnosis for 230,000 inpatient hospital stays and caused 3414 deaths (Sandler et al, 2002). In Western countries, diverticular disease chiefly affects the left colon, becomes more prevalent with increased age, and has been linked to a low dietary fiber intake. Right-sided diverticular disease is more common in Asian populations and affects younger clients, but its pathogenesis and relationship to left-sided diverticular disease remain unclear. Diverticular disease of the colon is the most common cause of acute lower gastrointestinal hemorrhage, which can be massive (Kang, Melville, and Maxwell, 2004).

Diverticulosis

The presence of diverticula is called **diverticulosis.** Diverticula often occur at the points at which blood vessels enter the intestinal muscle. A proposed causative factor in diverticulosis is the increased force needed to propel insufficient intestinal contents through the lumen. Often a

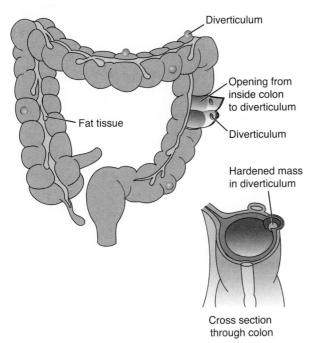

Figure **22–5** Diverticula of the transverse and descending colon. (Reprinted from Venes, D [ed]: Taber's Cyclopedic Medical Dictionary, ed 19. FA Davis, Philadelphia, 2001, p 600, by Beth Anne Willert, Dictionary Illustrator, with permission.)

person with diverticulosis has no signs or symptoms. Once an individual knows the diverticula are present, a high-fiber diet of 30 grams per day is advised. This should be accompanied by an adequate fluid intake.

Diverticulitis

When diverticula become inflamed, the condition is termed **diverticulitis.** Inflammation occurs in the elderly at about the same rate as in younger people with diverticulosis, 25 percent. Following the prescribed diet improves the condition of 85 percent of the clients.

Signs and symptoms of diverticulitis, with the exception of fever, occur in the abdomen. The client complains of cramps, pain in the lower left quadrant, dyspepsia, nausea and vomiting, distention and flatus, and alternating constipation and diarrhea. The inflammatory process can lead to adhesions or fistulas. A thickened intestinal wall from the scar tissue can cause an obstruction. Rupture of a diverticulum can initiate peritonitis. A quarter of clients with diverticulitis will develop potentially life-threatening complications, including perforation, fistulae, obstruction, or stricture (Kang, Melville, and Maxwell, 2004).

Initial therapy for uncomplicated diverticulitis is supportive, including monitoring, bowel rest, and antibiotics. While the inflammation is severe, elemental or predigested formulas or a low-fiber diet is given. After that, a high-fiber diet as for diverticulosis is prescribed. It is important that clients receive detailed instructions on the incorporation of fiber back into the diet after they have followed a low-fiber diet. Fiber should be reintroduced gradually to avoid the abdominal cramping, bloating, and gas pains that can occur with drastic changes in fiber intake. Although not proven to be helpful, avoiding foods with small seeds that could get caught in a diverticulum may be recommended.

Diseases of the Liver

Such an essential organ as the liver has sufficient reserve so that only 20 percent of its cells can carry out its functions satisfactorily (Patton and Aranda-Michel, 2002). The infiltration of liver cells by fat is called **fatty liver.** Many situations can cause fatty liver, including alcoholism and a low-protein or a starvation diet (because of the breakdown of adipose tissue for energy). Usually no harm occurs because of fatty liver unless it progresses. Treatment is to correct the cause. If it is alcohol consumption, abstinence reverses the pathology. More serious liver diseases are hepatitis and cirrhosis.

Hepatitis

Inflammation of the liver, or **hepatitis,** can result from viral infections, alcohol, drugs, or toxins. More than 50 percent of acute liver failure cases in the United States result from drug-induced injury to the liver that even occurs with therapeutic doses, most often involving a succession of unlikely events (Lee, 2003).

Three well-known viral infections are hepatitis A, hepatitis B, and hepatitis C. Hepatitis A is spread by the fecal-oral route and, rarely, by blood transfusion. It is included in Chapter 14. Hepatitis B, causing an estimated 70,000–80,000 infections yearly in the United States, is spread by body fluids such as blood, saliva, semen, and vaginal secretions and by contaminated inanimate objects. Thirty cases of acute hepatitis B, resulting in two fatalities, in three long-term care facilities in different states were traced primarily to breaks in technique for monitoring blood glucose levels. At one of the facilities, 89 percent of the residents tested by the nursing staff developed acute hepatitis B compare with 0 percent in residents who performed their own fingersticks (Centers for Disease Control, 2005).

Hepatitis C is primarily parenterally transmitted, with the highest incidence occurring in drug users and hemophilia clients. From 50 to 80 percent of persons infected with hepatitis C will develop chronic hepatitis, and 50 percent of those chronically infected develop cirrhosis or cancer of the liver (Heymann, 2004). Table 22–8 compares the occurrence, mode of transmission, high-risk populations, complications, and preventive vaccines for these three types of viral hepatitis.

Signs and Symptoms of Hepatitis

Regardless of type or cause, symptoms are anorexia, nausea, epigastric discomfort, fatigue, and weakness. Signs of hepatitis are vomiting, diarrhea, and jaundice caused by the inability of the liver to convert fat-soluble bilirubin to a water-soluble (conjugated) form. The degree of jaundice gives a rough estimate of the severity of the disease. Physical examination shows an enlarged and tender liver and an enlarged spleen.

Treatment of Hepatitis

No current medications can cure hepatitis, but combinations of interferon and antiviral drugs are being tested in

Table 22–8 Common Types of Viral Hepatitis

	HEPATITIS A	HEPATITIS B	HEPATITIS C
Occurrence	Worldwide, common in areas with poor sanitation	Worldwide, approximately 600,000 HBV-related deaths annually, about 21 percent the result of perinatal infection and 48 percent from early childhood infection	WHO estimates 2 to 3 percent of the world's population (130–170 million people) are chronically infected.
	Serologic evidence of prior infection in 33 percent of U.S. population		Estimated 12.6 million people in the Americas are serologically positive.
Usual mode of transmission	Fecal-oral: contaminated water, shellfish, raw produce	Body fluids	Parenteral equipment
	Rarely, blood products	Inanimate objects contaminated with body fluids including medical equipment, razors, toothbrushes, acupuncture and tattoo needles	Rarely, sexual contact or perinatal transmission
		Virus is stable on environmental surfaces at least 7 days	
High-risk populations	Household and sexual contacts of acute cases	Household and sexual contacts of infected persons, including perinatal	Individuals who share injecting equipment
	Contacts with diapered children in day care	Injecting drug users	Health-care workers using parenteral equipment (needle-stick accidents)
	Travelers to areas with endemic disease	Heterosexuals with multiple partners	
	Men who have sex with men	Men who have sex with men	
	Injecting drug users	Long-term international travelers in close contact with local people	
		Health-care and public-safety workers exposed to blood in their work	
		Hemodialysis clients	
Complications	Complete recovery usual but convalescence may be prolonged.	Estimated 15 to 25 percent of persons with chronic HBV will die prematurely from cirrhosis or hepatocellular carcinoma; may cause 80 percent of hepatocellular carcinoma worldwide	50 to 80 percent develop chronic infection, the progression of which is hastened by alcohol intake
	Case fatality rate: highest in adults older than 50 at 1.8 percent; about 100 deaths/year in U.S.	Case fatality rate: about 1 percent, higher in adults older than 40 years	50 percent of those chronically infected will develop cirrhosis or cancer of the liver
			HCV liver failure is the leading reason for liver transplants in the United States
Vaccine	Yes; products vary by manufacturer; none licensed for infants	Yes; believed effective for 15 years; WHO recommends universal infant vaccination with first dose within 24 hours of birth	No; the 6 genotypes and approximately 100 subtypes of the virus impedes development of effective vaccines.

SOURCE: Adapted from Bockhold, 2000; Centers for Disease Control, 2003, Heymann, 2004.

efforts to modify its course. Nevertheless, the cornerstones of treatment are bed rest, abstinence from alcohol, and optimum nutrition to permit the liver to heal. Convalescence may take from 3 weeks to 3 months. Clients on bed rest, especially debilitated clients, are more susceptible to pressure ulcers than the average client because of decreased synthesis of albumin and the globulins. If the client abstains from alcohol, the hepatitis is often reversible.

A high-kilocalorie, high-protein, moderate-fat diet is frequently prescribed for hepatitis clients. Energy intake should come from as much as 400 grams of carbohydrate daily. Protein in amounts up to 100 grams helps heal the liver. The client may tolerate emulsified fats in dairy products and eggs better than other fats. Up to 35 percent of kilocalories in fat can provide high energy in a lower volume of food. Fluid intake should be 3 to 3.5 liters per day.

Coaxing a person with hepatitis to accept such a substantial meal pattern is an enormous task because of the anorexia and nausea that accompany the disease. Since the nausea is often less in the morning than later in the day, hepatitis clients should be encouraged to eat a big breakfast. Polymeric oral feedings that are high in kilocalories and protein are widely used for between-meal feedings.

Cirrhosis of the Liver

The word cirrhosis comes from a French word for orange. In **cirrhosis** the liver becomes fibrous and contains orange-colored nodules that resemble the skin of an orange. Cirrhosis, most frequently caused by hepatitis C or alcoholism, was the twelfth leading cause of death in the United States in 2000, totaling 25,000 deaths (Gines et al, 2004). Other insults to the liver such as infection, biliary obstruction, and toxic chemicals, including drugs, may precede cirrhosis. The major nutritional effects of alcoholism are summarized in Clinical Application 22–6, and its connection to mortality is described in Clinical Application 22–7.

Several barriers interfere with alcoholism case-finding: (1) alcoholism's multiple and varied manifestations, (2) the health-care provider's personal definition and meaning of

---

Clinical Application 22–6

Nutritional Effects of Alcoholism

Alcoholism is a disease of alcohol consumption that produces tolerance, physical dependence, and characteristic organ pathology in the body. Ingestion of prodigious amounts of alcohol is not necessary for someone to become an alcoholic. The disease may be produced in some persons by 3 to 5 ounces per day of whiskey. The first notion to dispel is the cliché of the skid row alcoholic. There still are alcoholics on skid row, of course, but the disease is far more pervasive than that. In an affluent society, alcoholics may be obese, usually early in the disease rather than later, and may continue to function in several roles at work and in the family.

In the United States, alcoholism is the single most important factor in nutrient deficiencies. Associating the numerous functions of the liver with the fact that alcohol is toxic to all body cells, the nutritional havoc accompanying alcoholism becomes obvious. Even without liver damage, alcohol injures the intestine, thereby reducing absorption of vitamins A, D, K, thiamin, pyridoxine, folic acid, and B_{12}. Folic acid deficiency occurs in 50 to 80 percent of alcoholics.

The vitamin deficiency that is almost synonymous with alcoholism is that of thiamin because alcohol impedes the intestinal absorption of thiamin and in severe liver disease the metabolism and storage of thiamin is decreased. In the United States, thiamin deficiency affects 30 to 80 percent of alcoholics. The neurological symptoms of thiamin deficiency, called *dry beriberi*, present a disheartening picture. Clients have atrophy of many nerves, weakness in the ankles and toes, and numbness and tingling in the feet. Even more serious is wet beriberi, in which cardiac symptoms predominate. The severe form of wet beriberi, *shoshin wet beriberi*, can rapidly lead to heart failure and carries a high mortality rate (Smith, 1998).

The behavior of an intoxicated person readily shows that alcohol penetrates the blood-brain barrier. In fact, brain damage may occur before severe liver damage. The **Wernicke-Korsakoff syndrome** is a disorder of the central nervous system that is caused by thiamin deficiency and is diagnosed predominantly in alcoholics but also occasionally in malnourished clients with no history of alcohol abuse,

including women with hyperemesis gravidarum. Perhaps it is underdiagnosed in nonalcoholics because it is not considered. In one study, half the clients were not alcoholics and two of them were only diagnosed on autopsy (Ogershok et al, 2002). Clients with Wernicke-Korsakoff syndrome display disorientation, memory dysfunction, and **ataxia.** Weakness of the muscles that control the eyes produces double vision (*diplopia*) and abnormal movements of the eyeball (*nystagmus*). Thiamin is involved in the production of energy from glucose and helps oxidize glucose to form a compound that stores energy. This is a critical piece of information for health-care providers who care for alcoholic clients. Administering a simple solution of glucose intravenously can precipitate symptoms of Wernicke-Korsakoff syndrome if the client is thiamin-deficient. For this reason, thiamin is routinely administered parenterally to alcoholics. Because magnesium appears to be necessary for thiamin utilization, parenteral administration of this mineral is advised for shoshin wet beriberi (Smith, 1998).

Other vitamin deficiencies in alcoholics, in order of frequency after folic acid and thiamin, are of vitamin B_6, niacin, vitamin C, and vitamin A. Niacin deficiency occurs in one-third of alcoholics. Scurvy in the United States is almost exclusively found in alcoholics. Vitamin C, besides being necessary for tissue repair, plays a role in folic acid metabolism and in iron absorption. Storage of vitamin A in the liver is impaired. Visual impairment, abnormal adaptation to darkness, has been reported in 50 percent of alcoholics with cirrhosis and 15 percent of those without it (Feinman and Lieber, 1999).

Other nutritional effects possible in alcoholics are bone loss and bleeding tendencies. One-half of alcoholics show bone loss. Albumin carries calcium in the bloodstream. Hypoalbuminemia, reduced stores and faulty metabolism of vitamin D and vitamin K, low calcium intake, and steatorrhea causing binding of calcium in the intestine may all combine to produce bone loss. Several clotting factors, including prothrombin, are normally manufactured by the liver using vitamin K, but the process is impaired in alcoholism. Vitamin E deficiency, as well as thiamin deficiency, produces neurological changes, cerebellar degeneration, and peripheral neuropathy.

(Continued on the following page)

Nutritional Effects of Alcoholism

Potassium, phosphorus, and magnesium are the most common major mineral deficiencies in alcoholics. Electrolyte status should be monitored during treatment. (See refeeding syndrome in Chapter 24.) Insufficient magnesium impairs central nervous system activity and increases muscular excitability and therefore is suggested to exacerbate the increased neuroirritability displayed by clients in acute alcohol withdrawal. Iron and zinc are the trace minerals most often deficient in alcoholics. Low iron stores are related to gastrointestinal bleeding rather than poor absorption. Alcohol damages the intestinal mucosa and thereby permits increased absorption of iron. With low folic acid levels, however, red blood cell production cannot proceed normally. Anemia or bone marrow abnormalities have been found in 75 percent of clients hospitalized with alcoholism. Up to 50 percent of alcoholic clients are deficient in zinc. Zinc deficiency in alcoholic liver disease

has been associated with changes in smell, taste, and protein metabolism (Patton and Aranda-Michel, 2002). Zinc is needed for many enzymes that function in DNA and RNA metabolism, for the growth and repair of essential organs, and for the conversion of vitamin A to a functional form in the retina.

Finally, alcoholics suffer from protein-energy malnutrition. Even in early alcoholism, albumin levels are low-normal. The typical alcoholic consumes only 75 percent of required energy. The result of low-protein, low-energy intake is muscle wasting. Fat is not an adequate source of energy for alcoholics, owing to malabsorption as evidenced by steatorrhea that occurs in half the clients.

Awareness of the wide range of nutritional effects of alcoholism should help the nurse to focus on early case finding. Interruption of the downward spiral in health caused by alcohol could literally be lifesaving.

---

alcoholism, and (3) denial by the client and family. The CAGE questionnaire shown in Clinical Application 22–8 is a brief, effective screening tool to identify possible alcohol abusers.

Alcohol Contributes to Mortality

Excessive alcohol consumption is the third leading preventable cause of death in the United States and is associated with multiple adverse health consequences, including liver cirrhosis, various cancers, unintentional injuries, and violence. In 2001, excessive alcohol use was responsible for approximately 75,000 preventable deaths, including 13,674 from motor vehicle accidents, all of which were attributable to binge alcohol use defined as more than five drinks per occasion for men or four for women. In the same year, alcohol-attributable deaths included 7655 homicides, 6969 suicides, and 4766 due to falls (Centers for Disease Control, 2004a). Studies have shown that clients treated in general hospitals are unlikely to be diagnosed with an alcohol use disorder even when arriving at the hospital with a blood alcohol greater than 0.3 g/dL, more than three times the legal limit (Bostwick and Seaman, 2004; Smothers, Yahr, and Ruhl, 2004).

Alcohol can be immediately lethal if a large quantity of ethanol (or a smaller quantity of alcohols not intended for beverages) is consumed in a short period of time. Alcohol poisoning is especially heart-breaking when it kills a young person whose companions let the victim "sleep it off" through ignorance or fear of retribution. Teaching young people about the hazards of alcohol and counseling adult clients about the responsible use of alcohol are nursing functions in all settings. These interventions may be appropriate for friends and family members as well as for clients.

Pathophysiology

Alcohol needs no digestion. It is absorbed rapidly, 20 percent from the stomach and 80 percent from the small intestine. Immediately after absorption, the alcohol is carried throughout the body. In the liver, it is metabolized at the rate of 1/2 ounce of alcohol per hour. This refers to the alcohol content, not the whole beverage. This rate cannot be rushed, and giving coffee or other stimulants to an inebriated person induces not sobriety but merely wide-awake intoxication.

If the liver is not able to repair the damage, dying liver cells are replaced by scar tissue. Figure 22–6 traces the path from cell death to several cardinal signs of cirrhosis. Because the liver has multiple functions, one pathological change reinforces another. The **ascites** is worsened by hypoalbuminemia and is partly caused by and also worsened by sodium retention. Depressed plasma protein production, as evidenced by decreasing albumin levels, indicates a poor client outcome. A consideration in prescribing medications is the fact that the cirrhotic liver may reduce the rate of metabolism of drugs by as much as 50 percent (Lee, 2003).

Signs and Symptoms of Cirrhosis

Cirrhosis causes anorexia, epigastric pain, and nausea that worsens as the day goes on. Signs of the disease are abdominal distention, vomiting, steatorrhea, jaundice, ascites, edema, and gastrointestinal bleeding. Of clients with advanced cirrhosis, 70 percent develop esophageal varices (varicose veins of the esophagus) that cause hemorrhage in 25 to 35 percent of clients with cirrhosis. In as many as 30 percent of the clients, the first hemorrhage proves to be fatal (Sharara and Rockey, 2001). The muscle tremors that are seen frequently are attributed to hypomagnesemia. Laboratory tests show hypoglycemia and elevated serum triglyceride levels. The lack of enzymes for

CAGE Questionnaire for Identifying the Alcohol Abuser

The following instrument has been extensively validated against the psychiatric diagnostic criteria for alcoholism and alcohol abuse. Using one or more "yes" answers as indicative of alcohol abuse, the CAGE questionnaire's sensitivity was 86 percent and its specificity 93 percent in a walk-in clinic (Liskow et al, 1995). **Sensitivity** is the proportion of people correctly identified by the test as having the disease. **Specificity** is the proportion of people correctly identified by the test as not having the disease. Using two or more "yes" answers in hospitalized clients yielded a sensitivity of 76 percent and a specificity of 94 percent (Beresford et al, 1990). The designer of the questionnaire recommended that even one "yes" answer merits further inquiry (Ewing, 1984). Since the prevalence rate of alcoholism is 20 to 30 percent in clinical settings, a CAGE score of 1 is recommended there (Liskow et al, 1995). The CAGE questionnaire is a screening instrument to identify a need for a diagnostic workup. Its advantages are its simplicity and its proven accuracy in clinical studies.

C—Have you ever had a need to CUT BACK on your drinking?

A—Have people ANNOYED YOU with criticism about your drinking?

G—Have you ever felt GUILTY about your drinking?

E—Have you ever needed to start the day with a drink? (an EYE-OPENER)

Other screening instruments are available. No screening tool is perfect, but the key is to pick one and use it routinely since an estimated 10 percent of the population abuses drugs or alcohol (Mersy, 2003).

converting noncarbohydrate sources to energy causes hypoglycemia. Insufficient lipoprotein synthesis causes the elevated triglycerides and fatty liver. The end result of cirrhosis is liver failure, which leads to hepatic coma (Clinical Application 22–9).

Dietary Treatment of Cirrhosis

Abstinence from alcohol improves the outcome of all stages of alcoholic liver disease (Diehl, 2002). A protein-restricted diet may be prescribed when the liver cannot process the end products of protein metabolism but is used only in special circumstances such as hepatic encephalopathy. For the most part, clients with chronic liver disease are protein-depleted due to deranged metabolism, and the deficiency worsens as the disease progresses (Patton and Aranda-Michel, 2002) despite the body's need for protein to aid liver regeneration. Blood ammonia levels are tested frequently to assess the client's ability to metabolize dietary protein effectively. Sufficient kilocalories must be provided to prevent catabolism of tissue protein for energy. Simple carbohydrates are encouraged in frequent meals, including a midnight snack to

decrease overnight **gluconeogenesis** (Patton and Aranda-Michel, 2002). Enough fat is offered for palatability. Dietary fats that are already emulsified, such as those in homogenized milk and eggs, need less bile for digestion than other fats. Esophageal varices necessitate a soft diet.

Fluid and electrolyte balance demands ongoing attention. If the client has ascites, sodium probably will be restricted. A limitation of 600 to 800 milligrams per day is recommended because more stringent restriction is not well tolerated and, if the client has dilutional hyponatremia, fluid intake is also controlled (Gines et al, 2004). Monitoring the improvement or progression of ascites includes measuring abdominal girth and daily weighing. If the client has ascites without peripheral edema, a reasonable goal for weight loss is 0.5 kilogram (1.1 pounds) per day. If both ascites and peripheral edema are displayed, the goal for weight loss is 1 kilogram per day.

Table 22–9 displays various protein-controlled diets that assume the client tolerates fats. Extensive low-protein exchange lists have been developed to treat liver failure. The dietary management of these clients, particularly those with end-stage liver disease, is complex and constantly changing, requiring the services of a dietitian. Because of the high risk of vitamin deficiencies, cirrhosis clients are given pharmaceutical supplements. Up to five times the RDA of water-soluble vitamins may be necessary.

Gallbladder Disease

On the underside of the liver is a small pouch-like organ called the **gallbladder.** Its function is to concentrate and store bile until it is needed for digestion. The liver secretes 600 to 800 milliliters of bile per day that the gallbladder reduces to 60 to 160 milliliters.

Gallbladder disease was specified as the primary diagnosis for 434,000 hospital stays and caused 1143 deaths in 1998 (Sandler et al, 2002). The presence of gallstones is called **cholelithiasis.** One-fifth of adults over 40 years of age and one-third over 70 have gallstones, but one-third of these individuals with gallstones are asymptomatic. Most gallstones form when the bile is too scant or too concentrated or contains excessive cholesterol. When the gallbladder becomes inflamed (from irritation by the stones in 90 percent of the cases or by parasitic infection or prolonged fasting associated with TPN following severe injuries (termed *acalculous cholecystitis*), the condition is labeled **cholecystitis.**

Causative Factors

Heredity and hypercholesterolemia are associated with gallstones, whereas cardiovascular disease and diabetes mellitus, both related to heredity and hypercholesterolemia, are associated with gallbladder disease. Women are three times more likely than men to have gallbladder disease. A definite nutritional link is obesity, and a tentative link is the low serum levels of ascorbic acid found in women with gallbladder disease (Simon and Hudes, 2000). For both men and women nuts seem to have a protective effect in that consumption of 5 or more ounces of nuts per week was associated with decreased risk of symptomatic

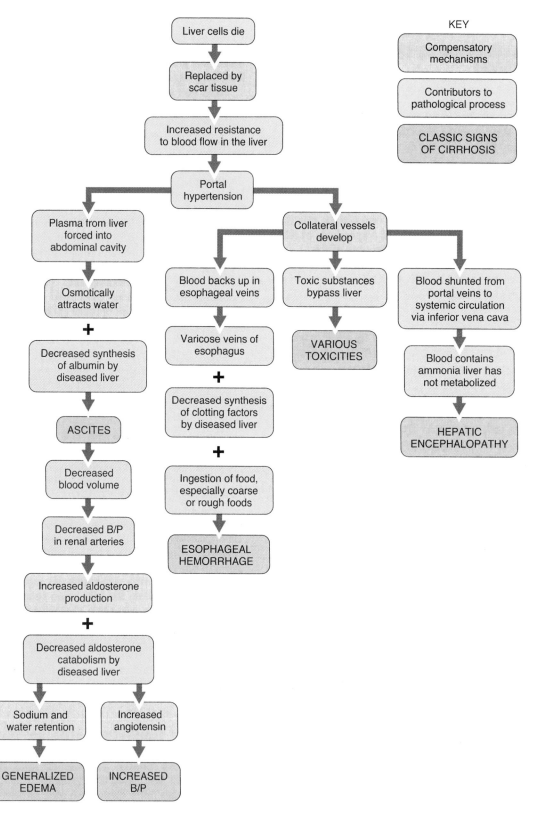

Figure 22–6 Progression of pathology leading to the classic signs and symptoms of cirrhosis of the liver. Many other manifestations appear given the multiple functions of the liver.

Hepatic Encephalopathy

Hepatic encephalopathy results from liver failure, but the precise mechanism involved in the pathology is uncertain; however, increased serum levels of ammonia and aromatic amino acids are associated with the disorder, and treatments to control one or both of these factors have been suggested. Because elevated serum ammonia levels interfere with normal mentation, the nurse should be cautious when interpreting interview data obtained from the client.

Ammonia is produced by intestinal bacteria and by digestive enzymes breaking down protein. Even if the person consumes no protein foods, the bacteria work on the cast-off cells of the gastrointestinal tract and on the blood from gastrointestinal bleeding, which is common in alcoholic cirrhosis. Ordinarily, the liver degrades ammonia to urea, which is then excreted in urine by the kidneys, but in liver failure, blood ammonia levels rise. Ammonia is toxic to all cells, including those of the liver and the brain. The laboratory values are not clearly correlated with the degree of encephalopathy, so a series of tests is necessary to monitor each client. Hypokalemia with resulting alkalosis, for instance, causes ammonia retention in the brain.

The liver normally breaks down amino acids. The client with liver failure exhibits a change in the ratio of aromatic amino acids (phenylalanine, tryptophan, and tyrosine) to branched-chain amino acids (leucine, isoleucine, lysine, and valine) because the branched-chain amino acids are not as dependent on liver metabolism as the aromatic amino acids are (Patton and Aranda-Michel, 2002). In the healthy client, this ratio is approximately 1:1, whereas in hepatic coma, it is 3:1 or higher, aromatic to branched-chain. The elevated levels of aromatic amino acids are thought to contribute to hepatic coma by interfering with the formation of the neurotransmitters dopamine and norepinephrine.

In hepatic encephalopathy, the damaged liver can no longer remove neurotoxic substances such as ammonia and manganese from the blood. When these molecules enter the brain, they can interfere with normal neurotransmitter activity, impair motor functions, and alter the structure of the **astrocytes** (Butterworth, 2003). Because of its clinical similarity to hepatic encephalopathy, manganese toxicity is proposed as a mechanism that contributes to the manifestations of both these conditions, and increased manganese levels in the brain have been recorded on autopsy of clients who succumbed to hepatic encephalopathy (Chetri and Choudhuri, 2003).

Some signs of hepatic encephalopathy can be observed before the onset of coma, including personality changes, irritability, weakness, apathy, confusion, and sleepiness. More specific signs are asterixis and fetor hepaticus. *Asterixis*, or liver flap, refers to involuntary jerking movements or a flapping of the hand when the arm is outstretched. *Fetor hepaticus* is a fecal odor to the breath. Finally, coma occurs.

Treatment consists of medications and dietary modifications, along with symptomatic care. Oral neomycin or metronidazole kill the bacteria in the intestine, thereby decreasing ammonia production, but this is short-term therapy due to side effects (Abou-Assi and Vlahcevic, 2001). Lactulose acidifies the large intestine, causing ammonia to be converted to ammonium ions, which are not absorbed but eliminated in the feces.

Limitation of protein in the diet to 40 to 60 grams of high-quality protein may be useful for short periods but is not recommended long-term because of potential worsening of already poor nutrition (Abou-Assi and Vlahcevic, 2001). The diet must be carefully planned. Some foods produce higher ammonia levels than most others. These include chicken, salami, ground beef, ham, gelatin, peanut butter, potatoes, onions, and buttermilk, as well as blue, American, and cheddar cheeses (Rudman et al, 1973). Because they contain fewer aromatic amino acids, vegetable proteins may be tolerated better than animal protein. Branched-chain amino acids have been administered orally or parenterally in attempts to treat hepatic encephalopathy. This therapy is not recommended routinely but may benefit protein-intolerant clients with chronic encephalopathy (Lieber, 1999) or children (Patton and Aranda-Michel, 2002). If enteral feeding is necessary, special preparations low in aromatic amino acids are available. Two of them are Hepatic-Aid II and Travasorb-Hepatic. Aspartame (NutraSweet) contains phenylalanine, an aromatic amino acid. If the theory holds, it too should be avoided.

---

gallstones in men and with decreased risk of cholecystectomy in women (Tsai et al, 2004a, 2004b).

Other risk factors for gallbladder disease include ileal disease or resection, long-term TPN, multiple pregnancies, and oral contraceptive use. Abnormal smooth musculature contractility, impaired gallbladder motility, and increased stasis contribute to the development of cholesterol gallstones (Portincasa, Di Ciaula, and vanBerge-Henegouwen, 2004). A long fast between the evening meal and the first meal of the next day could be modified by a light bedtime snack and/or by drinking two glasses of water on arising if breakfast will be delayed. Either practice stimulates the gallbladder to empty, thus decreasing the likelihood of very concentrated bile.

Symptoms and Treatment of Gallbladder Disease

The cardinal symptom of gallbladder disease is pain after ingestion of fat caused by spasms of the gallbladder. The pain is located in the right upper quadrant and often radiates to the right shoulder.

Asymptomatic gallstones are just observed except in certain situations thought to increase risk for gallbladder

Table 22–9 **Protein-Controlled Diets for Liver Disease**

DESCRIPTION	INDICATIONS	ADEQUACY
Although not the main therapy, these diets are prescribed to help attain and maintain normal amino acid balance, reduce blood ammonia levels, and improve clinical status. In addition to protein, sodium and fluid may be restricted. Branched chain amino acids that are chiefly metabolized in skeletal muscle may be given as a supplement.	These diets are used in severe liver disease such as acute hepatitis, advanced cirrhosis, or intractable hepatic encephalopathy.	The diets may not meet the RDA for B-complex vitamins, especially folic acid, calcium, and iron. Supplemental vitamins may be prescribed.

20-GRAM PROTEIN DIET (RARELY USED. MOST CLIENTS CAN TOLERATE AND NEED 40 TO 60 GRAMS.)

40-GRAM PROTEIN DIET

Meal Plan	Sample Menu	
Breakfast		To 20-Gram add:
1/2 cup milk	1/2 cup whole milk	1/2 cup milk
1 fruit	1/2 cup orange juice with 2 tbsp modular carbohydrate supplement†	2 meat exchanges
2 starches	1/2 cup Cream of Wheat with 1 tbsp modular carbohydrate supplement and 1 slice of toast with 1 tbsp margarine and jelly	1 starch exchange
		60-GRAM PROTEIN DIET
Fat (as tolerated)	2 tbsp cream	
Beverage	As tolerated and per fluid restriction	To 20-Gram add:
Lunch		2 cups milk
2 starches	1 cup rice with 1/4 cup unsalted tomato sauce and 1 tbsp olive oil	3 meat exchanges
Vegetable	1/2 cup green beans with 1 tsp margarine	1 starch exchange
Fruit	1/2 cup canned peaches with 1 tbsp modular carbohydrate supplement	1 vegetable exchange
		80-GRAM PROTEIN DIET
Beverage	As tolerated and per fluid restriction	
Dinner		To 20-Gram add:
2 starches	1 baked potato with 2 tbsp sour cream and 1 slice of bread with 1 tsp margarine and jelly	2 cups milk
Vegetable	1/2 cup mushrooms (for potato topping)	5 meat exchanges
Fruit	1/2 cup strawberries with 1 tbsp modular carbohydrate supplement	4 starch exchanges
Beverage	As tolerated and per fluid restriction	1 vegetable exchange

†Polycose, Sumacal, and Moducal are all modular carbohydrate supplements.

cancer: a calcified gallbladder, large gallstones, large polyps, and some Pima Indians (Simpson, Yen, and Ahmed, 2002). Surgery is the preferred option to treat symptomatic gallbladder disease, but medical management may be recommended for individuals who are poor surgical risks.

Dietary Modifications

During an acute attack, a full-liquid diet with minimal fat is recommended. For chronic gallbladder disease, the client should limit fat and obese clients should lose weight. Some clients obtain relief with the restriction of dietary fat; others do not. A reasonable approach to fat restriction is (1) to select skim milk dairy products, (2) to limit fats or oils to 3 teaspoons per day, and (3) to consume no more than 6 ounces of very lean meat per day. Gas-forming foods also are often poorly tolerated.

Another approach is to eliminate foods that cause symptoms. Clients usually can identify foods that cause them pain. Fried foods are the worst offenders. Table 22–10 identifies some foods that are low in fat and some that are high in fat.

Medical and Surgical Interventions

New procedures have been devised to treat gallstones without traditional surgery. One technique involves agents to dissolve the stones, some taken orally and some injected directly into the gallbladder. Another method is to break up the stones using shock waves through a procedure called *lithotripsy.* Clients and physicians still may opt for removal of the stones through an incision, a *cholecystotomy,* or for removal of the gallbladder, *cholecystectomy,* through a laparoscope or the traditional abdominal incision.

Postoperative diet routines are similar to those for other gastrointestinal surgery. When the client begins to take oral nourishment, clear liquids are given for 24 hours. The diet is progressed as tolerated. Because bile enters the duodenum continuously, balanced meals should be well tolerated. Many clients can eat a regular diet without diffi-

Table 22–10 **Comparison of Fat Content of Selected Foods**

LOW-FAT FOODS	FAT (g)	HIGH-FAT FOODS	FAT (g)
Starch/Breads			
Angel food cake, 1/12	<1	Pecan pie, 1/6 of pie	24
Italian bread, 1 slice	<1	Bread stuffing, 1/2 cup	13
English muffin, 1	1	Danish pastry	12
Raisin toast, 1 slice	1	Croissant, 1	12
Pancake, 4-inch, 1	2	Glazed raised doughnut, 1	13
Meats, Fish, and Poultry			
Beef round, 3 oz lean roasted	9	Beef prime rib, 3 oz lean only	24
Chicken breast, 3 oz roasted, without skin	9	Chicken, deep-fried thigh, 1	14
Boiled ham, 3 oz	9	Spare ribs, 3 oz	24
Tuna, 1/2 cup water-packed	6	Tuna, 1/2 cup oil-packed, drained	24
Fruits and Vegetables			
Banana, 8 3/4 inch long, 1	1	Avocado, 1	30
Raisins, 1 cup	1	Coconut, dried, 1 cup	50
Potato, baked, 1	<1	French fried potato, 2 × 3 1/2 inches, 15 pieces	12
Onion, raw, sliced, 1 cup	<1	French fried onion rings, 4	10
Milk Products			
Cottage cheese, 1 percent, 1/2 cup	1	Cottage cheese, 4 percent, 1/2 cup	5
Mozzarella, part skim, 1 oz	5	Cheddar, 1 oz	9
Skim milk, with added milk solids, 1 cup	1	Whole milk, 1 cup	8
Frozen yogurt, low-fat, 1 cup	4	Ice cream, regular, hard, vanilla, 1 cup	14
*Fast Foods**			
Arby's			
Junior Roast Beef sandwich	9	Beef 'n' Cheddar sandwich	21
McDonald's			
Hamburger	10	Quarter pounder with cheese	29
Subway			
6-inch Roast beef	5	6-inch Classic tuna	19
Wendy's			
Chicken Grill sandwich	7	Spicy Chicken Fillet sandwich	19

*Check with the restaurant. Recipes may be revised.

culty 1 month after surgery. Clients who become nauseated and suffer pain after eating certain foods preoperatively, however, may continue to avoid them postoperatively because of the association.

Diseases of the Pancreas

In addition to the endocrine secretions insulin, glucagon, and somatostatin, the **pancreas** secretes amylase, lipase, trypsin, and chymotrypsin. Pancreatic disease was recorded as the primary diagnosis for 211,000 inpatient hospital stays and caused 3195 deaths in 1998 (Sandler et al, 2002). Among the disorders of the pancreas are pancreatitis and cystic fibrosis.

Pancreatitis

When the blood vessels of the pancreas become abnormally permeable, plasma and plasma protein leak into the interstitial spaces. The resulting edema damages the pancreatic cells. Normally, the pancreatic enzymes necessary for digestion are inactive in the pancreas and become activated only upon entering the duodenum; otherwise, the active enzymes would digest the pancreas itself. In **pancre-**

atitis, the retained pancreatic enzymes, especially trypsin, become activated and do digest the pancreatic tissue.

Alcoholism is the most common cause of pancreatitis, generating up to 75 percent of the cases. Other conditions that can lead to pancreatitis are biliary tract disease or surgery; stomach surgery; and the administration of cancer chemotherapy, steroids, thiazides, or estrogens. In some cases, viral infection, pregnancy, or trauma has preceded pancreatitis. The characteristic symptom of pancreatitis is excruciating pain in the left upper quadrant. Nausea and vomiting accompany an attack. Laboratory tests reveal elevated levels of serum amylase and lipase.

In the treatment of pancreatitis, the client is advised to avoid alcohol. An acutely ill client is usually allowed nothing by mouth for 24 to 48 hours to reduce secretions. A nasogastric tube is used to suction stomach contents. Ice chips may be prescribed to lessen dryness of the mouth. Special ice chips may be made by freezing electrolyte solutions to circumvent the loss of gastric secretions that is stimulated by plain water or ice chips made with plain water. Increased secretions when administering gastric suction only escalates electrolyte losses. If necessary, the client is maintained on intravenous or TPN feedings until the acute phase subsides. Enteral administration of nutrients into the distal jejunum avoids the stimulation of pancreatic secretions and does not exacerbate the disease. Moreover, hypocaloric jejunal elemental enteral feeding was shown to be safer and less expensive than parenteral feeding and bowel rest in clients with acute pancreatitis, although enteral feeding was less effective in meeting estimated nutritional requirements (Abou-Assi, Craig, and O'Keefe, 2002).

When the pain subsides and bowel sounds return, oral intake is started. Clear liquids are given, progressing to a low-fat, high-carbohydrate diet. The use of elemental formulas may be necessary. Medium-chain triglycerides may be a better-tolerated source of fats than normal dietary fats. Six small meals per day constitute the usual pattern. The client's comfort level is monitored, and serum amylase concentrations are periodically checked. If the client's condition worsens, the acute-care regimen is reinstituted.

Acute pancreatitis may or may not progress to chronic pancreatitis. For chronic pancreatitis clients, alcohol is not recommended. Fat restriction similar to that for gallbladder disease may be helpful. Pancreatic enzymes can be given orally before or with meals to aid digestion. Because pancreatitis clients do not absorb vitamin B_{12} adequately, it is given parenterally.

Cystic Fibrosis

The most common cause of pancreatic insufficiency in children and young adults is **cystic fibrosis,** occurring in 1 of every 2500 live births. One in 20 whites carries the gene for this autosomal recessive disorder, which is the most common genetically inherited lethal disease in North America (Anselmo et al, 2004). This gene (*CFTR for cystic fibrosis transmembrane conductance regulator*) encodes for a protein that is thought to play a role in ion transport, mucus flow, inflammation, and bacterial adherence. More than 1,300 CRTR gene mutations have been associated with cystic fibrosis but the most common mutation is present in 90 percent of clients with cystic fibrosis in the United States (Rowe, Miller, and Sorscher, 2005). The FDA has approved the first DNA-based blood test to help detect cystic fibrosis but because the test detects a limited number of the more than 1300 genetic variations identified in the CFTR gene, the test should not be the sole measure used to diagnose cystic fibrosis (U.S. Food and Drug Administration, 2005).

The median estimated life expectancy of children with cystic fibrosis born in 1990 is 40 years, double the estimate of 20 years ago, and nearly half of all clients are now adults (Jaffe and Bush, 2001). In the United States, the median age of death from cystic fibrosis in 2000 was 24 years (Centers for Disease Control, 2004b). As a marker of mortality risk, height below the fifth percentile for age predicted significantly shorter lives than those attained by taller clients (Beker et al, 2001). Sometimes diagnosis is delayed until adulthood, when respiratory symptoms lead to a search for a definitive cause. As might be expected, those diagnosed after the age of 18 years suffer fewer complications and require less-intensive treatment than those diagnosed as children (Widerman et al, 2000).

Pathophysiology

The chief cause of morbidity and mortality in cystic fibrosis is obstruction of exocrine glands with mucus. Deficient chloride transport in the lungs is thought to result in the production of abnormally thick mucus (Centers for Disease Control, 2004b). The stagnant secretions then become a hospitable environment for bacteria. Fifty percent of children with cystic fibrosis have lung symptoms, and lung infection is the most common cause of death.

Pancreatic insufficiency, resulting from virtually absent pancreatic enzyme activity, is present at diagnosis among 80 percent or more of persons with cystic fibrosis and increases with age to 90 percent (Centers for Disease Control, 2004b). Pancreatic insufficiency causes fat and protein malabsorption, leading to stunted growth (deficit in height for age). The sign of cystic fibrosis related to the gastrointestinal tract is the passage of bulky, fatty, foul-smelling feces. This is caused by the impaired fat digestion. With increased life expectancy, more cystic fibrosis clients display hyperglycemia or diabetes mellitus.

The sweat of a cystic fibrosis client has more sodium chloride than normal. A sweat chloride level greater than 60 milliequivalents per liter is diagnostic of cystic fibrosis, but other criteria in combination also can be used (Centers for Disease Control, 2004b). The high electrolyte content of the sweat also puts the client at increased risk of imbalance during hot weather or fever.

Treatment of Cystic Fibrosis

Supportive care is the foundation of cystic fibrosis treatment. Pulmonary congestion and infections are treated as required. The client's energy needs may be double those of others the same age. When the lungs are involved, much of the client's energy is expended in respiratory effort. Because starches require amylase for digestion, carbohydrates in the form of simple sugars are a better source of energy. Even if the client also has diabetes mellitus, the diet will include more simple sugars than the usual diet for diabetes mellitus. Intensive therapy of the diabetes mellitus can be maintained with self-monitoring of blood glucose and multiple doses of insulin.

For cystic fibrosis clients, protein needs are double those of other individuals. Fat content should be as high as possible because it is a concentrated energy source. If necessary, medium-chain triglycerides can be used to increase fat intake without overtaxing the weak digestive system. Gastrostomy feedings, whether delivered continuously overnight or by bolus in daytime, produced significant improvements in weight and height in children (Rosenfeld et al, 1999).

Depending on the extent of pancreatic insufficiency, the client is given pancreatic enzymes orally. It is important to administer these enzyme-replacing drugs as directed with or before meals or snacks. Vitamin status can be monitored and supplementation tailored to the client's needs. Fat-soluble vitamins are supplemented in water-miscible form. Riboflavin needs are increased because of the client's high energy expenditure. Riboflavin deficiency manifesting as stomatitis was diagnosed in three children, 2 to 10 years old, with cystic fibrosis, two of whom had been receiving overnight gastrostomy feedings. In addition, the children had deficiencies of thiamin, pyridoxine, and iron (McCabe, 2001). Vitamin A should be readily available to help maintain the integrity of the respiratory and gastrointestinal mucosa. Vitamin K is required, because frequent courses of antibiotics kill the intestinal flora. Mineral intake is watched carefully if the weather is hot or the client is feverish. Extra salt is given if sweat losses are increased. Zinc levels often are low because of fecal losses, and deficiency of zinc contributes to failure of bone growth and to increased susceptibility to infection.

As of 2004, nine states (Colorado, Massachusetts, Mississippi, New Jersey, New York, Oklahoma, South Carolina, Wisconsin, and Wyoming) had implemented or planned to begin universal newborn screening programs for cystic fibrosis. Early diagnosis from screening produces long-term improvements in height for age and reductions in chronic malnutrition; however, screening tests are not perfect, so health-care providers need to be alert to the possibility of cystic fibrosis if the clinical signs and symptoms warrant, even if the screening test was negative (Centers for Disease Control, 2004b).

SUMMARY

Diseases of other body systems may be more immediately life threatening, but over the long term, gastrointestinal diseases can profoundly affect quality of life and life expectancy. Health-care workers should make nutrition a priority for clients undergoing diagnostic tests or surgery. Medications have revolutionized the treatment of peptic ulcers. If the client does have a gastrectomy and develops dumping syndrome, he or she should receive frequent dry meals that are low in simple sugars and should lie down after eating. Similar interventions are used for the elderly person with postprandial hypotension. In contrast, clients with hiatal hernias may be more comfortable if they remain upright after meals.

Celiac disease and cystic fibrosis are gastrointestinal diseases found in children as well as in adults. In celiac disease, gluten destroys the intestinal villi, causing major malabsorption problems. In cystic fibrosis, thick glandular secretions plug the pancreatic ducts, causing malabsorption, and the excessive mucus produced in the lungs is life threatening. Nourishing clients with Crohn's disease and ulcerative colitis poses significant challenges. Use of elemental formulas or total parenteral nutrition is sometimes necessary to permit healing. In intractable cases, colon resection and ileostomy or colostomy may be performed. This drastic surgery presents a new set of management problems, including fluid balance, odor control, and skin integrity.

Because of its multiple functions, the liver, when diseased, produces varied and severe consequences. The different types of hepatitis can be transmitted by food, by body fluids and wastes, and sometimes by inanimate objects. Complete recovery is the usual outcome of hepatitis A, but hepatitis B is thought to cause 80 percent of hepatocellular cancer. Vaccines are available to prevent these two types of hepatitis. Hepatitis C often progresses to a chronic infection that significantly increases the risk

of cancer of the liver or cirrhosis. In cirrhosis, the liver becomes scarred, hard, and increasingly nonfunctional. The result is portal hypertension, absorption of toxins through collateral channels, esophageal varices, ascites, bleeding problems, and possible hepatic coma. Alcohol abuse underlies most, but not all, cases of cirrhosis and pancreatitis. Treatment is abstinence and supportive therapy, with diet modifications geared to the client's current clinical status.

Of the major diseases included in this chapter, gallbladder disease is the most amenable to treatment. If a low-fat selective diet is not successful, medical and surgical techniques are available to remove the stones or the organ as necessary.

Wellness Tip 22–1 summarizes major guidelines to help maintain gastrointestinal health.

Wellness Tip **22–1** • Maximize nutrition 2 to 3 weeks before elective surgery. Be conscientious about consuming recommended amounts of foods high in protein, vitamins C and K, iron, and zinc.

- To avoid constipation, consume adequate fiber and fluid, obtain enough exercise, and schedule a regular time to defecate.
- Obtain appropriate hepatitis vaccinations. Implement safe food-handling practices. Wash hands thoroughly after using the toilet or changing diapers. Use universal precautions. Campaign for the adoption of safer needle systems. Report all needlestick injuries.
- Drink moderately (maximum of one drink/day for women, small men, and elderly and two drinks/day for average-size men), if at all. Teach young people the severe outcomes of acute alcohol poisoning.
- To avoid concentrated bile resulting from a long overnight fast that increases the risk of gallstones, eat breakfast or drink two glasses of water upon arising.

CASE STUDY 22-1

An outpatient, Ms. C, a 40-year-old white woman, has just been evaluated for right upper quadrant pain. The pain occurs after meals and radiates to the right shoulder. Ms. C has noticed her stools have become pale gray in the past 2 months. Ms. C is 5 ft 4 in tall, has a medium frame, and weighs 151 lb.

Ultrasound examination of the gallbladder showed the presence of numerous stones. None is obstructing the duct system yet.

(Continued on the following page)

CASE STUDY (Continued)

Ms. C is a single parent of four children, aged 4 to 17, and is employed as a secretary. If surgery does become necessary, she would like to delay it until the youngest child is in school. For that reason, she is electing medical management.

The nurse taking a dietary history discovers that Ms. C seldom eats breakfast, substituting a doughnut and coffee during her morning coffee break. Lunch is generally a bologna sandwich with chips. Dinner at home often consists of hamburgers, pizza, or macaroni and cheese. Ms. C told the nurse she does not know much about nutrition, that she shops as her mother did, and that she cooks food her children will eat.

NURSING CARE PLAN

SUBJECTIVE DATA Pain in right upper quadrant immediately after eating
Pale stools for 2 months by history
High-fat, low-fiber diet by history
Admitted lack of knowledge about nutrition

OBJECTIVE DATA Gallstones per ultrasound
115 percent of healthy body weight

NURSING DIAGNOSIS NANDA: Deficient Knowledge (NANDA, 2003, with permission) related to prescribed low-fat diet for cholecystitis as evidenced by admitted lack of knowledge about nutrition.

DESIRED OUTCOMES EVALUATION CRITERIA	NURSING ACTIONS/INTERVENTIONS	RATIONALE
NOC: Knowledge: Diet (Moorhead, Johnson, and Maas, 2004, with permission) Client will verbalize foods to avoid to maintain low-fat diet by end of teaching session.	NIC: Nutritional Counseling (Dochterman and Bulechek, 2004, with permission) Explain low-fat diet, adapting to client's lifestyle. Provide written instructions for client to take home.	Having written instructions available as a teaching tool structures the session and may stimulate questions the client would not think of otherwise. Taking the material home will reinforce the instruction.
Client will state means to modify meals to accommodate prescribed diet by end of teaching session.	Explore Ms. C's preferences for adding fiber to her diet.	Soluble fiber will combine with cholesterol, which comprises most gallstones, and carry it out of the body. Building on the client's choices increases chances of compliance.
	Obtain client's reaction to diet and offer alternatives to her present meal pattern.	Considering the client's wishes affirms her status as an individual. Personalizing the diet for her circumstances will increase the chances of success.
	Suggest Ms. C either eat breakfast or drink 2 glasses of water first thing in the morning.	Either of these actions will stimulate the gallbladder to empty and rid itself of the concentrated bile that has accumulated overnight.
Client will return to follow-up session in 1 week with report of the week's meals and any questions she may have.	Try to obtain a commitment to return for follow-up in 1 week.	This is quite a radical change from Ms. C's usual eating habits. Follow-up in 1 week will give the nurse an opportunity to reinforce the teaching, answer questions, and counsel the client to remain committed to the therapeutic regimen.

C T Q CRITICAL THINKING QUESTIONS

1. Expand this nursing care plan to a family case. What additional assessment data are needed? How might dietary interventions be modified for a 4-year-old and a 17-year-old?
2. What is your estimation of Ms. C's financial situation?

How would it impact on the implementation of the family care plan?
3. Critique the use of deficient knowledge as a long-term evaluative criterion.

⫸ CHAPTER REVIEW

1. Which of the following foods is allowed for a preoperative client on a low-residue diet?
   a. 8 ounces of milk with each of the three main meals
   b. Minestrone soup containing peas and lentils
   c. Broiled ground beef patty on a white bun
   d. A fresh fruit salad

2. The American Society of Anesthesiologists' guidelines suggest which of the following intakes is permissible for healthy individuals undergoing elective procedures?
   a. Water and apple juice until 1 hour before the procedure
   b. Plain tea and unbuttered toast with clear jelly 6 hours before scheduled surgery
   c. Infant formula or breast milk 4 hours before an elective procedure begins
   d. Light meal containing meat at 5 AM before a procedure scheduled for noon

3. Clients who have had resection of the ileum should be monitored for:
   a. Iron-deficiency anemia
   b. Fat-soluble vitamin deficiency
   c. Calcium and phosphorus deficiency
   d. Vitamin B_{12} deficiency

4. A client with cirrhosis of the liver should be asked if he or she experienced _____ before ordering a diet.
   a. Headache
   b. Vomiting of blood
   c. A recent course of antibiotic therapy
   d. Hives

5. Which of the following meal components is likely to lessen symptoms of the dumping syndrome?
   a. Mashed fresh strawberries
   b. Orange sherbet
   c. Salt-free tomato juice
   d. Whole-wheat toast with dietetic jelly

✚ CLINICAL ANALYSIS

Mr. W is a 55-year-old white man admitted to the acute care unit with jaundice and ascites secondary to cirrhosis of the liver. He has gained 15 pounds in the past 3 weeks, and his serum sodium is 125 mEq/L. He is a diagnosed alcoholic who has been through a detoxification program several times in the past 5 years. The dietitian has instructed Mr. W on a 1000-milligram sodium diet with a fluid restriction of 1000 milliliters per day.

1. When the nurse does the beginning of shift assessment, Mr. W says he tried "cutting down on salt" when he started gaining weight, but it didn't work. Which of the following statements best reflects a good understanding of Mr. W's pathology and treatment?
   a. Just cutting out added salt is not enough, because many foods are naturally high in sodium.
   b. Fluids are always restricted with a low-sodium diet.
   c. The ascites is caused by the inability of the liver to produce water-soluble bilirubin.
   d. Besides retaining sodium, Mr. W has ascites due to decreased blood pressure in the liver.

2. Mr. W vomits immediately after his next meal. The physician then orders a hydrating solution of 5-percent dextrose in water intravenously. If thiamin is not included in that order, the nurse should inquire about it because:
   a. Thiamin is necessary to predigest the dextrose for immediate absorption.
   b. Intravenous glucose without thiamin in the cirrhosis client can precipitate the Wernicke-Korsakoff syndrome.
   c. Thiamin prevents folic acid stores from being diluted by the hydrating solution.
   d. Deficiency of thiamin causes delirium tremens.

3. Mr. W's condition worsens. He is placed on a 40-gram protein diet. Mrs. W has been told the purpose of the protein restriction. The next day, Mrs. W asks the nurse, "If protein breakdown is causing the problem, why is he getting any at all?" Which of the following responses by the nurse would be most accurate?
   a. Some protein is necessary to spare glucose for basic energy needs.
   b. If the body receives no protein, it will destroy its own tissue to obtain it.
   c. The proteins in this diet are predigested and more easily absorbed than most.
   d. Protein is needed to feed the bacterial flora in the intestine.

REFERENCES

Abou-Assi, S, Craig, K, and O'Keefe, SJ: Hypocaloric jejunal feeding is better than total parenteral nutrition in acute pancreatitis: Results of a randomized comparative study. Am J Gastroenterol 97:2255, 2002.

Abou-Assi, S, and Vlahcevic, ZR: Hepatic encephalopathy: Metabolic consequence of cirrhosis often is reversible. Postgrad Med 109:52, 2001.

Allen, PLJ: Guidelines for the diagnosis and treatment of celiac disease in children. Pediatr Nurs 30:473, 2004.

American Society of Anesthesiologists Task Force on Preoperative Fasting: Practice guidelines for preoperative fasting and the use of pharmacologic agents to reduce the risk of pulmonary aspiration: Application to healthy patients undergoing elective procedures. Anesthesiology 90:896, 1999. Accessed September 22, 2004 at http://www.asahq.org/publicationsAndServices/NPO.pdf.

Andus, T, and Gross, V: Etiology and pathophysiology of inflammatory bowel disease—environmental factors. Hapatogastroenterology 47:29, 2000.

Anselmo, MA, et al: Cystic fibrosis on the Internet: a survey of site adherence to AMA guidelines. Pediatrics 114:100, 2004.

Aranda-Michel, J, and Giannella, RA: Acute diarrhea: A practical review. Am J Med 106:670, 1999.

Atkinson, W, et al: Food elimination based on IgG antibodies in irritable bowel syndrome: A randomised controlled trial. Gut 53:1459, 2004.

Bamba, T, et al: Dietary fat attenuates the benefits of an elemental diet in active Crohn's disease: A randomized, controlled trial. Eur J Gastroenterol Hepatol 15:151, 2003.

Beker, LT, et al: Stature as a prognostic factor in cystic fibrosis survival. J Am Diet Assoc 101:438, 2001.

Beresford, TP, et al: Comparison of CAGE questionnaire and computer-assisted laboratory profiles in screening for covert alcoholism. Lancet 336:482, 1990.

Bernstein, CN, et al: The incidence of fracture among patients with inflammatory bowel disease: A population-based cohort study. Ann Intern Med 133:795, 2000.

Bockhold, KM: Who's afraid of hepatitis C? Am J Nurs 100(5):26, 2000.

Bohmer, CJ, and Tuynman, HA: The effect of a lactose-restricted diet in patients with a positive lactose tolerance test, earlier diagnosed as irritable bowel syndrome: A 5-year follow-up study. Eur J Gastroenterol Hepatol 13:941, 2001.

Bostwick, JM, and Seaman, JS: Hospitalized patients and alcohol: Who is being missed? Gen Hosp Psychiatry 26:59, 2004.

Brown, JE: Nutrition Through the Life Cycle, ed 2. Thomson Wadsworth, Belmont, CA, 2005.

Bruun, LI, et al: Prevalence of malnutrition in surgical patients: Evaluation of nutritional support and documentation. Clin Nutr 18:141, 1999.

Bujanda, L: The effects of alcohol consumption upon the gastrointestinal tract. Am J Gastroenterol 95:2274, 2000.

Butterworth, RF: Hepatic encephalopathy: A serious complication of alcoholic liver disease. Alcohol Res Health 27:143, 2003.

Camilleri, M: Management of the irritable bowel syndrome. 120:652, 2001.

Camilleri, M, Heading, RC, and Thompson, WG: Clinical perspectives, mechanisms, diagnosis and management of irritable bowel syndrome. Aliment Pharmacol Ther 16:1407, 2002.

Carlson, E: Irritable bowel syndrome. Nurse Pract 23:82, 1998.

Centers for Disease Control: Alcohol-attributable deaths and years of potential life lost—United States, 2001. MMWR 53:866, 2004a. Accessed October 11, 2004 at http://www.cdc.gov/mmwr/preview/mmwrhtml/mm5337a2.htm.

Centers for Disease Control: Global progress toward universal childhood hepatitis B vaccination, 2003. MMWR 52:868, 2003. Accessed October 16, 2004 at http://www.cdc.gov/mmwr/preview/mmwrhtml/mm5236a5.htm.

Centers for Disease Control: Newborn screening for cystic fibrosis. MMWR 53:1, 2004b. Accessed October 16, 2004 at http://www.cdc.gov/mmwr/preview/mmwrhtml/rr5313a1.htm.

Centers for Disease Control: Transmission of Hepatitis B Virus Among Persons Undergoing Blood Glucose Monitoring in Long-Term—Care Facilities—Mississippi, North Carolina, and Los Angeles County, California, 2003—2004. MMWR 54:220, 2005. Accessed June 2, 2005 at http://www.cdc.gov/mmwr/preview/mmwrhtml/mm5409a2.htm.

Chetri, K, and Choudhuri, G: Role of trace elements in hepatic encephalopathy: Zinc and manganese. Indian J Gastroenterol 22:S28, 2003.

Collin, P, and Reunala, T: Recognition and management of the cutaneous manifestations of celiac disease: A guide for dermatologists. Am J Clin Dermatol 4:13, 2003.

Connon, JJ: Celiac disease. In Shils, ME, et al (eds): Modern Nutrition in Health and Disease, ed 9. Lippincott Williams & Wilkins, Philadelphia, 1999.

Connor, BA, and Landzberg, BR: Prevention and treatment of acute traveler's diarrhea. Infect Med 21:18, 2004.

Crenshaw, JT, and Winslow, EH: Preoperative fasting: Old habits die hard. Am J Nurs 102(5):36, 2002.

Diehl, AM: Liver disease in alcohol abusers: Clinical perspective. Alcohol 27:7, 2002.

Dochterman, J, and Bulechek, G (eds): Nursing Interventions Classification (NIC), ed 4. Mosby, St. Louis, 2004.

Ewing, JA: Detecting alcoholism: The CAGE questionnaire. JAMA 252:1905, 1984.

Faigel, DO: A clinical approach to constipation. Clin Cornerstone 4:11, 2002.

Famularo, G: Probiotic lactobacilli: A new perspective for the treatment of inflammatory bowel disease. Curr Pharm Des 9:1973, 2003.

Fasano, A, et al: Prevalence of celiac disease in at-risk and not-at-risk groups in the United States: a large multicenter study. Arch Intern Med 163:286, 2003.

Feinman, L, and Lieber, CS: Nutrition and diet in alcoholism. In Shils, ME, et al (eds): Modern Nutrition in Health and Disease, ed 9. Lippincott Williams & Wilkins, Philadelphia, 1999.

Fraser-Moodie, CA, et al: Weight loss has an independent beneficial effect on symptoms of gastro-oesophageal reflux in patients who are overweight. Scan J Gastroenterol 34:337, 1999.

Furrie, E, et al: Synbiotic therapy (Bifidobacterium longum/Synergy 1) initiates resolution of inflammation in patients with active ulcerative colitis: a randomised controlled pilot trial. Gut 54:242, 2005.

Gallagher-Allred, CR: Nutritional Care of the Terminally Ill. Aspen Publishers, Gaithersburg, MD, 1989.

Ghanchi, FD, and Rembacken, BJ: Inflammatory bowel disease and the eye. Surv Ophthalmol 48:663, 2003.

Ghanekar, A, and Grant, D: Small bowel transplantation. Curr Opin Crit Care 7:133, 2001.

Gines, P, et al: Management of cirrhosis and ascites. N Engl J Med 350:1646, 2004.

Graham, TO, and Kandil, HM: Nutritional factors in inflammatory bowel disease. Gastroenterol Clin North Am 31:203, 2002.

Griffiths, AM: Inflammatory Bowel Disease. In Shils, ME, et al (eds): Modern Nutrition in Health and Disease, ed 9. Lippincott Williams & Wilkins, Philadelphia, 1999.

Hervonen, K, et al: Concordance of dermatitis herpetiformis and celiac disease in monozygous twins. J Invest Dermatol 115:990, 2000.

Heyman, M: Effect of lactic acid bacterial on diarrheal diseases. J Am Coll Nutr 19:137S, 2000.

Heymann, DL (ed): Control of Communicable Diseases Manual, ed 18. American Public Health Association, Washington, DC, 2004.

Huang, JQ, Sridhar, S, and Hunt, RH: Role of Helicobacter pylori infection and non-steroidal anti-inflammatory drugs in peptic-ulcer disease: A meta-analysis. Lancet 359:14, 2002.

Huckleberry, Y: Nutritional support and the surgical patient. Am J Health Syst Pharm 61:671, 2004.

Hunter, JO: Nutritional factors in inflammatory bowel disease. Eur J Gastroenterol Hepatol 10:235, 1998.

Israel, EJ, et al: Case 3-2005: A 14-year-old boy with recent slowing of growth and delayed puberty. N Engl J Med 352:393, 2005.

Jaffe, A, and Bush, A: Cystic fibrosis: Review of the decade. Monaldi Arch Chest Dis 56:240, 2001.

Joachim, G: Responses of people with inflammatory bowel disease to foods consumed. Gastroenterol Nurs 23:160, 2000.

Jowett, SL, et al: Dietary beliefs of people with ulcerative colitis and their effect on relapse and nutrient intake. Clin Nutr 23:161, 2004a.

Jowett, SL, et al: Influence of dietary factors on the clinical course of ulcerative colitis: A prospective cohort study. Gut 53:1479, 2004b.

Kanauchi, O, et al: The beneficial effects of microflora, especially obligate anaerobes, and their products on the colonic environment in inflammatory bowel disease. Curr Pharm Des 11:1047, 2005.

Kang, JY, Melville, D, and Maxwell, JD: Epidemiology and management of diverticular disease of the colon. Drugs Aging 21:211, 2004.

Kemppainen, T, et al: Osteoporosis in adult patients with celiac disease. Bone 24:249, 1999.

Kudsk, KA, et al: Preoperative albumin and surgical site identify surgical risk for major postoperative complications. JPEN J Parenter Enteral Nutr 27:1, 2003.

Lam, SK: Differences in peptic ulcer between East and West. Baillieres Best Pract Res Clin Gastroenterol 14:41, 2000.

Lee, WM: Drug-induced hepatotoxicity. N Engl J Med 349:474, 2003.

Lichtenstein, GR: Evaluation of bone mineral density in inflammatory bowel disease: Current safety focus. Am J Gastroenterol 98:S24, 2003.

Lichtenstein, GR: Management of bone loss in inflammatory bowel disease. Semin Gastrointest Dis 12:275, 2001.

Lichtenstein, GR, and MacDermott, RP: Advances in the treatment of Crohn's disease: Focus on the biological approach. American College of Gastroenterology 66th Annual Scientific Meeting, October 22, 2001. Accessed November 17, 2001 at http://nurses.medscape.com/Medscape/CNO/2001/ACG/Story.cfm?story_id=2466.

Lieber, CS: Nutrition in liver disorders. In Shils, ME, et al (eds): Modern Nutrition in Health and Disease, ed 9. Lippincott Williams & Wilkins, Philadelphia, 1999.

Liskow, B, et al: Validity of the Cage questionnaire in screening for alcohol dependence in a walk-in (triage) clinic. J Stud Alcohol 56:277, 1995.

Lykins, TC, and Stockwell, J: Comprehensive modified diet simplifies nutrition management of adults with short-bowel syndrome. J Am Diet Assoc 98:309, 1998.

MacMillan, SL, et al: Early feeding and the incidence of gastrointestinal symptoms after major gynecologic surgery. Obstet Gynecol 96:604, 2000.

Magee, FA, et al: Contribution of dietary protein to sulfide production in the large intestine: An in vitro and a controlled feeding study in humans. Am J Clin Nutr 72:1488, 2000.

Malozemoff, W, and Gentlemen, B: When dinner's done—postprandial hypotension in older adults. Nursing Spectrum Midwest 5:18, 2004.

McCabe, H: Riboflavin deficiency in cystic fibrosis: Three case reports. J Hum Nutr Diet 14:365, 2001.

Mersy, DJ: Recognition of alcohol and substance abuse. Am Fam Physician 67:1529, 2003.

Moorhead, S, Johnson, M, and Maas, M (eds): Nursing Outcomes Classification (NOC), ed 3. Mosby, St. Louis, 2004.

Moses, PL, et al: Antineuronal antibodies in idiopathic achalasia and gastro-oesophageal reflux disease. Gut 52:629, 2003.

Musher, DM, and Musher, BL: Contagious acute gastrointestinal infections. N Engl J Med 351:2417, 2004.

NANDA International: Nursing Diagnoses: Definitions and Classification, 2003–2004. NANDA International, Philadelphia, 2003.

Nathens, AB, et al: Randomized, prospective trial of antioxidant supplementation in critically ill surgical patients. Ann Surg 236:814, 2002.

National Digestive Diseases Information Clearinghouse: Irritable bowel syndrome. National Institute of Diabetes and Digestive and Kidney Diseases, April 2003. Accessed September 28, 2004 at http://digestive.niddk.nih.gov/ddiseases/pubs/ibs/.

Ogershok, PR, et al: Wernicke encephalopathy in nonalcoholic patients. Am J Med Sci 323:107, 2002.

Parkman, HP, Hasler, WL, and Fisher, RS: American Gastroenterological Association medical position statement: Diagnosis and treatment of gastroparesis. Gastroenterology 127:1589, 2004.

Patton, KM, and Aranda-Michel, J: Nutritional aspects in liver disease and liver transplantation. Nutr Clin Pract 17:332, 2002.

Portincasa, P, Di Ciaula, A, and van Berge-Henegouwen, GP: Smooth muscle function and dysfunction in gallbladder disease. Curr Gastroenterol Rep 6:151, 2004.

Probert, CS, Jones, PR, and Ratcliffe, NM: A novel method for rapidly diagnosing the causes of diarrhoea. Gut 53:58, 2004.

Reid, CL: Nutritional requirements of surgical and critically-ill patients: Do we really know what they need? Proc Nutr Soc 63:467, 2004.

Rosenfeld, M, et al: Nutritional effects of long-term gastrostomy feedings in children with cystic fibrosis. J Am Diet Assoc 99:191, 1999.

Rowe, SM, Miller, S, and Sorscher, EJ: Cystic fibrosis. N Engl J Med 352:1992, 2005.

Rudman, D, et al: Ammonia content of food. Am J Clin Nutr 26:487, 1973.

Sandler, RS, et al: The burden of selected digestive diseases in the United States. Gastroenterology 122:1500, 2002.

Sharara, AI, and Rockey, DC: Gastroesophageal variceal hemorrhage. N Engl J Med 345:669, 2001.

Simon, JA, and Hudes, ES: Serum ascorbic acid and gallbladder disease prevalence among US adults. Arch Intern Med 160:931, 2000.

Simopoulos, AP: Omega-3 fatty acids in inflammation and autoimmune diseases. J Am Coll Nutr 21:495, 2002.

Simpson, ND, Yen, T, and Ahmed, A: Gallstones: Complications and management. Cyberounds Continuing Education. Accessed November 20, 2002 at http://www.cyberounds.com/conferences/gastroenterology/conferences/cu.../conference.htm.

Smith, DS, and Ferris, CD: Current concepts in diabetic gastroparesis. Drugs 63:1339, 2003.

Smith, SW: Severe acidosis and hyperdynamic circulation in a 39-year-old alcoholic. J Emerg Med 16:587, 1998.

Smothers, BA, Yahr, HT, and Ruhl, CE: Detection of alcohol use disorders in general hospital admissions in the United States. Arch Intern Med 164:749, 2004.

Spapen, H, et al: Soluble fiber reduces the incidence of diarrhea in septic patients receiving total enteral nutrition: A prospective, double-blind, randomized, and controlled trial. Clin Nutr 20:301, 2001.

Steed, HL, et al: A randomized controlled trial of early versus "traditional" postoperative oral intake after major abdominal gynecologic surgery. Am J Obstet Gynecol 186:861, 2002.

Stenson, WF: The esophagus and stomach. In Shils, ME, et al (eds): Modern Nutrition in Health and Disease, ed 9. Lippincott Williams & Wilkins, Philadelphia, 1999.

Svanes, C: Trends in perforated peptic ulcer: Incidence, etiology, treatment, and prognosis. World J Surg 24:277, 2000.

Talley, NJ, et al: Risk factors for chronic constipation based on a general practice sample. Am J Gastroenterol 98:1107, 2003.

Thompson, T: Gluten contamination of commercial oat products in the United States [Letter]. N Engl J Med 351:2021, 2004.

Thompson, T: Thiamin, riboflavin, and niacin contents of the gluten-free diet: Is there cause for concern? J Am Diet Assoc 99:858, 1999.

Tilg, H, and Kaser, A: Diet and relapsing ulcerative colitis: Take off the meat? Gut 53:1399, 2004.

Tsai, CJ, et al: Frequent nut consumption and decreased risk of cholecystectomy in women. Am J Clin Nutr 80:76, 2004a.

Tsai, C-J, et al: A prospective cohort study of nut consumption and the risk of gallstone disease in men. Am J Epidemiol 160:961, 2004b.

United States Food and Drug Administration: FDA Approves First DNA-based Test to Detect Cystic Fibrosis. FDA News. May 9, 2005. Accessed June 2, 2005 at http://www.fda.gov/bbs/topics/NEWS/2005/NEW01178.html

Wang, KY, et al: Effects of ingesting Lactobacillus- and Bifidobacterium-containing yogurt in subjects with colonized *Helicobacter pylori*. Am J Clin Nutr 80:737, 2004.

Widerman, E, et al: Health status and sociodemographic characteristics of adults receiving a cystic fibrosis diagnosis after age 18 years. Chest 118:427, 2000.

Williams, LS, and Hopper, PD: Understanding Medical Surgical Nursing, ed 2. FA Davis, Philadelphia, 2003.

Young, LS, and Thomas, KJ: Celiac sprue treatment in primary care. Nurse Pract 29:42, 2004.

CHAPTER 23

Diet and Cancer

Learning Objectives

After completing this chapter, the student should be able to:

1. List several correlations between dietary intake and cancers of specific sites.
2. Interpret dietary guidelines for the prevention of cancer.
3. Identify reasons that population correlations may not apply to subgroups or to individuals.
4. Name several factors thought to contribute to loss of appetite in cancer clients.
5. Discuss measures to increase oral intake for clients with cancer.

Cancer has been known and described for thousands of years. Amazingly, one substance now linked to prevention was used as a treatment in ancient Rome, where crushed cabbage leaves were applied to cancerous ulcers (Albert-Puleo, 1983). Now cabbage is one of the cruciferous vegetables in the diet associated with reduced risk of cancer.

Definitions and Statistics

Cancer means "crab," for the creeping way in which it spreads. Cancer is a general term for more than 100 types of malignant neoplastic disease.

Terminology

A **neoplasm,** is a new and abnormal formation of tissue (tumor) that grows at the expense of the healthy organism. Two main divisions of neoplasms are **malignant** or cancerous tumors, which infiltrate surrounding tissue and spread to distant sites of the body, and **benign** tumors, which are localized but potentially dangerous if located in vital organs.

Two of the chief types of cancer are sarcomas and carcinomas. **Sarcomas** arise from connective tissue, such as muscle or bone, and are more common in young people. **Carcinomas** occur in epithelial tissue, including cancers of the lung, breast, prostate, and colon, and are more com-

mon in older people. The characteristics common to all types of cancer are uncontrolled growth and the ability to spread to distant sites (**metastasize**). Clinical Application 23–1 summarizes the transformation of normal cells into cancer cells.

Occurrence and Mortality

Cancers in general are more common in older people. In 1999 to 2000, the prevalence of cancer by age group was as follows:

- Ages 18 to 44 years — 2 percent
- Ages 45 to 64 years — 7.4 percent,
- Ages 65 to 74 years — 17.3 percent,
- Ages 75 years or older — 22.8 percent (National Center, 2004).

Cancer is the second most common cause of death in the United States after diseases of the heart and is expected to become the leading cause of death in the next decade. In 2001, the age-adjusted death rate for cancer already exceeded that for heart disease in four states: Alaska, Minnesota, Montana, and Oregon. In 1990 to 2000, the five primary sites with the highest age-adjusted death rates for males were lung/bronchus, prostate, colon/rectum, pancreas, and leukemia; for females, lung/bronchus, breast, colon/rectum, pancreas, and ovary. Overall, cancer mortality is higher among men compared with women and higher among black populations compared with whites (Centers for Disease Control, 2004). The incidence of the five most common cancers for men and women is illustrated in Figure 23–1, which shows that lung cancer, colorectal cancer, and non-Hodgkin's lymphoma occupy the same ranks regardless of gender. Figure 23–2 exhibits the mortality rates by gender for whites and blacks for all cancers in the United States.

Clients who are alive and without recurrence of cancer 5 years after diagnosis are considered cured. This is termed the *5-year survival rate.* Depending on the site in which the cancer occurs, the survival rates vary greatly, but socioeconomic status affects the stage at which the cancer is diagnosed as well as survival rates. In a Michigan

Transformation of Normal Cells Into Cancer Cells

Cancer is basically uncontrolled replication of cells. Normal cells divide in the processes of growth and maintenance but stop dividing at appropriate points. Even in normal cell division, mistakes in deoxyribonucleic acid (DNA) transcription are made and corrected. Hundreds of incidents of oxidative damage to cell components, such as DNA, are estimated to occur in a cell daily, but this oxidative damage has not been directly linked to cancer. Obviously, not all of these mistakes go on to turn cells cancerous. Multiple enzyme systems inactivate the damaging elements, and various mechanisms repair the DNA (Slupphaug, Kavli, and Krokan, 2003). Deficiencies in DNA-damage signaling and repair pathways are fundamental to the etiology of most, if not all, human cancers (Khanna and Jackson, 2001). Several genes within a cell must be changed or **mutated** for cancer to occur.

Transformation of normal cells into cancer cells is a two-step process. The first step is **initiation.** The second step is promotion. Physical forces, chemicals, or biologic agents can damage genes. If the damage is not repairable, the gene has mutated, and if cancer develops later, the cancer cells are descendents of that mutated cell (Weinberg, 1996). The alteration may not be significant until the second step of the conversion to cancerous cells, **promotion,** takes place. The time period between initiation and promotion in some cases is 10 to 30 years but may be shorter if a mutated cancer-causing gene is inherited from a parent. Substances that enhance the expression of the altered gene are called promoters. They must be present at high levels for a prolonged period. Promoters are tissue specific, such as saccharin for cancer of the urinary bladder (in rats) and bile acids for colon cancer. In contrast to initiation, which results in permanent change, the process of promotion is reversible. Reducing exposure to high levels of promoters allows the body to repair the damaged cells.

Genes are carried in the DNA of the chromosomes in the cell nucleus. Two classes of genes play major roles in the life cycle of cells: **proto-oncogenes** and **tumor-suppressor genes**. In normal cells, proto-oncogenes support the growth and division of the cell, whereas tumor-suppressor genes inhibit those processes. Both proto-oncogenes and tumor-suppressor genes may be mutated and thus contribute to cancer development. The proto-oncogenes become carcinogenic **oncogenes** that stimulate excessive reproduction, and the tumor-suppressor genes become inactivated and unable to stop the multiplication of cells. As more is learned about the molecular basis of cancer, therapies can be developed that target the aberrant cells much more accurately than the treatments currently available. Several genes within a cell must undergo **mutation** for cancer to occur.

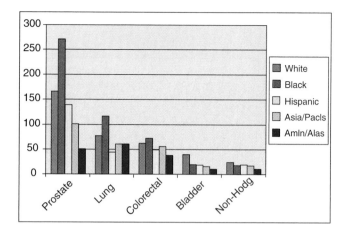

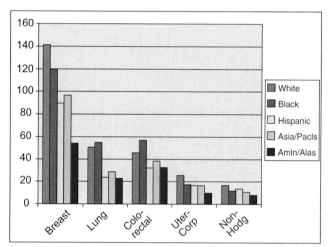

Figure **23–1** The five most common invasive cancers for men and women in the United States, 1997–2001. These are age-adjusted rates per 100,000 persons. Overall, about two-thirds of invasive cancers developed in the sites shown here. In men these sites are prostate, lung, colon and rectum, bladder, and non-Hodgkin's lymphoma; and in women, breast, lung, colon and rectum, corpus and uterus, and non-Hodgkin's lymphoma. The race/ethnicity groupings are white, black, Hispanic, Asian/Pacific Islander, and American Indian/Alaskan native. (Data derived from National Cancer Institute, 2004.)

study of female breast, cervix, lung, prostate, and colon carcinoma, persons over 65 years of age who were insured by Medicaid had the greatest risk of late-stage diagnosis and death (Bradley, Given, and Roberts, 2001). Similarly, national cervical cancer incidence and mortality rates increased with increasing poverty and decreasing education levels for the total population as well as for non-Hispanic white, black, American Indian, Asian/Pacific Islander, and Hispanic women. Patients in lower socioeconomic census tracts had significantly higher rates of late-stage cancer diagnosis and lower rates of cancer survival (Singh et al, 2004).

The causes of cancer are complex and often incompletely understood. Certain cancers appear in great numbers in particular countries. Clinical Application 23–2 summarizes some of these findings. In addition to people

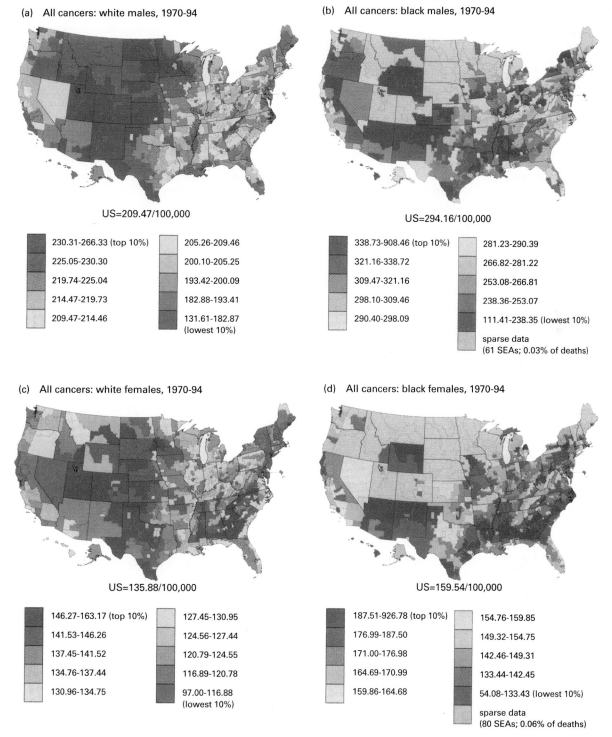

Cancer mortality rates by state economic area (age-adjusted 1970 US population)

(a) All cancers: white males, 1970-94

US=209.47/100,000

230.31-266.33 (top 10%)	205.26-209.46
225.05-230.30	200.10-205.25
219.74-225.04	193.42-200.09
214.47-219.73	182.88-193.41
209.47-214.46	131.61-182.87 (lowest 10%)

(b) All cancers: black males, 1970-94

US=294.16/100,000

338.73-908.46 (top 10%)	281.23-290.39
321.16-338.72	266.82-281.22
309.47-321.16	253.08-266.81
298.10-309.46	238.36-253.07
290.40-298.09	111.41-238.35 (lowest 10%)
	sparse data (61 SEAs; 0.03% of deaths)

(c) All cancers: white females, 1970-94

US=135.88/100,000

146.27-163.17 (top 10%)	127.45-130.95
141.53-146.26	124.56-127.44
137.45-141.52	120.79-124.55
134.76-137.44	116.89-120.78
130.96-134.75	97.00-116.88 (lowest 10%)

(d) All cancers: black females, 1970-94

US=159.54/100,000

187.51-926.78 (top 10%)	154.76-159.85
176.99-187.50	149.32-154.75
171.00-176.98	142.46-149.31
164.69-170.99	133.44-142.45
159.86-164.68	54.08-133.43 (lowest 10%)
	sparse data (80 SEAs; 0.06% of deaths)

Figure 23–2 Mortality rates for all cancers in the United States, 1970–1994, by race and sex. Depicted here are mortality rates for all cancers for (a) white males, (b) black males, (c) white females, and (d) black females. Note that the legend colors denote different rates per 100,000 age-adjusted population for each map. The brightest red is assigned to the highest 10 percent of each group, so that it indicates rates of 230 to 266/100,000 population for white males but 339 to 908/100,000 for black males. This Web site also contains maps of mortality rates for about 50 specific cancers, maps by county, and maps for the years 1950–1969 (Devesa et al, 1999).

History of Diet-Cancer Links in Various Populations

Particular cancers occur with greater frequency in some countries than others. When this was noted, the search began for dissimilarities in environment that could explain the differences. Because hereditary factors can confound the results when dissimilar populations are compared, the study of immigrants is especially enlightening.

In Japan there is more stomach cancer and less prostate and colon cancer than in the United States. In second-generation Japanese immigrants to the United States, however, the distribution of cancers becomes similar to that of other Americans. Similar findings are reported in Polish men for prostate cancer. On the other hand, migrants from Asia to the West, who maintain their traditional diet, do not have an increased risk of prostate cancer, attributed in part to phytoestrogens in vegetarian Asian diets (Vij and Kumar, 2004). See Clinical Application 23–6 for more information on phytoestrogens. Immigration, and presumed adoption of a Western diet, affects cancer development: age-adjusted breast cancer incidence rates per 100,000 Japanese women were 14 in Japan, 44 in Hawaii, and 57 in Los Angeles (Tomlinson, 1994).

Stomach and esophageal cancers are common where nitrates and nitrites are prevalent in food and water and where cured and pickled foods are popular. These areas include China, Japan, and Iceland. In Yangzhong, China, frequent intake of allium vegetables (garlic, onion, Welsh onion, and Chinese chives), raw vegetables, tomatoes, snap beans, and tea decreased the risk of stomach and esophageal cancer (Gao et al, 1999). Vitamins C and E and green tea can prevent formation of carcinogenic nitrosamines and nitrosamides (Greenwald, 1994; Ho et al, 1994; Kim et al, 1994). In Linxian County, China, where residents have one of the world's highest rates of esophageal and gastric **cardia** cancer; a 5-year trial of beta-carotene, vitamin E, and selenium reduced stomach cancer incidence by 20 percent and total mortality by 10 percent (Alberts and Garcia, 1995).

Elsewhere, a low rate of colon cancer is seen in Africa. The diet there is high in fiber, and the Africans pass bulky stools. The theory put forth was that the fiber both dilutes the carcinogens in the feces and pushes them out of the body faster than a low-fiber diet would. New research shows that black South Africans consume less than the RDA for fiber, so the low risk for colon cancer was then attributed to avoidance of excess animal protein and fat (O'Keefe et al, 1999). Avoidance is probably unintentional. The populations with high fiber intakes and low colon cancer rates also are seen in poor countries where obesity is uncommon, meat consumption is low, and physical activity is high.

This type of research is intriguing and offers a starting point for other investigations, but it cannot establish causation no matter how large the study.

in a given country possibly being influenced by similar environmental factors, including diet, they also may have **genes** that are similar compared with those found in people elsewhere. This chapter describes some examples of the associations that have been found and shows the difficulty of pinpointing the causative links and thus the difficulty of identifying a dietary behavior to adopt or to avoid with the goal of preventing cancer.

In the United States, about 33 percent of the 500,000 yearly cancer deaths are associated with cigarette smoking and about 33 percent with inappropriate nutritional and activity habits (Byers et al, 2002). This chapter considers diet and cancer. The relationship of diet to the development of cancer is explored first, followed by the nourishment of clients with cancer.

Dietary Components Associated With Cancer

It is difficult to assess the role of dietary components without also considering other factors that might contribute to the development of cancer. Outside of tobacco use, diet is probably the most important factor in the etiology of human cancer, thought to be responsible for about one-third of all cases in developed countries (Blackburn et al, 2003; Ferguson, 2002). Illustrating the limits of present knowledge, however, despite an overall healthy lifestyle and long life expectancy, Adventist populations have high rates of breast and prostate cancers (Willett, 2003). Over time, the relationship of diet to breast cancer has become clearer, and it is elaborated upon in Clinical Application 23–3.

Excesses of Certain Substances

Some substances and practices are associated with higher cancer rates. This is the case with energy and fatty acid intake, meat, alcohol, and certain cooking and preparation methods. These topics are addressed in the following section.

Energy and Fatty Acid Intake

Some of the end products of fat metabolism are thought to be carcinogenic, but dietary fat may contribute to the risk of cancer because of its energy density. Overweight and obesity increase the risk for cancers of the breast (postmenopausal), colon, endometrium, gallbladder, esophagus, pancreas, and kidney; however, moderate-to-vigorous exercise reduces colon and breast cancer risks independent of the effect of activity on weight (Byers et al, 2002). Obesity contributes to a poorer prognosis: men with BMIs of 40 or more had 52 percent higher death rates from all cancers than normal-weight men; for women, the corresponding rates were 62 percent higher (Calle et al, 2003).

Public health recommendations to decrease total fat intake for the prevention of cancer appear largely unwarranted (Kushi and Giovannucci, 2002), but additional information is needed regarding specific fatty acids in relation to causing or preventing cancer in particular sites. A high total fat intake is associated with a 24 percent increased risk of ovarian cancer whereas diets high in animal fat increased risk 70 percent, pointing out a need to clarify the

Breast Cancer and Diet

Mutations in certain genes greatly increase breast cancer risk, but these account for a minority of cases (Key, Verkasalo, and Banks, 2001). In fact, eight of nine women who develop breast cancer do not have an affected first-degree relative with the disease (Collaborative Group, 2001).

Large prospective studies have not found dietary fat per se or a diet high in red meats to be associated with breast cancer (Moyad, 2002; Terry, et al, 2001). Populations with high fat intakes generally have high rates of breast cancer, but studies of individual women have not confirmed an association of high-fat diets with breast cancer risk. The major risk factors for breast cancer are hormone-related, and the only generally recognized dietary risk factors are obesity and alcohol consumption.

Obesity increases breast cancer risk in postmenopausal women by about 30 percent, probably by increasing serum concentrations of bioavailable estradiol (Key et al, 2003). Breast cancer is associated with early menarche and late menopause, both effects of high estrogen levels, and with obesity in postmenopausal women since fat cells can produce estrogen. In Washington and New Mexico, women with BMIs above 30 had 130 percent higher concentrations of estradiol as those with BMIs lower than 22. Lastly, overweight and obese women with breast cancer have poorer survival compared with thinner women (McTiernan et al, 2003). Worldwide, 25 percent of breast cancer cases are due to overweight, obesity, and sedentary habits. Women who exercise 3 to 4 hours per week at a moderate to vigorous level have a 30 to 40 percent lower risk for breast cancer than sedentary women (McTiernan, 2003).

Moderate alcohol intakes increase breast cancer risk by about 7 percent per alcoholic drink per day, perhaps also by increasing estrogen levels (Key et al, 2003). Alcohol use, even at moderate levels (two drinks per day), increases risk for both premenopausal and postmenopausal breast cancer (McTiernan, 2003) because the metabolism of alcohol produces DNA-damaging reactive oxygen species that subject cells to oxidative stress (Ambrosone, 2000) and mediates an increase in estradiols that may be partly responsible for breast cancer risk (Poschl and Seitz, 2004). Adequate folate levels may be particularly important for women who are at higher risk of breast cancer because of high alcohol consumption (Zhang, 2004).

Specific dietary components have been investigated without changing the aforementioned relationships. No strong association was found between the ingestion of milk or other dairy products and breast cancer risk (Moorman and Terry, 2004). Similarly, analysis of eight prospective studies discerned no significant association between intakes of total meat, red meat, white meat, total dairy fluids, or total dairy solids and breast cancer risk and an inconsistent relationship was found between egg consumption and risk of breast cancer (Missmer et al, 2002). While high bone mineral density (BMD) in elderly women is related to higher rates of breast cancer, BMD is also regarded as a marker for lifetime estrogen exposure (Van der Klift et al, 2003).

Although not obtained through diet, some derivatives of vitamin D have been developed that may inhibit proliferation of cells, including those of breast cancer (O'Kelly and Koeffler, 2003). These synthetic products have the growth-regulating effects but not the calcium-mobilizing actions of vitamin D, thus avoiding the hypercalcemia caused by large doses of the natural vitamin (Colston and Hansen, 2002).

---

factors that might contribute to the disparity (Huncharek and Kupelnick, 2001). In the case of bowel cancer, for instance, increased concentrations of short-chain fatty acids and eicosanopentaenoic acid (EPA) seem to protect against colorectal cancer, but increased concentrations of medium-chain fatty acids and arachidonic acid (AA) may be associated with increased risk (Nkondjock et al, 2003). Long-chain omega-3 polyunsaturated fatty acids from fish show promise as nutrients to possibly prevent prostate cancer, but in contrast, another omega-3 PUFA, alpha-linolenic acid, might be a risk factor (Astorg, 2004). Consuming one or more servings of fish per week protected against digestive tract cancers in Italy (Fernandez et al, 1999); however, to what extent the fish-containing meals reduced meat consumption was not reported, but once again, the evidence supports the healthfulness of a varied diet.

Meat

Prolonged high consumption of red and processed meat may increase the risk of cancer in the distal portion of the large intestine. Over a ten year period, people consuming processed meat at the highest levels had a 50 percent higher risk of distal colon cancer than those consuming at the lowest levels. Likewise, high consumption of red meat was associated with a 40 percent higher risk of rectal cancer (Chao et al, 2005). Seventh Day Adventists and Mormons have a lower incidence of bowel cancer than other Americans, even when caffeine and alcohol differences between the study groups are equalized. Some Seventh Day Adventists eat meat, but those who did had higher rates of colon and prostate cancer than vegetarian members of the sect, and those who consumed the most beef had a higher risk of bladder cancer than those who consumed less (Fraser, 1999).

Alcohol

Alcohol intake greater than two drinks per day substantially increases risk for cancers of the mouth, pharynx, larynx, esophagus, liver, and breast and may be related to increased risk of colon cancer (Byers et al, 2002). Contrary to earlier reports linking alcohol to head and neck cancers only in smokers, new research suggests that chronic alcohol consumption increases the risk of those cancers regardless of exposure to tobacco smoke (Riedel, Goessler, and Hormann, 2003). Beyond its relationship to occurrence, even less than one drink per day was associated with up to a 30 percent increase in breast cancer mortality among postmenopausal women compared with nondrinkers (Feigelson et al, 2001). Although the exact mechanisms by which chronic alcohol ingestion stimulates carcinogenesis are not known, experimental studies in animals suggest that alcohol is a cocarcinogen and/or tumor promoter. The metabolism of alcohol leads to the generation of free radicals and acetaldehyde that binds to DNA and proteins, destroys folate, and seems to contribute to cirrhosis of the liver (Eriksson, 2001).

Another mechanism by which alcohol stimulates carcinogenesis is the induction of cytochrome P4502E1, which is associated with an increased production of free radicals and enhanced activation of procarcinogens found in alcoholic beverages. The consequences include nutritional deficiencies and alterations in the **immune system** resulting in an increased susceptibility to certain viruses such as hepatitis B and C viruses (Poschl and Seitz, 2004). Alcohol-induced cirrhosis, with resulting increased liver cell turnover, is associated with liver cancer. The combination of high alcohol and low folate intake increases the risk of colorectal tumors more than either factor alone. In addition, genetic variation in a gene necessary to folate metabolism that is found in Japanese people may explain the high rates of colorectal cancer in that population (Giovannucci, 2004).

Excessive beer consumption is associated with rectal cancer, possibly due to the formation of a nitrosamine compound during direct-fire drying of barley malt. This discovery led to modification of the brewing process (Sugimura and Wakabayashi, 1999). A possible pathophysiological reason for the correlation between alcohol and breast cancer is found in Clinical Application 23–3.

Certain Cooking and Preparation Methods

Temperatures at which food is cooked and at which it is consumed has been related to the occurrence of cancer. Other techniques of preserving food also have been linked to cancer in particular populations.

VERY HOT SERVING TEMPERATURES

Very hot drinks and foods probably increase the risk for cancers of the oral cavity, pharynx, and esophagus, so drinks and foods should not be consumed when they are scalding hot (Key et al, 2004). Indeed, consumption of high-temperature food was found to be an independent risk factor for stomach cancer and positively associated with esophageal cancer in India (Mathew et al, 2000; Phukan et al, 2001).

PRESERVATION METHODS

Epidemiological evidence supports an association between the risk of developing gastric cancer and the intake of salt and salt-preserved foods (Riboli and Norat,

2001). Additives used to preserve appearance and prevent bacterial contamination of processed meats, nitrites, when converted to nitrosamines in the stomach may increase risk of gastric cancer. Vitamin C-rich foods impede this conversion of nitrites and are suggested as a dietary means of modifying risk.

Cancers of the esophagus and stomach are correlated with large intakes of pickled and smoked foods. It is postulated that smoked foods may absorb tar similar to that in tobacco smoke. Charcoal broiling presents the same type of danger, in that **carcinogens** may be deposited on the surface of the food.

HIGH TEMPERATURE COOKING

Frying, broiling, and grilling meat, poultry, game, and fish produce carcinogens, substances known to cause cancer in animals when given at very high doses. These heterocyclic amines (HCAs) are produced by high temperature cooking of muscle meats. One kind of HCA has been on the Department of Health and Human Services' list of cancer-causing agents since 2002 and three more HCAs that arise from grilling meat were added to the list in 2005 (American Institute for Cancer Research, 2005). The amount of HCAs in cooked foods is small, but other components in the diet such as omega-6-polyunsaturated oils (see again Figure 20–6) have powerful promoting effects in target organs of HCAs. Conversely, foods containing antioxidants may decrease the action of HCAs (Weisburger, 2002).

Another class of carcinogens on the list of cancer-causing agents are polycyclic aromatic hydrocarbons (PAHs) that are formed when fat drips onto hot coals or stones. These potent carcinogens are deposited back onto food by smoke and flare-ups (American Institute for Cancer Research, 2005).

Low-temperature, high-moisture cooking, such as stewing and pot-roasting, does not produce the same level of carcinogens. Even when pan frying, using lower temperatures and turning ground beef patties every minute reduced the carcinogen levels while safely inactivating bacteria (Salmon et al, 2000). Marinades have been found to reduce the amount of HCAs, formed on grilled meats, by 92 to 99 percent, possibly by acting as a barrier to the flames or because of the vitamins C and E in the citrus juices and oils of the marinade (American Institute for Cancer Research, 2002). Although the amount of carcinogens in foods ordinarily consumed is low and insufficient to explain human cancer, some experts recommend avoiding exposure to these carcinogens or reducing their effects by cooking in microwave ovens (Sugimura et al, 2004).

INDIVIDUAL DIFFERENCES IN METABOLISM

Many studies related diet to risk of cancer, but frequently the follow-up intervention studies did not show the expected protection against cancer, possibly because the biological diversity of the participants was not controlled (Rennert, 2003). In the case of colon cancer, researchers have demonstrated genetic differences related to enzymes that catalyze the formation of carcinogens from meats cooked for a long time at high temperatures. People who were classified as *fast acetylators* based on these enzymes have shown a consistent trend towards higher risks for colorectal cancer with higher intakes of meat (Roberts-Thomson, Butler, and Ryan, 1999). Heterocyclic amines require activation by the enzymes CYP1A2 and N-acetyltransferase (NAT)2 or NAT1 before they can bind to DNA. Since smoking is known to induce CYP1A2, a study tested the relationships of smoking to preference for well-done meat and colorectal cancer. In people who had ever smoked, preference for well-done red meat was associated with an 8.8-fold increased risk of colorectal cancer among subjects with the NAT2 and CYP1A2 rapid phenotypes compared with smokers with low NAT2 and CYP1A2 activities who preferred their red meat rare or medium. No similar association was found in never-smokers, and there was no increased cancer risk associated with (1) well-done meat among smokers with a rapid phenotype for only one of these enzymes or (2) smokers with both rapid phenotypes who did not prefer their red meat well-done (Le Marchand et al, 2001).

The carcinogen does not have to be consumed. Even exposure to cooking oil fumes containing relatively high amounts of heterocyclic amines has been related to a greater than two-fold increase lung cancer occurrence in never-smoking females with NAT2 *fast acetylator* geno-type in Taiwan (Chiou et al, 2005).

Protective Dietary Components

A number of natural foodstuffs, especially fruits and vegetables, contain substances that have potential to prevent cancer. Antioxidants, such as vitamins C and E and beta-carotene, can reduce the risk of cancer. Besides the antioxidants, several other components in cruciferous vegetables protect against the effects of reactive oxygen species. Overall, cruciferous vegetables rank among the most promising dietary items to prevent cancer, and identification of active constituents may stimulate development of highly protective Brassica varieties (Steinkellner et al, 2001). In addition, legumes, grains, and green tea are under investigation as possibly containing substances protective against DNA damage (Abdulla and Gruber, 2000).

Fruits and Vegetables

Fruits and vegetables probably reduce the risk for cancers of the oral cavity, esophagus, stomach, and colorectum, and diets should include at least 400 grams per day of total fruits and vegetables (Key et al, 2004). That is not a huge quantity: one quarter-pound unpeeled apple is approximately 100 grams. Following are examples of research findings relating fruit and vegetable intake to various cancers. It is undoubtedly unrealistic to expect diet alone to prevent cancer, but it may contribute to a lessened risk.

BLADDER CANCER

Diets low in fruits increased the risk of bladder cancer by 40 percent, and low intakes of vegetables increased risk by 16 percent (Steinmaus, Nunez, and Smith, 2000). Cigarette smoking substantially increases the risk of bladder cancer, but total fruit consumption is probably associated with a small decrease in risk (Zeegers et al, 2004).

BREAST CANCER

Studies of foods and nutrients in relation to breast cancer showed high consumption of vegetables associated with a 25 percent decreased risk, of fruit with a 6 percent decrease, of vitamin C with a 20 percent decrease, and of beta-carotene with a 18 percent decrease (Gandini et al, 2000).

COLON CANCER

Epidemiologic, experimental (animal), and clinical investigations suggest that diets high in total fat, protein, kilocalories, alcohol, and meat (both red and white) and low in calcium and folate, are associated with an increased incidence of colorectal cancer (National Cancer Institute, 2005). Folate from dietary sources alone was related to a modest reduction in risk for colon cancer. Research most strongly supports high folic acid intake as reducing risks of colon and breast cancers, possibly explained by a variation in the gene for an enzyme involved in folic acid metabolism that is associated with colon cancer (Willett, 2000).

LUNG CANCER

A 50 percent decreased risk of lung cancer was associated with higher intake of white grapefruit and onions and a 40 percent decreased risk was associated with apples, all attributed to the flavonoids contained in the foods (Le Marchand et al, 2000). Among male smokers, higher consumption of fruits and vegetables was associated with a 27 percent lower risk of lung cancer, with the greatest effect from **lycopene** (Holick et al, 2002). As became evident in the Alpha-Tocopherol study (1994), beta-carotene can have pro-oxidant effects under certain conditions, such as high oxygen pressures and oxidative stress found in the lungs of smokers (Kamat and Lamm, 2002). In sum, the best preventive strategy for lung cancer is smoking cessation.

ORAL, PHARYNGEAL, AND ESOPHAGEAL CANCER

Vegetable intake, including green vegetables, cruciferous vegetables, and yellow vegetables, total fruit intake, and citrus fruit intake are protective against these cancers. Specifically, carotene, vitamins C and E, and selenium are protective, most likely in combination with each other and other micronutrients (Chainani-Wu, 2002). In a study of British women, a high BMI in early adulthood and low consumption of fruit were risk factors for adenocarcinoma of the esophagus (Cheng et al, 2000).

OVARIAN CANCER

Of ovarian cancer cases in 50-year-old or older Italian women, 24 percent were attributed to of low intake of green vegetables (Parazzini, et al, 2000). Moreover, supplements of vitamins C and E reduced the risk of ovarian cancer by 60 and 67 percent respectively (Fleischauer et al, 2001) and high dietary intake of beta-carotene was associated with a 16 percent decrease in ovarian cancer risk (Huncharek, Klassen, and Kupelnick, 2001).

PROSTATE CANCER

Studies have shown that tomato products may help prevent prostate cancer. Consuming large amounts of raw tomato reduced its risk 11 percent, and consuming large amounts of cooked tomato products reduced its risk 19 percent (Etminan, Takkouche, and Caamano-Isorna, 2004). Cooking breaks open the tomato cells and evaporates water to increase the concentration of lycopene. Additionally, ingestion of three servings per week of cruciferous vegetables, compared with less than one serving per week, was associated with a 41 percent decrease in prostate cancer (Cohen, Kristal, and Stanford, 2000).

A VARIETY OF WHOLE FOODS

It is possible that all the micronutrients and phytochemicals in fruits and vegetables have not been identified or that several of the components produce synergistic effects. A deficiency of eight nutrients (folic acid, vitamin B_{12}, vitamin B_6, niacin, vitamin C, vitamin E, iron, or zinc) mimics the radiation damage to DNA. Micronutrient deficiency may help to explain why the quarter of the population that eats the fewest fruits and vegetables has about double the rate for most types of cancer compared with the quarter of the people with the highest intake. A level of folate deficiency causing chromosome breaks was found in approximately 10 percent of the United States' population, with a much higher percentage in the poor (Ames, 2001). At this stage of understanding, however, eating a variety of whole foods, not individual micronutrients, is the appropriate formula to decrease the risk of cancer. Clinical Application 23–4 elaborates upon vegetable intake in relation to cancer, but Clinical Application 23–5 cautions against overenthusiastic supplementation.

Fiber and Fluid

The relationship of dietary fiber to colon cancer has been studied for 30 years without clear-cut conclusions, possibly because separate fiber sources were not considered and colon cancers were not defined by location (Hill, 2003). Colon cancers are not identical in pathology, and all fiber may not be equally protective. A Cochrane Review reported that there is currently no evidence from randomized controlled trials to suggest that increased dietary fiber will reduce the incidence or recurrence of adenomatous polyps (precursor of colon cancer) within a 2- to 4-year period (Asano and McLeod, 2002). Conversely, studies show that highest intakes of dietary fiber (which were still below the recommended 25 grams per day) reduced the risk of colon cancer by 42 percent, with the greatest effect displayed in the left colon and the least effect in the rectum (Bingham et al, 2003).

Regarding a different site, a high intake of cereal fiber may significantly decrease the risk of gastric cardia cancer (Roth and Mobarhan, 2001). Whether fiber offers specific protection from cancer or not, adequate intake contributes

---

Clinical Application 23–4

The Role of Vegetables in Cancer Prevention

Low intakes of vegetables have been associated with stomach and colon cancers. In Japan, smokers who ingested yellow or green vegetables every day had 20 to 30 percent lower lung cancer rates than smokers who did not consume those vegetables every day. Vegetables contain many substances that may contribute to cancer prevention. Some of these substances are carotene, indoles, and antioxidants.

Carotene, the precursor of vitamin A, is present in many green and deep-yellow vegetables. Vitamin A helps to maintain epithelial tissue, protects against oxidation, may influence host **immune** defenses, and assists in the control of cellular differentiation, a process that is faulty in the rapidly growing cancer cell. Thus, an adequate intake of carotene may be instrumental in preventing cancer. The fact that beta-carotene *supplements* were associated with increased morbidity and mortality from lung cancer (Clinical Application 23–5) should not deter someone from consuming vegetables rich in this nutrient (Alpha-Tocopherol, 1994).

Cruciferous vegetables, those of the cabbage family, are correlated with the prevention cancer in many organs (Murillo and Mehta, 2001). Among the phytochemicals that these vegetables contain are **indoles** that activate enzymes to destroy carcinogens. Members of the cruciferous family include broccoli, Brussels sprouts, cabbage, cauliflower, collards, kohlrabi, and kale.

Antioxidants prevent oxidation of molecules by becoming oxidized themselves. Some molecules become very unstable when oxidized and damage nearby molecules. This reaction could modify a cell's DNA to set in motion the uncontrolled reproduction of cancer cells. Many vegetables contain carotene and vitamin C, which are antioxidants. Additionally, some spices have antioxidant capability. From the most active to the least active are cloves, cinnamon, pepper, ginger, and garlic. Curcumin, the active ingredient in turmeric, is reported to be several times more potent than vitamin E as a free radical scavenger (Lampe, 2003). More is not better, however, because high intakes of very spicy foods and chili were found to be risk factors for esophageal and stomach cancers in India (Mathew et al, 2000; Phukan et al, 2001).

It is unclear which of these substances contributes the most to cancer prevention. Indeed, several of them may work together more effectively than individually or may work in different ways to halt carcinogenesis. Perhaps another, yet untested substance in the vegetables is more valuable for cancer prevention than those mentioned here. For these reasons, taking supplements is not recommended. Eating a variety of vegetables, including those linked to low cancer incidence, is the better method of protecting a person's health.

More Is Not Better: Beta-Carotene and Lung Cancer

Evidence from observational studies linking lower rates of lung cancer to people eating more fruits and vegetables and people having higher serum beta-carotene concentrations stimulated clinical trials with supplements. In Finland, when testing beta-carotene and vitamin E as cancer-preventive agents for lung cancer, the intervention produced the surprising finding of a 16 percent *increase* in lung cancer and an 8 percent *increase* in total mortality in the beta-carotene group (Alpha-Tocopherol, 1994). Similar results occurred, a 28 percent higher than expected incidence of lung cancer and 17 percent higher mortality, when beta-carotene and retinol were given to men and women who had been heavy smokers and to men with extensive occupational asbestos exposure (Omenn et al, 1994 and 1996).

to lipid and weight control and can be recommended on that basis.

Although essential with a high fiber diet, fluid alone has been associated with health benefits. Drinking 2531 milliliters of fluid daily compared with 1290 milliliters was linked to a 49 percent decrease in bladder cancer (Kamat and Lamm, 2002). Next to water, tea is the most popular beverage in the world, and the cancer-preventive effects of this beverage have been suggested related to the antioxidant polyphenols it contains. Epidemiological studies have shown decreased cancer occurrence in individuals who drink green tea regularly (Kazi et al, 2002), and drinking up to 1.5 cups of tea daily was linked to a 43 percent decrease in the risk of colon cancer, with greater effects seen in men (Su and Arab, 2002). In animal studies, some teas, including green, have reduced cancer risk, but the effect is unproven in humans (Byers et al, 2002).

Vitamin E

Vitamin E and selenium are both antioxidants that protect cells against breakdown. These two nutrients can substitute for one another, so relating one alone to cancer is a complicated process. Prospective studies are consistent with a protective role for selenium, and possibly vitamin E, in the etiology of prostate cancer (Dagnelie et al, 2004). The Alpha-Tocopherol study mentioned earlier also showed 34 percent fewer cases of prostate cancer and 16 percent fewer cases of colorectal cancer than expected in the men receiving vitamin E (Greenwald and McDonald, 1997), but an adverse effect was the increased deaths from hemorrhagic stroke in those receiving vitamin E (Alpha-Tocopherol, 1994).

Calcium

In both animals and humans, calcium seems to protect against some colon cancers. Higher calcium intake was associated with a 27 percent reduction in distal colon cancer in women and a 42 percent reduction in men but was not associated with reductions in proximal colon cancer (Wu et al, 2002). Experts theorize that calcium reduces cell turnover rates and chemically interferes with bile acids and fatty acids to possibly reduce their toxicity. Many studies use colorectal adenomatous polyps as an endpoint due to the large number of patients and the long follow-up required if colon cancer were the endpoint. Calcium supplements of 1200 to 2000 milligrams per day for 3 to 4 years resulted in a 26 percent reduction in recurrent adenomatous polyps; however, general use is not recommended (Weingarten, Zalmanovici, and Yaphe, 2004).

On the other hand, a very high calcium intake, more than 2000 milligrams per day, appears to increase the risk of prostate cancer (Dagnelie et al, 2004). A component of foods recently receiving attention as having a possible role in cancer prevention is phytoestrogens or plant estrogens. These substances, found in a variety of foodstuffs, are considered in Clinical Application 23–6.

Questionable Relationships to Cancer

Studies have produced inconclusive data or conflicting reports on the relationship of certain substances to cancer. These include coffee, caffeine and aflatoxin-contaminated peanuts or corn.

In Massachusetts and New Hampshire, *increased* risk for epithelial ovarian cancer was associated with consumption of coffee and caffeine but only among premenopausal women (Kuper et al, 2000). In contrast, an Australian study found that compared to no intake, consumption of four or more cups of coffee daily was associated with a 49 percent

Phytoestrogens

These naturally occurring compounds, including several groups of nonsteroidal estrogens, such as isoflavones and lignans, are widely distributed in plants. There is evidence to suggest that they have a protective effect against prostate tumors (Vij and Kumar, 2004). The few studies conducted in humans clearly confirm that soy isoflavones can exert hormonal effects that may help prevent breast and prostate cancers; however, there are few guidelines on optimal doses for specific health outcomes (Cassidy, 2003).

Some experts warn that caution is warranted because studies do not unequivocally support benefits from soy isoflavones. Breast cancer survivors in particular are advised to consume only moderate amounts of soy foods and to avoid high levels and concentrated sources of soy (Byers et al, 2002). The role of isoflavones in cancer prevention, particularly of tumors under endocrine control (breast, prostate, and others), is only supported by weak to nonexistent clinical evidence. In addition, disturbing data have been reported on potential negative effects of soy isoflavones on cognitive function in the aged, particularly regarding tofu intake (Sirtori, 2001).

decrease in risk of epithelial ovarian cancer but was not attributable to caffeine (Jordan et al, 2004).

Again, the explanation may involve genetics, illustrating that general dietary advice may not be appropriate for everyone. In Hawaii, regular coffee, but not tea or soda, was associated with an 80 percent increase in the risk of ovarian cancer, an association that may be modified by CYP1A2 genotype and exposures, such as cruciferous vegetable consumption, that influence CYP1A2 expression. CYP1A2 is a key enzyme in the metabolism of coffee and in the activation of heterocyclic aromatic compounds that may be carcinogenic so that somewhat stronger relationships of coffee and caffeine intake to increased risk were found among women with cruciferous vegetable consumption above the median (Goodman et al, 2003).

In contrast, breast cancer was unrelated to coffee or caffeine. In Sweden, the country with the world's highest per capita coffee consumption, a study of 59,036 women showed no association between intake of coffee, tea, and caffeine and breast cancer incidence (Michels et al, 2002).

Aflatoxins, contaminants of improperly stored food caused by molds, are inconclusively linked to cancer as sole risk factors. Aflatoxin contamination of peanuts and corn is related to primary liver cancer, especially in Africa and Asia, but interpreting this information is complicated because hepatitis B is endemic to both continents. The cancer may be caused by the aflatoxins, by hepatitis B virus, or by both since they act synergistically to amplify risk (Kensler et al, 2004). No evidence relates aflatoxins to cancer risk in the United States. A brief summary of the work on cancer vaccines appears in Box 23–1.

Dietary Practices to Reduce Cancer Risk

Cancer evolves from genetic and environmental factors, of which diet is only one. Nevertheless, certain dietary practices are widely recommended to decrease the risk of cancer. For the most part, these practices have been incorporated into the Dietary Guidelines and MyPyramid and are exemplified in the New American Plate (Fig. 23–3), an educational tool from the American Institute for Cancer Research. Previous chapters detailed the extent to which Americans are not complying with dietary recommendations. The AICR sponsors research, disseminates findings, and offers educational materials, including recipes, to health professionals and the public. Its Web site is http://www.aicr.org.

Good evidence supports the possible or probable benefit of fruits and vegetables in minimizing cancer risk. Other desirable food practices relate to red meat consumption and the choice of beverages. Lastly, physical activity and weight control offer a means to decrease cancer risk.

Increase Fruit and Vegetable Intake

Without question, the predominant advice emphasizes fruit and vegetable intake for prevention of many types of cancer. A variety of fruits and vegetables should be the goal but regular consumption of cruciferous vegetables might be a step toward the goal. Fruits and vegetables rich in Vitamin C could possibly mitigate the undesirable effects of processed meats.

A logo developed for a California program to increase fruits, vegetables, and fiber intake is shown in Figure 23–4. That campaign used broadcast and print media and point-of-sale reminders, posters, and recipes to educate consumers (Foerster et al, 1995).

Prudent Meat Selection and Preparation

Red meat should be limited to small, lean portions. Poultry, fish, and legumes should be primary protein

Box 23–1

Vaccines in Cancer

Several cancers are related to viruses: primary liver cancer to hepatitis B virus and hepatitis C virus, cervical cancer to human papillomavirus, lymphoma to Epstein-Barr virus, Kaposi sarcoma (see Chapter 25) to certain types of human herpesvirus, and leukemia and lymphoma to human T-cell lymphotrophic virus. In the case of cervical cancer, the human papillomavirus is considered to be a necessary cause and evidence is mounting as to viral causation in some of the other conditions (Heymann, 2004). A logical question becomes, why not vaccinate against these viruses? In fact, vaccination against hepatitis B has greatly reduced the incidence of hepatocellular cancer in southeast Asia (King, 2004).

One reason vaccines are slow in coming relates to the same reason influenza vaccine is redesigned every year. Viruses can mutate or change characteristics so the antibodies produced by an old vaccine are no longer effective. Tumor cells also can change their characteristics slightly to avoid detection by the immune system. In addition, to illustrate the size of the problem, more than

500 tumor antigens have been identified. In spite of this, Canada has approved one vaccine for stage IV melanoma (King, 2004).

To take advantage of the interaction between antigens and the immune system, therapeutic cancer vaccines are being developed to treat disease by stimulating both **cellular immunity** and **humoral immunity** and show promise but thus far, have not improved survival or freedom from disease (King, 2004). Development of cancer vaccines is proceeding on two fronts: *allogeneic vaccines* that are manufactured from tumor cells of several people and *autologous vaccines* made from the client's own tumor cells. The process is exacting and may require fresh tumor tissue transported on ice overnight to the manufacturer. Even if DNA or RNA samples are used, at most they can only be preserved by freezing and cannot be treated with paraffin or formalin (King, 2004). Comprehensive information on clinical trials and other subjects can be found on the National Cancer Institute's Web site accessed at http://www.cancer.gov/cancertopics/pdq/cancerdatabase.

Table **23–1** **Dietary Interventions That May Contribute to Reduced Cancer Risk**

	CHOOSE	LIMIT
Fruits and vegetables	5 or more daily servings Regular consumption of cruciferous vegetables If juices taken, choose 100% juice	Fried vegetables High-fat snacks Refined carbohydrates
Grains	Whole grains	Sugar
Meats	Fish, poultry, legumes Small portions of lean meat Vitamin C-rich foods with grilled or processed meats Microwaved, baked, broiled, poached, low-temperature, or marinated cooking methods	Red meat Processed meats Fried foods Charbroiled foods High-temperature cooking Heavy salt use Alcohol
Beverages	Water Tea, especially green	Sweetened drinks Scalding hot beverages and foods Sitting Riding
Activity	30 minutes 5 days/week	
Weight Control	See Chapter 18	

sources. Processed meats and salted meats should be consumed very occasionally.

Slow, moist, low temperature cooking methods are preferred. To minimize the heterocyclic amines (HCAs) in grilled or fried meats and fish, briefly microwave them before frying or broiling. Marinades decrease HCA formation and grilling on foil or dampening flare-ups with water spray decrease PAH formation (American Institute for Cancer Research, 2001). Food safety dictates basting marinade be fresh, not that in which the raw meat was soaked.

Lastly, trimming off and discarding charred portions is a healthful practice.

Choose Beverages Carefully

Alcohol consumption should be limited to two standard drinks per day for men and one standard drink per day for women and lighter weight men. Water and green tea may be preferable to coffee. Regardless, scalding hot beverages should be avoided.

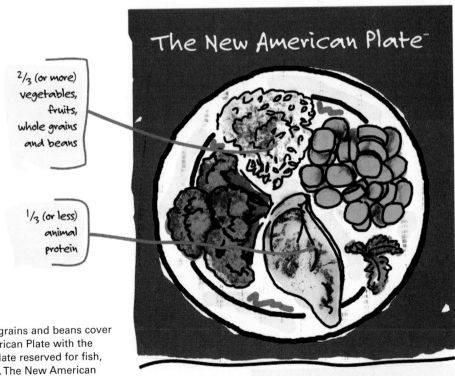

The New American Plate

2/3 (or more) vegetables, fruits, whole grains and beans

1/3 (or less) animal protein

Figure **23–3** Vegetables, fruits, whole grains and beans cover two-thirds (or more) of the New American Plate with the remaining one-third (or less) of the plate reserved for fish, poultry, meat, and lowfat dairy foods. The New American Plate® is a registered trademark of the American Institute for Cancer Research, 2000 (reprinted with permission).

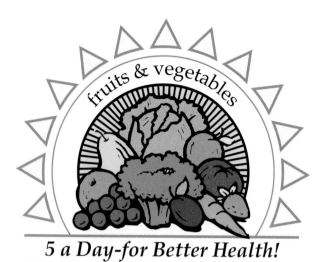

fruits & vegetables

5 a Day-for Better Health!

Figure **23–4** National 5-a-Day program logo. The program logo and slogan are registered service marks. To use them, food industry and state health authority partners sign a license agreement to follow guidelines that maintain the scientific integrity of all messages and other communications to the public. (Reprinted from Foerster et al, 1995, with permission.)

Control Weight Through Physical Activity

Changing behavior to avoid a possible future illness is difficult but avoiding recurrence of cancer should provide strong motivation. In fact, walking just 3 to 5 hours per week at an average pace after a diagnosis of breast cancer reduced the risk of death from the disease (Holmes et al, 2005). Nevertheless, overweight and obese women diagnosed with breast cancer reported low **self-efficacy** for exercise and eating, suggesting that interventions should focus on increasing self-efficacy to encourage behavior change (Pinto et al, 2002). The most important incentives to exercise in women with a history of breast cancer were

expectation of benefit and sense of responsibility, whereas the most important barriers were lack of time and inertia (Leddy, 1997).

Box 23–2 outlines some of the factors to consider when confronted with research findings concerning nutrition. There are no guarantees, even with an optimal diet and favorable lifestyle, that one will not develop cancer. Nevertheless, the general guidelines for a healthy diet are nearly congruent for preventing the two major causes of death in the United States, heart disease and cancer. Table 23–2 summarizes the benefit versus risk evaluation by the American Cancer Society of the evidence available pertaining to dietary interventions to prevent various cancers. A somewhat different interpretation of the evidence for antioxidant supplementation came from the U.S. Preventive Services Task Force (2003) that declared the evidence was insufficient to recommend for or against the use of antioxidant vitamin supplements to prevent cardiovascular disease or cancer. It did specifically recommend against using beta-carotene supplements because of lack of benefit to middle-aged and older adults as well as demonstrated associations with higher incidence of lung cancer and higher all-cause mortality in heavy smokers.

Nutrition for Cancer Clients

Once a person has cancer, nutrition becomes part of the treatment. Despite the possible role of diet in preventing cancer, dietary manipulation has not been shown to cure cancer. The dietary goal is to maintain the client's strength to endure the treatment of the cancer. Energy needs based on body weight are 25 to 35 kcal/kg/day including 1 to 2 g/kg/day of protein (Wilkes, 2000). A study in Germany found 24.2 percent of hospitalized clients to be malnourished, with significantly higher prevalence in those with malignant disease and older clients. Malnourished clients also had 40 percent longer hospital stays (Pirlich et al, 2003). Optimal nutrition may enhance medical treatment,

---

Box 23–2 **Research Findings: Probabilities Not Certainties**

There is a natural progression in research from descriptive to experimental studies that reflects increasing certainty that the findings display reality. Unfortunately, the significance and practical applications of research results are often overstated and publicized in the general press before being reviewed and replicated by other scientists. A single study may be interesting but should not be the basis for radical behavior changes. Peer scientists should examine all research for its strengths and weaknesses. Possible shortcomings affecting all research include:

- Inaccurate measurements. Recall data from questionnaires, although showing statistical differences in large studies may not accurately reflect dietary intake or other behaviors. Even blood levels may be insensitive to small differences and may not correlate with cellular levels in certain organs.
- Imperfect statistical controls. Although extraneous variables are often held constant by statistical manipu-

lation, the process is not perfect and all extraneous variables may not be considered.
- Incorrect assumptions. An underlying physiological basis for a given effect increases the credibility of research. New methods to test physiological effects often challenge earlier assumptions and conclusions. For instance, the mechanism supporting the value of cranberry juice in decreasing bladder infections was determined to be inhibition of *E. coli*. The earlier anecdotal evidence regarding cranberry juice was dismissed by scientists who assumed that the mechanism of action would have to be acidification of the urine and cranberry juice did not make that much difference in pH.

The following table lists some of types of studies (under three major categories—descriptive, correlational, and experimental), their distinguishing qualities, and examples of individual studies focusing on nutrition and cancer.

TYPE OF STUDY	CHARACTERISTICS	APPLICATION TO NUTRITION	LIMITATIONS	EXAMPLE
DESCRIPTIVE (Observational)	Reports naturally occurring events	Examines a population in relation to presence of risk factors, average intake of nutrients, cancer rates and mortality, utilization of health care, etc.	Cannot establish causation. Diet is just one of many influences on health outcomes. Even less certainty results if the population is diverse (Heaney, 2000).	In a 1999 United States Renal Data System survey of 3468 new dialysis patients, 46 percent indicated that they had not consulted with a dietitian before the initiation of dialysis (Moore et al, 2003).
CORRELATIONAL	Compares phenomena in groups with particular outcomes.	Determines the existence of systematic relationships between consumption of specific foods or supplements and cancer occurrence.	Correlation does not establish causation. An untested variable may be causing the relationship.	
Cross-Sectional	Compares behavior of different groups using the same measures at one point in time.		The point in time may not be typical.	In 35,955 subjects from 10 European countries, total fish consumption varied six- to seven-fold, with the lowest consumption in Germany and the highest in Spain (Welch, 2002).
Case Control	Compares reported behavior by cancer clients with reported behavior by a control group of similar people without cancer.		Controls may differ from cases in significant ways that were not considered and in ability to recall behavior accurately.	Increased risk for epithelial ovarian cancer was associated with consumption of coffee and caffeine but only among premenopausal women (Kuper et al, 2000).
Prospective (Cohort)	Measures phenomena of interest in a large population. Much later compares those with particular outcome to those without it in relation to the earlier determined practice.	Determines usual diet and other pertinent traits of large group of people at Point A. Waits until illness of interest develops in an adequate number of the people. Compares the groups with disease and without it in relation to the early diet.	Requires very large groups to obtain sufficient cases. May take years for illness of interest to develop, and diet may have changed in the interim.	Coffee, tea, and caffeine was not associated with breast cancer incidence in 59,036 Swedish women (Michels, 2002).
EXPERIMENTAL	Compares results of an intervention administered to one group but not to another.	Administers vitamin or specific food to one group, placebo or none to another. Measures changes in illness, symptoms, blood levels, etc.	Component selected for intervention may not be the one that gave the effect when whole foods were investigated.	

(Continued on the following page)

Box 23–2 **Research Findings: Probabilities Not Certainties** *(Continued)*

TYPE OF STUDY	CHARACTERISTICS	APPLICATION TO NUTRITION	LIMITATIONS	EXAMPLE
Cell and Tissue Cultures			Laboratory results may not be duplicated in animals or humans.	A flavonoid fraction from cranberry extract inhibited proliferation of eight human tumor cell lines of multiple origins (Ferguson et al, 2004).
Animals			Very large doses may be used that are unrealistic to extrapolate to humans.	Adequate intakes of vitamin E and protein prevent increases of oxidative damage to DNA, lipids, and protein induced by total body irradiation in mice (Shin and Yamada, 2002).
Humans			Difficult to shield participant from knowing their intervention or control status. May take a long time to see an effect. Ethical considerations limit the withholding of treatment from the control group.	Ten days of preoperative and 9 days of postoperative TPN reduced the complication rate by approximately one-third and prevented mortality in patients with gastric or colorectal tumors and preoperative weight loss of 10 percent or more (Bozzetti et al, 2000).

In summary, careful reading of research reports is required to make wise judgments about the applicability to health practices. Occasionally, an intervention trial is terminated early to permit an obviously effective treatment to be extended to the control group, as in the folic acid–neural tube defect study (MRC Vitamin Study Research Group, 1991), or to prevent harm, as in the beta-carotene/vitamin A–lung cancer trial (Redlich et al, 1998). Even in these rare situations, the complete reasons for the effect shown by the overwhelming evidence are not always clear. A broad perspective is necessary to guide a person's behavior toward healthy choices for a lifetime.

Table 23–2 **Benefit Versus Risk Evaluation by the American Cancer Society (for the General Public)**

INTERVENTION	BLADDER	BREAST	COLORECTAL	ENDOMETRIAL	ORAL OR ESOPHAGEAL	PANCREAS	PROSTATE	STOMACH
Increased fruit and vegetable intake	A3	A3	A2	A3	A2	A3	A3	A2
Limited red meat intake	C	B	A2	B	B	A3	A3	C
Increased physical activity	B	A1	A1	A2	B	B	B	C
Overweight avoidance	C	A1	A1	A1	A2	B	B	B
Limited alcohol intake	C	A2	A3	B	A1	A3	C	C
Soy food consumption	B	B	B	B	B	B	C	C
Beta-carotene supplements	B	B	B	B	B	B	B	B
Vitamin E supplements	B	B	B	B	B	B	C	B
Vitamin C supplements	B	B	B	B	B	B	A3	B
Folic acid supplements	B	A3	A3	B	B	B	B	B
Selenium supplements	B	B	A3	B	B	B	A3	B

A1 = convincing evidence of benefit; A2 = probable benefit; A3 = possible benefit; B = insufficient evidence of benefit or risk; C = evidence of lack of benefit; D = evidence of harm.

The few instances of *convincing evidence of benefit* show there is much research remaining to be done. Perhaps, for many reasons, some of them ethical, definitive answers may not be found. Adapted from Byers et al, 2002.

although conclusive evidence is lacking. A review of studies of pelvic radiotherapy found no evidence to support the effectiveness of nutritional interventions in controlling bowel symptoms; however, further research was recommended into low-fat diets, probiotic supplements, and elemental diets (McGough et al, 2004).

With modern treatment, many people are cancer survivors. In the United States, approximately 9.5 million persons are cancer survivors, and 62 percent of Americans with cancer survive more than 5 years after diagnosis (Brown et al, 2003). These individuals may be especially motivated to improve their lifestyles to prevent recurrences or new primary cancers. A summary of the benefits or risks of some interventions possible for cancer survivors is listed in Table 23–3. There is less empirical evidence pertaining to surviving cancer than there is regarding preventing it, but still some rationale exists for particular choices. No consensus has been reached regarding antioxidant supplementation because some experts believe antioxidants could be used by the tumor cells to repair damage by treatments whereas other experts believe the benefit to bolstering normal cells would outweigh the theoretical assistance to the cancer cells. Nevertheless, a prudent course would be to confine antioxidant intakes to the ULs or less when receiving therapy (Brown et al, 2003).

Cachexia

A state of malnutrition and wasting is called **cachexia.** Often seen in up to two-thirds of cancer clients, it is also associated with other diseases, including AIDS, alcoholism, heart failure, malaria, rheumatoid arthritis, and tuberculosis. The client loses weight involving both adipose tissue and skeletal muscle, but the wasting is not due to malnutrition, which preferentially depletes lipids from adipose tissue (see Chapter 24). Overall skeletal muscle protein breakdown rates in cancer patients have not been found to be different from controls, but the rate of muscle protein synthesis is reduced, thereby producing net muscle protein loss (Barber and Rogers, 2002). In cancer, cachexia occurs, despite efforts to nourish the client, because of the tumor's effects on the client's metabolism in which increased resting energy expenditure can occur despite the reduced dietary intake, indicating a malfunction of metabolism that rarely can be explained by the actual energy demands of the tumor (Plata-Salaman, 2000). Several substances produced by the tumor have been identified as mediators of tissue wasting in cachexia. A lipid-mobilizing factor stimulates lipolysis and increases energy expenditure. Cachexia-inducing tumors also produce a chemical that causes protein catabolism in skeletal muscle, while visceral protein is preserved (Tisdale, 2001b). Of particular relevance to nutrition is that a polyunsaturated fatty acid, *eicosapentaenoic acid (EPA)*, weakens the activity of this proteolytic-inducing factor and prevents loss of skeletal muscle (Tisdale, 2001a). Specifically, fish oil-enriched nutritional supplements given to clients with pancreatic cancer produced a median weight gain of 1 kilogram over 3 weeks and significantly affected serum mediators of catabolism (Barber et al, 2001). Ross

Table 23–3 **Benefit Versus Risk Evaluation for Cancer Survivors by the American Cancer Society**

	Breast		Colorectal		Lung		Prostate	
	RECURRENCE	QUALITY OF LIFE	RECURRENCE	QUALITY OF LIFE	RECURRENCE	QUALITY OF LIFE	RECURRENCE	QUALITY OF LIFE
Striving for HBW during treatment	A3	B	A3	B	A3	A2	B	B
Striving for HBW after treatment	A2	A2	A3	A2	A3	A3	B	A3
Increasing physical activity* during treatment	B	A2	B	A2	B	B	B	A3
Increasing physical activity* after treatment	A3	A2	A3	A2	B	A3	B	A2
Limiting total fat	B	B	B	B	B	B	B	B
Limiting saturated fat	B	A3	A3	B	B	B	A3	B
Increasing fruits and vegetables	A3	B	A3	B	A2	B	A3	A3
Increasing fiber	B	B	B	B	B	B	B	B
Increasing omega-3 fatty acids	B	B	B	B	B	B	B	B
Increasing soy	B†	B†	B	B	B	B	B	B

A1 = convincing evidence of benefit; A2 = probable benefit; A3 = possible benefit; B = insufficient evidence of benefit or risk; C = evidence of lack of benefit; D = evidence of harm**.
*What is low-intensity exercise for a healthy person may be high-intensity for the cancer survivor.
†Avoid concentrated sources of soy and soy isoflavones.
**For the factors and cancers listed, there is no convincing evidence of benefit to clients during or after treatment for cancer, but neither is there evidence of lack of benefit or of harm.
SOURCE: Adapted from Brown et al, 2003.

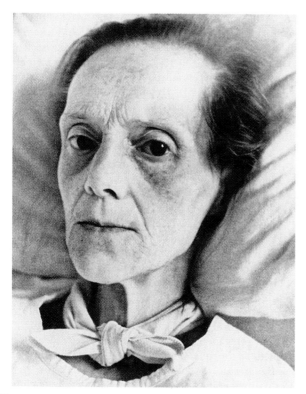

Figure **23–5** This woman is cachectic, showing signs of malnutrition and wasting. (Reproduced from Nutrition Today, 16(3), cover, © Williams & Wilkins, 1981, with permission.)

Laboratories has marketed a nutritional supplement for cancer clients containing EPA (ProSure(R) Shake); however, instructions state it should be used under medical supervision even though it is an over-the-counter product. Figure 23–5 shows a woman with cachexia.

Cancer also changes the client's carbohydrate metabolism. Insulin resistance is common. The client can no longer produce glucose efficiently from carbohydrate but instead uses tissue protein for energy. In traumatized non-cancer clients, catabolism of fat for fuel gradually replaces protein breakdown, but the cancer client's body does not make this adaptive change. By contrast, see starvation in Chapter 24.

Another likely causative factor in cachexia is the body's inflammatory response to the tumor. Treatment with anti-inflammatory drugs seems to have an anabolic effect (Barber, 2002).

Assessment Considerations

Unexplained weight loss is one of the seven danger signals of cancer, but it is not a universal sign. Compared to 80 percent of clients with cancers of the stomach and pancreas who experienced weight loss, just 31 to 40 percent of those with breast or hematologic cancers or sarcomas and 54 to 64 percent of those with cancers of the colon, lung, and prostate were so affected. Anorexia and changes in the sense of taste often precede the diagnosis of cancer. Because the tumor alters the person's metabolism, it is possible for weight loss to occur without a reduction in

food intake. Involuntary weight loss of more than 10 percent is associated with poorer survival rates (Shils and Shike, 1999), and percentage of weight loss is a sensitive and specific tool that can effectively screen and identify malnutrition in cancer clients (Ravasco et al, 2003). In addition, compared to 10 percent of those remaining disease-free, unexplained weight loss occurred in 84 percent of breast cancer clients who developed recurrences, and the weight loss preceded the diagnosis of recurrence by 4 to 12 months (Marinho, Rettori, and Vieira-Matos, 2001). As cancer clients often develop ascites as well as other third-space sequestering of fluids, interpreting the weight gain or loss may be difficult. Nevertheless, weight is an important measure of progress in treating ascites.

Serum proteins, particularly albumin, reflect skeletal muscle and visceral protein status. Increased breakdown of the body's tissues and catabolism of the albumin produces low serum albumin levels. Hypoalbuminemia also may be caused by nephrotic syndrome or loss of proteins from removal of third-space fluids. Serum transferrin is also used as a marker for protein status. Because its half-life is 8 days, compared with 20 days for albumin, serum transferrin levels reflect the client's responses to stress or to nutritional support faster than serum albumin levels.

Common Nutritional Problems in Cancer Clients

Some nutritional problems in cancer clients are due to the disease, and others are due to treatment modalities. Common problems affecting the consumption of meals and nourishment of cancer clients are early satiety and anorexia, taste alterations, local effects in the mouth, nausea, vomiting and diarrhea, and altered immune response.

Early Satiety and Anorexia

Although they may look starved, cancer clients may take a few bites of food and declare that they are full. They may say that they have no appetite at all. The main source of this symptom is the cancer itself, by mechanisms that are beginning to be understood. Control of the disease improves the appetite. Sometimes, though, the physical pressure from the tumor or third-space fluid accumulation may give a feeling of fullness. Relieving that problem may improve food intake.

Some additional factors may interfere with appetite. The psychological stress of dealing with cancer may produce anxiety or depression. The person may be grappling with a body image change or may be going through the grieving process for the loss of a body function or the potential loss of life itself.

Taste Alterations

Cancer clients often have changes in taste perceptions, particularly a decreased threshold for bitterness. Accordingly, they will often say that beef and pork taste bitter or metallic. Some clients report a decreased sensation of sweet, salty, and sour tastes, and they desire increased seasonings. These taste changes are caused by the cancer and the various modes of therapy.

Local Effects in the Mouth

Clients who are being treated with radiation for head and neck cancers often experience mouth ulcers, decreased and thick saliva, and swallowing difficulty. Any of these may interfere with nutritional intake.

Nausea, Vomiting, and Diarrhea

This triad of symptoms often accompanies radiation treatment or chemotherapy, as well as certain types of tumors. Since the gastrointestinal tract cells normally are replaced every few days, these rapidly dividing cells are more vulnerable to the cancer treatments than are more slowly reproducing body cells. Not all clients suffer these side effects to the same extent, and they generally cease when the treatment is completed.

Radiation enteritis involves injury to the intestine. Clients at greater risk of radiation enteritis are those who are thin; who have had previous abdominal surgery; who have hypertension, diabetes mellitus, or pelvic inflammatory disease; or who receive chemotherapy along with the radiation. Delays in onset of symptoms of 20 years have been reported (Turtel and Shike, 1999). A case was reported of a client whose anal ulcer caused by radiotherapy was healed in 7 weeks with oral vitamin A (Levitsky et al, 2003).

Altered Immune Response

Sometimes, antineoplastic agents also suppress the client's immune system. Clients receiving them are at risk of overwhelming infections from organisms that would not affect other persons. Clients receiving radiation therapy or radiation as part of bone marrow transplantation also are at high risk of infections and need to be protected from all organisms, even those that are harmless to most healthy people. Clinical Application 23–7 details the role of the immune system in preventing cancer.

Nutritional Interventions

Based on the problem areas just listed, dietary alterations are suggested. Parenteral therapy and tube feedings are covered in detail in Chapter 15, and dietary management of a long list of symptoms common in terminally ill clients is included in Box 26–2.

For Early Satiety and Anorexia

Many nutrient-dense feedings are offered to the cancer client. For instance, adding 1 1/3 cups of instant dry skim milk powder to 1 quart of liquid milk increases the nutrient density, with little or no change in palatability. Similarly, 1 tablespoon of dry skim milk powder can be added to foods such as mashed potatoes and puddings.

Cancer clients should be encouraged to eat whether they are hungry or not. Appropriate exercise before meals may help to stimulate appetite. Attractively prepared food served in a pleasant environment is enticing. Very small servings, offered frequently, may increase the client's intake. For clients in the hospital or hospice, receiving favorite foods from home or sharing a meal with the family

---

Clinical Application 23–7

Role of the Immune System in Cancer

The immune system can recognize and eliminate tumor cells, but the tumors also can interfere with and evade immune responses by multiple mechanisms (Blattman and Greenberg, 2004; Rodriguez, Zea, and Ochoa, 2003). The increased incidence of cancer in AIDS clients and in organ transplant clients on immunosuppressive drugs demonstrates the consequence of a weakened immune system.

Part of the body's immune defense is provided by certain white blood cells called **T-lymphocytes.** These cells have the task of recognizing foreign materials, including cancer cells, as "non-self" and acting to destroy the invaders. Some of the T-lymphocytes develop into killer cells, which bind to the foreign cell membrane and release lysosomal enzymes into the cancer cell that destroys it. The T-lymphocytes mature in the **thymus** gland in the chest, hence the name, thymic lymphocytes. Contributing to the development of cancer in the elderly is the deterioration of the immune system, since the thymus gland begins to shrink at sexual maturity and by age 50 only 10 percent of the original gland remains.

The gastrointestinal system encompasses almost 50 percent of the mass of the immune system and 70 to 80 percent of immunologic-secreting cells and yet can be affected not only by tumor growth but by cancer treatments (Bloch, 2003). Consequently, efforts to maintain the integrity of gastrointestinal tract could contribute to the person's health in ways that go beyond nutrition.

---

may help overcome the client's aversion to food and offer the family the opportunity to contribute to a loved one's care. Unfortunately the case was not proved in one study that found neither calorie nor protein intake differed significantly between two groups of pediatric oncology clients eating with their caregivers versus alone, but satisfaction with food service was significantly higher in the social dining group (Williams et al, 2004). Children sometimes can be coaxed to eat by decorating their food with faces or serving it in the form of designs such as cars or dolls or the child's name. Involving the child in food preparation or in choosing the menu can help to stimulate the appetite. Reorganizing a pediatric oncology unit to provide "room service" improved the children's energy intake significantly and their protein intake by 18 percent as well as their satisfaction with the hospital food service (Williams, Virtue, and Adkins, 1998).

For the severely anorexic client, offering 1 ounce of a complete nutritional supplement every hour can be effective in promoting nourishment. Clients with severe, chronic anorexia who can tolerate oral intake may benefit from drug therapy with *megestrol acetate*, a semi-synthetic progesterone, one of the most effective appetite stimulants for clients with cancer anorexia. Despite the fact that weight gain stimulated by progestational agents is primarily fat and not lean body mass (MacDonald, 2003), overall quality of life was improved in most clients with cancer who took megestrol for 2 to 8 weeks (Tomiska et al, 2003). When treating a terminally ill client, improving quality of life through some enjoyment of food and family is an appropriate goal. Nourishing the terminally ill client is the subject of Chapter 26.

To Combat Bitter or Metallic Tastes

Oral hygiene before meals freshens the mouth. Sometimes lemon-flavored beverages improve taste sensations. Cooking in a microwave oven or in glass utensils may minimize the metallic taste. Experiment with plastic table service if metal utensils are a problem. As protein sources, eggs, fish, poultry, and dairy products may be better received than beef or pork. Serving meat cold or at room temperature lessens the bitter taste. Sweet sauces and marinades added to the meat may improve its palatability.

For Local Effects About the Mouth

A single canker sore can be remarkably painful. A cancer client with multiple oral ulcerations may complain of severe pain on food ingestion. In addition, some clients also have a dry mouth and difficulty swallowing. For all of these problems, good oral hygiene, before and after meals, is essential.

MOUTH ULCERATIONS

Foods should be soft and mild. Sauces, gravies, and dressings may make foods easier to eat. Cream soups and milk provide much nutrition for the volume ingested. Cold foods have a somewhat numbing effect and may be better tolerated than hot food. Taking liquids with meals helps wash down the food. Drinking straws may help get the liquids past mouth ulcerations. Substances likely to irritate the mouth ulcerations should be avoided. These may include hot items, salty or spicy foods, acidic juices, and alcohol (even in mouthwash). To maintain oral intake, it may be necessary to resort to an anesthetic mouthwash. If the mouth is anesthetized, clients should be instructed to chew slowly and carefully to avoid biting their lips, tongue, or cheeks.

DRY MOUTH

Adequate hydration helps keep the mouth moist. Food lubricants can be of value: gravy, butter, margarine, milk, beer, or bouillon may aid in consuming a near-adequate diet when the mouth is dry. Synthetic salivas are available also, but they have caused allergic reactions (Kandala and Playfor, 2003). In addition, many clients prefer sips of water to the synthetic products. Sugarless hard candy, chewing gum, or popsicles also may stimulate saliva production.

SWALLOWING DIFFICULTY

This problem may linger throughout a course of treatment. To combat it, clients should make swallowing a conscious act. They should inhale, swallow, and exhale. They should experiment with head position. Tilting the head backward or forward may help. Foods for these clients should be nonsticky and of even consistency. Lumpy gravy and mixed vegetables, for example, are hard to manage.

Dunking bread products in beverages helps lubricate the passage.

For Nausea, Vomiting, and Diarrhea

Antiemetic medications should be given an appropriate number of hours before chemotherapy begins and continued on a regular schedule. These drugs are most effective if given prophylactically before the client becomes nauseated. Identifying the pathway inducing nausea and vomiting helps to select effective medications, which might include a derivative of marijuana, *dronabinol* (Haughney, 2004). Similarly, medications for pain and insomnia must be given liberally, but an opioid regimen also necessitates measures to prevent constipation. Because nausea and vomiting frequently accompany pain in clients without cancer, so, too, controlling the cancer client's pain may alleviate nausea. In addition to administering antiemetic drugs, the nurse should monitor the client's hydration and electrolyte status.

As with morning sickness, eating dry crackers before arising may alleviate the nausea. Liquids taken between meals, rather than with them, reduce the volume in the stomach. Similarly, a low-fat diet is digested faster, leaving less content in the stomach to cause nausea or to be vomited. Clients should eat slowly and chew thoroughly. Resting after eating and taking liquids 30 to 60 minutes after solid food helps to control nausea. Foods the client especially likes should be saved for times when the client feels well, so that these favorite foods do not become associated with vomiting and are thereafter avoided. Food aversions develop in more than half of chemotherapy clients, usually involving two to four foods, but they may be accepted several weeks or months after the completion of therapy (Utermohlen, 1999).

Avoid strong cooking odors by selecting milder foods, ventilating the kitchen, and using microwave or boil-in-bag preparation. As with the client who has gastrointestinal upset, clear liquids should be tried first, after vomiting ceases, and the diet progressed as tolerated. Unconventional mealtimes may be instituted to ensure that the client receives nourishment when nausea is minimal. If this means that breakfast is eaten at 2 AM and lunch at 6 AM, so be it. This accommodation is truly individualized care.

Maintenance of fluid and electrolyte intake is critical in the client with diarrhea, and early recognition and treatment can modify this complication. Among the dietary modifications that may be used are the following:

- Adding pectin-containing foods to the client's intake
- Implementing a low-residue diet
- Testing for and treating lactose intolerance
- Restoring intestinal bacteria with active cultures of yogurt

A concentrated freeze-dried living bacteria compound was effective in preventing diarrhea in clients receiving 6 to 7 weeks of pelvic radiation (Delia et al, 2002). Pancreatic secretions and bile acids in the bowel seem to increase the susceptibility of the small bowel to radiation. Nourishing clients enterally with amino acids or partially digested protein and very little fat helped to decrease diarrhea and weight loss and to minimize interruptions to the treatment schedule. Such feedings are not recommended routinely because of the inconvenience but may be appropriate for malnourished clients or those with severe radiation toxicity (Turtel and Shike, 1999).

For Altered Immune Response

Clients may be placed in protective isolation to minimize their exposure to microorganisms. As for dietary interventions, fresh fruits and fresh vegetables may be restricted since they cannot be disinfected adequately. Raw and undercooked entrees and appetizers such as smoked and pickled fish as well as unpasteurized foods may be off limits. Yogurt also may have to be avoided because of the possibility of translocation of bacteria from the intestine to the bloodstream. Other measures are similar to those taken to protect AIDS clients and are included in Chapter 25.

Total Parenteral Nutrition or Tube Feedings

The principles of tube feeding and total parenteral nutrition (TPN) apply to cancer clients as well as to clients generally. Clients should be started on appropriate feeding methods before they become severely malnourished. A client whose weight is 5 kilograms below a healthy body weight and whose serum albumin is less than 3 grams per 100 milliliters should be considered as a candidate for intensive nutritional support. Other individuals deserve early interventions because of the location of the cancer. As an example, increased dietitian supervision of clients with head and neck cancer, including the time between surgery and the start of chemotherapy, reduced the weight loss these clients sustained (Dawson et al, 2001). The Charting Tip in Box 23–3 advocates forethought when documenting cancer clients' at-home treatments and diet plans.

Other Nursing Interventions

Oral hygiene before and after meals may help clients to eat better. Oral hygiene with isotonic saline alone or combined with soda bicarbonate is recommended. Alcohol and glycerin products dry the mucosa, and hydrogen peroxide damages new tissue.

Physical therapy may prevent further loss of muscle tissue due to weight loss. Massage and relaxation exercises may assist clients in coping. Depending on the techniques

| Box 23–3 | **Charting Tip** |

- When admitting a client who provides much of his or her own care at home, try to learn all about treatments and dietary preferences and document them. If the client becomes less self-sufficient after surgery or after beginning cancer therapy, the staff will not have to ask multiple questions before providing care. Recording this information ensures that others besides the nurse who obtained it will be able to meet the client's needs.

used, massage can either stimulate or relax a person. Besides the local effects, the client receives the benefit of touch from another person. This can be very valuable, because cancer clients sometimes feel, rightly or wrongly, that they are being shunned. In one type of relaxation exercise, clients are coached to relax areas of the body in sequence. Others focus the client's mind on controlled breathing or mental images. These procedures have the added advantage of assisting the client to achieve some control over an oppressive situation. Clients respond differently to nursing interventions. No single technique works in every situation.

Music therapy has been effective in alleviating the distress of cancer clients and has the advantage of not requiring training or active participation to implement. A comparison of routine hospice care with or without music therapy affirmed the value of music to an improved quality of life (Hilliard, 2003). Moreover, clients receiving a music intervention in addition to other antiemetic treatments during high-dose chemotherapy experienced less nausea and fewer instances of vomiting than those who did not receive the music (Ezzone et al, 1998).

Nursing cancer clients requires creativity and patience. It also exemplifies one of the most satisfying rewards of nursing. By entering clients' lives at critical times, the nurse often shares their hopes and fears and memories. As often as not, we can learn as much from them as they can from us. Cancer clients, by confronting a potentially fatal disease, can teach themselves, their families, and their caregivers the truth of the adage that life is a journey, not a destination.

SUMMARY

Cancer is the second leading cause of death in the United States. Many different kinds of cancer exist, but all occur when normal cells reproduce uncontrollably both at the site of origin and in metastatic sites of the body. The two-step process of cancer development may evolve over decades, involving initiators that alter a cell's genes and promoters that then activate the altered genes to begin their unruly growth. As more is discovered about the molecular basis of cancer, more refined and individualized treatments will be possible.

Dietary guidelines to prevent cancer are similar to those included throughout this book. People should avoid obesity through controlled consumption of the energy nutrients and should limit intakes of alcohol, fat, and meats, especially those that are cured, smoked, or charbroiled. Positive dietary steps are to maintain generous intakes of fruits, vegetables, fiber, and fluid and adequate but not excessive intakes of vitamin E and calcium. Wellness Tip 23–1 summarizes general guidelines.

(Continued on the following page)

SUMMARY *(Continued)*

Cancer clients often present difficult nutritional challenges. Both the disease and its treatment can cause early satiety and anorexia, taste alterations, local effects in the mouth, nausea, vomiting, diarrhea, and altered immune responses. Creative interventions for these problems help make the client's life significantly more comfortable and can give a sense of accomplishment to the nurse and provide solace to the family.

Wellness Tip **23–1** • Do not smoke.
• Choose a wide variety of fruits and vegetables. Eight to 10 servings a day as recommended in the DASH Diet for hypertension would also be suitable in attempts to minimize cancer risk.
• Choose whole grains, cereals, and legumes to provide half the kilocalories in the daily diet.

• Eat small portions (3 ounces/day) of fish, poultry, or meat and limit intake of cured, smoked, and charbroiled foods.
• Limit consumption of saturated fats in favor of monounsaturated and polyunsaturated forms.
• Confine salt intake to less than 6 grams (about 1 teaspoon) per day.
• Cook foods at low temperatures instead of frying or grilling.
• If alcohol is consumed, restrict it to one to two standard drinks per day, depending on age, gender, and body size.
• If a supplemental vitamins and minerals are desired, pick a multivitamin/mineral product containing the nutrients at RDA levels rather than individual products.
• Avoid excess body weight.
• Exercise regularly.

CASE STUDY 23-1

Ms. X is admitted to the hospital for a third course of chemotherapy. She is divorced, with no children, and lives with her mother, who is very supportive. Hopeful that this therapy will stem the cancer, Ms. X is determined to complete the prescribed treatments. Nausea and vomiting in the past two courses of chemotherapy caused her to suspend treatment before it was completed.

Ms. X is 42 years old, 5 ft 5 in tall, and weighs 119 lb. Her elbow breadth is 2 1/4 in. The mucous membranes of her oral cavity are intact. Her favorite foods are ice cream and steak, although for the past 2 months beef has tasted bitter to her. A 24-hour recall indicated she consumed a relatively balanced diet that totaled approximately 1800 kilocalories.

NURSING CARE PLAN

SUBJECTIVE DATA History of intolerance to chemotherapy due to excessive nausea and vomiting
Taste alteration for beef
Stated determination to complete treatment
Estimated deficit of 400 kilocalories for previous day

OBJECTIVE DATA 94 percent healthy body weight (127 lb)
No breaks in mucous membranes of mouth

NURSING DIAGNOSIS NANDA: Imbalanced Nutrition: Less than Body Requirements (NANDA, 2003, with permission) related to side effects of chemotherapy as evidenced by body weight 6 percent under healthy body weight for height

DESIRED OUTCOMES EVALUATION CRITERIA	NURSING ACTIONS/INTERVENTIONS	RATIONALE
NOC: Nutritional Status (Moorhead, Johnson, and Maas, 2004, with permission.)	NIC: Nutrition Therapy (Dochterman and Bulechek, 2004, with permission.)	
Client will maintain current weight during chemotherapy treatments.	Give antiemetics on scheduled basis for maximum effectiveness.	Antiemetics work better as preventive medicine than as curative.
	Assess daily the times nausea occurs. Schedule meals at other times.	Individualizing meal schedules for clients at high risk of malnutrition should increase dietary intake.
	Offer dry crackers whenever nausea occurs.	Some clients have received relief from nausea by eating dry crackers.
	Give gentle oral hygiene every 4 hours.	Keeping the oral cavity clean and fresh helps to maintain intake.

DESIRED OUTCOMES EVALUATION CRITERIA	NURSING ACTIONS/INTERVENTIONS	RATIONALE
	Encourage client to eat slowly and chew thoroughly.	Eating slowly and chewing thoroughly reduce the incidence and severity of nausea.
	Provide a back rub and quiet time after meals.	Rest after eating will lessen pressure on stomach and intestines. Appropriate massage induces relaxation.
	Help client to select music that will relax her during treatments.	Music therapy has improved the effectiveness of an antiemetic regimen in chemotherapy clients.
	Teach relaxation exercises and controlled breathing to be used when nausea occurs.	These exercises give the client some control over her environment. Teaching the exercises before treatments begin will be more effective than trying to interrupt the cycle of nausea and vomiting once begun.
	If vomiting occurs, monitor weight, hydration, and electrolyte status.	Early identification and interruption of a pathological process permits easier and less invasive treatments. Loss of gastric secretions can cause fluid volume deficit and alkalosis.
	Consult with clinical dietitian and physician regarding supplements, high-protein, low-fat diet, enteral feeding, or TPN.	Although this client is not 10 percent below minimum body weight, if she loses an additional 5 lb, she will reach that benchmark. Aggressive nutritional support should begin before the client becomes severely malnourished.

C T Q CRITICAL THINKING QUESTIONS

1. What additional assessment data might impact the design of Ms. X's nursing care plan?
2. How could you involve the client's mother in her care?
3. Later, the physician's chart notes indicate Ms. X's cancer has not responded to treatment. Ms. X is aware of her situation. She tells the nurse, "If this doesn't work, I'm going to starve it out by fasting and purging." How should the nurse respond?

⟫ CHAPTER REVIEW

1. Research has identified which of the following factors as possibly explaining the conflicting results reported concerning dietary intakes and cancer development?
   a. Erroneous classification of the tumor types
   b. Genetic differences in the metabolism of the people studied
   c. A time frame that extends over too many years
   d. Too large a sample of people recruited to the study

2. Cruciferous vegetables that are specifically thought to protect against cancer are:
   a. Corn, lima beans, and peas
   b. Carrots, green beans, and tomatoes
   c. Brussels sprouts, bean sprouts, and water chestnuts
   d. Broccoli, cauliflower, and cabbage

3. Which of the following foods is likely to be well received by a cancer client with mouth ulcerations?
   a. Hot chicken noodle soup
   b. Orange juice with orange sherbet
   c. Vanilla milkshake
   d. Soda crackers with cream cheese

4. Which of the following is the best advice to increase oral intake for a chemotherapy client who suffers from nausea and vomiting?
   a. Drink plenty of fluids with the meal
   b. Eat high-fat, high-protein meals
   c. Take only foods that are well liked
   d. Eat slowly and chew thoroughly

5. If visitors brought all of the following to a client in protective isolation, which should the nurse question?
   a. Fruit basket
   b. Homemade vegetable soup
   c. Apple pie
   d. Malted milk and French fries

CLINICAL ANALYSIS

Ms. R is a 70-year-old widow under treatment for breast cancer. She is being cared for by her daughter, Ms. S, with assistance from a home healthcare service. Despite fairly good oral intake at the daughter's urging, Ms. R continues to lose weight and now carries 95 pounds on her 5-foot, 4-inch frame. Her main complaint regarding food is its bitter taste.

1. Ms. S asks why her mother continues to lose weight when she is taking half the meals and more than half the supplements offered. Which of the following replies by the nurse would be most appropriate?
   a. "Your mother must be too active and using more calories than she is taking in."
   b. "Probably the medications are dehydrating her. We should increase her fluid intake."
   c. "Frequently the tumor short-circuits the body's metabolism so that nutrients cannot be used normally."
   d. "She doesn't take in enough protein to prevent loss of muscle. We should try supplements of amino acid powders."

2. Ms. S expressed interest in learning what she could do to lessen her own chances of developing a malignancy of the breast. Which of the following suggestions have the best evidence for preventing breast cancer?
   a. Limit intake of red, processed, or charbroiled meats
   b. Maintain a normal weight and minimize or avoid alcohol intake
   c. Gradually increase fiber intake to 25 grams per day, accompanied by adequate fluid intake
   d. Eat a variety of colorful fruits and vegetables every day

3. Which of the following interventions could alleviate the bitter tastes Ms. R is experiencing?
   a. Serving meats cold or microwaved in glass dishes
   b. Limiting the intake of dairy products
   c. Avoiding sauces and marinades that could increase the bitter taste
   d. All of the above

REFERENCES

Abdulla, M, and Gruber, P: Role of diet modification in cancer prevention. Biofactors 12:45, 2000.

Albert-Puleo, M: Physiological effects of cabbage with reference to its potential as a dietary cancer-inhibitor and its use in ancient medicine. J Ethnopharmacol 9:261, 1983.

Alberts, DS, and Garcia, DJ: An overview of clinical cancer chemoprevention studies with emphasis on positive phase III studies. J Nutr 125:692S, 1995.

Alpha-Tocopherol, Beta-carotene Cancer Prevention Study Group: Effect of vitamin E and beta-carotene on the incidence of lung cancer and other cancers in male smokers. N Engl J Med 330:1029, 1994.

Ambrosone, CB: Oxidants and antioxidants in breast cancer. Antioxid Redox Signal 2:903, 2000.

American Institute for Cancer Research: Experts reissue warning about grilling. May 23, 2005. Accessed May 25, 2005 at http://www.aicr.org/press/pubsearchdetail.lasso?index=2026

American Institute for Cancer Research: The Facts About Grilling. AICR, Washington, DC, 2001. Accessed May 25, 2005 at http://www.aicr.org/publications/brochures/online/nap.pdf

American Institute for Cancer Research: Caveat grilling debate. Newsletter 6:1, 2002.

American Institute for Cancer Research: The New American Plate. AICR, Washington, DC, 2000. Accessed May 25, 2005 at http://www.aicr.org/publications/brochures/online/nap.pdf

Ames, BN: DNA damage from micronutrient deficiencies is likely to be a major cause of cancer. Mutat Res 475:7, 2001.

Ansano, T, and McLeod, RS: Dietary fibre for the prevention of colorectal adenomas and carcinomas. Cochrane Database Syst Rev z: CD003430, 2002.

Astorg, P: Dietary N-6 and N-3 polyunsaturated fatty acids and prostate cancer risk: A review of epidemiological and experimental evidence. Cancer Causes Control 15:367, 2004.

Barber, MD, et al: Effect of a fish oil-enriched nutritional supplement on metabolic mediators in patients with pancreatic cancer cachexia. Nutr Cancer 40:118, 2001.

Barber, MD: The pathophysiology and treatment of cancer cachexia. Nutr Clin Prac 17:203, 2002.

Barber, MD, and Rogers, BB: Advances in the management of tumor-induced weight loss. Medscape Nursing Continuing Education, 2002. Accessed November 17, 2004 at http://www.medscape.com/viewprogram/2008_pnt.

Bingham, SA: Dietary fibre in food and protection against colorectal cancer in the European Prospective Investigation into Cancer and Nutrition (EPIC): An observational study. Lancet 361:1496, 2003.

Blackburn, GL, et al: Diet and breast cancer. J Womens Health 12:183, 2003.

Blattman, JN, and Greenberg, PD: Cancer immunotherapy: A treatment for the masses. Science 305:200, 2004.

Bloch, AS: Special considerations for nutrition interventions with oncology patients. Oncology 17(suppl 2):17, 2003.

Bozzetti, F, et al: Perioperative total parenteral nutrition in malnourished, gastrointestinal cancer patients: A randomized, clinical trial. JPEN J Parenter Enteral Nutr 24:7, 2000.

Bradley, CJ, Given, CW, and Roberts, C: Disparities in cancer diagnosis and survival. Cancer 91:178, 2001.

Brown, JK, et al: Nutrition and physical activity during and after cancer treatment: An American Cancer Society guide for informed choices. CA Cancer J Clin 53:268, 2003.

Byers, T, et al: American Cancer Society guidelines on nutrition and physical activity for cancer prevention. CA Cancer J Clin 52:92, 2002.

Calle, EE, et al: Overweight, obesity, and mortality from cancer in a prospectively studied cohort of U.S. adults. N Engl J Med 348:1625, 2003.

Cassidy, A: Potential risks and benefits of phytoestrogen-rich diets. Int J Vitam Nutr Res 73:120, 2003.

Centers for Disease Control: Cancer mortality surveillance—United States, 1990–2000. MMWR 53(SS03):1, 2004. Accessed May 24, 2005 at http://www.cdc.gov/mmwr/preview/mmwrhtml/ss5303a1.htm.

Chainani-Wu, N: Diet and oral, pharyngeal, and esophageal cancer. Nutr Cancer 44:104, 2002.

Chao, A, et al: Meat Consumption and Risk of Colorectal Cancer. JAMA 293:172, 2005.

Cheng, KK, et al: A case-control study of oesophageal adenocarcinoma in women: A preventable disease. Br J Cancer 83:127, 2000.

Chiou, HL, et al: NAT2 fast acetylator genotype is associated with an increased risk of lung cancer among never-smoking women in Taiwan. Cancer Lett 223:93, 2005.

Collaborative Group on Hormonal Factors in Breast Cancer: Familial breast cancer: Collaborative reanalysis of individual data from 52 epidemiological studies including 58 209 women with breast cancer and 101 986 women without the disease. Lancet 358:1389, 2001.

Colston, KW, and Hansen, CM: Mechanisms implicated in the growth regulatory effects of vitamin D in breast cancer. Endocr Relat Cancer 9:45, 2002.

Cohen, JH, Kristal, AR, and Stanford, JL: Fruit and vegetable intakes and prostate cancer risk. J Natl Cancer Inst 92:61, 2000.

Cross, AJ, and Sinha, R: Meat-related mutagens/carcinogens in the etiology of colorectal cancer. Environ Mol Mutagen 44:44, 2004.

Dagnelie, PC, et al: Diet, anthropometric measures and prostate cancer risk: A review of prospective cohort and intervention studies. BJU Int 93:1139, 2004.

Dawson, ER, et al: Increasing dietary supervision can reduce weight loss in oral cancer patients. Nutr Cancer 41:70, 2001.

Delia, P, et al: Prophylaxis of diarrhoea in patients submitted to radiotherapeutic treatment on pelvic district: Personal experience. Dig Liver Dis 34:S84, 2002.

Devesa, SS, et al: Atlas of cancer mortality in the United States, 1950–1994. Publication No NIH 99-4564. U.S. Government Printing Office, Washington, DC, 1999. Accessed November 05, 2004 at http://dceg.cancer.gov/cgi-bin/atlas/avail-maps?site=acc.

Dochterman, J, and Bulechek, G (eds): Nursing Interventions Classification (NIC), ed 4. Mosby, St. Louis, 2004.

Eriksson, CJ: The role of acetaldehyde in the actions of alcohol (update 2000). Alcohol Clin Exp Res 25:15S, 2001.

Etminan, M, Takkouche, B, and Caamano-Isorna, F: The role of tomato products and lycopene in the prevention of prostate cancer: a meta-analysis of observational studies. Cancer Epidemiol Biomarkers Prev 13:340, 2004.

Ezzone, S, et al: Music as an adjunct to antiemetic therapy. Oncol Nurs Forum 25:1551, 1998.

Feigelson, HS, et al: Alcohol consumption increases the risk of fatal breast cancer (United States). Cancer Causes Control 12:895, 2001.

Ferguson, LR: Natural and human-made mutagens and carcinogens in the human diet. Toxicology 27:181, 2002.

Ferguson, PJ, et al: A flavonoid fraction from cranberry extract inhibits proliferation of human tumor cell lines. J Nutr 134:1529, 2004.

Fernandez, et al: Fish consumption and cancer risk. Am J Clin Nutr 70:85, 1999.

Fleischauer, AT, et al: Dietary antioxidants, supplements, and risk of epithelial ovarian cancer. Nutr Cancer 40:92, 2001.

Foerster, SB, et al: California's "5 a Day—for Better Health" campaign: An innovative population-based effort to effect large-scale dietary change. Am J Prev Med 11:124, 1995.

Fraser, GE: Associations between diet and cancer, ischemic heart disease, and all-cause mortality in non-Hispanic white California Seventh-day Adventists. Am J Clin Nutr 70(suppl 3):532S, 1999.

Gandini, S, et al: Meta-analysis of studies on breast cancer risk and diet: The role of fruit and vegetable consumption and the intake of associated micronutrients. Eur J Cancer 36:636, 2000.

Gao, CM, et al: Protective effect of allium vegetables against both esophageal and stomach cancer: A simultaneous case-referent study of a high-epidemic area in Jiangsu Province, China. Jpn J Cancer Res 90:614, 1999.

Giovannucci, E: Alcohol, one-carbon metabolism, and colorectal cancer: Recent insights from molecular studies. J Nutr 134:2475S, 2004.

Goodman, MT, et al: Association of caffeine intake and CYP1A2 genotype with ovarian cancer. Nutr Cancer 46:23, 2003.

Greenwald, P: Antioxidant vitamins and cancer risk. Nutrition 10:433, 1994.

Greenwald, P, and McDonald, SS: Cancer prevention: The roles of diet and chemoprevention. Cancer Control: J Moffitt Cancer Center 4:118, 1997.

Haughney, A: Nausea and vomiting in end-stage cancer. Am J Nurs 104(11):40, 2004.

Heaney, RP: Calcium, dairy products, and osteoporosis. J Am Coll Nutr 19:83S, 2000.

Heymann, DL(ed): Control of Communicable Diseases Manual, ed 18. American Public Health Association, Washington, DC, 2004.

Hill, M: Dietary fibre and colon cancer: Where do we go from here? Proc Nutr Soc 62:63, 2003.

Hilliard, RE: The effects of music therapy on the quality and length of life of people diagnosed with terminal cancer. J Music Ther 40:113, 2003.

Ho, C-T, et al: Phytochemicals in teas and rosemary and their cancer-preventive properties. In Huang, M-T, et al (eds): Food Phytochemicals II: Teas, Spices, and Herbs. American Chemical Society, Washington, DC, 1994.

Holick, CN, et al: Dietary carotenoids, serum B-carotene, and retinol and risk of lung cancer in the Alpha-Tocopherol, Beta-carotene Cohort Study. Am J Epidemiol 156:536, 2002.

Holmes, MD, et al: Physical activity and survival after breast cancer diagnosis. JAMA 293:2479, 2005.

Huncharek, M, Klassen, H, and Kupelnick, B: Dietary beta-carotene intake and the risk of epithelial ovarian cancer: A meta-analysis of 3,782 subjects from five observational studies. In Vivo 15:339, 2001.

Huncharek, M, and Kupelnick, B: Dietary fat intake and risk of epithelial ovarian cancer: a meta-analysis of 6,689 subjects from 8 observational studies. Nutr Cancer 40:87, 2001.

Jordan, SJ, et al: Coffee, tea and caffeine and risk of epithelial ovarian cancer. Cancer Causes Control 15:359, 2004.

Kamat, AM, and Lamm, DL: Chemoprevention of bladder cancer. Urol Clin North Am 29:157, 2002.

Kandala, V, and Playfor, S: Massive tongue swelling following the use of synthetic saliva. Paediatr Anaesth 13:827, 2003.

Kazi, A, et al: Potential molecular targets of tea polyphenols in human tumor cells: Significance in cancer prevention. In Vivo 16:397, 2002.

Kensler, TW, et al: Chemoprevention of hepatocellular carcinoma in aflatoxin endemic areas. Gastroenterology 127:S310, 2004.

Key, TJ, et al: Diet, nutrition and the prevention of cancer. Public Health Nutr 7:187, 2004.

Key, TJ, et al: Nutrition and breast cancer. Breast 12:412, 2003.

Key, TJ, Verkasalo, PK, and Banks, E: Epidemiology of breast cancer. Lancet Oncol 2:133, 2001.

Khanna, KK, and Jackson, SP: DNA double-strand breaks: Signaling, repair and the cancer connection. Nat Genet 27:247, 2001.

Kim, M, et al: Preventive effect of green tea polyphenols on colon Carcinogenesis. In Huang, M-T, et al (eds): Food Phytochemicals II: Teas; Spices, and Herbs. American Chemical Society Washington, DC, 1994.

King, SE: Therapeutic cancer vaccines: An emerging treatment option. Clin J Oncol Nurs 8:271, 2004.

Kuper, H, et al: Population based study of coffee, alcohol and tobacco use and risk of ovarian cancer. Int J Cancer 88:313, 2000.

Kushi, L, and Giovannucci, E: Dietary fat and cancer. Am J Med 113:63S, 2002.

Lampe, JW: Spicing up a vegetarian diet: Chemopreventive effects of phytochemicals. Am J Clin Nutr 78:579S, 2003.

Leddy, SK: Incentives and barriers to exercise in women with a history of breast cancer. Oncol Nurs Forum 24:885, 1997.

Le Marchand, L, et al: Combined effects of well-done red meat, smoking, and rapid N-acetyltransferase 2 and CYP1A2 phenotypes in increasing colorectal cancer risk. Cancer Epidemiol Biomarkers Prev 10:1259, 2001.

Le Marchand, L, et al: Intake of flavonoids and lung cancer. J Natl Cancer Inst 92:154, 2000.

Levitsky, J, et al: Oral vitamin A therapy for a patient with a severely symptomatic postradiation anal ulceration: Report of a case. Dis Colon Rectum 46:679, 2003.

MacDonald, N: Nutrition as an integral component of supportive care. Oncology 17(suppl 2): 8, 2003.

Marinho, LA, Rettori, O, and Vieira-Matos, AN: Body weight loss as an indicator of breast cancer recurrence. Acta Oncol 40:832, 2001.

Mathew, A, et al: Diet and stomach cancer: A case-control study in South India. Eur J Cancer Prev 9:89, 2000.

McGough, C, et al: Role of nutritional intervention in patients treated with radiotherapy for pelvic malignancy. Br J Cancer 90:2278, 2004.

McTiernan, A, et al: Adiposity and sex hormones in post-menopausal breast cancer survivors. J Clin Oncol 21:1961, 2003.

McTiernan, A: Behavioral risk factors in breast cancer: Can risk be modified? Oncologist 8:326, 2003.

Michels, KB, et al: Coffee, tea, and caffeine consumption and breast cancer incidence in a cohort of Swedish women. Ann Epidemiol 12:21, 2002.

Missmer, SA, et al: Meat and dairy food consumption and breast cancer: A pooled analysis of cohort studies. Int J Epidemiol 31:79, 2002.

Moore, H, et al: National Kidney Foundation Council on Renal Nutrition survey: Past-present clinical practices and future strategic planning. J Ren Nutr 13:233, 2003.

Moorhead, S, Johnson, M, and Maas, M (eds): Nursing Outcomes Classification (NOC), ed 3. Mosby, St. Louis, 2004.

Moorman, PG, and Terry, PD: Consumption of dairy products and the risk of breast cancer: A review of the literature. Am J Clin Nutr 80:5, 2004.

Moyad, MA: Dietary fat reduction to reduce prostate cancer risk: Controlled enthusiasm, learning a lesson from breast of other cancers, and the big picture. Urology 59(suppl 1):51, 2002.

MRC Vitamin Study Research Group: Prevention of neural tube defects: Results of the Medical Research Council Vitamin Study. Lancet 338:131, 1991.

Murillo, G, and Mehta, RG: Cruciferous vegetables and cancer prevention. Nutr Cancer 41:17, 2001.

NANDA International: Nursing Diagnoses: Definitions and Classification, 2003–2004. NANDA International, Philadelphia, 2003.

National Cancer Institute: Colorectal cancer (PDQ®): Prevention. 02/16/2005. Accessed May 26, 2005 at http://www.cancer.gov/cancertopics/pdq/prevention/colorectal/healthprofessional

National Cancer Institute: SEER Cancer Statistics Review, 1975–2001. 2004. Accessed October 31, 2004 at http://seer.cancer.gov/csr/1975_2001/results_merged/topic_race_ethnicity.pdf.

National Center for Health Statistics: NCHS Data on Cancer. Accessed October 19, 2004 at http://cdc.gov/nchs/data/factsheets/cancer.pdf.

Nkondjock, A, et al: Specific fatty acids and human colorectal cancer: An overview. Cancer Detect Prev 27:55, 2003.

O'Keefe, SJ, et al: Rarity of colon cancer in Africans is associated with low animal product consumption, not fiber. Am J Gastroenterol 94:1373, 1999.

O'Kelly, J, and Koeffler, HP: Vitamin D analogs and breast cancer. Recent Results Cancer Res 164:333, 2003.

Omenn, GS, et al: Risk factors for lung cancer and for intervention effects in CARET, the Beta-Carotene and Retinol Efficacy Trial. J Natl Cancer Inst 98:1550, 1996.

Omenn, GS, et al: The beta-carotene and retinol efficacy trial (CARET) for chemoprevention of lung cancer in high risk populations: Smokers and asbestos-exposed workers. Cancer Res 54:2038S, 1994.

Parazzini, F, et al: Population attributable risk for ovarian cancer. Eur J Cancer 36:520, 2000.

Phukan, RK, et al: Role of dietary habits in the development of esophageal cancer in Assam, the north-eastern region of India. Nutr Cancer 39:204, 2001.

Pinto, BM, et al: Motivation to modify lifestyle risk behaviors in women treated for breast cancer. Mayo Clin Proc 77:122, 2002.

Pirlich, M, et al: Prevalence of malnutrition in hospitalized medical patients: Impact of underlying disease. Dig Dis 21:245, 2003.

Plata-Salaman, CR: Central nervous system mechanisms contributing to the cachexia-anorexia syndrome. Nutrition 16:1009, 2000.

Poschl, G, and Seitz, HK: Alcohol and cancer. Alcohol 30:155, 2004.

Ravasco, P, et al: Nutritional deterioration in cancer: The role of disease and diet. Clin Oncol 15:443, 2003.

Redlich, CA, et al: Effect of supplementation with beta-carotene and vitamin A on lung nutrient levels. Cancer Epidemiol Biomarkers Prev 7:211, 1998.

Rennert, G: Diet and cancer: Where are we and where are we going? Proc Nutr Soc 62:59, 2003.

Riboli, E, and Norat, T: Cancer prevention and diet: Opportunities in Europe. Public Health Nutr 4:475, 2001.

Riedel, F, Goessler, U, and Hormann, K: Alcohol-related diseases of the mouth and throat. Best Pract Res Clin Gastroenterol 17:543, 2003.

Roberts-Thomson, IC, Butler, WJ, and Ryan, P: Meat, metabolic genotypes and risk for colorectal cancer. Eur J Cancer Prev 8:207, 1999.

Rodriguez, PC, Zea, AH, and Ochoa, AC: Mechanisms of tumor evasion from the immune response. Cancer Chemother Biol Response Modif 21:351, 2003.

Roth, J, and Mobarhan, S: Preventive role of dietary fiber in gastric cardia cancers. Nutr Rev 59:372, 2001.

Salmon, CP, et al: Minimization of heterocyclic amines and thermal inactivation of *Escherichia coli* in fried ground beef. J Nat Cancer Inst 92:1773, 2000.

Shils, ME, and Shike, M: Nutritional support of the cancer patient. In Shils, ME, et al (eds): Modern Nutrition in Health and Disease, ed 9. Lippincott Williams & Wilkins, Philadelphia, 1999.

Shin, SJ, and Yamada, K: Adequate intakes of vitamin E and protein prevent increases of oxidative damage to DNA, lipids, and protein induced by total body irradiation in mice. Nutr Cancer 44:169, 2002.

Singh, GK, et al: Persistent area socioeconomic disparities in U.S. incidence of cervical cancer, mortality, stage, and survival, 1975–2000. Cancer 101:1051, 2004.

Sirtori, CR: Risks and benefits of soy phytoestrogens in cardiovascular diseases, cancer, climacteric symptoms and osteoporosis. Drug Saf 24:665, 2001.

Slupphaug, G, Kavli, B, and Krokan, HE: The interacting pathways for prevention and repair of oxidative DNA damage. Mutat Res 531:231, 2003.

Steinkellner, H, et al: Effects of cruciferous vegetables and their constituents on drug metabolizing enzymes involved in the bioactivation of DNA-reactive dietary carcinogens. Mutat Res 480:285, 2001.

Steinmaus, CM, Nunez, S, and Smith, AH: Diet and bladder cancer: a meta-analysis of six dietary variables. Am J Epidemiol 151:693, 2000.

Su, LJ, and Arab, L: Tea consumption and the reduced risk of colon cancer: Results from a national prospective cohort study. Public Health Nutr 5:419, 2002.

Sugimura, T, and Wakabayashi, K: Carcinogens in foods. In Shils, ME, et al (eds): Modern Nutrition in Health and Disease, ed 9. Lippincott Williams & Wilkins, Philadelphia, 1999.

Sugimura, T, et al: Heterocyclic amines: Mutagens/carcinogens produced during cooking of meat and fish. Cancer Sci 95:290, 2004.

Terry, P, et al: A prospective study of major dietary patterns and the risk of breast cancer. Cancer Epidemiol Biomarkers Prev 10:1281, 2001.

Tisdale, MJ: Cancer anorexia and cachexia. Nutrition 17:438, 2001a.

Tisdale, MJ: Loss of skeletal muscle in cancer: Biochemical mechanisms. Front Biosci 6:D164, 2001b.

Tomiska, M, et al: Palliative treatment of cancer anorexia with oral suspension of megestrol acetate. Neoplasma 50:227, 2003.

Tomlinson, SS: Dietary and lifestyle factors associated with breast cancer rates. J Am Acad Phys Assist 7:622, 1994.

Truswell, AS: Meat consumption and cancer of the large bowel. Eur J Clin Nutr 56:S19, 2002.

Turtel, PS, and Shike, M: Diseases of the small bowel. In Shils, ME, et al (eds): Modern Nutrition in Health and Disease, ed 9. Lippincott Williams & Wilkins, Philadelphia, 1999.

Utermohlen, V: Diet, nutrition, and drug interactions. In Shils, ME, et al (eds): Modern Nutrition in Health and Disease, ed 9. Lippincott Williams & Wilkins, Philadelphia, 1999.

United States Preventive Services Task Force: Vitamin supplementation to prevent cancer and cardiovascular disease. United States Department of Health and Human Services, Rockville, MD, 2003. Accessed September 2, 2004 at http://www.ahrq.gov/clinic/uspstf/uspsvita.htm.

van der Klift, M, et al: Bone mineral density and the risk of breast cancer: The Rotterdam Study. Bone 32:211, 2003.

Vij, U, and Kumar, A: Phyto-oestrogens and prostatic growth. Natl Med J India 17:22, 2004.

Weinberg, RA: How cancer arises. Sci Am 275:62, 1996. Accessed June 27, 2000 at http://www.sciam.com/0996issue/0996 weinberg.html.

Weingarten, MA, Zalmanovici, A, and Yaphe, J: Dietary calcium supplementation for preventing colorectal cancer and adenomatous polyps. Cochrane Database Syst Rev 1: CD003548, 2004.

Weisburger, JH: Comments on the history and importance of aromatic and heterocyclic amines in public health. Mutat Res 506:9, 2002.

Welch, AA, et al: Variability of fish consumption within the 10 European countries participating in the European Investigation into Cancer and Nutrition (EPIC) study. Public Health Nutr 5:1273, 2002.

Wilkes, G: Nutrition: The forgotten ingredient in cancer care. Am J Nurs 100(4):46, 2000.

Willett, WC: Diet and cancer. Oncologist 5:393, 2000.

Willett, W: Lessons from dietary studies in Adventists and questions for the future. Am J Clin Nutr 78:539S, 2003.

Williams, R, et al: A comparison of calorie and protein intake in hospitalized pediatric oncology patients dining with a caregiver versus patients dining alone: A randomized, prospective clinical trial. J Pediatr Oncol Nurs 21:223, 2004.

Williams, R, Virtue, K, and Adkins, A: Clinical issues: Room service improves patient food intake and satisfaction with hospital food. J Pediatr Oncol Nurs 15:183, 1998.

Wu, K, et al: Calcium intake and risk of colon cancer in women and men. J Natl Cancer Inst 94:437, 2002.

Zeegers, MP, et al: The association between smoking, beverage consumption, diet and bladder cancer: A systematic literature review. World J Urol 21:392, 2004.

Zhang, SM: Role of vitamins in the risk, prevention, and treatment of breast cancer. Curr Opin Obstet Gynecol 16:19, 2004.

CHAPTER 24

Nutrition During Stress

Learning Objectives

After completing this chapter, the student should be able to:

1. Explain how people can protect themselves nutritionally from the effects of excessive mental stress.
2. List four hypermetabolic conditions that increase resting energy expenditure and, hence, kilocaloric requirements.
3. Describe how metabolism differs in starvation and hypermetabolism.
4. Discuss the effects of impaired respiratory function on nutritional status and appropriate nutritional therapy.
5. List six recommendations for the safe refeeding of malnourished clients.

Stress is any stimulus or condition that threatens the body's mental or physical well-being. This chapter discusses how the body responds to four distinct types of stress and how these conditions impact nutritional needs. The chapter begins with a discussion of mental stress experienced by physically healthy persons. The body's response to mental stress differs markedly from the response to starvation. Starvation is the second type of stress discussed in this chapter. The third type of stress discussed is that caused by a severe physical injury such as a motor vehicle accident, gunshot or stab wound, a burn, or severe fracture. A severe physical stress invokes a hypermetabolic response. A discussion of medical nutrition therapy for the client with severe pulmonary disease follows. Each of these stressors may cause a different metabolic response and require slightly different nutritional care. The chapter concludes with a discussion of the principles for safely refeeding nutritionally deprived clients.

Nutrition and Mental Stress

The effects of mental stress cannot be isolated easily from the effects of physical stress. The physical self and the mental self are structurally related. For example, in the presence of danger, a series of chemical reactions occurs that are associated with our feeling of fear. Hormones mediate the fight-or-flight response, discussed in Chapter 1, Evolution and the Science of Nutrition. In other words, the fear (mental factor) triggers the hormones (physical factors). Despite the relationship between mental and physical stress, no reliable evidence shows that mental stress increases the need for kilocalories or nutrients.

Not All Stress Is Negative

A balanced amount of stress maximizes health. Human beings need some stress for mental well-being. For example, boredom is stressful for many people. Mental stresses related to ambition, drive, and desire may in fact be perceived as positive. Stress, such as strain, tension, and/or anxiety, is commonly perceived as negative. Most people perceive the death of a spouse, divorce, unemployment, financial problems, and personal injury as negative. Clearly, we cannot control all the events that affect us. However, we do have some control over how we respond to such events. The relationship between nutritional status and people's response to emotional stress has not been completely researched.

Chronic Disease

Mental stress is related to the incidence of cancer, cardiovascular disease, hypertension, and some forms of gastrointestinal diseases. All of these chronic diseases are related to nutrition. Epidemiological evidence indicates that diets that contain recommended amounts of fruits, vegetables, and grains are associated with a lower incidence of heart disease and certain cancers. But it is not known which, if any, specific substances in the diet are responsible or whether taking more than the DRI doses of supplements may do more harm than good (Quandt, 1999). A healthy mental state is known to be important for reducing the risk of heart disease. People who are ordinarily tense, impatient, and ambitious tend to have a high serum cholesterol level. Clients with diabetes report that emotional stress increases their blood glucose levels.

The dietary treatments for chronic diseases should focus on dietary components that are known to be related to health outcomes. For example, clients who have diabetes benefit the most from a carbohydrate-, fat-, and kilocalorie-controlled diet to normalize blood and lipid levels and maintain or lose body weight. Maintenance of body weight by both diet and exercise has been shown to help prevent cancer, diabetes, hypertension, and heart disease. Sodium-restricted diets have been shown to help control hypertension.

Gastrointestinal Complication

Ulcers and some intestinal diseases are aggravated by perceived excessive mental stress. A client may report that he or she has specific food intolerances when under emotional stress but that the same food is easily tolerated in the absence of stress. This is partially due to impairment of gastrointestinal function during episodes of stress. Decreased motility can cause the development of anorexia, abdominal distention, gas pains, and constipation. These symptoms may contribute to food intolerances or reduced food intake. Fear, anger, and worry also stimulates the hypothalamus to activate the autonomic nervous system, which depresses secretions, inhibits peristalsis, and slows propulsion of food by increasing sphincter tone (Bray, 2000). Thus, the effects of emotional stress, including food intolerances, can vary not only from person to person but also in the same person at different times dependant on the extent of activation of the autonomic nervous system.

Food Intake

The volume of food a client consumes and the desire to prepare food are sometimes affected by emotional stress. Some people respond to stress by eating more; others respond by eating less. Mental stress can cause a person to lose interest in food preparation. Thus, mental stress can lead to either overnutrition or undernutrition. An individual's perceived stress should always be taken into consideration when formulating the nutritional component of a care plan.

The time at which food is eaten also may be important. Undernutrition is related to cognition. Extensive evidence indicates that relatively modest increases in circulating glucose concentrations enhance learning and memory processes in rats and humans. For example, students who eat breakfast score higher on examinations than those who do not (Gold, 1995). Dietary carbohydrate is necessary for optimal cognitive function.

Requirements for Nutrients

Nutrition experts believe the need for most nutrients is not increased above DRIs solely as a result of excessive mental activity. The needs for kilocalories, amino acids, and vitamins in healthy individuals have all received some attention from scientists.

Kilocalories

Mental stress alone does not increase our need for kilocalories. For example, mental effort used in studying demands few, if any, additional kilocalories. Likewise, a single person coping with financial problems, a job, and child-rearing does not require extra kilocalories solely as a result of excessive mental activity. Because mental stress does not require additional kilocalories, our requirement for certain vitamins is not increased solely as a result of mental activity. Thiamin, riboflavin, and niacin requirements are based on kilocalorie or protein requirements; if the need for kilocalories (protein) is not increased, neither is the requirement for these vitamins.

A person who responds to mental stress with increased physical movement or muscle activity requires additional kilocalories to maintain his or her body weight. Mental stress may cause a person to sleep less, walk more, tremble, fidget, or otherwise increase the work of the muscles. In this situation, additional kilocalories are needed in underweight clients. Observe clients' body language during encounters.

Amino Acids

Research has failed to show a relationship between amino acids and stress in healthy individuals. Recently, many health-food manufacturers have developed erogenic aids (amino acid supplements) that falsely claim to increase stamina, endurance, and muscle development by releasing growth hormone. There is no scientific evidence that these products actually release growth hormone, which is fortunate because if they did, acromegaly might result (Barrett and Herbert, 1999). **Acromegaly** is a disease marked by elongation and enlargement of facial and extremity bones. This condition is often associated with somnolence, moodiness, and decreased libido. The Federation of American Societies for Experimental Biology (FASEB) has criticized the widespread use of amino acids in supplements because little scientific literature exists about most amino acid supplements taken by healthy persons, because no scientific rationale has been presented to justify the use of amino acid supplements by healthy individuals, and because safety levels for amino acid supplements have not been established (Barrett and Herbert, 1999).

Vitamins and Minerals

Most evidence gathered thus far indicates that vitamins in excess of the DRIs do not counterbalance the negative effects of mental stress. Manufacturers of nutritional supplements for "stress" have yet to produce valid scientific evidence that their products have a health benefit. In 1990, the Federal Trade Commission (FTC) barred a large manufacturer from making unsubstantiated claims that any vitamin product is needed to replace nutrients lost as a result of athletic activity or the stress of daily living (Barrett and Herbert, 1999). A healthy, well-balanced diet with adequate protein, fiber, minerals, and vitamins is the best nutritional insurance against excessive stress. Maintenance of a healthy body weight is an indication that kilocaloric intake is appropriate.

The Stress of Starvation

The physical stress of starvation does alter nutrient needs. Biologically, our bodies evolved to cope with periods of feast or famine. Our response to the stress of starvation evolved slowly over the course of millions of years. The human body's response to food deprivation differs from the body's response to other forms of stress. **Uncomplicated starvation** means that the client is experiencing food deprivation without an underlying disease state. During uncomplicated starvation, clients expend about 70 percent of the kilocalories they normally need to maintain body weight. Because of the biochemical adaptation to starvation, these clients require fewer kilocalories than is normal for their height and weight.

The human body has a well-defined response to starvation. The breakdown or catabolism of nutrient stores to meet energy needs characterizes our response. Every cell within the human body needs a constant supply of energy to function. During starvation, a series of chemical reactions occurs to meet each cell's energy needs. A summary of these chemical reactions follows:

1. *Glycogenolysis* is the breakdown of glycogen (the liver's carbohydrate stores). This releases glucose into the bloodstream. However, the body's limited glycogen stores last only a few hours.
2. *Gluconeogenesis* is the production of glucose from non-carbohydrate stores (only the glycerol portion of triglycerides and amino acids derived from proteins in muscle and organ mass). The primary source of glucose in early starvation is the increased rate of gluconeogenesis. This results in a reduction of lean body mass (LBM).

3. *Lipolysis* is the breakdown of adipose tissue for energy. This releases free fatty acids into the bloodstream. In prolonged starvation, adaptive mechanisms conserve body protein stores by enabling a greater proportion of energy needs to be met by increased fatty acids, with a decreased requirement for glucose.
4. *Ketosis* is the accumulation in the body of the ketone bodies: acetone, beta-hydroxybutyric acid, and acetoacetic acid. Ketosis results from the incomplete metabolism of fatty acids, generally from carbohydrate deficiency, and occurs commonly in starvation. The body utilizes some ketone bodies for energy during prolonged starvation to meet the central nervous system's need for glucose. This reduces, but does not eliminate, the need for glucose.

Prolonged starvation, in sum, is characterized by decreased energy expenditure, diminished gluconeogenesis, and increased ketone production (Winkler and Malone, 2004). These chemical reactions are summarized in Figure 24–1.

Each body cell needs glucose, fatty acids, or the end products of fatty acids and amino acids for energy. Body cells need fuel constantly. Amino acids can be utilized for energy, but only after the liver converts them into glucose or fat. Specific organs have a preference for glucose as a fuel source. (The medical literature uses the word *preference* in this context; the word *affinity* may be substituted

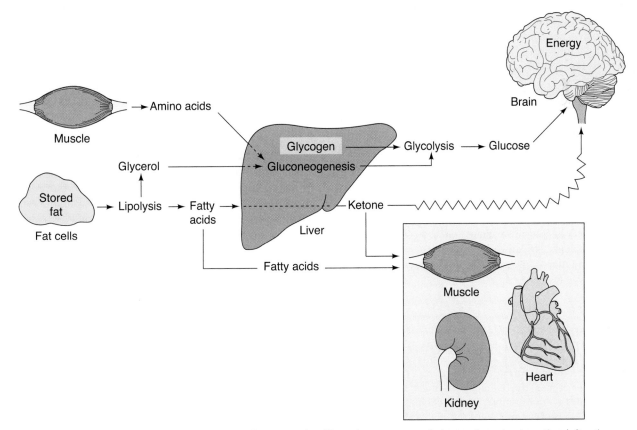

Figure **24–1** Origin of fuel and fuel consumption during starvation. The primary source of glucose in early starvation (after the depletion of glycogen stores) is the increased rate of gluconeogensis. In prolonged starvation, adaptive mechanisms conserve protein by enabling a greater proportion of energy needs to be met by ketone bodies, with a decreased requirement for glucose.

for preference.) The brain prefers glucose for energy. Some cells can also utilize ketone bodies for energy. The brain will use ketone bodies but prefers glucose. For the most part, the human body can use only a very small part of the fat molecule, the glycerol portion, to manufacture glucose. This means that body protein stores must be continually broken down to supply the brain with glucose during starvation after the liver's glycogen stores are depleted.

The heart, kidney, and skeletal muscle tissues prefer fatty acids and/or ketone bodies for their fuel sources. This means that even if a starving person is fed glucose (as in intravenous feeding), some fat is still needed to prevent the breakdown of adipose tissue. A balance of the end products of fat and carbohydrate metabolism is necessary for survival.

In prolonged starvation, most body organs switch to a less-preferred fuel source. Even the brain increasingly begins to utilize more ketone bodies for energy after adaptation to starvation than before. The breakdown of muscle tissue continues in prolonged starvation but at a much lower rate than previously. The human body also becomes more efficient in reusing amino acids for protein synthesis. Thus, urea nitrogen excretion decreases during prolonged starvation. The rate of tissue breakdown in prolonged starvation also decreases because the metabolic rate and total energy expenditure decrease to conserve energy and prolong life. The catabolic or starved individual spontaneously decreases physical activity, increases sleep, and has a lower body temperature. All of these adaptations during prolonged starvation serve one purpose—to prolong life. The human body gets "more miles per gallon" as a result of individual body organs switching to a less-preferred fuel source.

The Stress Response

A severe physical assault to the body invokes a different metabolic response called hypermetabolism. The term **hypermetabolism** refers to major changes in how energy is utilized after severe injury, illness, or infection. Kilocaloric needs decrease during uncomplicated starvation and increase (sometimes markedly) as a result of bodily response to a severe physical assault. This stress response is a dynamic process that has an ebb phase, a flow phase, and an anabolic phase. A client can progress or regress from one phase to another during his or her clinical course. The need for protein varies according to the client's stress level.

Ebb Phase

The **ebb phase** begins with an initial stress stimulus and typically lasts for approximately 24 hours. Blood pressure, cardiac output, body temperature, and oxygen consumption are all reduced during the ebb phase. The body does this so that it has the capacity to meet the increased demands of the environment. These clients require about 1.5 grams of protein per kilogram of body weight per day. The stress response is activated by hormonal and cell mediators—counter-regulatory hormones such as

Table 24–1	Hormonal Secretion During Phase Two of the Stress Response and the Metabolic Effect of These Hormones*
HORMONAL SECRETIONS	**EFFECT OF METABOLISM**
Increased **epinephrine**	Rate of lipolysis increased
	Rate of glycolysis increased
	Rate of gluconeogenesis increased
Decreased insulin	Storage of glucose, fatty acids, and amino acids ceases. Glucose delivery to the cells thus decreases. For this reason, hyperglycemia is commonly seen in stressed clients.
Increased glucagons	Rate of gluconeogenesis increases
Increased antidiuretic hormone	Increase in water retention
Increased aldosterone	Increase in sodium retention

*Net effect: decrease in body protein and fat stores.

catecholamines, cortisol, and growth hormone (Winkler and Malone, 2004).

Flow Phase

Increased cardiac output, oxygen consumption, body temperature, energy expenditure, urinary nitrogen losses and altered glucose metabolism, and accelerated catabolism characterize the **flow phase**. In addition, the flow phase is marked by pronounced hormonal changes. Table 24–1 lists hormones secreted during this stage of the stress response and describes the impact these hormones have on metabolism. These hormonal conditions favor the breakdown of body protein stores to provide glucose. This leads to a rapid loss of nitrogen in the urine as lean body mass is broken down to furnish the cells with glucose. Box 24–1 discusses the benefits of intensive insulin therapy in critically ill patients. The need for protein is about 2 grams per kilogram of body weight during the flow phase but is highly dependent on the severity of the injury. The administration of elevated levels of protein may contribute to a high renal

Box 24–1	Intensive Insulin Therapy in Critically Ill Patients

Hyperglycemia and insulin resistance are common in critically ill patients because of hormonal response to a severe stress. Even if a patient has not had diabetes prior to the stressor, hyperglycemia frequently becomes problematic. Intensive insulin therapy to maintain blood glucose at or below 110 mg per deciliter reduces morbidity and mortality among critically ill patients in the surgical intensive care unit (Van der Berge, 2005). This level of glucose control is only possible with close monitoring and an insulin drip.

load, especially in infants and elderly adults, dictating routine monitoring of fluid status, blood urea nitrogen, and serum creatinine levels (Skipper, 1998). The first emphasis of care is fluid and electrolyte resuscitation.

Blood flow to the gastrointestinal tract is often diminished during this phase of the stress response. This reduced flow decreases the supply of both oxygen and nutrients to the gastrointestinal tract. The secretion of mucus is diminished, and the secretion of gastric acid is increased. Cells that line the gastrointestinal tract waste away and die as a result of these changes. The client may complain of diarrhea and bloating.

Recovery or Anabolic Phase

The third stage of the stress response, the **anabolic phase**, is also marked by changes in hormonal secretions. Insulin and growth hormone increase in the bloodstream during the anabolic phases. Secretion of most of the other hormones decreases. The building up of body tissue and nutrient stores (anabolism) characterizes this phase. Protein need during the anabolic phase is 2 to 3 grams per kilogram of body weight but depends on the severity of the injury.

It is obviously desirable for a client to progress to the third phase of the stress stage as rapidly as possible. Tissue building, or anabolism, is beneficial. The ability of a client to rebuild tissue after a physical stress depends on several factors. Age is one factor. The client's prior nutritional status and the severity and duration of the stress particularly influence tissue growth. Clients who have ample nutrient stores to draw on during stress are better able to tolerate the negative effects of the stress. Good nutrition is a form of insurance, because the nutrient stores are available to be used if an unexpected stress occurs.

Nutrition and Metabolic Stress From Illness, Trauma, and Infection

Cancer, major surgery, burns, infections, and trauma are the physical stressors that have the greatest impact on metabolism. The needs of clients with cancer are described in Chapter 23. This section of this chapter focuses on the nutritional needs of clients experiencing surgery, burns, infections and fevers, and trauma. Nutritional support during extreme stress is needed to decrease the length of the stress, prevent complications, and minimize human suffering.

Hypermetabolism

Hypermetabolism is an abnormal increase in the rate at which fuel or kilocalories are burned. Hypermetabolism can be identified by an increased metabolic rate, negative nitrogen balance, hyperglycemia, and increased oxygen consumption. The body increasingly uses protein obtained from internal body stores (lean body mass) to meet energy needs. This may deplete lean body mass. A loss of 40 percent of lean body mass is fatal (Demling and DeSanti, 2001).

Protein Needs

Protein needs are elevated during hypermetabolism. Injury or illness requires active protein formation. Surgical wound healing, tissue repair, replacement of red blood cells and plasma protein lost in hemorrhage, and the immune response to infection all require a constant supply of protein. For these reasons, a client who is hypermetabolic has an increased need for protein. A hypermetabolic client may lose as much as 3 kg of LBM per day (Mason and Epstein, 2003). This is caused by a marked increase in catecholamines and other stress hormones. The extent of hypermetabolism and catabolism depends on the degree of injury and patient response to the injury.

URINE ASSESSMENT OF PROTEIN STATUS

Total urinary excretion of nitrogen increases with the client's stress level. Urinary creatinine measurements may be used to estimate muscle protein reserves. One problem common to the use of all urinary measurements is the completion of an accurate 24-hour urine collection. Nurses are typically responsible for collecting a 24-hour urine specimen from the client. If even one voiding is discarded, the measurement will be inaccurate.

Kilocalories and Hypermetabolic Stress

Clients who are hypermetabolic have an increased need for kilocalories. The negative nitrogen balance observed in hypermetabolic clients may be the result of inadequate kilocaloric intake rather than of insufficient protein intake or the result of both. Patients lose weight because an increased need for energy coupled with a possibly inadequate energy intake and/or protein intake promotes weight loss.

EARLY FEEDING

The use of early nutritional support has been studied. The use of enteral nutrition shortly after the event that precipitated the stress may be advantageous because it supplies essential nutrients, keeps the gastrointestinal tract active, and halts the elevation of levels of catabolic stress hormones. Enteral feeding has been found to directly nourish the gastrointestinal tract and may help reverse the defective gut barrier that accompanies burn shock. The use of enteral nutrition as opposed to parenteral nutrition also results in an important decrease in the incidence of infectious complications in the critically ill (Gramlich, 2004). In contrast, intravenous nutritional support appears to lack effectiveness in burn patients and may actually increase morbidity and mortality (Hansbrough, 1998).

Although early enteral feeding offers many advantages, the introduction of nutrients into the gastrointestinal tract needs to be evaluated on an individual basis. Low mesenteric blood flow (commonly referring to the peritoneal fold that encircles the small intestine), severe tachycardia, hypotension, a volume deficit, and multisystem organ failure preclude the use of enteral feedings. For these patients, intravenous nutrition is often obligatory.

KILOCALORIE NEEDS

Energy expenditure is the number of kilocalories that an individual uses to meet the body's demand for fuel. There is no universally accepted method to estimate a given patient's energy expenditure. Each organization usually has a protocol to follow to calculate the number of kilocalories to be initially delivered via nutritional support. The patient is then monitored closely to determine metabolic response to the initial kilocalorie estimate.

It is vital to follow an institution's nutrition support protocol to have internal consistency within the organization. Many different team members, including several physicians, often provide care to one patient in a critical care unit. A protocol for nutrition support is usually written by the registered dietitian and carefully approved by a medical staff committee and then approved further by the chief of the medical staff. Deviations from the protocol, although sometimes clinically appropriate, are subject to review by the assigned medical committee and third party payers.

Two different methods to calculate energy expenditure are discussed in this text. The first method is the least complex. Energy needs are calculated as follows:

Critical care: 20 to 30 kcal/kg* (25 to 35 for ventilated patients)

Non-critical care: 25 to 35 kcal/kg

If overweight, use maximum IBW:

F = 100 pounds for 5 feet and 5# for each inch over 5 feet + or − 10%

M = 106 for 5 feet and 6# for each inch over 5 feet + or − 10%

Parenteral guidelines for macronutrient distribution include:

Dextrose:

1. Initiate at 3 grams/kg or 300 mL D$_{70}$ (210 grams)
2. Maximum of 5 grams/kg in stressed patients
3. Maximum of 7 to 8 grams/kg in non-stressed patients
4. Assess tolerance with repeated blood glucose monitoring

Lipids:

1. Initiate with 30% of total kcal as fat
2. Maximum of 0.5 to 1.0 gram/kg in stressed patients
3. Maximum of 2.5 gram/kg in non-stressed patients
4. Maximum of 40 50% of total kcal in any patient.
5. Assess tolerance with triglyceride levels and if greater than 300, hold lipid

Protein:

1. Give full protein requirement the first day in patients without hepatic or renal impairment

HARRIS-BENEDICT EQUATION

The second method discussed in this text to estimate kilocalorie need is the Harris-Benedict equation because it is still widely used to estimate REE for critically ill clients. The Harris-Benedict equation is presented in Clinical Calculation 24–1, along with an example of these

---

Clinical Calculation 24–1

Calculation of Kilocaloric Need for Both a Male and a Female

MALE CLIENT

Energy Need = REE × Activity Factor × Stress Factor

Step 1: Use the following **Harris-Benedict equation** to calculate the male client's resting energy expenditure:

$$REE = 66 + (13.7 \times weight\ in\ kg) + (5 \times height\ in\ cm) - (6.8 \times age)$$

Step 2: Multiply an activity factor by the client's REE (Table 24–2).

Step 3: Multiply the answer obtained in step 2 by the appropriate stress factor (Table 24–3).

FEMALE CLIENT

Energy Need = REE × Activity Factor × Stress Factor

Step 1: Use the following Harris-Benedict equation to calculate the female client's resting energy expenditure:

$$REE = 655 + (9.6 \times weight\ in\ kg) + (1.7 \times height\ in\ cm) - (4.7 \times age)$$

Step 2: Multiply an activity factor by the client's REE (Table 24–2).

REE 3 Activity Factor

Step 3: Multiply the answer obtained in step 2 by the appropriate stress factor (Table 24–3).

REE × Activity Factor × Stress Factor

EXAMPLE CALCULATION

Assume you need to estimate the kilocalorie need of a 154-lb (70-kg) male who is 5 ft 5 in (165 cm) tall and 25 years old. Assume he is confined to bed and has a fractured long bone.

Sample calculation for step 1:

70-kg male who is 165 cm tall and 25 years old
REE = 66 + (13.7 × 70) + (5 × 165) − (6.8 × 25)
REE = 66 + 959 + 825 − 170
REE = 1680

Sample calculation for step 2:

REE × Activity Factor
1680 × 1.2
2016

Sample calculation for step 3:

Answer from step 2 × Stress Factor
2016 × 1.35
2721.6 = client's estimated energy need

Table 24–2 **Activity Factors Commonly Used to Calculate a Client's Activity Kilocalories**

For a client confined to bed	0.2, or 20 percent
For a client out of bed	0.3, or 30 percent

calculations. Note that different equations are used for male and female clients. The Harris-Benedict equation allows the health-care provider to calculate estimated kilocalorie needs based on an individual client's height, age, and weight. This method calculates resting energy expenditure using the Harris-Benedict equation and then determines additional kilocalories needed for both activity and stress.

ACTIVITY FACTOR

The Harris-Benedict equation calculates the patient's REE. Physical activity is not included in the REE and must be calculated. Table 24–2 shows activity factors for clients confined to bed as 0.20, or 20 percent, and for those not confined to bed as 0.30, or 30 percent.

STRESS FACTOR

Research has shown that different types of stress increase kilocaloric needs differently. A **stress factor** is a number assigned to a given pathological state to predict how much a client's kilocaloric need has increased as a result of the type of stress the client is experiencing from that stress state. Table 24–3 lists various types of physical stress and the stress factor used for each disease state.

As you can see in the table, a client with burns over 50 percent of his or her body has a stress factor of 2.0. This means kilocaloric need is twice (200 percent) his or her resting energy expenditure. In contrast, the stress factor after minor surgery is 1.05. This means a client who has had minor surgery needs only 5 percent more kilocalories than his or her REE multiplied by the previously determined physical activity factor. Stress factors are convenient to use in estimating kilocaloric needs.

Table 24–3 **Stress Factors Commonly Used to Determine a Client's Need for Kilocalories**

STRESSOR	FACTOR
Uncomplicated minor surgery	1.05
Starvation	0.70
For each degree F above 98.6	1.07
Cancer	1.1–1.45
Soft tissue trauma	1.14–1.37
Skeletal trauma (fracture)	1.35
Burns (10–30 percent of body surface area)	1.5
Burns (30–50 percent of body surface area)	1.75
Burns (>50 percent of body surface area)	2.0
Peritonitis	1.2–1.5
Major sepsis	1.4–1.8

Protein Needs

The protocol to calculate a patient's protein requirement varies from one institution to the next. For non-critical care patients the 0.8 to 1.2 grams/kg of ideal body weight (IBW) formula is often used. For critical care patients the 1.2 to 1.5 grams/kg of IBW is often used. These calculations have replaced the kilocalorie:nitrogen (Kcal:N) ratios (discussed below).

Ratios of Kilocalorie to Nitrogen in the Hypermetabolic Client

Protein requirements cannot be totally separated from energy requirements because protein is used as an energy source in the absence of adequate kilocalories. The current practice is to calculate **kilocalorie:nitrogen ratios** for hypermetabolic clients. As a rule, the average healthy person needs 1 gram of nitrogen per 300 kilocalories (range, 1:300 to 350). One gram of nitrogen is derived from 6.25 grams of protein. A hypermetabolic client needs approximately 1 gram of nitrogen per 100 to 150 kilocalories (range, 100 to 200) (Souba and Wilmore, 1999). A hypermetabolic client needs about twice as much protein as a client not in a state of hypermetabolism. Clinical Calculation 24–2 demonstrates the calculation of kilocalorie:nitrogen ratios in a TPN solution. Most nutritional supplements have the kilocalorie:nitrogen ratio of the product listed either on the label or in a package insert.

Vitamin and Mineral Needs

The hypermetabolic client usually requires increased B vitamins, vitamin A, and zinc (Skipper, 1998). The B vitamins help release the chemical energy stored in foods. Whenever a client requires increased kilocalories, the need for the B-vitamin complex automatically increases. When anabolism or the building of body tissue is indicated, vitamin C requirements are increased. Hypermetabolic clients usually need to build up depleted tissue stores. Catabolism with a loss of lean body mass increases the loss of potassium, magnesium, phosphorus, and zinc (Winkler and Malone, 2004). These may be provided either in the diet or, more commonly, intravenously.

Examples of Hypermetabolic Conditions

The hypermetabolic conditions that influence nutritional needs most profoundly are major surgery, burns, infections and fevers, and trauma. All of these conditions increase resting energy expenditure and therefore kilocaloric requirements. The following sections discuss these conditions.

Surgery

Uncomplicated minor surgery increases the surgical client's kilocaloric requirement by only 5 percent. Surgery needed to repair soft tissue trauma requires a 14- to 37-percent increase in kilocalories. A surgical client with complications may require a large increase in kilocalories (Table 24–3).

Clinical Calculation 24–2

Calculation of a Sample TPN Solution

Please calculate the total kilocalories, nonprotein calories, grams of nitrogen, calorie/nitrogen ratio, and percent calories from fat in the following TPN solution: 500 cc D_{50}, 500 cc amino acids 10 percent, 250 cc lipid 10 percent.

DEXTROSE

$$D_{50} = 0.50 \times 500 \text{ cc} = 250 \text{ g dextrose}$$
$$250 \text{ g} \times 3.4 \text{ kcal/g} = 850 \text{ kcal}$$

AMINO ACIDS

$$500 \text{ cc} \times 0.10 = 50 \text{ g protein}$$
$$50 \text{ g protein} \times 4 \text{ kcal/g} = 200 \text{ kcal}$$

LIPIDS

$$250 \text{ cc} \times 1.1 \text{ kcal/cc} = 275 \text{ kcal}$$

TOTAL CALORIES

$$850 \text{ from dextrose} + 200 \text{ from protein}$$
$$+ 275 \text{ from lipid} = 1325 \text{ kcal}$$

NONPROTEIN CALORIES

$$\text{Kcal from dextrose } 850 + \text{ kcal from lipid } 275 =$$
$$1125 \text{ nonprotein kcal}$$

GRAMS OF NITROGEN

$$50 \text{ divided by } 6.25 = 8.0 \text{ g nitrogen}$$

CALORIE:NITROGEN RATIO

$$850 \text{ (from dextrose)} + 275 \text{ (from lipid)}$$
$$= 1125 \text{ nonprotein kcal}$$
$$1125 \text{ divided by } 8.0 \text{ g nitrogen} = 141$$
$$\text{Calorie:nitrogen ratio} = 141 \text{ to } 1$$

PERCENT KILOCALORIES FROM FAT

$$\text{Kcal from fat divided by total kcal}$$
$$275 \text{ kcal from fat divided by } 1325 \text{ total kcal} = 21 \text{ percent}$$

Burns

Major burns are the most extreme state of stress a client can sustain. They produce a hypermetabolic state that raises kilocaloric needs higher than those of most other stress states. Kilocaloric requirements may be as high as 8000 kilocalories per day. Even a client who was well nourished before becoming burned may rapidly develop protein-kilocalorie malnutrition. As indicated in Table 24–3, the degree to which the metabolic rate increases is directly related to the body surface area burned. The percentage of body surface area burned is determined by totaling the individual percentages given in Figure 24–2A. Although it is not reflected in the stress factors listed in the table, the deeper the burn, the higher is the client's kilo-

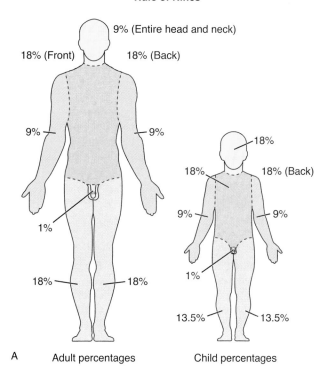

Rule of Nines

9% (Entire head and neck)

18% (Front) 18% (Back)

9% 9%

1%

18% 18%

A Adult percentages

18%

18% 18% (Back)

9% 9%

1%

13.5% 13.5%

Child percentages

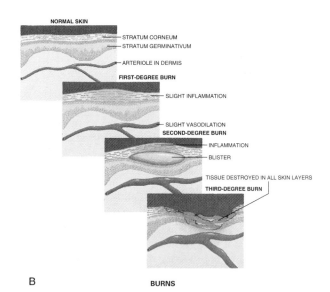

NORMAL SKIN
STRATUM CORNEUM
STRATUM GERMINATIVUM
ARTERIOLE IN DERMIS
FIRST-DEGREE BURN
SLIGHT INFLAMMATION
SLIGHT VASODILATION
SECOND-DEGREE BURN
INFLAMMATION
BLISTER
TISSUE DESTROYED IN ALL SKIN LAYERS
THIRD-DEGREE BURN

B **BURNS**

Figure **24–2** A, The percentage of body surface area burned is determined by comparing the body surface area of the client's burns to the percentages given in the chart. For example, if a client has extensive burns over both legs, the total body surface area burned would be 36 percent (18 percent for the first leg plus 18 percent for the second leg). (Reprinted from Venus, D [ed]: Taber's Cyclopedic Medical Dictionary, ed 19. FA Davis, Philadelphia, 2001, p 296, by Beth Anne Willert, MS, Illustrator, with permission.) B, Burns are classified as first-degree, second-degree, and third-degree. (Reprinted from Thomas, CL [ed]: Taber's Cyclopedic Medical Dictionary, ed 18. FA Davis, Philadelphia, 1997, p 278, by Beth Anne Willert, MS, Illustrator, with permission.)

caloric need. Figure 24–2B illustrates first-, second-, and third-degree burns. Burn clients may remain in a hypermetabolic state for many weeks.

The increased load of waste products produced in some clients with burns is one reason for an increase in fluid requirements. Extra fluids help the kidneys eliminate these waste products. Capillary permeability is increased in burn clients; thus, plasma proteins, fluids, and electrolytes escape into the burn area and interstitial space. This shift reduces the volume of the plasma, so fluid volume needs to be replaced.

Physicians disagree on the best time to begin feeding burn clients. Some physicians keep the client NPO for the first 24 to 72 hours, and others initiate tube feedings within 4 hours following a burn injury. Here, an important consideration is that **peristalsis,** the wavelike motion that propels food through the gastrointestinal tract, ceases in some burn clients. Until peristalsis returns, the client's stomach should not be the site of choice for a tube feeding. The patient may also have an ileus caused by muscle paralysis or an obstruction. Physicians who do feed patients early insert the feeding tube into the client's intestines past the ileus and deliver a very slow, continuous-drip feeding. The slow, continuous drip minimizes the likelihood of the feeding collecting in the intestines because it is readily absorbed.

The rationale for early feeding in these patients follows. If the small intestine *maintains its digestive and absorptive properties,* enteral support is the preferred method of nutrient delivery. Several studies have shown that enteral nutrition initiated within 24 hours of injury was well tolerated and resulted in a statistically significant lower incidence of postoperative pneumonia, intra-abdominal abscess, and catheter sepsis (Souba and Wilmore, 1999). No evidence supports a delay in enteral feeding until the resuscitation period has ended (Skipper, 1998). Patients with burns of less than 20 percent of total body surface area are usually capable of orally consuming sufficient nutrients (Skipper, 1998).

Rather than beginning feedings on the day of injury, some physicians resume oral feeding of the client with the return of normal bowel activity. For most clients, this is 2 to 4 days after the initial burn. Burn clients are usually allowed a clear- or full-liquid diet at this time. Dietary progression begins 4 to 10 days after the injury, as tolerated.

Burn clients are particularly susceptible to **sepsis,** the state in which disease-producing organisms are present in the blood. Major sepsis further increases a client's metabolic rate. See Table 24–3 for the stress factor to use in determining kilocaloric needs during sepsis. Clients with Foley catheters and intravenous lines are at risk for sepsis.

Stress factors can be multiplied by each other. For example, the formula to use for a client with greater than 50 percent burns over the body surface area and major sepsis is:

$$\text{Kilocalorie Need} = \text{REE} \times \text{Activity Factor} \times \text{Stress Factor No. 1 (2.0 for 50 percent burn)} \times \text{Stress Factor No. 2 (1.5 for major sepsis)}$$

Sepsis, of course, is not limited to burn clients; surgical and trauma clients may also suffer from sepsis.

For all burn clients, a nutritional assessment is essential to minimize complications and allow nutritional therapy to be effectively evaluated. The food intake of these clients should be monitored and documented. The kilocalories, grams of protein, kilocalorie:nitrogen ratio, grams of nitrogen (N), and percent of kilocalories from fat consumed or taken intravenously should be charted daily.

A high-protein, high-kilocalorie diet is ordered for most burn clients; often the diet is initially offered in six small meals. Complete nutritional oral supplements are commonly used to increase the client's kilocaloric and protein intake. The protein content of the diet can be increased by providing a between-meal feeding high in protein, a serving of two eggs at breakfast, and a large serving of meat at both lunch and supper. If the client drinks a full 8 ounces of milk with each meal, this further increases the protein content of the diet.

Infections and Fever

Malnutrition decreases resistance to infection, and infection aggravates malnutrition by depleting body nutrient stores. Fever characteristically accompanies infection but can also result from a variety of causes. The body needs extra kilocalories and fluids during fever because it takes more energy to support the higher metabolic rate. Infection often results in decreased food intake and absorption of nutrients, altered metabolism, and increased excretion of nutrients. In any hypermetabolic state, such as fever or infection, extra kilocalories are needed because the client's REE increases. Table 24–3 shows a stress factor of $1 + 0.07$ for each degree Fahrenheit the client's temperature exceeds normal. For example, to determine the kilocaloric need of a client with a prolonged fever of 104.6°F, the stress factor is 1.49 ($1 + 7$ degrees $\times 0.07$). Protein and fluid requirements are increased for clients with an infection. Extra protein is also needed to enable the body to produce antibodies and white blood cells to fight the infection. Perspiration entails a loss of fluids from the body, and many clients with fever have increased perspiration. Fluid may also be lost in vomiting and diarrhea, and this fluid needs to be replaced.

Trauma

Trauma may be defined as a physical injury or wound caused by an external source of violence. Stab and gunshot wounds, multiple fractures, and injuries acquired in motor vehicle accidents are examples of trauma. Victims of traumas may become hypermetabolic, depending on the severity of the injury. Vitamin supplements may be necessary. Vitamin C plays a role in wound healing, and its administration restores healing. Vitamin C functions as a cofactor in the hydroxylation of proline into collagen and enhances cellular and humoral response to stress. Doses as high as 500 to 1000 mg per day have been recommended (Skipper, 1998). Vitamin A, calcium, and zinc are also important in wound healing. Vitamin A enhances fibroplasia and collagen accumulation in wounds. Calcium is needed for calcium-dependent collagenases, iron for the formation of collagen, and zinc as a cofactor for enzymes responsible for cellular proliferation. These clients are at nutritional risk and may need extra kilocalories and protein.

Nutrition and Respiration

The scientific literature addresses the relationship between good nutrition and **respiration.** Respiration refers to the exchange of gases (oxygen and carbon dioxide) between a living organism and its environment. The air or oxygen inhaled and the carbon dioxide exhaled is the act of **ventilation.** Ventilation means breathing. **Pulmonary** means concerning or involving the lungs. **Chronic obstructive pulmonary disease (COPD)** refers to a group of lung diseases with a common characteristic of chronic airflow obstruction. COPD has become the fourth leading cause of death in the United States. **Respiratory failure** is an acute or chronic disease caused by an imbalance between the amount of gases entering the lungs and the demand of body cells for gases, resulting in tissue hypoxia. Acute respiratory failure is an imbalance as a result of a disease that affects ventilation in a client who has a healthy lung and normal alveoli. Chronic respiratory failure results from a disease in the bronchial structures and/or functioning (alveoli) structures of the lung. Malnutrition is commonly seen in clients with respiratory diseases.

Effects of Impaired Nutritional Status on Respiratory Function

Poor nutrition is related to inadequate pulmonary function in five important ways. First, clients with respiratory diseases or inadequate respiratory function frequently have an inadequate food intake, which is related to anorexia, shortness of breath, and/or gastrointestinal distress. Shortness of breath during food preparation and consumption of meals may limit kilocaloric intake. Inadequate oxygen delivery to the cells causes fatigue. Impaired gastrointestinal tract motility is common in clients with respiratory diseases (see the following section).

Second, kilocaloric requirements are often increased in clients with pulmonary disease. Research has estimated that although the number of kilocalories needed to breathe ranges from 36 to 72 kilocalories per day in normal individuals, the kilocaloric cost of breathing increases to 430 to 720 kilocalories per day in clients with COPD (Brown and Light, 1983). Kilocalorie requirements can be estimated at 25 kcal/kg of body weight for maintenance therapy and 35 kcal/kg for repletion therapy (Skipper, 1998). As a result of the combined effects of decreased food intake and increased energy requirements, weight loss is commonly seen in these clients.

The third important relationship between nutrition and pulmonary function is the effect of catabolism. When kilocaloric intake is decreased, the body begins to break down muscle stores, including those of the respiratory muscles. A loss in the lean mass of any muscle affects the muscle's function. The lung's structure itself is thus affected as a result of catabolism. Malnutrition may also result in decreased lung-tissue cell replacement or growth.

Gastrointestinal distress is common in clients with pul-

monary disease and is related to malnutrition. A loss of gastrointestinal structure including muscle mass may lead to hemorrhage and paralytic ileus. **Paralytic ileus** is the temporary cessation of peristalsis. This contributes to decreased food intake and the feeling of anorexia. In addition, paralytic ileus may lead to a translocation of bacteria. Decreased peristalsis in the GI tract fosters the movement (translocation) of bacteria from the GI tract into the bloodstream. This, in turn, leads to sepsis, or blood-borne infection, a sometimes fatal complication.

The fourth important relationship between nutrition and pulmonary function is that malnutrition increases the risk of respiratory tract infections. Lung infection is frequently the cause of death in pulmonary clients. In a state of malnutrition, the body decreases the production of antibodies, which are necessary to fight infection. Also, as a result of starvation, the lungs decrease production of pulmonary phospholipid (a fat-like substance). Phospholipids assist in keeping the lung tissue lubricated and help to protect the lungs from any disease-producing organisms that are inhaled.

The fifth important relationship between nutrition and pulmonary function is that improved nutritional status has been shown to be associated with a better ability to wean clients from ventilators. A ventilator is a machine that provides gases under pressure to clients who are unable to breathe on their own because of an insufficient number of ventilations or inspired volume amounts for cellular respiration. Clients on ventilators do not have to use their respiratory muscles to breathe. Active muscle movement stimulates muscle growth through protein stimulus. This is the same principle that applied to physical exercise increasing muscle size. To some extent, all the respiratory muscles **atrophy,** or waste away, due to inactivity while a client is artificially breathing.

Clients on ventilators are usually weaned slowly from these machines as their conditions improve. Some experts have attributed clients' ability to be successfully weaned from ventilators to an increase in protein synthesis. Good nutrition stimulates respiratory muscle growth. By correcting for infections, inflammations, and injuries, avoiding iatrogenic complications, and devoting careful attention to nutritional status, patients with chronic critical illnesses can potentially overcome their pulmonary conditions and debilitated states, to fully recover (Mechanick, and Brett, 2005).

In mechanically ventilated patients, there is good data to indicate that once a patient is extubated, swallowing dysfunction and a real risk of aspiration is present in most patients and my last up to several days. Patients who have been intubated for more than 48 hours are especially prone to aspiration (Ajemian, 2001).

Nutritional Therapy

Respiratory disease can affect both food intake and nutrient utilization. Many clients with respiratory diseases also have problems with water balance.

Energy Nutrient Utilization

Many clients with COPD suffer from carbon dioxide retention and oxygen depletion. Such clients are said to be carbon dioxide retainers. The medical goal for these clients is to decrease their blood level of carbon dioxide. The following formula helps explain this concept:

Protein (or Carbohydrate or Fat) + Oxygen = Heat Energy + Water + Carbon Dioxide

Fat kilocalories produce less carbon dioxide than carbohydrate kilocalories. For this reason, a diet high in fat is often used for carbon dioxide retainers. A high-fat diet may also assist the client with respiratory failure who must be weaned from mechanical ventilation. A high-fat diet may provide as much as 50 percent of the kilocalories in the form of fat. Figure 24–3 illustrates the relationship between nutrition and respiratory status in clients with pulmonary insufficiency and shows the influence of high-carbohydrate and high-fat diets.

Some physicians oppose the use of a high-fat diet for carbon dioxide retainers. Their opposition is based on research that has shown that a high-fat intake may be immunosuppressive in some clients (Juskelis, 1991). For this reason, fat in excess of 50 percent of total kilocalories is rarely prescribed.

Care must be taken not to overfeed clients with reduced respiratory function. Excess intake can raise the demand for oxygen and the production of carbon dioxide beyond the clients' capacity. The total number of kilocalories fed to the pulmonary client should be closely monitored. A nutritional assessment helps estimate the client's kilocaloric need and assists in therapy. Several companies market complete nutritional supplements targeted to clients who need a greater percentage of kilocalories provided from fat. However, recent data suggests no conclusive benefit for the routine use of high-fat formulas in mechanically ventilated patients (Malone, 2004).

Vitamins and Minerals

An assumption can be made that vitamins and minerals need to be supplied at least at levels of the DRI plus repletion because specific requirements for respiratory failure are unknown (Mueller, 2004). Usually electrolyte levels are closely monitored in ICU patients because of fluid imbalances and the occurrence of **respiratory acidosis** and **respiratory alkalosis.** Some patients' intravenous solutions require daily manipulation to correct imbalances of electrolytes.

An adequate intake of vitamins A and C is essential for helping to prevent pulmonary infections and decrease the extent of lung tissue damage. Foods high in vitamin A, such as fortified milk, dark green or yellow fruits and vegetables, some breakfast cereals (check the label), cheese, and eggs, should be included in the diet. Foods high in vitamin C, such as citrus fruits and juices, strawberries, and fortified breakfast cereals (check the label), should also be included. Sources of vitamins A and C should be carefully chosen to ensure that they do not contribute to gas production.

Water, Phosphorus, and Magnesium

Water balance and serum phosphorus levels need to be closely monitored in these clients. Clients with COPD and acute respiratory failure often need fluid restriction. Fluid

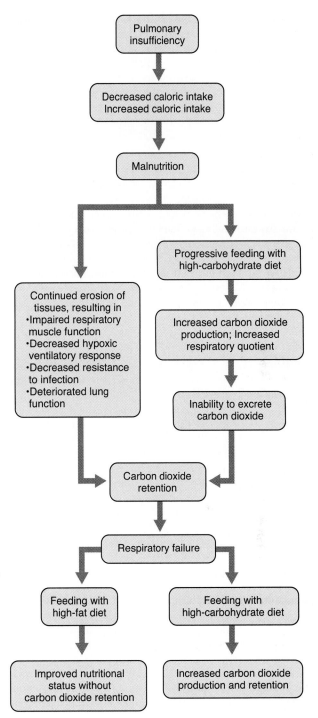

Figure 24–3 Interrelationship between nutrition and respiratory status in clients with pulmonary insufficiency. Influence of high-carbohydrate and high-fat diets is shown. (Reprinted from Specialized Nutrition for Pulmonary Patients, December 1984, p 14, Ross Laboratories, with permission.)

restriction assists in the control of **pulmonary edema** or a movement of fluid into interstitial lung tissue. Low serum phosphorus levels or hypophosphatemia are often seen in clients who are respirator-dependent. Phosphorus leaves the intracellular space and moves into the extracellular space during starvation. Serum phosphorus levels are in the normal or near-normal range at this point. With refeeding, phosphate moves back into the intracellular space. At this point, the serum phosphorus level may drop below normal. If this occurs, it is crucial that the client receive phosphate therapy. Because acute hypophosphatemia has been reported to cause respiratory failure, serum phosphorus levels should be monitored in all clients receiving aggressive nutritional support. A magnesium deficiency appears to cause a loss of muscle strength (American Dietetic Association, 2000).

Feeding Techniques

Many of these clients lack the energy to eat. Complaints of fatigue are common. The gastrointestinal distress experienced by these clients contributes to the anorexia. Foods from the cabbage family such as broccoli, cabbage, and Brussels sprouts may produce gas and contribute to gastrointestinal distress. Small, frequent feedings of foods with a high-nutrient density should be encouraged. Serving food items that require little or no chewing may help with difficulties chewing, breathlessness, and swallowing.

Refeeding Syndrome

Refeeding is the reintroduction of kilocalories and nutrients by oral or other routes into a patient. **Refeeding syndrome** is a detrimental state that results when a previously severely malnourished person is reintroduced to food and nutrients improperly. Complications with refeeding can occur regardless of the route by which nutrients are delivered—oral, enteral, and/or parenteral.

The term *refeeding syndrome* has been used to describe a series of metabolic and physiological reactions that occur in some malnourished clients when nutritional rehabilitation is begun. Improper refeeding of a chronically malnourished client can result in congestive heart failure (CHF) and respiratory failure. Clients at risk include those with alcoholism, chronic weight loss, hyperglycemia, or insulin-dependent diabetes mellitus and clients on chronic antacid or diuretic therapy. Elderly persons living alone who choose not to eat or are unable to eat because of progressive infirmity are likely candidates. Any incompetent mentally or physically challenged adult or abused child who has not been eating either by choice or neglect is also likely to experience refeeding syndrome.

Starvation leads to both a loss of the lean body mass in the heart and respiratory muscles and decreased insulin secretion. When carbohydrate intake is low, the pancreas adapts by decreasing insulin secretion. With the reintroduction of carbohydrates into the diet, insulin secretion will increase. The increased insulin secretion is associated with increased sodium and water retention. Other hormones are also activated with carbohydrate feeding. As a result of hormone action, increases in metabolic rate, oxygen consumption, and carbon dioxide production occur. The net effect of these metabolic changes is an increased workload for the cardiopulmonary system. Refeeding may increase the work of the cardiopulmonary system beyond its diminished capacity (due to the loss of lean body mass) and cause CHF and respiratory failure.

Starvation also leads to an increase in extracellular fluid and an increased loss of intracellular phosphorus, potassium, and magnesium. The degree of intracellular loss of these minerals reflects the degree of loss of lean body mass. Before refeeding, serum phosphorus and magnesium levels may remain in the lower range of normal, whereas the intracellular and total body stores of these minerals are depleted. After refeeding, these minerals are redistributed from the extracellular to the intracellular compartments. Repeated laboratory measurements taken after refeeding is started may show low serum levels of phosphorus, magnesium, and potassium. Failure to correct for these mineral deficiencies may be fatal for the client.

Principles of Safe Refeeding of the Malnourished Client

Health-care workers need to be aware of the dangers of refeeding a severely malnourished or starved client. Starved or severely malnourished clients may be seen in outpatient settings as well as in hospital intensive care units and long-term care facilities. A high prevalence of malnutrition is common in outpatient settings. The following recommendations may help the health-care worker avoid the refeeding syndrome in malnourished clients.

1. Recognize clients at risk. Refeeding syndrome occurs in clients with frank starvation, including war victims undergoing repletion, chronically ill clients who are malnourished, clients on prolonged intravenous dextrose solutions without other modes of nutritional support, hypermetabolic clients who have not received nutritional support for 1 to 2 weeks, clients who report prolonged fasting, obese clients who report a recent loss of a considerable amount of weight, chronic alcoholics, and clients with anorexia nervosa.

2. Health-care workers practicing in outpatient settings not directly under the supervision of a physician need to develop a referral plan in the event they suspect a client is a likely candidate for refeeding syndrome. These clients require the expertise of a physician.

3. A physician needs to test for and correct all electrolyte abnormalities before initiating nutritional support, whether by the oral, enteral, or parenteral route. Many physicians depend on other health-care workers to assist in the monitoring of serum phosphorus, magnesium, and potassium values. For nurses practicing within hospitals, this means notifying the physician on receipt of laboratory test results showing low serum levels of these minerals. It is especially important to notify the physician before implementing changes in tube feedings, oral diets, or the rate of hyperalimentation. In larger hospitals, the nutrition support service performs this service.

4. The physician needs to restore circulatory volume and to monitor pulse rate and intake and output before initiating nutritional support. Again, many physicians depend on nurses and other health-care workers to assist in monitoring these signs.

5. The kilocaloric delivery to a previously starved

client should be slow. Tube-fed and parenterally fed clients need to be closely monitored. The rate, total volume, and concentration of kilocalories delivered should be carefully monitored and documented. The concentration, volume, and rate of kilocaloric intake should be increased one at a time. Stepwise advancement to a higher kilocalorie intake should not occur unless the client is metabolically and physiologically stable.

6. Electrolytes should be monitored before nutritional support is started and at designed intervals thereafter.

Refeeding the malnourished client requires a team effort. A careful diet history taken by the dietitian can assist in the identification of clients likely to become victims of the refeeding syndrome. Changes in taste, appetite, intake, weight, or consumption of a special diet may indicate significantly altered status. Correction of electrolyte abnormalities by the physician before implementing nutritional support can prevent death. Careful observation and monitoring by the nutritional support service can identify early signs of this syndrome. Open and prompt communication among all health-care team members may be crucial to the client's survival.

SUMMARY

Stress is defined as any condition that threatens the body's mental or physical well-being. The best nutritional insurance against unexpected stress is good nutrient stores developed from a well-balanced diet. The use of supplemental vitamins, minerals, and amino acids in healthy individuals for excessive mental activity or stress has not been proved to provide a health benefit. However, a well-balanced diet or diet therapy for the treatment and prevention of chronic diseases exacerbated by mental stress has been shown to provide a health benefit.

The physical stress of hypermetabolism invokes the stress response and alters nutritional requirements for kilocalories, protein, and micronutrients. The stress response has three well-defined phases, which are mediated by hormones: the ebb phase, the flow phase, and the recovery (or anabolic) phase. Hypermetabolism differs from starvation in that resting energy expenditure (REE) increases during hypermetabolism and decreases during

a prolonged state of starvation. Major surgery, severe infections, fever, major burns, and severe trauma are all examples of hypermetabolic states.

Respiratory status profoundly affects nutrient need and utilization as well as food intake. Nutritional support can decrease catabolism of the respiratory muscles, improve immune function, minimize carbon dioxide production, and improve the likelihood of successfully weaning clients who are on mechanical **respirators.**

Refeeding a previously starved client involves some risks. Refeeding may increase the work of the cardiorespiratory system beyond its diminished capacity and cause congestive heart failure and respiratory failure. Refeeding syndrome is a series of metabolic reactions seen in some malnourished clients when they are re-fed. All health-care workers have a responsibility to understand this syndrome. A team approach to refeeding the malnourished client is necessary to prevent tragic complications.

CASE STUDY 24-1

Mr. X is a 42-year-old man who was admitted to the intensive care unit (ICU) with a diagnosis of acute bronchitis. He has a known history of carbon dioxide retention and chronic obstructive pulmonary disease. Mr. X is 5 ft 11 in (180 cm), 140 lbs (63.6 kg), and has a medium body frame (HBW = 87.5 percent; BMI = 19.5). He reports a recent 9-lb weight loss over a 3-week period. The client is on a mechanical ventilator. The physician's goal is to wean the client from the ventilator as soon as possible. Mr. X complains of fatigue, gas pains, anorexia, **dyspnea** (difficulty breathing), and early satiety. The client consumed a cup of coffee and one slice of toast for breakfast before falling asleep. The physician has ordered a 50-percent fat high-kilocalorie, high-protein diet.

NURSING CARE PLAN

SUBJECTIVE DATA Reports a 3-lb/week loss over the last 3 weeks.
Complains of fatigue, gas pains, anorexia, dyspnea, and early satiety.

OBJECTIVE DATA 87.5 percent HBW; BMI = 19.5
Observed low-food intake
Known history of COPD with carbon dioxide retention

NURSING DIAGNOSIS NANDA: Dysfunctional Ventilatory Weaning Response (NANDA, 2003, with permission) related to inadequate nutrition, recent weight loss, fatigue, gas pains, anorexia, dyspnea, and early satiety as evidenced by 87.5 percent HBW and known history of COPD and carbon dioxide retention.

(Continued on the following page)

CASE STUDY (Continued)

DESIRED OUTCOMES EVALUATION CRITERIA	NURSING ACTIONS/INTERVENTIONS	RATIONALE
NOC: Nutritional Status (Moorhead, Johnson, and Maas, 2004, with permission)	NIC: Nutrition Management (Dochterman and Bulechek, 2004, with permission)	
States that good nutrition is important to independent respiration in 1 day.	Emphasizes the importance of the prescribed diet to independent respiration.	Successful weaning to independent respiration is enhanced by good nutrition. Good nutrition decreases respiratory muscle catabolism, fosters protein synthesis, and facilitates production of pulmonary phospholipids.
Consumes an appropriate food intake in 3 days.	Consult with the dietitian to set a nutritional goal for the client based on the client's estimated energy expenditure using the Harris-Benedict formula, total energy requirements, and protein requirements.	The pulmonary client should not be overfed or underfed. Determination of the client's energy and protein requirements will provide baseline information to determine nutritional needs. Kilocalories and carbohydrates in excess will increase carbon dioxide retention. A deficiency of kilocalories and protein will increase catabolism of the respiratory muscles.
	Promote a pleasant, relaxed environment, including socialization, if possible, at mealtime.	Eating is both a social and biological experience. Kilocalorie intake will be greater if an attempt is made to provide a pleasant eating environment.
	Consult with the dietitian to provide a diet with modifications that meet the needs, such as:	Clients with pulmonary disease are often too tired to eat and may have gastrointestinal complaints. Small frequent meals, easily chewed foods, and reduction of empty kilocalories may assist in helping the client to meet estimated kilocalorie and protein needs.
	Texture and modification as necessary. Avoidance of foods not tolerated due to questionable limited GI tract motility such as gassy vegetables, spicy foods, milk products (secondary to lactase deficiency), etc.	
	Between-meal supplements that are acceptable to the client.	Documentation of food intake with subsequent analysis of protein and kilocalorie content will provide an objective measure of nursing care plan effectiveness. The results of the analysis can be used to provide feedback to the client.

C T Q CRITICAL THINKING QUESTIONS

1. After 2 days of monitoring the patient's kilocalorie and protein intake and despite encouragement to eat from the nurses and the dietitian, the patient refuses to eat much food. His kilocalorie intake is less than 500, with only 12 grams of protein. What would you recommend?

2. The patient's physician has ordered a fluid restriction of 800 mL qd plus output. The patient is angry and wants more fluids. How would you handle this situation?

3. You question the client's mental competence. What should you do?

⫸ CHAPTER REVIEW

1. Clients who complain about excessive mental stress benefit the most by counseling to:
   a. Supplement their diet with thiamin
   b. Drink extra fluids
   c. Eat a balanced diet
   d. Increase their protein intake

2. Which of these conditions does not increase a client's resting energy expenditure?
   a. Infection
   b. Chronic obstructive pulmonary disease
   c. Starvation
   d. Burn

3. A burn client's need for kilocalories is related to:
   a. The amount of protein eaten
   b. The total body surface area burned
   c. The volume of food tolerated
   d. Existing nutrient stores

4. Malnutrition is commonly seen in clients with pulmonary disease for all but one of the following reasons. Identify the exception.
   a. Many of these clients have a decreased food intake.
   b. Many of these clients expend more kilocalories to breathe.
   c. Many of these clients have impaired gastrointestinal tract function.
   d. Many of these clients have an extraordinary ability to fight infection.

5. Experts advocate the following when refeeding a malnourished client:
   a. Immediately pushing kilocalories and protein to replenish lost stores
   b. Progressing the rate, volume, and concentration of a tube feeding as rapidly as possible
   c. Full participation of all members of the health-care team to manage commonly seen metabolic abnormalities
   d. Correction of the hyperphosphatemia seen during the refeeding of a malnourished client

✤ CLINICAL ANALYSIS

1. Mr. X is suffering from second- and third-degree burns over 40 percent of his body. His physician has decided to use topical agents and leave the wound open to air. In the first 30 to 40 days postburn, the health-care team is planning nutritional support. The best supplemental feedings for the client would use:
   a. A modular feeding with a kilocalorie:nitrogen ratio of 150:1
   b. A modular feeding with a kilocalorie:nitrogen ratio of 300:1
   c. A polymeric (complete nutritional) supplement that is acceptable to the client
   d. High-kilocalorie desserts such as apple pie, cake, and ice cream

2. Mrs. J is an alcoholic who has previously reported that she has not eaten "food" for at least the last 3 months. She stated that her sole source of kilocalories had been in the form of alcohol. She was recently transferred to the unit in which you work after her treatment for alcohol withdrawal on another unit. The physician has ordered a high-kilocalorie, high-protein diet. So far, she has eaten 100 percent of the three high-kilocalorie, high-protein trays she has received while on your unit. While reviewing the client's laboratory values, you notice her serum phosphorus, magnesium, and calcium levels are decreased. Mrs. J's depressed phosphorus values may be related to:
   a. A movement of phosphorus into the extracellular space
   b. A total compartmental depletion of phosphorus
   c. A lack of phosphorus in Mrs. J's present dietary intake
   d. A movement of phosphorus into the intracellular space

3. Mr. C is a heavy smoker. He was recently admitted to your unit with carbon dioxide retention and a diagnosis of chronic obstructive pulmonary disease. He complains of gas pains. The client may derive benefit from:
   a. Caffeinated beverages
   b. Broccoli, onions, peas, melons, and cabbage
   c. Six small meals
   d. Custard, hot cooked cereals, bananas, ground meats, and mashed potatoes

REFERENCES

Ajemian, MS, et al: Routine fiberoptic endoscopic evaluation of swallowing following prolonged intubation: Implications for management. Arch Surg 136:437, 2001.

American Dietetic Association: Manual of Clinical Dietetics, ed 6. American Dietetic Association, Chicago, 2000.

Barrett, S, and Herbert, V: Fads, frauds, and quackery. In Shils, ME, et al (eds): Modern Nutrition in Health and Disease, ed 9. Williams & Wilkins, Baltimore, 1999.

Bray, GA: Afferent signals regulating food intake. Proc Nutr Soc 59:373, 2000.

Brown, SE, and Light, RW: What is now known about protein-energy depletion: When COPD patients are malnourished. J Respir Dis May:36, 1983.

Demling, RH, and DeSanti, L: Involuntary weight loss and protein-energy malnutrition: Diagnosis and treatment. www.medscape, accessed May, 2005

Dochterman, JC, and Bulechek, GM: Nursing Interventions Classification (NIC), ed 3. Mosby, Philadelphia, 2004.

Gold, PE: Role of glucose in regulating brain and cognition. Am J Clin Nutr 61(suppl):9875, 1995.

Gramlich, L, et al: Does enteral nutrition compared to parenteral nutrition result in better outcomes in critically ill adult patient? A systematic review of the literature. Nutrition. 10:843, 2004.

Hansbrough, JF: Enteral nutritional support in burn patients. Gastrointest Endosc Clin N Am 8:645, 1998.

Juskelis, D: Starvation in patients: Guidelines for refeeding. Registered Dietitian Clinical Interactions 11:2, 1991.

Malone, AM: The use of specialized enteral formulas in pulmonary disease. Nutr Clin Prac. 19:557–562, 2004.

Mason, J, and Epstein, S: Nutritional management of the patient with acute respiratory failure. www.cyberounds, accessed May, 2005

Mechanick, JL and Brett, EM: Nutrition and the chronically critically ill patient. Curr Opin Clin Nut Metab Care. 8(1):33, Jan, 2005.

Moorhead, S, Johnson, M, and Maas, M (eds): Nursing Outcomes Classification (NOC), ed 3. Mosby, Philadelphia, 2004.

Mueller, DH: Medical Nutrition Therapy for Pulmonary Disease in Food, Nutrition, and Diet Therapy, ed 11. Saunders, Philadelphia, 2004.

NANDA International: Nursing Diagnoses: Definitions and Classification, 2003–2004. NANDA International, Philadelphia, 2003.

Quandt, SA: Cultural influences on food consumption and nutritional status. In Shils, ME, et al (eds): Modern Nutrition in Health and Disease, ed 9. Williams & Wilkins, Baltimore, 1999.

Skipper, A: Dietitian's Handbook of Enteral and Parenteral Nutrition, ed 2. Aspen Publishing, Gaithersburg, MD, 1998.

Souba, WW, and Wilmore, D: Diet and nutrition in the care of the patient with surgery, trauma, and sepsis. In Shils, ME, et al (eds): Modern Nutrition in Health and Disease, ed 9. Williams & Wilkins, Baltimore, 1999.

Thomas, CL (ed): Taber's Cyclopedic Medical Dictionary, ed 18. FA Davis, Philadelphia, 1997.

Van den Berg, G, et al: Intensive insulin therapy in critically ill patients. N Eng J Med. 345:1359–1367, 2001.

Venus, D (ed): Taber's Cyclopedic Medical Dictionary, ed 19. FA Davis, Philadelphia, 2001.

Winkler, MF, and Malone, AM: Medical Nutrition therapy for Metabolic Stress: Sepsis, Trauma, Burns, and Surgery in Food, Nutrition, and Diet Therapy. Saunders, Philadelphia, 2004, p 1062.

Diet in HIV and AIDS

After completing this chapter, the student should be able to:

1. Define AIDS and HIV and list transmission routes for the virus.
2. List nutrition-related complications seen in clients infected with HIV and, for each complication, describe interventions to improve nutritional status.
3. Discuss why malnutrition is commonly seen in clients with HIV or AIDS.
4. Describe why each client with AIDS needs an individualized nutritional assessment.

Acquired immune deficiency syndrome (AIDS) is a life-threatening disease and a major public health issue. The **human immunodeficiency virus (HIV)** causes AIDS. The impact of this virus on our society is and will continue to be a challenge. This chapter discusses the prevention, diagnosis, and treatment of HIV **infection.** HIV is complicated by the side effects of medications, coinfections with other infections, and disease, wasting, and lipodystrophy. The course of acquired immune deficiency syndrome is often complicated by malnutrition. For these reasons, a major portion of this chapter is devoted to the nutritional care of clients infected with HIV.

Human Immunodeficiency Virus

The human immunodeficiency virus attacks both the immune system and the nervous system. **Immunity** refers to resistance to or protection against a specified disease. When the AIDS virus enters the bloodstream, it begins to attack cells with a specific protein called CD_4 on their surfaces. CD_4 is present on lymphocytes. Lymphocytes are the main source of the body's immune capability, which involves humoral immunity produced by B cells and cell-mediated immunity produced by T cells. CD_4 levels decrease as the HIV disease progresses. A healthy, uninfected person usually has 500 to 1500 CD_{4+} cells per cubic millimeter of blood (Ungvarski and Flaskerud, 1999).

The HIV virus enters the cell, conscripts its DNA, and reprograms it to reproduce the virus. Loss of CD_4 function leaves an individual susceptible to infections and certain cancers. Evidence shows that the AIDS virus may also attack the nervous system, causing damage to the brain.

Acquired Immune Deficiency Syndrome

AIDS is a disease complex characterized by a collapse of the body's natural immunity against disease. Every part of the human body may be affected. The disease is progressive but runs an unpredictable course with periods of remission. On average it takes about 10 years for HIV to progress to AIDS. This disease is often diagnosed after certain indicator-opportunistic diseases occur, such as infection, tumor, wasting, or dementia. The Centers for Disease Control has published a specific list of infections and cancers that are used to diagnose AIDS. This list is constantly being reviewed and revised as more information is gathered on the course of this disease. The World Health Organization defines AIDS more simply (Box 25–1).

No Known Cure

Dramatic but expensive treatment advances have changed the health-care community's view of AIDS. The use of highly active antiretroviral therapy (HAART) has decreased mortality rates. However, findings indicate that in the vast majority of patients receiving HAART who had undetectable levels of HIV-1 RNA in plasma, the virus has not been eradicated. Also, HAART is not a treatment option for much of the world's population. Sadly, the medications are too costly.

Signs and Symptoms

The natural history of HIV infection is divided into three phases: early symptomatic phase, clinical latency, and advanced HIV disease (or AIDS).

Early Symptomatic Phase

The HIV-infected individual may develop an acute flu-like illness, with symptoms appearing about 2 to 6 weeks after

Box 25–1 **World Health Organization's Case Definition of Adult AIDS***

Major Signs

Weight loss of greater than 10 percent of body weight
Chronic diarrhea of longer than 1 month's duration
Fever of longer than 1 month's duration, either intermittent or constant

Minor Signs

Persistent cough for greater than 1 month
General pruritic dermatitis (severe itching due to inflammation of the skin)
Recurrent herpes zoster (recurrent infectious disease caused by the varicella-zoster virus)
Oropharyngeal candidiasis (infection of the throat with any species of Candida)
Chronic progressive and disseminated herpes simplex infections (an acute infectious disease caused by the herpes simplex virus type I)
Generalized lymphadenopathy (disease of the lymph nodes)

*AIDS in an adult is diagnosed if at least two major and one minor signs are present in the absence of a known cause of immunosuppression, such as cancer or severe malnutrition.

exposure to the virus. Typically, the symptoms are not severe enough for the client to seek medical attention.

Clinical Latency

After this phase, the individual may be **asymptomatic** for years. Most HIV-infected persons have no symptoms, and many are not even aware that they are infected. The danger lies in their ability to infect other people unknowingly. Some people remain symptom-free for years after infection with the HIV virus. Even though the client is symptom-free, viral replication continues. If untreated, there is a steady decline in CD_{4+} cells during this stage (about 40 to 80 cells per cubic millimeter of blood) for each year of infection (Ungvarski and Flasterud, 1999).

Viral load tests are also used to measure and monitor disease progression in clients who have been diagnosed. Amplicor HIV-1, better known as the PCR test, is used to determine the likelihood of disease progression. The higher the viral load, the more likely the chance of disease progression. People who began studies with a viral load of less than 20,000 had only a 1 percent chance of experiencing disease progression during the following 60 weeks compared with 24 percent of people who started with a viral load over 200,000 (www.aidsinfonyc.org).

Advanced HIV Disease Phase (AIDS)

After a period of 2 to 10 or more years, without treatment, the CD_4 count drops to less than half the normal value, the viral load increases, and the immune system begins to fail, permitting opportunistic infections and other conditions characteristic of AIDS (Batterham, 1999). When the CD_4 cell count drops to less than 50, there is an increasing chance

of treatment failure. Death becomes likely, usually within 1 year (Ungvarski and Flaskerud, 1999).

The Epidemic

AIDS Worldwide

The AIDS **epidemic** started about 24 years ago, and the number of people living with HIV continues to increase steadily. Sixty-six percent of infected people are in Africa, and 20 percent are in Asia. By the end of 2003, an estimated 34.6 to 42.3 million people throughout the world were living with HIV infection and more than twenty million had died of AIDS (Steinbrook, 2004). More than 95 percent of new infections occur in the developing world, where access to therapy is limited (Batterham, Brown, and Garcia, 2001). Globally, the AIDS epidemic shows no signs of abating.

AIDS in the United States

The Centers for Disease Control and Prevention cites the following figures for the United States (Centers for Disease Control, 2004):

- During 1981 to 2001, 1.3 to 1.4 million persons in United States infected with HIV
- 816,149 living with AIDS
- 467,910 deaths

The epidemic increasingly affects women, minorities, persons infected through heterosexual contact, and the poor. These affected groups are usually diagnosed at a later stage of infection when related disease is present and often delay care for themselves because they must care for others or have competing subsistence needs for their time and resources (Stein et al, 2000).

Transmittal Routes

The human immunodeficiency virus is not easily transmissible. Evidence indicates that the AIDS virus is spread through blood and body fluids. Direct contact of blood to blood or of virus to mucous membrane must occur for disease transmittal. In practical terms, there are three transmittal routes: blood-borne, perinatal, and sexual.

Blood-Borne Route

HIV may be transmitted by exposure to contaminated blood or blood products through transfusion, sharing of drug apparatus, and injuries to health-care workers from needles and other sharp objects. Box 25–2 outlines precautions to prevent needlestick injuries. Intravenous drug abusers often share needles and other equipment for drug injection. This practice can result in a minute amount of blood from an infected person being injected into the bloodstream of the next user. In addition, cases of AIDS have been linked with receipt of blood products from HIV-infected donors (before donated blood was routinely tested for the HIV virus), acupuncture treatments performed with improperly sterilized needles, and receipt of transplanted organs from a person later discovered to have been HIV infected.

Box 25–2 Needlestick Injuries

To prevent needlestick injuries, needles should not be:

- Recapped
- Purposely bent or broken by hand
- Removed from disposable syringes
- Otherwise manipulated by hand

Guidelines for disposal of syringes, needles, scalpel blades, and other sharp objects include:

- Placing them in a puncture-resistant container located as close to the area of use as is practical
- Placing large-bore reusable needles in a puncture-resistant container for transport to the processing area (Figure 25–1 illustrates a health-care worker disposing a needle into an appropriate container.)

Perinatal Transmission

Most children with AIDS contract the virus from their infected mothers through blood-to-blood transmission before or at birth. Breast-feeding has been implicated in transmission, since HIV has been isolated from breast milk. In the United States, the Centers for Disease Control advise HIV-positive women against breast-feeding. On the other hand, in developing countries, breast-feeding is still advocated by WHO because of the concern about infant morbidity and mortality due to poor sanitation.

Sexual Transmission

The most likely way to become infected with HIV is to have unprotected sexual contact with an infected individual's blood, semen, and possibly vaginal secretions. The virus enters a person's bloodstream through the rectum, vagina, or penis. Small tears in the surface lining of the vagina or rectum may occur during insertion of the penis, fingers, or other objects, thus opening an avenue for entrance of the virus directly into the bloodstream. Both homosexual and heterosexual persons are at risk for AIDS. The only people not at risk of infection by this route are celibate individu-

als and couples who have maintained mutually faithful monogamous relationships (only one continuing sexual partner) for at least 15 years.

AIDS: You Can Protect Yourself

The best advice for avoiding infection is to avoid direct contact with anyone's blood or body fluids. This involves practicing safer sexual behaviors and following universal precautions or body substance isolation procedures. Nurses need to advise clients to adopt safer sexual practices. Many resources are available describing precautions to prevent sexual transmission.

Universal Precautions or Body Substance Isolation

Health-care workers need to consider all clients as potentially infected with HIV and/or other blood-borne pathogens. **Universal precautions** dictate that every client and every client's blood and certain body fluids should be considered contaminated and treated as such. **Body substance isolation** procedures are used when all body fluids should be considered contaminated and treated as such. Body substance isolation is thus more comprehensive than universal precautions. Whether universal precautions or body substance isolation procedures are followed in a given facility varies. Clinical Application 25–1 discusses the myth of transmission via casual contact.

Test Screening

Antibodies to HIV are diagnosed initially by enzyme-linked immunosorbent assays (ELISA) and agglutination assays and are confirmed by Western blot or more specific tests. The accuracy of existing HIV tests is limited because new strains of the virus are still being discovered that may not be identified by current tests. Negative results also can occur in infected individuals because of lack of antibody formation early in the disease and in late stages because of loss of ability to produce antibodies (Watson and Jaffe, 1995).

Complications of HIV Infection

AIDS is characterized by weakness, anorexia, diarrhea, weight loss, fever, and a decreased white blood cell count, or **leukopenia**. Common problems associated with AIDS include opportunistic infections, gastrointestinal dysfunction, tumors, AIDS dementia complex (ADC), and organ dysfunction. In the last years, several clients have developed a

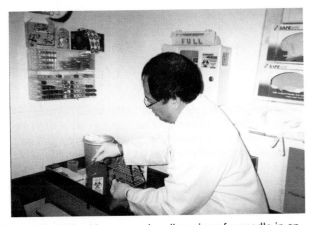

Figure 25–1 A health-care worker disposing of a needle in an approved sharps container. Note that he is wearing gloves.

Clinical Application 25–1

No Risk of AIDS From Casual Contact

Most infected people contracted the virus through intimate sexual contact. No cases have been found where AIDS has been transmitted through casual (nonsexual) contact with a household member, relative, coworker, or friend. Casual contact includes sneezing, coughing, eating or drinking from common utensils, or merely being around an infected person.

syndrome of lipodystrophy that is characterized by peripheral and facial wasting, in which all the veins in the extremities are prominent and the abdomen is enlarged (Batterham, 1999).

Opportunistic Infections

Parasitic, bacterial, viral, and fungal organisms are everywhere in our environment. The healthy person's immune system keeps these organisms in check and under control. AIDS places the client at high risk for certain infections, called **opportunistic infections.** Some of the infections these clients develop were rarely seen in the United States before the onset of the AIDS epidemic. Four opportunistic infections are commonly seen in AIDS clients: thrush, tuberculosis, pneumocystis pneumonia, and **cryptosporidiosis.**

Thrush

A physical assessment may show signs of **thrush,** which produces a thick whitish coating on the tongue or in the throat and may be accompanied by sore throat. See Figure 25–2. Thrush is a fungal infection that can cause oral ulcers, frequent fevers, and gastrointestinal inflammation. Basic teaching for mouth care by the health educator should include:

- Keep the mouth clean by rinsing with a dilute solution of hydrogen peroxide and water at least three times a day, especially after eating. Instruct clients not to swallow the solution.
- Use a cotton swab instead of a toothbrush if brushing is painful or causes bleeding. Commercial mouthwash may cause discomfort or pain.
- Avoid hot foods.
- Try soft foods, such as scrambled eggs, cottage cheese, mashed potatoes, mashed winter squash, puddings, custards, milk, juices (not citrus), canned fruits such as peaches, pears, and apricots, and bananas.
- Cut meat into small pieces or grind or blend it.
- Supplement diet with a complete oral nutritional supplement.
- Use a straw.
- Tilt head forward or backward to ease swallowing.
- Avoid any food that causes discomfort. Fried, spicy, sour, salty, and sticky foods may not be tolerated, such as chips, nuts, seeds, raw vegetables, peanut butter, pickles, citrus fruits and juices, and tomatoes.

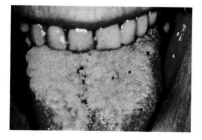

CANDIDIASIS

Figure **25–2** Thrush with mouth pain may interfere with nutritional intake. A soft diet may be helpful.

Tuberculosis

Tuberculosis (TB) is spread from person to person through tiny airborne particles. By sharing surroundings with a person who has active pulmonary TB, a susceptible person may inhale the disease-producing bacteria. Fortunately, most people who have inhaled these particles never become contagious or develop active TB. Even a healthy immune system cannot kill all the particles. HIV infection weakens the body's immune system and makes it more likely that the individual who has inhaled TB-related particles will develop active TB.

Pneumocystis Pneumonia

Pneumonia, characterized by shortness of breath, fatigue, and anorexia, is also common in AIDS clients. About 60 percent of AIDS clients are infected with one type of pneumonia-causing organism, called *Pneumocystis carinii*, hence the name **pneumocystis pneumonia.** The organisms settle in the person's lungs, causing progressively worsening breathing problems and eventually leading to death.

Cryptosporidiosis

Persons with HIV are at a high risk for food-borne illnesses. Food safety and sanitation should always be a part of client education in this population. Because of the gastrointestinal infections acquired by immunosuppressed clients, an additional safety precaution has been recommended. Because of outbreaks of **cryptosporidiosis** in public drinking water, the Centers for Chronic Disease Control (CDC) has suggested that people with HIV infection and AIDS drink sterilized water and avoid tap water (American Dietetic Association, 1995).

Gastrointestinal Dysfunction

The gastrointestinal tract is a common site for expression of HIV-related symptoms. The client may feel pain in the mouth or esophagus due to the growth of opportunistic infections. The client may have difficulty swallowing because of open lesions or sores. AIDS commonly affects both the small and large intestine. The enzymes necessary for digestion and absorption in the wall of the small intestine may be lacking or present in insufficient amounts. Malabsorption may occur with diarrhea. Gut failure may follow. The medications these clients receive to control their infections also contribute to the gastrointestinal dysfunction.

AIDS Dementia Complex

AIDS dementia complex (ADC) is the most common HIV-caused central nervous system illness associated with AIDS. It is estimated that at least 40 to 50 percent of adults with AIDS have some neurological dysfunction. Experts believe ADC frequently is misdiagnosed as Alzheimer's disease in persons over 50. This dysfunction is usually chronic and progressive. Early symptoms of ADC are difficulty in concentration, slowness in thinking and response, and memory impairment. Behavioral symptoms include social withdrawal, apathy, and personality changes. Such symptoms may be interpreted solely as a psychiatric disorder.

Motor symptoms include clumsiness of gait, difficulty with fine motor movements, and poor balance and coordination.

Tumors

Kaposi's sarcoma is the most frequently seen malignancy among AIDS clients. The most common manifestation of Kaposi's sarcoma is single or multiple lesions appearing on the lower extremities and especially on the feet and ankles. These open areas appear reddish, purple, or brown. Treatment consists of radiation, surgery, and/or chemotherapy.

Organ Dysfunction

AIDS affects many organs in the body, leading to organ dysfunction. Diseases of the gallbladder, liver, and kidneys are seen in some AIDS clients. **Cholecystitis,** inflammation of the gallbladder, can occur in conjunction with certain opportunistic infections seen in AIDS patients. **Hepatomegaly,** an enlarged liver, is frequently seen with pain, fever, and abnormal liver function test results, especially of the alkaline phosphatase level. **Pancreatitis,** inflammation of the pancreas, has also been noted in some infected clients. AIDS can lead to **end-stage renal failure** within weeks.

Clearly, AIDS has many complications. Ongoing research has yet to discover a cure for this terrible disease.

Lipodystrophy

Since February 1998, reports from France, Spain, Switzerland, Hong Kong, Australia, and the United States of an odd redistribution of fat, called lipodystrophy, have been received. Lipodystrophy, now preferably called fat redistribution syndrome, is characterized by increasing abdominal girth, decreasing fat mass in the extremities and face, the advent of a "buffalo hump," and breast enlargement in patients with HIV, especially those on HAART with a protease inhibitor. Also seen are increased serum triglyceride, glucose, and insulin levels and, sometimes, increased blood pressure (Batterham, Brown, and Garcia, 2001).

Treatment

A variety of new medications show some promise of killing or inhibiting the activity of the HIV virus. Clinical Application 25–2 discusses drug treatment for AIDS. Research has shown has shown that progressive resistance training or weightlifting may protect lean body mass

---

Clinical Application 25–2

Medications Used for HIV and Aids

Drug therapy for clients with HIV has increased in complexity. There are currently four classes of antiretroviral medications: nucleoside reverse transcriptase inhibitors, nonnucloside reverse transcriptase inhibitors, protease inhibitors, and fusion inhibitors (Am Diet Assoc, 2004). Lifelong medication therapy with combinations of these medications may be required for management. This presents challenges to nutritional status by introducing

potential interactions with food, body metabolism, and side effects. Clients must often take different medications each day to suppress opportunistic infections and control symptoms. Medications that increase blood lipid levels and promote diarrhea may require the patient to further modify his or her diet. The following table lists common medications used in HIV/AIDS, typical dosing, and food tips.

Protease Inhibitors

MEDICATION	GENERIC NAME	DOSING	FOOD TIPS
Indinavir	Crixivan	BID, every 12 hours TID, every 8 hours	Take on an empty stomach to enhance absorption. Take with a light snack that contains 300 kcal, 6 grams of protein, and 2 grams of fat to reduce stomach upset. Drink at least 1 cup of water or juice (not grapefruit) with each dose. Drink a total of 10 cups of water and/or juice every day to prevent kidney stones.
Ritonavir	Norvir	BID	Take with a full meal. Complications may include diarrhea, lipodystrophy, and elevated lipids. Avoid alcohol.
Saquinavir	Fortovase (Invirase)	BID or TID	Take within 2 hours of a high-fat meal or snack. This will increase the drug's absorption by 5 to 10 times. A high-fat meal should contain about 55 grams of fat. Possible complications include lipodystrophy and elevated lipids.
Nelfinavir	Viracept	TID Doses should not exceed 12 hours	Take with food. Possible complications include diarrhea, lipodystrophy, and elevated lipids.

(Continued on the following page)

Clinical Application 25–2 *(Continued)*

Protease Inhibitors

MEDICATION	GENERIC NAME	DOSING	FOOD TIPS
Didanosine (ddl)	Videx	Once per day	Take on an empty stomach. Do not take with other medications.
Lamivudine (3TC)	Epivir	BID	With or without food.
Stavudine (d4T)	Zerit	BID	Take with or without food.
Zalcitibine (ddC)	Hivid	TID	Take with or without food.
Zidovudine (AZT)	Retrovir	BID	Take with food, preferably nonfat. Take 400 IU vitamin E qd to decrease bone marrow suppression.
Abacavir	1592U89	BID	Take with or without food.
Nevirapine	Viramune	BID	No food restriction.
Delavirdine	Efavirenz	Once a day at bedtime	No food restriction.

How are the drugs mentioned in this table combined? Typically a protease inhibitor is combined with two nonnucleoside reverse transcriptase inhibitors. For example, Crixivan is combined with AZT and DDL. This requires following a tight schedule. Here is a sample schedule:

6:00 AM	Indinavir
7:00 AM	Breakfast and AZT
9:00 AM	DDL on an empty stomach
11:00 AM	Lunch
2:00 PM	Indinavir
5:00 PM	Dinner and AZT
8:00 PM	Snack
10:00 PM	Indinavir
12:00 AM	DDL on an empty stomach

Other medications may be useful in reversing the nutritional decline and sequelae associated with AIDS. Marinal, dronabinal, and megace have all been shown to have significant efficacy in appetite stimulation, increased kilocalorie intake, reversing weight loss, and improving patient's sense of well-being. Meal plans to support medication regimens include not only meal timing but also macronutrient and micronutrient modulation and symptoms management strategies.

and reduce visceral adiposity. Progressive resistance training or weightlifting can increase lean mass without the potential side effects and expenses of pharmacologic treatments. Realistically, health-care intervention can only suppress most infections for these clients, not cure them.

Prevention and Counseling

Notification of a positive HIV test finding creates a crisis for the individual. A person who has had pretest counseling is more prepared and likely to cope better. Counseling the individual on how best to fight the virus is important; for example, the HIV-positive individual needs to receive all current immunizations to boost his or her immunity. Behaviors that interfere with wellness and reduce immunity, such as drinking alcohol, smoking, and illegal drug use, should be discouraged. Adequate rest, good nutrition, and exercise all can improve general good health and should be encouraged.

Nutrition and HIV Infection

Food and nutrition security have been linked worldwide to both the transmission of HIV and poor outcomes related to HIV disease. Food security is defined as having access by all people at all times to sufficient food for an active and healthy life and includes, at a minimum, a ready availabil-

ity of nutritionally adequate and safe foods and an assured ability to acquire food in socially acceptable ways (American Dietetic Association, 2002). Nutrition security may be defined as the provision of an environment that encourages and motivates society to make food choices consistent with short- and long-term health (American Dietetic Association, 2003). Food and nutrition insecurity lead some people to survival strategies that expose them to a greater risk of HIV infection. Among these strategies are migration to urban slums and involvement in the sex trade. Lack of infrastructure precluding access to health-care services compounds the problem. Children lose educational opportunities when they stay at home to provide basic care for malnourished and infected family members. Adults responsible for children become sick and die, and the social and economic infrastructures diminish. Lack of education, food, economic support, and access to health-care services may increase the risk of malnutrition (American Dietetic Association, 2004).

Nutritional management is both a preventive and a therapeutic treatment in HIV infection. Malnutrition is a major mediator and predictor of death from AIDS (Solomons, 1999). A malnourished client has a limited ability to fight infection. Well-nourished individuals infected with the HIV virus are better able to offer some resistance to opportunistic infections and tolerate the side effects of treatment. Good nutritional status may influence response to medications by decreasing the incidence of adverse drug reactions, providing available raw materials for reactions evoked by medications, and supporting organ functions. Because these patients take multiple prescribed medications, almost all need extensive counseling on food and medication interactions.

One study found the use of a multivitamin supplement delayed the onset of advanced disease and the need for antiretroviral therapy in HIV-positive people (Fawzi et al, 2004). Worldwide, few people who have advanced disease are receiving antiretroviral treatment. Micronutrient supplements have been proposed as a low-cost intervention that may slow the progression of HIV disease. The impact of micronutrient supplementation may be less in the developed nations of the world because the general population is far less likely to be malnourished.

Some experts believe that the most effective medical intervention involves the prevention, early identification, and early treatment of enteric infections and malabsorption. Keeping AIDS clients well nourished is often a challenge because of their numerous medical complications. Dietary modifications are frequently indicated for many of them.

Nutrition and Immunity

The function of the immune system is to protect the body against foreign invasion. Foreign invaders include viruses, bacteria, tumor cells, fungi, and transplant material. Studies have shown that a deficiency of almost any nutrient affects a cell's ability to fight infection and handle foreign invaders. Therefore, malnutrition itself can result in an immune deficiency. Many experts believe that malnutrition aggravates AIDS and may suppress any residual immune function. Deficiencies of iron, zinc, pyridoxine, folic acid, and vitamins B_{12}, C, and A are associated with immunologic changes. Malnourished clients with AIDS have minimal internal resources to fight opportunistic infections.

Malnutrition in AIDS Clients

Malnutrition causes a number of physiological alterations that may lead to decreased resistance to infection. For example, malnutrition can cause increased gut permeability, which allows more alien material to be absorbed into the body. Malnutrition may also result in decreased intestinal secretions. Some of these secretions are necessary for the proper digestion and absorption of food. Malnutrition may also cause a change in intestinal flora. This may affect the utilization of nutrients. Malnutrition may lead to hormonal imbalances and a decreased ability to repair tissue. The body ceases to replace and repair tissue because it lacks the raw materials to do so. A well-balanced diet is essential to optimal immune function.

Some HIV-positive clients need an additional 400 kilocalories per day to maintain their weight and prevent wasting. Wasting is a loss of both body fat and lean body mass and always accompanies an inadequate intake of kilocalories and protein. Wasting has been shown to increase mortality and shorten life.

Cachexia is a loss of lean body mass without a weight loss. Weight can be rising while lean body mass is decreasing. This happens because cachexia occurs when the body's immune response is turned on and certain catabolic cytokines, such as interleukin-1 and tumor necrosis factor, are also turned on. These cytokines alter metabolism in such a way that protein is utilized excessively and fat is utilized insufficiently. Thus, the protein compartment of the body declines and the fat compartment is relatively spared (Mason and Roubenoff, 1999). Cachexia is a slower process than wasting, and life can be sustained for quite a period of time during the process. Death results when approximately 40 percent of baseline lean body mass is lost. Clients with HIV should be alerted to this phenomenon and have their body composition monitored. Nutrition education is indicated (Box 25–3). Also, exercise has been shown to help conserve lean body mass.

Malabsorption

Diarrhea and malabsorption are probably the major nutrition-related problems for AIDS clients. Diarrhea is also commonly listed as a side effect of antiretroviral medications (Brown and Batterham, 2001). Mucosal atrophy and decreased digestive enzyme activity contribute to the malabsorption seen in persons with AIDS. Carbohydrate malabsorption and steatorrhea are frequently seen in

Box 25–3   **Counseling the Client With HIV and AIDS**

1. Offer nutrition education soon after the initial diagnosis.
2. Review the principles of safe food handling and storage with the client.
3. Closely monitor the client's blood lipids, triglyceride, glucose, and cholesterol levels and recommend modification of the diet as indicated.
4. Consider multivitamin and mineral supplement.
5. Discourage inappropriate weight loss as many HIV clients lose lean body mass first and fat second. Address prevention, restoration, and maintenance of optimal body composition with emphasis on lean tissue. Encourage physical activity.
6. If indicated, encourage more and frequent meals to increase energy intake. Snacks, complete nutritional supplements, and intravenous feedings may be necessary.
7. Soluble-fiber supplementation has been shown to be an effective treatment for diarrhea (Brown and Batterham, 2001).
8. Evaluate signs and symptoms and tailor counseling to client's unique needs.
9. Discuss potential medication-nutrition interactions.
10. Review use of nutrient supplements and potential interactions with nonprescription and herbal supplements.
11. Address food and nutrition security issues. Refer to social worker if client lacks enough food.

AIDS clients with diarrhea. Gastrointestinal problems such as diarrhea may occur in children with HIV infection due to disaccharide intolerance rather than to enteric infection with known pathogens. Malabsorption of fat, simple sugars, and vitamin B_{12} is known to occur in clients with intestinal infections. AIDS clients who have diarrhea or malabsorption clearly have additional vitamin and mineral needs. Clinicians measure 25-hydroxy–vitamin D levels (as an indicator of fat-soluble vitamin absorption) and folate or zinc (as an indicator of water-soluble vitamin status) (Mason and Roubenoff, 1999).

Other factors may contribute to the diarrhea seen in these clients. Malnutrition can cause a decrease in pancreatic secretions, decreased levels of the enzymes found in the walls of the small intestine (lactase, sucrase, and maltase), villous atrophy, and decreased absorptive surfaces. Side effects of medication therapy may be related to malabsorption. For example, bacterial overgrowth of organisms that are not susceptible to the chosen antibiotic may occur with long-term anti-infective therapy. The colon contains colonies of bacteria that aid in food digestion. Whenever an individual takes an antibiotic, these helpful bacterial colonies are disrupted and may permit overgrowth of other relatively resistant bacteria that promote diarrhea.

Initially, dietary treatment involves identification of the cause of the diarrhea and a determination of which nutrients the client cannot absorb. The concentration of hydrogen in the breath can be measured after oral lactose or sucrose administration to determine whether the client is intolerant to either of these sugars. An elevated breath hydrogen level implies intolerance, because the hydrogen is primarily a product of metabolism of these sugars by colon bacteria. Fecal microbiologic evaluations and intestinal biopsies are used to determine absorptive capability. In some clients infected with HIV, malabsorption of sucrose, maltose, lactose, and fat has been documented, even in the absence of diarrhea.

Clients with a form of carbohydrate intolerance may benefit from either a lactose-restricted or a disaccharide-free diet. A disaccharide-free diet is indicated for severe intolerance to sugar. Sucrose needs to be broken down into glucose and fructose (lactose into glucose and galactose; maltose into glucose and glucose) before absorption is possible. A disaccharide-free diet excludes most fruits and vegetables and many starches and is nutritionally inadequate. Vitamin C is deficient, and daily supplementation is recommended. Some of these clients may tolerate a small amount of sugar, but they usually need assistance in understanding their tolerance level. A lactose-free diet may be sufficient for clients who are deficient only in lactase.

A low-fat diet may be necessary to control steatorrhea. In cases of severe fat intolerance, medium-chain triglycerides are more readily absorbed. Clinical Application 25–3 discusses several ways in which medium-chain triglycerides can be incorporated into table foods. Usually the physician prescribes this diet as needed.

Several additional meal-planning tips are suggested to promote the client's well-being and to control the malabsorption:

Clinical Application 25–3

Incorporating Medium-Chain Triglyceride Oil Into Table Foods

Medium-chain triglyceride (MCT) oil can replace vegetable oil in most recipes with satisfactory results. The easiest ways to introduce MCT oil in food preparation are in salad dressings, blended with milk (pretreated with lactase enzyme if necessary) or fruit juices, and in sautéed foods. MCT oil can be used to make cookies, bread, pancakes, French toast, muffins, and pie crusts. MCT oil is made by Mead-Johnson and can usually be purchased from a pharmacy.

1. Fluids should be encouraged to maintain hydration when large fluid volume is lost in stools.
2. Yogurt and other foods that contain the *Lactobacillus acidophilus* culture may be helpful if bacteria overgrowth is a problem secondary to long-term anti-infective use.
3. Small, frequent meals make the best use of a limited absorptive capacity of the gut.
4. A multivitamin supplement is indicated to increase the amount of vitamin available for absorption.
5. An elemental formula for medical use or parenteral nutrition may be necessary during severe bouts of malabsorption. An elemental formula for medical use contains partially digested nutrients. Promising studies have shown that clients experienced increased weight gain and good tolerance when this type of formula was given at home (Trujillo et al, 1992).
6. Avoidance of sorbital, which is used as a sweetening agent in both sugar-free candies and some medications, has been shown to cause diarrhea and should be avoided.

In some situations, the malabsorption is highly resistant to any treatment. Nutritional therapy goals should maximize client comfort. Fiber-containing supplements or foods high in fiber may be beneficial for decreasing diarrhea; eliminating caffeine intake also may help control it. The benefits of overly restricting the client's diet may not suffice to offset the resulting loss in client comfort in an incurable situation.

Increased Nutritional Requirements

Several studies suggest that the resting energy expenditure (REE) is elevated in patients with early HIV infection and increases with subsequent AIDS (Smith and Lowry, 1999). Fever and infection increase kilocaloric, protein, and certain mineral and vitamin requirements. Dietitians frequently use the **Harris-Benedict equation** and multiply by appropriate stress and activity factors to determine kilocaloric requirements. Energy needs are 10 to 15 percent higher than predicted by the Harris-Benedict equation and should be taken into account by the appropriate stress factor when estimating energy requirements (Wafaie et al, 2004).

Not all patients with AIDS become hypermetabolic. Studies have indicated that a small percentage of the AIDS population without secondary infection may be hypometabolic and demonstrate a response similar to that seen in starvation (Smith and Lowry, 1999). Hypometabolic patients need a gradual increase in kilocalories and a lower kilocalorie:nitrogen ratio. These patients should also be monitored for refeeding syndrome.

Decreased Food Intake

Anorexia can be a major problem for many clients with AIDS. A poor food intake may be the result of fever, respiratory infections, drug side effects, gastrointestinal complications, oral and esophageal pain, and emotional stress. Clients with ADC may experience mechanical problems with eating. Some drugs used in these clients, such as bactrim and pentamine, may cause nausea, vomiting, and taste changes that decrease the client's desire to eat. Interaction with the client to encourage food intake is particularly important when the person is feeling relatively well.

Nutritional Care in AIDS

Manifestations of the HIV virus vary greatly from one client to another. Therefore, nutritional care must be tailored to each client's unique set of symptoms. Quality nutritional care starts with screening.

Screening

Screening HIV-infected clients for nutritional problems is a crucial component of quality client care. Early indicators of decreased nutritional status include decreases in body weight, percent body fat, a low albumin level, and body mass index (BMI). Dietary assessment of persons living with HIV is important at all stages of the disease in order to identify those 25 to 35 percent with inadequate intake who require counseling (Woods et al, 2002). A baseline measure of percent body fat and lean body mass helps monitor disease progression. The recent food intake is particularly important to include as part of the screening and assessment process. Barriers the client may have to safe nutritious food should be evaluated as part of the nutrition screening process. Lack of food and poor food choices are linked to transmission of HIV infection and a poor response to treatment. Referral to a social worker is always indicated to address these challenging issues.

Planning Nutrient Delivery

In keeping with the general principle "if the gut works, use it," every effort should be made to feed the client orally. The anorexia commonly seen in AIDS clients can sometimes be resolved by changing the meal plan. Try offering smaller, frequent feedings. Serving food cold or at room temperature may help some clients consume more kilocalories. Modification of seasonings and kilocaloric density may also improve intake. Modification of texture may assist the client with poor chewing ability or oral lesions.

The Centers for Disease Control recommends the use of regular dishware for clients with blood-borne diseases. Because AIDS is not transmitted through food, food handling, or dishes, regular dishes and utensils may be used without risk. This means an isolation setup is not necessary. Historically, an isolation setup included only disposable dishware, a cardboard tray, and plastic utensils. Disposable dishware compounds the client's feelings of social isolation. Regular dishware provides better quality food at appropriate temperatures and allows the food to appear more appetizing. However, many health-care institutions require all workers to wear protective gloves when handling soiled dishes to protect them from infection with opportunistic organisms.

If the client is unable to consume sufficient nutrients from table foods, supplemental feedings and/or other enteral feedings should be considered. The type of malnutrition should influence the food and supplements offered, which the dietitian usually determines. For example, if the client's protein status is adequate but the client has an energy deficit, a carbohydrate and/or fat supplement may be the best choice. In such a situation, the client's serum albumin level is normal but the client still may be losing weight. On the other hand, if the client's albumin is low but his or her body weight is stable, a protein supplement would be preferable. Of course, water balance also influences body weight, so this example is necessarily an oversimplification. The point is that not all supplemental feedings are equally desirable at any given stage of illness. Clients are encouraged to consume particular nutrients based on individual assessment data.

If the client is unable to consume sufficient nutrients orally and the gut is working, a tube feeding may be considered. If the gut is not functioning properly, PPN or TPN may be considered. The goal with these clients should always be to prolong living, not to prolong dying. A client has the right to refuse any alternative-feeding route offered.

Monitoring

To ensure that adequate nutrients are being consumed, the client must be evaluated periodically. Body weight and nutritional intake should be monitored frequently. BMI and percent body fat should be monitored every few weeks. The loss of lean tissue central to body metabolism may be present throughout the disease process, regardless of weight maintenance, suggesting that weight is not a good early indicator of declining nutritional status (Ott et al, 1993). Throughout this process, health-care workers should maintain a supportive, nonjudgmental approach, which is the key to establishing a trusting relationship.

Client Teaching

Nutritional education is an important part of total client care. All AIDS clients need instruction on food safety because low immune system functioning makes them much more susceptible to food-borne illnesses. This will minimize the likelihood of opportunistic infection. Instructions on dietary modifications and the use of supplemental feedings are also indicated. Many of these clients need instruction on the importance of good nutrition and how to prepare nutrient-dense meals. An assessment of the client's knowledge level and understanding of the individualized meal plan is appropriate. Food tips for travelers with HIV are discussed in Box 25–4.

Box 25–4 **Food Tips for Travelers With HIV Infection**

Travel, particularly to third-world countries, may carry a significant risk for the exposure of HIV-infected persons to opportunistic pathogens. For this reason, HIV-infected travelers should be counseled on the following before departure from home:

- Raw or undercooked seafood, eggs (Caesar dressings), and poultry should be avoided.
- Unpasteurized milk and dairy products should be avoided.
- Items purchased from street vendors should be avoided.
- Tap water and ice made from tap water should be avoided. Hot coffee or tea, beer, wine, or water brought to a rolling boil for 1 minute is preferable.

Treatment of water with iodine or chlorine may not be as effective as boiling but can be used, perhaps in conjunction with filtration, when boiling is not practical.
- Items generally considered safe include steaming hot foods served, fruits peeled by the traveler, and bottled (especially carbonated) beverages.
- Accidental ingestion of lake or river water while swimming or engaging in other recreational activities may carry a risk. In the severely immunocompromised client, an additional restriction may be necessary. Some soft cheese and ready-to-eat foods (e.g., hot dogs and cold cuts from delicatessen counters) have been known to cause listeriosis. These foods should be reheated until they are steaming hot before ingestion.

FOOD FADDISM AND QUACKERY

Some clients with AIDS are vulnerable to both food faddism and quackery because they become desperate enough to try anything that arouses hope. **Food faddism** is an unusual pattern of food behavior enthusiastically adapted by its adherents. **Food quackery** is the promotion for profit of a medical scheme or remedy that is unproved or known to be false (Barrett and Herbet, 1999).

Health-care educators need to carefully balance and consider the danger of unusual food behaviors versus taking away any hope the client may have. Clients may tune out educators if they perceive that their beliefs and feelings are discounted without sensitivity. Some unusual food behaviors are not harmful, and some food behaviors can result in negative health consequences. The client with limited resources who spends all of his or her money on dietary supplements and herbal products with limited health benefits and very little or no money on food will develop malnutrition. A reliable desktop reference and carefully chosen Internet sites can help the health educator determine what is inappropriate. Care must be taken not to use Internet sites that sell questionable products.

Follow-Up Care

The nutritional status of a client often depends on appropriate follow-up care. A referral to a community agency, a home health-care program, an outpatient clinic, or a dietitian should be made to provide continuity of care.

SUMMARY

The AIDS epidemic is worldwide. Although HAART and protease inhibitors have reduced mortality rates, no cure has been found for AIDS. Known transmittal routes include blood-to-blood, perinatal, and sexual contact. As health-care professionals, we can all protect ourselves from AIDS by using extreme care when handling blood and equipment that has been in contact with blood and as private individuals by practicing safe sexual behaviors. HIV attacks the immune system and leaves its victims defenseless against opportunistic infections. AIDS is a disease with many clinical complications. Nutritional management is both a preventive and a therapeutic treatment in clients infected with HIV. Increased nutrient needs, decreased food intake, and impaired nutrient absorption contribute to the malnutrition seen in AIDS clients.

CASE STUDY 25-1

Ms. S is a 30-year-old woman who acquired HIV from her drug-abusing husband and subsequently infected their son in utero. She could not believe the test results when she was first told. Now she is seeking nutritional information to allow her to increase her chance for a quality life and her son's chance to survive infancy. Her knowledge of basic nutrition is good.

NURSING CARE PLAN

SUBJECTIVE DATA Lack of information on relationship of nutrition to AIDS
Concrete goals established

OBJECTIVE DATA HIV-positive tests, both mother and infant
Percent body fat, 25

NURSING DIAGNOSIS NANDA: Deficient knowledge (NANDA, 2003, with permission) related to AIDS progression and verbal statements

DESIRED OUTCOMES EVALUATION CRITERIA	NURSING ACTIONS/INTERVENTIONS	RATIONALE
NOC: Knowledge: disease process (Moorhead, Johnson, and Maas, 2004, with permission)	NIC: Teaching: Disease Process (Dochterman and Bulechek, 2004)	
Client will verbalize areas in which nutrition could affect AIDS development.	Reinforce need for regular, balanced meals. Emphasize adequate kilocalories.	The stress of receiving this diagnosis may impede use of previously learned information.
	Instruct Ms. S to keep home environment clean, especially kitchen, bathroom, and basements where molds and fungi could thrive.	Organisms that are harmless to persons with normal immune systems can cause opportunistic infections in HIV-infected persons.
	Teach client to monitor herself and her son for changes in health related to food intake or digestion.	Discovering beginning malabsorption problems would permit treatment before malnutrition becomes apparent.
Client will monitor her percent body fat	Explain the relationships among percent body fat, percent lean body mass, and exercise.	Exercise can prevent a loss of lean body mass.
		Weight can be stable but body fat content can increase.

C T Q CRITICAL THINKING QUESTIONS

1. The client has developed mouth sores from thrush and would like you to arrange for her to have TPN. She claims it is just too painful to eat. What would you recommend?
2. The client's child has been diagnosed HIV positive. During a home visit, you notice the kitchen is filthy. You instruct the client on food safety and sanitation. On a return visit, despite prior instruction on food safety, you notice that the client's kitchen is still not clean. The client claims she is too tired to clean. What do you do?
3. The client went to a health food store and purchased several bottles of vitamin pills and herbal supplements. She believes she can take these in lieu of eating. What should you do?

⟩⟩⟩ CHAPTER REVIEW

1. The health-care worker's best insurance against HIV transmission on the job is:
   a. Frequent hand washing
   b. Universal precautions
   c. Body substance isolation
   d. Adherence to all food safety policies and procedures

2. A client on HAART can partially compensate for fat redistribution syndrome by:
   a. Taking medications as prescribed
   b. Taking supplemental vitamins and minerals
   c. Consuming a low-fat diet
   d. Exercising

3. Compared to wasting, cachexia is:
   a. A slower process
   b. The result of both a protein and kilocalorie deficit
   c. Always the result of a poor food intake
   d. Best treated by the inclusion of 400 additional kilocalories per day

4. Clinicians measure _____ as an indicator of fat-soluble vitamin absorption.
   a. Folate
   b. Zinc
   c. 25-hyroxy–vitamin D
   d. Glucose

5. Educating an AIDS client about food safety is important:
   a. to minimize the risk of rare tumors
   b. to prevent body fat redistribution
   c. to enhance renal function
   d. to prevent opportunistic infections

CLINICAL ANALYSIS

1. Mr. Y, a 45-year-old black male, was diagnosed as HIV-positive 1 month ago. His height is 6 feet 0 inches, and his weight is 178 pounds and stable. He reports no signs or symptoms and has not seen a physician yet. He wants to know what he should eat. As the nurse during this first visit, it may be appropriate to discuss:
   a. The many benefits of HAART
   b. Food safety, exercise, good nutrition, and the importance of follow-up with a physician
   c. The expected outcome and potential complications
   d. Vitamin-mineral supplementation, increased kilocalorie needs, and the treatment for malabsorption

2. Carlos, a 25-year-old Hispanic male, presents with severe diarrhea. He was diagnosed with HIV about 8 years ago. He has five to six watery stools each day that do not appear to be related to his medications. His height is 5 feet 10 inches, and his weight is 140 pounds (usual weight is 175 pounds). He is an inpatient, and the physician has ordered a stool culture but the results are not back. You recommend:
   a. Extra fluids with meals to prevent dehydration
   b. A clear-liquid, complete nutritional supplement
   c. A high-fat and high-fiber diet to provide both kilocalories and bulk to his diet
   d. Six small meals with a milkshake between meals to push kilocalories and protein

3. Dave, a 36-year-old white male, complains of fatigue. He is often too tired to cook and has little interest in food. He lives alone and is on disability. His CD_4 cell count is 400, and his viral load is 100,000. You recommend:
   a. A tube feeding
   b. Referral to a social service agency for a friendly visitor
   c. Meals-on-Wheels
   d. Six small meals daily

REFERENCES

American Dietetic Association: Position of the American Dietetic and Canadian Dietetic Associations: Nutrition intervention in the care of persons with human immunodeficiency virus. J Am Diet Assoc 104:1425, 2004.

American Dietetic Association: Addressing world hunger, malnutrition, and food insecurity [position paper]. J Am Diet Assoc 103:1046, 2003.

Position of the American Dietetic Association: Domestic food and nutrition security [position paper]. J Am Diet Assoc 102:1840, 2002.

American Dietetic Association: Manual of Clinical Dietetics, ed 6. American Dietetic Association, Chicago, 2000.

Barrett, S, and Herbet, V: Fads, frauds, and quackery. In Shils, ME, et al (eds): Modern Nutrition in Health and Disease, ed 9. Williams & Wilkins, Baltimore, 1999.

Batterham, M: Lipodystrophy—a side effect of protease inhibitor therapy. Positive Communications: A publication of the HIV/AIDS dietetic practice group. American Dietetic Association, Chicago, 1998.

Batterham, M, Brown, D, and Garcia, R: Nutritional management of HIV/AIDS in the era of highly active antiretroviral therapy: A review. Aust J Nutr Diet 58:211, 2001.

Benatar, SR: Health care reform and crisis of HIV and AIDS in South Africa. N Engl J Med 351:81, 2004.

Brown, D, and Batterham, M: Nutritional management in the era of highly active antiretroviral therapy: A review of treatment strategy. Aust J Nutr Diet 58:224, 2001.

Centers for Disease Control: Health, United States, 2004. Atlanta. Available at www.cdc/nchs/data/hus04trend, accessed May, 2005.

Dochterman, JC, and Bulechek, GM: Nursing Interventions Classification (NIC), ed 4. Mosby, Philadelphia, 2004.

Fawzi, W, et al: A randomized trial of multivitamin supplements and HIV disease progression and mortality. N Engl J Med. 351:23, 2004.

HIV/AIDS in the era of highly active antiretroviral therapy: A review. Aust J Nutr Diet 58:211, 2001.

Kruzich, LA, et al: US youth in the early stages of HIV disease have low intakes of some micronutrients important for optimal immune function. J Am Diet Assoc 104:1095, 2004.

Mason, J, and Roubenoff, R: Nutritional issues of clinical concern in HIV patients. Accessed July 28, 1999 at http://www.cyberounds.com/conferences/0499/conference.html.

Moorhead, S, Johnson, M, and Maas, M: Nursing Outcomes Classification (NOC), ed 3. Mosby, Philadelphia, 2004.

NANDA International: Nursing Diagnoses: Definitions and Classification, 2003–2004. NANDA International, Philadelphia, 2003.

Ott, M, et al: Early changes of body composition in human immunodeficiency virus-infected patients: Tetrapolar body impedance and analysis indicates significant malnutrition. Am J Clin Nutr 57:15, 1993.

Skinbrook, R: The AIDS epidemic in 2004. N Engl J Med 351:115, 2004.

Smith, MK, and Lowry, SF: The hypermetabolic state. In Shils, ME, et al (eds): Modern Nutrition in Health and Disease, ed 9. Williams & Wilkins, Baltimore, 1999.

Solomons, NE: International priorities for clinical and therapeutic nutrition in the context of public relations. In Shils, ME, Olson, JE, Shikes, M, and Ross, CA (eds): Modern Nutrition in Health and Disease, ed 9. Williams & Wilkins, Baltimore, 1999.

Stein, MD, et al: Delays in seeking HIV care due to competing caregiver responsibilities. Am J Public Health 90:1108, 2000.

Steinbrook, R: The AIDS epidemic in 2004. N Engl J Med 351:115, 2004.

Trujillo, EB, et al: Assessment of nutritional status, nutrient intake, and nutrition support in AIDS patients. J Am Diet Assoc 92:477, 1992.

Ungvarski, PJ, and Flaskerud, JH: HIV/AIDS: A Guide to Primary Care Management. WB Saunders, Philadelphia, 1999.

Viral load tests. Accessed May 2000 at www.aidsinfonyc.org.

Volberding, PA: Improving the outcomes of care for patients with human immunodeficiency virus infection. N Engl J Med 334:729, 1996.

Wafaie, FW, et al: A randomized trial of multivitamin supplements and HIV disease progression and mortality. N Engl J Med 351:23, 2004.

Watson, J, and Jaffe, MS: Nurse's Manual of Laboratory and Diagnostic Tests, ed 2. FA Davis, Philadelphia, 1995.

Woods, MN, et al: Nutrient intake and body weight in a large HIV cohort that includes women and minorities. J Am Diet Assoc 102:203, 2002.

CHAPTER 26

Nutritional Care of the Terminally Ill

Learning Objectives

After completing this chapter, the student should be able to:

1. Differentiate between palliative and curative nutritional care.
2. State appropriate nutritional screening questions for the terminally ill client.
3. List at least two appropriate dietary management techniques for symptom control for each of the following: anemia, anorexia, bowel obstruction, cachexia, constipation, cough, dehydration, diarrhea, dysgeusia, esophageal reflux, fever, fluid accumulation, hiccups, incontinence, jaundice and hepatic encephalopathy, migraine headache, nausea and vomiting, pruritus, stomatitis, weakness, wounds and pressure sores, and **xerostomia.**
4. State appropriate assessment questions for a terminally ill client.
5. Discuss the ethical and legal considerations for feeding a terminally ill client.

This chapter discusses clients who have been certified by physicians to be terminally ill. An individual is considered terminally ill if he or she has a medical prognosis of 6 months or less based on the usual disease progression. Although a physician can estimate life expectancy based on disease progression, this is not an exact science. A client diagnosed with a terminal disease may live longer or less long than predicted because the disease may not follow its usual progression. Individuals who have been certified by a physician as terminally ill can elect the Hospice benefit under federal guidelines (www.ncfa.gov/medicaid). Hospice is the major health-care program for the terminally ill in the United States.

Dealing With Death

Our culture emphasizes the enjoyment of life. At the beginning of this century, most people died at home, and many died young. Death was a part of everyday life. In the past 50 years, most people have died in hospitals or long-term care facilities. Often an ambulance is called if a person is dying. Although health-care workers have received much training on how to reverse the effects of disease, we have received much less training on how to assist our clients with dying. With changes in the health-care system bringing decreased lengths of hospital stays, an increasing number of clients will again be cared for in their homes. Training health-care workers to provide home care for terminally ill clients is becoming essential.

To help the dying, health-care workers must first contemplate and then accept their own mortality. Nurses, physicians, and other health-care workers tend to deny death as much as lay people do. One study showed that basic interventions to maintain comfort were often not provided in hospitals. Oral hygiene was often poor, thirst remained unquenched, little assistance was given to encourage eating, contact between nurses and dying patients was minimal and distancing between nurses and dying patients was evident, with this isolation increasing as death approached (Mills, Davies, and Macrae, 1994). Health-care providers may also become attached to particular clients and become overwhelmed by feelings, thereby becoming ineffective as helping caregivers. Nutritional and dietary issues are at the center of some ethical questions concerning the care of these clients. Becoming an advocate for clients' best interests is a priority when providing quality care to the dying. Health-care professionals need to address patients' values, goals of care, and preferences with regard to treatment to truly become patient advocates.

The Dying Process

Death is an unavoidable part of the life cycle. Both physiological and psychological changes occur as part of the dying process. The client's age, diagnosis, and physical condition influence physiological changes. Regardless of the underlying disease, cardiopulmonary failure is the final cause of death. Pulmonary and circulatory failure may be gradual or sudden. The major signs and symptoms in the final days and hours of life include cessation of eating and drinking, oliguria and incontinence, muscle weakness, difficulty in breathing, cyanosis, decreased mental alertness, and changes in vital signs.

Hospice team members may describe clients with a terminal diagnosis as actively dying. An actively dying client has a life expectancy of a few hours or a few days. The reason for the actively dying designation is to determine staff needs. The following sections discuss the criteria team members use to determine the actively dying status.

Cessation of Eating and Drinking

Life will soon cease when a client's eating and drinking diminishes critically. One study reported that 8 percent of clients with cancer completely cease to eat and/or drink (Feuz and Rapin, 1994). Oral intake dwindles because a client has no desire to eat or because disease prevents digestion. This greatly decreased oral intake is often worrisome to family members. Health-care workers need to counsel family members that dehydration at this time is believed to have a euphoric effect and is not painful. Clinical Application 26–1 discusses the physiological responses to fluid restriction. Fluids and comfort care such as ice chips, lubricating the lips, and small amounts of food and water reduce the thirst sensations from dehydration. Withholding and minimizing hydration can have the desirable effect of reducing disturbing oral and bronchial secretions, need for frequent urination, and reducing cough from diminished pulmonary congestion (American Dietetic

---

Clinical Application 26–1

Physiological Response to Fluid Restriction

Young, healthy, active individuals who are deprived of water develop thirst, dry mouth, and headache, followed by fatigue; cognitive impairment occurs as dehydration progresses and becomes severe with abnormal electrolytes, rising blood urea nitrogen, and hemoconcentration (Shils, 1999). If water is not taken, renal failure is likely.

Hospice workers taking care of terminally ill clients report the following (Junkerman and Schiedermayer, 1998):

- Actively dying clients often voluntarily stop eating and drinking and do not tolerate a substantial amount of tube feedings.
- Actively dying clients who are given normal fluid replacement commonly show signs of fluid overload, including pulmonary edema.
- Actively dying clients almost never report feelings of hunger or thirst.
- Dehydration results in less vomiting and diarrhea, less need to suction secretions, less dyspnea, and peripheral edema.

Hospice discourages the use of tube feedings and orally administered fluids for dying patients. However, fluids should be offered to clients and given if requested by clients. There is growing support in clinical literature for the position that neither nutrition nor hydration in terminal patients increases comfort or the quality of life.

Association, 2002). It is unkind to force food or fluids on a client who is actively dying.

Oliguria and Incontinence

Because oral intake is usually decreased for several days before death, urine output is often diminished and may cease. The color of the urine may become very dark. A period of incontinence often precedes the oliguria, and anuria occurs. General fatigue, muscle weakness, and decreased mental acuity are among the reasons for the incontinence. Bedding should be changed as quickly as possible to avoid skin irritation. Death usually occurs within 48 to 72 hours after urine output stops.

Difficulty in Breathing

Most clients have some difficulty breathing before death. Caregivers may become alarmed when they hear a loud, hoarse, and bubbling sound. This sound is caused by the passage of breath through pharyngeal and pulmonary secretions that lodge at the back of the client's throat. Atropine is often administered to decrease the secretions. Elevating the head of the bed, gentle suctioning, and positioning the client on his or her side help maintain a clear airway. All terminally ill clients do not have these sounds with respiration. Some clients experience apnea (a temporary cessation of breathing). A change such as these in breathing is an indicator that life will soon cease.

Cyanosis

Slightly bluish, grayish, or dark purple discoloration of the skin caused by poor oxygenation is called **cyanosis.** The client's feet, legs, hands, and groin feel cold. Many health-care workers believe this is one of the most useful indicators that the end of life is approaching. Slowed circulation and decreased tissue perfusion cause these signs.

Decreased Mental Alertness

The amount of blood reaching the brain, lungs, liver, and kidneys decreases as general circulation slows. Sleepiness, apathy, disorientation, confusion, restlessness, and finally a decreased level of consciousness that frequently progresses to a sleep-like state are among the signs that death is imminent.

Changes in Vital Signs

A decrease in body temperature, an increase in pulse rate, a rise and then a decrease in respirations, and a fall in blood pressure are signs of impending death. Death occurs when there is no pulse and respiration ceases.

Family members and caregivers of terminally ill clients often express fear at the thought of being alone with an actively dying client. For this reason, health-care workers often remain with the client and their loved ones during this time. Some nurses resist working with the terminally ill because they think that they cannot cope with this experience. However, death is not always a painful experience. Death can provide an opportunity for personal growth, joyous affirmation of life, and meaningful attachments. Health-care workers who share the death experience with a client and the client's family often describe the experience as rewarding and profound.

Palliative Versus Curative Care

Palliative care has been defined as the active total care of an individual when curative measures are no longer considered an option by either the medical team or the patient (Cox and McCallum, 2000). The goal of curative care is arresting the disease. The goal of palliative care is the relief of symptoms to alleviate or ease pain and discomfort. Emphasis in palliative care is placed on addressing the problems of pain, loneliness, and loss of control that are common in dying clients. Palliative care programs address and/or include the client and family members in the plan of care.

Hospice is a concept that dates back to medieval times. During the crusades, travelers needed a place to stop for comfort. The Knights of Hospitallers of the Order of St. John of Jerusalem in the twelfth century sheltered sick and religious pilgrims. They established hospices in England, Germany, Italy, Cyprus, and Rhodes. The soul, the mind, and the spirit were considered as much in need of help as the body. Around the fifteenth century, anatomic and surgical practices developed. Physicians moved into hospitals that emphasized curative treatments. Monks and nuns remained in cloisters and cared for the people the physicians could not heal, including the disabled, the chronically ill, and the terminally ill. During the eighteenth and nineteenth centuries, great advances in curative treatments occurred, and hospitals became highly specialized in acute life-threatening situations. Hospitals were less able to offer shelter to people nearing life's end. At the same time, caring for the terminally ill became less a private or religious function and more a public and governmental one.

The modern hospice has its roots in the late nineteenth century, when a place of shelter for the incurable ill was founded in Dublin. The British physician Dr. Cicely Saunders inspired the hospice movement in the United States. Dr. Saunders is noted for her work in pain control and for the founding of St. Christopher's Hospice in London in 1967. The first operational hospice program in the United States was established in New Haven, Connecticut, in the early 1970s.

Hospice philosophy includes the belief that death is a natural aspect of life. Hospice is committed to the philosophy that persons have the right to die in the setting of their choice and to be as comfortable as possible. Central to the hospice philosophy is the idea that palliative care is appropriate when treatment of the client's disease becomes ineffective and irrelevant. Studies suggest that medical care for patients with serious advanced illnesses is characterized by undertreatment of symptoms, conflict about who should make decisions about patient care, impairments in caregivers' physical and psychological health, and depletion of family resources (Morrison and Meiser, 2004).

Nutrition Screening

All palliative care begins with the establishment of the goals of care. Studies suggest that what terminally ill patients want is to have their pain and other symptoms relieved, improve their quality of life, avoid being a burden to their family, have a close relationship with loved ones, and maintain a sense of control (Steinhauser et al, 2000). The goal of palliative nutritional care is to assist the client and/or caregiver with any food-related concerns. These difficulties may be related to uncomfortable symptoms and/or attitudes and beliefs held about food. Screening the client with a terminal illness for food-related concerns is the first step. There are major differences between screening a client who is undergoing curative and/or preventive treatment and screening a terminally ill client who is receiving palliative care. First, the health-care worker needs to ascertain if the client has any symptoms that may be diminished by nutritional intervention. Second, the attitudes and beliefs of the client and/or caregiver about food need to be examined. Some clients and their caregivers have difficulty accepting that the terminally ill client frequently eats much less than is needed to sustain life. Box 26–1 is an example of a nutrition screening form for the client with a terminal condition.

Health-care professionals, patients, and family members frequently want to discuss the use of a intravenous or tube feedings in a terminally ill patient during the screening process. The frequency of percutaneous endoscopic

---

Box 26–1 **A Sample Nutrition Screening Form for the Client With a Terminal Condition**

Name _____ Caregiver's Name _____

Date _____ Diagnosis _____

1. Have you had any concerns about weight changes or food intake?
   _____ No _____ Yes   Describe _____
2. For clients on tube feedings or parenteral feedings only: Have your feedings created or increased discomfort, diarrhea, distension, etc.?
   Type: _____ Amount _____ Infusion rate _____
3. Do you feel your symptoms could be decreased/controlled through dietary change?
   _____ No _____ Yes   Describe _____
4. Do you feel diet or nutritional supplement would benefit you or your disease process?
   _____ No _____ Yes   Type _____
5. Do you believe that your diet caused your disease or will slow the progression of your disease?
   _____ No _____ Yes   Describe _____
6. Do you find eating enhances comfort? _____ No _____ Yes
7. What concerns do you have regarding your diet intake? _____
8. Would you (client or caregiver) like to discuss food-related concerns with the dietitian? _____ No _____ Yes

gastrostomy (PEG) tube use has increased from 15,000 in 1989 to 123,000 in 1995 (American Dietetic Association, 2002). The use of any artificial feeding should always be considered but is often inconsistent with treatment goals. For example, in the case of a patient with end-stage dementia who has dysphagia, placement of a PEG tube may be considered (Morrison and Meier, 2004). If the treatment goal of the patient is to reduce suffering and enhance the quality of life, a PEG tube is unlikely to meet this goal. A PEG tube placement requires a painful invasive procedure, eliminates the pleasurable oral sensations of eating and drinking, is associated with an increased use of restraints, can cause cellulites, vomiting, diarrhea, and fluid imbalances, and is unlikely to reduce the risk of aspiration (Singer, Martin, and Kelner, 1999). Even if the goal is survival, no survival benefits have been shown in observational studies in which patient with dementia received tube feedings compared with similar patients who did not receive tube feedings (Finucane, Christmas, and Travis, 1999).

Assessment

During the nutritional assessment, it is important that every question posed to the client and/or caregiver has a purpose. Health-care workers generally need to know the results of laboratory tests, diagnostic procedures, physical examinations, and anthropometric measures as well as the level of immune function and food intake information to determine a client's nutritional status. These nutritional parameters may have no value in the provision of nutritional care for a terminally ill client, however. For example, why ask if a client drinks milk? Is it to estimate if the client is meeting the calcium, riboflavin, and vitamin D allowances? If it is determined that the client's milk intake is suboptimal, would anything be done about the inadequacy? If the client has diarrhea with severe abdominal cramping after the ingestion of milk, however, a recommendation to drink lactose-free milk would be appropriate. Unless the client will experience relief from bothersome symptoms, it is best not to recommend behavioral changes that may be difficult for the client to make. On the other hand, if the client expresses concern about the nutritional adequacy of his or her diet, nutrition education is not contraindicated. Communication with the client is a core skill of palliative medicine.

Intervention and Symptom Control

Box 26–2 describes appropriate dietary management for symptom control for a client with a terminal illness. If a

---

Box 26–2 **Dietary Management for Symptom Control**

Anemia

1. Recommend vitamin C source with red meats and iron-fortified foods.
2. Discourage use of coffee, tea, and chocolate if the client has gastrointestinal bleeding.
3. Recommend multivitamin supplement if client desires, but avoid megadose vitamins.

Anorexia

1. Discuss practical issues with client and/or caregiver, such as food attitudes, social aspects of eating, food preferences, and beliefs about food.
2. Encourage concentration on the sensual pleasure of eating, such as table setting, garnishes, smells, and socialization.
3. Evaluate client's desire for a sense of well-being.
4. Suggest use of small, frequent feedings.
5. Educate caregiver to recognize early signs of malnutrition and provide protein supplements, make food accessible, and encourage eating as desired by the client and/or caregiver if the client's prognosis is more than a few weeks.
6. Evaluate client acceptance of a liquid diet and recommend complete oral nutritional supplements.
7. Teach caregiver that the client has the right to self-determination and may refuse to eat and/or drink when actively dying. The caregiver should continue to offer nourishment as a sign of love and caring but not harass the client to eat or drink.

Bowel Obstruction

1. NPO may be indicated; limited clear liquids may be possible.

2. Encourage small meals low in fiber and residue if oral intake is not contraindicated.
3. Encourage the client to eat slowly, chew food well, and rest after each meal if oral intake is not contraindicated.
4. Recommend dry feedings if oral intake is not contraindicated.
5. Recommend avoidance of sugary fatty foods, alcohol, and foods with a strong odor.

Cachexia

1. Teach relaxation techniques and encourage use before mealtime.
2. Encourage client and/or caregiver to concentrate on the sensual pleasures of eating such as setting an attractive table and plate, the use of food garnishes, and the importance of an appetizing eating environment (remove bedpans and emesis basin, etc., before serving the food).
3. Evaluate client for dysgeusia and dysphagia and xerostomia. Refer to symptoms and definitions of terms on this table.

Constipation

1. Encourage high-fiber foods (bran, whole grains, fruits, vegetables, nuts, and legumes) if an adequate fluid intake can be maintained.
2. Instruct the client to avoid high-fiber foods if dehydration or an obstruction is suspected or anticipated.
3. Assess the client's fluid intake and recommend an increased intake if needed.
4. Recommend taking 1 to 2 oz with the evening meal of a special recipe: 2 cups applesauce, 2 cups

unprocessed bran (All-bran), and 1 cup of 100-percent prune juice (Gallagher-Allred, 1989). Refrigerate this mixture between uses and discard after 5 days if not used.
5. Suggest limiting cheese and high-fat, sugary foods (doughnuts, cakes, pies, cookies) that may be constipating.
6. Discontinue calcium and iron supplements if contributing to constipation.
7. Review the client's medications. If the client is taking bulking agents (milk of magnesia, magnesium citrate, Metamucil, or Golytely), a large fluid intake is essential. Suggest the client and/or caregiver mask the taste of these medications in applesauce, mashed potatoes, gravy, orange juice, and nectars.

Cough

1. Encourage fluids and ice chips.
2. Recommend hard candy, including sour balls.
3. Have the client try tea and coffee to dilate pulmonary vessels.

Dehydration

1. Encourage fluids such as juices, ice cream, gelatin, custards, puddings, and soups if the client's life expectancy is more than a few days.
2. Encourage the client to try creative beverages such as orange sherbet and milk shake.
3. Consider a nasogastric tube feeding for fluid delivery only after a discussion with other team members, client, and caregivers. Plain water and foods high in electrolytes can be delivered via a tube feeding.
4. Consider a parenteral line only after a tube feeding is considered and rejected and after an in depth discussion with the team members, client, and family. Client goals, expectations, and quality-of-life issues should all be very carefully considered. Parenteral lines for the delivery of nutrients and water are rarely indicated in terminally ill clients.
5. There is strong clinical, ethical, and legal support for and against the administration of food and water when issues arise regarding what is and is not wanted by the patient and what is or is not warranted by empirical and clinical evidence (ADA, 2002).

Diarrhea

1. Consider modification of diet to omit lactose, gluten, or fat if related to diarrhea.
2. Suggest a decrease in dietary fiber content.
3. Consider the omission of gas-forming vegetables if an association between the consumption of these foods and diarrhea can be ascertained.
4. Consider the use of a low-residue diet.
5. Encourage high-potassium foods (bananas, tomato juice, orange juice, potatoes, etc.) if the client is dehydrated.
6. Recommend dry feedings (drink fluids 1 hour before or 30 to 60 minutes after meals).
7. Encourage intake of medium-chain triglycerides and a diet high in protein and carbohydrates for steatorrhea due to pancreatic insufficiency.
8. Consider the use of a complete oral nutritional supplement to provide adequate nutrient composition while helping the client overcome mild-to-moderate malabsorption.
9. For copious diarrhea and/or diarrhea combined with a decubitus on the coccyx, consider use of a clear-liquid complete nutritional supplement or a predigested oral nutritional supplement.

Disgeusia (abnormal taste)

1. Encourage oral care before mealtime.
2. Evaluate whether client experiences a bitter, sweet, or no taste after food consumption.

If foods taste bitter, encourage consumption of poultry, fish, milk and milk products, and legumes. Recommend the use of marinated meats and poultry in juices or wine. Sour and salty foods are generally not liked when a client experiences a bitter taste. Cook food in a glass or porcelain container to improve taste. Recommend a decreased use of red meats, sour juices, coffee, tea, tomatoes, and chocolate. The use of a modular protein supplement may be helpful if the client's protein intake is suboptimal.

If food has no taste, recommend foods served at room temperature, highly seasoned foods, and sugary foods.

If foods have a sweet taste, recommend sour juices, tart foods, lemon juice, vinegar, pickles, spices, herbs, and the use of a modular carbohydrate supplement.

Dyspnea (difficulty breathing)

1. Encourage coffee, tea, carbonated beverages, and chocolate. These foods are bronchodilators that increase blood pressure, dilate pulmonary vessels, increase glomerular filtration rate, and thereby break up and expel pulmonary secretions and fluids (Gallagher-Allred, 1989).
2. Encourage use of a soft diet. Liquids are usually better tolerated than solids. Cold foods are often better accepted than hot foods.
3. Recommend small, frequent feedings.
4. Encourage ice chips, frozen fruit juices, and popsicles; these are often well accepted.
5. Consider the use of a complete high-fat, low-carbohydrate nutritional supplement. This decreases carbon dioxide retention and assists in breathing.

Esophageal Reflux

1. Recommend small feedings.
2. Discourage foods that lower esophageal sphincter pressure, such as high-fat foods, chocolate, peppermint, spearmint, and alcohol.
3. Encourage client to sit up while eating and for 1 hour afterward.
4. Recommend avoidance of food within 3 hours before bedtime.
5. Teach relaxation techniques.

(Continued on the following page)

Box 26–2 **Dietary Management for Symptom Control** *(Continued)*

Fever

1. Recommend a high fluid intake.
2. Consider a tube feeding for severe dehydration to maintain hydration after a discussion with team members. This is not recommended if death is imminent (hours/days).
3. Recommend high-protein, high-caloric foods.

Fluid Accumulation

1. Recommend a mild sodium restriction (3 to 4 g/day). Recommend a lower sodium restriction only if this is the wish of the client.
2. Discourage a fluid restriction unless the client has significant hyponatremia.
3. Provide a list of foods high in protein and potassium.

Hiccups

1. Recommend smaller meals and slow eating.
2. Discourage the use of a straw.
3. Add peppermint to food to decrease gastric distention (Gallagher-Allred, 1989).
4. Recommend client swallow a large teaspoon of granulated sugar.

Hypoglycemia

1. Assess the client's and/or caregiver's knowledge about diabetes and hypoglycemia.
2. Determine if the client is truly insulin dependent as part of the admission assessment process. The following suggest true insulin-dependence:
   - The introduction of insulin soon after the diagnosis
   - A history of previous ketoacidosis
   - Use of more than one daily dose of insulin fo years
3. Evaluate the client's expressed desire for extent of medical care. The primary guide for determining the level of nutritional intervention is the wish of the client.
4. Determine the last time the client experienced the signs of a hypoglycemic episode. Many of these clients have deficiencies in the counterregulatory hormones, especially epinephrine, and may lapse into a coma without any warning signs. Caregivers need to be informed of this potential complication. Educate the client and/or caregiver on the treatment of hypoglycemia (15-15 rule, "Diet in Diabetes Mellitus and Hypoglycemia").
5. Monitor client's blood glucose level. A suitable range for blood sugars would be 127 to 309 mg/dL in the hospice population (Boyd, 1993).
6. Encourage 30 to 50 g of carbohydrate every 3 hours to prevent starvation ketosis. Each of the following is equal to 30 to 50 g of carbohydrate: 3/4 cup Carnation Instant Breakfast, 1 cup regular gelatin, 1 cup vanilla ice cream, 1 1/2 cups ginger ale, 1 cup orange juice, 1 cup apple juice.

Incontinence

1. Discourage intake of coffee, tea, and carbonated beverages containing caffeine, especially before bedtime.
2. Continue to encourage adequate fluid intake.

Jaundice and Hepatic Encephalopathy

1. Encourage a high-carbohydrate diet.
2. Encourage a protein-restricted diet only if the client desires.
3. Specialized oral nutritional supplements for clients with liver disease are often ineffective for the terminally ill but may be beneficial when the client desires to "live long enough to _____."
4. Evaluate presence of esophageal varices. If present, provide soft foods.

Nausea and Vomiting

1. Discuss practical issues with client and/or caregiver such as food attitudes, social aspects of eating, and unpredictable food preferences (Dietitians Association of Australia, 1992).
2. Recommend client restrict fluids to 1 hour before or after meals to prevent early satiety.
3. Assess if sweet, fried, or fatty foods are poorly tolerated; recommend avoidance if necessary.
4. Evaluate if starchy foods such as crackers, breads, potatoes, rice, and pasta are better tolerated. Encourage increased consumption if helpful.
5. Encourage the client to eat slowly, chew feed well, and rest after each meal as these behaviors may increase food intake.
6. Recommend the client avoid offensive odors during food preparation.
7. Recommend that the person who has recently experienced severe nausea and vomiting try 1 to 2 bites of food per hour.
8. Emphasize the sensual aspects of food, including appearance (serve garnished food on attractive tableware), odor of environment (remove bedpans and emesis basins from room), taste (cater to the client's likes and dislikes), and the importance of companionship during mealtime.
9. Recommend the avoidance of food if nausea and vomiting become severe and food makes the client feel worse. Feeding may not be desirable if death is expected within hours or a few days and the effects of partial dehydration or the withdrawal of nutrition support will not adversely alter client comfort (American Dietetic Association, 1987).

Migraine Headaches

1. Recommend that the client eat at regular intervals. Hunger or missed meals can trigger a migraine headache.
2. Recommend that the highly motivated client keep a food diary and record the onset of any headaches.

Migraine headaches can be triggered by one or many foods. Common food offenders include many common food additives, processed meats, peanuts and peanut products, soybeans, yeast, chocolate, aged cheeses, seasonings, caffeine, some types of alcohol, and flavorings.

Pruritus (severe itching)

1. Recommend avoidance of known allergy foods.
2. Encourage fluid intake for clients receiving antihistamines.
3. Recommend avoidance of coffee, tea, carbonated beverages containing caffeine, alcohol, and cocoa that can cause vasodilation and itching.

Stomatitis (inflammation of the mouth)

1. Consider multivitamin supplement with folic acid and vitamin B_{12}.
2. Recommend avoidance of spicy, acidic, rough, hot, and salty foods.
3. Recommend a consistency modification, such as pureed, soft, or liquid.
4. Consider the use of a complete nutritional supplement.
5. Recommend creamy foods, whites sauces, and gravies.
6. Consider between-meal supplements, such as milkshakes, eggnogs, and puddings.
7. Recommend caregiver add sugar to acid or salty foods to alter the food's taste.
8. Recommend meals be served when the client's pain is under control.
9. Recommend good oral care before and after meals.

Weakness

1. Recommend multivitamin-mineral supplement with folic acid, vitamin B_{12}, and iron.
2. Encourage high-potassium foods (bananas, cantaloupe, milk, baked winter squash, etc.) if client vomits easily.

3. Recommend a modification in the food's consistency (mechanical soft or full liquid) to decrease the energy cost of eating.

Wounds and Pressure Sores

1. Recommend caregiver cater to the client's food preferences.
2. Use of aggressive nutritional support is rarely effective but may be appropriate if the client and family desire quantity. For example, "I want to live and see my _____ ."
3. Correct elevated glucose levels to decrease risk of infection.
4. Evaluate the use of a multivitamin and mineral supplement that contains zinc and vitamin C. As excess dietary zinc impedes healing, do not routinely recommend a zinc supplement without assessment information.
5. Encourage protein and caloric intake equal to estimated needs only if the client desires and is able.
6. Encourage client to dip foods in gravy, margarine, butter, and olive oil to increase calorie intake.

Xerostomia (dry mouth)

1. Encourage frequent sips of water, fruit juices, ice chips, popsicles, ice cream, and sherbet.
2. Recommend the use of hard candy.
3. Consider a modification of food consistency such as soft, mechanical soft, or full liquids.
4. Recommend avoidance of extremely hot or cold foods. Foods served at room temperature are generally better tolerated.
5. Recommend creamy foods, white sauces, and gravies.
6. Encourage the client to dip foods in gravy, margarine, butter, olive oil, coffee, and broth.
7. Consider the need for a complete liquid nutritional supplement between meals.

---

nurse feels uncomfortable discussing these issues with the client or lacks the time to counsel the client, a referral to the dietitian is indicated.

Ethical and Legal Considerations

Many of the legal and ethical issues concerning health-care delivery and health-care provider-client relations involve the provision of nutrition and hydration. In the past, before the development of tube feedings and intravenous feedings, the inability to eat and drink by mouth meant death from progressive body wasting. Stopping food or water inevitably leads to death within 14 days from dehydration (Wade, 2001). Now a decision needs to be made whether to feed a client. A client may experience a more comfortable death if he or she is slightly dehydrated. On the other

hand, efforts to hydrate some clients (not those actively dying) may offer a benefit. This is controversial. Death from dehydration precludes the use of any organs for transplantation (Wade, 2001). Some clients feel strongly a need to be an organ donor. Sometimes a client, significant other, or physician thinks that artificial hydration may promote client comfort and prolong life in a given situation. Perhaps a client's vital signs had been fluctuating and are now stable. Ethicists use rational processes for determining the most morally desirable course of action in the face of conflicting value choices. The process of choosing an ethical course of action involves medical goals and proportionality, client preferences, quality of life, and contextual features. Contextual features are the characteristics of a given situation.

Medical Care Goals and Proportionality

The medical care goals that apply to the client with a terminal illness include:

- Relieving symptoms, pain, and suffering
- Preventing untimely death ("I want to live long enough to....")
- Improving functional status or maintaining compromised status
- Educating and counseling the client and his or her significant others regarding the client's condition and prognosis
- Avoiding harming the client in the course of care
- Promoting health and preventing disease not related to the terminal disease

The physician is responsible for the initial education and counseling of clients regarding their condition and prognosis.

The principle of proportionality is an important ethical consideration in the treatment of terminally ill clients. **Proportionality** means a medical treatment is ethically mandatory to the extent that it is likely to confer greater benefits than burdens to the client. For example, many experts believe that a client who is actively dying and is slightly dehydrated has a more comfortable death. Dehydration has been reported to reduce a client's secretions and excretions, thus decreasing breathing problems, emesis, and incontinence. Dehydration can sedate the brain just before death. Greatly diminished oral intake or its cessation is one of the signs that death is imminent. In another context, a client who is terminally ill but whose condition is stable and enjoys many activities of daily living may appreciate or request education on how to maintain hydration. A nutritional intervention is appropriate if the client would receive greater benefits than burdens.

Client Preference

The most important ethical principle to consider is the client's right to self-determination. Some individuals may perceive suffering as an important means of personal growth or a religious experience. Other individuals may hope a miracle cure will be discovered for his or her disease. Others may be ready for and accepting of death. Health-care workers have a responsibility to provide a combination of emotional support and technical nutritional advice on how best to achieve each client's goals.

Quality of Life

The most fundamental goal of medical care is an improvement in the quality of life for those who seek care. If improvement is not possible, a goal of medical care is maintenance of the same quality of life or slowing a decline in quality of life. Oral feeding is part of being human and associated with human dignity. One study found that 92 percent of all cancer clients could eat and/or drink until the day they died (Feuz and Rapin, 1994). These clients derived some pleasure from the sensual aspect of food and the socialization that accompanies meals. Food conveys emotional, spiritual, sociological, and biologic meanings. If food remains enjoyable for a client with a terminal illness, the health-care worker should encourage mealtimes to be shared with loved ones. If eating is not a pleasant experience, however, it should not be overemphasized.

Contextual

Every terminally ill client has his or her own story, with both a history and a future. A client's decision to eat or not to eat is part of his or her narrative. Two examples can illustrate why eating issues should always be given consideration when formulating a care plan. Client 1 lives in a rooming house without air conditioning; his family does not want to get involved; he does not have cooking facilities; he refuses to eat the meals delivered to him from the Senior Nutrition Center; and he insists that he wants to die at home. Client 2 lives with his male companion in a beach house; his friend carries him every day to the beach to watch the sunset; meals are prepared for him by his boyfriend and many other neighbors and friends. Client 1 refuses to eat. Client 2 tries to eat a small amount at least six times a day. The willingness to eat is part of each man's story.

The contextual features in a patient's situation often relate to food acceptance. In Client 1's situation, the health-care worker may offer a valuable service by reassuring the client that he will not be abandoned because he refuses to eat. The fear of abandonment is among the most frequently cited apprehensions of dying (American Dietetic Association, 1987). Even if a client refuses to eat, health-care workers should remain supportive. The client may change his or her mind. The health-care worker should not consider the rejection of food as a sign of personal or professional failure.

A consideration of a client's medical goals, preferences, quality of life, and contextual features may provide a framework for resolution of ethical dietary issues. Hospice programs have interdisciplinary care teams, and the interdisciplinary team conference is the best arena in which to discuss ethical feeding conflicts.

Legal Issues

The issue of whether to discontinue food and fluid to a client with a terminal illness first emerged in the 1960s. Clients have the legal right to refuse treatment, including artificial feedings. This right is based on the Fourteenth Amendment to the Constitution, which refers to the right to liberty, including the right to be left alone and not invaded or treated against one's will. Courts have recognized that competent adults have the right to refuse treatment, including artificial feeding. The state may exert its authority to expand the individual's right to liberty, however, based on other concepts. The preservation of life, the prevention of suicide, the protection of innocent third parties (such as minor children), and the protection of the ethical integrity and professional discretion of the medical profession are among these concepts. Health-care workers need to be familiar with the laws in their individual states and the policies and procedures of the organization for which they work. They should also know their professional organization's standards of practice. In some states, a charge of battery can be made if a client is fed artificially against his or her wishes. In some states, a charge of negligence can be made if clients are allowed to intentionally starve themselves to death. Situations such as these should be discussed at the interdisciplinary team meeting or brought to the risk manager's attention. (The risk manager is hired by a health-care organization to identify, evaluate, and correct potential risks of injuring clients, staff, visitors, or property.)

With incompetent adult clients, caretakers and family should try to ascertain the client's wishes from past written and oral statements and actions. State laws differ as to whether nutrition and hydration are medically obligatory or medically optional. Some clients may wish for the withdrawal of antibiotics and ventilators but wish to continue nutritional support. This situation may occur when an individual has a permanent feeding tube in place because of an inability to swallow, such as may occur with cancer of the esophagus. What can the nurse legally do if the client is incompetent and the family wants the feeding tube removed? What can the nurse legally do if family members disagree about whether to have the feeding tube removed? When in doubt, the best advice is to continue to feed the client until the health-care team, the institution's ethics committee, or the facility's risk manager reviews the case. The artificial feeding can be stopped at a future time if the decision is changed, but a deceased person cannot be brought back to life.

Individuals may make their wishes known in writing through advanced directives, such as a living will or durable power of attorney. An **advanced directive** is a signed document in which the client has specified what type of medical care is desired should he or she lose the ability to make decisions. A **durable power of attorney** for health care is a document in which the client gives another person power to make medical treatment and related personal care decisions for him or her. It can be used as an addition to the advanced directive. Health-care workers are responsible for becoming familiar with a client's advanced directive, durable power of attorney, and living will. In the event that a client does not have a written directive, the next of kin or guardian should be consulted about probable preference for the level of nutritional intervention (American Dietetic Association, 1987).

General Considerations

Oral feedings should be advocated over tube and intravenous feedings for terminally ill clients. Food and control of food intake can be one of life's last pleasures. The client's decision to eat or not to eat is his or her right. If the client chooses to eat, wants to maintain or achieve a reasonable body weight, and wants to maintain muscle mass, it is essential to try to provide adequate nutrition. An effort should be made to enhance the individual's enjoyment of food. A pleasant dining environment that includes a cheerful attitude by caregivers may encourage food intake. The use of complete oral nutrition supplements may provide some relief from symptoms associated with hunger, thirst, and malnutrition. Previously prescribed dietary restrictions should be reevaluated and liberalized. The client's right to self-determination should guide the health-care worker in determining whether to allow foods that are not permitted within the diet prescription.

Palliative care does not automatically preclude aggressive nutritional support. The client's informed preference for the level of nutrition intervention is important. If the client wants maximal nutrition support and the policy of the organization is not to provide hyperalimentation or tube feedings for terminally ill clients, the client has the right to be informed of the name of a facility that will provide this service. Artificial feeding is generally not desirable if death is expected within hours or a few days. The effects of partial dehydration and the withdrawal of nutritional support will not adversely alter the client's comfort. Enteral or parenteral feeding would probably worsen the client's condition, symptoms, or discomfort when shock, pulmonary edema, diarrhea, or aspiration is a potential or actual complication. The client or surrogate needs to be informed of these facts when he or she requests maximal support.

SUMMARY

Death is an aspect of life. If we want to help the dying, we must examine our own attitudes toward death. Treatment for terminally ill clients is palliative. The goal of care is symptomatic relief to reduce or alleviate pain. Nutritional intervention can frequently alleviate or reduce the pain and suffering of a terminally ill client. The use of oral feedings should always be given preferential consideration over tube and parenteral feedings. Oral feeding is ordinary care, whereas tube feedings and hyperalimentation are considered by some to be extraordinary care.

In the United States, the client's expressed desire is the primary guide for determining the extent of nutritional and hydration therapy. Our Constitution guarantees clients the right to self-determination. Ethical and legal dilemmas should be brought to the attention of the interdisciplinary team, the risk manager, or the facility's ethics committee promptly. Artificial feeding should never be stopped unless one of these parties has investigated the situation and made a legal and ethical determination that the feeding should cease. A health-care worker has an obligation to know his or her client's advanced directive, durable power of attorneys, and living will documentation.

CASE STUDY 26-1

Ms. Z is a 60-year-old woman who has a diagnosis of amyotrophic lateral sclerosis (ALS), also called Lou Gehrig's disease, with a prognosis of less than 6 months. The client has at least two swallowing impediments. She is unable to dislodge food that collects under her tongue, in cheeks, and on her hard palate. She does not have adequate swallow control (the bolus goes down before she wants it to). Because of these impediments, Ms. Z is unable to tolerate thin liquids, and the maintenance of hydration and aspiration are of concern to the caregiver. Ms. Z is alert, oriented, and highly educated. She saw a television program that led her to believe that a high-protein diet would delay the progression of ALS. She would like instruction on a high-protein diet.

NURSING CARE PLAN

SUBJECTIVE DATA Client believes a high-protein diet will delay the progression of her ALS
Caregiver is concerned about the danger of aspiration and the maintenance of hydration

OBJECTIVE DATA Diagnosis: ALS with a prognosis of less than 6 months
Lack of swallowing control

NURSING DIAGNOSIS NANDA: Deficient knowledge (NANDA, 2003, with permission) related to lack of desired information about foods high in protein as evidenced by verbal statements. Deficient knowledge related to a lack of understanding of how to increase and/or maintain hydration with the client's swallowing impediments as evidenced by the caregiver's verbal statements

DESIRED OUTCOMES EVALUATION CRITERIA	NURSING ACTIONS/INTERVENTIONS	RATIONALE
NOC: Knowledge: Diet (Moorhead Johnson, and Maas, 2004, with permission)	NIC: Diet (Dochterman and Bulechek, 2004, with permission)	
The client will indicate how she can incorporate foods high in protein and of semisolid or pureed consistency into her diet.	Plan a 70- to 80-g protein semiliquid/ pureed diet (2 cups thickened milk, 6 oz meat or equivalent, 2 vegetables, and 6 starches) for the client or refer the client to the dietitian to plan and instruct the client and/or caregiver on the diet.	Because a 70- to 80-g protein diet would most likely not harm the client and would make her feel in control, instruction on the diet is appropriate.
The caregiver will verbalize how to reduce the likelihood of aspiration by following safety precautions for clients with dysphagia.	Discuss feeding issues with the caregiver such as the correct body positioning and eating conditions	The risk of aspiration is high in clients with dysphagia.
	Eliminate distractions.	
	Position individual in an upright position (90 degrees at the hip) with feet flat on floor.	
	Give semiliquids in very small amounts (syringe) and only after food has been cleared from the mouth.	
	Feed the client very small bites.	
	Encourage several dry swallows between bites of food.	
	If the Adam's apple rises, it is likely the food is being swallowed and not deposited in the cheeks.	
	A wet-sounding voice with a gurgle may mean food is resting on the vocal cords.	

C T Q CRITICAL THINKING QUESTIONS

1. The client's swallowing disorders are becoming more severe. Ms. Z is capable of eating only very small bites of food very slowly. The client's daughter is her caregiver, and she states, "It has been taking me 2 hours to feed my mother each meal. If I go any faster, she chokes. My husband is becoming very resentful and has asked me to make a decision. He says I can't continue to spend all day with my mother and ignore him." What would you say to this caregiver?

2. The caregiver believes the client is still mentally alert and oriented, although the client cannot communicate. The client has progressed to the point where she has lost all motor function. She cannot talk or walk and has lost the use of her hands. The client's physician now believes Ms. Z has an ileus (paralysis of the bowel). Why does this mean the patient cannot be fed orally? What are the treatment options? Who needs to be informed of the treatment options?

⫸ CHAPTER REVIEW

1. A diet prescription consistent with palliative care goals is:
   a. 40 grams of protein for liver failure
   b. Low-cholesterol, low-saturated-fat diet for hyperlipoproteinemia
   c. Gluten-free diet for diarrhea and celiac disease
   d. High-calorie, high-protein diet for anorexia in an actively dying client

2. An appropriate nutritional screening question for a client with a terminal illness is:
   a. "How many times a day do you eat?"
   b. "How much weight have you lost in the past month?"
   c. "Do you look forward to meals?"
   d. "Do you include a green or yellow vegetable in your diet each day?"

3. The most important ethical principle to consider when a decision must be made about whether or not to feed a client is:
   a. The client's right to self-determination
   b. Proportionality
   c. Medical goals
   d. The client's quality of life

4. Which recommendation would be appropriate for a client with end-stage congestive heart failure who requests dietary advice?
   a. Recommend a low-potassium diet
   b. Recommend a 1000-cc fluid restriction
   c. Monitor the client's fluid intake and output
   d. Recommend a 3- or 4-gram sodium diet

5. The intervention appropriate for a terminally ill client with dyspnea who requests dietary treatment is:
   a. Encourage a high-fiber diet
   b. Consider a high-fat, low-carbohydrate complete nutritional supplement
   c. Recommend fresh fruits, whole grains, and vegetables
   d. Encourage avoidance of caffeine

✚ CLINICAL ANALYSIS

1. Mr. O is actively dying. Mr. O's wife is concerned because her husband adamantly refuses all food and fluids. The nurse should:
   a. Call the doctor and request an order for a tube feeding
   b. Call the doctor and request an order for an intravenous feeding
   c. Instruct the caregiver to be more creative in the type of food and fluids she gives the client
   d. Counsel the caregiver that oral intake often ceases near the end of life

2. Mrs. P has diagnoses of brain cancer and insulin-dependent diabetes mellitus and a prognosis of a few days. She and her caregiver have been self-monitoring her blood glucose levels. The caregiver is quite concerned because Mrs. P's blood glucose levels are running between 400 to 500 milligrams per deciliter. Historically, the client claims to have followed her 1200-calorie diet faithfully. Recently, her appetite is markedly reduced and her blood glucose levels are elevated (hypermetabolism). The physician has been contacted and refuses to increase the client's insulin further but recommends to Mrs.

P's caregiver to stop monitoring the client's blood glucose levels. The nurse should:
   a. Encourage the caregiver to offer Mrs. P frequent sips of clear liquid fruit juices (about 30 grams of carbohydrate every 3 hours)
   b. Encourage the caregiver to continue to offer the client the 1200-calorie diet to avoid a hypoglycemic episode
   c. Recommend the caregiver look for a new doctor because obviously the doctor does not know how to treat clients with insulin-dependent diabetes
   d. Contact the hospice medical director and ask for an order to increase the client's insulin

3. Mr. J has a partial bowel obstruction and shows signs of dehydration. He has an order for Metamucil prn. The nurse should immediately recommend:
   a. High-fiber foods such as bran, whole grains, fruits, and vegetables
   b. Discontinuation of the Metamucil
   c. Increasing the dose of Metamucil
   d. Cheese, cakes, pies, cookies, and doughnuts

REFERENCES

American Dietetic Association: Manual of Clinical Dietetics, ed 6. American Dietetic Association, Chicago, 2000.

American Dietetic Association: Migraine headaches and food: The "trigger" factor. J Am Diet Assoc 95:1240, 1995.

American Dietetic Association: Position of the American Dietetic Association: Ethical and legal issues in nutrition, hydration, and feeding. J Am Diet Assoc 102:716, 2002.

American Dietetic Association: Position of the American Dietetic Association: Issues in feeding the terminally ill adult. J Am Diet Assoc 87:76, 1987.

Boyd, K: Diabetes mellitus in hospice patients: Some guidelines. Palliative Med 7:163, 1993.

Cox, A, and McCallum, PD: Medical nutrition therapy in palliative care. In McCallum, PD, Polisena, CG (eds): The Clinical Guide to Oncology Nutrition. American Dietetic Association, Chicago, 2000.

Dietitians Association of Australia: Position Paper: Nutrition priorities in palliative care of oncology patients. Dietitians Association of Australia 92–93, 1992.

Dochterman, J, and Bulechek, GM: Nursing Interventions Classification (NIC), ed 4. Mosby, Philadelphia, 2004.

Feuz, A, and Rapin, C: An observational study of the role of pain management and food adaptation of elderly patients with terminal cancer. J Am Diet Assoc 94:767, 1994.

Finucane, TE, Christmas, C, and Travis, K: Tube feeding in patients with advanced dementia. JAMA 14:282, 1999.

Gallagher-Allred, CR: Nutritional Care of the Terminally Ill. Aspen Publishers, Gaithersburg, MD, 1989.

Junkerman, C, and Schiedermayer, D: Practical Ethics for Student, Interns, and Residents, ed 2. University Publishing Group, Fredrick, MD, 1998.

Mills, M, Davies, HTO, and Macrae, WA: Care of dying patients in hospital. Br Med J 309:583, 1994.

Moorhead, S, Johnson, M, and Maas, M: Nursing Outcomes Classification (NOC), ed 3. Mosby, Philadelphia, 2004.

Morrison, RD, and Meier, DE: Palliative care. N Engl J Med. 350: 2582, 2004.

NANDA International: Nursing Diagnoses: Definitions and Classification, 2003–2004. NANDA International, Philadelphia, 2003.

Nenner, F: Listen to voices. BMJ 322:372, 2001.

Shils, ME: Nutrition and medical ethics: The interplay of medical decisions, patients rights, and the judicial system. In Shils, ME, et al (eds): Modern Nutrition in Health and Disease, ed 9. Williams & Wilkins, Baltimore, 1999.

Singer, PA, Martin, DK, Kelner, M: Quality of end-of-life care: Patient perspectives. JAMA. 281:163, 1999.

Steinhauser, KE, et al: Factors considered important at the end of life by patients, family, physicians, and other care providers. JAMA 284:2476, 2000.

Wade, DT: Ethical issues in diagnoses and management of patients in permanent vegetative state. BMJ 322:352, 2001.

Exchange Lists of the American Dietetic and American Diabetes Associations

Starch List

One starch exchange equals 15 g carbohydrate, 3 g protein, 0–1 g fat, and 80 cal.

Bread

Bagel	1/2 (1 oz)
Bread, reduced-calorie	2 slices (1 1/2 oz)
Bread, white, whole-wheat, pumpernickel, rye	1 slice (1 oz)
Bread sticks, crisp, 4 in long 3 1/2 in	2 (2/3 oz)
English muffin	1/2
Hot dog or hamburger bun	1/2 (1 oz)
Pita, 6 in across	1/2
Roll, plain, small	1 (1 oz)
Raisin bread, unfrosted	1 slice (1 oz)
Tortilla, corn, 6 in across	1
Tortilla, flour, 7–8 in across	1
Waffle, 4 1/2 in square, reduced-fat	1

Cereals and Grains

Bran cereals	1/3 cup
Bulgur	1/2 cup
Cereals, cooked	1/2 cup
Cereals, unsweetened, ready-to-eat	3/4 cup
Cornmeal (dry)	3 tbsp
Couscous	1/3 cup
Flour (dry)	3 tbsp
Granola, low-fat	1/4 cup
Grape-Nuts	1/4 cup
Grits	1/2 cup
Kasha	1/2 cup
Millet	1/4 cup
Muesli	1/4 cup
Saltine-type crackers	6
Snack chips, fat-free (tortilla, potato)	15–20 (3/4 oz)
Whole-wheat crackers, no fat added	2–4 (3/4 oz)

Oats	1/2 cup
Pasta (cooked)	1/2 cup
Puffed cereal	1 1/2 cups
Rice milk	1/2 cup
Rice, white or brown	1/3 cup
Shredded Wheat	1/2 cup
Sugar-Frosted cereal	1/2 cup
Wheat germ	3 tbsp

Starchy Vegetables

Baked beans	1/3 cup
Corn	1/2 cup
Corn on cob, medium	1 (5 oz)
Mixed vegetables with corn, peas, or pasta	1 cup
Peas, green	1/2 cup
Plantain	1/2 cup
Potato, baked or boiled	1 small (3 oz)
Potato, mashed	1/2 cup
Squash, winter (acorn, butternut)	1 cup
Yam, sweet potato, plain	1/3 cup

Crackers and Snacks

Animal crackers	8
Graham crackers, 2 1/2 in square	3
Matzoh	3/4 oz
Melba toast	5 slices
Oyster crackers	24
Popcorn (popped, no fat added or low-fat microwave)	3 cups
Pretzels	3/4 oz
Rice cakes, 4 in across	2
Chow mein noodles	1/2 cup

Dried Beans, Peas, and Lentils (Count as 1 starch exchange, plus 1 very lean meat exchange.)

Beans and Peas (garbanzo, pinto, kidney, white, split, black-eyed)	1/2 cup
Lima beans	1/2 cup
Lentils	1/2 cup
Misc*	3 tbsp

Starchy Foods Prepared with Fat (Count as 1 starch exchange, plus 1 fat exchange.)

Biscuit, 2 1/2 in across	1

*400 mg or more of sodium per serving.

Corn bread, 2 in cube	1 (2 oz)
Crackers, round butter type	6
Croutons	1 cup
French-fried potatoes	10 (1 1/2 oz)
Granola	1/4 cup
Muffin, small	1 (1 1/2 oz)
Pancake, 4 in across	2
Popcorn, microwave	3 cups
Sandwich crackers, cheese or peanut butter filling	3
Stuffing, bread (prepared)	1/4 cup
Taco shell, 6 in across	2
Waffle, 4 1/2 in square	1
Whole-wheat crackers, fat added	4–6 (1 oz)

Fruit List

One fruit exchange equals 15 g carbohydrate and 60 cal. The weight includes skin, core, seeds, and rind.

Fruit

Apple, unpeeled, small	1 (4 oz)
Applesauce, unsweetened	1/2 cup
Apples, dried	4 rings
Apricots, fresh	4 whole (5 1/2 oz)
Apricots, dried	8 halves
Apricots, canned	1/2 cup
Banana, small	1 (4 oz)
Blackberries	3/4 cup
Blueberries	3/4 cup
Cantaloupe, small	1/3 melon (11 oz) or 1 cup cubes
Cherries, sweet, fresh	12 (3 oz)
Cherries, sweet, canned	1/2 cup
Dates	3
Figs, fresh	1 1/2 large or 2 medium (3 1/2 oz)
Figs, dried	1 1/2
Fruit cocktail	1/2 cup
Grapefruit, lg	1/2 (11 oz)
Grapefruit sections, canned	3/4 cup
Grapes, small	17 (3 oz)
Honeydew melon	1 slice (10 oz) or 1 cup cubes
Kiwi	1 (3 1/2 oz)
Mandarin oranges, canned	3/4 cup
Mango, small	1/2 fruit (5 1/2 oz) or 1/2 cup
Nectarine, small	1 (5 oz)
Orange, small	1 (6 1/2 oz)
Papaya	1 cup cubes or 1/2 fruit

Peach, medium, fresh	1 (6 oz)
Peaches, canned	1/2 cup
Pear, lg, fresh	1/2 (4 oz)
Pears, canned	1/2 cup
Pineapple, fresh	3/4 cup
Pineapple, canned	1/3 cup
Plums, small	2 (5 oz)
Plums, canned	1/2 cup
Prunes, dried	3
Raisins	2 tbsp
Raspberries	1 cup
Strawberries	1 1/4 cup whole berries
Tangerines, small	2 (8 oz)
Watermelon	1 slice (13 1/2 oz) or 1 1/4 cup cubes

Fruit Juice

Apple juice/cider	1/2 cup
Cranberry juice cocktail	1/3 cup
Cranberry juice cocktail reduced-calorie	1 cup
Fruit juice blends, 100 percent juice	1/3 cup
Grape juice	1/3 cup
Grapefruit juice	1/2 cup
Orange juice	1/2 cup
Pineapple juice	1/2 cup
Prune juice	1/3 cup

Milk List

One milk exchange equals 12 g carbohydrate and 8 g protein.
Skim and Very Low-Fat Milk

(0–3 g fat per serving)

Skim milk	1 cup	Nonfat or low-fat buttermilk	1 cup
1/2 percent milk	1 cup	Evaporated skim milk	1/2 cup
1 percent milk	1 cup	Nonfat dry milk	1/3 cup dry

| Plain nonfat yogurt | 3/4 cup |
| Nonfat or low-fat fruit-flavored yogurt sweetened with aspartame or with a nonnutritive sweetener | 1 cup |

Low-Fat (5 g fat per serving)

| 2 percent milk | 1 cup |

| Plain low-fat yogurt | 8 oz |
| Sweet acidophilus milk | 1 cup |

Whole Milk (8 g fat per serving)

Whole milk	1 cup
Evaporated whole milk	1/2 cup
Goat's milk	1 cup
Kefir	1 cup

Other Carbohydrates List

One exchange equals 15 g carbohydrate, or 1 starch, or 1 fruit, or 1 milk.

FOOD	SERVING SIZE	EXCHANGES PER SERVING
Angel food cake, unfrosted	1/12th cake	2 carbohydrates
Brownie, small, unfrosted	2 in square	1 carbohydrate, 1 fat
Cake, unfrosted	2 in square	1 carbohydrate, 1 fat
Cake, frosted	2 in square	2 carbohydrates, 1 fat
Cookie, fat-free	2 small	1 carbohydrate
Cookie or sandwich cookie with creme filling	2 small	1 carbohydrate, 1 fat
Cupcake, frosted	1 small	2 carbohydrates, 1 fat
Cranberry sauce, jellied	1/4 cup	2 carbohydrates
Doughnut, plain cake	1 medium (1 1/2 oz)	1 1/2 carbohydrates, 2 fat
Doughnut, glazed	3 3/4 in across (2 oz)	2 carbohydrates, 2 fats
Fruit juice bars, frozen, 100 percent juice	1 bar (3 oz)	1 carbohydrate
Fruit snacks, chewy (pureed fruit concentrate)	1 roll (3/4 oz)	1 carbohydrate
Fruit spreads, 100 percent fruit	1 tbsp	1 carbohydrate
Gelatin, regular	1/2 cup	1 carbohydrate
Gingersnaps	3	1 carbohydrate
Granola bar	1 bar	1 carbohydrate, 1 fat
Granola bar, fat-free	1 bar	2 carbohydrates
Hummus	1/3 cup	1 carbohydrate, 1 fat
Ice cream	1/2 cup	1 carbohydrate, 2 fats
Ice cream, light	1/2 cup	1 carbohydrate, 1 fat
Ice cream, fat-free, no sugar added	1/2 cup	1 carbohydrate
Jam or jelly, regular	1 tbsp	1 carbohydrate
Milk, chocolate, whole	1 cup	2 carbohydrates, 1 fat
Pie, fruit, 2 crusts	1/6 pie	3 carbohydrates, 2 fats
Pie, pumpkin or custard	1/8 pie	1 carbohydrate, 2 fats
Potato chips	12–18 (1 oz)	1 carbohydrate, 2 fats
Pudding, regular (made with low-fat milk)	1/2 cup	2 carbohydrates
Pudding, sugar-free (made with low-fat milk)	1/2 cup	1 carbohydrate
Salad dressing, fat-free*	1/4 cup	1 carbohydrate
Sherbet, sorbet	1/2 cup	2 carbohydrates
Spaghetti or pasta sauce, canned*	1/2 cup	1 carbohydrate, 1 fat
Sweet roll or Danish	1 (2 1/2 oz)	2 1/2 carbohydrates, 2 fats
Syrup, light	2 tbsp	1 carbohydrate
Syrup, regular	1 tbsp	1 carbohydrate
Syrup, regular	1/4 cup	4 carbohydrates
Tortilla chips	6–12 (1 oz)	1 carbohydrate, 2 fats
Yogurt, frozen, low-fat, fat-free	1/3 cup	1 carbohydrate, 0–1 fat
Yogurt, frozen, fat-free no sugar added	1/2 cup	1 carbohydrate
Yogurt, low-fat with fruit	1 cup	3 carbohydrates, 0–1 fat
Vanilla wafers	5	1 carbohydrate, 1 fat

*400 mg or more sodium per exchange.

Vegetable List

In general, one vegetable exchange is 1/2 cup cooked vegetable or juice or 1 cup raw vegetable.
One vegetable exchange equals 5 g carbohydrate, 2 g protein, 0 g fat, and 25 cal.

Artichoke	Mushrooms
Artichoke hearts	Okra
Asparagus	Onions
Beans (green, wax, Italian)	Pea pods
Bean sprouts	Peppers (all varieties)
Beets	Radishes
Broccoli	Salad greens (endive, escarole, lettuce, romaine,
Brussels sprouts	spinach)
Cabbage	Sauerkraut*
Carrots	Spinach
Cauliflower	Summer squash
Celery	Tomato
Cucumber	Tomatoes, canned
Eggplant	Tomato sauce*
Green onions or scallions	Tomato/vegetable juice*
Greens (collard, kale, mustard, turnip)	Turnips
Kohlrabi	Water chestnuts
Leeks	Watercress
Mixed vegetables (without corn, peas, or pasta)	Zucchini

*400 mg or more sodium per exchange.

Meat and Meat Substitutes List

Very Lean Meat and Substitutes List

One exchange equals 0 g carbohydrate, 7 g protein, 0–1 g fat, and 35 cal. One very lean meat exchange is equal to any one of the following items.

Poultry: Chicken or turkey (white meat, no skin), Cornish hen (no skin)	1 oz
Fish: Fresh or frozen cod, flounder, haddock, halibut, trout; tuna fresh or canned in water	1 oz
Shellfish: Clams, crab, lobster, scallops, shrimp, imitation shellfish	1 oz
Game: Duck or pheasant (no skin), venison, buffalo, ostrich	1 oz
Cheese with 1 g or less fat per ounce:	
Nonfat or low-fat cottage cheese	3/4 cup
Fat-free cheese	1 oz
Other: Processed sandwich meats with 1 g or less fat per ounce, such as deli thin, shaved meats, chipped beef,* turkey ham	1 oz
Egg whites	2
Egg substitutes, plain	1/4 cup
Hot dogs with 1 g or less fat per ounce*	1 oz
Kidney (high in cholesterol)	1 oz
Sausage with 1 g or less fat per ounce	1 oz
Count as one very lean meat and one starch exchange.	
Dried beans, peas, lentils (cooked)	1/2 cup

Lean Meat and Substitutes List

One exchange equals 0 g carbohydrate, 7 g protein, 3 g fat, and 55 cal. One lean meat exchange is equal to any one of the following items.

Beef: USDA Select or Choice grades of lean beef trimmed of fat, such as round, sirloin, and flank steak; tenderloin; roast (rib, chuck, rump); steak (T-bone, porterhouse, cubed), ground round	1 oz
Pork: Lean pork, such as fresh ham; canned, cured, or boiled ham; Canadian bacon*; tenderloin, center loin chop	1 oz
Lamb: Roast, chop, leg	1 oz
Veal: Lean chop, roast	1 oz
Poultry: Chicken, turkey (dark meat, no skin), chicken white meat (with skin), domestic duck or goose (well drained of fat, no skin)	1 oz
Fish:	
Herring (uncreamed or smoked)	1 oz
Oysters	6 medium
Salmon (fresh or canned), catfish	1 oz
Sardines (canned)	2 medium
Tuna (canned in oil, drained)	1 oz
Game: Goose (no skin), rabbit	1 oz
Cheese:	
4.5 percent fat cottage cheese	1/2 cup
Granted Parmesan	2 tbsp

Cheeses with 3 g or less fat per ounce	1 oz
Other:	
Hot dogs with 3 g or less fat per ounce*	1 1/2 oz
Processed sandwich meat with 3 g or less fat per ounce, such as turkey pastrami or kielbasa	1 oz
Liver, heart (high in cholesterol)	1 oz

Medium-Fat Meat and Substitutes List

One exchange equals 0 g carbohydrate, 7 g protein, 5 g fat, and 75 cal. One medium-fat meat exchange is equal to any one of the following items.

Beef: Most beef products fall into this category (ground beef, meatloaf, corned beef, short ribs, Prime grades of meat trimmed of fat, such as prime rib)	1 oz
Pork: Top loin, chop, Boston butt, cutlet	1 oz
Lamb: Rib roast, ground	1 oz
Veal: Cutlet (ground or cubed, unbreaded)	1 oz
Poulty: Chicken dark meat (with skin), ground turkey or ground chicken, fried chicken (with skin)	1 oz
Fish: Any fried fish product	1 oz
Cheese: With 5 g or less fat per ounce	
Feta	1 oz
Mozzarella	1 oz
Ricotta	1/4 cup
Other: Egg (high in cholesterol, limit to 4 per week)	1
Sausage with 5 g or less fat per ounce	1 oz

Soy milk	1 cup
Tempeh	1/4 cup
Tofu	4 oz

High-Fat Meat and Substitutes List

One exchange equals 0 g carbohydrate, 7 g protein, 8 g fat, and 100 cal. Remember these items are high in saturated fat, cholesterol, and c and may raise blood cholesterol levels if eaten on a regular basi high-fat meat exchange is equal to any one of the following item

Pork: Spareribs, ground pork, pork sausage	1 oz
Cheese: All regular cheese, such as American*, cheddar, Monterey Jack, Swiss	1 oz
Other: Processed sandwich meats with 8 g or less fat per ounce, such as bologna, pimento loaf, salami	1 oz
Sausage, such as bratwurst, Italian, knockwurst, Polish, smoked	1 oz
Hot dog (turkey or chicken)*	1 (10/1b)
Bacon	3 slices
Count as one high-fat meat plus one fat exchange.	
Hot dog (beef, pork, or combination)*	1 (10/1b)
Peanut butter (contains unsaturated fat)	2 tbsp

*400 mg or more sodium per exchange.

Fat List

Monounsaturated Fats List

One fat exchange equals 5 g fat and 45 cal.

Avocado, medium	1/8 (1 oz)
Oil (canola, olive, peanut)	1 tsp
Olives: ripe (black)	8 large
green, stuffed*	10 large
Nuts	
almonds, cashews	6 nuts
mixed (50 % peanuts)	6 nuts
peanuts	10 nuts
pecans	4 halves
Peanut butter, smooth or crunchy	2 tsp
Sesame seeds	1 tbsp
Tahini paste	2 tsp

Polyunsaturated Fats List

One fat exchange equals 5 g fat and 45 cal.

Margarine: stick, tub, or squeeze	1 tsp
lower-fat (30 percent to 50 percent vegetable oil)	1 tbsp
Mayo: regular	1 tsp
reduced-fat	1 tbsp

Nuts, walnuts, English	4 halves
Oil (corn, safflower, soybean)	1 tsp
Salad dressing: regular*	1 tbsp
reduced-fat	2 tbsp
Miracle Whip Salad Dressing®:	
regular	2 tsp
reduced-fat	1 tbsp
Seeds: pumpkin, sunflower	1 tbsp

Saturated Fats List†

One fat exchange equals 5 g of fat and 45 cal.

Bacon, cooked	1 slice (20 slices/lb)
Bacon, grease	1 tsp
Butter: stick	1 tsp
whipped	2 tsp
reduced-fat	1 tbsp
Chitterlings, boiled	2 tbsp (1/2 oz)
Coconut, sweetened, shredded	2 tbsp
Cream, half and half	2 tbsp

Cream cheese: regular	1 tbsp (1/2 oz)	Fatback or salt pork, see below	1 tsp
		Shortening or lard	2 tbsp
reduced-fat	2 tbsp (1 oz)	Sour cream: regular	3 tbsp
		reduced-fat	

*400 mg or more sodium per exchange.
†Saturated fats can raise blood cholesterol levels.

Free Foods List

A *free food* is any food or drink that contains less than 20 cal or less than 5 g of carbohydrate per serving. Foods with a serving size listed should be limited to three servings per day. Be sure to spread them out throughout the day. If you eat all three servings at one time, it could affect your blood glucose level. Foods listed without a serving size can be eaten as often as you like.

Fat-Free or Reduced-Fat Foods

Cream cheese, fat-free	1 tbsp
Creamers, nondairy, liquid	1 tbsp
Creamers, nondairy, powdered	2 tsp
Mayo, fat-free	1 tbsp
Mayo, reduced-fat	1 tsp
Margarine, fat-free	4 tbsp
Margarine, reduced-fat	1 tsp
Miracle Whip®, nonfat	1 tbsp
Miracle Whip®, reduced-fat	1 tsp
Nonstick cooking spray	
Salad dressing, fat-free	1 tbsp
Salad dressing, fat-free, Italian	2 tbsp
Salsa	1/4 cup
Sour cream, fat-free, reduced-fat	1 tbsp
Whipped topping, regular or light	2 tbsp

Sugar-Free or Low-Sugar Foods

Candy, hard, sugar-free	1 candy
Gelatin dessert, sugar-free	2 tsp
Gelatin, unflavored	
Gum, sugar-free	
Jam or jelly, low-sugar or light	
Sugar substitutes*	
Syrup, sugar-free	2 tbsp

Drinks

Bouillon, broth, consommé†	1 tbsp
Bouillon or broth, low-sodium	
Carbonated or mineral water	
Cocoa powder, unsweetened	

Coffee
Club soda
Diet soft drinks, sugar-free
Drink mixes, sugar-free
Tea
Tonic water, sugar-free

Condiments

Catsup	1 tbsp
Horseradish	
Lemon juice	
Lime juice	
Mustard	
Pickles, dill†	1 1/2 large
Soy sauce, regular or light†	
Taco sauce	
Vinegar	1 tbsp

Seasonings

Be careful with seasonings that contain sodium or are salts, such as garlic or celery salt, and lemon pepper.
Flavoring extracts
Garlic
Herbs, fresh or dried
Pimento
Spices
Tabasco® or hot pepper sauce
Wine, used in cooking
Worcestershire sauce

*Sugar substitutes, alternatives, or replacements that are approved by the Food and Drug Administration (FDA) are safe to use. Common brand names include: Equal® (aspartame), Sprinkle Sweet® (saccharin), Sweet One® (acesulfame K), Sweet-10® (saccharin), Sugar Twin® (saccharin), Sweet 'n Low® (saccharin).
†400 mg or more of sodium per choice.

Combination Foods List

Many of the foods we eat are mixed together in various combinations. These combination foods do not fit into any one exchange list. Often it is hard to tell what is in a casserole dish or prepared food item. This is a list of exchanges for some typical combination foods. This list will help you fit these foods into your meal plan. Ask your dietitian for information about any other combination foods you would like to eat.

FOOD	SERVING SIZE	EXCHANGES PER SERVING
Entrees		
Tuna noodle casserole, lasagna, spaghetti with meatballs, chilli with beans, macaroni and cheese*	1 cup (8 oz)	2 carbohydrates, 2 medium-fat meats
Chow mein (without noodles or rice)	2 cups (16 oz)	1 carbohydrate, 2 lean meats
Pizza, cheese, thin crust*	1/4 of 10 in (5 oz)	2 carbohydrates, 2 medium-fat meats, 1 fat
Pizza, meat topping, thin crust*	1/4 of 10 in (5 oz)	2 carbohydrates, 2 medium-fat meats, 2 fats
Pot pie*	1 (7 oz)	2 carbohydrates, 1 medium-fat meat, 4 fats
Frozen entrees		
Salisbury steak with gravy, mashed potato*	1 (11 oz)	2 carbohydrates, 3 medium-fat meats, 3–4 fats
Turkey with gravy, mashed potato, dressing*	1 (11 oz)	2 carbohydrates, 2 medium-fat meats, 2 fats
Entree with less than 300 cal*	1 (8 oz)	2 carbohydrates, 3 lean meats
Soups		
Bean*	1 cup	1 carbohydrate, 1 very lean meat, 1 vegetable
Cream (made with water)*	1 cup (8 oz)	1 carbohydrate, 1 fat
Split pea (made with water)*	1/2 cup (4 oz)	1 carbohydrate
Tomato (made with water)*	1 cup (8 oz)	1 carbohydrate
Vegetable beef, chicken noodle, or other broth-type*	1 cup (8 oz)	1 carbohydrate

*400 mg or more of sodium per choice.

Fast Foods*

FOOD	SERVING SIZE	EXCHANGES PER SERVING
Burritos with beef†	2	4 carbohydrates, 2 medium-fat meats, 2 fats
Chicken nuggets†	6	1 carbohydrate, 2 medium-fat meats, 1 fat
Chicken breast and wing, breaded and fried†	1 ea.	1 carbohydrate, 4 medium-fat meats, 2 fats
Fish sandwich/tartar sauce†	1	3 carbohydrates, 1 medium-fat meat, 3 fats
French fries, thin	20–25	2 carbohydrates, 2 fats
Hamburger, regular	1	2 carbohydrates, 2 medium-fat meats
Hamburger, large†	1	2 carbohydrates, 3 medium-fat meats, 1 fat
Hot dog with bun†	1	1 carbohydrate, 1 high-fat meat, 1 fat
Individual pan pizza†	1	5 carbohydrates, 3 medium-fat meats, 3 fats
Soft-serve cone	1 medium	2 carbohydrates, 1 fat
Submarine sandwich†	1 sub (6 in)	3 carbohydrates, 1 vegetable, 2 medium-fat meats, 1 fat
Taco, hard shell†	1 (6 oz)	2 carbohydrates, 2 medium-fat meats, 2 fats
Taco, soft shell†	1 (3 oz)	1 carbohydrate, 1 medium-fat meat, 1 fat

*400mg or more sodium per exchange.
†Ask at your fast-food restaurant for nutrition information about your favorite fast foods.

Using Food Labels

Nutrition facts on food labels can help you with choices. These labels are required by law for most foods and are based on standard serving sizes. However, these serving sizes may not always be the same as the serving sizes in this booklet.

- Check the serving size on the label. Is it nearly the same size as the food exchange? You may need to adjust the size of the serving to fit your meal plan.

- Look at the grams of carbohydrate in the serving size. (One starch, fruit, milk, or other carbohydrate has about 15 grams of carbohydrate.) So, if 1 cup of cereal has 30 grams of carbohydrate, it will count as 2 starch choices in your meal plan. You may need to adjust the size of the serving so it contains the number of carbohydrate choices you have for a meal or a snack.

- Look at the grams of protein in the serving size. (One

meat choice has 7 grams of protein.) If the food has more than 7 grams of protein in a serving, you can figure out the number of meat choices by dividing the grams of protein by 7. Meats generally contain fat, too.

- Look at the grams of fat in the serving size. (One fat choice has 5 grams of fat.) If one waffle has 15 grams of carbohydrate and 5 grams of fat, it counts as 1 starch choice and 1 fat choice.
- Look at the number of calories in the serving size. If there are less than 20 calories per serving, it is a free food. However, if it has more than 20 calories, follow the preceding steps to count the food choices.

Ask your dietitian for help using information on food labels. Some food labels may also give exchanges. These are based on information in this appendix.

CHILI WITH BEANS NUTRITION FACTS	
Serving Size 1 cup (253 g) Servings Per Container 2	
Amount Per Serving	
Calories 260 Calories from Fat 72	
	% Daily Value
Total Fat 8 g	13%
Saturated Fat 3 g	17%
Cholesterol 130 mg	44%
Sodium 1010 mg	42%
Total Carbohydrate 22 g	7%
Dietary Fiber 9 g	36%
Sugars 4 g	
Protein 25 g	

The Exchange Lists are the basis of a meal-planning system designed by a committee of the American Diabetes Association and the American Dietetic Association. While designed primarily for people with diabetes and others who must follow special diets, the Exchange Lists are based on principles of good nutrition that apply to everyone. Copied with permission.

SOURCE: Adapted from Exchange Lists for Meal Planning © 1995, American Diabetes Association, The American Dietetic Association.

Caffeine and Nutritive Values of Foods (Abridged)

Caffeine Values: Caffeine is a compound found mostly in coffee, tea, cola, cocoa, chocolate, and in foods containing these. This table lists the amounts of caffeine found in these beverages and foods.

FOOD	SERVING SIZE	CAFFEINE (mg)
BEVERAGES		
Chocolate milk, includes malted milk	8 fl oz	5–8
Chocolate shake	16 fl oz	8
Cocoa, prepared from powder		
Regular	6 fl oz	4–6
Sugar-free	6 fl oz	15
Coffee, regular		
Brewed	6 fl oz	103
Prepared from instant	6 fl oz	57
Coffee, decaffeinated		
Brewed	6 fl oz	2
Prepared from instant	6 fl oz	2
Coffee liqueur	1.5 fl oz	14
Cola or pepper-type, with caffeine	12 fl oz	37
Diet cola, with caffeine	12 fl oz	50
Tea, regular		
Brewed	6 fl oz	36
Instant, prepared	8 fl oz	26–36
Tea, decaffeinated, brewed	6 fl oz	2
CHOCOLATE FOODS		
Baking chocolate, unsweetened	1 square (1 oz)	58
Brownies	1	1–3
Candies		
Dark chocolate	1.45-oz bar	30
Milk chocolate bar	1.55-oz bar	11
Semisweet chocolate chips	1/4 cup	26–28
Chocolate with other ingredients (nuts, crisped rice, etc.)	about 1.5 oz	3–11
Cereal (containing cocoa)	1 oz	1
Cocoa powder, unsweetened	1 tbsp	12
Cookies (chocolate chip, devil's food, chocolate sandwich)	1	1
Chocolate cupcake with chocolate frosting	1	1–2
Frosting	1/12 pkg (2 tbsp)	1–2
Fudge	1 piece (about 3/4 oz)	2–3
Ice cream/frozen yogurt	1/2 cup	2
Pudding		
Prepared from dry mix	1/2 cup	3
Ready-to-eat	4 oz	6
Syrup		
Thin-type	1 tbsp	3
Fudge-type	1 tbsp	1

SOURCE: U.S. Department of Agriculture, Agricultural Research Service (2000).

Nutritive Value of the Edible Part of Food

FOOD DESCRIPTION	MEASURE OF EDIBLE PORTION	WEIGHT (g)	WATER (%)	CALORIES (kcal)	PROTEIN (g)	TOTAL (g)	FATTY ACIDS SATU-RATED FAT (g)	MONO-UNSATU-RATED (g)	POLY-UNSATU-RATED (g)
BEVERAGES									
Alcoholic									
Beer									
Regular	12 fl oz	355	92	146	1	0	0.0	0.0	0.0
Light	12 fl oz	354	95	99	1	0	0.0	0.0	0.0
Gin, rum, vodka, whiskey									
80 proof	1.5 fl oz	42	67	97	0	0	0.0	0.0	0.0
Mixed drinks, prepared from recipe									
Daiquiri	2 fl oz	60	70	112	Tr	Tr	Tr	Tr	Tr
Pina colada	4.5 fl oz	141	65	262	1	3	1.2	0.2	0.5
Wine									
Red	3.5 fl oz	103	89	74	Tr	0	0.0	0.0	0.0
White	3.5 fl oz	103	90	70	Tr	0	0.0	0.0	0.0
Carbonated*									
Club soda	12 fl oz	355	100	0	0	0	0.0	0.0	0.0
Cola type	12 fl oz	370	89	152	0	0	0.0	0.0	0.0
Diet, sweetened with aspartame									
Cola	12 fl oz	355	100	4	Tr	0	0.0	0.0	0.0
Other than cola or pepper type	12 fl oz	355	100	0	Tr	0	0.0	0.0	0.0
Grape	12 fl oz	372	89	160	0	0	0.0	0.0	0.0
Root beer	12 fl oz	370	89	152	0	0	0.0	0.0	0.0
Chocolate-flavored beverage mix									
Powder	2–3 heaping tsp	22	1	75	1	1	0.4	0.2	Tr
Cocoa									
Powder containing nonfat dry milk									
Prepared (6 oz water plus 1 oz powder)	1 serving	206	86	103	3	1	0.7	0.4	Tr
Coffee									
Brewed	6 fl oz	178	99	4	Tr	0	Tr	0.0	Tr
Instant, prepared (1 rounded tsp powder plus 6 fl oz water)	6 fl oz	179	99	4	Tr	0	Tr	0.0	Tr

Tr indicates trace.

*Mineral content varies depending on water source.

CHOLESTEROL (mg)	CARBOHYDRATE (g)	TOTAL DIETARY FIBER (g)	CALCIUM (mg)	IRON (mg)	POTASSIUM (mg)	SODIUM (mg)	VITAMIN A (IU)	(RE)	THIAMIN (mg)	RIBOFLAVIN (mg)	NIACIN (mg)	ASCORBIC ACID (mg)
0	13	0.7	18	0.1	89	18	0	0	0.02	0.09	1.6	0
0	5	0.0	18	0.1	64	11	0	0	0.03	0.11	1.4	0
0	0	0.0	0	Tr	1	Tr	0	0	Tr	Tr	Tr	0
0	4	0.0	2	0.1	13	3	2	0	0.01	Tr	Tr	1
0	40	0.8	11	0.3	100	8	3	0	0.04	0.02	0.2	7
0	2	0.0	8	0.4	115	5	0	0	0.01	0.03	0.1	0
0	1	0.0	9	0.3	82	5	0	0	Tr	0.01	0.1	0
0	0	0.0	18	Tr	7	75	0	0	0.00	0.00	0.0	0
0	38	0.0	11	0.1	4	15	0	0	0.00	0.00	0.0	0
0	Tr	0.0	14	0.1	0	21	0	0	0.02	0.08	0.0	0
0	0	0.0	14	0.1	7	21	0	0	0.00	0.00	0.0	0
0	32	0.0	11	0.7	4	26	0	0	0.00	0.00	0.0	0
0	39	0.0	19	0.2	4	48	0	0	0.00	0.00	0.0	0
0	20	1.3	8	0.7	128	45	4	Tr	0.01	0.03	0.1	Tr
2	22	2.5	97	0.4	202	148	4	0	0.03	0.16	0.2	Tr
0	1	0.0	4	0.1	96	4	0	0	0.00	0.00	0.4	0
0	1	0.0	5	0.1	64	5	0	0	0.00	Tr	0.5	0

(continued on the following page)

Nutritive Value of the Edible Part of Food

FOOD DESCRIPTION	MEASURE OF EDIBLE PORTION	WEIGHT (g)	WATER (%)	CALORIES (kcal)	PROTEIN (g)	TOTAL FAT (g)	FATTY ACIDS SATU-RATED (g)	MONO-UNSATU-RATED (g)	POLY-UNSATU-RATED (g)
Fruit drinks, noncar-bonated, canned or bottled, with added ascorbic acid									
Cranberry juice cocktail	8 fl oz	253	86	144	0	Tr	Tr	Tr	0.1
Fruit punch drink	8 fl oz	248	88	117	0	0	Tr	Tr	Tr
Grape drink	8 fl oz	250	88	113	0	0	Tr	0.0	Tr
Lemonade									
Frozen concentrate, prepared	8 fl oz	248	89	99	Tr	0	Tr	Tr	Tr
Powder, prepared with water									
Regular	8 fl oz	266	89	112	0	0	Tr	Tr	Tr
Low calorie, sweetened with aspartame	8 fl oz	237	99	5	0	0	0.0	0.0	0.0
Malted milk, with added nutrients									
Chocolate									
Powder	3 heaping tsp	21	3	75	1	1	0.4	0.2	0.1
Milk and milk beverages. See Dairy products.									
Soy milk. See Legumes, nuts, and seeds.									
Tea									
Brewed									
Black	6 fl oz	178	100	2	0	0	Tr	Tr	Tr
DAIRY PRODUCTS									
Butter. See Fats and oils.									
Cheese									
Natural									
Blue	1 oz	28	42	100	6	8	5.3	2.2	0.2
Camembert (3 wedges per 4-oz container)	1 wedge	38	52	114	8	9	5.8	2.7	0.3
Cheddar									
Cut pieces	1 oz	28	37	114	7	9	6.0	2.7	0.3
Shredded	1 cup	113	37	455	28	37	23.8	10.6	1.1
Cottage									
Creamed (4% fat)									
Large curd	1 cup	255	79	233	28	10	6.4	2.9	0.3
Small curd	1 cup	210	79	217	26	9	6.0	2.7	0.3
Low fat (2%)	1 cup	226	79	203	31	4	2.8	1.2	0.1
Low fat (1%)	1 cup	226	82	164	28	2	1.5	0.7	0.1
Cream									
Regular	1 tbsp	15	54	51	1	5	3.2	1.4	0.2
Low fat	1 tbsp	15	64	35	2	3	1.7	0.7	0.1
Feta	1 oz	28	55	75	4	6	4.2	1.3	0.2
Low fat, cheddar or colby	1 oz	28	63	49	7	2	1.2	0.6	0.1
Mozzarella, made with									
Whole milk	1 oz	28	54	80	6	6	3.7	1.9	0.2
Part-skim milk (low moisture)	1 oz	28	49	79	8	5	3.1	1.4	0.1

CHOLESTEROL (mg)	CARBOHYDRATE (g)	TOTAL DIETARY FIBER (g)	CALCIUM (mg)	IRON (mg)	POTASSIUM (mg)	SODIUM (mg)	VITAMIN A (IU)	VITAMIN A (RE)	THIAMIN (mg)	RIBOFLAVIN (mg)	NIACIN (mg)	ASCORBIC ACID (mg)
0	36	0.3	8	0.4	46	5	10	0	0.02	0.02	0.1	90
0	30	0.2	20	0.5	62	55	35	2	0.05	0.06	0.1	73
0	29	0.0	8	0.4	13	15	3	0	0.01	0.01	0.1	85
0	26	0.2	7	0.4	37	7	52	5	0.01	0.05	Tr	10
0	29	0.0	29	0.1	3	19	0	0	0.00	Tr	0.0	34
0	1	0.0	50	0.1	0	7	0	0	0.00	0.00	0.0	6
1	18	0.2	93	3.6	251	125	2,751	824	0.64	0.86	10.7	32
0	1	0.0	0	Tr	66	5	0	0	0.00	0.02	0.0	0
21	1	0.0	150	0.1	73	396	204	65	0.01	0.11	0.3	0
27	Tr	0.0	147	0.1	71	320	351	96	0.01	0.19	0.2	0
30	Tr	0.0	204	0.2	28	176	300	79	0.01	0.11	Tr	0
119	1	0.0	815	0.8	111	701	1,197	314	0.03	0.42	0.1	0
34	6	0.0	135	0.3	190	911	367	108	0.05	0.37	0.3	0
31	6	0.0	126	0.3	177	850	342	101	0.04	0.34	0.3	0
19	8	0.0	155	0.4	217	918	158	45	0.05	0.42	0.3	0
10	6	0.0	138	0.3	193	918	84	25	0.05	0.37	0.3	0
16	Tr	0.0	12	0.2	17	43	207	55	Tr	0.03	Tr	0
8	1	0.0	17	0.3	25	44	108	33	Tr	0.04	Tr	0
25	1	0.0	140	0.2	18	316	127	36	0.04	0.24	0.3	0
6	1	0.0	118	0.1	19	174	66	18	Tr	0.06	Tr	0
22	1	0.0	147	0.1	19	106	255	68	Tr	0.07	Tr	0
15	1	0.0	207	0.1	27	150	199	54	0.01	0.10	Tr	0

(continued on the following page)

Nutritive Value of the Edible Part of Food

FOOD DESCRIPTION	MEASURE OF EDIBLE PORTION	WEIGHT (g)	WATER (%)	CALORIES (kcal)	PROTEIN (g)	TOTAL FAT (g)	FATTY ACIDS SATU-RATED (g)	MONO-UNSATU-RATED (g)	POLY-UNSATU-RATED (g)
DAIRY PRODUCTS *(Continued)*									
Muenster	1 oz	28	42	104	7	9	5.4	2.5	0.2
Neufchatel	1 oz	28	62	74	3	7	4.2	1.9	0.2
Parmesan, grated									
	1 tbsp	5	18	23	2	2	1.0	0.4	Tr
	1 oz	28	18	129	12	9	5.4	2.5	0.2
Provolone	1 oz	28	41	100	7	8	4.8	2.1	0.2
Ricotta, made with									
Whole milk	1 cup	246	72	428	28	32	20.4	8.9	0.9
Part skim milk	1 cup	246	74	340	28	19	12.1	5.7	0.6
Swiss	1 oz	28	37	107	8	8	5.0	2.1	0.3
Pasteurized processed cheese									
American									
Regular	1 oz	28	39	106	6	9	5.6	2.5	0.3
Fat free	1 slice	21	57	31	5	Tr	0.1	Tr	Tr
Swiss	1 oz	28	42	95	7	7	4.5	2.0	0.2
Pasteurized processed cheese spread,									
American	1 oz	28	48	82	5	6	3.8	1.8	0.2
Cream, sweet									
Half and half (cream and milk)	1 tbsp	15	81	20	Tr	2	1.1	0.5	0.1
Light, coffee, or table	1 tbsp	15	74	29	Tr	3	1.8	0.8	0.1
Whipping, unwhipped (volume about double when whipped)									
Light	1 cup	239	64	699	5	74	46.2	21.7	2.1
Heavy	1 cup	238	58	821	5	88	54.8	25.4	3.3
Whipped topping (pressurized)	1 tbsp	3	61	8	Tr	1	0.4	0.2	Tr
Cream, sour									
Regular	1 tbsp	12	71	26	Tr	3	1.6	0.7	0.1
Reduced fat	1 tbsp	15	80	20	Tr	2	1.1	0.5	0.1
Fat free	1 tbsp	16	81	12	Tr	0	0.0	0.0	0.0
Cream Product, imitation (made with vegetable fat)									
Sweet									
Creamer									
Liquid (frozen)	1 tbsp	15	77	20	Tr	1	0.3	1.1	Tr
Powdered	1 tsp	2	2	11	Tr	1	0.7	Tr	Tr
Whipped topping									
Frozen	1 cup	75	50	239	1	19	16.3	1.2	0.4
Powdered, prepared with whole milk	1 cup	80	67	151	3	10	8.5	0.7	0.2
	1 tbsp	4	60	11	Tr	1	0.8	0.1	Tr
Frozen dessert									
Frozen yogurt, soft serve									
Chocolate	1/2 cup	72	64	115	3	4	2.6	1.3	0.2
Vanilla	1/2 cup	72	65	114	3	4	2.5	1.1	0.2
Ice cream									
Regular									
Chocolate	1/2 cup	66	56	143	3	7	4.5	2.1	0.3
Vanilla	1/2 cup	66	61	133	2	7	4.5	2.1	0.3

†The vitamin A values listed for imitation sweet cream products are mostly from beta-carotene added for coloring.

CHOLES-TEROL (mg)	CARBO-HYDRATE (g)	TOTAL DIETARY FIBER (g)	CALCIUM (mg)	IRON (mg)	POTAS-SIUM (mg)	SODIUM (mg)	VITAMIN A (IU)	VITAMIN A (RE)	THIAMIN (mg)	RIBO-FLAVIN (mg)	NIACIN (mg)	ASCOR-BIC ACID (mg)
27	Tr	0.0	203	0.1	38	178	318	90	Tr	0.09	Tr	0
22	1	0.0	21	0.1	32	113	321	85	Tr	0.06	Tr	0
4	Tr	0.0	69	Tr	5	93	35	9	Tr	0.02	Tr	0
22	1	0.0	390	0.3	30	528	199	49	0.01	0.11	0.1	0
20	1	0.0	214	0.1	39	248	231	75	0.01	0.09	Tr	0
124	7	0.0	509	0.9	257	207	1205	330	0.03	0.48	0.3	0
76	13	0.0	669	1.1	308	307	1063	278	0.05	0.46	0.2	0
26	1	0.0	272	Tr	31	74	240	72	0.01	0.10	Tr	0
27	Tr	0.0	174	0.1	46	406	343	82	0.01	0.10	Tr	0
2	3	0.0	145	0.1	60	321	308	92	0.01	0.10	Tr	0
24	1	0.0	219	0.2	61	388	229	65	Tr	0.08	Tr	0
16	2	0.0	159	0.1	69	381	223	54	0.01	0.12	Tr	0
6	1	0.0	16	Tr	19	6	65	16	0.01	0.02	Tr	Tr
10	1	0.0	14	Tr	18	6	95	27	Tr	0.02	Tr	Tr
265	7	0.0	166	0.1	231	82	2694	705	0.06	0.30	0.1	1
326	7	0.0	154	0.1	179	89	3499	1002	0.05	0.26	0.1	1
2	Tr	0.0	3	Tr	4	4	25	6	Tr	Tr	Tr	0
5	1	0.0	14	Tr	17	6	95	23	Tr	0.02	Tr	Tr
6	1	0.0	16	Tr	19	6	68	17	0.01	0.02	Tr	Tr
1	2	0.0	20	0.0	21	23	100	13	0.01	0.02	Tr	0
0	2	0.0	1	Tr	29	12	13†	1†	0.00	0.00	0.0	0
0	1	0.0	Tr	Tr	16	4	4	Tr	0.00	Tr	0.0	0
0	17	0.0	5	0.1	14	19	646†	65†	0.00	0.00	0.0	0
8	13	0.0	72	Tr	121	53	289*	39*	0.02	0.09	Tr	1
0	1	0.0	Tr	Tr	1	2	19†	2†	0.00	0.00	0.0	0
4	18	1.6	106	0.9	188	71	115	31	0.03	0.15	0.2	Tr
1	17	0.0	103	0.2	152	63	153	41	0.03	0.16	0.2	1
22	19	0.8	72	0.6	164	50	275	79	0.03	0.13	0.1	Tr
29	16	0.0	84	0.1	131	53	270	77	0.03	0.16	0.1	Tr

(continued on the following page)

							FATTY ACIDS		
FOOD DESCRIPTION	**MEASURE OF EDIBLE PORTION**	**WEIGHT (g)**	**WATER (%)**	**CALORIES (kcal)**	**PROTEIN (g)**	**TOTAL FAT (g)**	**SATU-RATED (g)**	**MONO-UNSATU-RATED (g)**	**POLY-UNSATU-RATED (g))**
DAIRY PRODUCTS *(Continued)*									
Light (50% reduced fat), vanilla	1/2 cup	66	68	92	3	3	1.7	0.8	0.1
Soft serve, french vanilla	1/2 cup	86	60	185	4	11	6.4	3.0	0.4
Sherbet, orange	1/2 cup	74	66	102	1	1	0.9	0.4	0.1
Milk									
Fluid, no milk solids added									
Whole (3.3% fat)	1 cup	244	88	150	8	8	5.1	2.4	0.3
Reduced fat (2%)	1 cup	244	89	121	8	5	2.9	1.4	0.2
Lowfat (1%)	1 cup	244	90	102	8	3	1.6	0.7	0.1
Nonfat (skim)	1 cup	245	91	86	8	Tr	0.3	0.1	Tr
Buttermilk	1 cup	245	90	99	8	2	1.3	0.6	0.1
Canned									
Condensed, sweetened	1 cup	306	27	982	24	27	16.8	7.4	1.0
Evaporated									
Whole milk	1 cup	252	74	339	17	19	11.6	5.9	0.6
Skim milk	1 cup	256	79	199	19	1	0.3	0.2	Tr
Dried									
Nonfat, instant, with added vitamin A	1 cup	68	4	244	24	Tr	0.3	0.1	Tr
Milk beverage									
Chocolate milk (commercial)									
Whole	1 cup	250	82	208	8	8	5.3	2.5	0.3
Reduced fat (2%)	1 cup	250	84	179	8	5	3.1	1.5	0.2
Lowfat (1%)	1 cup	250	85	158	8	3	1.5	0.8	0.1
Sherbet. See Dairy Products, frozen dessert.									
Yogurt									
With added milk solids									
Made with lowfat milk									
Fruit flavored	8-oz container	227	74	231	10	2	1.6	0.7	0.1
Plain	8-oz container	227	85	144	12	4	2.3	1.0	0.1
Made with nonfat milk									
Fruit flavored	8-oz container	227	75	213	10	Tr	0.3	0.1	Tr
Plain	8-oz container	227	85	127	13	Tr	0.3	0.1	Tr
EGGS									
Egg									
Raw									
Whole	1 medium	44	75	66	5	4	1.4	1.7	0.6
White									
Yolk									
Cooked, whole									
Fried, in margarine, with salt	1 large	46	69	92	6	7	1.9	2.7	1.3
Hard cooked, shell removed	1 large	50	75	78	6	5	1.6	2.0	0.7
Scrambled, in margarine, with whole milk, salt	1 large	61	73	101	7	7	2.2	2.9	1.3
Egg substitute, liquid	1/4 cup	63	83	53	8	2	0.4	0.6	1.0

CHOLES-TEROL (mg)	CARBO-HYDRATE (g)	TOTAL DIETARY FIBER (g)	CALCIUM (mg)	IRON (mg)	POTAS-SIUM (mg)	SODIUM (mg)	VITAMIN A (IU)	(RE)	THIAMIN (mg)	RIBO-FLAVIN (mg)	NIACIN (mg)	ASCOR-BIC ACID (mg)
9	15	0.0	92	0.1	139	56	109	31	0.04	0.17	0.1	1
78	19	0.0	113	0.2	152	52	464	132	0.04	0.16	0.1	1
4	22	0.0	40	0.1	71	34	56	10	0.02	0.06	Tr	2
33	11	0.0	291	0.1	370	120	307	76	0.09	0.40	0.2	2
18	12	0.0	297	0.1	377	122	500	139	0.10	0.40	0.2	2
10	12	0.0	300	0.1	381	123	500	144	0.10	0.41	0.2	2
4	12	0.0	302	0.1	406	126	500	149	0.09	0.34	0.2	2
9	12	0.0	285	0.1	371	257	81	20	0.08	0.38	0.1	2
104	166	0.0	868	0.6	1136	389	1004	248	0.28	1.27	0.6	8
74	25	0.0	657	0.5	764	267	612	136	0.12	0.80	0.5	5
9	29	0.0	741	0.7	849	294	1004	300	0.12	0.79	0.4	3
12	35	0.0	837	0.2	1160	373	1612	483	0.28	1.19	0.6	4
31	26	2.0	280	0.6	417	149	303	73	0.09	0.41	0.3	2
17	26	1.3	284	0.6	422	151	500	143	0.09	0.41	0.3	2
7	26	1.3	287	0.6	426	152	500	148	0.10	0.42	0.3	2
10	43	0.0	345	0.2	442	133	104	25	0.08	0.40	0.2	1
14	16	0.0	415	0.2	531	159	150	36	0.10	0.49	0.3	2
5	43	0.0	345	0.2	440	132	16	5	0.09	0.41	0.2	2
4	17	0.0	452	0.2	579	174	16	5	0.11	0.53	0.3	2
187	1	0.0	22	0.6	53	55	279	84	0.03	0.22	Tr	0
211	1	0.0	25	0.7	61	162	394	114	0.03	0.24	Tr	0
212	1	0.0	25	0.6	63	62	280	84	0.03	0.26	Tr	0
215	1	0.0	43	0.7	84	171	416	119	0.03	0.27	Tr	Tr
1	Tr	0.0	33	1.3	208	112	1361	136	0.07	0.19	0.1	0

(continued on the following page)

Nutritive Value of the Edible Part of Food

FOOD DESCRIPTION	MEASURE OF EDIBLE PORTION	WEIGHT (g)	WATER (%)	CALORIES (kcal)	PROTEIN (g)	TOTAL FAT (g)	FATTY ACIDS SATU-RATED (g)	FATTY ACIDS MONO-UNSATU-RATED (g)	FATTY ACIDS POLY-UNSATU-RATED (g)
FATS AND OILS									
Butter (4 sticks per lb)									
Salted	1 stick	113	16	813	1	92	57.3	26.6	3.4
	1 tsp	5	16	36	Tr	4	2.5	1.2	0.2
Unsalted	1 stick	113	18	813	1	92	57.3	26.6	3.4
Lard	1 cup	205	0	1849	0	205	80.4	92.5	23.0
Margarine, vitamin A-fortified, salt added									
Regular (about 80% fat)									
Hard (4 sticks per lb)	1 stick	113	16	815	1	91	17.9	40.6	28.8
	1 tsp	5	16	34	Tr	4	0.7	1.7	1.2
Soft									
	1 tsp	5	16	34	Tr	4	0.6	1.3	1.6
Spread (about 60% fat)									
Hard (4 sticks per lb)	1 stick	115	37	621	1	70	16.2	29.9	20.8
	1 tsp	5	37	26	Tr	3	0.7	1.2	0.9
Soft	1 cup	229	37	1236	1	139	29.3	72.1	31.6
	1 tsp	5	37	26	Tr	3	0.6	1.5	0.7
Spread (about 40% fat)	1 cup	232	58	801	1	90	17.9	36.4	32.0
	1 tsp	5	58	17	Tr	2	0.4	0.8	0.7
Margarine butter blend	1 stick	113	16	811	1	91	32.1	37.0	18.0
	1 tbsp	14	16	102	Tr	11	4.0	4.7	2.3
Oils, salad or cooking									
Canola	1 cup	218	0	1927	0	218	15.5	128.4	64.5
Corn	1 cup	218	0	1927	0	218	27.7	52.8	128.0
Olive	1 cup	216	0	1909	0	216	29.2	159.2	18.1
Peanut	1 cup	216	0	1909	0	216	36.5	99.8	69.1
Safflower, high oleic	1 cup	218	0	1927	0	218	13.5	162.7	31.3
Sesame	1 cup	218	0	1927	0	218	13.0	86.5	90.9
Soybean, hydrogenated	1 cup	218	0	1927	0	218	32.5	93.7	82.0
Soybean, hydrogenated and cottonseed oil blend	1 cup	218	0	1927	0	218	39.2	64.3	104.9
Sunflower	1 cup	218	0	1927	0	218	22.5	42.5	143.2
Salad dressings									
Commercial									
Blue cheese									
Regular	1 tbsp	15	32	77	1	8	1.5	1.9	4.3
Low calorie	1 tbsp	15	80	15	1	1	0.4	0.3	0.4
Caesar									
Regular	1 tbsp	15	34	78	Tr	8	1.3	2.0	4.8
Low calorie	1 tbsp	15	73	17	Tr	1	0.1	0.2	0.4
French									
Regular	1 tbsp	16	38	67	Tr	6	1.5	1.2	3.4
Low calorie	1 tbsp	16	69	22	Tr	1	0.1	0.2	0.6
Italian									
Regular	1 tbsp	15	38	69	Tr	7	1.0	1.6	4.1
Low calorie	1 tbsp	15	82	16	Tr	1	0.2	0.3	0.9
Mayonnaise									
Regular	1 tbsp	14	15	99	Tr	11	1.6	3.1	5.7
Fat free	1 tbsp	16	84	12	0	Tr	0.1	0.1	0.2
Russian									
Regular	1 tbsp	15	35	76	Tr	8	1.1	1.8	4.5
Low calorie	1 tbsp	16	65	23	Tr	1	0.1	0.1	0.4
Thousand island									
Regular	1 tbsp	16	46	59	Tr	6	0.9	1.3	3.1
Low calorie	1 tbsp	15	69	24	Tr	2	0.2	0.4	0.9

CHOLES-TEROL (mg)	CARBO-HYDRATE (g)	TOTAL DIETARY FIBER (g)	CALCIUM (mg)	IRON (mg)	POTAS-SIUM (mg)	SODIUM (mg)	VITAMIN A (IU)	VITAMIN A (RE)	THIAMIN (mg)	RIBO-FLAVIN (mg)	NIACIN (mg)	ASCOR-BIC ACID (mg)
248	Tr	0.0	27	0.2	29	937	3468	855	0.01	0.04	Tr	0
11	Tr	0.0	1	Tr	1	41	153	38	Tr	Tr	Tr	0
248	Tr	0.0	27	0.2	29	12	3468	855	0.01	0.04	Tr	0
195	0	0.0	Tr	0.0	Tr	Tr	0	0	0.00	0.00	0.0	0
0	1	0.0	34	0.1	48	1070	4050	906	0.01	0.04	Tr	Tr
0	Tr	0.0	1	Tr	2	44	168	38	Tr	Tr	Tr	Tr
0	Tr	0.0	1	0.0	2	51	168	38	Tr	Tr	Tr	Tr
0	0	0.0	24	0.0	34	1143	4107	919	0.01	0.03	Tr	Tr
0	0	0.0	1	0.0	1	48	171	38	Tr	Tr	Tr	Tr
0	0	0.0	48	0.0	68	2276	8178	1830	0.02	0.06	Tr	Tr
0	0	0.0	1	0.0	1	48	171	38	Tr	Tr	Tr	Tr
0	1	0.0	41	0.0	59	2226	8285	1854	0.01	0.05	Tr	Tr
0	Tr	0.0	1	0.0	1	46	171	38	Tr	Tr	Tr	Tr
99	1	0.0	32	0.0	41	1014	4035	903	0.01	0.04	Tr	Tr
12	Tr	0.0	4	Tr	5	127	507	113	Tr	Tr	Tr	Tr
0	0	0.0	0	0.0	0	0	0	0	0.00	0.00	0.0	0
0	0	0.0	0	0.0	0	0	0	0	0.00	0.00	0.0	0
0	0	0.0	Tr	0.8	0	Tr	0	0	0.00	0.00	0.0	0
0	0	0.0	Tr	0.1	Tr	Tr	0	0	0.00	0.00	0.0	0
0	0	0.0	0	0.0	0	0	0	0	0.00	0.00	0.0	0
0	0	0.0	0	0.0	0	0	0	0	0.00	0.00	0.0	0
0	0	0.0	0	0.0	0	0	0	0	0.00	0.00	0.0	0
0	0	0.0	0	0.0	0	0	0	0	0.00	0.00	0.0	0
0	0	0.0	0	0.0	0	0	0	0	0.00	0.00	0.0	0
3	1	0.0	12	Tr	6	167	32	10	Tr	0.02	Tr	Tr
Tr	Tr	0.0	14	0.1	1	184	2	Tr	Tr	0.02	Tr	Tr
Tr	Tr	Tr	4	Tr	4	158	3	Tr	Tr	Tr	Tr	0
Tr	3	Tr	4	Tr	4	162	3	Tr	Tr	Tr	Tr	0
0	3	0.0	2	0.1	12	214	203	20	Tr	Tr	Tr	0
0	4	0.0	2	0.1	13	128	212	21	0.00	0.00	0.0	0
0	1	0.0	1	Tr	2	116	11	4	Tr	Tr	Tr	0
1	1	Tr	Tr	Tr	2	118	0	0	0.00	0.00	0.0	0
8	Tr	0.0	2	0.1	5	78	39	12	0.00	0.00	Tr	0
0	2	0.6	0	0.0	15	190	0	0	0.00	0.00	0.0	0
3	2	0.0	3	0.1	24	133	106	32	0.01	0.01	0.1	1
1	4	Tr	3	0.1	26	141	9	3	Tr	Tr	Tr	1
4	2	0.0	2	0.1	18	109	50	15	Tr	Tr	Tr	0
2	2	0.2	2	0.1	17	153	49	15	Tr	Tr	Tr	0

(continued on the following page)

Nutritive Value of the Edible Part of Food

FOOD DESCRIPTION	MEASURE OF EDIBLE PORTION	WEIGHT (g)	WATER (%)	CALORIES (kcal)	PROTEIN (g)	TOTAL FAT (g)	FATTY ACIDS SATU-RATED (g)	MONO-UNSATU-RATED (g)	POLY-UNSATU-RATED (g)
Shortening (hydrogenated soybean and cottonseed oils)	1 cup	205	0	1812	0	205	51.3	91.2	53.5
FISH AND SHELLFISH									
Catfish, breaded, fried	3oz	85	59	195	15	11	2.8	4.8	2.8
Clam									
Raw, meat only	3 oz	85	82	63	11	1	0.1	0.1	0.2
	1 medium	15	82	11	2	Tr	Tr	Tr	Tr
Breaded, fried	3/4 cup	115	29	451	13	26	6.6	11.4	6.8
Canned, drained solids	3 oz	85	64	126	22	2	0.2	0.1	0.5
	1 cup	106	64	237	41	3	0.3	0.3	0.9
Cod									
Baked or broiled	3 oz	85	76	89	20	1	0.1	0.1	0.3
	1 fillet	90	76	95	21	1	0.1	0.1	0.3
Canned, solids and liquid	3 oz	85	76	89	19	1	0.1	0.1	0.2
Crab									
Alaska king									
Steamed	1 leg	134	78	130	26	2	0.2	0.2	0.7
Imitation, from surimi	3 oz	85	74	87	10	1	0.2	0.2	0.6
Blue									
Steamed	3 oz	85	77	87	17	2	0.2	0.2	0.6
Canned crabmeat	1 cup	135	76	134	28	2	0.3	0.3	0.6
Crab cake, with egg, onion, fried in margarine	1 cake	60	71	93	12	5	0.9	1.7	1.4
Fish fillet, battered or breaded, fried	1 fillet	91	54	211	13	11	2.6	2.3	5.7
Fish stick breaded, frozen, reheated	1 stick (4 x 1 x 1/2 inches)	28	46	76	4	3	0.9	1.4	0.9
Flounder or sole, baked or broiled	3 oz	85	73	99	21	1	0.3	0.2	0.5
Haddock, baked or broiled	3 oz	85	74	95	21	1	0.1	0.1	0.3
Halibut, baked or broiled	3 oz	85	72	119	23	2	0.4	0.8	0.8
Herring, pickled	3 oz	85	55	223	12	15	2.0	10.2	1.4
Lobster, steamed	3 oz	85	76	83	17	1	0.1	0.1	0.1
Ocean perch, baked or broiled	3 oz	85	73	103	20	2	0.3	0.7	0.5
Oyster									
Raw, meat only	1 cup	248	85	169	17	6	0.9	0.8	2.4
	6 medium	84	85	57	6	2	0.6	0.3	0.8
Breaded, fried	3 oz	85	65	167	7	11	2.7	4.0	2.8
Pollock, baked or broiled	3 oz	85	74	96	20	1	0.2	0.1	0.4
Rockfish, baked or broiled	3 oz	85	73	103	20	2	0.4	0.4	0.5
Roughy, orange, baked or broiled	3 oz	85	69	76	16	1	Tr	0.5	Tr
Salmon									
Baked or broiled (red)	3 oz	85	62	184	23	9	1.6	4.5	2.0
Canned (pink), solids and liquid (includes bones)	3 oz	85	69	118	17	5	1.3	1.5	1.7
Smoked (chinook)	3 oz	85	72	99	16	4	0.8	1.7	0.8
Sardine, Atlantic, canned in oil, drained solids (includes bones)	3 oz	85	60	177	21	10	1.3	3.3	4.4
Scallop, cooked									
Breaded, fried	6 large	93	58	200	17	10	2.5	4.2	2.7
Steamed	3 oz	85	73	95	20	1	0.1	0.1	0.4

CHOLES-TEROL (mg)	CARBO-HYDRATE (g)	TOTAL DIETARY FIBER (g)	CALCIUM (mg)	IRON (mg)	POTAS-SIUM (mg)	SODIUM (mg)	VITAMIN A (IU)	VITAMIN A (RE)	THIAMIN (mg)	RIBO-FLAVIN (mg)	NIACIN (mg)	ASCOR-BIC ACID (mg)
0	0	0.0	0	0.0	0	0	0	0	0.00	0.00	0.0	0
69	7	0.6	37	1.2	289	238	24	7	0.06	0.11	1.9	0
29	2	0.0	39	11.9	267	48	255	77	0.07	0.18	1.5	11
5	Tr	0.0	7	2.0	46	8	44	13	0.01	0.03	0.3	2
87	39	0.3	21	3.0	266	834	122	37	0.21	0.26	2.9	0
57	4	0.0	78	23.8	534	95	485	145	0.13	0.36	2.9	19
107	8	0.0	147	44.7	1005	179	912	274	0.24	0.68	5.4	35
40	0	0.0	8	0.3	439	77	27	9	0.02	0.04	2.1	3
47	0	0.0	18	0.4	449	185	39	12	0.07	0.07	2.1	1
71	0	0.0	79	1.0	351	1436	39	12	0.07	0.07	1.8	10
17	9	0.0	11	0.3	77	715	56	17	0.03	0.02	0.2	0
85	0	0.0	88	0.8	275	237	5	2	0.09	0.04	2.8	3
120	0	0.0	136	1.1	505	450	7	3	0.11	0.11	1.8	4
90	Tr	0.0	63	0.6	194	198	151	49	0.05	0.05	1.7	2
31	15	0.5	16	1.9	291	484	35	11	0.10	0.10	1.9	0
31	7	0.0	6	0.2	73	163	30	9	0.04	0.05	0.6	0
58	0	0.0	15	0.3	292	89	32	9	0.07	0.10	1.9	0
63	0	0.0	36	1.1	339	74	54	16	0.03	0.04	3.9	0
111	0	0.0	63	2.0	599	131	95	29	0.06	0.07	6.9	0
35	0	0.0	51	0.9	490	59	152	46	0.06	0.08	6.1	0
11	8	0.0	65	1.0	59	740	732	219	0.03	0.12	2.8	0
61	1	0.0	52	0.3	299	323	74	22	0.01	0.06	0.9	0
46	0	0.0	116	1.0	298	82	39	12	0.11	0.11	2.1	1
131	10	0.0	112	16.5	387	523	248	74	0.25	0.24	3.4	9
45	3	0.0	38	5.6	131	177	84	25	0.08	0.08	1.2	3
69	10	0.2	53	5.9	207	354	257	77	0.13	0.17	1.4	3
82	0	0.0	5	0.2	329	99	65	20	0.06	0.06	1.4	0
37	0	0.0	10	0.5	442	65	186	56	0.04	0.07	3.3	0
22	0	0.0	32	0.2	327	69	69	20	0.10	0.16	3.1	0
74	0	0.0	6	0.5	319	56	178	54	0.18	0.15	5.7	0
47	0	0.0	181	0.7	277	471	47	14	0.02	0.16	5.6	0
20	0	0.0	9	0.7	149	666	75	22	0.02	0.09	4.0	0
121	0	0.0	325	2.5	337	429	190	57	0.07	0.19	4.5	0
57	9	0.2	39	0.8	310	432	70	20	0.04	0.10	1.4	2
45	3	0.0	98	2.6	405	225	85	26	0.09	0.05	1.1	0

(continued on the following page)

FOOD DESCRIPTION	MEASURE OF EDIBLE PORTION	WEIGHT (g)	WATER (%)	CALORIES (kcal)	PROTEIN (g)	TOTAL FAT (g)	FATTY ACIDS		
							SATU-RATED (g)	MONO-UNSATU-RATED (g)	POLY-UNSATU-RATED (g)
FISH AND SHELLFISH									
(continued)									
Shrimp									
Breaded, fried	3 oz	85	53	206	18	10	1.8	3.2	4.3
	6 large	45	53	109	10	6	0.9	1.7	2.3
Canned, drained solids	3 oz	85	73	102	20	2	0.3	0.2	0.6
Swordfish, baked or broiled	3 oz	85	69	132	22	4	1.2	1.7	1.0
Trout, baked or broiled	3 oz	85	68	144	21	6	1.8	1.8	2.0
Tuna									
Baked or broiled	3 oz	85	63	118	25	1	0.3	0.2	0.3
Canned, drained solids									
Oil pack, chunk light	3 oz	85	60	168	25	7	1.3	2.5	2.5
Water pack, chunk light	3 oz	85	75	99	22	1	0.2	0.1	0.3
Water pack, solid white	3 oz	85	73	109	20	3	0.7	0.7	0.9
Tuna salad: light tuna in oil, pickle relish, mayo-type salad dressing	1 cup	205	63	383	33	19	3.2	5.9	8.5
FRUITS AND FRUIT JUICES									
Apples									
Raw									
Unpeeled, 2 3/4-inch diameter (about 3 per lb)	1 apple	138	84	81	Tr	Tr	0.1	Tr	0.1
Apple juice, bottled or canned	1 cup	248	88	117	Tr	Tr	Tr	Tr	0.1
Apple pie filling, canned	1/8 of 21-oz can	74	73	75	Tr	Tr	Tr	0.0	Tr
Applesauce, canned									
Sweetened	1 cup	255	80	194	Tr	Tr	0.1	Tr	0.1
Unsweetened	1 cup	244	88	105	Tr	Tr	Tr	Tr	Tr
Apricots									
Raw, without pits (about 12 per lb with pits)	1 apricot	35	86	17	Tr	Tr	Tr	0.1	Tr
Canned, halves, fruit and liquid									
Heavy syrup pack	1 cup	258	78	214	1	Tr	Tr	0.1	Tr
Juice pack	1 cup	244	87	117	2	Tr	Tr	Tr	Tr
Dried, sulfured	10 halves	35	31	83	1	Tr	Tr	0.1	Tr
Apricot nectar, canned, with added ascorbic acid	1 cup	251	85	141	1	Tr	Tr	0.1	Tr
Avocados, raw, without skin and seed									
California (about 1/5 whole)	1 oz	28	73	50	1	5	0.7	3.2	0.6
Bananas, raw									
Whole, medium (7 to 7 7/8 inches long)	1 banana	118	74	109	1	1	0.2	Tr	0.1
Sliced									
Blackberries, raw	1 cup	144	86	75	1	1	Tr	0.1	0.3
Blueberries									
Raw	1 cup	154	85	81	1	1	Tr	0.1	0.2
Frozen, sweetened, thawed	1 cup	230	77	186	1	Tr	Tr	Tr	0.1
Cantaloupe. See Melons.									
Cherries									
Sweet, raw, without pits and stems	10 cherries	68	81	49	1	1	0.1	0.2	0.2
Cherry pie filling, canned	1/5 of 21-oz can	74	71	85	Tr	Tr	Tr	Tr	Tr

CHOLES-TEROL (mg)	CARBO-HYDRATE (g)	TOTAL DIETARY FIBER (g)	CALCIUM (mg)	IRON (mg)	POTAS-SIUM (mg)	SODIUM (mg)	VITAMIN A (IU)	(RE)	THIAMIN (mg)	RIBO-FLAVIN (mg)	NIACIN (mg)	ASCOR-BIC ACID (mg)
150	10	0.3	57	1.1	191	292	161	48	0.11	0.12	2.6	1
80	5	0.2	30	0.6	101	155	85	25	0.06	0.06	1.4	1
147	1	0.0	50	2.3	179	144	51	15	0.02	0.03	2.3	2
43	0	0.0	5	0.9	314	98	116	35	0.04	0.10	10.0	1
58	0	0.0	73	0.3	375	36	244	73	0.20	0.07	7.5	3
49	0	0.0	18	0.8	484	40	58	17	0.43	0.05	10.1	1
15	0	0.0	11	1.2	176	301	66	20	0.03	0.10	10.5	0
26	0	0.0	9	1.3	201	287	48	14	0.03	0.06	11.3	0
36	0	0.0	12	0.8	201	320	16	5	0.01	0.04	4.9	0
27	19	0.0	35	2.1	365	824	199	55	0.06	0.14	13.7	5
0	21	3.7	10	0.2	159	0	73	7	0.02	0.02	0.1	8
0	29	0.2	17	0.9	295	7	2	0	0.05	0.04	0.2	2
0	19	0.7	3	0.2	33	33	10	1	0.01	0.01	Tr	1
0	51	3.1	10	0.9	156	8	28	3	0.03	0.07	0.5	4
0	28	2.9	7	0.3	183	5	71	7	0.03	0.06	0.5	3
0	4	0.8	5	0.2	104	Tr	914	91	0.01	0.01	0.2	4
0	55	4.1	23	0.8	361	10	3173	137	0.05	0.06	1.0	8
0	30	3.9	29	0.7	403	10	4126	412	0.04	0.05	0.8	12
0	22	3.2	16	1.6	482	4	2534	253	Tr	0.05	1.0	1
0	36	1.5	18	1.0	286	8	3303	331	0.02	0.04	0.7	137
0	2	1.4	3	0.3	180	3	174	17	0.03	0.03	0.5	2
0	28	2.8	7	0.4	467	1	96	9	0.05	0.12	0.6	11
0	18	7.6	46	0.8	282	0	238	23	0.04	0.06	0.6	30
0	50	4.8	14	0.9	138	2	101	9	0.05	0.12	0.6	2
0	7	2.5	4	0.2	148	2	449	45	0.03	0.02	0.4	19
0	8	2.9	4	0.3	176	2	532	53	0.03	0.03	0.4	23
0	11	0.6	10	0.3	152	0	146	14	0.03	0.04	0.3	5
0	21	0.4	8	0.2	78	13	152	16	0.02	0.01	0.1	3

(continued on the following page)

Nutritive Value of the Edible Part of Food

FOOD DESCRIPTION	MEASURE OF EDIBLE PORTION	WEIGHT (g)	WATER (%)	CALORIES (kcal)	PROTEIN (g)	TOTAL FAT (g)	FATTY ACIDS		
							SATURATED (g)	MONO-UNSATURATED (g)	POLY-UNSATURATED (g)
FRUITS AND FRUIT JUICES									
(continued)									
Cranberry sauce, sweetened, canned (about 8 slices per can)	1 slice	57	61	86	Tr	Tr	Tr	Tr	Tr
Dates, without pits									
Whole	5 dates	42	23	116	1	Tr	0.1	0.1	Tr
Figs, dried	2 figs	38	28	97	1	Tr	0.1	0.1	0.2
Fruit cocktail, canned, fruit and liquid									
Heavy syrup pack	1 cup	248	80	181	1	Tr	Tr	Tr	0.1
Juice pack	1 cup	237	87	109	1	Tr	Tr	Tr	Tr
Grapefruit									
Raw, without peel, membrane and seeds (3 3/4-inch diameter)									
Pink or red	1/2 grapefruit	123	91	37	1	Tr	Tr	Tr	Tr
White	1/2 grapefruit	118	90	39	1	Tr	Tr	Tr	Tr
Canned, sections with light syrup	1 cup	254	84	152	1	Tr	Tr	Tr	0.1
Grapefruit juice									
Raw									
White	1 cup	247	90	96	1	Tr	Tr	Tr	0.1
Canned									
Unsweetened	1 cup	247	90	94	1	Tr	Tr	Tr	0.1
Sweetened	1 cup	250	87	115	1	Tr	Tr	Tr	0.1
Frozen concentrate, unsweetened									
Diluted with 3 parts water by volume	1 cup	247	89	101	1	Tr	Tr	Tr	0.1
Grapes, seedless, raw	10 grapes	50	81	36	Tr	Tr	0.1	Tr	0.1
Grape juice									
Canned or bottled	1 cup	253	84	154	1	Tr	0.1	Tr	0.1
Frozen concentrate, sweetened, with added vitamin C									
Diluted with 3 parts water by volume	1 cup	250	87	128	Tr	Tr	0.1	Tr	0.1
Kiwi fruit, raw, without skin (about 5 per lb with skin)	1 medium	76	83	46	1	Tr	Tr	Tr	0.2
Lemons, raw, without peel (2 1/8-inch diameter with peel)	1 lemon	58	89	17	1	Tr	Tr	Tr	0.1
Lemon juice									
Raw (from 2 1/8-inch diameter lemon)	juice of 1 lemon	47	91	12	Tr	0	0.0	0.0	0.0
Canned or bottled, unsweetened	1 cup	244	92	51	1	1	0.1	Tr	0.2
Lime juice									
Raw (from 2-inch diameter lime)	juice of 1 lime	38	90	10	Tr	Tr	Tr	Tr	Tr
Canned, unsweetened	1 cup	246	93	52	1	1	0.1	0.1	0.2
Mangos, raw, without skin and seed (about 1 1/2 per lb with skin and seed)									
Sliced	1 cup	165	82	107	1	Tr	0.1	0.2	0.1

†Sodium benzoate and sodium bisulfite added as preservatives.

CHOLESTEROL (mg)	CARBOHYDRATE (g)	TOTAL DIETARY FIBER (g)	CALCIUM (mg)	IRON (mg)	POTASSIUM (mg)	SODIUM (mg)	VITAMIN A (IU)	VITAMIN A (RE)	THIAMIN (mg)	RIBOFLAVIN (mg)	NIACIN (mg)	ASCORBIC ACID (mg)
0	22	0.6	2	0.1	15	17	11	1	0.01	0.01	0.1	1
0	31	3.2	13	0.5	274	1	21	2	0.04	0.04	0.9	0
0	25	4.6	55	0.8	271	4	51	5	0.03	0.03	0.3	Tr
0	47	2.5	15	0.7	218	15	508	50	0.04	0.05	0.9	5
0	28	2.4	19	0.5	225	9	723	73	0.03	0.04	1.0	6
0	9	1.4	14	0.1	159	0	319	32	0.04	0.02	0.2	47
0	10	1.3	14	0.1	175	0	12	1	0.04	0.02	0.3	39
0	39	1.0	36	1.0	328	5	0	0	0.10	0.05	0.6	54
0	23	0.2	22	0.5	400	2	25	2	0.10	0.05	0.5	94
0	22	0.2	17	0.5	378	2	17	2	0.10	0.05	0.6	72
0	28	0.3	20	0.9	405	5	0	0	0.10	0.06	0.8	67
0	24	0.2	20	0.3	336	2	22	2	0.10	0.05	0.5	83
0	9	0.5	6	0.1	93	1	37	4	0.05	0.03	0.2	5
0	38	0.3	23	0.6	334	8	20	3	0.07	0.09	0.7	Tr
0	32	0.3	10	0.3	53	5	20	3	0.04	0.07	0.3	60
0	11	2.6	20	0.3	252	4	133	14	0.02	0.04	0.4	74
0	5	1.6	15	0.3	80	1	17	2	0.02	0.01	0.1	31
0	4	0.2	3	Tr	58	Tr	9	1	0.01	Tr	Tr	22
0	16	1.0	27	0.3	249	51†	37	5	0.10	0.02	0.5	61
0	3	0.2	3	Tr	41	Tr	4	Tr	0.01	Tr	Tr	11
0	16	1.0	30	0.6	185	39†	39	5	0.08	0.01	0.4	16
0	35	3.7	21	0.3	323	4	8061	805	0.12	0.12	1.2	57
0	28	3.0	17	0.2	257	3	6425	642	0.10	0.09	1.0	46

(continued on the following page)

FOOD DESCRIPTION	MEASURE OF EDIBLE PORTION	WEIGHT (g)	WATER (%)	CALORIES (kcal)	PROTEIN (g)	TOTAL FAT (g)	FATTY ACIDS		
							SATU-RATED (g)	MONO-UNSATU-RATED (g)	POLY-UNSATU-RATED (g)

FRUITS AND FRUIT JUICES
(continued)

FOOD DESCRIPTION	MEASURE OF EDIBLE PORTION	WEIGHT (g)	WATER (%)	CALORIES (kcal)	PROTEIN (g)	TOTAL FAT (g)	SATU-RATED (g)	MONO-UNSATU-RATED (g)	POLY-UNSATU-RATED (g)
Melons, raw, without rind and cavity contents									
Cantaloupe (5-inch diameter)									
Wedge									
Cubes	1 cup	160	90	56	1	Tr	0.1	Tr	0.2
Honeydew (6- to- 7-inch diameter)									
Wedge									
Diced (about 20 pieces per cup)	1 cup	170	90	60	1	Tr	Tr	Tr	0.1
Mixed fruit, frozen, sweetened, thawed (peach, cherry, raspberry, grape and boysenberry)	1 cup	250	74	245	4	Tr	0.1	0.1	0.2
Nectarines, raw (2 1/2-inch diameter)	1 nectarine	136	86	67	1	1	0.1	0.2	0.3
Oranges, raw									
Whole, without peel and seeds (2 5/8-inch diameter)	1 orange	131	87	62	1	Tr	Tr	Tr	Tr
Orange juice									
Raw, all varieties	1 cup	248	88	112	2	Tr	0.1	0.1	0.1
Canned, unsweetened	1 cup	249	89	105	1	Tr	Tr	0.1	0.1
Chilled (refrigerator case)	1 cup	249	88	110	2	1	0.1	0.1	0.2
Frozen concentrate									
Diluted with 3 parts water by volume	1 cup	249	88	112	2	Tr	Tr	Tr	Tr
Papayas, raw 1/2-inch cubes	1 cup	140	89	55	1	Tr	0.1	0.1	Tr
Peaches									
Raw									
Whole, 2 1/2-inch diameter pitted (about 4 per lb)	1 peach	98	88	42	1	Tr	Tr	Tr	Tr
Canned, fruit and liquid									
Heavy syrup pack	1 cup	262	79	194	1	Tr	Tr	0.1	0.1
Juice pack	1 cup	248	87	109	2	Tr	Tr	Tr	Tr
Dried, sulfured	3 halves	39	32	93	1	Tr	Tr	0.1	0.1
Frozen, sliced, sweetened, with added ascorbic acid, thawed	1 cup	250	75	235	2	Tr	Tr	0.1	0.2
Pears									
Raw, with skin, cored, 2 1/2-inch diameter	1 pear	166	84	98	1	1	Tr	0.1	0.2
Canned, fruit and liquid									
Heavy syrup pack	1 cup	266	80	197	1	Tr	Tr	0.1	0.1
Juice pack	1 cup	248	86	124	1	Tr	Tr	Tr	Tr
Pineapple									
Raw, diced	1 cup	155	87	76	1	1	Tr	0.1	0.2
Canned, fruit and liquid									
Heavy syrup pack									
Crushed, sliced, or chunks	1 cup	254	79	198	1	Tr	Tr	Tr	0.1

CHOLES-TEROL (mg)	CARBO-HYDRATE (g)	TOTAL DIETARY FIBER (g)	CALCIUM (mg)	IRON (mg)	POTAS-SIUM (mg)	SODIUM (mg)	VITAMIN A (IU)	VITAMIN A (RE)	THIAMIN (mg)	RIBO-FLAVIN (mg)	NIACIN (mg)	ASCOR-BIC ACID (mg)
0	13	1.3	18	0.3	494	14	5158	515	0.06	0.03	0.9	68
0	16	1.0	10	0.1	461	17	68	7	0.13	0.03	1.0	42
0	61	4.8	18	0.7	328	8	805	80	0.04	0.09	1.0	188
0	16	2.2	7	0.2	288	0	1001	101	0.02	0.06	1.3	7
0	15	3.1	52	0.1	237	0	269	28	0.11	0.05	0.4	70
0	26	0.5	27	0.5	496	2	496	50	0.22	0.07	1.0	124
0	25	0.5	20	1.1	436	5	436	45	0.15	0.07	0.8	86
0	25	0.5	25	0.4	473	2	194	20	0.28	0.05	0.7	82
0	27	0.5	22	0.2	473	2	194	20	0.02	0.04	0.5	97
0	14	2.5	34	0.1	360	4	398	39	0.04	0.04	0.5	87
0	11	2.0	5	0.1	193	1	524	53	0.02	0.04	1.0	6
0	52	3.4	8	0.7	241	16	870	86	0.03	0.06	1.6	7
0	29	3.2	15	0.7	317	10	945	94	0.02	0.04	1.4	9
0	24	3.2	11	1.6	388	3	844	84	Tr	0.08	1.7	2
0	60	4.5	8	0.9	325	15	710	70	0.03	0.09	1.6	236
0	25	4.0	18	0.4	208	0	33	3	0.03	0.07	0.2	7
0	51	4.3	13	0.6	173	13	0	0	0.03	0.06	0.6	3
0	32	4.0	22	0.7	238	10	15	2	0.03	0.03	0.5	4
0	19	1.9	11	0.6	175	2	36	3	0.14	0.06	0.7	24
0	51	2.0	36	1.0	264	3	36	3	0.23	0.06	0.7	19

(continued on the following page)

FOOD DESCRIPTION	MEASURE OF EDIBLE PORTION	WEIGHT (g)	WATER (%)	CALORIES (kcal)	PROTEIN (g)	TOTAL FAT (g)	FATTY ACIDS SATU-RATED (g)	MONO-UNSATU-RATED (g)	POLY-UNSATU-RATED (g)
FRUITS AND FRUIT JUICES									
(continued)									
Juice pack									
Crushed, sliced, or chunks	1 cup	249	84	149	1	Tr	Tr	Tr	0.1
Pineapple juice, unsweetened, canned	1 cup	250	86	140	1	Tr	Tr	Tr	0.1
Plums									
Raw (2 1/8-inch diameter)	1 plum	66	85	36	1	Tr	Tr	0.3	0.1
Canned, purple, fruit and liquid									
Heavy syrup pack	1 cup	258	76	230	1	Tr	Tr	0.2	0.1
Juice pack	1 cup	252	84	146	1	Tr	Tr	Tr	Tr
Prunes, dried, pitted									
Uncooked	5 prunes	42	32	100	1	Tr	Tr	0.1	Tr
Stewed, unsweetened, fruit and liquid	1 cup	248	70	265	3	1	Tr	0.4	0.1
Prune juice, canned or bottled	1 cup	256	81	182	2	Tr	Tr	0.1	Tr
Raisins, seedless									
Cup, not packed	1 cup	145	15	435	5	1	0.2	Tr	0.2
Raspberries									
Raw	1 cup	123	87	60	1	1	Tr	0.1	0.4
Frozen, sweetened, thawed	1 cup	250	73	258	2	Tr	Tr	Tr	0.2
Rhubarb, frozen, cooked, with sugar	1 cup	240	68	278	1	Tr	Tr	Tr	0.1
Strawberries									
Raw									
Sliced	1 cup	166	92	50	1	1	Tr	0.1	0.3
Frozen, sweetened, sliced, thawed	1 cup	255	73	245	1	Tr	Tr	Tr	0.2
Tangerines									
Raw, without peel and seeds (2 3/8-inch diameter)	1 tangerine	84	88	37	1	Tr	Tr	Tr	Tr
Canned (mandarin oranges), light syrup, fruit and liquid	1 cup	252	83	154	1	Tr	Tr	Tr	0.1
Watermelon, raw (15-inches long x 7 1/2-inch diameter)									
Diced	1 cup	152	92	49	1	1	0.1	0.2	0.2
GRAIN PRODUCTS									
Bagels, enriched									
Plain	3 1/2-inch bagel	71	33	195	7	1	0.2	0.1	0.5
Cinnamon raisin	3 1/2-inch bagel	71	32	195	7	1	0.2	0.1	0.5
Egg	3 1/2-inch bagel	71	33	197	8	1	0.3	0.3	0.5
Banana bread, prepared from recipe, with margarine	1 slice	60	29	196	3	6	1.3	2.7	1.9
Barley, pearled									
Uncooked									
Cooked	1 cup	157	69	193	4	1	0.1	0.1	0.3
Biscuits, plain or buttermilk, enriched									

CHOLES-TEROL (mg)	CARBO-HYDRATE (g)	TOTAL DIETARY FIBER (g)	CALCIUM (mg)	IRON (mg)	POTAS-SIUM (mg)	SODIUM (mg)	VITAMIN A		THIAMIN (mg)	RIBO-FLAVIN (mg)	NIACIN (mg)	ASCOR-BIC ACID (mg)
							(IU)	(RE)				
0	39	2.0	35	0.7	304	2	95	10	0.24	0.05	0.7	24
0	34	0.5	43	0.7	335	3	13	0	0.14	0.06	0.6	27
0	48	3.5	3	0.9	716	8	1400	140	0.07	0.08	1.2	17
0	9	1.0	3	0.1	114	0	213	21	0.03	0.06	0.3	6
0	60	2.6	23	2.2	235	49	668	67	0.04	0.10	0.8	1
0	38	2.5	25	0.9	388	3	2543	255	0.06	0.15	1.2	7
0	26	3.0	21	1.0	313	2	835	84	0.03	0.07	0.8	1
0	70	16.4	57	2.8	828	5	759	77	0.06	0.25	1.8	7
0	45	2.6	31	3.0	707	10	8	0	0.04	0.18	2.0	10
0	115	5.8	71	3.0	1089	17	12	1	0.23	0.13	1.2	5
0	14	8.4	27	0.7	187	0	160	16	0.04	0.11	1.1	31
0	65	11.0	38	1.6	285	3	150	15	0.05	0.11	0.6	41
0	75	4.8	348	0.5	230	2	166	17	0.04	0.06	0.5	8
0	12	3.8	23	0.6	276	2	45	5	0.03	0.11	0.4	94
0	66	4.8	28	1.5	250	8	61	5	0.04	0.13	1.0	106
0	9	1.9	12	0.1	132	1	773	77	0.09	0.02	0.1	26
0	41	1.8	18	0.9	197	15	2117	212	0.13	0.11	1.1	50
0	30	0.5	45	0.5	443	2	1046	105	0.15	0.05	0.2	55
0	11	0.8	12	0.3	176	3	556	56	0.12	0.03	0.3	15
0	38	1.6	53	2.5	72	379	0	0	0.38	0.22	3.2	0
0	39	1.6	13	2.7	105	229	52	0	0.27	0.20	2.2	Tr
0	38	1.6	9	2.8	48	359	77	23	0.38	0.17	2.4	Tr
26	33	0.7	13	0.8	80	181	278	72	0.10	0.12	0.9	1
0	44	6.0	17	2.1	146	5	11	2	0.13	0.10	3.2	0

(continued on the following page)

FOOD DESCRIPTION	MEASURE OF EDIBLE PORTION	WEIGHT (g)	WATER (%)	CALORIES (kcal)	PROTEIN (g)	TOTAL FAT (g)	FATTY ACIDS SATURATED (g)	MONO-UNSATURATED (g)	POLY-UNSATURATED (g)
GRAIN PRODUCTS									
(continued)									
Prepared from recipe,									
with 2% milk	2 1/2 -inch biscuit	60	29	212	4	10	2.6	4.2	2.5
	4" biscuit	101	29	358	7	16	4.4	7.0	4.2
Refrigerated dough, baked									
Regular	2 1/2-inch biscuit	27	28	93	2	4	1.0	2.2	0.5
Lower fat	2 1/4-inch biscuit	21	28	63	2	1	0.3	0.6	0.2
Breads, enriched									
Cracked wheat	1 slice	25	36	65	2	1	0.2	0.5	0.2
Egg bread (challah)	1/2-inch slice	40	35	115	4	2	0.6	0.9	0.4
French or vienna									
(includes sourdough)	1/2-inch slice	25	34	69	2	1	0.2	0.3	0.2
Indian fry (Navajo) bread	5-inch bread	90	27	296	6	9	2.1	3.6	2.3
Italian	1 slice	20	36	54	2	1	0.2	0.2	0.3
Mixed grain									
Untoasted	1 slice	26	38	65	3	1	0.2	0.4	0.2
Oatmeal									
Untoasted	1 slice	27	37	73	2	1	0.2	0.4	0.5
Pita	4-inch pita	28	32	77	3	Tr	Tr	Tr	0.1
	6 1/2-inch pita	60	32	165	5	1	0.1	0.1	0.3
Pumpernickel									
Untoasted	1 slice	32	38	80	3	1	0.1	0.3	0.4
Raisin									
Untoasted	1 slice	26	34	71	2	1	0.3	0.6	0.2
Rye									
Untoasted	1 slice	32	37	83	3	1	0.2	0.4	0.3
Wheat									
Untoasted	1 slice	25	37	65	2	1	0.2	0.4	0.2
Wheat, reduced calorie	1 slice	23	43	46	2	1	0.1	0.1	0.2
White									
Untoasted	1 slice	25	37	67	2	1	0.1	0.2	0.5
Soft crumbs	1 cup	45	37	120	4	2	0.2	0.3	0.9
White, reduced calorie	1 slice	23	43	48	2	1	0.1	0.2	0.1
Bread, whole wheat									
Untoasted	1 slice	28	38	69	3	1	0.3	0.5	0.3
Bread crumbs, dry, grated									
Plain, enriched	1 cup	108	6	427	14	6	1.3	2.6	1.2
Seasoned, unenriched	1 cup	120	6	440	17	3	0.9	1.2	0.8
Bread crumbs, soft. See White bread.									
Bread stuffing, prepared from dry mix	1/2 cup	100	65	178	3	9	1.7	3.8	2.6
Breakfast bar, cereal crust with fruit filling, fat free	1 bar	37	14	121	2	Tr	Tr	Tr	0.1
Breakfast cereals									
Hot type, cooked									
Corn (hominy) grits									
Regular or quick, enriched									
White	1 cup	242	85	145	3	Tr	0.1	0.1	0.2
Yellow	1 cup	242	82	145	3	Tr	0.1	0.1	0.2
Instant, plain	1 packet	137	82	89	2	Tr	Tr	Tr	0.1
Cream of Wheat									
Regular	1 cup	251	87	133	4	1	0.1	0.1	0.3
Quick	1 cup	239	87	129	4	Tr	0.1	0.1	0.3

CHOLES-TEROL (mg)	CARBO-HYDRATE (g)	TOTAL DIETARY FIBER (g)	CALCIUM (mg)	IRON (mg)	POTAS-SIUM (mg)	SODIUM (mg)	VITAMIN A (IU)	(RE)	THIAMIN (mg)	RIBO-FLAVIN (mg)	NIACIN (mg)	ASCOR-BIC ACID (mg)
2	27	0.9	141	1.7	73	348	49	14	0.21	0.19	1.8	Tr
3	45	1.5	237	2.9	122	586	83	23	0.36	0.31	3.0	Tr
0	13	0.4	5	0.7	42	325	0	0	0.09	0.06	0.8	0
0	12	0.4	4	0.6	39	305	0	0	0.09	0.05	0.7	0
0	12	1.4	11	0.7	44	135	0	0	0.09	0.06	0.9	0
20	19	0.9	37	1.2	46	197	30	9	0.18	0.17	1.9	0
0	13	0.8	19	0.6	28	152	0	0	0.13	0.08	1.2	0
0	48	1.6	210	3.2	67	626	0	0	0.39	0.27	3.3	0
0	10	0.5	16	0.6	22	117	0	0	0.09	0.06	0.9	0
0	12	1.7	24	0.9	53	127	0	0	0.11	0.09	1.1	Tr
0	13	1.1	18	0.7	38	162	4	1	0.11	0.06	0.8	0
0	16	0.6	24	0.7	34	150	0	0	0.17	0.09	1.3	0
0	33	1.3	52	1.6	72	322	0	0	0.36	0.20	2.8	0
0	15	2.1	22	0.9	67	215	0	0	0.10	0.10	1.0	0
0	14	1.1	17	0.8	59	101	0	0	0.09	0.10	0.9	Tr
0	15	1.9	23	0.9	53	211	2	Tr	0.14	0.11	1.2	Tr
0	12	1.1	26	0.8	50	133	0	0	0.10	0.07	1.0	0
0	10	2.8	18	0.7	28	118	0	0	0.10	0.07	0.9	Tr
Tr	12	0.6	27	0.8	30	135	0	0	0.12	0.09	1.0	0
Tr	22	1.0	49	1.4	54	242	0	0	0.21	0.15	1.8	0
0	10	2.2	22	0.7	17	104	1	Tr	0.09	0.07	0.8	Tr
0	13	1.9	20	0.9	71	148	0	0	0.10	0.06	1.1	
0	78	2.6	245	6.6	239	931	1	0	0.83	0.47	7.4	0
1	84	5.0	119	3.8	324	3,180	16	4	0.19	0.20	3.3	Tr
0	22	2.9	32	1.1	74	543	313	81	0.14	0.11	1.5	0
Tr	28	0.8	49	4.5	92	203	1249	125	1.01	0.42	5.0	1
0	31	0.5	0	1.5	53	0	0	0	0.24	0.15	2.0	0
0	31	0.5	0	1.5	53	0	145	15	0.24	0.15	2.0	0
0	21	1.2	8	8.2	38	289	0	0	0.15	0.08	1.4	0
0	28	1.8	50	10.3	43	3	0	0	0.25	0.00	1.5	0
0	27	1.2	50	10.3	45	139	0	0	0.24	0.00	1.4	0

(continued on the following page)

FOOD DESCRIPTION	MEASURE OF EDIBLE PORTION	WEIGHT (g)	WATER (%)	CALORIES (kcal)	PROTEIN (g)	TOTAL FAT (g)	FATTY ACIDS SATU-RATED (g)	MONO-UNSATU-RATED (g)	POLY-UNSATU-RATED (g)
GRAIN PRODUCTS									
(continued)									
Mix'n Eat, plain	1 packet	142	82	102	3	Tr	Tr	Tr	0.2
Malt O Meal	1 cup	240	88	122	4	Tr	0.1	0.1	Tr
Oatmeal									
Regular, quick or instant, plain, nonfortified	1 cup	234	85	145	6	2	0.4	0.7	0.9
Instant, fortified, plain	1 packet	177	86	104	4	2	0.3	0.6	0.7
Quaker instant									
Apples and cinnamon	1 packet	149	79	125	3	1	0.3	0.5	0.6
Maple and brown sugar	1 packet	155	75	153	4	2	0.4	0.6	0.7
Ready to eat									
All Bran	1/2 cup	30	3	79	4	1	0.2	0.2	0.5
Apple Cinnamon Cheerios	3/4 cup	30	3	118	2	2	0.3	0.6	0.2
Apple Jacks	1 cup	30	3	116	1	Tr	0.1	0.1	0.2
Berry Berry Kix	3/4 cup	30	2	120	1	1	0.2	0.5	0.1
Cap'n Crunch	3/4 cup	27	2	107	1	1	0.4	0.3	0.2
Cheerios	1 cup	30	3	110	3	2	0.4	0.6	0.2
Chex									
Corn	1 cup	30	3	113	2	Tr	0.1	0.1	0.2
Honey nut	3/4 cup	30	2	117	2	1	0.1	0.4	0.2
Multi bran	1 cup	49	3	165	4	1	0.2	0.3	0.5
Rice	1 1/4 cup	31	3	117	2	Tr	Tr	Tr	Tr
Wheat	1 cup	30	3	104	3	1	0.1	0.1	0.3
Cinnamon Life	1 cup	50	4	190	4	2	0.3	0.6	0.8
Cocoa Krispies	3/4 cup	31	2	120	2	1	0.6	0.1	0.1
Corn flakes									
General Mills, Total	1 1/3 cup	30	3	112	2	Tr	0.2	0.1	Tr
Kellogg's	1 cup	28	3	102	2	Tr	0.1	Tr	0.1
Froot Loops	1 cup	30	2	117	1	1	0.4	0.2	0.3
Frosted Flakes	3/4 cup	31	3	119	1	Tr	0.1	Tr	0.1
Frosted Mini Wheats									
Regular	1 cup	51	5	173	5	1	0.2	0.1	0.6
Bite size	1 cup	55	5	187	5	1	0.2	0.2	0.6
Golden Grahams	3/4 cup	30	3	116	2	1	0.2	0.3	0.2
Honey Frosted Wheaties	3/4 cup	30	3	110	2	Tr	0.1	Tr	Tr
Honey Nut Cheerios	1 cup	30	2	115	3	1	0.2	0.5	0.2
Kix	1 1/3 cup	30	2	114	2	1	0.2	0.1	Tr
Life	3/4 cup	32	4	121	3	1	0.2	0.4	0.6
Lucky Charms	1 cup	30	2	116	2	1	0.2	0.4	0.2
Nature Valley Granola	3/4 cup	55	4	248	6	10	1.3	6.5	1.9
100% Natural cereal									
With oats, honey, and raisins	1/2 cup	51	4	218	5	7	3.2	3.2	0.8
With raisins, low fat	1/2 cup	50	4	195	4	3	0.8	1.3	0.5
Product 19	1 cup	30	3	110	3	Tr	Tr	0.2	0.2
Puffed rice	1 cup	14	3	56	1	Tr	Tr	Tr	Tr
Puffed wheat	1 cup	12	3	44	2	Tr	Tr	Tr	Tr
Raisin bran									
General Mills, Total	1 cup	55	9	175	4	1	0.2	0.2	0.2
Kellogg's	1 cup	61	8	186	6	1	0.0	0.2	0.8

CHOLESTEROL (mg)	CARBOHYDRATE (g)	TOTAL DIETARY FIBER (g)	CALCIUM (mg)	IRON (mg)	POTASSIUM (mg)	SODIUM (mg)	VITAMIN A (IU)	VITAMIN A (RE)	THIAMIN (mg)	RIBOFLAVIN (mg)	NIACIN (mg)	ASCORBIC ACID (mg)
0	21	0.4	20	8.1	38	241	1252	376	0.43	0.28	5.0	0
0	26	1.0	5	9.6	31	2	0	0	0.48	0.24	5.8	0
0	25	4.0	19	1.6	131	2	37	5	0.26	0.05	0.3	0
0	18	33.0	163	6.3	99	258	1510	453	0.53	0.28	5.5	0
0	26	2.5	104	3.9	106	121	1019	305	0.30	0.35	4.1	Tr
0	31	2.6	105	3.9	112	234	1008	302	0.30	0.34	4.0	0
0	23	9.7	106	4.5	342	61	750	225	0.39	0.42	5.0	15
0	25	1.6	35	4.5	60	1580	750	225	0.38	0.43	5.0	15
0	27	0.6	3	4.5	32	134	750	225	0.39	0.42	5.0	15
0	26	0.2	66	4.5	24	185	750	225	0.38	0.43	5.0	15
0	23	0.9	5	4.5	35	208	36	4	0.38	0.42	5.0	0
0	23	2.6	55	8.1	89	284	1250	375	0.38	0.43	5.0	15
0	26	0.5	100	9.0	32	289	0	0	0.38	0.00	5.0	6
0	26	0.4	102	9.0	27	224	0	0	0.38	0.44	5.0	6
0	41	6.4	95	13.7	191	325	0	0	0.32	0.00	4.4	5
0	27	0.3	104	9.0	36	291	0	0	0.38	0.02	5.0	6
0	24	3.3	60	9.0	116	269	0	0	0.23	0.04	3.0	4
0	40	3.0	135	7.5	113	220	16	2	0.63	0.71	8.4	Tr
0	27	0.4	4	1.8	60	210	750	225	0.37	0.43	5.0	15
0	26	0.8	237	18.0	34	203	1250	375	1.50	1.70	20.1	60
0	24	0.8	1	8.7	25	298	700	210	0.36	0.39	4.7	14
0	26	0.6	3	4.2	32	141	703	211	0.39	0.42	5.0	14
0	28	0.6	1	4.5	20	200	750	225	0.37	0.43	5.0	15
0	42	5.5	18	14.3	170	2	0	0	0.36	0.41	5.0	0
0	45	5.9	0	15.4	186	2	0	0	0.33	0.39	4.7	0
0	26	0.9	14	4.5	53	275	750	225	0.38	0.43	5.0	15
0	26	1.5	8	4.5	56	211	750	225	0.38	0.43	5.0	15
0	24	1.6	20	4.5	85	259	750	225	0.38	0.43	5.0	15
0	26	0.8	44	8.1	41	263	1250	375	0.38	0.43	5.0	15
0	25	2.0	98	9.0	79	174	12	1	0.40	0.45	5.3	0
0	25	1.2	32	4.5	54	203	750	225	0.38	0.43	5.0	15
0	36	3.5	41	1.47	183	89	0	0	0.17	0.06	0.6	0
1	36	3.7	39	1.7	214	11	4	1	0.14	0.09	0.8	Tr
1	40	3.0	30	1.3	169	129	9	1	0.15	0.06	0.9	Tr
0	25	1.0	3	18.0	41	216	750	225	1.50	1.71	20.0	60
0	13	0.2	1	4.4	16	Tr	0	0	0.36	0.25	4.9	0
0	10	0.5	3	3.8	42	Tr	0	0	0.31	0.22	4.2	0
0	43	5.0	238	18.0	287	240	1250	375	1.50	1.70	20.0	0
0	47	8.2	35	5.0	437	354	832	250	0.43	0.49	5.6	0

(continued on the following page)

FOOD DESCRIPTION	MEASURE OF EDIBLE PORTION	WEIGHT (g)	WATER (%)	CALORIES (kcal)	PROTEIN (g)	TOTAL FAT (g)	FATTY ACIDS		
							SATU- RATED (g)	MONO- UNSATU- RATED (g)	POLY- UNSATU- RATED (g)
GRAIN PRODUCTS									
(continued)									
Raisin Nut Bran	1 cup	55	5	209	5	4	0.7	1.9	0.5
Reese's Peanut									
Butter Puffs	3/4 cup	30	2	129	3	3	0.6	1.4	0.6
Rice Krispies	1 1/4 cup	33	3	124	2	Tr	0.1	0.1	0.2
Rice Krispies									
Treats cereal	3/4 cup	30	4	120	1	2	0.4	1.0	0.2
Shredded Wheat	2 biscuits	46	4	156	5	1	0.1	NA	NA
Special K	1 cup	31	3	115	6	Tr	0.0	0.0	0.2
Quaker Toasted Oatmeal,									
Honey Nut	1 cup	49	3	191	5	3	0.5	1.2	0.7
Total, Whole Grain	3/4 cup	30	3	105	3	1	0.5	0.1	0.1
Trix	1 cup	30	2	122	1	2	0.4	0.9	0.3
Wheaties	1 cup	30	3	110	3	1	0.2	0.2	0.2
Brownies, without icing									
Commercially prepared									
Regular, large (2 3/4-inch									
sq x 7/8-inch thick)	1 brownie	56	14	227	3	9	2.4	8.0	1.3
Fat free, 2-inch sq	1 brownie	28	12	89	1	Tr	0.2	0.1	Tr
Bulgur									
Cooked	1 cup	182	78	151	6	Tr	0.1	0.1	0.2
Cakes, prepared from dry mix									
Angel food (1/12 of 10-inch									
diameter)	1 piece	50	33	129	3	Tr	Tr	Tr	0.1
Yellow, light, with water,									
egg whites, no frosting									
(1/12 of 9-inch diameter	1 piece	69	37	181	3	2	1.1	0.9	0.2
Cakes, prepared from recipe									
Chocolate, without frosting									
(1/12 of 9-inch diameter)	1 piece	95	24	340	5	14	5.2	5.7	2.6
Gingerbread (1/2 of 8-inch									
square)	1 piece	74	28	263	3	12	3.1	5.3	3.1
White									
Without frosting (1/12 of									
9-inch diameter)	1 piece	74	23	264	4	9	2.4	3.9	2.3
Cakes, commercially prepared									
Angelfood (1/12 of 12-oz cake)	1 piece	28	33	72	2	Tr	Tr	Tr	0.1
Chocolate with chocolate									
frosting (1/8 of 18-oz cake)	1 piece	64	23	235	3	10	3.1	5.6	1.2
Fruitcake	1 piece	43	25	139	1	4	0.5	1.8	1.4
Snack cakes									
Chocolate, creme-filled,									
with frosting	1 cupcake	50	20	188	2	7	1.4	2.8	2.6
Chocolate, with frosting,									
low fat	1 cupcake	43	23	131	2	2	0.5	0.8	0.2
Sponge, creme-filled	1 cake	43	20	155	1	5	1.1	1.7	1.4
Sponge, individual shortcake	1 shortcake	30	30	87	2	1	0.2	0.3	0.1
Yellow									
With vanilla frosting	1 piece	64	22	239	2	9	1.5	3.9	3.3
Cheesecake (1/6 of 17-oz cake)	1 piece	80	46	257	4	18	7.9	6.9	1.3
Cookies									
Butter, commercially									
prepared	1 cookie	5	5	23	Tr	1	0.6	0.3	Tr
Chocolate chip, medium									
(2 1/4-to 2 1/2-inch diameter)									
Commercially prepared									
Regular	1 cookie	10	4	48	1	2	0.7	1.2	0.2

CHOLES-TEROL (mg)	CARBO-HYDRATE (g)	TOTAL DIETARY FIBER (g)	CALCIUM (mg)	IRON (mg)	POTAS-SIUM (mg)	SODIUM (mg)	VITAMIN A		THIAMIN (mg)	RIBO-FLAVIN (mg)	NIACIN (mg)	ASCOR-BIC ACID (mg)
							(IU)	(RE)				
0	41	5.1	74	4.5	218	246	0	0	0.37	0.42	5.0	0
0	23	0.4	21	4.5	62	177	750	225	0.38	0.43	5.0	15
0	29	0.4	3	2.0	42	354	825	248	0.43	0.46	5.5	17
0	26	0.3	2	1.8	19	190	750	225	0.39	0.42	5.0	15
0	38	5.3	20	1.4	196	3	0	NA	0.12	0.05	2.6	0
0	22	1.0	5	8.7	55	250	750	225	0.53	0.59	7.0	15
Tr	39	3.3	27	4.5	185	166	500	150	0.37	0.42	5.0	6
0	24	2.6	258	18.0	97	199	1250	375	1.50	1.70	20.1	60
0	26	0.7	32	4.5	18	197	750	225	0.38	0.43	5.0	15
0	24	2.1	55	8.1	104	222	750	225	0.38	0.43	5.0	150
10	36	1.2	16	1.3	83	175	39	3	0.14	0.12	1.0	0
0	22	1.0	17	0.7	89	90	1	Tr	0.03	0.04	0.3	Tr
0	34	8.2	18	1.7	124	9	0	0	0.10	0.5	0.8	0
0	29	0.1	42	0.1	68	255	0	0	0.05	0.10	0.1	0
0	37	0.6	69	0.6	41	279	6	1	0.06	0.12	0.6	0
55	51	1.5	57	1.5	133	299	133	38	0.13	0.20	1.1	Tr
24	36	0.7	53	2.1	325	242	36	10	0.14	0.12	1.3	Tr
1	42	0.6	96	1.1	70	242	41	12	0.14	0.18	1.1	Tr
0	16	0.4	39	0.1	26	210	0	0	0.03	0.14	0.2	0
27	35	1.8	28	1.4	128	214	54	16	0.02	0.09	0.4	Tr
2	26	1.6	14	0.9	66	116	9	2	0.02	0.04	0.3	Tr
9	30	0.4	37	1.7	61	213	9	3	0.11	0.15	1.2	0
0	29	1.8	15	0.7	96	178	0	0	0.02	0.06	0.3	0
7	27	0.2	19	0.5	37	155	7	2	0.07	0.06	0.5	Tr
31	18	0.2	21	0.8	30	73	46	14	0.07	0.08	0.6	0
35	38	0.2	40	0.7	34	220	40	12	0.06	0.04	0.3	0
44	20	0.3	41	0.5	72	166	438	117	0.02	0.15	0.2	Tr
6	3	Tr	1	0.1	6	18	34	8	0.02	0.02	0.2	0
0	7	0.3	3	0.3	14	32	Tr	0	0.02	0.03	0.3	0

(continued on the following page)

						FATTY ACIDS		
FOOD DESCRIPTION	MEASURE OF EDIBLE PORTION	WEIGHT (g)	WATER (%)	CALORIES (kcal)	PROTEIN (g)	TOTAL FAT (g)	SATU- RATED (g)	MONO- UNSATU- RATED (g)	POLY- UNSATU- RATED (g)

GRAIN PRODUCTS
(continued)

FOOD DESCRIPTION	MEASURE	WEIGHT	WATER	CALORIES	PROTEIN	TOTAL FAT	SATURATED	MONO	POLY
Reduced fat	1 cookie	10	4	45	1	2	0.4	0.6	0.5
Prepared from recipe, with margarine	1 cookie	16	6	78	1	5	1.3	1.7	1.3
Fig bar	1 cookie	16	17	56	1	1	0.2	0.5	0.4
Molasses									
Medium	1 cookie	15	6	65	1	2	0.5	1.1	0.3
Oatmeal									
Commercially prepared, with or without raisins									
Regular, large	1 cookie	25	6	113	2	5	1.1	2.5	0.6
Fat free	1 cookie	11	13	36	1	Tr	Tr	Tr	0.1
Prepared from recipe, with raisins (2 5/8-inch diameter)	1 cookie	15	6	65	1	2	0.5	1.0	0.8
Peanut butter									
Commercially prepared	1 cookie	15	6	72	1	4	0.7	1.9	0.8
Prepared from recipe, with margarine (3-inch diameter)	1 cookie	20	6	95	2	5	0.9	2.2	1.4
Sandwich type, with creme filling									
Chocolate cookie	1 cookie	10	2	47	Tr	2	0.4	0.9	0.7
Vanilla cookie									
Round	1 cookie	10	2	48	Tr	2	0.3	0.8	0.8
Shortbread, commercially prepared									
Plain (1 5/8-inch diameter sq)	1 cookie	8	4	40	Tr	2	0.5	1.1	0.3
Pecan									
Regular (2-inch diameter)	1 cookie	14	3	76	1	5	1.1	2.6	0.6
Sugar									
Commercially prepared	1 cookie	15	5	72	1	3	0.8	1.8	0.4
Prepared from recipe, with margarine (3-inch diameter)	1 cookie	14	9	66	1	3	0.7	1.4	1.0
Vanilla wafer, lower fat, medium size	1 cookie	4	5	18	Tr	1	0.2	0.3	0.2
Corn chips									
Plain	1 oz	28	1	153	2	9	1.3	2.7	4.7
Cornbread									
Prepared from mix, piece 3 3/4 x 2 1/2 x 3/4 inches	1 piece	60	32	188	4	6	1.6	3.1	0.7
Prepared from recipe, with 2% milk, piece 2 1/2-inch sq x 1 1/2-inches	1 piece	65	39	173	4	5	1.0	1.2	2.1
Cornmeal, yellow, dry form									
Cornstarch	1 tbsp	8	8	30	Tr	Tr	Tr	Tr	Tr
Couscous									
Cooked	1 cup	157	73	176	6	Tr	Tr	Tr	0.1

CHOLESTEROL (mg)	CARBO-HYDRATE (g)	TOTAL DIETARY FIBER (g)	CALCIUM (mg)	IRON (mg)	POTAS-SIUM (mg)	SODIUM (mg)	VITAMIN A		THIAMIN (mg)	RIBO-FLAVIN (mg)	NIACIN (mg)	ASCOR-BIC ACID (mg)
							(IU)	(RE)				
0	7	0.4	2	0.3	12	38	Tr	0	0.03	0.03	0.3	0
5	9	0.4	6	0.4	36	58	102	26	0.03	0.03	0.2	Tr
0	11	0.7	10	0.5	33	56	5	1	0.03	0.03	0.3	Tr
0	11	0.1	11	1.0	52	69	0	0	0.05	0.04	0.5	0
0	17	0.7	9	0.6	36	96	5	1	0.07	0.06	0.6	Tr
0	9	0.8	4	0.2	23	33	0	0	0.02	0.03	0.1	0
5	10	0.5	15	0.4	36	81	96	25	0.04	0.02	0.2	Tr
Tr	9	0.3	5	0.4	25	62	1	Tr	0.03	0.03	0.6	0
6	12	0.4	8	0.4	46	104	120	31	0.04	0.04	0.7	Tr
0	7	0.3	3	0.4	18	60	Tr	0	0.01	0.02	0.2	0
0	7	0.2	3	0.2	9	35	0	0	0.03	0.02	0.3	0
2	5	0.1	3	0.2	8	36	7	1	0.03	0.03	0.3	0
5	8	0.3	4	0.3	10	39	Tr	Tr	0.04	0.03	0.3	0
8	10	0.1	3	0.3	9	54	14	4	0.03	0.03	0.4	Tr
4	8	0.2	10	0.3	11	69	135	35	0.04	0.04	0.3	Tr
2	3	0.1	2	0.1	4	12	1	Tr	0.01	0.01	0.1	0
0	16	1.4	36	0.4	40	179	27	3	0.01	0.04	0.3	0
37	29	1.4	44	1.1	77	467	123	26	0.15	0.16	1.2	Tr
26	28	1.9	162	1.6	96	428	180	35	0.19	0.19	1.5	Tr
0	7	0.1	Tr	Tr	Tr	1	0	0	0.00	0.00	0.0	0
0	36	2.2	13	0.6	91	8	0	0	0.10	0.04	1.5	0

(continued on the following page)

Nutritive Value of the Edible Part of Food

FOOD DESCRIPTION	MEASURE OF EDIBLE PORTION	WEIGHT (g)	WATER (%)	CALORIES (kcal)	PROTEIN (g)	TOTAL FAT (g)	FATTY ACIDS SATU-RATED (g)	MONO-UNSATU-RATED (g)	POLY-UNSATU-RATED (g)
GRAIN PRODUCTS									
(continued)									
Crackers									
Cheese, 1-inch sq	10 crackers	10	3	50	1	3	0.9	1.2	0.2
Graham, plain									
2 1/2-inch sq	2 squares	14	4	59	1	1	0.2	0.6	0.5
Melba toast, plain	4 pieces	20	5	78	2	1	0.1	0.2	0.3
Rye wafer, whole grain,									
plain	1 wafer	11	5	37	1	Tr	Tr	Tr	Tr
Saltine									
Square	4 crackers	12	4	52	1	1	0.4	0.8	0.2
Oyster-type	1 cup	45	4	195	4	5	1.3	2.9	0.8
Sandwich-type									
Wheat with cheese	1 sandwich	7	4	33	1	1	0.4	0.8	0.2
Cheese with peanut									
butter	1 sandwich	7	4	34	1	2	0.4	0.8	0.3
Standard snack-type									
Bite size	1 cup	62	4	311	5	16	2.3	6.6	5.9
Round	4 crackers	12	4	60	1	3	0.5	1.3	1.1
Wheat, thin square	4 crackers	8	3	38	1	2	0.4	0.9	0.2
Whole wheat	4 crackers	16	3	71	1	3	0.5	0.9	1.1
Croissant, butter	1 croissant	57	23	231	5	12	6.6	3.1	0.6
Croutons, seasoned	1 cup	40	4	186	4	7	2.1	3.8	0.9
Danish pastry, enriched									
Cheese filled	1 danish	71	31	266	6	16	4.8	8.0	1.8
Fruit filled	1 danish	71	27	263	4	13	3.5	7.1	1.7
Doughnuts									
Cake-type	1 hole	14	21	59	1	3	0.5	1.3	1.1
	1 medium	47	21	198	2	11	1.7	4.4	3.7
Yeast leavened, glazed	1 hole	13	25	52	1	3	0.8	1.7	0.4
	1 medium	60	25	242	4	14	3.5	7.7	1.7
Eclair, prepared from recipe,									
5 x 2 x 1 3/4 inches	1 eclair	100	52	262	6	16	4.1	6.5	3.9
English muffin, plain,									
enriched									
Untoasted	1 muffin	57	42	134	4	1	0.1	0.2	0.5
French toast									
Prepared from recipe,									
with 2% milk, fried in									
margarine	1 slice	65	55	149	5	7	1.8	2.9	1.7
Granola bar									
Hard, plain	1 bar	28	4	134	3	6	0.7	1.2	3.4
Soft, uncoated									
Chocolate chip	1 bar	28	5	119	2	5	2.9	1.0	0.6
Raisin	1 bar	28	6	127	2	5	2.7	0.8	0.9
Macaroni (elbows), enriched,									
cooked	1 cup	140	66	197	7	1	0.1	0.1	0.4
Muffins									
Blueberry									
Prepared from mix (2 1/4 -inch diameter x 1 3/4 inches)	1 muffin	50	36	150	3	4	0.7	1.8	1.5
Prepared from recipe, with 2% milk	1 muffin	57	40	162	4	6	1.2	1.5	3.1
Bran with raisins, toaster type, toasted	1 muffin	34	27	106	2	3	0.5	0.8	1.7

CHOLES-TEROL (mg)	CARBO-HYDRATE (g)	TOTAL DIETARY FIBER (g)	CALCIUM (mg)	IRON (mg)	POTAS-SIUM (mg)	SODIUM (mg)	VITAMIN A (IU)	VITAMIN A (RE)	THIAMIN (mg)	RIBO-FLAVIN (mg)	NIACIN (mg)	ASCOR-BIC ACID (mg)
1	6	0.2	15	0.5	15	100	16	3	0.06	0.04	0.5	0
0	11	0.4	3	0.5	19	85	0	0	0.03	0.04	0.6	0
0	15	1.3	19	0.7	40	166	0	0	0.08	0.05	0.8	0
0	9	2.5	4	0.7	54	87	1	0	0.05	0.03	0.2	Tr
0	9	0.4	14	0.6	15	156	0	0	0.07	0.06	0.6	0
0	32	1.4	54	2.4	58	586	0	0	0.25	0.21	2.4	0
Tr	4	0.1	18	0.2	30	98	5	1	0.03	0.05	0.3	Tr
Tr	4	0.2	6	0.2	17	69	22	2	0.03	0.02	0.5	Tr
0	38	1.0	74	2.2	82	525	0	0	0.25	0.21	2.5	0
0	7	0.2	14	0.4	16	102	0	0	0.05	0.04	0.5	0
0	5	0.4	4	0.4	15	64	0	0	0.04	0.03	0.4	0
0	11	1.7	8	0.5	48	105	0	0	0.03	0.02	0.7	0
38	26	1.5	21	1.2	67	424	424	106	0.22	0.14	1.2	Tr
3	25	2.0	38	1.1	72	495	16	4	0.20	0.17	1.9	0
11	26	0.7	25	1.1	70	320	104	32	0.13	0.18	1.4	Tr
81	34	1.3	33	1.3	59	251	53	16	0.19	0.16	1.4	3
5	7	0.2	6	0.3	18	76	8	2	0.03	0.03	0.3	Tr
17	23	0.7	21	0.9	60	257	27	8	0.10	0.11	0.9	Tr
1	6	0.2	6	0.3	14	44	2	1	0.05	0.03	0.4	Tr
4	27	0.7	26	1.2	65	205	8	2	0.22	0.13	1.7	Tr
127	24	0.6	63	1.2	117	337	718	191	0.12	0.27	0.8	Tr
0	26	1.5	99	1.4	75	264	0	0	0.25	0.16	2.2	0
75	16	0.7	65	1.1	87	311	315	86	0.13	0.21	1.1	Tr
0	18	1.5	17	0.8	95	83	43	4	0.07	0.03	0.4	Tr
Tr	20	1.4	26	0.7	96	77	12	1	0.06	0.04	0.3	0
Tr	19	1.2	29	0.7	103	80	0	0	0.07	0.05	0.3	0
0	40	1.8	10	2.0	43	1	0	0	0.29	0.14	2.3	0
23	24	0.6	13	0.6	39	219	39	11	0.07	0.16	1.1	1
21	23	1.1	108	1.3	70	251	80	22	0.16	0.16	1.3	1
3	19	2.8	13	1.0	60	179	58	16	0.07	0.10	0.8	0

(continued on the following page)

FOOD DESCRIPTION	MEASURE OF EDIBLE PORTION	WEIGHT (g)	WATER (%)	CALORIES (kcal)	PROTEIN (g)	TOTAL FAT (g)	FATTY ACIDS		
							SATU-RATED (g)	MONO-UNSATU-RATED (g)	POLY-UNSATU-RATED (g)
GRAIN PRODUCTS									
(continued)									
Corn									
Prepared from mix									
(2 1/4-inch diameter x									
1 1/2-inches)	1 muffin	50	31	161	4	5	1.4	2.6	0.6
Noodles, chow mein, canned	1 cup	45	1	237	4	14	2.0	3.5	7.8
Noodles (egg noodles),									
enriched, cooked									
Regular	1 cup	160	69	213	8	2	0.5	0.7	0.7
Pancakes, plain (4-inch									
diameter)									
Frozen, ready to heat	1 pancake	36	45	82	2	1	0.3	0.4	0.3
Prepared from complete									
mix	1 pancake	38	53	74	2	1	0.2	0.3	0.3
Pie crust, baked									
Standard type									
From recipe	1 pie shell	180	10	949	12	62	15.5	27.3	16.4
Graham cracker	1 pie shell	239	4	1181	10	60	12.4	27.2	16.5
Pies									
Commercially prepared (1/6									
of 8-inch diameter)									
Apple	1 piece	117	52	277	2	13	4.4	5.1	2.6
Blueberry	1 piece	117	53	271	2	12	2.0	5.0	4.1
Cherry	1 piece	117	46	304	2	13	3.0	6.8	2.4
Pecan	1 piece	113	19	452	5	21	4.0	12.1	3.6
Pumpkin	1 piece	109	58	229	4	10	1.9	4.4	3.4
Popcorn									
Air popped, unsalted	1 cup	8	4	31	1	Tr	Tr	0.1	0.2
Oil popped, salted	1 cup	11	3	55	1	3	0.5	0.9	1.5
Caramel coated									
With peanuts	1 cup	42	3	168	3	3	0.4	1.1	1.4
Without peanuts	1 cup	35	3	152	1	5	1.3	1.0	1.6
Cheese flavor	1 cup	11	3	58	1	4	0.7	1.1	1.7
Pretzels, made with									
enriched flour									
Stick, 2 1/4-inch long	10 pretzels	3	3	11	Tr	Tr	Tr	Tr	Tr
Twisted, regular	10 pretzels	60	3	229	5	2	0.5	0.8	0.7
Twisted, dutch, 2 3/4 x									
2 5/8-inches	1 pretzel	16	3	61	1	1	0.1	0.2	0.2
Rice									
Brown, long grain, cooked	1 cup	195	73	216	5	2	0.4	0.6	0.6
White, long grain, enriched									
Regular									
Cooked	1 cup	158	68	205	4	Tr	0.1	0.1	0.1
Instant, prepared	1 cup	165	76	162	3	Tr	0.1	0.1	0.1
Parboiled									
Cooked	1 cup	175	72	200	4	Tr	0.1	0.1	0.1
Wild, cooked	1 cup	164	74	166	7	1	0.1	0.1	0.3
Rice cake, brown rice, plain	1 cake	9	6	35	1	Tr	0.1	0.1	0.1
Rice Krispies Treat squares	1 bar	22	6	91	1	2	0.3	0.6	1.1
Rolls									
Dinner	1 roll	28	32	84	2	2	0.5	1.0	0.3
Hamburger or hot dog	1 roll	43	34	123	4	2	0.5	0.4	1.1
Hard, kaiser	1 roll	57	31	167	6	2	0.3	0.6	1.0

CHOLESTEROL (mg)	CARBOHYDRATE (g)	TOTAL DIETARY FIBER (g)	CALCIUM (mg)	IRON (mg)	POTASSIUM (mg)	SODIUM (mg)	VITAMIN A		THIAMIN (mg)	RIBOFLAVIN (mg)	NIACIN (mg)	ASCORBIC ACID (mg)
							(IU)	(RE)				
31	25	1.2	38	1.0	66	398	105	23	0.12	0.14	1.1	Tr
0	26	1.8	9	2.1	54	198	38	4	0.26	0.19	2.7	0
53	40	1.8	19	2.5	45	11	32	10	0.30	0.13	2.4	08
3	16	0.6	22	1.3	26	183	36	10	0.14	0.17	1.4	Tr
5	14	0.5	48	0.6	67	239	12	3	0.08	0.08	0.7	Tr
0	86	3.0	18	5.2	121	976	0	0	0.70	0.50	6.0	0
0	156	3.6	50	5.2	210	1365	1876	483	0.25	0.42	5.1	0
0	40	1.9	13	0.5	76	311	145	35	0.03	0.03	0.3	4
0	41	1.2	9	0.4	59	380	164	40	0.01	0.04	0.4	3
0	47	0.9	14	0.6	95	288	329	63	0.03	0.03	0.2	1
36	65	4.0	19	1.2	84	479	198	53	0.10	0.14	0.3	1
22	30	2.9	65	0.9	168	307	3743	405	0.06	0.17	0.2	1
0	6	1.2	1	0.2	24	Tr	16	2	0.02	0.02	0.2	0
0	6	1.1	1	0.3	25	97	17	2	0.01	0.01	0.2	Tr
0	34	1.6	28	1.6	149	124	27	3	0.02	0.05	0.8	0
2	28	1.8	15	0.6	38	73	18	4	0.02	0.02	0.8	0
1	6	1.1	12	0.2	29	98	27	5	0.01	0.03	0.2	Tr
0	2	0.1	1	0.1	4	51	0	0	0.01	0.02	0.2	0
0	48	1.9	22	2.6	55	1029	0	0	0.28	0.37	3.2	0
0	13	0.5	6	0.7	23	274	0	0	0.07	0.10	0.8	0
0	45	3.5	20	0.8	84	10	0	0	0.19	0.05	3.0	0
0	45	0.6	16	1.9	55	2	0	0	0.26	0.02	2.3	0
0	35	1.0	13	1.0	7	5	0	0	0.12	0.08	1.5	0
0	43	0.7	33	2.0	65	5	0	0	0.44	0.03	2.5	0
0	35	3.0	5	1.0	166	5	0	0	0.09	0.14	2.1	0
0	7	0.4	1	0.1	26	29	4	Tr	0.01	0.01	0.7	0
0	18	0.1	1	0.5	9	77	200	60	0.15	0.18	2.0	0
Tr	14	0.8	33	0.9	37	146	0	0	0.14	0.09	1.1	Tr
0	22	1.2	60	1.4	61	241	0	0	0.21	0.13	1.7	Tr
0	30	1.3	54	1.9	62	310	0	0	0.27	0.19	2.4	0

(continued on the following page)

| | | | | | | FATTY ACIDS | | |
FOOD DESCRIPTION	MEASURE OF EDIBLE PORTION	WEIGHT (g)	WATER (%)	CALORIES (kcal)	PROTEIN (g)	TOTAL FAT (g)	SATU-RATED (g)	MONO-UNSATU-RATED (g)	POLY-UNSATU-RATED (g)
GRAIN PRODUCTS									
(continued)									
Spaghetti, cooked									
Enriched	1 cup	140	66	197	7	1	0.1	0.1	0.4
Whole wheat	1 cup	140	67	174	7	1	0.1	0.1	0.3
Sweet rolls, cinnamon									
Commercial, with raisins	1 roll	60	25	223	4	10	1.8	2.9	4.5
Refrigerated dough, baked, with frosting	1 roll	30	23	109	2	4	1.0	2.2	0.5
Taco shell, baked	1 medium	13	6	62	1	3	0.4	1.2	1.1
Tapioca, pearl, dry	1 cup	152	11	544	Tr	Tr	Tr	Tr	Tr
Toaster pastries									
Fruit filled	1 pastry	52	12	204	2	5	0.8	2.2	2.0
Low fat	1 pastry	52	12	193	2	3	0.7	1.7	0.5
Tortilla chips									
Plain									
Regular	1 oz	28	2	142	2	7	1.4	4.4	1.0
Low fat, baked	10 chips	14	2	54	2	1	0.1	0.2	0.4
Tortillas, ready to cook (about 6-inch diameter)									
Corn	1 tortilla	26	44	58	1	1	0.1	0.2	0.3
Flour	1 tortilla	32	27	104	3	2	0.6	1.2	0.3
Waffles, plain									
Prepared from recipe, 7-inch diameter	1 waffle	75	42	218	6	11	2.1	2.6	5.1
Low fat, 4-inch diameter	1 waffle	35	43	83	2	1	0.3	0.4	0.4
Wheat flours									
All purpose, enriched									
Sifted, spooned	1 cup	115	12	419	12	1	0.2	0.1	0.5
Unsifted, spooned	1 cup	125	12	455	13	1	0.2	0.1	0.5
Bread, enriched	1 cup	137	13	495	16	2	0.3	0.2	1.0
Self rising, enriched, unsifted, spooned	1 cup	125	11	443	12	1	0.2	0.1	0.5
Whole wheat, from hard wheats, stirred, spooned	1 cup	120	10	407	16	2	0.4	0.3	0.9
Wheat germ, toasted, plain	1 tbsp	7	6	27	2	1	0.1	0.1	0.5
LEGUMES, NUTS, AND SEEDS									
Almonds, shelled									
Whole	1 oz (24 nuts)	28	5	164	6	14	1.1	9.1	3.5
Beans, dry									
Cooked									
Black	1 cup	172	66	277	15	1	0.2	0.1	0.4
Great Northern	1 cup	177	69	209	15	1	0.2	Tr	0.3
Kidney, red	1 cup	177	67	225	15	1	0.1	0.1	0.5
Lima, large	1 cup	188	70	216	15	1	0.2	0.1	0.3
Pea (navy)	1 cup	182	63	258	16	1	0.3	0.1	0.4
Pinto	1 cup	171	64	234	14	1	0.2	0.2	0.3
Canned, solids and liquid									
Baked beans									
Plain or vegetarian	1 cup	254	73	236	12	1	0.3	0.1	0.5
Kidney, red	1 cup	256	77	218	13	1	0.1	0.1	0.5
Lima, large	1 cup	241	77	190	12	Tr	0.1	Tr	0.2
White	1 cup	262	70	307	19	1	0.2	0.1	0.3

CHOLESTEROL (mg)	CARBOHYDRATE (g)	TOTAL DIETARY FIBER (g)	CALCIUM (mg)	IRON (mg)	POTASSIUM (mg)	SODIUM (mg)	VITAMIN A (IU)	VITAMIN A (RE)	THIAMIN (mg)	RIBOFLAVIN (mg)	NIACIN (mg)	ASCORBIC ACID (mg)
0	40	2.4	10	2.0	43	1	0	0	0.29	0.14	2.3	0
0	37	6.3	21	1.5	62	4	0	0	0.15	0.06	1.0	0
40	31	1.4	43	1.0	67	230	129	38	0.19	0.16	1.4	1
0	17	0.6	10	0.8	19	250	1	0	0.12	0.07	1.1	Tr
0	8	1.0	21	0.3	24	49	0	0	0.03	0.01	0.2	0
0	135	1.4	30	2.4	17	2	0	0	0.01	0.00	0.0	0
0	37	1.1	14	1.8	58	218	501	2	0.15	0.19	2.0	Tr
0	40	0.8	23	1.8	34	131	494	49	0.15	0.29	2.0	2
0	18	1.8	44	0.4	56	150	56	6	0.02	0.05	0.4	0
0	11	0.7	22	0.2	37	57	52	6	0.03	0.04	0.1	Tr
0	12	1.4	46	0.4	40	42	0	0	0.03	0.02	0.4	0
0	18	1.1	40	1.1	42	153	0	0	0.17	0.09	1.1	0
52	25	0.7	191	1.7	119	383	171	49	0.20	0.26	1.6	Tr
9	15	0.4	20	1.9	50	155	506	NA	0.31	0.26	2.6	0
0	88	3.1	17	5.3	123	2	0	0	0.90	0.57	6.8	0
0	95	3.4	19	5.8	134	3	0	0	0.98	0.62	7.4	0
0	99	3.3	21	6.0	137	3	0	0	1.11	0.70	10.3	0
0	93	3.4	423	5.8	155	1588	0	0	0.84	0.52	7.3	0
0	87	14.6	41	4.7	486	6	0	0	0.54	0.26	7.6	0
0	3	0.9	3	0.6	66	Tr	0	0	0.12	0.06	0.4	Tr
0	6	3.3	70	1.2	206	Tr	3	Tr	0.07	0.23	1.1	0
0	41	15.0	46	3.6	611	2	1.0	2	0.42	0.10	0.9	0
0	37	12.4	120	3.8	692	4	2	0	0.28	0.10	1.2	2
0	40	13.1	50	5.2	713	4	0	0	0.28	0.10	1.0	2
0	39	13.2	32	4.5	955	4	0	0	0.30	0.10	0.8	0
0	48	11.6	127	4.5	670	2	4	0	0.37	0.11	1.0	2
0	44	14.7	82	4.5	800	3	3	0	0.32	0.16	0.7	4
0	52	12.7	127	0.7	752	1008	434	43	0.39	0.15	1.1	8
0	40	16.4	61	3.2	658	873	0	0	0.27	0.23	1.2	3
0	36	11.6	51	4.4	530	810	0	0	0.13	0.08	0.6	0
0	57	12.6	191	7.8	1189	13	0	0	0.25	0.10	0.3	0

(continued on the following page)

Nutritive Value of the Edible Part of Food

FOOD DESCRIPTION	MEASURE OF EDIBLE PORTION	WEIGHT (g)	WATER (%)	CALORIES (kcal)	PROTEIN (g)	TOTAL FAT (g)	FATTY ACIDS		
							SATU- RATED (g)	MONO- UNSATU- RATED (g)	POLY- UNSATU- RATED (g)
LEGUMES, NUTS, AND SEEDS									
(continued)									
Black-eyed peas, dry									
Cooked	1 cup	172	70	200	13	1	0.2	0.1	0.4
Brazil nuts, shelled	1 oz (6–8 nuts)	28	3	186	4	19	4.6	6.5	6.8
Cashews, salted									
Oil roasted	1 cup	130	4	749	21	63	12.4	36.9	10.6
Chickpeas, dry									
Cooked	1 cup	164	60	269	15	4	0.4	1.0	1.9
Canned, solids and liquid	1 cup	240	70	286	12	3	0.3	0.6	1.2
Coconut									
Raw									
Piece, about 2 x 2 x 1/2 inches	1 piece	45	47	159	1	15	13.4	0.6	0.2
Dried, sweetened, shredded	1 cup	93	13	466	3	33	29.3	1.4	0.4
Hazelnuts (filberts), chopped	1 cup	115	5	722	17	70	5.1	52.5	9.1
Hummus, commercial	1 tbsp	14	67	23	1	1	0.2	0.6	0.5
Lentils, dry, cooked	1 cup	198	70	230	18	1	0.1	0.1	0.3
Macadamia nuts, dry-roasted, salted	1 cup	134	2	959	10	102	16.0	79.4	2.0
Mixed nuts, with peanuts, salted									
Dry-roasted	1 oz	28	2	168	5	15	2.0	8.9	3.1
Oil-roasted									
Peanuts									
Dry-roasted									
Salted	1 oz (about 28)	28	2	166	7	14	2.0	7.0	4.4
Unsalted									
Oil-roasted, salted	1 cup	144	2	837	38	71	9.9	35.2	22.4
Peanut butter									
Regular									
Smooth style	1 tbsp	16	1	95	4	8	1.7	3.9	2.2
Chunk style	1 tbsp	16	1	94	4	8	1.5	3.8	2.3
Reduced fat, smooth	1 tbsp	18	1	94	5	6	1.3	2.9	1.8
Peas, split, dry, cooked	1 cup	196	69	231	16	1	0.1	0.2	0.3
Pecans, halves	1 cup	108	4	746	10	78	6.7	44.0	23.3
Pistachio nuts, dry-roasted, with salt, shelled	1 oz (47 nuts)	28	2	161	6	13	1.6	6.8	3.9
Refried beans, canned	1 cup	252	76	237	14	3	1.2	1.4	0.4
Sesame seeds	1 tbsp	8	5	47	2	4	0.6	1.7	1.9
Soybeans, dry, cooked	1 cup	172	63	298	29	15	2.2	3.4	8.7
Soy products									
Miso	1 cup	275	41	567	32	17	2.4	3.7	9.4
Soy milk	1 cup	245	93	81	7	5	0.5	0.8	2.0
Tofu									
Firm	1/4 block	81	8	62	7	4	0.5	0.8	2.0
Soft, piece 2 1/2 x 2 3/4 x 1 inches	1 piece	120	87	73	8	4	0.6	1.0	2.5
Sunflower seed kernels, dry-roasted, with salt	1/4 cup	32	1	186	6	16	1.7	3.0	10.5
Walnuts, English	1 cup chopped	120	4	785	18	78	7.4	10.7	56.6
	1 oz (14 halves)	28	4	185	4	18	1.7	2.5	13.4

CHOLES-TEROL (mg)	CARBO-HYDRATE (g)	TOTAL DIETARY FIBER (g)	CALCIUM (mg)	IRON (mg)	POTAS-SIUM (mg)	SODIUM (mg)	VITAMIN A (IU)	(RE)	THIAMIN (mg)	RIBO-FLAVIN (mg)	NIACIN (mg)	ASCOR-BIC ACID (mg)
0	36	11.2	41	4.3	478	7	26	3	0.35	0.09	0.9	1
0	4	1.5	50	1.0	170	1	0	0	0.28	0.03	0.5	Tr
0	37	4.9	53	5.3	689	814	0	0	0.55	0.23	2.3	0
0	45	12.5	80	4.7	477	11	44	5	0.19	0.10	0.9	2
0	54	10.6	77	3.2	413	718	58	5	0.07	0.08	0.3	9
0	7	4.1	6	1.1	160	9	0	0	0.03	0.01	0.2	1
0	44	4.2	14	1.8	313	244	0	0	0.03	0.02	0.4	1
0	19	11.2	131	5.4	782	0	46	5	0.74	0.13	2.1	7
0	2	0.8	5	0.3	32	53	4	Tr	0.03	0.01	0.1	0
0	40	15.6	38	6.6	731	4	16	2	0.33	0.14	2.1	3
0	17	10.7	94	3.6	486	355	0	0	0.95	0.12	3.0	1
0	7	2.6	20	1.0	169	190	4	Tr	0.06	0.06	1.3	Tr
0	6	2.3	15	0.6	187	230	0	0	0.12	0.03	3.8	0
0	27	13.2	127	2.6	982	624	0	0	0.36	0.16	20.6	0
0	3	0.9	6	0.3	107	75	0	0	0.01	0.02	2.1	0
0	3	1.1	7	0.3	120	78	0	0	0.02	0.02	2.2	0
0	6	0.9	6	0.3	120	97	0	0	0.05	0.01	2.6	0
0	41	16.3	27	2.5	710	4	14	2	0.37	0.11	1.7	1
0	15	10.4	76	2.7	443	0	83	9	0.71	0.14	1.3	1
0	8	2.9	31	1.2	293	121	151	15	0.24	0.04	0.4	1
20	39	13.4	88	4.2	673	753	0	0	0.07	0.04	0.8	15
0	1	0.9	10	0.6	33	3	5	1	0.06	0.01	0.4	0
0	17	10.3	175	8.8	886	2	15	2	0.27	0.49	0.7	3
0	77	14.9	182	7.5	451	10,029	239	25	0.27	0.69	2.4	0
0	4	3.2	10	1.4	345	29	78	7	0.39	0.17	0.4	0
0	2	0.3	131	1.2	143	6	6	1	0.08	0.08	Tr	Tr
0	2	0.2	133	1.3	144	10	8	1	0.06	0.04	0.6	Tr
0	8	2.9	22	1.2	272	250	0	0	0.03	0.08	2.3	Tr
0	16	8.0	125	3.5	529	2	49	5	0.41	0.18	2.3	2
0	4	1.9	29	0.8	125	1	12	1	0.10	0.04	0.5	Tr

(continued on the following page)

FOOD DESCRIPTION	MEASURE OF EDIBLE PORTION	WEIGHT (g)	WATER (%)	CALORIES (kcal)	PROTEIN (g)	TOTAL FAT (g)	FATTY ACIDS		
							SATU-RATED (g)	MONO-UNSATU-RATED (g)	POLY-UNSATU-RATED (g)
MEAT AND MEAT PRODUCTS									
Beef, cooked									
Cuts braised, simmered, or pot roasted									
Relatively fat, such as chuck blade, piece, 2 1/2 x 2 1/2 x 3/4 inches									
Lean and fat	3 oz	85	47	293	23	22	8.7	9.4	0.8
Ground beef, broiled									
83% lean	3 oz	85	57	218	22	14	5.5	6.1	0.5
73% lean	3 oz	85	54	246	20	18	6.9	7.7	0.7
Liver, fried, slice, 6 1/2 x 2 3/8 x 3/8 inches	3 oz	85	56	184	23	7	2.3	1.4	1.5
Roast, oven cooked, no liquid added									
Relatively lean, such as eye of round, 2 pieces, 2 1/2 x 2 1/2 x 3/8 inches									
Steak, sirloin, broiled, piece, 2 1/2 x 2 1/2 x 3/4 inches									
Lean and fat	3 oz	85	57	219	24	13	5.2	5.6	0.5
Lean only	3 oz	85	62	166	26	6	2.4	2.6	0.2
Beef, dried, chipped	1 oz	28	57	47	8	1	0.5	0.5	0.1
Lamb, cooked									
Chops									
Loin, broiled									
Lean, and fat	3 oz	85	52	269	21	20	8.4	8.2	1.4
Lean only	3 oz	85	61	184	25	8	3.0	3.6	0.5
Leg, roasted, 2 pieces, 4 1/8 x 2 1/4 x 1/4 inches									
Lean and fat	3 oz	85	57	219	22	14	5.9	5.9	1.0
Lean only	3 oz	85	64	162	24	7	2.3	2.9	0.4
Pork, cured, cooked									
Bacon									
Regular	3 medium slices	19	13	109	6	9	3.3	4.5	1.1
Canadian style (6 slices per 6-oz pkg)	2 slices	47	62	86	11	4	1.3	1.9	0.4
Ham, canned, roasted 2 pieces, 4 1/8 x 2 1/4 x 1/4 inches	3 oz	85	67	142	18	7	2.4	3.5	0.8
Pork, fresh, cooked									
Chop, loin (cut 3 per lb with bone)									
Broiled									
Lean and fat	3 oz	85	58	204	24	11	4.1	5.0	0.8
Lean only	3 oz	85	61	172	26	7	2.5	3.1	0.5
Pan fried									
Lean and fat	3 oz	85	53	235	25	14	5.1	6.0	1.6
Lean only	3 oz	85	57	197	27	9	3.1	3.8	1.1
Sausages and luncheon meats									
Bologna, beef and pork (8 slices per 8-oz pkg)	2 slices	57	54	180	7	16	6.1	7.6	1.4

CHOLES-TEROL (mg)	CARBO-HYDRATE (g)	TOTAL DIETARY FIBER (g)	CALCIUM (mg)	IRON (mg)	POTAS-SIUM (mg)	SODIUM (mg)	VITAMIN A (IU)	VITAMIN A (RE)	THIAMIN (mg)	RIBO-FLAVIN (mg)	NIACIN (mg)	ASCOR-BIC ACID (mg)
88	0	0.0	11	2.6	196	54	0	0	0.06	0.20	2.1	0
71	0	0.0	6	2.0	266	60	0	0	0.05	0.23	4.2	0
77	0	0.0	9	2.1	248	71	0	0	0.03	0.16	4.9	0
410	7	0.0	9	5.3	309	90	30,689	9120	0.18	3.52	12.3	20
77	0	0.0	9	2.6	311	54	0	0	0.09	0.23	3.3	0
76	0	0.0	9	2.9	343	56	0	0	0.11	0.25	3.6	0
12	Tr	0.0	2	1.3	126	984	0	0	0.02	0.06	1.5	0
85	0	0.0	17	1.5	278	65	0	0	0.09	0.21	6.0	0
81	0	0.0	16	1.7	320	71	0	0	0.09	0.24	5.8	0
79	0	0.0	9	1.7	266	56	0	0	0.09	0.23	5.6	0
76	0	0.0	7	1.8	287	58	0	0	0.09	0.25	5.4	0
16	Tr	0.0	2	0.3	92	303	0	0	0.13	0.05	1.4	0
27	1	0.0	5	0.4	181	719	0	0	0.38	0.09	3.2	0
35	Tr	0.0	6	0.9	298	9.8	0	0	0.82	0.21	4.3	0
70	0	0.0	28	0.7	304	49	8	3	0.91	0.24	4.5	Tr
70	0	0.0	26	0.7	319	51	7	2	0.98	0.26	4.7	Tr
78	0	0.0	23	0.8	361	68	7	2	0.97	0.26	4.8	1
78	0	0.0	20	0.8	382	73	7	2	1.06	0.28	5.1	1
31	2	0.0	7	0.9	103	581	0	0	0.10	0.08	1.5	0

(continued on the following page)

FOOD DESCRIPTION	MEASURE OF EDIBLE PORTION	WEIGHT (g)	WATER (%)	CALORIES (kcal)	PROTEIN (g)	TOTAL FAT (g)	FATTY ACIDS		
							SATU-RATED (g)	MONO-UNSATU-RATED (g)	POLY-UNSATU-RATED (g)
MEAT AND MEAT PRODUCTS									
(continued)									
Braunschweiger									
(6 slices per 6-oz pkg)	2 slices	57	48	205	8	18	6.2	8.5	2.1
Brown and serve, cooked,									
link, 4 x 7/8 inches raw	2 links	26	45	103	4	9	3.4	4.5	1.0
Canned, minced luncheon meat									
Pork with ham (12 slices									
per 12-oz can)	2 slices	57	52	188	8	17	5.7	7.7	1.2
Pork and chicken (12 slices									
per 12-oz can)	2 slices	57	64	117	9	8	2.7	3.8	0.8
Chopped ham (8 slices									
per 6-oz pkg)	2 slices	21	64	48	4	4	1.2	1.7	0.4
Cooked ham (8 slices									
per 8-oz pkg)									
Regular	2 slices	57	65	104	10	6	1.9	2.8	0.7
Extra lean	2 slices	57	71	75	11	3	0.9	1.3	0.3
Frankfurter (10 per 1-lb pkg), heated									
Beef and pork	1 frank	45	54	144	5	13	4.8	6.2	1.2
Pork sausage, fresh, cooked									
Link (4 x 7/8 inches raw)	2 links	26	45	96	5	8	2.8	3.6	1.0
Patty (3 7/8 x 1/4 inches raw)	1 patty	27	45	100	5	8	2.9	3.8	1.0
Salami, beef and pork									
Cooked type (8 slices									
per 8-oz pkg)	2 slices	57	60	143	8	11	4.6	5.2	1.2
Vienna sausage (7 per									
4-oz can)	1 sausage	16	60	45	2	4	1.5	2.0	0.3
Veal, lean and fat, cooked									
Cutlet, braised, 4 1/8 x									
2 1/4 x 1/2 inches	3 oz	85	55	179	31	5	2.2	2.0	0.4
Rib, roasted, 2 pieces,									
4 1/8 x 2 1/4 x 1/4 inches	3 oz	85	60	194	20	12	4.6	4.6	0.8
MIXED DISHES AND FAST FOODS									
Mixed dishes									
Beef macaroni, frozen,									
Healthy Choice	1 package	240	78	211	14	2	0.7	1.2	0.3
Beef stew, canned	1 cup	232	82	218	11	12	5.2	5.5	0.5
Chicken pot pie, frozen	1 small pie	217	60	484	13	29	9.7	12.5	4.5
Chili con carne with beans,									
canned	1 cup	222	74	255	20	8	2.1	2.2	1.4
Macaroni and cheese,									
canned, made with									
corn oil	1 cup	252	82	199	8	6	3.0	NA	1.3
Meatless burger patty,									
frozen,									
Morningstar									
Farms	1 patty	85	71	91	14	1	0.1	0.3	0.2
Pasta with meatballs in									
tomato sauce, canned	1 cup	252	78	260	11	10	4.0	4.2	0.6
Spaghetti in tomato sauce									
with cheese, canned	1 cup	252	80	192	6	2	0.7	0.3	0.3
Tortellini, pasta with	3/4 cup								
cheese filling, frozen	(yields 1 cup								
	cooked)	81	31	249	11	6	2.9	1.7	0.4

CHOLESTEROL (mg)	CARBOHYDRATE (g)	TOTAL DIETARY FIBER (g)	CALCIUM (mg)	IRON (mg)	POTASSIUM (mg)	SODIUM (mg)	VITAMIN A (IU)	VITAMIN A (RE)	THIAMIN (mg)	RIBOFLAVIN (mg)	NIACIN (mg)	ASCORBIC ACID (mg)
89	2	0.0	5	5.3	113	652	8009	2405	0.14	0.87	4.8	0
18	1	0.0	3	0.3	49	209	0	0	0.09	0.04	0.9	0
40	1	0.0	0	0.4	233	758	0	0	0.18	0.10	2.0	0
43	1	0.0	0	0.7	352	539	0	0	0.10	0.12	2.0	18
11	0	0.0	1	0.2	67	288	0	0	0.13	0.04	0.8	0
32	2	0.0	4	0.6	189	751	0	0	0.49	0.14	3.0	0
27	1	0.0	4	0.4	200	815	0	0	0.53	0.13	2.8	0
23	1	0.0	5	0.5	75	504	0	0	0.09	0.05	1.2	0
22	Tr	0.0	8	0.3	94	336	0	0	0.19	0.07	1.2	1
22	Tr	0.0	9	0.3	97	349	0	0	0.20	0.07	1.2	1
37	1	0.0	7	1.5	113	607	0	0	0.14	0.21	2.0	0
8	Tr	0.0	2	0.1	16	152	0	0	0.01	0.02	0.3	0
114	0	0.0	7	1.1	326	57	0	0	0.05	0.30	9.0	0
94	0	0.0	9	0.8	251	78	0	0	0.04	0.23	5.9	0
14	33	4.6	46	2.7	365	444	514	50	0.28	0.16	3.1	58
37	16	3.5	28	1.6	404	947	3860	494	0.17	0.14	2.9	10
41	43	1.7	33	2.1	256	857	2285	343	0.25	0.36	4.1	2
24	24	8.2	67	3..3	608	1058	884	93	0.15	0.15	2.1	1
8	29	3.0	113	2.0	123	1058	713	NA	0.28	0.25	2.5	0
0	8	4.3	87	2.9	434	383	0	0	0.26	0.55	4.1	0
20	31	6.8	28	2.3	416	1053	920	93	0.19	0.16	3.3	8
8	39	7.8	40	2.8	302	963	932	58	0.35	0.28	4.5	10
34	38	1.5	123	1.2	72	279	50	13	0.25	0.25	2.2	0

(continued on the following page)

Nutritive Value of the Edible Part of Food

FOOD DESCRIPTION	MEASURE OF EDIBLE PORTION	WEIGHT (g)	WATER (%)	CALORIES (kcal)	PROTEIN (g)	TOTAL FAT (g)	SATURATED (g)	MONO-UNSATURATED (g)	POLY-UNSATURATED (g)
MIXED DISHES AND FAST FOODS									
(continued)									
Fast foods									
Breakfast items									
Biscuit with egg and sausage	1 biscuit	180	43	581	19	39	15.0	16.4	4.4
Croissant with egg, cheese, bacon	1 croissant	129	44	413	16	28	15.4	9.2	1.8
Danish pastry									
Cheese-filled	1 pastry	91	34	353	6	25	5.1	15.6	2.4
Fruit-filled	1 pastry	94	29	335	5	16	3.3	10.1	1.6
English muffin with egg, cheese, Canadian bacon	1 muffin	137	57	289	17	13	4.7	4.7	1.6
French toast sticks	5 sticks	141	30	513	8	29	4.7	12.6	9.9
Hashed brown potatoes	1/2 cup	72	60	151	2	9	4.3	3.9	0.5
Pancakes with butter, syrup	2 pancakes	232	50	520	8	14	5.9	5.3	2.0
Burrito									
With beans and cheese	1 burrito	93	54	189	8	6	3.4	1.2	0.9
With beans and meat	1 burrito	116	52	255	11	9	4.2	3.5	0.6
Cheeseburger									
Regular size, with condiments									
Double patty with mayo-type dressing, vegetables	1 sandwich	166	51	417	21	21	8.7	7.8	2.7
Single patty	1 sandwich	113	48	295	16	14	6.3	5.3	1.1
Large, with condiments									
Single patty with mayo-type dressing, vegetables	1 sandwich	219	53	563	28	33	15.0	12.6	2.0
Single patty with bacon	1 sandwich	195	44	608	32	37	16.2	14.5	2.7
Chicken fillet (breaded and fried) sandwich, plain	1 sandwich	182	47	515	24	29	8.5	10.4	8.4
Chili con carne	1 cup	253	77	256	25	8	3.4	3.4	0.5
Chimichanga with beef	1 chimichanga	174	51	425	20	20	8.5	8.1	1.1
Coleslaw	3/4 cup	99	74	147	1	11	1.6	2.4	6.4
Desserts									
Ice milk, soft, vanilla, in cone	1 cone	103	65	164	4	6	3.5	1.8	0.4
Pie, fried, with fruit filling (5 x 3 3/4 inches)	1 pie	128	38	404	4	21	3.1	9.5	6.9
Sundae, hot fudge	1 sundae	158	60	284	6	9	5.0	2.3	0.8
Enchilada with cheese	1 enchilada	163	63	319	10	19	10.6	6.3	0.8
Fish sandwich, with tartar sauce and cheese	1 sandwich	183	45	523	21	29	8.1	8.9	9.4
French fries	1 small	85	35	291	4	16	3.3	9.0	2.7
	1 medium	134	35	458	6	25	5.2	14.3	4.2
	1 large	169	35	578	7	31	6.5	18.0	5.3
Frijoles (refried beans, chili sauce, cheese)	1 cup	167	69	225	11	8	4.1	2.6	0.7
Hamburger									
Regular size, with condiments									
Double patty	1 sandwich	215	51	576	32	32	12.0	14.1	2.8
Single patty	1 sandwich	106	45	272	12	10	3.6	3.4	1.0

CHOLES-TEROL (mg)	CARBO-HYDRATE (g)	TOTAL DIETARY FIBER (g)	CALCIUM (mg)	IRON (mg)	POTAS-SIUM (mg)	SODIUM (mg)	VITAMIN A (IU)	(RE)	THIAMIN (mg)	RIBO-FLAVIN (mg)	NIACIN (mg)	ASCOR-BIC ACID (mg)
302	41	0.9	155	4.0	320	1141	635	164	0.50	0.45	3.6	0
215	24	Na	151	2.2	201	889	472	120	0.35	0.34	2.2	0
20	29	NA	70	1.8	116	319	155	43	0.26	0.21	2.5	3
19	45	NA	22	1.4	110	333	86	24	0.29	0.21	1.8	2
234	27	1.5	151	2.4	199	729	586	156	0.49	0.45	3.3	0
75	58	2.7	78	3.0	127	499	45	13	0.23	0.25	3.0	0
9	16	NA	7	0.5	267	290	18	3	0.08	0.01	1.1	5
58	91	NA	128	2.6	251	1104	281	70	0.39	0.56	3.4	3
14	27	NA	107	1.1	248	583	625	119	0.11	0.35	1.8	1
24	33	NA	53	2.5	329	670	319	32	0.27	0.42	2.7	1
60	35	NA	171	3.4	335	1051	398	65	0.35	0.28	8.1	2
37	27	NA	111	2.4	223	616	462	94	0.25	0.23	3.7	2
88	38	NA	206	4.7	445	1108	613	129	0.39	0.46	7.4	8
111	37	NA	162	4.7	332	1043	406	80	0.31	0.41	6.6	2
60	39	NA	60	4.7	353	957	100	31	0.33	0.24	6.8	9
134	22	NA	68	5.2	691	1007	1662	167	0.13	1.14	2.5	2
9	43	NA	63	4.5	586	910	146	16	0.49	0.64	5.8	5
5	13	NA	34	0.7	177	267	338	50	0.04	0.03	0.1	8
28	24	0.1	153	0.2	169	92	211	52	0.05	0.26	0.3	1
0	55	3.3	28	1.6	83	479	35	4	0.18	0.14	1.8	2
21	48	0.0	207	0.6	395	182	221	57	0.06	0.30	1.1	2
4	29	NA	324	1.3	240	784	1161	186	0.08	0.42	1.9	1
68	48	NA	185	3.5	353	939	432	97	0.46	0.42	4.2	3
0	34	3.0	12	0.7	586	168	0	0	0.07	0.03	2.4	10
0	53	4.7	19	1.0	923	265	0	0	0.11	0.05	3.8	16
0	67	5.9	24	1.3	1164	335	0	0	0.14	0.07	4.8	20
37	29	NA	189	2.2	605	882	456	70	0.13	0.33	1.5	2
103	39	NA	92	5.5	527	742	54	4	0.34	0.41	6.7	1
30	34	2.3	126	2.7	251	534	74	10	0.29	0.24	3.9	2

(continued on the following page)

FOOD DESCRIPTION	MEASURE OF EDIBLE PORTION	WEIGHT (g)	WATER (%)	CALORIES (kcal)	PROTEIN (g)	TOTAL FAT (g)	FATTY ACIDS		
							SATU- RATED (g)	MONO- UNSATU- RATED (g)	POLY- UNSATU- RATED (g)
MIXED DISHES AND FAST FOODS									
(continued)									
Large, with condiments, mayo-type dressing, and vegetables									
Double patty	1 sandwich	226	54	540	34	27	10.5	10.3	2.8
Single patty	1 sandwich	218	56	512	26	27	10.4	11.4	2.2
Hot dog									
Plain	1 sandwich	98	54	242	10	15	5.1	6.9	1.7
With chili	1 sandwich	114	48	296	14	13	4.9	6.6	1.2
With corn flour coating (corndog)	1 corndog	175	47	460	17	19	5.2	9.1	3.5
Mashed potatoes	1/3 cup	80	79	66	2	1	0.4	0.3	0.2
Nachos, with cheese sauce	6–8 nachos	113	40	346	9	19	7.8	8.0	2.2
Onion rings, breaded and fried	8–9 rings	83	37	276	4	16	7.0	6.7	0.7
Pizza (slice = 1/8 of 12-inch pizza)									
Cheese	1 slice	63	48	140	8	3	1.5	1.0	0.5
Pepperoni	1 slice	71	47	181	10	7	2.2	3.1	1.2
Roast beef sandwich, plain	1 sandwich	139	49	346	22	14	3.6	6.8	1.7
Salad, tossed, with chicken, no dressing	1 1/2 cups	218	87	105	17	2	0.6	0.7	0.6
Shake									
Chocolate	16 fl oz	333	72	423	11	12	7.7	3.6	0.5
Vanilla	16 fl oz	333	75	370	12	10	6.2	2.9	0.4
Shrimp, breaded and fried	6–8 shrimp	164	48	454	19	25	5.4	17.4	0.6
Submarine sandwich (6'-inches long), with oil and vinegar									
Cold cuts (with lettuce, cheese, salami, ham, tomato, onion)	1 sandwich	228	58	456	22	19	6.8	8.2	2.3
Roast beef (with tomato, lettuce, mayo)	1 sandwich	216	59	410	29	13	7.1	1.8	2.6
Tuna salad (with mayo, lettuce)	1 sandwich	256	54	584	30	28	5.3	13.4	7.3
Taco, beef	1 small	171	58	369	21	21	11.4	6.6	1.0
	1 large	263	58	568	32	32	17.5	10.1	1.5
Taco salad (with ground beef, cheese, taco shell)	1 1/2 cups	198	72	279	13	15	6.8	5.2	1.7
Tostada (with cheese, tomato, lettuce)									
With beans and beef	1 tostada	225	70	333	16	17	11.5	3.5	0.6
With guacamole	1 tostada	131	73	181	6	12	5.0	4.3	1.5
POULTRY AND POULTRY PRODUCTS									
Chicken									
Fried in vegetable shortening, meat with skin									
Batter dipped									
Breast, 1/2 breast (5.6 oz with bones)	1/2 breast	140	52	364	35	18	4.9	7.6	4.3
Drumstick (3.4 oz with bones)	1 drumstick	72	53	193	16	11	3.0	4.6	2.7
Flour coated									
Breast, 1/2 breast (4.2 oz with bones)	1/2 breast	98	57	218	31	9	2.4	3.4	1.9

CHOLES-TEROL (mg)	CARBO-HYDRATE (g)	TOTAL DIETARY FIBER (g)	CALCIUM (mg)	IRON (mg)	POTAS-SIUM (mg)	SODIUM (mg)	VITAMIN A (IU)	VITAMIN A (RE)	THIAMIN (mg)	RIBO-FLAVIN (mg)	NIACIN (mg)	ASCOR-BIC ACID (mg)
122	40	NA	102	5.9	570	791	102	11	0.36	0.38	7.6	1
87	40	NA	96	4.9	480	824	312	33	0.41	0.37	7.3	3
44	18	NA	24	2.3	143	670	0	0	0.24	0.27	3.6	Tr
51	31	NA	19	3.3	166	480	58	6	0.22	0.40	3.7	3
79	56	NA	102	6.2	263	973	207	37	0.28	0.70	4.2	0
2	13	NA	17	0.4	235	182	33	8	0.07	0.04	1.0	Tr
18	36	NA	272	1.3	172	816	559	92	0.19	0.37	1.5	1
14	31	NA	73	0.8	129	430	8	1	0.08	0.10	0.9	1
9	21	NA	117	0.6	110	336	382	74	0.18	0.16	2.5	1
14	20	NA	65	0.9	153	267	282	55	0.13	0.23	3.0	2
51	33	NA	54	4.2	316	792	210	21	0.38	0.31	5.9	2
72	4	NA	37	1.1	447	209	935	96	0.11	0.13	5.9	17
43	68	2.7	376	1.0	666	323	310	77	0.19	0.82	0.5	1
37	60	1.3	406	0.3	579	273	433	107	0.15	0.61	0.6	3
200	40	NA	84	3.0	184	1446	120	36	0.21	0.90	0.0	0
36	51	NA	189	2.5	394	1651	424	80	1.00	0.80	5.5	12
73	44	NA	41	2.8	330	845	413	50	0.41	0.41	6.0	6
49	55	NA	74	2.6	335	1293	187	41	0.46	0.33	11.3	4
56	27	NA	221	2.4	474	802	855	147	0.15	0.44	3.2	2
87	41	NA	339	3.7	729	1233	1315	226	0.24	0.68	4.9	3
44	24	NA	192	2.3	416	762	588	77	0.10	0.36	2.5	4
74	30	NA	189	2.5	491	871	1276	173	0.09	0.50	2.9	4
20	16	NA	212	0.8	326	401	879	109	0.07	0.29	1.0	2
119	13	0.4	28	1.8	281	385	94	28	0.16	0.20	14.7	0
62	6	0.2	12	1.0	134	194	62	19	0.08	0.15	3.7	0
87	2	0.1	16	1.2	254	74	49	15	0.08	0.13	13.5	0

(continued on the following page)

FOOD DESCRIPTION	MEASURE OF EDIBLE PORTION	WEIGHT (g)	WATER (%)	CALORIES (kcal)	PROTEIN (g)	TOTAL FAT (g)	FATTY ACIDS		
							SATU-RATED (g)	MONO-UNSATU-RATED (g)	POLY-UNSATU-RATED (g)
POULTRY AND POULTRY PRODUCTS									
(continued)									
Drumstick (2.6 oz with bones)	1 drumstick	49	57	120	13	7	1.8	2.7	1.6
Roasted, meat only									
Breast, 1/2 breast (4.2 oz with bone and skin)	1/2 breast	86	65	142	27	3	0.9	1.1	0.7
Drumstick (2.9 oz with bone and skin)	1 drumstick	44	67	76	12	2	0.7	0.8	0.6
Duck, roasted, flesh only	1/2 duck	221	64	444	52	25	9.2	8.2	3.2
Turkey									
Roasted, meat only									
Dark meat	3 oz	85	63	159	24	6	2.1	1.4	1.8
Light meat	3 oz	85	66	133	25	3	0.9	0.5	0.7
Ground, cooked									
Poultry food products									
Chicken									
Canned, boneless	5 oz	142	69	234	31	11	3.1	4.5	2.5
Frankfurter (10 per 1-lb pkg)	1 frank	45	58	116	6	9	2.5	3.8	1.8
Roll, light meat (6 slices per 6-oz pkg)	2 slices	57	69	90	11	4	1.1	1.7	0.9
Turkey									
Gravy and turkey, frozen	5-oz package	142	85	95	8	4	1.2	1.4	0.7
Patties, breaded or battered, fried (2.25 oz)	1 patty	64	50	181	9	12	3.0	4.8	3.0
SOUPS, SAUCES, AND GRAVIES									
Soups									
Canned, condensed									
Prepared with equal volume of whole milk									
Clam chowder, New England	1 cup	248	85	164	9	7	3.0	2.3	1.1
Cream of chicken	1 cup	248	85	191	7	11	4.6	4.5	1.6
Cream of mushroom	1 cup	248	85	203	6	14	5.1	3.0	4.6
Tomato	1 cup	248	85	161	6	6	2.9	1.6	1.1
Prepared with equal volume of water									
Bean with pork	1 cup	253	84	172	8	6	1.5	2.2	1.8
Beef broth, bouillon, consomme	1 cup	241	96	29	5	0	0.0	0.0	0.0
Beef noodle	1 cup	244	92	83	5	3	1.1	1.2	0.5
Chicken noodle	1 cup	241	92	75	4	2	0.7	1.1	0.6
Chicken and rice	1 cup	241	94	60	4	2	0.5	0.9	0.4
Clam chowder, Manhattan	1 cup	244	92	78	2	2	0.4	0.4	1.3
Cream of chicken	1 cup	244	91	117	3	7	2.1	3.3	1.5
Cream of mushroom	1 cup	244	90	129	2	9	2.4	1.7	4.2
Minestrone	1 cup	241	91	82	4	3	0.6	0.7	1.1
Pea, green	1 cup	250	83	165	9	3	1.4	1.0	0.4
Tomato	1 cup	244	90	85	2	2	0.4	0.4	1.0
Vegetable beef	1 cup	244	92	78	6	2	0.9	0.8	0.1
Vegetarian vegetable	1 cup	241	92	72	2	2	0.3	0.8	0.7
Canned, ready to serve, low fat, reduced sodium									
Chicken broth	1 cup	240	97	17	3	0	0.0	0.0	0.0

CHOLESTEROL (mg)	CARBOHYDRATE (g)	TOTAL DIETARY FIBER (g)	CALCIUM (mg)	IRON (mg)	POTASSIUM (mg)	SODIUM (mg)	VITAMIN A (IU)	VITAMIN A (RE)	THIAMIN (mg)	RIBOFLAVIN (mg)	NIACIN (mg)	ASCORBIC ACID (mg)
44	1	Tr	6	0.7	112	44	41	12	0.04	0.11	3.0	0
73	0	0.0	13	0.9	220	64	18	5	0.06	0.10	11.8	0
41	0	0.0	5	0.6	108	42	26	8	0.03	0.10	2.7	0
197	0	0.0	27	6.0	557	144	170	51	0.57	1.04	11.3	0
72	0	0.0	27	2.0	247	67	0	0	0.05	0.21	3.1	0
59	0	0.0	16	1.1	259	54	0	0	0.05	0.11	5.8	0
88	0	0.0	20	2.2	196	714	166	48	0.02	0.18	9.0	3
45	3	0.0	43	0.9	38	617	59	17	0.03	0.05	1.4	0
28	1	0.0	24	0.5	129	331	46	14	0.04	0.07	3.0	0
26	7	0.0	20	1.3	87	787	60	18	0.03	0.18	2.6	0
40	10	0.3	9	1.4	176	512	24	7	0.06	0.12	1.5	0
22	17	1.5	186	1.5	300	992	164	40	0.07	0.24	1.0	3
27	15	0.2	181	0.7	273	1047	714	94	0.07	0.26	0.9	1
20	15	0.5	179	0.6	270	918	154	37	0.08	0.28	0.9	2
17	22	2.7	159	1.8	449	744	848	109	0.13	0.25	1.5	68
3	23	8.6	81	2.0	402	951	888	89	0.09	0.03	0.6	2
0	2	0.0	10	0.5	154	636	0	0	0.02	0.03	0.7	1
5	9	0.7	15	1.1	100	952	630	63	0.07	0.06	1.1	Tr
7	9	0.7	17	0.8	55	1106	711	72	0.05	0.06	1.4	Tr
7	7	0.7	17	0.7	101	815	660	65	0.02	0.02	1.1	Tr
2	12	1.5	27	1.6	188	578	964	98	0.03	0.04	0.8	4
10	9	0.2	34	0.6	88	986	561	56	0.03	0.06	0.8	Tr
2	9	0.5	46	0.5	100	881	0	0	0.05	0.09	0.7	1
2	11	1.0	34	0.9	313	911	2338	234	0.05	0.04	0.9	1
0	27	2.8	28	2.0	190	918	203	20	0.11	0.07	1.2	2
0	17	0.5	12	1.8	264	695	688	68	0.09	0.05	1.4	66
5	10	0.5	17	1.1	173	791	1891	190	0.04	0.05	1.0	2
0	12	0.5	22	1.1	210	822	3005	301	0.05	0.05	0.9	1
0	1	0.0	19	0.6	204	554	0	0	Tr	0.03	1.6	1

(continued on the following page)

FOOD DESCRIPTION	MEASURE OF EDIBLE PORTION	WEIGHT (g)	WATER (%)	CALORIES (kcal)	PROTEIN (g)	TOTAL FAT (g)	FATTY ACIDS SATU-RATED (g)	MONO-UNSATU-RATED (g)	POLY-UNSATU-RATED (g)
SOUPS, SAUCES, AND GRAVIES									
(continued)									
Chicken noodle	1 cup	237	92	76	6	2	0.4	0.6	0.4
Chicken and rice	1 cup	241	88	116	7	3	0.9	1.3	0.7
Chicken and rice with vegetables	1 cup	239	91	88	6	1	0.4	0.5	0.5
Clam chowder, New England	1 cup	244	89	117	5	2	0.5	0.7	0.4
Lentil	1 cup	242	88	126	8	2	0.3	0.8	0.2
Minestrone	1 cup	241	87	123	5	3	0.4	0.9	1.0
Vegetable	1 cup	238	91	81	4	1	0.3	0.4	0.3
Ready-to-serve									
Barbecue	1 tbsp	16	81	12	Tr	Tr	Tr	0.1	0.1
Cheese	1/4 cup	63	71	110	4	8	3.8	2.4	1.6
Hoisin	1 tbsp	16	44	35	1	1	0.1	0.2	0.3
Nacho cheese	1/4 cup	63	70	119	5	10	4.2	3.1	2.1
Pepper or hot	1 tsp	5	90	1	Tr	Tr	Tr	Tr	Tr
Salsa	1 tbsp	16	90	4	Tr	Tr	Tr	Tr	Tr
Soy	1 tbsp	16	69	9	1	Tr	Tr	Tr	Tr
Spaghetti/marinara/pasta	1 cup	250	87	143	4	5	0.7	2.2	1.8
Teriyaki	1 tbsp	18	68	15	1	0	0.0	0.0	0.0
Worcestershire	1 tbsp	17	70	11	0	0	0.0	0.0	0.0
Gravies, canned									
Beef	1/4 cup	58	87	31	2	1	0.7	0.6	Tr
Chicken	1/4 cup	60	85	47	1	3	0.8	1.5	0.9
SUGARS AND SWEETS									
Candy									
Chocolate, milk									
Plain	1 bar (1.55 oz)	44	1	226	3	14	8.1	4.4	0.5
With almonds	1 bar (1.45 oz)	41	2	216	4	14	7.0	5.5	0.9
With peanuts, Mr. Goodbar (Hershey)	1 bar (1.75 oz)	49	1	267	5	17	7.3	5.7	2.4
With rice, cereal, Nestle Crunch	1 bar (1.55 oz)	44	1	230	3	12	6.7	3.8	0.4
Chocolate chips									
Milk	1 cup	168	1	862	12	52	31.0	16.7	1.8
Semisweet	1 cup	168	1	805	7	50	29.8	16.7	1.6
White	1 cup	170	1	916	10	55	33.0	15.5	1.7
Fudge, prepared from recipe									
Chocolate									
Plain	1 piece	17	10	65	Tr	1	0.9	0.4	0.1
With nuts	1 piece	19	7	81	1	3	1.1	0.8	1.0
Gumdrops/gummy candies									
Gumdrops (3/4-inch diameter)	1 cup	182	1	703	0	0	0.0	0.0	0.0
	1 medium	4	1	16	0	0	0.0	0.0	0.0
Hard candy	1 piece	6	1	24	0	Tr	0.0	0.0	0.0
	1 small piece	3	1	12	0	Tr	0.0	0.0	0.0
Jelly beans	10 large	28	6	104	0	Tr	Tr	0.1	Tr
	10 small	11	6	40	0	Tr	Tr	Tr	Tr
Marshmallows									
Miniature	1 cup	50	16	159	1	Tr	Tr	Tr	Tr
Regular	1 regular	7	16	23	Tr	Tr	Tr	Tr	Tr
Special Dark sweet choclate (Hershey)	1 miniature	8	1	46	Tr	3	1.7	0.9	0.1
Frosting, ready-to-eat									
Chocolate	1/12 package	38	17	151	Tr	7	2.1	3.4	0.8
Vanilla	1/12 package	38	13	159	Tr	6	1.9	3.3	0.9

CHOLES-TEROL (mg)	CARBO-HYDRATE (g)	TOTAL DIETARY FIBER (g)	CALCIUM (mg)	IRON (mg)	POTAS-SIUM (mg)	SODIUM (mg)	VITAMIN A (IU)	VITAMIN A (RE)	THIAMIN (mg)	RIBO-FLAVIN (mg)	NIACIN (mg)	ASCOR-BIC ACID (mg)
19	9	1.2	19	1.1	209	460	920	95	0.11	0.11	3.4	1
14	14	0.7	22	1.0	422	482	2010	202	0.05	0.13	5.0	2
17	12	0.7	24	1.2	275	459	1644	165	0.12	0.07	2.6	1
5	20	1.2	17	0.9	283	529	244	59	0.05	0.09	0.9	5
0	20	5.6	41	2.7	336	443	951	94	0.11	0.09	0.7	1
0	20	1.2	39	1.7	306	170	1357	135	0.15	0.08	1.0	1
5	13	1.4	31	1.5	290	466	3196	319	0.08	0.07	1.8	1
0	2	0.2	3	0.1	28	130	139	14	Tr	Tr	0.1	1
18	4	0.3	116	0.1	19	522	199	40	Tr	0.07	Tr	Tr
Tr	7	0.4	5	0.2	19	258	2	Tr	Tr	0.03	0.2	Tr
20	3	0.5	118	0.2	20	492	128	32	Tr	0.08	Tr	Tr
0	Tr	0.1	Tr	Tr	7	124	14	1	Tr	Tr	Tr	4
0	1	0.3	5	0.2	34	69	96	10	0.01	0.01	0.1	2
0	1	0.1	3	0.3	64	871	0	0	0.01	0.03	0.4	0
0	21	4.0	55	1.8	738	1030	938	95	0.14	0.10	2.7	20
0	3	Tr	5	0.3	41	690	0	0	0.01	0.01	0.2	0
0	3	0.0	18	0.9	136	167	18	2	0.01	0.02	0.1	2
2	3	0.2	3	0.4	47	325	0	0	0.02	0.02	0.4	0
1	3	0.2	12	0.3	65	346	221	67	0.01	0.03	0.3	0
10	26	1.5	84	0.6	169	36	81	24	0.03	0.13	0.1	Tr
8	22	2.5	92	0.7	182	30	30	6	0.02	0.18	0.3	Tr
4	25	1.7	53	0.6	219	73	70	18	0.08	0.12	1.6	Tr
6	29	1.1	74	0.2	151	59	30	9	0.15	0.25	1.7	Tr
37	99	5.7	321	2.3	647	138	311	92	0.13	0.51	0.5	1
0	106	9.9	54	5.3	613	18	35	3	0.09	0.15	0.7	0
36	101	0.0	338	0.4	486	153	60	2	0.11	0.48	1.3	1
2	14	0.1	7	0.1	18	11	32	8	Tr	0.01	Tr	Tr
3	14	0.2	10	0.1	30	11	38	9	0.01	0.02	Tr	Tr
0	180	0.0	5	0.7	9	80	0	0	0.00	Tr	Tr	0
0	4	0.0	Tr	Tr	Tr	2	0	0	0.00	Tr	Tr	0
0	6	0.0	Tr	Tr	Tr	2	0	0	Tr	Tr	Tr	0
0	3	0.0	Tr	Tr	Tr	1	0	0	Tr	Tr	Tr	0
0	26	0.0	1	0.3	10	7	0	0	0.00	0.00	0.0	0
0	10	0.0	Tr	0.1	4	3	0	0	0.00	0.00	0.0	0
0	41	0.1	2	0.1	3	24	1	0	Tr	Tr	Tr	0
0	6	Tr	Tr	Tr	Tr	3	Tr	0	Tr	Tr	Tr	0
Tr	5	0.4	2	0.2	25	1	3	Tr	Tr	0.01	Tr	0
0	24	0.2	3	0.5	74	70	249	75	Tr	0.01	Tr	0
0	26	Tr	1	Tr	14	34	283	86	0.00	Tr	Tr	0

(continued on the following page)

FOOD DESCRIPTION	MEASURE OF EDIBLE PORTION	WEIGHT (g)	WATER (%)	CALORIES (kcal)	PROTEIN (g)	TOTAL FAT (g)	FATTY ACIDS		
							SATU-RATED (g)	MONO-UNSATU-RATED (g)	POLY-UNSATU-RATED (g)
SUGARS AND SWEETS									
(continued)									
Gelatin dessert, prepared with gelatin dessert powder and water									
Regular	1/2 cup	135	85	80	2	0	0.0	0.0	0.0
Reduced calorie (with aspartame)	1/2 cup	117	98	8	1	0	0.0	0.0	0.0
Honey, strained or extracted	1 tbsp	21	17	64	Tr	0	0.0	0.0	0.0
Jams and preserves	1 tbsp	20	30	56	Tr	Tr	Tr	Tr	0.0
Jellies	1 tbsp	19	29	54	Tr	Tr	Tr	Tr	Tr
Puddings									
Prepared with dry mix and 2% milk									
Chocolate									
Instant	1/2 cup	147	75	150	5	3	1.6	0.9	0.2
Regular (cooked)	1/2 cup	142	74	151	5	3	1.8	0.8	0.1
Vanilla									
Instant	1/2 cup	142	75	148	4	2	1.4	0.7	0.1
Regular (cooked)	1/2 cup	140	76	141	4	2	1.5	0.7	0.1
Sugar									
Brown									
Packed	1 cup	220	2	827	0	0	0.0	0.0	0.0
Unpacked	1 tbsp	9	2	34	0	0	0.0	0.0	0.0
White									
Granulated	1 tsp	4	0	16	0	0	0.0	0.0	0.0
	1 cup	200	0	774	0	0	0.0	0.0	0.0
Powdered, unsifted	1 tbsp	8	Tr	31	0	Tr	Tr	Tr	Tr
	1 cup	120	Tr	467	0	Tr	Tr	Tr	0.1
Syrup									
Chocolate-flavored syrup or topping									
Thin-type	1 tbsp	19	31	53	Tr	Tr	0.1	0.1	Tr
Fudge-type	1 tbsp	19	22	67	1	2	0.8	0.7	0.1
Corn, light	1 tbsp	20	23	56	0	0	0.0	0.0	0.0
Maple	1 tbsp	20	32	52	0	Tr	Tr	Tr	Tr
Molasses, blackstrap	1 tbsp	20	29	47	0	0	0.0	0.0	0.0
Table blend, pancake									
Regular	1 tbsp	20	24	57	0	0	0.0	0.0	0.0
Reduced calorie	1 tbsp	15	55	25	0	0	0.0	0.0	0.0
VEGETABLES AND VEGETABLE PRODUCTS									
Alfalfa sprouts, raw	1 cup	33	91	10	1	Tr	Tr	Tr	0.1
Artichokes, globe or French, cooked, drained	1 cup	168	84	84	6	Tr	0.1	Tr	0.1
	1 medium	120	84	60	4	Tr	Tr	Tr	0.1
Asparagus, green									
Cooked, drained									
From raw	1 cup	180	92	43	5	1	0.1	Tr	0.2
	4 spears	60	92	14	2	Tr	Tr	Tr	0.1
From frozen	1 cup	180	91	50	5	1	0.2	Tr	0.3
	4 spears	60	91	17	2	Tr	0.1	Tr	0.1
	4 spears	72	94	14	2	Tr	0.1	Tr	0.2
Bamboo shoots, canned, drained	1 cup	131	94	25	2	1	0.1	Tr	0.2
Beans									
Lima, immature seeds, frozen, cooked, drained									
Baby limas	1 cup	180	72	189	12	1	0.1	Tr	0.3

CHOLESTEROL (mg)	CARBOHYDRATE (g)	TOTAL DIETARY FIBER (g)	CALCIUM (mg)	IRON (mg)	POTASSIUM (mg)	SODIUM (mg)	VITAMIN A (IU)	VITAMIN A (RE)	THIAMIN (mg)	RIBOFLAVIN (mg)	NIACIN (mg)	ASCORBIC ACID (mg)
0	19	0.0	3	Tr	1	57	0	0	0.00	Tr	Tr	0
0	1	0.0	2	Tr	0	56	0	0	0.00	Tr	Tr	0
0	17	Tr	1	0.1	11	1	0	0	0.00	0.01	Tr	Tr
0	14	0.2	4	0.1	15	6	2	Tr	0.00	Tr	Tr	2
0	13	0.2	2	Tr	12	5	3	Tr	Tr	Tr	Tr	Tr
9	28	0.6	153	0.4	247	417	253	56	0.05	0.21	0.1	1
10	28	0.4	160	0.5	240	149	253	68	0.05	0.21	0.2	1
9	28	0.0	146	0.1	185	406	241	64	0.05	0.20	0.1	1
10	26	0.0	153	0.1	193	224	252	70	0.04	0.20	0.1	1
0	214	0.0	187	4.2	761	86	0	0	0.02	0.02	0.2	0
0	9	0.0	8	0.2	31	4	0	0	Tr	Tr	Tr	0
0	4	0.0	Tr	Tr	Tr	Tr	0	0	0.00	Tr	0.0	0
0	200	0.0	2	0.1	4	2	0	0	0.00	0.04	0.0	0
0	8	0.0	Tr	Tr	Tr	Tr	0	0	0.00	0.00	0.0	0
0	119	0.0	1	0.1	2	1	0	0	0.00	0.00	0.0	0
0	12	0.3	3	0.4	43	14	6	1	Tr	0.01	0.1	Tr
Tr	12	0.5	15	0.2	69	66	3	1	0.01	0.0	0.1	Tr
0	15	0.0	1	Tr	1	24	0	0	Tr	Tr	Tr	0
0	13	0.0	13	0.2	41	2	0	0	Tr	Tr	Tr	0
0	12	0.0	172	3.5	498	11	0	0	0.01	0.01	0.2	0
0	15	0.0	Tr	Tr	Tr	17	0	0	Tr	Tr	Tr	0
0	7	0.0	Tr	Tr	Tr	30	0	0	Tr	Tr	Tr	0
0	1	0.8	11	0.3	26	2	51	5	0.03	0.04	0.2	3
0	19	9.1	76	2.2	595	160	297	30	0.11	0.11	1.7	17
0	13	6.5	54	1.5	425	114	212	22	0.08	0.08	1.2	12
0	8	2.9	36	1.3	288	20	970	97	0.22	0.23	1.9	19
0	3	1.0	12	0.4	96	7	323	32	0.07	0.08	0.6	6
0	9	2.9	41	1.2	392	7	1472	148	0.12	0.19	1.9	44
0	3	1.0	14	0.4	131	2	491	49	0.04	0.06	0.6	15
0	2	1.2	12	1.3	124	207	382	38	0.04	0.07	0.7	13
0	4	1.8	10	0.4	105	9	10	1	0.03	0.03	0.2	1
0	35	10.8	50	3.5	740	52	301	31	0.13	0.10	1.4	10

(continued on the following page)

FOOD DESCRIPTION	MEASURE OF EDIBLE PORTION	WEIGHT (g)	WATER (%)	CALORIES (kcal)	PROTEIN (g)	TOTAL FAT (g)	FATTY ACIDS		
							SATU-RATED (g)	MONO-UNSATU-RATED (g)	POLY-UNSATU-RATED (g)

VEGETABLES AND VEGETABLE PRODUCTS
(continued)

FOOD DESCRIPTION	MEASURE	WEIGHT	WATER	CALORIES	PROTEIN	TOTAL FAT	SATU-RATED	MONO	POLY
Snap, cut									
Cooked, drained									
From raw									
Green	1 cup	125	89	44	2	Tr	0.1	Tr	0.2
Yellow	1 cup	125	89	44	2	Tr	0.1	Tr	0.2
From frozen									
Green	1 cup	135	91	38	2	Tr	0.1	Tr	0.1
Yellow	1 cup	135	91	38	2	Tr	0.1	Tr	0.1
Canned, drained									
Green	1 cup	135	93	27	2	Tr	Tr	Tr	0.1
Yellow	1 cup	135	93	27	2	Tr	Tr	Tr	0.1
Beans, dry. See Legumes.									
Bean sprouts (mung)									
Raw	1 cup	104	90	31	3	Tr	Tr	Tr	0.1
Cooked, drained	1 cup	124	93	26	3	Tr	Tr	Tr	Tr
Beets									
Cooked, drained									
Slices	1 cup	170	87	75	3	Tr	Tr	0.1	0.1
Canned, drained									
Slices	1 cup	170	91	53	2	Tr	Tr	Tr	0.1
Beet greens, leaves and stems, cooked, drained, 1-inch pieces	1 cup	144	89	39	4	Tr	Tr	0.1	0.1
Black-eyed peas, immature seeds, cooked, drained									
From raw	1 cup	165	75	160	5	1	0.2	0.1	0.3
From frozen	1 cup	170	66	224	14	1	0.3	0.1	0.5
Broccoli									
Raw									
Chopped or diced	1 cup	88	91	25	3	Tr	Tr	Tr	0.1
Spear, about 5 inches long	1 spear	31	91	9	1	Tr	Tr	Tr	0.1
Flower cluster	1 floweret	11	91	3	Tr	Tr	Tr	Tr	Tr
Brussels sprouts, cooked, drained									
From raw	1 cup	156	87	61	4	1	0.2	0.1	0.4
From frozen	1 cup	155	87	65	6	1	0.1	Tr	0.3
Cabbage, common varieties, shredded									
Raw	1 cup	70	92	18	1	Tr	Tr	Tr	0.1
Cooked, drained	1 cup	150	94	33	2	1	0.1	Tr	0.3
Cabbage, Chinese, shredded, cooked, drained									
Pak choi or bok choy	1 cup	170	96	20	3	Tr	Tr	Tr	0.1
Cabbage, red, raw, shredded	1 cup	70	92	17	1	Tr	Tr	Tr	0.1
Cabbage, savoy, raw, shredded	1 cup	70	92	19	1	Tr	Tr	Tr	Tr
Carrot juice									
Carrots									
Raw									
Whole, 7 1/2 inches long	1 carrot	72	88	31	1	Tr	Tr	Tr	0.1
Grated	1 cup	110	88	47	1	Tr	Tr	Tr	0.1
Cauliflower									
Raw	1 floweret	13	92	3	Tr	Tr	Tr	Tr	Tr
	1 cup	100	92	25	2	Tr	Tr	Tr	0.1

CHOLESTEROL (mg)	CARBO-HYDRATE (g)	TOTAL DIETARY FIBER (g)	CALCIUM (mg)	IRON (mg)	POTAS-SIUM (mg)	SODIUM (mg)	VITAMIN A (IU)	VITAMIN A (RE)	THIAMIN (mg)	RIBO-FLAVIN (mg)	NIACIN (mg)	ASCOR-BIC ACID (mg)
0	10	4.0	58	1.6	374	4	833	84	0.09	0.12	0.8	12
0	10	4.1	58	1.6	374	4	101	10	0.09	0.12	0.8	12
0	9	4.1	66	1.2	170	12	841	54	0.05	0.12	0.5	6
0	9	4.1	66	1.2	170	12	151	15	0.05	0.12	0.5	6
0	6	2.6	35	1.2	147	354	471	47	0.02	0.08	0.3	6
0	6	1.8	35	1.2	147	339	142	15	0.02	0.08	0.3	6
0	6	1.9	14	0.9	155	6	22	2	0.09	0.13	0.8	14
0	5	1.5	15	0.8	125	12	17	1	0.06	0.13	1.0	14
0	17	3.4	27	1.3	519	131	60	7	0.05	0.07	0.6	6
0	12	2.9	26	3.1	252	330	19	2	0.02	0.07	0.3	7
0	8	4.2	164	2.7	1309	347	7344	734	0.17	0.42	0.7	36
0	34	8.3	211	1.8	690	7	1305	130	0.17	0.24	2.3	4
0	40	10.9	39	3.6	638	9	128	14	0.44	0.11	1.2	4
0	5	2.6	42	0.8	286	24	1357	136	0.06	0.10	0.6	82
0	2	0.9	15	0.3	101	8	478	48	0.02	0.04	0.2	29
0	1	0.3	5	0.1	36	3	330	33	0.01	0.01	0.1	10
0	14	4.1	56	1.9	495	33	1122	112	0.17	0.12	0.9	97
0	13	6.4	37	1.1	504	36	913	91	0.16	0.18	0.8	71
0	4	1.6	33	0.4	172	13	93	9	0.04	0.03	0.2	23
0	7	3.5	47	0.3	146	12	198	20	0.09	0.08	0.4	30
0	3	2.7	158	1.8	631	58	4366	437	0.05	0.11	0.7	44
0	4	1.4	36	0.3	144	8	28	3	0.04	0.02	0.2	40
0	4	2.2	25	0.3	161	20	700	70	0.05	0.02	0.2	22
0	7	2.2	19	0.4	233	25	20,253	2025	0.07	0.04	0.7	7
0	11	3.3	30	0.6	355	39	30,942	3094	0.11	0.06	1.0	10
0	1	0.3	3	0.1	39	4	2	Tr	0.01	0.01	0.1	6
0	5	2.5	22	0.4	303	30	19	2	0.06	0.06	0.5	46

(continued on the following page)

FOOD DESCRIPTION	MEASURE OF EDIBLE PORTION	WEIGHT (g)	WATER (%)	CALORIES (kcal)	PROTEIN (g)	TOTAL FAT (g)	FATTY ACIDS		
							SATU-RATED (g)	MONO-UNSATU-RATED (g)	POLY-UNSATU-RATED (g)
VEGETABLES AND VEGETABLE PRODUCTS									
(continued)									
Cooked, drained, 1 inch pieces									
From raw	1 cup	124	93	29	2	1	0.1	Tr	0.3
	3 flowerets	54	93	12	1	Tr	Tr	Tr	0.1
From frozen	1 cup	180	94	34	3	Tr	0.1	Tr	0.2
Celery									
Raw									
Stalk, 7 1/2 to 8 inches long	1 stalk	40	95	6	Tr	Tr	Tr	Tr	Tr
Pieces, diced	1 cup	120	95	19	1	Tr	Tr	Tr	0.1
Chives, raw, chopped	1 tbsp	3	91	1	Tr	Tr	Tr	Tr	Tr
Cilantro, raw	1 tsp	2	92	Tr	Tr	Tr	Tr	Tr	Tr
Coleslaw, home prepared	1 cup	120	82	83	2	3	0.5	0.8	1.6
Collards, cooked, drained, chopped									
From raw	1 cup	190	92	49	4	1	0.1	Tr	0.3
From frozen	1 cup	170	88	61	5	1	0.1	Tr	0.4
Corn, sweet, yellow									
Cooked, drained									
From raw, kernels on cob	1 ear	77	70	83	3	1	0.2	0.3	0.5
From frozen									
Kernels on cob	1 ear	63	73	59	2	Tr	0.1	0.1	0.2
Kernels	1 cup	164	77	131	5	1	0.1	0.2	0.3
Canned									
Cream style	1 cup	256	79	184	4	1	0.2	0.3	0.5
Whole kernel, vacuum pack	1 cup	210	77	166	5	1	0.2	0.3	0.5
Cucumber									
Peeled									
Sliced	1 cup	119	96	14	1	Tr	Tr	Tr	0.1
Unpeeled									
Sliced	1 cup	104	96	14	1	Tr	Tr	Tr	0.1
Eggplant, cooked, drained	1 cup	99	92	28	1	Tr	Tr	Tr	0.1
Endive, curly (including escarole), raw, small pieces	1 cup	50	94	9	1	Tr	Tr	Tr	Tr
Garlic, raw	1 clove	3	59	4	Tr	Tr	Tr	Tr	Tr
Jerusalem artichoke, raw, sliced	1 cup	150	78	114	3	Tr	0.0	Tr	Tr
Kale, cooked, drained, chopped									
From raw	1 cup	130	91	36	2	1	0.1	Tr	0.3
From frozen	1 cup	130	91	39	4	1	0.1	Tr	0.3
Kohlrabi, cooked, drained, slices	1 cup	165	90	48	3	Tr	Tr	Tr	0.1
Leeks, bulb and lower leaf portion, chopped or diced, cooked, drained	1 cup	104	91	32	1	Tr	Tr	Tr	0.1
Lettuce, raw									
Butterhead, as Boston types									
Leaf	1 medium leaf	8	96	1	Tr	Tr	Tr	Tr	Tr
Head, 5-inch diameter	1 head	163	96	21	2	Tr	Tr	Tr	0.2

§White varieties contain only a trace amount of vitamin A; other nutrients are the same.

CHOLES-TEROL (mg)	CARBO-HYDRATE (g)	TOTAL DIETARY FIBER (g)	CALCIUM (mg)	IRON (mg)	POTAS-SIUM (mg)	SODIUM (mg)	VITAMIN A (IU)	VITAMIN A (RE)	THIAMIN (mg)	RIBO-FLAVIN (mg)	NIACIN (mg)	ASCOR-BIC ACID (mg)
0	5	3.3	20	0.4	176	19	21	2	0.05	0.06	0.5	55
0	2	1.5	9	0.2	77	8	9	1	0.02	0.03	0.2	24
0	7	4.9	31	0.7	250	32	40	4	0.07	0.10	0.6	56
0	1	0.7	16	0.2	115	35	54	5	0.02	0.02	0.1	3
0	4	2.0	48	0.5	344	104	161	16	0.06	0.05	0.4	8
0	Tr	0.1	3	Tr	9	Tr	131	13	Tr	Tr	Tr	2
0	Tr	Tr	1	Tr	8	1	98	10	Tr	Tr	Tr	0
10	15	1.8	54	0.7	217	28	762	98	0.08	0.07	0.3	39
0	9	5.3	226	0.9	494	17	5945	595	0.08	0.20	1.1	35
0	12	4.8	357	1.9	427	85	10,168	1017	0.08	0.20	1.1	45
0	19	2.2	2	0.5	192	13	167	17	0.17	0.06	1.5	5
0	14	1.8	2	0.4	158	3	133§	13§	0.11	0.04	1.0	3
0	32	3.9	7	0.6	241	8	361§	36§	0.14	0.12	2.1	5
0	46	3.1	8	1.0	343	730	248§	26§	0.06	0.14	2.5	12
0	41	4.2	11	0.9	391	571	506§	50§	0.09	0.15	2.5	17
0	3	0.8	17	0.2	176	2	88	8	0.02	0.01	0.1	3
0	3	0.8	15	0.3	150	2	224	22	0.02	0.02	0.2	6
0	7	2.5	6	0.3	246	3	63	6	0.08	0.02	0.6	1
0	2	1.6	26	0.4	157	11	1025	103	0.04	0.04	0.2	3
0	1	0.1	5	0.1	12	1	0	0	0.01	Tr	Tr	1
0	26	2.4	21	5.1	644	6	30	3	0.30	0.09	2.0	6
0	7	2.6	94	1.2	296	30	9620	962	0.07	0.09	0.7	53
0	7	2.6	179	1.2	417	20	8260	826	0.06	0.15	0.9	35
0	11	1.8	41	0.7	561	35	58	7	0.07	0.03	0.6	89
0	8	1.0	31	1.1	90	10	48	5	0.03	0.02	0.2	4
0	Tr	0.1	2	Tr	19	Tr	73	7	Tr	Tr	Tr	1
0	4	1.6	52	0.5	419	8	1581	158	0.10	0.10	0.5	13

(continued on the following page)

FOOD DESCRIPTION	MEASURE OF EDIBLE PORTION	WEIGHT (g)	WATER (%)	CALORIES (kcal)	PROTEIN (g)	TOTAL FAT (g)	FATTY ACIDS		
							SATU- RATED (g)	MONO- UNSATU- RATED (g)	POLY- UNSATU- RATED (g)
VEGETABLES AND VEGETABLE PRODUCTS									
(continued)									
Crisphead, as iceberg									
Leaf	1 medium	8	96	1	Tr	Tr	Tr	Tr	Tr
Head, 6-inch diameter	1 head	539	96	65	5	1	0.1	Tr	0.5
Pieces, shredded or chopped	1 cup	55	96	7	1	Tr	Tr	Tr	0.1
Romaine or cos									
Innerleaf	1 leaf	10	95	1	Tr	Tr	Tr	Tr	Tr
Pieces, shredded	1 cup	56	95	8	1	Tr	Tr	Tr	0.1
Mushrooms									
Raw, pieces or slices	1 cup	70	92	18	2	Tr	Tr	Tr	0.1
Canned, drained, pieces	1 cup	156	91	37	3	Tr	0.1	Tr	0.2
Mustard greens, cooked, drained	1 cup	140	94	21	3	Tr	Tr	0.2	0.1
Okra, sliced, cooked, drained									
From frozen	1 cup	184	91	52	4	1	0.1	0.1	0.1
Onions									
Raw									
Chopped	1 cup	160	90	61	2	Tr	Tr	Tr	0.1
Cooked (whole or sliced), drained	1 cup	210	88	92	3	Tr	0.1	0.1	0.2
	1 medium	94	88	41	1	Tr	Tr	Tr	0.1
Dehydrated flakes	1 tbsp	5	4	17	Tr	Tr	Tr	Tr	Tr
Onions, spring, raw, top and bulb									
Chopped	1 cup	100	90	32	2	Tr	Tr	Tr	0.1
Whole, medium, 4 1/8 inches long	1 whole	15	90	5	Tr	Tr	Tr	Tr	Tr
Onion rings, 2- to- 3-inch diameter breaded, par fried, frozen, oven heated	10 rings	60	29	244	3	16	5.2	6.5	3.1
Parsley, raw	10 springs	10	88	4	Tr	Tr	Tr	Tr	Tr
Parsnips, sliced, cooked, drained	1 cup	156	78	126	2	Tr	0.1	0.2	0.1
Peas, edible pod, cooked, drained									
From raw	1 cup	160	89	67	5	Tr	0.1	Tr	0.2
Peas, green									
Canned, drained	1 cup	170	82	117	8	1	0.1	0.1	0.3
Frozen, boiled, drained	1 cup	160	80	125	8	Tr	0.1	Tr	0.2
Peppers									
Hot chili, raw									
Green	1 pepper	45	88	18	1	Tr	Tr	Tr	Tr
Red	1 pepper	45	88	18	1	Tr	Tr	Tr	Tr
Jalapeno, canned, sliced, solids and liquids	1/4 cup	26	89	7	Tr	Tr	Tr	Tr	0.1
Sweet (2 3/4 inches long, 2 1/2-inch diameter)									
Raw									
Green									
Chopped	1 cup	149	92	40	1	Tr	Tr	Tr	0.2
Red									
Chopped	1 cup	149	92	40	1	Tr	Tr	Tr	0.2
Cooked, drained, chopped									
Green	1 cup	136	92	38	1	Tr	Tr	Tr	0.1

CHOLESTEROL (mg)	CARBOHYDRATE (g)	TOTAL DIETARY FIBER (g)	CALCIUM (mg)	IRON (mg)	POTASSIUM (mg)	SODIUM (mg)	VITAMIN A (IU)	VITAMIN A (RE)	THIAMIN (mg)	RIBOFLAVIN (mg)	NIACIN (mg)	ASCORBIC ACID (mg)
0	Tr	0.1	2	Tr	13	1	26	3	Tr	Tr	Tr	Tr
0	11	7.5	102	2.7	852	49	1779	178	0.25	0.16	1.0	21
0	1	0.8	10	0.3	87	5	182	18	0.03	0.02	0.1	2
0	Tr	0.2	4	0.1	29	1	260	26	0.01	0.01	0.1	2
0	1	1.0	20	0.6	162	4	1456	146	0.06	0.06	0.3	13
0	3	0.8	4	0.7	259	3	0	0	0.06	0.30	2.8	2
0	8	3.7	17	1.2	201	663	0	0	0.13	0.03	2.5	0
0	3	2.8	104	1.0	283	22	4243	424	0.06	0.09	0.6	35
0	11	5.2	177	1.2	431	6	946	94	0.18	0.23	1.4	22
0	14	2.9	32	0.4	251	5	0	0	0.07	0.03	0.2	10
0	21	2.9	46	0.5	349	6	0	0	0.09	0.05	0.3	11
0	10	1.3	21	0.2	156	3	0	0	0.04	0.02	0.2	5
0	4	0.5	13	0.1	81	1	0	0	0.03	0.01	Tr	4
0	7	2.6	72	1.5	276	16	385	39	0.06	0.08	0.5	19
0	1	0.4	11	0.2	41	2	58	6	0.01	0.01	0.1	3
0	23	0.8	19	1.0	77	225	135	14	0.17	0.08	2.2	1
0	1	0.3	14	0.6	55	6	520	52	0.01	0.01	0.1	13
0	30	6.2	58	0.9	573	16	0	0	0.13	0.08	1.1	20
0	11	4.5	67	3.2	384	6	210	21	0.20	0.12	0.9	77
0	21	7.0	34	1.6	294	428	1306	131	0.21	0.13	1.2	16
0	23	8.8	38	2.5	269	139	1069	107	0.45	0.16	2.4	16
0	4	0.7	8	0.5	153	3	347	35	0.04	0.04	0.4	109
0	4	0.7	8	0.5	153	3	4838	484	0.04	0.04	0.4	109
0	1	0.7	6	0.5	50	434	442	44	0.01	0.01	0.1	3
0	10	2.7	13	0.7	264	3	942	94	0.10	0.04	0.8	133
0	10	3.0	13	0.7	264	3	8493	849	0.10	0.04	0.8	283
0	8	2.4	11	0.5	211	2	6783	678	0.08	0.04	0.6	226
0	9	1.6	12	0.6	226	3	805	80	0.08	0.04	0.6	101

(continued on the following page)

| | | | | | | FATTY ACIDS | | |
| | | | | | | SATU-RATED (g) | MONO-UNSATU-RATED (g) | POLY-UNSATU-RATED (g) |
FOOD DESCRIPTION	MEASURE OF EDIBLE PORTION	WEIGHT (g)	WATER (%)	CALORIES (kcal)	PROTEIN (g)	TOTAL FAT (g)			
VEGETABLES AND VEGETABLE PRODUCTS									
(continued)									
Pimento, canned	1 tbsp	12	93	3	Tr	Tr	Tr	Tr	Tr
Potatoes									
Baked (2 1/3 x 4 3/4 inches)									
With skin	1 potato	202	71	220	5	Tr	0.1	Tr	0.1
Flesh only	1 potato	156	75	145	3	Tr	Tr	Tr	0.1
Boiled (2 1/2-inch diameter)									
Peeled after boiling	1 potato	136	77	118	3	Tr	Tr	Tr	0.1
	1 cup	156	77	134	3	Tr	Tr	Tr	0.1
Potato products, prepared									
Au gratin									
From home recipe, with butter	1 cup	245	74	323	12	19	11.6	5.3	0.7
Hashed brown									
From frozen (about 3 x 1 1/2 x 1/2 inches)	1 patty	29	56	63	1	3	1.3	1.5	0.4
Mashed									
From dehydrated flakes (without milk); whole milk, butter, and salt added	1 cup	210	76	237	4	12	7.2	3.3	0.5
From home recipe									
With whole milk	1 cup	210	78	162	4	1	0.7	0.3	0.1
Potato puffs, from frozen	10 puffs	79	53	175	3	8	4.0	3.4	0.6
Potato salad, home-prepared	1 cup	250	76	358	7	21	3.6	6.2	9.3
Scalloped									
From home recipe, with butter	1 cup	245	81	211	7	9	5.5	2.5	0.4
Pumpkin									
Cooked, mashed	1 cup	245	94	49	2	Tr	0.1	Tr	Tr
Radishes, raw (3/4-inch to 1-inch diameter)	1 radish	5	95	1	Tr	Tr	Tr	Tr	Tr
Rutabagas, cooked, drained, cubes	1 cup	170	89	66	2	Tr	Tr	Tr	0.2
Sauerkraut, canned, solids and liquid	1 cup	236	93	45	2	Tr	0.1	Tr	0.1
Seaweed									
Kelp, raw	2 tbsp	10	82	4	Tr	Tr	Tr	Tr	Tr
Spirulina, dried	1 tbsp	1	5	3	1	Tr	Tr	Tr	Tr
Shallots, raw, chopped	1 tbsp	10	80	7	Tr	Tr	Tr	Tr	Tr
Soybeans, green, cooked, drained	1 cup	180	69	254	22	12	1.3	2.2	5.4
Spinach									
Raw									
Chopped	1 cup	30	92	7	1	Tr	Tr	Tr	Tr
Cooked, drained									
From frozen (chopped or leaf)	1 cup	190	90	53	6	Tr	0.1	Tr	0.2
Canned, drained	1 cup	214	92	49	6	1	0.2	Tr	0.4
Squash									
Summer (all varieties), sliced									
Raw	1 cup	113	94	23	1	Tr	Tr	Tr	0.1
Winter, (all varieties), baked, cubes	1 cup	205	89	80	2	1	0.3	0.1	0.5

CHOLESTEROL (mg)	CARBOHYDRATE (g)	TOTAL DIETARY FIBER (g)	CALCIUM (mg)	IRON (mg)	POTASSIUM (mg)	SODIUM (mg)	VITAMIN A (IU)	VITAMIN A (RE)	THIAMIN (mg)	RIBOFLAVIN (mg)	NIACIN (mg)	ASCORBIC ACID (mg)
0	1	0.2	1	0.2	19	2	319	32	Tr	0.01	0.1	10
0	51	4.8	20	2.7	844	16	0	0	0.22	0.07	3.3	26
0	34	2.3	8	0.5	610	8	0	0	0.16	0.03	2.2	20
0	27	2.4	7	0.4	515	5	0	0	0.14	0.03	2.0	18
0	31	2.8	12	0.5	512	8	1	1	0.15	0.03	2.0	12
56	28	4.4	292	1.6	970	1061	647	93	0.16	0.28	2.4	24
0	8	0.6	4	0.4	126	10	0	0	0.03	0.01	0.7	2
4	37	4.2	55	0.6	628	636	40	13	0.18	0.08	2.3	14
0	24	2.5	24	1.2	300	589	13	2	0.15	0.06	1.7	5
170	28	3.3	48	1.6	635	1323	523	83	0.19	0.15	2.2	25
29	26	4.7	140	1.4	926	821	331	47	0.17	0.23	2.6	26
0	12	2.7	37	1.4	564	2	2651	265	0.08	0.19	1.0	12
0	Tr	0.1	1	Tr	10	1	Tr	Tr	Tr	Tr	Tr	1
0	15	3.1	82	0.9	54	34	954	95	0.14	0.07	1.2	32
0	10	5.9	71	3.5	401	1560	42	5	0.05	0.05	0.3	35
0	1	0.1	17	0.3	9	23	12	1	0.01	0.02	Tr	Tr
0	Tr	Tr	1	0.3	14	10	6	1	0.02	0.04	0.1	Tr
0	2	0.2	4	0.1	33	1	119	12	0.01	Tr	Tr	1
0	20	7.6	261	4.5	970	25	281	29	0.47	0.28	2.3	31
0	1	0.8	30	0.8	167	24	2015	202	0.02	0.06	0.2	8
0	10	5.7	277	2.9	566	163	14,790	1478	0.11	0.32	0.8	23
0	7	5.1	272	4.9	740	58	18,781	1879	0.03	0.30	0.8	31
0	5	2.1	23	0.5	220	2	221	23	0.07	0.04	0.6	17
0	18	5.7	29	0.7	896	2	7292	730	0.17	0.05	1.4	20

(continued on the following page)

FOOD DESCRIPTION	MEASURE OF EDIBLE PORTION	WEIGHT (g)	WATER (%)	CALORIES (kcal)	PROTEIN (g)	TOTAL FAT (g)	FATTY ACIDS SATU-RATED (g)	MONO-UNSATU-RATED (g)	POLY-UNSATU-RATED (g)
VEGETABLES AND VEGETABLE PRODUCTS									
(continued)									
Winter, butternut, frozen, cooked, mashed	1 cup	240	88	94	3	Tr	Tr	Tr	0.1
Sweetpotatoes									
Cooked (2-inch diameter 5 inches long raw)									
Baked, with skin	1 potato	146	73	150	3	Tr	Tr	Tr	0.1
Boiled, without skin	1 potato	156	73	164	3	Tr	0.1	Tr	0.2
Candied (2 1/2 x 2-inch piece)	1 piece	105	67	144	1	3	1.4	0.7	0.2
Canned									
Vacuum pack, mashed	1 cup	255	76	232	4	1	0.1	Tr	0.2
Tomatillos, raw	1 medium	34	92	11	Tr	Tr	Tr	0.1	0.1
Tomatoes									
Raw, year round average									
Chopped or sliced	1 cup	180	94	38	2	1	0.1	0.1	0.2
Whole									
Cherry	1 cherry	17	94	4	Tr	Tr	Tr	Tr	Tr
Canned, solids and liquid	1 cup	240	94	46	2	Tr	Tr	Tr	0.1
Sun dried									
Plain	1 piece	2	15	5	Tr	Tr	Tr	Tr	Tr
Tomato juice, canned, with salt added	1 cup	243	94	41	2	Tr	Tr	Tr	0.1
Tomato products, canned									
Paste	1 cup	262	74	215	10	1	0.2	0.2	0.6
Puree	1 cup	250	87	100	4	Tr	0.1	0.1	0.2
Sauce	1 cup	245	89	74	3	Tr	0.1	0.1	0.2
Spaghetti/marinara/pasta sauce. See Soups, Sauces, and Gravies.									
Stewed	1 cup	255	91	71	2	Tr	Tr	0.1	0.1
Turnips, cooked, cubes	1 cup	156	94	33	1	Tr	Tr	Tr	0.1
Turnip greens, cooked, drained									
From raw (leaves and stems)	1 cup	144	93	29	2	Tr	0.1	Tr	0.1
From frozen (chopped)	1 cup	164	90	49	5	1	0.2	Tr	0.3
Vegetable juice cocktail, canned	1 cup	242	94	46	2	Tr	Tr	Tr	0.1
Vegetables, mixed									
Canned, drained	1 cup	163	87	77	4	Tr	0.1	Tr	0.2
Frozen, cooked, drained	1 cup	182	83	107	5	Tr	0.1	Tr	0.1
Waterchestnuts, canned, slices, solids and liquids	1 cup	140	86	70	1	Tr	Tr	Tr	Tr
MISCELLANEOUS ITEMS									
Bacon bits, meatless	1 tbsp	7	8	31	2	2	0.3	0.4	0.9
Baking soda	1 tsp	5	Tr	0	0	0	0.0	0.0	0.0
Beef jerky	1 large piece	20	23	81	7	5	2.1	2.2	0.2
Catsup	1 cup	240	67	250	4	1	0.1	0.1	0.4
	1 tbsp	15	67	16	Tr	Tr	Tr	Tr	Tr
Celery seed	1 tsp	2	6	8	Tr	1	Tr	0.3	0.1
Chili powder	1 tsp	3	8	8	Tr	Tr	0.1	0.1	0.2
Chocolate, unsweetened, baking									
Solid	1 square	28	1	148	3	16	9.2	5.2	0.5
Liquid	1 oz	28	1	134	3	14	7.2	2.6	3.0

|| For product with no salt added: If salt added, consult the nutrition label for sodium value.

CHOLES-TEROL (mg)	CARBO-HYDRATE (g)	TOTAL DIETARY FIBER (g)	CALCIUM (mg)	IRON (mg)	POTAS-SIUM (mg)	SODIUM (mg)	VITAMIN A (IU)	VITAMIN A (RE)	THIAMIN (mg)	RIBO-FLAVIN (mg)	NIACIN (mg)	ASCOR-BIC ACID (mg)
0	24	2.2	46	1.4	319	5	8014	802	0.12	0.09	1.1	8
0	35	4.4	41	0.7	508	15	31,860	3186	0.11	0.19	0.9	36
0	38	2.8	33	0.9	287	20	26,604	2660	0.08	0.22	1.0	27
8	29	2.5	27	1.2	198	74	4398	440	0.02	0.04	0.4	7
0	54	4.6	56	2.3	796	135	20,357	2035	0.09	0.15	1.9	67
0	2	0.6	2	0.2	91	Tr	39	4	0.01	0.01	0.6	4
0	8	2.0	9	0.8	400	16	1121	112	0.11	0.09	1.1	34
0	1	0.2	1	0.1	38	2	106	11	0.01	0.01	0.1	3
0	10	2.4	72	1.3	530	355	1428	144	0.11	0.07	1.8	34
0	1	0.2	2	0.2	69	42	17	2	0.01	0.01	0.2	1
0	10	1.0	22	1.4	535	877	1351	136	0.11	0.08	1.6	44
0	51	10.7	92	5.1	2455	231	6406	639	0.41	0.50	8.4	111
0	24	5.0	43	3.1	1065	85‖	3188	320	0.18	0.14	4.3	26
0	18	3.4	34	1.9	909	1482	2399	240	0.16	0.14	2.8	32
0	17	2.6	84	1.9	607	564	1380	138	0.12	0.09	1.8	29
0	8	3.1	34	0.3	211	78	0	0	0.04	0.04	0.5	18
0	6	5.0	197	1.2	292	42	7917	792	0.06	0.10	0.6	39
0	8	5.6	249	3.2	367	25	13,079	1309	0.09	0.12	0.8	36
0	11	1.9	27	1.0	467	653	2831	283	0.10	0.07	1.8	67
0	15	4.9	44	1.7	474	243	18,985	1899	0.07	0.08	0.9	8
0	24	8.0	46	1.5	308	64	7784	779	0.13	0.22	1.5	6
0	17	3.5	6	1.2	165	11	6	0	0.02	0.03	0.5	2
0	2	0.7	7	0.1	10	124	0	0	0.04	Tr	0.1	Tr
0	0	0.0	0	0.0	0	1259	0	0	0.00	0.00	0.0	0
10	2	0.4	4	1.1	118	438	0	0	0.03	0.03	0.3	0
0	65	3.1	46	1.7	1154	2846	2438	245	0.21	0.18	3.3	36
0	4	0.2	3	0.1	72	178	152	15	0.01	0.01	0.2	2
0	1	0.2	35	0.9	28	3	1	Tr	0.01	0.01	0.1	Tr
0	1	0.9	7	0.4	50	26	908	91	0.01	0.02	0.2	2
0	8	4.4	21	1.8	236	4	28	3	0.02	0.05	0.3	0
0	10	5.1	15	1.2	331	3	3	Tr	0.01	0.08	0.6	0

(continued on the following page)

Nutritive Value of the Edible Part of Food

FOOD DESCRIPTION	MEASURE OF EDIBLE PORTION	WEIGHT (g)	WATER (%)	CALORIES (kcal)	PROTEIN (g)	TOTAL FAT (g)	FATTY ACIDS SATU-RATED (g)	MONO-UNSATU-RATED (g)	POLY-UNSATU-RATED (g)
MISCELLANEOUS ITEMS									
(continued)									
Cinnamon	1 tsp	2	10	6	Tr	Tr	Tr	Tr	Tr
Cocoa powder,									
unsweetened	1 cup	86	3	197	17	12	6.9	3.9	0.4
Cream of tartar	1 tsp	3	2	8	0	0	0.0	0.0	0.0
Curry powder	1 tsp	2	10	7	Tr	Tr	Tr	0.1	0.1
Garlic powder	1 tsp	3	6	9	Tr	Tr	Tr	Tr	Tr
Horseradish, prepared	1 tsp	5	85	2	Tr	Tr	Tr	Tr	Tr
Mustard, prepared, yellow	1 tsp or 1 packet	5	82	3	Tr	Tr	Tr	0.1	Tr
Olives, canned									
Pickled, green	5 medium	17	78	20	Tr	2	0.3	1.6	0.2
Ripe, black	5 large	22	80	25	Tr	2	0.3	1.7	0.2
Onion powder	1 tsp	2	5	7	Tr	Tr	Tr	Tr	Tr
Oregano, ground	1 tsp	2	7	5	Tr	Tr	Tr	Tr	0.1
Paprika	1 tsp	2	10	6	Tr	Tr	Tr	Tr	0.2
Parsley, dried	1 tbsp	1	9	4	Tr	Tr	Tr	Tr	Tr
Pepper, black	1 tsp	2	11	5	Tr	Tr	Tr	Tr	Tr
Pickles, cucumber									
Dill, whole, medium (3 3/4 inches long)	1 pickle	65	92	12	Tr	Tr	Tr	Tr	0.1
Fresh (bread and butter pickles), slices 1 1/2-inch diameter 1/4-inch thick	3 slices	24	79	18	Tr	Tr	Tr	Tr	Tr
Pickle relish, sweet	1 tbsp	15	62	20	Tr	Tr	Tr	Tr	Tr
Potato chips									
Regular									
Plain									
Salted	1 oz	28	2	152	2	10	3.1	2.8	3.5
Unsalted	1 oz	28	2	152	2	10	3.1	2.8	3.5
Reduced fat	1 oz	28	1	134	2	6	1.2	1.4	3.1
Fat free, made with olestra	1 oz	28	2	75	2	Tr	Tr	0.1	0.1
Made from dried potatoes									
Trail mix									
Regular, with raisins, chocolate chips, salted nuts and seeds	1 cup	146	7	707	21	47	8.9	19.8	16.5
Vanilla extract	1 tsp	4	53	12	Tr	Tr	Tr	Tr	Tr
Vinegar									
Cider	1 tbsp	15	94	2	0	0	0.0	0.0	0.0
Distilled	1 tbsp	17	95	2	0	0	0.0	0.0	0.0
Yeast, baker's									
Dry, active	1 pkg	7	8	21	3	Tr	Tr	0.2	Tr
Compressed	1 cake	17	69	18	1	Tr	Tr	0.2	Tr

CHOLES-TEROL (mg)	CARBO-HYDRATE (g)	TOTAL DIETARY FIBER (g)	CALCIUM (mg)	IRON (mg)	POTAS-SIUM (mg)	SODIUM (mg)	VITAMIN A		THIAMIN (mg)	RIBO-FLAVIN (mg)	NIACIN (mg)	ASCOR-BIC ACID (mg)
							(IU)	(RE)				
0	2	1.2	28	0.9	11	1	6	1	Tr	Tr	Tr	1
0	47	28.6	110	11.9	1311	18	17	2	0.07	0.21	1.9	0
0	2	Tr	Tr	0.1	495	2	0	0	0.00	0.00	0.0	0
0	1	0.7	10	0.6	31	1	20	2	0.01	0.01	0.1	Tr
0	2	0.3	2	0.1	31	1	0	0	0.01	Tr	Tr	1
0	1	0.2	3	Tr	12	16	Tr	0	Tr	Tr	Tr	1
0	Tr	0.2	4	0.1	8	56	7	1	Tr	Tr	Tr	Tr
0	Tr	0.2	10	0.3	9	408	51	5	0.00	0.00	Tr	0
0	1	0.7	19	0.7	2	192	89	9	Tr	0.00	Tr	Tr
0	2	0.1	8	0.1	20	1	0	0	0.01	Tr	Tr	Tr
0	1	0.6	24	0.7	25	Tr	104	10	0.01	Tr	0.1	1
0	1	0.4	4	0.5	49	1	1273	127	0.01	0.04	0.3	1
0	1	0.4	19	1.3	49	6	303	30	Tr	0.02	0.1	2
0	1	0.6	9	0.6	26	1	4	Tr	Tr	0.01	Tr	Tr
0	3	0.8	6	0.3	75	833	214	21	0.01	0.02	Tr	1
0	4	0.4	8	0.1	48	162	34	3	0.00	0.01	0.0	2
0	5	0.2	Tr	0.1	4	122	23	2	0.00	Tr	Tr	Tr
0	15	1.3	7	0.5	361	168	0	0	0.05	0.06	1.1	9
0	15	1.4	7	0.5	361	2	0	0	0.05	0.06	1.1	9
0	19	1.7	6	0.4	494	139	0	0	0.06	0.08	2.0	7
0	17	1.1	10	0.4	366	185	1469	441	0.10	0.02	1.3	8
6	66	8.8	159	4.9	946	177	64	7	0.60	0.33	6.4	2
0	1	0.0	Tr	Tr	6	Tr	0	0	Tr	Tr	Tr	0
0	1	0.0	1	0.1	15	Tr	0	0	0.00	0.00	0.0	0
0	1	0.0	0	0.0	2	Tr	0	0	0.00	0.00	0.0	0
0	3	1.5	4	1.2	140	4	Tr	0	0.17	0.38	2.8	Tr
0	3	1.4	3	0.6	102	5	0	0	0.32	0.19	2.1	Tr

C Nutritional Assessment Tools

The Warning Signs of poor nutritional health are often overlooked. Use this checklist to find out if you or someone you know is at nutritional risk.

Read the statements below. Circle the number in the yes column for those that apply to you or someone you know. For each yes answer, score the number in the box. Total your nutritional score.

DETERMINE YOUR NUTRITIONAL HEALTH

		YES
*D	I have an illness or condition that made me change the kind and/or amount of food I eat.	2
E	I eat fewer than 2 meals per day.	3
	I eat few fruits or vegetables, or milk products.	2
	I have 3 or more drinks of beer, liquor or wine almost every day.	2
T	I have tooth or mouth problems that make it hard for me to eat.	2
E	I don't always have enough money to buy the food I need.	4
R	I eat alone most of the time.	1
M	I take 3 or more different prescribed or over-the-counter drugs a day.	1
I	Without wanting to, I have lost or gained 10 pounds in the last 6 months.	2
N	I am not always physically able to shop, cook and/or feed myself.	2
E	Age_____ Today's Date_____	**TOTAL**

NAME _____   SEX _____   PHONE # _____

ADDRESS _____   CITY _____   STATE _____   ZIP CODE _____

Total Your Nutritional Score. If it's...

0-2 **Good!** Recheck your nutritional score in 6 months.

3-5 **You are at moderate nutritional risk.** See what can be done to improve your eating habits and lifestyle. Your office of aging, senior nutrition program, senior citizens center or health department can help. Recheck your nutritional score in 3 months.

6 or more **You are at high nutritional risk.** Bring this checklist the next time you see your doctor, dietitian or other qualified health or social service professional. Talk with them about any problems you may have. Ask for help to improve your nutritional health.

These materials developed and distributed by the Nutrition Screening Initiative, a project of:
AMERICAN ACADEMY OF FAMILY PHYSICIANS
THE AMERICAN DIETETIC ASSOCIATION
NATIONAL COUNCIL ON THE AGING, INC.

FOR OFFICE USE ONLY
- - - - - - - - - - - - - - - - - - - -
INTERVENTION RECOMMENDED
- ☐ Social Service   ☐ Medication Use
- ☐ Nutrition Education/   ☐ Oral Health
  Counseling   ☐ Nutrition Support
- ☐ MentalHealth

Remember that warning signs suggest risk but do not represent diagnosis of any condition.
See below to learn more about the warning signs of poor nutritional health.

Disease

Any disease, illness, or chronic condition that causes you to change the way you eat or makes it hard for you to eat puts your nutritional health at risk. Four out of five adults have chronic diseases that are affected by diet. Confusion or memory loss that keeps getting worse is estimated to affect one out of five or more of older adults. This can make it hard to remember what, when, or if you've eaten. Feeling sad or depressed, which happens to about one in eight older adults, can cause big changes in appetite, digestion, energy level, weight, and well-being.

Eating Poorly

Eating too little and eating too much both lead to poor health. Eating the same foods day after day or not eating fruit, vegetables, and milk products daily will also cause poor nutritional health. One in five adults skips meals daily. Only 13 percent of adults eat the minimum amount of fruit and vegetables needed. One in four older adults drinks too much alcohol. Many health problems become worse if you drink more than one or two alcoholic beverages per day.

Tooth Loss/Mouth Pain

A healthy mouth, teeth, and gums are needed to eat. Missing, loose, or rotten teeth or dentures that do not fit well or cause mouth sores make it hard to eat.

Economic Hardship

As many as 40 percent of older Americans have incomes of less than $6000 per year. Having less—or choosing to spend less—than $25–30 per week for food makes it very hard to get the foods you need to stay healthy.

Reduced Social Contact

One-third of all older people live alone. Being with people daily has a positive effect on morale, well-being, and eating.

Multiple Medicines

Many older Americans must take medicines for health problems. Almost half of older Americans take multiple medicines daily. Growing old may change the way we respond to drugs. The more medicines you take, the greater the chance for side effects such as increased or decreased appetite, change in taste, constipation, weakness, drowsiness, diarrhea, nausea, and others. Vitamins or minerals when taken in large doses act like drugs and can cause harm. Alert your doctor to everything you take.

Involuntary Weight Loss/Gain

Losing or gaining a lot of weight when you are not trying to do so is an important warning sign that must not be ignored. Being overweight or underweight also increases your chance of poor health.

Needs Assistance in Self-Care

Although most older people are able to eat, one of every five has trouble walking, shopping, and buying and cooking food, especially as they get older.

Elder Years Above Age 80

Most older people lead full and productive lives. But as age increases, risk of frailty and health problems increase. Checking your nutritional health regularly makes good sense.

Level 1 Screen

Body Weight

Measure height to the nearest inch and weight to the nearest pound. Record the values below and mark them on the Body Mass Index (BMI) scale to the right. Then use a straight edge (ruler) to connect the two points and circle the spot where the straight line crosses the center line (body mass index). Record the number below.

Healthy older adults should have a BMI between 24 and 27.

Height (in): _____
Weight (lbs): _____
Body Mass Index: _____
(number from center column)

Check any that are true for the individual:

☐ Has lost or gained 10 pounds (or more) in the past
6 months
☐ Body mass index <24
☐ Body mass index >27

For the remaining sections, please ask the individual which of the statements (if any) is true for him or her and place a check by each that applies.

Eating Habits

☐ Does not have enough food to eat each day
☐ Usually eats alone
☐ Does not eat anything on one or more days each
month
☐ Has poor appetite
☐ Is on a special diet
☐ Eats vegetables two or fewer times a day
☐ Eats milk or milk products once or not at all daily
☐ Eats fruit or drinks fruit juice once or not at all
daily

SOURCE: Reprinted with permission by the Nutrition Screening Initiative, a project of the American Academy of Family Physicians, the American Dietetic Association, and the National Council on the Aging, Inc., and funded in part by a grant from Ross Products Division, Abbott Laboratories.

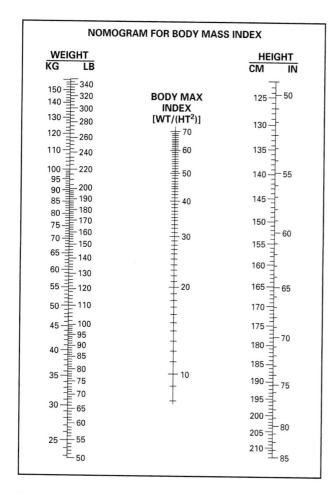

NOMOGRAM FOR BODY MASS INDEX

WEIGHT
KG   LB

BODY MAX
INDEX
[WT/(HT²)]

HEIGHT
CM   IN

Living Environment

☐ Lives on an income of less than $6000 per year (per individual in the household)
☐ Lives alone
☐ Is housebound
☐ Is concerned about home security
☐ Lives in a home with inadequate heating or cooling
☐ Does not have a stove and/or refrigerator
☐ Is unable or prefers not to spend money on food (<$25–30 per person spent on food each week)

Functional Status

Usually or always needs assistance with (check each that applies):

☐ Bathing
☐ Dressing
☐ Grooming
☐ Toileting
☐ Eating
☐ Walking or moving about
☐ Traveling (outside the home)
☐ Preparing food
☐ Shopping for food or other necessities

If you have checked one or more statements on this list, the individual you have interviewed may be at risk for poor nutritional status. Please refer this individual to the appropriate health-care or social-service professional in your area. For example, a dietitian should be contacted for problems with selecting, preparing, or eating a healthy diet, or a dentist if the individual experiences pain or difficulty when chewing or swallowing. Those individuals whose income, lifestyle, or functional status may endanger their nutritional and overall health should be referred to available community services: home-delivered meals, congregate meal programs, transportation services, counseling services (alcohol abuse, depression, bereavement, etc.), home health-care agencies, day-care programs, etc.

Please repeat this screen at least once each year—sooner if the individual has a major change in his or her health, income, immediate family (e.g., spouse dies), or functional status.

☐ Eats breads, cereals, pasta, rice, or other grains five or fewer times daily
☐ Has difficulty chewing or swallowing
☐ Has more than one alcoholic drink per day (if woman); more than two drinks per day (if man)
☐ Has pain in mouth, teeth, or gums

A physician should be contacted if the individual has gained or lost 10 pounds unexpectedly or without intending to during the past 6 months. A physician should also be notified if the individual's body mass index is above 27 or below 22.

Figure 2 Level I Screen. (From the Nutrition Screening Initiative: A project of the American Academy of Family Physicians, The American Dietetic Association, and the National Council on the Aging, Inc. and funded in part by a grant from Ross Laboratories, a division of Abbott laboratories, with permission.)

FEATURES OF SUBJECTIVE GLOBAL ASSESSMENT (SGA)

Select appropriate category with a check mark or enter numerical value.

A. History
    1. Weight change
       —Overall loss in past 6 months: amount = _____ kg; % loss = _____
       —Change in past 2 weeks: _____ increase
                       _____ no change
                       _____ decrease

    2. Dietary intake change (relative to normal)
       _____ No change
       _____ Change _____ duration = _____ weeks
                     _____ type: _____ suboptimal solid diet _____ full liquid diet
                                    _____ hypocaloric liquids _____ starvation

    3. Gastrointestinal symptoms (that persisted for >2 weeks)
       _____ none _____ nausea _____ vomiting _____ diarrhea _____ anorexia

    4. Functional capacity
       _____ No dysfunction (eg, full capacity)
       _____ Dysfunction _____ duration = _____ weeks
                     _____ type: _____ working suboptimally
                                 _____ ambulatory
                                 _____ bedridden

    5. Disease and its relation to nutritional requirements
       Primary diagnosis (specify): _____
       Metabolic demand (stress): _____ no stress _____ low stress
                             _____ moderate stress _____ high stress

B. Physical (for each trait, specify: 0 = normal, 1+ = mild, 2+ = moderate, 3+ = severe)
    _____ loss of subcutaneous fat (triceps, chest)
    _____ muscle wasting (quadriceps, deltoids)
    _____ ankle edema
    _____ sacral edema
    _____ ascites

C. SGA rating (select one):
    _____ A = Well nourished (<5% wt. loss or if >5% with recent gain and improved appetite)
    _____ B = Moderately (or suspected of being) malnourished (5–10% wt. loss, no gain, mild subQ loss)
    _____ C = Severely malnourished (>10% wt. loss, severe subQ loss, muscle wasting)

SOURCE: Detsky et al: What is subjective global assessment? JPEN 11:8, 1987, with permission.

Nutritional Screening Form

Name _____ Date _____ Adm. Date _____

Sex _____ Birthdate _____ Physician's Name _____

Adm. Dx. _____

Diet Information   Diet order _____ Date prescribed _____

Accepts all major groups _____

Feeds self _____ Type of assistance needed _____

Physical   Height _____ Weight _____ Healthy body weight % _____

Weight change in last 3 months _____ Chewing ability _____

Weight history _____ Swallowing ability _____

Hearing _____ Vision _____ Bowel function _____

Bladder function _____ Edema _____ Nausea _____

Pressure ulcer _____ Stage _____ Allergies _____

Laboratory   Blood glucose _____ Albumin _____ Potassium _____

Lymphocytes _____ Hemoglobin _____ Hematocrit _____

Cholesterol _____

Medications   Insulin _____ Diuretics _____ Laxatives _____

Vit/min supp _____ Antibiotics _____ Thyroid _____

Anticoagulants _____ Antidepressants (MAO) _____

Antabuse _____ Flagyl _____ Lithium _____

If the above identifies a problem, continue with in-depth assessment.

_____ (Signature) _____ (Date)

Growth Charts for Boys and Girls Birth to 20 Years

Growth charts, such as the six that follow, are used to evaluate growth in infants, children, and adolescents. The charts are a valuable tool in nutritional assessment. The charts permit use of weight, length or stature, age, head circumference, body mass index (BMI), and gender to document an individual's status. The charts, and other versions showing different percentiles, can be downloaded from http://www.cdc.gov/nchs/about/major/nhanes/ growthcharts/ clinical_charts.htm.

To use a chart, select the appropriate one for the characteristics you wish to plot. For example, for a male infant weighing 28 lb at 15 months of age, the correct chart is labeled "Birth to 36 months: Boys Length-for-age and Weight-for-age percentiles." By following the lines for 28 pounds at the right and 15 months on the bottom, you see that the two lines intersect about at the curved line marked "90th." This indicates the boy is heavier than 90 percent of 15-month-old males. The heavy dark line marked "50th" is the point at which half the 15-month-old boys are heavier and half are lighter than 24.5 lb.

A child's progress can be plotted on a chart to immediately see if there have been drastic changes in the growth pattern. The physician will probably want to know about a child above the 95th percentile or below the 5th percentile or one with rapid changes above the 75th or below the 25th percentiles.

Birth to 36 months: Boys
Length-for-age and Weight-for-age percentiles

NAME _____

RECORD # _____

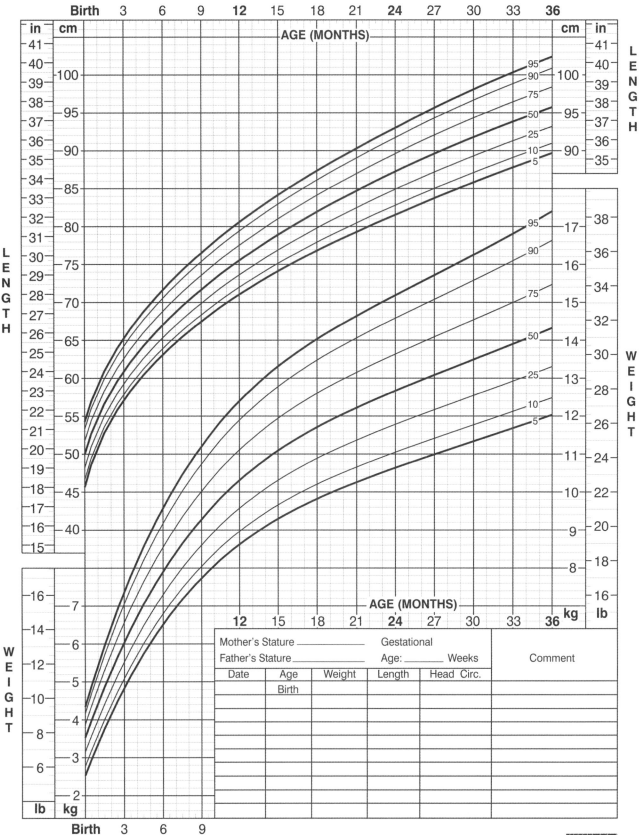

Published May 30, 2000 (modified 4/20/01).
SOURCE: Developed by the National Center for Health Statistics in collaboration with
   the National Center for Chronic Disease Prevention and Health Promotion (2000).
   http://www.cdc.gov/growthcharts

SAFER · HEALTHIER · PEOPLE™

Birth to 36 months: Boys
Head circumference-for-age and
Weight-for-length percentiles

NAME _____

RECORD # _____

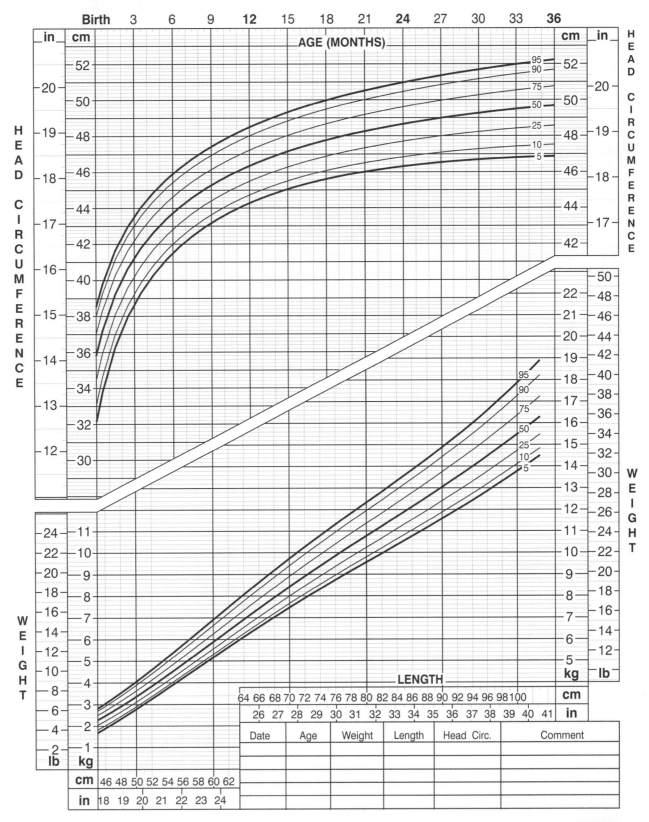

Date	Age	Weight	Length	Head Circ.	Comment

Published May 30, 2000 (modified 10/16/00).
SOURCE: Developed by the National Center for Health Statistics in collaboration with
the National Center for Chronic Disease Prevention and Health Promotion (2000).
http://www.cdc.gov/growthcharts

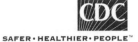

SAFER • HEALTHIER • PEOPLE™

647

2 to 20 years: Boys
Body mass index-for-age percentiles

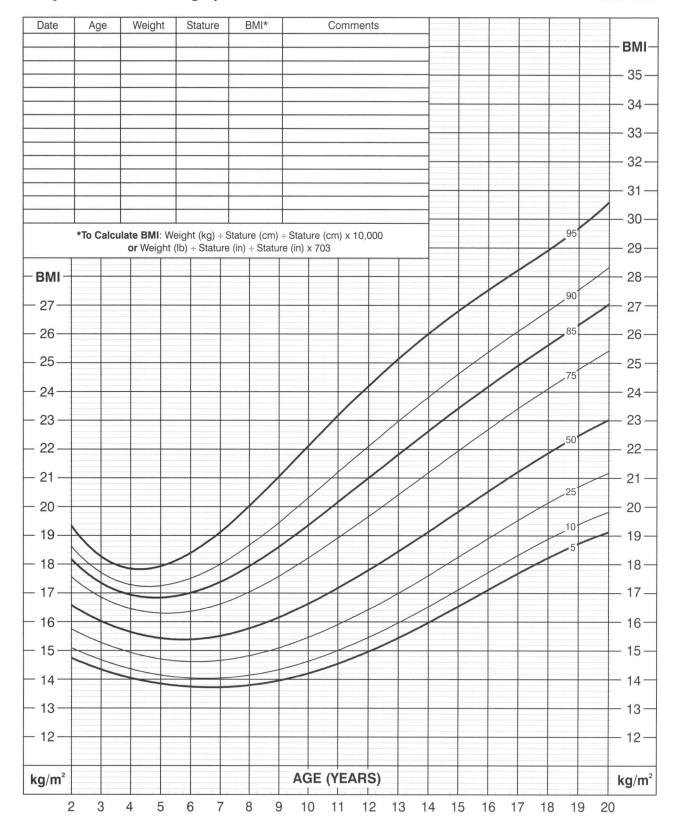

Date	Age	Weight	Stature	BMI*	Comments

*To Calculate BMI: Weight (kg) ÷ Stature (cm) ÷ Stature (cm) x 10,000
or Weight (lb) ÷ Stature (in) ÷ Stature (in) x 703

AGE (YEARS)

kg/m²

BMI

Published May 30, 2000 (modified 10/16/00).

SOURCE: Developed by the National Center for Health Statistics in collaboration with
the National Center for Chronic Disease Prevention and Health Promotion (2000).
http://www.cdc.gov/growthcharts

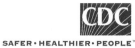

SAFER · HEALTHIER · PEOPLE™

Birth to 36 months: Girls
Length-for-age and Weight-for-age percentiles

NAME _____

RECORD # _____

AGE (MONTHS)

Birth 3 6 9 12 15 18 21 24 27 30 33 36

in	cm		cm	in

LENGTH

41, 40, 39, 38, 37, 36, 35, 34, 33, 32, 31, 30, 29, 28, 27, 26, 25, 24, 23, 22, 21, 20, 19, 18, 17, 16, 15

100, 95, 90, 85, 80, 75, 70, 65, 60, 55, 50, 45, 40

95, 90, 75, 50, 25, 10, 5

WEIGHT

17, 16, 15, 14, 13, 12, 11, 10, 9, 8

95, 90, 75, 50, 25, 10, 5

38, 36, 34, 32, 30, 28, 26, 24, 22, 20, 18, 16

AGE (MONTHS)

12 15 18 21 24 27 30 33 36

kg lb

16, 7, 14, 6, 12, 5, 10, 4, 8, 3, 6, 2

WEIGHT

Mother's Stature _____	Gestational	
Father's Stature _____	Age: _____ Weeks	Comment

Date	Age	Weight	Length	Head Circ.	
	Birth				

lb kg

Birth 3 6 9

Published May 30, 2000 (modified 4/20/01).
SOURCE: Developed by the National Center for Health Statistics in collaboration with
the National Center for Chronic Disease Prevention and Health Promotion (2000).
http://www.cdc.gov/growthcharts

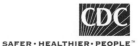

SAFER · HEALTHIER · PEOPLE™

649

Birth to 36 months: Girls
Head circumference-for-age and
Weight-for-length percentiles

NAME _____

RECORD # _____

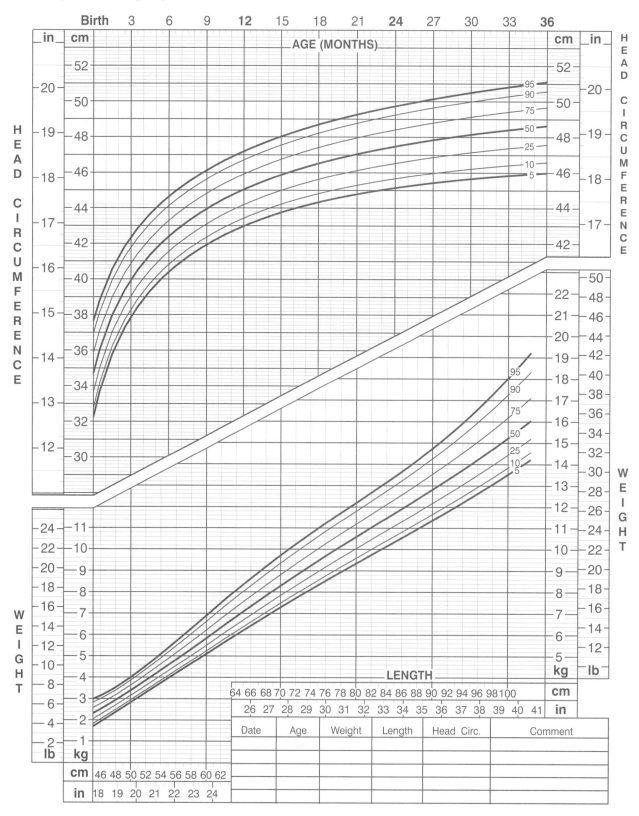

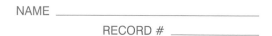

AGE (MONTHS)

Birth 3 6 9 12 15 18 21 24 27 30 33 36

Date	Age	Weight	Length	Head Circ.	Comment

Published May 30, 2000 (modified 10/16/00).
SOURCE: Developed by the National Center for Health Statistics in collaboration with
the National Center for Chronic Disease Prevention and Health Promotion (2000).
http://www.cdc.gov/growthcharts

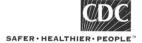

SAFER · HEALTHIER · PEOPLE™

650

2 to 20 years: Girls
Body mass index-for-age percentiles

NAME _____

RECORD # _____

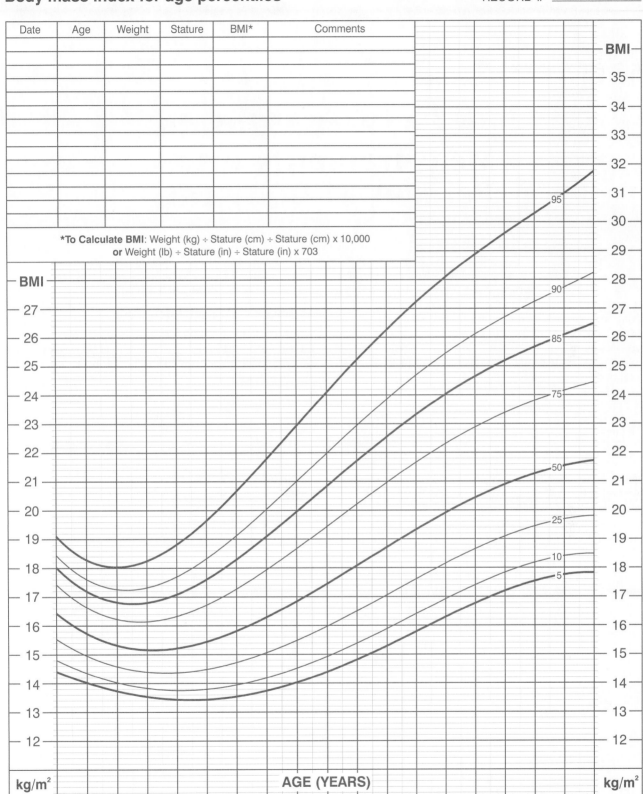

Date	Age	Weight	Stature	BMI*	Comments

*To Calculate BMI: Weight (kg) ÷ Stature (cm) ÷ Stature (cm) x 10,000
or Weight (lb) ÷ Stature (in) ÷ Stature (in) x 703

BMI

27
26
25
24
23
22
21
20
19
18
17
16
15
14
13
12

kg/m²

AGE (YEARS)

2 3 4 5 6 7 8 9 10 11 12 13 14 15 16 17 18 19 20

BMI

35
34
33
32
31
30
29
28
27
26
25
24
23
22
21
20
19
18
17
16
15
14
13
12

kg/m²

95
90
85
75
50
25
10
5

Published May 30, 2000 (modified 10/16/00).
SOURCE: Developed by the National Center for Health Statistics in collaboration with
the National Center for Chronic Disease Prevention and Health Promotion (2000).
http://www.cdc.gov/growthcharts

CDC
SAFER · HEALTHIER · PEOPLE™

651

To Convert Skinfold Measurements Into Percent of Body Fat

Add the averages of all skinfold sites to arrive at a total skinfold measurement. Take the measurement to charts for determining percent of body fat.

Using the Tables:

Adults: Tables A and B: Read sum of four skinfolds in far left column. Read across the line to appropriate age column. Figure in that column indicates what percentage of total body weight is fat.

Youth: Tables C and D: Same as above, except read sum of two skinfolds—Triceps and Subscapular.

Body Fat and Skinfolds

The equivalent fat content, as a percentage of body weight, for a range of values for the sum of four skinfolds (biceps, triceps, subscapular, and suprailiac) of males and females of different ages.

Table A

SKINFOLDS (mm)	Males			
	Ages			
	17–29	30–39	40–49	50+
15	4.8	—	—	—
20	8.1	12.2	12.2	12.6
25	10.5	14.2	15.0	15.6
30	12.9	16.2	17.7	18.6
35	14.7	17.7	19.6	20.8
40	16.4	19.2	21.4	22.9
45	17.7	20.4	23.0	24.7
50	19.0	21.5	24.6	26.5
55	20.1	22.5	25.9	27.9
60	21.2	23.5	27.1	29.2
65	22.2	24.3	28.2	30.4
70	23.1	25.1	29.3	31.6
75	24.0	25.9	30.3	32.7
80	24.8	26.6	31.2	33.8
85	25.5	27.2	32.1	34.8
90	26.2	27.8	33.0	35.8
95	26.9	28.4	33.7	36.6
100	27.6	29.0	34.4	37.4
105	28.2	29.6	35.1	38.2
110	28.8	30.1	35.8	39.0
115	29.4	30.6	36.4	39.7
120	30.0	31.1	37.0	40.4
125	30.5	31.5	37.6	41.1
130	31.0	31.9	38.2	41.8
135	31.5	32.3	38.7	42.4
140	32.0	32.7	39.2	43.0
145	32.5	33.1	39.7	43.6

Table B

SKINFOLDS (mm)	Females			
	Ages			
	16–29	30–39	40–49	50+
15	10.5	—	—	—
20	14.1	17.0	19.8	21.4
25	16.8	19.4	22.2	24.0
30	19.5	21.8	24.5	26.6
35	21.5	23.7	26.4	28.5
40	23.4	25.5	28.2	30.3
45	25.0	26.9	29.6	31.9
50	26.5	28.2	31.0	33.4
55	27.8	29.4	32.1	34.6
60	29.1	30.6	33.2	35.7
65	30.2	31.6	34.1	36.7
70	31.2	32.5	35.0	37.7
75	32.2	33.4	35.9	38.7
80	33.1	34.3	36.7	39.6
85	34.0	35.1	37.5	40.4
90	34.8	35.8	38.3	41.2
95	35.6	36.5	39.0	41.9
100	36.4	37.2	39.7	42.6
105	37.1	37.9	40.4	43.3
110	37.8	38.6	41.0	43.9
115	38.4	39.1	41.5	44.5
120	39.0	39.6	42.0	45.1
125	39.6	40.1	42.5	45.7
130	40.2	40.6	43.0	46.2
135	40.8	41.1	43.5	46.7
140	41.3	41.6	44.0	47.2
145	41.8	42.1	44.5	47.7

(Continued on the following page)

Males					Females				
SKINFOLDS (mm)	Ages				**SKINFOLDS (mm)**	Ages			
	17–29	**30–39**	**40–49**	**50+**		**16–29**	**30–39**	**40–49**	**50+**
150	32.9	33.5	40.2	44.1	150	42.3	42.6	45.0	48.2
155	33.3	33.9	40.7	44.6	155	42.8	43.1	45.4	48.7
160	33.7	34.3	41.2	45.1	160	43.3	43.6	45.8	49.2
165	34.1	34.6	41.6	45.6	165	43.7	44.0	46.2	49.6
170	34.5	34.8	42.0	46.1	170	44.1	44.4	46.6	50.0
175	34.9	—	—	—	175	—	44.8	47.0	50.4
180	35.3	—	—	—	180	—	45.2	47.4	50.8
185	35.6	—	—	—	185	—	45.6	47.8	51.2
190	35.9	—	—	—	190	—	45.9	48.2	51.6
195	—	—	—	—	195	—	46.2	48.5	52.0
200	—	—	—	—	200	—	46.5	48.8	52.4
205	—	—	—	—	205	—	—	49.1	52.7
210	—	—	—	—	210	—	—	49.4	53.0

In two-thirds of the instances, the error was within ±3.5 percent of the body weight as fat for the women and ±5 percent for the men.

Modified from Durnin, JVGA, and Womersley, J: Body fat assessed from total body density and its estimation from skinfold thickness: Measurements on 481 men and women aged from 16 to 72 years. Br J Nutr 32:77, 1974. By permission of the Nutritional Society.

Tables from the Mayo Clinic Diet Manual, Fifth Edition, Published by W.B. Saunders Company of Philadelphia, 1981; by permission of Mayo Foundation, and Cambridge University Press, publishers of the British Journal of Nutrition.

The relationship of skinfold thickness to body fat in children and individuals under 17 is addressed by The American Alliance for Health, Physical Education, Recreation and Dance in the publication, Lifetime Health Related Physical Fitness Test Manual. They suggest that national percentile norms provide the best reference. They further suggest that the ideal is at the 50th percentile. Those below 25 percent should be encouraged to reduce amount of body fat, while those above 90 percentile should not be encouraged to lose body fat.

Table C

Percentile Norms. Ages 6–18* for Sum of Triceps Plus Subscapular Skinfolds (mm) for Boys†

AGE	6	7	8	9	10	11	12	13	14	15	16	17
PERCENTILE												
99	7	7	7	7	7	8	8	7	7	8	8	8
95	8	9	9	9	9	9	9	9	9	9	9	9
90	9	9	9	10	10	10	10	10	9	10	10	10
85	10	10	10	10	11	11	10	11	10	11	11	11
80	10	10	10	11	11	12	11	11	11	11	11	12
75	11	11	11	11	12	12	11	12	11	12	12	12
70	11	11	11	12	12	12	12	12	12	12	12	13
65	11	11	12	12	13	13	13	12	12	13	13	13
60	12	12	12	13	13	14	13	13	13	13	13	14
55	12	12	13	13	14	15	14	14	13	14	14	14
50	12	12	13	14	14	16	15	15	14	14	14	15
45	13	13	14	14	15	16	15	16	14	15	15	16
40	13	13	14	15	16	17	16	17	15	16	16	16
35	13	14	15	16	17	19	17	18	16	18	17	17
30	14	14	16	17	18	20	19	19	18	18	18	19
25	14	15	17	18	19	22	21	22	20	20	20	21
20	15	16	18	20	21	24	24	25	23	22	22	24
15	16	17	19	23	24	28	27	29	27	25	24	26
10	18	18	21	26	28	33	33	36	31	30	29	30
5	20	24	28	34	33	38	44	46	37	40	37	38

*The norms for age 17 may be used for age 18.

†Based on data from Johnston, FE, DV Hamill, and S Lemeshow. (1) Skinfold Thickness of Children 6–11 Years (Series II, No. 120, 1972), and (2) Skinfold Thickness of Youths 12–17 Years (Series II, No. 132, 1974). U.S. National Center for Health Statistics, U.S. Department of HEW, Washington, DC

Table D

Percentile Norms. Ages 6–18* for Sum of Triceps Plus Subscapular Skinfolds (mm) for Girls†

AGE	6	7	8	9	10	11	12	13	14	15	16	17
PERCENTILE												
99	8	8	8	9	9	8	9	10	10	11	11	12
95	9	10	10	10	10	11	11	12	13	14	14	15
90	10	11	11	12	12	12	12	13	15	16	16	16
85	11	12	12	12	13	13	13	14	16	17	18	18
80	12	12	12	13	13	14	14	15	17	18	19	19
75	12	12	13	14	14	15	15	16	18	20	20	20
70	12	13	14	15	15	16	16	17	19	21	21	22
65	13	13	14	15	16	16	17	18	20	22	22	23
60	13	14	15	16	17	17	17	19	21	23	23	24
55	14	15	16	16	18	18	19	20	22	24	24	26
50	14	15	16	17	18	19	19	20	24	28	25	27
45	15	16	17	18	20	20	21	22	25	26	27	28
40	15	16	18	19	20	21	22	23	26	28	29	30
35	16	17	19	20	22	22	24	25	27	29	30	32
30	17	18	20	22	24	23	25	27	30	32	32	34
25	18	19	21	24	25	25	27	30	32	34	34	36
20	18	20	23	26	28	28	31	33	35	37	37	40
15	19	22	25	29	31	31	35	39	39	42	42	42
10	22	25	30	34	35	36	40	43	42	48	46	46
5	26	28	36	40	41	42	48	51	52	56	57	58

*The norms for age 17 may be used for age 18.
†Based on data from Johnston, FE, DV Hamill, and S Lemeshow. (1) Skinfold Thickness of Children 6–11 Years (Series II, No. 120, 1972), and (2) Skinfold
   Thickness of Youths 12–17 Years (Series II, No. 132, 1974). U.S. National Center for Health Statistics, U.S. Department of HEW, Washington, DC
Tables from Lifetime Health Related Physical Fitness Test Manual, AAHPERD, Reston, VA, 1980. With permission of the American Alliance for Health,
   Physical Education, Recreation and Dance.

Dietary Reference Intakes for Individuals: Vitamins and Minerals, RDAs, and AIs

Dietary Reference Intakes (DRIs): Recommended Intakes for Individuals, Vitamins Food and Nutrition Board, Institute of Medicine, National Academies

LIFE-STAGE GROUP	VITAMIN A (µg/d)[a]	VITAMIN C (mg/d)	VITAMIN D (µg/d)[b,c]	VITAMIN E (mg/d)[d]	VITAMIN K (µg/d)	THIAMIN (mg/d)	RIBOFLAVIN (mg/d)	NIACIN (mg/d)[e]	VITAMIN B$_6$ (mg/d)	FOLATE (µg/d)[f]	VITAMIN B$_{12}$ (µg/d)	PANTOTHENIC Acid (mg/d)	BIOTIN (µg/d)	CHOLINE (mg/d)[g]
Infants														
0–6 mo	400*	40*	5*	4*	2.0*	0.2*	0.3*	2*	0.1*	65*	0.4*	1.7*	5*	125*
7–12 mo	500*	50*	5*	5*	2.5*	0.3*	0.4*	4*	0.3*	80*	0.5*	1.8*	6*	150*
Children														
1–3 yr	300	15	5*	6	30*	0.5	0.5	6	0.5	150	0.9	2*	8*	200*
4–8 yr	400	25	5*	7	55*	0.6	0.6	8	0.6	200	1.2	3*	12*	250*
Males														
9–13 yr	600	45	5*	11	60*	0.9	0.9	12	1.0	300	1.8	4*	20*	375*
14–18 yr	900	75	5*	15	75*	1.2	1.3	16	1.3	400	2.4	5*	25*	550*
19–30 yr	900	90	5*	15	120*	1.2	1.3	16	1.3	400	2.4	5*	30*	550*
31–50 yr	900	90	5*	15	120*	1.2	1.3	16	1.3	400	2.4	5*	30*	550*
51–70 yr	900	90	10*	15	120*	1.2	1.3	16	1.7	400	2.4[h]	5*	30*	550*
>70 yr	900	90	15*	15	120*	1.2	1.3	16	1.7	400	2.4[h]	5*	30*	550*
Females														
9–13 yr	600	45	5*	11	60*	0.9	0.9	12	1.0	300	1.8	4*	20*	375*
14–18 yr	700	65	5*	15	75*	1.0	1.0	14	1.2	400[f]	2.4	5*	25*	400*
19–30 yr	700	75	5*	15	90*	1.1	1.1	14	1.3	400[f]	2.4	5*	30*	425*
31–50 yr	700	75	5*	15	90*	1.1	1.1	14	1.3	400[f]	2.4	5*	30*	425*
51–70 yr	700	75	10*	15	90*	1.1	1.1	14	1.5	400	2.4[h]	5*	30*	425*
>70 yr	700	75	15*	15	90*	1.1	1.1	14	1.5	400	2.4[h]	5*	30*	425*
Pregnancy														
≤18 yr	750	80	5*	15	75*	1.4	1.4	18	1.9	600[f]	2.6	6*	30*	450*
19–30 yr	770	85	5*	15	90*	1.4	1.4	18	1.9	600[f]	2.6	6*	30*	450*
31–50 yr	770	85	5*	15	90*	1.4	1.4	18	1.9	600[f]	2.6	6*	30*	450*
Lactation														
≤18 yr	1200	115	5*	19	75*	1.4	1.6	17	2.0	500	2.8	7*	35*	550*
19–30 yr	1300	120	5*	19	90*	1.4	1.6	17	2.0	500	2.8	7*	35*	550*
31–50 yr	1300	120	5*	19	90*	1.4	1.6	17	2.0	500	2.8	7*	35*	550*

SOURCES: Dietary Reference Intakes for Calcium, Phosphorous, Magnesium, Vitamin D, and Fluoride (1997); Dietary Reference Intakes for Thiamin, Riboflavin, Niacin, Vitamin B$_6$, Folate, Vitamin B$_{12}$, Pantothenic Acid, Biotin, and Choline (1998); Dietary Reference Intakes for Vitamin C, Vitamin E, Selenium, and Carotenoids (2000); and Dietary Reference Intakes for Vitamin A, Vitamin K, Arsenic, Boron, Chromium, Copper, Iodine, Iron, Manganese, Molybdenum, Nickel, Silicon, Vanadium, and Zinc (2001). These reports may be accessed via www.nap.edu. Copyright 2001 by the National Academy of Sciences. All rights reserved.

Note: This table (taken from the DRI reports, see www.nap.edu) presents Recommended Dietary Allowances (RDAs) in bold type and Adequate Intakes (AIs) in ordinary type followed by an asterisk (*). RDAs and AIs may both be used as goals for individual intake. RDAs are set to meet the needs of almost all (97%–98%) individuals in a group. For healthy breastfed infants, the AI is the mean intake. The AI for other life-stage and gender groups is believed to cover needs of all individuals in the group, but lack of data or uncertainty in the data prevent being able to specify with confidence the percentage of individuals covered by this intake.

[a]As retinol activity equivalents (RAEs). 1 RAE = 1 µg retinol, 12 µg β-carotene, 24 µg α-carotene, or 24 µg β-cryptoxanthin. To calculate RAEs from REs of provitamin A carotenoids in foods, divide the REs by 2. For preformed vitamin A in foods or supplements and for provitamin A carotenoids in supplements, 1 RE = 1 RAE.

[b]Calciferol 1 µg calciferol = 40 IU vitamin D.

[c]In the absence of adequate exposure to sunlight.

[d]As α-tocopherol. α-Tocopherol includes *RRR*-α-tocopherol, the only form of α-tocopherol that occurs naturally in foods, and the *2R*-stereoisometric forms of α-tocopherol (*RRR*-, *RSR*-, *RRS*-, and *RSS*-α-tocopherol) that occur in fortified foods and supplements. It does not include the *2S*-stereoisometric forms of α-tocopherol (*SRR*-, *SSR*-, *SR*-, and *SSS*- a tocopherol), also found in fortified foods and supplements.

[e]As niacin equivalents (NE). 1 mg of niacin = 60 mg of tryptophan; 0–6 months = preformed niacin (not NE).

[f]As dietary folate equivalents (DFE). 1 DFE = 1 µg food folate = 0.6 µg of folic acid from fortified food or as a supplement consumed with food = 0.5 µg of a supplement taken on an empty stomach.

[g]Although AIs have been set for choline, few data assess whether a dietary supply of choline is needed at all stages of the life cycle, and it may be that the choline requirement can be met by endogenous synthesis at some of these stages.

[h]Because 10 to 30 percent of older people may malabsorb food-bound B$_{12}$, it is advisable for those older than 50 years to meet their RDA mainly by consuming foods fortified with B$_{12}$ or a supplement containing B$_{12}$.

[i]In view of evidence linking folate intake with neural tube defects in the fetus, it is recommended that all women capable of becoming pregnant consume 400 µg from supplements or fortified foods in addition to intake of food folate from a varied diet.

[i]It is assumed that women will continue consuming 400 µg from supplements or fortified food until their pregnancy is confirmed and they enter prenatal care, which ordinarily occurs after the end of the periconceptional period—the critical time for formation of the neural tube.

SOURCE: Tables compiled and copied with permission from Mahon, KL and Escott-Stump: Krause's Food, Nutrition, and Diet Therapy, ed 11. Elsevier, Philadelphia, 2004.

Dietary Reference Intakes (DRIs): Recommended Intakes for Individuals, Minerals Food and Nutrition Board, Institute of Medicine, National Academies

LIFE-STAGE GROUP	CALCIUM (mg/d)	CHROMIUM (μg/d)	COPPER (μg/d)	FLUORIDE (mg/d)	IODINE (μg/d)	IRON (mg/d)	MAGNESIUM (mg/d)	MANGANESE (mg/d)	MOLYBDENUM (μg/d)	PHOSPHORUS (mg)	SELENIUM (μg/d)	ZINC (mg/d)
Infants												
0–6 mo	210*	0.2*	200*	0.01*	110*	0.27*	30*	0.003*	2*	100*	15*	2*
7–12 mo	270*	5.5*	220*	0.5*	130*	11	75*	0.6*	3*	275*	20*	3
Children												
1–3 yr	500*	11*	340	0.7*	90	7	80	1.2*	17	460	20	3
4–8 yr	800*	15*	440	1*	90	10	130	1.5*	22	500	30	5
Males												
9–13 yr	1300*	25*	700	2*	120	8	240	1.9*	34	1250	40	8
14–18 yr	1300*	35*	890	3*	150	11	410	2.2*	43	1250	55	11
19–30 yr	1000*	35*	900	4*	150	8	400	2.3*	45	700	55	11
31–50 yr	1000*	35*	900	4*	150	8	420	2.3*	45	700	55	11
51–70 yr	1200*	30*	900	4*	150	8	420	2.3*	45	700	55	11
>70 yr	1200*	30*	900	4*	150	8	420	2.3*	45	700	55	11
Females												
9–13 yr	1300*	21*	700	2*	120	8	240	1.6*	34	1250	40	8
14–18 yr	1300*	24*	890	3*	150	15	360	1.6*	43	1250	55	9
19–30 yr	1000*	25*	900	3*	150	18	310	1.8*	45	700	55	8
31–50 yr	1000*	25*	900	3*	150	18	320	1.8*	45	700	55	8
51–70 yr	1200*	20*	900	3*	150	8	320	1.8*	45	700	55	8
>70 yr	1200*	20*	900	3*	150	8	320	1.8*	45	700	55	8
Pregnancy												
≤18 yr	1300*	29*	1000	3*	220	27	400	2.0*	50	1250	60	13
19–30 yr	1000*	30*	1000	3*	220	27	350	2.0*	50	700	60	11
31–50 yr	1000*	30*	1000	3*	220	27	360	2.0*	50	700	60	11
Lactation												
≤18 yr	1300*	44*	1300	3*	290	10	360	2.6*	50	1250	70	14
19–30 yr	1000*	45*	1300	3*	290	9	310	2.6*	50	700	70	12
31–50 yr	1000*	45*	1300	3*	290	9	320	2.6*	50	700	70	12

SOURCES: Dietary Reference Intakes for Calcium, Phosphorus, Magnesium, Vitamin D, and Fluoride (1997); Dietary Reference Intakes for Thiamin, Riboflavin, Niacin, Vitamin B$_6$, Folate, Vitamin B$_{12}$, Pantothenic Acid, Biotin, and Choline (1998); Dietary Reference Intakes for Vitamin C, Vitamin E, Selenium, and Carotenoids (2000); and Dietary Reference Intakes for Vitamin A, Vitamin K, Arsenic, Boron, Chromium, Copper, Iodine, Iron, Manganese, Molybdenum, Nickel, Silicon, Vanadium, and Zinc (2001). Copyright 2001 by the National Academy of Sciences. All rights reserved.

Note: This table presents Recommended Dietary Allowances (RDAs) in bold type and Adequate Intakes (AIs) in ordinary type followed by an asterisk (*). RDAs and AIs may both be used as goals for individual intake. RDAs are set to meet the needs of almost all (97%–98%) individuals in a group. For healthy breastfed infants, the AI is the mean intake. The AI for other life-stage and gender groups is believed to cover needs of all individuals in the group, but lack of data or uncertainty in the data prevent being able to specify with confidence the percentage of individuals covered by this intake.

SOURCE: Tables compiled and copied with permission from Mahon, KL and Escott-Stump: Krause's Food, Nutrition, and Diet Therapy, ed 11. Elsevier, Philadelphia, 2004.

G

Dietary Reference Intakes: Tolerable Upper Intake Levels for Vitamins and Minerals

Dietary Reference Intakes (DRIs): Tolerable Upper Intake Levels (UL[a]), Vitamins Food and Nutrition Board, Institute of Medicine, National Academies

LIFE-STAGE GROUP	VITAMIN A (µg/d)[b]	VITAMIN C (mg/d)	VITAMIN D (µg/d)	VITAMIN E (mg/d)[c,d]	VITAMIN K	THIAMIN	RIBOFLAVIN	NIACIN (mg/d)[d]	VITAMIN B$_6$ (mg/d)[d]	FOLATE (µg/d)[d]	VITAMIN B$_{12}$	PANTO- THENIC ACID	BIOTIN	CHOLINE (g/d)	CAROTE- NOIDS[e]
Infants															
0–6 mo	600	ND[f]	25	ND	ND	ND	ND	ND	ND	ND	ND	ND	ND	ND	ND
7–12 mo	600	ND	25	ND	ND	ND	ND	ND	ND	ND	ND	ND	ND	ND	ND
Children															
1–3 yr	600	400	50	200	ND	ND	ND	10	30	300	ND	ND	ND	1.0	ND
4–8 yr	900	650	50	300	ND	ND	ND	15	40	400	ND	ND	ND	1.0	ND
Males, Females															
9–13 yr	1700	1200	50	600	ND	ND	ND	20	60	600	ND	ND	ND	2.0	ND
14–18 yr	2800	1800	50	800	ND	ND	ND	30	80	800	ND	ND	ND	3.0	ND
19–70 yr	3000	2000	50	1000	ND	ND	ND	35	100	1000	ND	ND	ND	3.5	ND
>70 yr	3000	2000	50	1000	ND	ND	ND	35	100	1000	ND	ND	ND	3.5	ND
Pregnancy															
≤18 yr	2800	1800	50	800	ND	ND	ND	30	80	800	ND	ND	ND	3.0	ND
19–50 yr	3000	2000	50	1000	ND	ND	ND	35	100	1000	ND	ND	ND	3.5	ND
Lactation															
18 yr	2800	1800	50	800	ND	ND	ND	30	80	800	ND	ND	ND	3.0	ND
19–50 yr	3000	2000	50	1000	ND	ND	ND	35	100	1000	ND	ND	ND	3.5	ND

SOURCES: Dietary Reference Intakes for Calcium, Phosphorous, Magnesium, Vitamin D, and Fluoride (1997); Dietary Reference Intakes for Thiamin, Riboflavin, Niacin, Vitamin B$_6$, Folate, Vitamin B$_{12}$, Pantothenic Acid, Biotin, and Choline (1998); Dietary Reference Intakes for Vitamin C, Vitamin E, Selenium, and Carotenoids (2000); and Dietary Reference Intakes for Vitamin A, Vitamin K, Arsenic, Boron, Chromium, Copper, Iodine, Iron, Manganese, Molybdenum, Nickel, Silicon, Vanadium, and Zinc (2001). These reports may be accessed via www.nap.edu. Copyright 2001 by the National Academy of Sciences. All rights reserved.

[a]UL = The maximum level of daily nutrient intake that is likely to pose no risk of adverse effects. Unless otherwise specified, the UL represents total intake from food, water, and supplements. Due to lack of suitable data, ULs could not be established for vitamin K, thiamin, riboflavin, vitamin B$_{12}$, pantothenic acid, biotin, or carotenoids. In the absence of ULs, extra caution may be warranted in consuming levels above recommended intakes.

[b]As preformed vitamin A only.

[c]As α-tocopherol; applies to any form of supplemental α-tocopherol.

[d]The ULs for vitamin E, niacin, and folate apply to synthetic forms obtained from supplements, fortified foods, or a combination of the two.

[e]β-Carotene supplements are advised only to serve as a provitamin A source for individuals at risk of vitamin A deficiency.

[f]ND = Not determinable due to lack of data of adverse effects in this age group and concern with regard to lack of ability to handle excess amounts. Source of intake should be from food only to prevent high levels of intake.

SOURCE: Tables compiled and copied with permission from Mahon, KL and Escott-Stump: Krause's Food, Nutrition, and Diet Therapy, ed. 11, Elsevier, Philadelphia, 2004.

Dietary Reference Intakes (DRIs): Tolerable Upper Intake Levels (UL[a]), Minerals Food and Nutrition Board, Institute of Medicine, National Academies

LIFE-STAGE GROUP	ARSENIC[b]	BORON (mg/d)	CALCIUM (g/d)	CHROMIUM	COPPER (μg/d)	FLUORIDE (mg/d)	IODINE (μg/d)	IRON (mg/d)	MAGNESIUM (mg/d)[c]	MANGANESE (mg/d)	MOLYBDENUM (μg/d)	NICKEL (mg/d)	PHOSPHORUS (g/d)	SELENIUM (μg/d)	SILICON[d]	VANADIUM (mg/d)[e]	ZINC (mg/d)
Infants																	
0–6 mo	ND[f]	ND	ND	ND	ND	0.7	ND	40	ND	ND	ND	ND	ND	45	ND	ND	4
7–12 mo	ND	ND	ND	ND	ND	0.9	ND	40	ND	ND	ND	ND	ND	60	ND	ND	5
Children																	
1–3 yr	ND	3	2.5	ND	1000	1.3	200	40	65	2	300	0.2	3	90	ND	ND	7
4–8 yr	ND	6	2.5	ND	3000	2.2	300	40	110	3	600	0.3	3	150	ND	ND	12
Males, Females																	
9–13 yr	ND	11	2.5	ND	5000	10	600	40	350	6	1100	0.6	4	280	ND	ND	23
14–18 yr	ND	17	2.5	ND	8000	10	900	45	350	9	1700	1.0	4	400	ND	ND	34
19–70 yr	ND	20	2.5	ND	10,000	10	1100	45	350	11	2000	1.0	4	400	ND	1.8	40
>70 yr	ND	20	2.5	ND	10,000	10	1100	45	350	11	2000	1.0	3	400	ND	1.8	40
Pregnancy																	
≤18 yr	ND	17	2.5	ND	8000	10	900	45	350	9	1700	1.0	3.5	400	ND	ND	34
19–50 yr	ND	20	2.5	ND	10,000	10	1100	45	350	11	2000	1.0	3.5	400	ND	ND	40
Lactation																	
≤18 yr	ND	17	2.5	ND	8000	10	900	45	350	9	1700	1.0	4	400	ND	ND	34
19–50 yr	ND	20	2.5	ND	10,000	10	1100	45	350	11	2000	1.0	4	400	ND	ND	40

SOURCES: Dietary Reference Intakes for Calcium, Phosphorous, Magnesium, Vitamin D, and Fluoride (1997); Dietary Reference Intakes for Thiamin, Riboflavin, Niacin, Vitamin B₆, Folate, Vitamin B₁₂, Pantothenic Acid, Biotin, and Choline (1998); Dietary Reference Intakes for Vitamin C, Vitamin E, Selenium, and Carotenoids (2000); and Dietary Reference Intakes for Vitamin A, Vitamin K, Arsenic, Boron, Chromium, Copper, Iodine, Iron, Manganese, Molybdenum, Nickel, Silicon, Vanadium, and Zinc (2001). These reports may be accessed via www.nep.edu. Copyright 2001 by the National Academy of Sciences. All rights reserved.

[a]UL = The maximum level of daily nutrient intake that is likely to pose no risk of adverse effects. Unless otherwise specified, the UL represents total intake from food, water, and supplements. Due to lack of suitable data, ULs could not be established for arsenic, chromium, and silicon. In the absence of ULs, extra caution may be warranted in consuming levels above recommended intakes.

[b]Although the UL was not determined for arsenic, there is no justification for adding arsenic to food or supplements.

[c]The ULs for magnesium represent intake from a pharmacologic agent only and do not include intake from food and water.

[d]Although silicon has not been shown to cause adverse effects in humans, there is no justification for adding silicon to supplements.

[e]Although vanadium in food has not been shown to cause adverse effects in humans, there is no justification for adding vanadium to food, and vanadium supplements should be used with caution. The UL is based on adverse effects in laboratory animals, and this data could be used to set a UL for adults but not children and adolescents.

[f]ND = Not determinable due to lack of data of adverse effects in this age group and concern with regard to lack of ability to handle excess amounts. Source of intake should be from food only to prevent high levels of intake.

SOURCE: Tables compiled and copied with permission from Mahon, KL and Escott-Stump: Krause's Food, Nutrition, and Diet Therapy, ed. 11, Elsevier, Philadelphia, 2004.

Dietary Reference Intakes: Recommended Intakes for Individuals, Macronutrients

Dietary Reference Intakes (DRIs): Recommended Intakes for Individuals, Macronutrients Food and Nutrition Board, Institute of Medicine, National Academies

LIFE-STAGE GROUP	PROTEIN RDA/AI g/day[a]	PROTEIN AMDR[b]	CARBOHYDRATE RDA/AI g/day	CARBOHYDRATE AMDR	FIBER RDA/AI g/day	FIBER AMDR	FAT RDA/AI g/day*	FAT AMDR	n-6 POLYUNSATURATED FATTY ACIDS (LINOLEIC ACID) RDA/AI g/day*	n-6 AMDR	n-3 POLYUNSATURATED FATTY ACIDS (α-LINOLENIC ACID) RDA/AI g/day*	n-3 AMDR[d]	SATURATED AND TRANS FATTY ACIDS AND CHOLESTEROL RDA/AI g/day	SAT AMDR
Infants														
0–6 mo	9.1*	ND[c]	60*	ND	ND		31*		4.4	ND	0.5	ND	ND	
7–12 mo	**13.5**	ND	95*	ND	ND		30*		4.6	ND	0.5	ND	ND	
Children														
1–3 yr	**13**	**5–20**	**130**	45–65	19			30–40	7	5–10	0.7	0.6–1.2		
4–8 yr	**19**	**10–30**	**130**	45–65	25			25–35	10	5–10	0.9	0.6–1.2		
Males														
9–13 yr	**34**	**10–30**	**130**	45–65	31			25–35	12	5–10	1.2	0.6–1.2		
14–18 yr	**52**	**10–30**	**130**	45–65	38			25–35	16	5–10	1.6	0.6–1.2		
19–30 yr	**56**	**10–35**	**130**	45–65	38			20–35	17	5–10	1.6	0.6–1.2		
31–50 yr	**56**	**10–35**	**130**	45–65	38			20–35	17	5–10	1.6	0.6–1.2		
50–70 yr	**56**	**10–35**	**130**	45–65	30			20–35	14	5–10	1.6	0.6–1.2		
>70 yr	**56**	**10–35**	**130**	45–65	30			20–35	14	5–10	1.6	0.6–1.2		
Females														
9–13 yr	**34**	**10–30**	**130**	45–65	26			25–35	10	5–10	1.0	0.6–1.2		
14–18 yr	**46**	**10–30**	**130**	45–65	26			25–35	11	5–10	1.1	0.6–1.2		
19–30 yr	**46**	**10–35**	**130**	45–65	25			20–35	12	5–10	1.1	0.6–1.2		
31–50 yr	**46**	**10–35**	**130**	45–65	25			20–35	12	5–10	1.1	0.6–1.2		
50–70 yr	**46**	**10–35**	**130**	45–65	21			20–35	11	5–10	1.1	0.6–1.2		
>70 yr	**46**	**10–35**	**130**	45–65	21			20–35	11	5–10	1.1	0.6–1.2		
Pregnant														
≤18 yr	**71**	**10–35**	**175**	45–65	28			20–35	13	5–10	1.4	0.6–1.2		
19–30 yr	**71**	**10–35**	**175**	45–65	28			20–35	13	5–10	1.4	0.6–1.2		
31–50 yr	**71**	**10–35**	**175**	45–65	28			20–35	13	5–10	1.4	0.6–1.2		
Lactating														
≤18 yr	**71**	**10–35**	**210**	45–65	29			20–35	13	5–10	1.3	0.6–1.2		
19–30 yr	**71**	**10–35**	**210**	45–65	29			20–35	13	5–10	1.3	0.6–1.2		
31–50 yr	**71**	**10–35**	**210**	45–65	29			20–35	13	5–10	1.3	0.6–1.2		

Data from *Dietary reference intakes for energy, carbohydrate, fiber, fat, fatty acids, cholesterol, protein, and amino acids,* Washington, DC, 2002, The National Academies Press.

Note: This table represents Recommended Dietary Allowances (RDAs) in bold type and Adequate Intakes (AIs) in ordinary type. RDAs and AIs may both be used as goals for individual intake. RDAs are set to meet the needs of almost all (97%–98%) individuals in a group. For healthy breastfed infants, the AI is the mean intake. The AI for other life-stage and gender groups is believed to cover the needs of all individuals in the group, but lack of data prevents being able to specify with confidence the percentage of individuals covered by this intake.

[a] Based on 1.5 g/kg/day for infants, 1.1 g/kg/day for 1–3 yr, 0.95 g/kg/day for 4–13 yr, 0.85 g/kg/day for 14–18 yr, 0.8 g/kg/day for adults, and 1.1 g/kg/day for pregnant (using prepregnancy weight) and lactating women.

[b] Acceptable Macronutrient Distribution Range (AMDR) is the range of intake for a particular energy source that is associated with reduced risk of chronic disease while providing intakes of essential nutrients. If an individual has consumed in excess of the AMDR, there is a potential of increasing the risk of chronic diseases and insufficient intakes of essential nutrients.

[c] ND = Not determinable due to lack of data of adverse effects in this age group and concern with regard to lack of ability to handle excess amounts. Source of intake should be from food only to prevent high levels of intake.

[d] Approximately 10% of the total can come from longer-chain, *n-3* fatty acids.

SOURCE: Tables compiled and copied with permission from Mahon, KL and Escott-Stump: Krause's Food, Nutrition, and Diet Therapy, ed 11. Elsevier, Philadelphia, 2004.

Dietary Reference Intakes for Water, Potassium, Sodium, Chloride, and Sulfate

Water

| AI | men 19–30 yrs | 3.7 liters |
| AI | women 19–30 yrs | 2.7 liters |

Potassium

| AI | 4.7 grams adults |
| UL | not established |

Sodium

AI*	1.5 grams/day	younger adults
AI	1.3 grams/day	men and women 50–70 yrs
AI	1.2 grams/day	men and women ≥71 yrs
UL†	2.3 grams/day	younger adults

Sulfate

| EAR | not established |
| UL | not established |

Sulfate requirements are met when intakes include recommended levels for sulfur-containing amino acids

Chloride

AI	2.3 grams/day	younger adults
AI	2.0 grams/day	50–70 yrs
AI	1.8 grams/day	≥71 yrs

*AI does not apply to highly active such as endurance athletes.

†The UL may be lower among certain groups of individuals who are most sensitive to blood pressure effects of increased sodium intake (e.g., older persons, African Americans, and individuals with hypertension, diabetes, or chronic kidney disease). In contrast, for individuals who are unacclimatized to prolonged physical activity in a hot environment, their needs may exceed the UL because of sodium sweat loss.

SOURCE: Institute of Medicine of the National Academies, Dietary References for Energy, Carbohydrate, Fiber, Fat, Fatty Acids, Cholesterol, Protein, and Amino Acids, The National Academy. Washington DC, 2002.

J

Reference Intake Values for Energy for Active Individuals*

LIFE-STAGE GROUP	Healthy, Physically Active, Total Energy Expenditure (EER) kcal/day	
	MALES	FEMALES
INFANTS		
0–6 mo	570	520 (3 mo)
7–12 mo	743	676 (9 mo)
CHILDREN		
1–2 yr	1046	992 (24 mo)
3–8 yr	1742	1642 (yr)
9–13 yr	2279	2071 (11 yr)
14–18 yr	3152	2368 (16 yr)
ADULTS		
>18 yr	3067*	2403 (19 yr)*
PREGNANT WOMEN		
14–18 yr		
First trimester		2368 (16 yr)
Second trimester		2708 (16 yr)
Third trimester		2855 (19 yr)
19–50 yr		
First trimester		2403 (19 yr)*
Second trimester		2743 (19 yr)*
Third trimester		2855 (19 yr)*
LACTATING WOMEN		
14–18 yr		2698 (16 yr)
First 6 mo		2768 (16 yr)
Second 6 mo		
19–50 yr		
First 6 mo		2733 (19 yr)*
Second 6 mo		2803 (19 yr)*

*Subtract 10 kcal/day for men and 7 kcal/day for women for each year above 19.

SOURCE: Institute of Medicine of the National Academies, Dietary Reference for Energy, Carbohydrate, Fiber, Fat, Fatty Acids, Cholesterol, Protein, and Amino Acids. The National Academy Press, Washington, DC, 2002.

Medical Nutritional Formulas

Modular Formulas

A modular formula contains only one nutrient and can be used to supplement the diet orally or as an additional component of a tube feeding.

NUTRIENT	FORMULA	COMMENTS
Protein	Casec ProMod Propac Pro-Mix	Orally best used as an additive to soups, beverages, cooked cereals, canned fruits, and gravies. Used when protein intake is inadequate to meet need.
Carbohydrate	Polycose Moducal Sumacal Nutrisource	Orally best added to fruits and fruit juices. Frequently used for protein-fat-electrolyte–restricted diets to boost kcalories.
Fat	MCT oil	Orally best used in milkshakes and hot cereals and as an oil. Contains medium-chain triglycerides and is used for lipid malabsorption.

Selected Elemental Formulas

Elemental formulas are designed for metabolically stressed patients with impaired GI function. Most of the nutrients are pre-digested.

FORMULA	DESCRIPTION	COMMENTS

Sandosource
  Peptide
Tolerex
Vivonex Plus
Vivonex TEN
Crucial
Peptamen
Peptamen VHP
Reabilian
Criticare HN
Vivionex
  Pediatric
Vital HN
	Complete nutritional supplements are formulated to serve as a meal replacement.	Expensive—should only be used if indicated.
		May be given orally or as a tube feeding. Not acceptable orally to many patients.

Complete Nutritional Supplements

Complete nutritional supplements (CNS) contain all the essential nutrients in a specified volume. There are dozens of these products. Some of these products are designed for oral use, and some are designed for tube feedings. Most health-care facilities select only one or two of these formulas to use as the standard in-house formula.

PRODUCT	MANUFACTURER	DESCRIPTION	VOLUME FOR 100% DRI (mL)	MOsm/kg WATER	kcal/mL	PROTEIN grams/ 1000 ml
Boost	Mead Johnson	Oral supplement intact protein	1180	590–670	1.01	42
Nutren	Nestle	Oral supplement intact protein	1500	590–670 (varies by flavor)	1.0	40
Ensure	Ross Products, Abbott Laboratories	Oral supplement intact protein	948	590	1.06	37
Ensure Plus	Ross Products, Abbott Laboratories	Oral supplement intact protein	1185	680	1.5	55
Ensure Plus High Nitrogen	Ross Products, Abbott Laboratories	Oral supplement intact protein	1000	525	1.5	63
Boost with Fiber	Novartis	Oral/tube feeding with fiber	1080	480	1.01	43
Ensure High Protein	Ross Products, Abbott Laboratories	High-protein intact protein oral supplement	948	610	0.95	51
Jevity 1 cal	Ross Products, Abbott Laboratories	Tube feeding intact protein fiber-containing	1321	300	1.06	44
Jevity 1.5	Ross Products, Abbott Laboratories	Tube feeding intact protein fiber-containing	1000	525	1.5	64
FiberSource HN	Novartis	Tube feeding intact fiber	1165	490	1.2	53

Specialized Formulas

PRODUCT	MANUFACTURER	DESCRIPTION	VOLUME FOR 100% RDI FOR AT LEAST 19 KEY NUTRIENTS	MOsm/kg WATER	KCALORIES PER mL	PROTEIN gram/ 1000 kcal
Nepro	Ross Products, Abbott Laboratories	Renal dialysis	947	665	2.0	70
Suplena	Ross Products, Abbott Laboratories	Renal insufficiency	947	600	2.0	30
Adverat	Ross Products Abbott Laboratories	HIV/AIDS	1184	680	1.28	60
Impact	Novartis	Critical care healing support diets	1500	375	1.0	56
TraumaCal	Novartis	Critical care healing support	2000	560	1.5	82
Glytrol	Nestle	Glucose intolerance	1400	280 (unflavored)	1.0	45
Glucerna	Ross Products, Abbott Laboratories	Glucose intolerance	1422	355	1.0	42
NutriHep	Nestle Laboratories	Hepatic	1000	790	1.5	40
PediaSure	Ross Products, Abbott Laboratories	Pediatric	1000 (children 1–6) 1300 (children 7–10)	345	1.0	30
Kindercal	Mead Johnson	Pediatric	946	440 (Van)	1.06	30
Pulmocare	Ross Products, Abbott Laboratories	Pulmonary	947	475	1.5	63

Values taken from: www.novartisnutrition.com/us/home accessed, May, 2005.

Client Teaching Aids

1200-Calorie Simplified Meal Plan

Breakfast:

1/2 cup orange juice or 1/2 banana or 1 fresh orange
1 small bagel or 2 slices of toast or 1 slice of toast and 1/2 cup cooked cereal
1 egg or 1 oz low-fat cheese
1 cup of skim milk

Lunch and Dinner:

2 oz of processed lunch meat with 3 grams of fat or less per oz or 1/2 cup water-packed tuna or 1/2 cup of cottage cheese or 2 oz of any lean meat

1 slice of bread or 6 small crackers or 1/2 cup of cooked pasta or 3/4 oz matzoh or 1/3 cup couscous or 1/2 cup of rice
1/2 to 1 cup of vegetables
1 small piece of fresh fruit or 1/2 cup of 100-percent fruit juice or 1 1/4 cup of fresh berries or melon
1 of margarine or 1 tbsp of salad dressing or 2 tbsp of reduced-fat salad dressing or 1 tsp olive or canola oil or 5 large olives or 2 whole walnuts

Snack:

1 cup of skim milk
1 small piece of fresh fruit or 1/2 cup of 100 percent fruit juice or 1 1/4 cup of fresh berries or melon

1500-Calorie Simplified Meal Plan

Breakfast:

1 cup orange juice or 1 banana or 1/4 cup of raisins

1/2 of a small bagel or 1 slice of toast or 1/2 cup cooked cereal

1 cup of skim milk

2 tsp of margarine or 2 tbsp of cream cheese

Lunch and Dinner:

3 oz of processed lunch meat with 3 grams of fat or less per oz or 3/4 cup water-packed tuna or 3/4 cup of cottage cheese or 3 oz of any lean meat or 1 cup of tofu

2 slices of bread or 12 small crackers or 1 cup of cooked pasta or 1 1/2 oz matzoh or 2/3 cup couscous or 2/3 cup of rice or 1 small baked potato

1/2 to 1 cup of vegetables

1 small piece of fresh fruit or 1/2 cup of 100 percent fruit juice or 1 1/4 cup of fresh berries or melon

1 tsp of margarine or 1 tbsp of salad dressing or 2 tbsp of reduced-fat salad dressing or 1 tsp olive or canola oil or 5 large olives or 2 whole walnuts

Snack:

1 cup of skim milk or 1 cup of plain unsweetened yogurt

1 slice of bread or 5 small crackers or 3/4 cup of unsweetened cold cereal or 1 1/2 cup of fat-free popcorn

1 small piece of fresh fruit or 1/2 cup of 100 percent fruit juice or 1 1/4 cup of fresh berries or melon

Sodium-Restricted Diet

Description

A sodium-restricted diet is often recommended to assist in the control of blood pressure and/or prevent water retention. The level of restriction (measured in grams or miligrams of sodium) depends on individual tolerance for sodium.

Sodium is in table salt, foods, medications, and water. Approximately one-half of salt is sodium. A sodium-restricted diet restricts the use of table salt and many foods processed with salt and sodium. Food naturally contains sodium. Sometimes a recommendation is made to restrict the intake of milk, regular salted breads, cereal, meat, and salted fats. If this is your situation, please consult a registered dietitian to prevent a nutritional deficiency. Local water supplies and water that has been chemically softened may contain considerable sodium. Sometimes a recommendation is made to drink bottled sodium-free water. Read food and medication labels and avoid those products that contain excessive amounts of sodium.

Nutritional Adequacy

The suggested meal plan provides foods in amounts that meet the recommended standards for all nutrients (except iron for females) for a 2000 kcalorie diet.

FOOD GROUP	FOODS RECOMMENDED	FOODS NOT RECOMMENDED	HINTS
Grain Group: 6 oz (1/2 whole grains)	Bread products without salted tops Cooked cereals Cold cereals without excessive added sodium (check label or speak with a dietitian) Puffed Wheat, Puffed Rice, and Shredded Wheat Homemade bread products without excessive added salt Rice and pasta To lower sodium further, purchase bread products made without any salt, soda, and baking powder (not necessary for all individuals on sodium-restricted diets)	Bread products that look salty Instant hot cereals Seasoned pasta and rice mixes	Choose whole grains whenever possible The first ingredient on the food label after the word *ingredient* should be whole wheat or whole grain
Vegetable Group: 2 1/2 cups per day	Vegetables are naturally low in sodium Fresh, frozen, or unsalted canned vegetables	Most canned vegetables, unless labeled unsalted, are higher in sodium than those recommended Sauerkraut Vegetable juices can contain excessive sodium Frozen convenience vegetable casseroles frequently contain excessive sodium	Try to eat at least three servings per day—most people do not eat enough vegetables Try to include a green or yellow vegetable each day
Fruits: 2 cups per day	Fruits are naturally low in sodium	Some dried fruits contain sodium preservatives and should be avoided	Remember to include a source of vitamin C each day (citrus, cantaloupe, strawberries)
Milk: 3 cups per day	Most	Buttermilk is higher in sodium than other milk products Malted milk and other milk mixes may contain appreciable amounts of sodium	Many individuals' diets lack sufficient calcium, which is essential for healthy bones, because they do not drink milk
Meat and Meat Substitute Group: 5.5 oz equivalents per day	Unprocessed meat, fish, and poultry Eggs Low-sodium peanut butter Dried peas and beans Tofu	Processed meats: canned, salted, smoked, and cured, including lunch meats, bacon, ham, sausage, hot dogs Many convenience meat products—check labels Salted nuts	Frozen convenience meat products that contain more than 500 mg of sodium per serving should be used infrequently Many low- and reduced-sodium meat products are available, such as reduced-sodium hot dogs
Others: Oils, sweets, and desserts Oils = 6 teaspoons sweets + dessert per MyPyramid discretionary allowance	Lemons, limes, cornstarch, flour, unsalted popcorn, vinegar, low-sodium catsup, low-sodium mustard, cocoa powder, cream of tartar, homemade unsalted gravies, unsalted broth and bouillon	Olives, salted condiments such as catsup, mustard, mayonnaise, relishes, steak sauces, barbecue sauce, soy sauce, monosodium glutamate (MSG), Worcestershire sauce, bacon bits, prepared horseradish sauce, dill pickles	There are many salt-free seasoning mixes in the grocery store Remember sodium is an acquired taste and most people can adjust to a lower sodium intake in time. Many people find the use of highly salted foods objectionable, especially after they have followed a sodium-restricted diet for some time. Avoid seasonings with the word salt such as celery salt. Use celery powder instead. Salted snack foods such as potato chips and salted pretzels are very high in sodium Rarely

Meal Plan—Approximately 1250 mg of Sodium

Breakfast

1 cup skim milk
Banana
1/2 cup unsalted oatmeal
1 slice of whole-grain bread
1 teaspoon of margarine and jelly
1 cup of orange juice
Coffee, if desired

Lunch and Dinner

2–3 oz of unsalted unprocessed meat or meat substitute

1/2 cup of low-sodium and unsalted whole grain pasta or rice
1 cup of an unsalted vegetable
1 cup skim milk
Fresh fruit
Whole-grain dinner roll
1 teaspoon of margarine
Green leafy salad with an unsalted salad dressing or vinegar and monounsaturated oil
1 cup of skim milk at one meal
Coffee or tea, if desired
To decrease sodium further, encourage the use of unsalted bread and margarine
To increase sodium further, increase the servings of whole grains from 3 to 6 per day and margarine from 3 to 5 tsp

What to Consider Before Taking Dietary Supplements

Items sold as dietary supplements in the United States do not receive the same oversight from the Food and Drug Administration as that given to food and prescription or over-the-counter drugs. Nevertheless, many supplements have effects equal in power to those of drugs.

Some people have experienced problems because of the lack of product standardization, poor quality control, and contamination with harmful substances.
If you decide to take dietary supplements:

- Discuss your desires and plans with your primary health-care provider.
- Treat the supplement as medicine. You are expecting medicinal results.
- Store the supplements in childproof containers.
- Take the product as directed.
- Add just one supplement at a time. Observe for desired actions and for side effects.
- Discontinue use and report to your primary health-care provider if desired effects do not occur or if new symptoms appear.
- Use the supplements for short periods of time only.
- Inform surgeons and anesthesiologists of your intake.

They may want you to stop taking supplements 2–3 weeks before scheduled surgery.
- Purchase the products from a reputable supplier. Use the same brand consistently. European sources are preferable to Asian ones.

Cautions:

- Do not give supplements or medicinal teas to infants or children.
- Do not consume supplements if you are pregnant, planning to become pregnant, or breast-feeding.
- Do not take supplements if you are elderly.
- Do not use supplements if you are subject to allergies, except with careful investigation and extreme caution.
- Do not add to your treatment plan any products with the same effects as other drugs you are taking, particularly blood thinners or aspirin and other nonsteroidal anti-inflammatory drugs (NSAIDS).

It is best to avoid the following botanicals: borage, chaparral, comfrey, ephedra, germander, kombucha, lobelia, pennyroyal, sassafras, and wormwood.

Monitor for side effects and report them to your primary healthcare provider or to the **FDA's MEDWATCH at 1-800-FDA-1088** or on the Internet at http://www.fda.gov/medwatch/report/consumer/consumer.htm.

Survival Skills for Patients with Diabetes on Medication

Acceptable Blood Glucose Levels

A normal blood glucose level is between 60 and 120 mg/dL before a meal and less than 140 mg/dL 2 hours after a meal. Glycosylated hemoglobin is a test that measures the average blood glucose for the past 60 days. The physician typically determines acceptable blood glucose and glycosylated hemoglobin for clients with diabetes. Here are some guidelines:

- *Intensive Treatment*: 70–140 mg/dL before meals; less than 180 mg/dL 2 hours after meals; glycosylated hemoglobin within 1 percent of normal.
- *Average Treatment*: 80–160 mg/dL before meals; less than 200 mg/dL 2 hours after meals; glycosylated hemoglobin within 2 percent of normal

Hyperglycemia (Blood Glucose Greater Than 250 mg/dL)

Controlling your diabetes means dealing with your blood glucose when it is too high. This condition can occur rapidly or gradually. Usually, you will be able to lower your own blood glucose. There are times, however, when emergency care is needed.

Causes

- Too little insulin or oral medication
- Too much food
- Less activity or exercise than usual
- More stress than usual
- Illness, infection, or injury

Symptoms

- Fatigue
- Increased thirst
- Unexplained weight loss
- Blurry vision
- Increased hunger
- Dry mouth and skin
- Increased urination

Treatment

- Check your blood glucose more frequently.
- **Take your insulin or oral medication as prescribed (adjust dosage only if told to do so by your doctor).**
- Follow your meal plan, adding more calorie-free liquids.
- Follow the four sick day rules listed below.

Hypoglycemia (Blood Glucose Less Than 60 mg/dL)

Controlling blood glucose means dealing with your blood glucose when it drops too low. This condition is called hypoglycemia.

Causes of Hypoglycemia

- Too much insulin or oral medication
- More exercise or activity than usual
- Skipping or delaying meals or snacks or eating less food than usual

Signs

- Slurred speech
- Headache
- Tingling of lips
- Coma
- Weakness
- Nervousness
- Sweating
- Tremors
- Hunger
- Rapid heart beat
- Confusion/disorientation

Treatment

1. Test your blood glucose immediately.
2. Quickly take 15 grams of carbohydrate; 15 grams of carbohydrate is equal to any of the foods listed in the Food Substitutions When Ill section or:

3 glucose tabs (from pharmacy)	6 hard candies
1 tube of glucose gel (from pharmacy)	1 fruit exchange
8 oz of skim milk (no fat)	1 starch exchange
4 oz juice or regular cola	

3. Test your blood glucose again 15 minutes later.
4. If your blood glucose has not risen, take another glucose dose as above.
5. Treatment of low blood glucose should not take the place of a meal or snack.
6. Eat a meal.

Exercise Guidelines

Before beginning any exercise program, consult your doctor, especially if you are over age 40 or have had diabetes for 10 years or longer.

General Recommendations

1. Type of exercise: Aerobic, high repetitions, low-weight-bearing
2. Frequency: Daily exercise aids blood glucose control
3. Duration: 40–60 minutes; longer than 40 minutes is required to begin breakdown of body fat
4. Timing: 60–90 minutes after meals when the blood glucose level is highest; consistency in time of day will assist in the regulation of blood glucose levels

Benefits of Exercise

- Helps your body use insulin more effectively
- Can lower blood glucose levels
- Strengthens heart and lungs
- Reduces body fat and increases muscle
- Assists with weight control
- Helps you cope with stress
- Helps improve body image
- Lowers blood pressure

Risks of Exercise

- Certain types of exercise may worsen eye, kidney, or nerve problems.
- Blood pressure may rise higher during exercise in people with diabetes than in those without diabetes.
- People with diabetes are at increased risk for heart problems. **Stop exercising and consult your doctor if you have any of the following symptoms: chest pain,**

unusual fatigue, dizziness, visual disturbances, or nausea.

- Know how to prevent hypoglycemia if you take insulin or diabetes pills.
- Wear your diabetes ID during exercise.

Special Considerations for Patients with Type 2 Diabetes

- Food intake must be regulated and maintained, not increased, despite increased appetite.
- Check your blood glucose level before and after exercise.
- Exercise is most beneficial when the blood glucose level is below 200 mg/dL.
- Exercise in the evening may benefit blood glucose levels the next morning.
- Regular exercise is more beneficial than sporadic exercise.
- Exercise is best done 60–90 minutes after eating.

Sick Day Guidelines

Illness, such as a cold or flu, can cause serious problems with diabetes control. The four main rules for sick day management are:

1. Continue to take the insulin or diabetes pill prescribed.
2. Test blood glucose frequently (every 2–4 hours); record results.
3. Frequent fluid intake is recommended (8–12 oz/hour).
4. Try to eat the usual amount of carbohydrate (milk, fruit, and starch exchanges), divided into smaller meals and snacks if necessary; if blood glucose is 250 mg/dL or higher, all of the usual amount of carbohydrate is not necessary. **Call your doctor if your blood glucose is higher than 250 mg/dL for more than two tests in a row.**

Food Substitutions When Ill

Each of the following may be substituted for a fruit or starch exchange on sick days:

1/2 cup regular gelatin	1/2 cup ice cream
1/4 cup sherbet	1/4 cup plain pudding
4 oz cola	1 cup cream soup
6 oz ginger ale	1 cup yogurt
1 Tbs honey	1 Tbs corn syrup
1 Tbs brown sugar	

Meal Plan

What and when you eat influences your blood glucose levels. For this reason, it is necessary that you follow some type of meal plan. Many different types of meal plans are available for you to choose from, including:

1. American Dietetic Association Food Exchange Lists
2. *Month of Meals*—menus for 1 month
3. Food Pyramid and Healthy Food Choices
4. Carbohydrate counting

The dietitian will assist you in the selection of an appropriate meal-planning system. The effectiveness of any diet is objectively evaluated by consistently monitoring lipid, glycosylated hemoglobin, and blood glucose levels as well as body weight.

Eating Out

With the help of a meal plan, the person with diabetes can enjoy eating in restaurants. Care must be taken not to consume more fat and calories than usual. Some patients save their daily fat calories and use them at the meal that they plan to eat in the restaurant. Here is a list of suggestions for reducing fat and calories:

- Order salad dressings on the side
- Ask that broiled, grilled, or baked entrees be prepared without added oil, butter, or margarine.
- Request that vegetables, rice, potatoes, and pasta be prepared without fat.
- Select raw vegetables, fresh fruit, crackers, and diet dressing from salad bars.
- The key to reducing fat in a fast-food restaurant is to buy a small, plain hamburger, side salad, fruit juice, and skimmed milk.

Snacking

For persons with type 2 diabetes, snacking is discouraged. Snacking prevents normalization of glucose levels during the day. Also, most persons with type 2 diabetes are overweight, and weight reduction assists in the control of blood glucose levels. Some overweight people are unable to stop eating once they start.

Some people with type 2 diabetes have a long history of snacking and are not willing to change their usual pattern of eating. For these individuals, snacks that contain less than 20 calories per serving may be the most feasible approach to weight control. Following is a list of low-calorie snacks:

Raw vegetables
3 mini rice cakes
1 cup air-popped popcorn
1/2 cup unsweetened cranberries
1/2 cup unsweetened rhubarb
1 dill pickle (high in sodium)
7 pretzel sticks
2 vanilla wafers
2 gingersnaps

Additional Tips

1. Drink alcohol in moderation only when your blood glucose has been in good control. Do *not* drink alcohol on an empty stomach if you take insulin or oral diabetes medication. It may cause a low blood sugar reaction.
2. Have an annual exam with a board-certified ophthalmologist (a doctor specializing in eye care).
3. Over the long term, diabetes can lead to foot problems, including infection and amputation. Check your feet (and legs) daily. Look between toes and on bottoms for sores, redness, infection, drainage, swelling, or bruises. Report problems to your doctor early. Keep your feet clean and wear clean, dry socks. Never go barefoot. Protect any area where sensation is lost.

4. Communicate with your family doctor. Maintain good daily records of your food intake, medication schedule, and blood glucose levels. Share these with your doctor.
5. Join the local chapter of the American Diabetes Association.
6. Eliminating smoking and controlling blood pressure and elevated blood cholesterol levels are important for reducing the risk of heart and circulatory problems. Controlling high blood pressure reduces the chance of having heart attacks, strokes, and kidney disease. Have your blood pressure checked at least once a year, and take blood pressure medication as prescribed.
7. A physician should promptly treat urinary tract infections. Contact your physician if you experience pain, burning, or urgency on urination. Frequent urination is also a symptom of a urinary tract infection.
8. Keep up to date on immunizations.

Survival Skills for Patients with Type 2 Diabetes Diet Controlled

Acceptable Blood Glucose Levels

A normal blood glucose level is 60–120 mg/dL before a meal and less than 140 mg/dL after a meal. A glycosylated hemoglobin measures your average blood glucose for the past 60 days. Acceptable blood glucose and glycosylated hemoglobin levels for patients with diabetes are typically within 1 percent of normal.

Exercise Guidelines

Before beginning any exercise program, consult your doctor, especially if you are over age 40 or have had diabetes for 10 years or longer.

General Recommendations

Type of Exercise: Aerobic, high repetitions, low-weight-bearing
Frequency: Daily frequency aids blood glucose control
Duration: 40–60 minutes; longer than 40 minutes is required to begin breakdown of body fat
Timing: 60–90 minutes after meals when the blood glucose level is highest
Consistency in time of day will assist in the regulation of blood glucose levels

Benefits of Exercise

- Helps your body use insulin more effectively
- Can lower blood glucose levels
- Strengthens heart and lungs
- Reduces body fat and increases muscle
- Assists with weight control
- Helps you to cope with stress
- Helps improve body image
- Lowers blood pressure

Risks of Exercise

Certain types of exercise may worsen eye, kidney, or nerve problems. Blood pressure may rise higher during exercise in people with diabetes than in those without diabetes.

People with diabetes are at increased risk for heart problems. **Stop exercising and consult your doctor if you have any of the following symptoms: chest pain, unusual fatigue, dizziness, visual disturbances, or nausea.**

Wear your diabetes ID during exercise.

Special Considerations for Patients with Type 2 Diabetes

- Food intake must be regulated and maintained, not increased despite increased appetite.
- Check your blood glucose level before and after exercise.
- Exercise is the most beneficial if your blood glucose is below 200 mg/dL.
- Exercise in the evening may benefit blood glucose levels the next morning.
- Regular exercise is more beneficial than sporadic exercise.
- Exercise is best done 60–90 minutes after eating.

Hyperglycemia (Blood Glucose Greater Than 250 mg/dL)

Controlling your diabetes means dealing with your blood glucose when it is too high. This condition can occur rapidly or gradually. Usually, you will be able to lower your own blood glucose. There are times, however, when emergency care is needed.

Causes

- Too much food
- More stress than usual
- Less activity or exercise than usual
- Illness, infection, or injury

Symptoms

- Fatigue
- Blurry vision
- Dry mouth and skin
- Increased thirst
- Increased hunger
- Increased urination
- Unexplained weight loss

Treatment

- Check your blood glucose more frequently
- Follow your meal plan, adding more calorie-free liquids
- Follow your exercise plan only if blood glucose level is less than 250 mg/dL

Meal Plan

Nutrition is an essential component of management for all persons with diabetes because diabetes is directly related to how the body uses food. Patients report improved health, better control over body weight, and improved control of blood glucose and lipid levels when they adhere to dietary recommendations.

For all of these reasons, it is necessary to follow some type of meal plan. Many different types of meal plans are available for you to choose from, including:

1. American Dietetic Association Food Exchange Lists
2. *Month of Meals*—menus for one month
3. Food Pyramid and "Healthy Food Choices"

The patient needs to select and follow an appropriate meal-planning system. The effectiveness of any diet can be objectively evaluated by consistently monitoring lipid, glycosylated hemoglobin, and blood glucose levels and body weight. All meal-planning systems are based on the *Dietary Guidelines for Healthy Americans*.

Eating Out

With the help of a meal plan, the person with diabetes can enjoy eating in restaurants. Care must be taken not to consume more fat and calories than usual. Some patients save their daily fat calories and use them at the meal that they plan to eat in the restaurant. Here is a list of suggestions for reducing fat and calories:

- Order salad dressings on the side
- Ask that broiled, grilled, or baked entrees be prepared without additional oil, butter, and margarine

- Request that vegetables, rice, potatoes, and pasta is prepared without fat
- Select raw vegetables, fresh fruit, crackers, and diet dressing from salad bars

The key to reducing fat in a fast food restaurant is to buy a small, plain hamburger, side salad, fruit juice, and skimmed milk.

Snacking

For persons with type 2 diabetes, snacking is discouraged. Snacking prevents normalization of glucose levels during the day. Also, most persons with type 2 diabetes are overweight, and weight reduction assists in the control of blood glucose levels. Some overweight people are unable to stop eating once they start.

Some people with type 2 diabetes have a long history of snacking and are not willing to change their usual pattern of eating. For these individuals, snacks, which contain less than 20 calories per serving, may be the most feasible approach to weight control. Following is a list of low-calorie snacks:

Raw vegetables
1-cup air-popped popcorn
1/2 cup unsweetened cranberries
3 mini rice cakes
1/2 cup unsweetened rhubarb
2 gingersnaps
1 dill pickle (high in sodium)
7 pretzel sticks
2 vanilla wafers

Additional Tips

1. Drink alcohol in moderation only when your blood glucose has been in good control. Do **not** drink alcohol on an empty stomach as it may cause a low blood sugar reaction. Visible medical identification should be carried or worn when drinking away from home.
2. Have an annual exam with a board-certified ophthalmologist (a doctor specializing in eye care)
3. Over the long term, diabetes can lead to foot problems, including infection and amputation. Check your feet (and legs) daily. Look between toes and on bottoms for sores, redness, infection, drainage, swelling or bruises. Report problems to your doctor early. Keep your feet clean and wear clean dry socks. Never go barefoot. Protect any area where sensation is lost.
4. Eliminating smoking and controlling blood pressure and elevated blood cholesterol levels are important for reducing the risk of heart and circulatory problems. Controlling high blood pressure reduces the chance of having heart attacks, strokes, and kidney disease. Have your blood pressure checked at least once a year and take blood pressure medication as prescribed.
5. Urinary tract infections should be promptly treated by a physician. Contact your physician if you experience pain, burning, or urgency on urination. Frequent urination is also a symptom of a urinary tract infection.
6. Keep up to date on immunizations.

Tips for Safe Swallowing

- Eat slowly
- Avoid distractions while eating
- Do not talk while eating
- Remove loose dentures
- Sit up while eating with hips at a 90 degree angle, shoulder slightly forward, and feet flat on the floor or firmly supported
- Position head correctly
- Use a teaspoon and take only one-half a teaspoon of food or fluids at a time
- Swallow completely between bites
- Select foods and fluids of appropriate consistency
- Do not use liquids to clear the mouth after a swallow unless instructed to do so

- Remain upright for 30 minutes after eating
- Mealtime should be pleasant—socialization is important to enhance awareness and stimulate the appetite
- Frequent dry swallows help clear the mouth

Foods may be thickened with

- A commercial thickener like "Thick-It"
- Instant mashed potatoes
- Pureed fruits and vegetables
- Finely chopped crackers
- Powdered dry milk
- Pureed tofu
- Heavy cream
- Banana flakes
- Bread crumbs

Answers to Questions

Chapter 1
Chapter Review
1. b   2. c   3. a   4. b   5. d
Clinical Analysis
1. d   2. a   3. d

Chapter 2
Chapter Review
1. b   2. b   3. c   4. a   5. c
Clinical Analysis
1. d   2. b   3. a

Chapter 3
Chapter Review
1. b   2. c   3. c   4. d   5. a
Clinical Analysis
1. c   2. d   3. a

Chapter 4
Chapter Review
1. c   2. b   3. c   4. b   5. c
Clinical Analysis
1. d   2. a   3. c

Chapter 5
Chapter Review
1. a   2. c   3. b   4. b   5. d
Clinical Analysis
1. d   2. c   3. a

Chapter 6
Chapter Review
1. c   2. a   3. c   4. b   5. d
Clinical Analysis
1. d   2. d   3. b

Chapter 7
Chapter Review
1. c   2. d   3. a   4. a   5. b
Clinical Analysis
1. d   2. c   3. b

Chapter 8
Chapter Review
1. b   2. b   3. c   4. a   5. c
Clinical Analysis
1. b   2. a   3. b

Chapter 9
Chapter Review
1. c.   2. d   3. b   4. a   5. d
Clinical Analysis
1. a   2. d   3. c

Chapter 10
Chapter Review
1. d   2. a   3. c   4. b   5. b
Clinical Analysis
1. a   2. d   3. a

Chapter 11
Chapter Review
1. b   2. a   3. c   4. a   5. d
Clinical Analysis
1. c   2. b.   3. d

Chapter 12
Chapter Review
1. c   2. b   3. c   4. b   5. d
Clinical Analysis
1. d   2. c   3. a

Chapter 13
Chapter Review
1. b   2. d   3. b   4. a   5. d
Clinical Analysis
1. b   2. b   3. c

Chapter 14
Chapter Review
1. c   2. a   3. d   4. b   5. a
Clinical Analysis
1. b   2. a   3. c

Chapter 15
Chapter Review
1. c   2. a   3. c   4. b   5. a
Clinical Analysis
1. c   2. c   3. a

Chapter 16
Chapter Review
1. c   2. a   3. b   4. b   5. a
Clinical Analysis
1. c   2. d   3. d

Chapter 17
Chapter Review
1. b   **2.** e   **3.** c   **4.** d   **5.** a
Clinical Analysis
1. c   **2.** c   **3.** a

Chapter 18
Chapter Review
1. a   **2.** b   **3.** d   **4.** b   **5.** b
Clinical Analysis
1. a   **2.** b   **3.** c

Chapter 19
Chapter Review
1. a   **2.** b   **3.** d   **4.** b   **5.** a
Clinical Analysis
1. c   **2.** a   **3.** b

Chapter 20
Chapter Review
1. a   **2.** c   **3.** d   **4.** b   **5.** d
Clinical Analysis
1. b   **2.** d   **3.** c

Chapter 21
Chapter Review
1. b   **2.** b   **3.** d   **4.** a   **5.** d
Clinical Analysis
1. c   **2.** b   **3.** a

Chapter 22
Chapter Review
1. c   **2.** b   **3.** d   **4.** b   **5.** d
Clinical Analysis
1. a   **2.** b   **3.** b

Chapter 23
Chapter Review
1. b   **2.** d   **3.** c   **4.** d   **5.** a
Clinical Analysis
1. c   **2.** b   **3.** a

Chapter 24
Chapter Review
1. c   **2.** c   **3.** b   **4.** d   **5.** c
Clinical Analysis
1. c   **2.** d   **3.** b

Chapter 25
Chapter Review
1. b   **2.** d   **3.** a   **4.** c   **5.** d
Clinical Analysis
1. b   **2.** b   **3.** b

Chapter 26
Chapter Review
1. c   **2.** c   **3.** a   **4.** d   **5.** b
Clinical Analysis
1. d   **2.** a   **3.** b

Glossary

Commonly used terms and terms that appear in **boldface** in the chapters can be found in this glossary. After each definition, the chapter or chapters in which the term is either introduced or discussed extensively are identified numerically in parentheses.

Abdominal circumference (girth)—Distance around the trunk at the umbilicus. (2)

Abdominal obesity—Excess body fat located between the chest and pelvis. (18)

Abortifacient—Anything used to cause or induce an abortion. (16)

Absorption—The movement of the end products of digestion from the gastrointestinal tract into the blood and/or lymphatic system. (10)

Accreditation—Process by which a nongovernmental agency recognizes an institution for meeting established criteria of quality. (2)

Acculturation—Process of adopting the values, attitudes, and behaviors of another culture. (2)

Acetone—A ketone body found in urine, which can be due to the excessive breakdown of stored body fat. (3)

Acetylcholine—A chemical necessary for the transmission of nervous impulses. (7)

Acetyl CoA—Important intermediate byproduct in metabolism formed from the breakdown of glucose, fatty acids, and certain amino acids. (10)

Achalasia—Failure of the gastrointestinal muscle fibers to relax where one part joins another. (22)

Achlorhydria—Absence of free hydrochloric acid in the stomach. (13)

Acidosis—Condition that results when the pH of the blood falls below 7.35; may be caused by diarrhea, uremia, diabetes mellitus, respiratory depression, and certain drug therapies. (9)

Acquired immune deficiency syndrome (AIDS)—A disease complex caused by a virus that attacks the immune system and causes neurological disease and permits opportunistic infections and malignancies. (25)

Acrodermatitis enteropathica—Rare autosomal-recessive disease that causes zinc deficiency through an unknown mechanism of absorptive failure; fatal if untreated. (8)

Acute illness—A sickness characterized by rapid onset, severe symptoms, and a short course. (15)

Acute renal failure—Condition that occurs suddenly, in which the kidneys are unable to perform essential functions; usually temporary. (21)

Adaptive thermogenesis—The adjustment in energy expenditure the body makes to a large increase or decrease in kilocalorie intake of several days' duration. (6)

Additive—A substance added to food to increase its flavor, shelf life, and/or characteristics such as texture, color, and aroma. (14)

Adequate Intake (AI)—The average observed or experimentally defined intake by a defined population or subgroup that appears to sustain a defined nutritional state; incorporates information on the reduction of disease risk; may be used as a goal for an individual's nutrient intake if an EAR or RDA cannot be set. (2)

Adipose cells—Cells in the human body that store fat. (4)

Adipose tissue—Tissue containing masses of fat cells. (4)

Adolescence—Time from the onset of puberty until full growth is reached. (12)

Adenosine diphosphate (ADP)—A substance present in all cells involved in energy metabolism. Energy is released when molecules of ATP, another compound in cells, release a phosphoric acid chain and become ADP. The opposite chemical reaction of adding the third phosphoric acid group to ADP requires much energy. (8)

Adrenal glands—Small organs on the superior surface of the kidneys that secrete many hormones, including epinephrine (adrenalin) and aldosterone. (7)

Aerobic exercise—Training methods such as running or swimming that require continuous inspired oxygen. (6)

Afferent—Proceeding toward a center, as arteries, veins, lymphatic vessels, and nerves. (18)

Afferent arteriole—Small blood vessel by which blood enters the glomerulus (functional unit of the kidney). (21)

Aflatoxin—A naturally occurring food contaminant produced by some strains of *Aspergillus* molds found especially on peanuts and peanut products. (14, 23)

AIDS dementia complex (ADC)—A central nervous system disorder caused by the human immunodeficiency virus. (25)

Albumin—A plasma protein responsible for much of the colloidal osmotic pressure of the blood. (9)

Aldosterone—An adrenocorticoid hormone that increases sodium and water retention by the kidneys. (9)

Alimentary canal—The digestive tube extending from the mouth to the anus. (10)

Alkaline phosphatase—An enzyme found in highest concentration in the liver, biliary tract epithelium, and bones; enzyme levels are elevated in liver, bone, and biliary disease. (14)

Alkalosis—Condition that results when the pH of the blood rises above 7.45; may be caused by vomiting, nasogastric suctioning, or hyperventilation. (8)

Allele—One of two or more different genes containing specific inheritable characteristics that occupy corresponding positions (loci) on paired chromosomes; an individual possessing a pair of identical alleles, either dominant or recessive, is homozygous for this gene. (11)

Allergen—Substance that provokes an abnormal, individual hypersensitivity. (12)

Allergy—State of abnormal, individual hypersensitivity to a substance. (10)

Alopecia—Hair loss, especially of the head; baldness. (8)

Alpha-tocopherol equivalent (α-TE)—The measure of vitamin E; 1 milligram of alpha-tocopherol equivalent equals 1.4 International Units of natural alpha-tocopherol or 1 IU of synthetic vitamin. (7)

Amenorrhea—Absence of menstruation; normally occurs before puberty, after menopause, and during pregnancy and lactation. (12)

Amino acids—Organic compounds that are the building blocks of protein; also the end products of protein digestion. (5)

Amniotic fluid—Albuminous liquid that surrounds and protects the fetus throughout pregnancy. (11)

Amylase—A class of enzymes that splits starches; for example, salivary amylase, pancreatic amylase. (10)

Anabolic phase—The third and last phase of stress; characterized by the building up of body tissue and nutrient stores; also called recovery phase. (24)

Anabolism—The building up of body compounds or tissues by the synthesis of more complex substances from simpler ones; the constructive phase of metabolism. (5, 8)

Anaerobic exercise—A form of physical activity such as weight lifting or sprinting that does not rely on continuous inspired oxygen. (6)

Anaphylaxis—Exaggerated, life-threatening hypersensitivity response to a previously encountered antigen; in severe cases, produces bronchospasm, vascular collapse, and shock. (12)

Anastomosis—The surgical connection between tubular structures. (22)

Anemia—Condition of less-than-normal values for red blood cells or hemoglobin, or both; result is decreased effectiveness in oxygen transport; causes may include inadequate iron intake, malabsorption, and chronic or acute blood loss. (7, 8, 11)

Anencephaly—Congenital absence of the brain; cerebral hemispheres missing or reduced to small masses; fatal within a few weeks. (11)

Angina pectoris—Severe pain and a sense of constriction about the heart caused by lack of oxygen to the heart muscle. (20)

Angiotensin II—End product of complex reaction in response to low blood pressure; effect is vasoconstriction and aldosterone secretion. (9)

Anorexia—Loss of appetite. (13)

Anorexia of aging—Loss of appetite in an elderly individual related to physiologic, social, psychological, or medical causes. (13)

Anion—An ion with a negative charge. (9)

Antagonist—A substance that counteracts the action of another substance. (7)

Anthropometry—The science of measuring the human body. (2)

Anti-insulin antibodies (AIAs)—A protein found to be elevated in persons with insulin-dependent diabetes mellitus. (19)

Anorexia nervosa—A mental disorder characterized by a 25-percent loss of usual body weight, an intense fear of becoming obese, and self-starvation. (18)

Anorexigenic—Causing loss of appetite. (18)

Anthropometric measurements—Physical measurements of the human body such as height, weight, and skinfold thickness; used to determine body composition and growth. (2)

Anthropometry—Science of measuring the body. (2)

Antibody—A specific protein developed in the body in response to a substance that the body senses to be foreign. (5)

Anticholinergic—An agent that blocks parasympathetic nerve impulses, thereby causing dry mouth, blurred vision due to dilated pupils, and decreased gastrointestinal and bronchial secretions. (16)

Antidiuretic hormone (ADH)—Hormone formed in the hypothalamus and released from the posterior pituitary in response to blood that is too concentrated; effect is return of water to the bloodstream by the kidney. (9, 19)

Antigen—Protein or oligosaccharide marker on surface of cells; body can detect foreign antigens on organisms, foods, and transplanted tissues. (12)

Antineoplastic drug—A drug that combats tumors. (17)

Antioxidant—A substance that prevents or inhibits the uptake of oxygen; in the body, antioxidants prevent tissue damage; in foods, antioxidants prevent deterioration. (1, 7)

Anuria—A total lack of urine output. (21)

Apoferritin—A protein found in intestinal mucosal cells that combines with iron to form ferritin; it is always found attached to iron in the body. (8)

Apolipoproteins—Protein components of lipoproteins that assist in regulating lipid metabolism; apo A, the primary HDL apoprotein, is inversely related to the risk for developing coronary artery disease. (20)

Appetite—A strong desire for food or for a pleasant sensation, based on previous experience, that causes one to seek food for the purpose of tasting and enjoying. (6)

Aquaporin—Water transport proteins, found in many cell membranes, that serve as water-selective channels and explain the speed at which water moves across cell membranes. (9)

Arachidonic acid—An omega-6 polyunsaturated fatty acid present in peanuts; precursor of prostaglandins. (12)

Ariboflavinosis—Condition arising from a deficiency of riboflavin in the diet. (7)

Arrhythmia—Irregular heartbeat. (20)

Arteriosclerosis—Common arterial disorder characterized by thickening, hardening, and loss of elasticity of the arterial walls; also called "hardening of the arteries." (20)

Arthritis—Inflammatory condition of the joints, usually accompanied by pain and swelling. (13)

Ascites—Accumulation of serous fluid in the peritoneal (abdominal) cavity. (9, 22)

Ascorbic acid—Vitamin C; *ascorbic* literally means "without scurvy." (7)

Ash—The residue that remains after an item is burned; usually refers to the mineral content of the human body. (1)

Aspartame—Artificial sweetener composed of aspartic acid and phenylalanine; 180 times sweeter than sucrose; brand names: Equal, Nutrasweet. (5)

Aspergillus—Genus of molds that produce aflatoxins. (14)

Aspiration—The state whereby a substance has been drawn into the nose, throat, or lungs. (15)

Assessment—An organized procedure to gather pertinent facts. (2)

Astrocyte—A supporting cell of the central nervous system that contributes to the blood-brain barrier. (22)

Asymptomatic—Without symptoms. (25)

Ataxia—Defective muscular coordination, especially seen in voluntary movement attempts. (22)

Atherosclerosis—A form of arteriosclerosis characterized by the deposit of fatty material inside the arteries; major factor contributing to heart disease. (20)

Atom—Smallest particle of an element that has all the properties of the element. An atom consists of the nucleus, which contains protons (positively charged particles), neutrons (particles with no electrical charge), and surrounding electrons (negatively charged particles). (3, 9)

Atopy—Genetic predisposition to develop allergy primarily involving IgE antibodies; the tendency is inherited but the specific clinical form (hay fever, asthma, dermatitis) is not; a child with two atopic parents has a 75-percent chance of developing allergies; a child with one topic parent has a 50-percent chance. (12)

ATP (adenosine triphosphate)—Compound in cells, especially muscle cells, that stores energy; when needed, enzymes break off one phosphoric acid group, which releases energy for muscle contraction. (8)

Atrophy—Decrease in size of a normally developed organ or tissue. (24)

Autoimmune disease—A disorder in which the body produces an immunologic response against itself. (19)

Autonomy—Achieving independence; the psychosocial developmental task of the toddler. (12)

Autosomal recessive inheritance—Non-sex-linked pattern of inheritance in which an affected gene must be received from both parents for the individual to be affected; examples: cystic fibrosis, PKU, galactosemia, sickle cell disease. (5)

Avidin—Protein in raw egg white that inhibits the B vitamin biotin. (7)

Bacteria—Single-celled microorganisms that lack a true nucleus; may be either harmless to humans or disease producing. (3)

Balanced diet—One including sufficient foods from each of the major food groups daily; one containing all the essential nutrients in required amounts. (2)

Barium enema—Series of x-ray studies of the colon used to demonstrate the presence and location of polyps, tumors, diverticula, or positional abnormalities. The client is first administered an enema containing a radioopaque substance (barium) that enhances visualization when the film is exposed. (15)

Barium swallow—The primary diagnostic tool for direct visualization of the swallowing mechanism is called the *cookie swallow* or *modified barium swallow*. During this procedure, the client consumes three items of different viscosities. Each item contains a contrast medium that allows all phases of the swallowing mechanism to be visualized in x-rays. A physician is always present during this procedure. (10)

Basal ganglia—Four masses of gray matter located in the cerebrum; contribute to the subconscious aspects of voluntary movement; inhibit tremors. (8)

Benign—Not recurrent or progressive; nonmalignant; benign tumor may be life-threatening in crucial tissue such as the brain. (23)

Beriberi—Disease caused by deficiency of vitamin B_1 (thiamin). (7)

Beta-carotene—Carotenoid with the greatest provitamin A activity.

Beta-endorphin—Chemical released in the brain during exercise that produces a state of relaxation. (6)

Bicarbonate—Any salt containing the HCO_3 anion; blood bicarbonate is a measure of alkali (base) reserve of the body; bicarbonate of soda is sodium bicarbonate ($NaHCO_3$). (9)

Bile—Yellow secretion of the liver that alkalinizes the intestine and breaks large fat globules into smaller ones to facilitate enzyme digestive action. (10)

Binging—Eating to excess; eating from 5,000 to 20,000 kilocalories per day. (18)

Bioavailability—The rate and extent to which an active drug or nutrient or metabolite enters the general circulation, permitting access to the site of action; measured by concentration of the drug in body fluids or by the magnitude of the pharmacologic response. (14, 17)

Bioelectric impedance—Indirect measure of body fatness based on differences in electrical conductivity of fat, muscle, and bone. (2)

Biologic value—Scoring system of how well food proteins can be converted into body protein; eggs are norm of 100 percent of nitrogen being retained. (5)

Biotin—B-complex vitamin widely available in foods. (7)

Bladder—A body organ, also called the urinary bladder, that receives urine from the kidneys and discharges it through the urethra. (10)

Blood pressure—Force exerted against the walls of blood vessels by the pumping action of the heart. (20)

Blood urea nitrogen (BUN)—The amount of nitrogen present in the blood as urea, often elevated in renal disorders; may be referred to as serum urea nitrogen (SUN). (13, 21)

Body frame size—Designation of a person's skeletal structure as small, medium, or large; used to determine healthy body weight (HBW). (2)

Body image—The mental image a person has of himself or herself. (18)

Body mass index (BMI)—Weight in kilograms divided by the square of height in meters; BMIs of 19 to 24 are considered normal. (2)

Body substance isolation—A situation in which all body fluids should be considered contaminated and treated as such by all health-care workers. (25)

Bolus—A mass of food that is ready to be swallowed or a single dose of feeding or medication. (10, 15)

Bolus feeding—Giving a 4- to 6-hour volume of a tube feeding within a few minutes. (15)

Bomb calorimeter—A device used to measure the energy content of food. (6)

Botulism—An often fatal form of food intoxication caused by the ingestion of food containing poisonous toxins produced by the microorganism *Clostridium botulinum*. (14)

Bowman's capsule—The cuplike top of an individual nephron; functions as a filter in the formation of urine. (21)

Buffer—A substance that can react to offset excess acid or excess alkali (base) in a solution; blood buffers include carbonic acid, bicarbonate, phosphates, and proteins, including hemoglobin. (9)

Bulimia—Excessive food intake followed by extreme methods, such as self-induced vomiting and the use of laxatives, to rid the body of the foods eaten. (18)

C-reactive protein (CRP)—An abnormal protein produced by the liver in response to acute inflammation that is strongly associated with future vascular events. (20)

Cachexia—State of malnutrition and wasting seen in chronic conditions such as cancer, AIDS, malaria, tuberculosis, and pituitary disease. (23)

Calcidiol—Inactive form of vitamin D produced by the liver; half-life about 3 weeks; main storage site is the blood. (7)

Calcification—Process in which tissue becomes hardened with calcium deposits; necessary for bone anabolism; pathological in vitamin D toxicity. (7)

Calcitonin—Hormone produced by the thyroid gland that slows the release of calcium from the bone when serum calcium levels are high. (8)

Calcitriol—The activated form of vitamin D, 1,25-dihydroxycholecalciferol. (7, 21)

Calorie—A measurement unit of energy; unit equaling the amount of heat required to raise the temperature of 1 gram of water 1 degree Celsius; laypersons' term for kilocalorie. (6)

Campylobacter—Flagellated, gram-negative bacteria; important cause of diarrheal illnesses. (14)

Candida albicans—Microscopic fungal organism normally present on skin and mucous membranes of healthy people; cause of thrush, vaginitis, opportunistic infections. (25)

Capillary—Minute vessel connecting arteriole and venule; vessel wall acts as semipermeable membrane to exchange substances between blood and lymph and interstitial fluid. (10)

Carbohydrate—Any of a group of organic compounds, including sugar, starch, and cellulose, that contains only carbon, oxygen, and hydrogen. (3)

Carbonic acid—Aqueous solution of carbon dioxide; carbon dioxide in solution or in blood is carbonic acid. (9)

Carcinogen—Any substance or agent that causes the development of or increases the risk of cancer. (23)

Carcinoma—A malignant neoplasm that occurs in epithelial tissue. (23)

Cardia—Upper orifice of the stomach connecting with the esophagus. (23)

Cardiac arrhythmia—Irregular heartbeat. (18)

Cardiac output—Volume of blood ejected by the heart in 1 minute. (20)

Cardiac sphincter—Smooth muscle band at the lower end of the esophagus; prevents reflux of stomach contents. (10, 22)

Cardiomyopathy—Disease of heart muscle; may be primary due to unknown cause or secondary to another cardiac disorder or systemic disease. (8)

Carotene—One of several yellow to red antioxidant pigments that are precursors to vitamin A. (7)

Carotenemia—Excess carotene in the blood, producing yellow skin but not discoloring the whites of the eyes. (7)

Carotenoid—Group of more than 500 red, orange, or yellow pigments found in fruits and vegetables, about 50 of which are precursors of vitamin A; includes carotene, which is such a precursor, and lycopene, which is not. (7, 22)

Casein—Principal protein in cow's milk. (12)

Catabolism—The breaking down of body compounds or tissues into simpler substances; the destructive phase of metabolism. (5)

Catalyst—A substance that speeds up a chemical reaction without entering into or being changed by the reaction. (5)

Cataract—Clouding of the lens of the eye. (13)

Cation—An ion with a positive charge. (9)

Cecum—The first portion of the large intestine between the ileum and the ascending colon. (10)

Celiac disease (gluten-sensitive enteropathy)—An intolerance to dietary gluten, which damages the intestine and produces diarrhea and malabsorption. (10, 22)

Cell—The smallest functional unit of structure in all plants and animals. (10)

Cellular immunity—Delayed immune response produced by T-lymphocytes, which mature in the thymus gland; examples of this type of response are rejection of transplanted organs and some autoimmune diseases. (23)

Cerebrovascular accident (CVA)—An abnormal condition in which the brain's blood vessels are occluded by a thrombus, an embolus, or hemorrhage, resulting in damaged brain tissue; stroke. (20)

Chelating agent—A chemical compound that binds metallic ions into a ring structure, inactivating them; used to remove poisonous metals from the body. (8)

Chemical digestion—Digestive process that involves the splitting of complex molecules into simpler forms. (10)

Chemical reaction—The process of combining or breaking down substances to obtain different substances. (10)

Chlorophyll—The green plant pigment necessary for the manufacture of carbohydrates. (3)

Cholecalciferol—Vitamin D_3, formed when the skin is exposed to sunlight; further processed by the liver and kidneys; may be reported as serum 25-hydroxy-cholecalciferol. (7)

Cholecystitis—Inflammation of the gallbladder. (22, 25)

Cholecystokinin—A hormone secreted by the duodenum; stimulates contraction of the gallbladder (releases bile) and the secretion of pancreatic juice. (10)

Cholelithiasis—The presence of gallstones. (22)

Cholestasis—Blockage of the flow of bile; due to liver disease or obstructions in the duct system. (8)

Cholesterol—A fat-like substance made in the human body and found in foods of animal origin; associated with an increased risk of heart disease. (4, 20)

Choline—Vitamin-like organic compound recognized as an essential nutrient; required for normal carbohydrate and fat metabolism and involved in protein metabolism. (7)

Chronic illness—A sickness persisting for a long period that shows little change or a slow progression over time. (15)

Chronic obstructive pulmonary disease (COPD)—A group of chronic diseases with a common characteristic of chronic airflow obstruction. (24)

Chronic renal failure—An irreversible condition in which the kidneys cannot perform vital functions. (21)

Chvostek's sign—Spasm of facial muscles following a tap over the facial nerve in front of the ear; indication of tetany. (8)

Chylomicron—A lipoprotein that carries triglycerides in the bloodstream after meals. (10, 20)

Chyme—The mixture of partly digested food and digestive secretions found in the stomach and small intestine during digestion of a meal. (10)

Chymotrypsin—A protein-splitting enzyme produced by the pancreas; active in the intestine. (10)

Cirrhosis—Chronic disease of the liver in which functioning cells degenerate and are replaced by fibrosed connective tissue. (22)

Client-care conference—A meeting that includes all health-care team members and may include the client or a significant other to review and update the client's nursing care plan. (15)

Clostridium botulinum—An anaerobic (grows without air) organism that produces a poisonous toxin; the cause of botulism. (14)

Clostridium perfringens—A bacterium that produces a poisonous toxin that causes a food intoxication; the symptoms are generally mild and of short duration and include intestinal disorders. (14)

Coenzyme—A substance that combines with an enzyme to activate it. (7)

Cognitive—Referring to or associated with the act of knowing. (12, 18)

Colectomy—Surgical removal of part or all of the colon. (22)

Collagen—Fibrous insoluble protein found in connective tissue. (7)

Collecting tubule—The last segment of the renal tubule; follows the distal convoluted tubule. Several nephrons usually share a single collecting tubule. (21)

Colloidal osmotic pressure—Pressure produced by plasma and cellular proteins. (9)

Colon—The large intestine from the end of the small intestine to the rectum. (10)

Colostomy—Surgical procedure in which an opening to the large intestine is constructed on the abdomen. (22)

Comorbidity—A disease coexisting with the primary disease. (18)

Complementation—Principle of meal planning advocating combining plant foods within a meal so that it contains all the essential amino acids; now applied to daily intake rather than to single meals. (5)

Complete protein—A protein containing all essential amino acids that humans need; usually found in animal sources such as milk, meat, eggs, and fish. (5)

Complex carbohydrate—A carbohydrate composed of many molecules of $C_6H_{12}O_6$ joined together; polysaccharide; includes starch, glycogen, and fiber. (3)

Compound—Two or more elements united chemically in specific proportions. (9)

Compound fat—Substance obtained when one of the fatty acids joined to the glycerol molecule is replaced by another molecule, such as a protein. (4)

Congestive heart failure (CHF)—Condition resulting from the failure of the heart to maintain adequate blood circulation; due to complex reactive mechanisms, fluid is retained in the body's tissues. (20)

Constipation—Decrease in a person's normal frequency of defecation; stool often hard, dry, or difficult to expel. (22)

Contamination iron—Iron that leaches from cookware into the food; in special circumstances, can become hazardous. (8)

Continuous ambulatory peritoneal dialysis (CAPD)—A form of self-dialysis in which the dialysate is allowed to remain in the abdominal cavity for 4–6 hours before replacement. (21)

Continuous feeding—Enteral feeding in which the formula drips slowly throughout the prescribed time span. (15)

Contraindication—Any circumstance under which treatment should not be given. (15)

Coronary heart disease (CHD)—Disease resulting from the decreased flow of blood through the coronary arteries to the heart muscle. (20)

Coronary occlusion—Blockage of one or more branches of the coronary arteries, which supply the heart muscle with oxygen and nutrients. (20)

Creatine—Nonprotein substance synthesized in the body from arginine, glycine, and methionine; combines with phosphate to form creatine phosphate, which is stored in muscle tissue as an energy source. (13, 16)

Creatinine—Nonprotein nitrogenous end product of creatine metabolism; because creatinine is excreted by the kidneys, serum creatinine levels are used to detect and monitor renal disease and to estimate muscle protein reserves. (13, 21)

Cretinism—A congenital condition resulting from a lack of thyroid secretions; characterized by a stunted and malformed body and arrested mental development. (8)

Crohn's disease—Inflammatory disease appearing in any area of the bowel in which diseased areas can be found alternating with healthy tissue. (22)

Cross-contamination—The spreading of a disease-producing organism from one food, person, or object to another food, person, or object. (14)

Cruciferous—Belonging to a botanical mustard family; includes broccoli, Brussels sprouts, cabbage, cauliflower, kale, kohlrabi, and swiss chard. (23)

Crystalluria—The presence of crystals in the urine; may be caused by the administration of sulfonamides. (17)

Culture—The learned, shared, and transmitted values, beliefs, and norms of a particular group that guides its thinking, decisions, and actions in patterned ways. (2)

Cyanocobalamin—Vitamin B_{12}; essential for proper blood formation. (7)

Cyclical variation—A recurring series of events during a specified period. (1)

Cystic fibrosis—Hereditary disease often affecting the lungs and pancreas in which glandular secretions are abnormally thick. (22)

Cystitis—Inflammation of the bladder. (21)

Cytochrome P450 enzyme—Group of genetically determined enzymes that help to metabolize fat-soluble vitamins, steroids, fatty acids, and other substances and to detoxify drugs and environmental pollutants. (16, 17)

Deamination—Metabolic process whereby nitrogen is removed from an amino acid. (10)

Deciliter (dL)—100 milliliters or 1/10 liter. (19)

Decubitus ulcer—A pressure sore on the lower back, such as a bedsore. (13, 15)

Degenerative joint disease (DJD)—Osteoarthritis. (13)

Dehiscence—Separation of the edges of a surgical incision. (22)

Delusion—False belief that is firmly maintained despite obvious proof to the contrary. (7)

Dementia—The impairment of intellectual function that usually is progressive and interferes with normal social and occupational activities. (1)

Dental caries—The gradual decay and disintegration of the teeth; a dental cavity is a hole in a tooth caused by dental caries. (3)

Dental plaque—Colorless and transparent gummy mass of microorganisms that grows on the teeth, predisposing them to decay. (3)

Deoxyribonucleic acid (DNA)—Protein substance in the cell nucleus that directs all the cell's activities, including reproduction. (5)

Desirable body weight—A person's body weight as compared with the 1959 Desirable Height/Weight Table. (18)

Desired outcome—The behavioral or physical change in a client that indicates the achievement of a nursing goal. (2)

Development—Gradual process of changing from a simple to a more complex organism; involves psychosocial and physical changes, not only an increase in size. (12)

Dextrose—Another name for the simple sugar glucose. (3)

Diabetes incipidus—Increased water intake and increased urine output resulting from inadequate secretion of antidiuretic hormone (ADH) by the posterior pituitary or by failure of the kidney tubules to respond to ADH; underlying causes can be tumor, surgery, trauma, infection, radiation injury, or congenital anomaly. (9)

Diabetes mellitus—Disease caused by insufficient insulin secretion by the pancreas or insulin resistance by body tissues causing excess glucose in the blood and deranged carbohydrate, fat, and protein metabolism. (19)

Diabetic neuropathy—Degeneration of peripheral nerves occurring in diabetes; possible causes are microscopic changes in blood vessels or metabolic defects in nerve tissue. (19)

Diacetic acid—A ketone body found in the urine, which can be due to the excessive breakdown of stored body fat. (3)

Diagnostic—Relating to scientific and skillful methods to establish the cause and nature of a sick person's illness. (15)

Dialysate—In renal failure, the fluid used to remove or deliver compounds or electrolytes that the failing kidney cannot excrete or retain in proper concentrations. (21)

Dialysis—The process of diffusing blood across a semipermeable membrane to remove toxic materials and to maintain fluid, electrolyte, and acid-base balances in cases of impaired kidney function or absence of the kidneys. (21)

Dialysis dementia—A neurological disturbance seen in clients who have been on dialysis for a number of years. (21)

Diastolic pressure—Pressure exerted against the arteries between heart beats; the lower number of a blood pressure reading. (9, 20)

Dietary fiber—Material in foods, mostly from plants, that the human body cannot break down or digest. (3)

Dietary recall, 24-hour—Description of what a person has eaten for the previous 24 hours. (2)

Dietary Reference Intake (DRI)—Four nutrient-based reference values that can be used for assessing and planning diets for the healthy general population; refer to average daily intakes for 1 or more weeks; include Estimated Average Requirements (EARs), Recommended Dietary Allowances (RDAs), Adequate Intakes (AIs), and Tolerable Upper Intake Levels (ULs). (2)

Dietary status—Description of what a person has been eating; his or her usual intake. (2)

Digestion—The process by which food is broken down mechanically and chemically in the gastrointestinal tract into forms simple enough for intestinal absorption. (10)

Diglyceride—Two fatty acids joined to a glycerol molecule. (4)

Dilutional hyponatremia—Serum sodium that is low, not because of an absolute lack of sodium but because of an excess of water. (8)

Disaccharide—A simple sugar composed of two units of $C_6H_{12}O_6$ joined together; examples include sucrose, lactose, and maltose. (3)

Disulfide linkage—Specific chemical bond joining amino acids; in hair, skin, and nails, holds amino acids in their distinct shapes. (8)

Diverticulitis—Inflammation of a diverticulum. (22)

Diverticulosis—Presence of one or more diverticula. (22)

Diverticulum—A sac or pouch in the walls of a tubular organ; pl., diverticula. (22)

Docosahexaenoic acid (DHA)—Omega-3 polyunsaturated fatty acid found in fish oils. (4, 12, 20)

Dopamine—Catecholamine synthesized by the adrenals; immediate precursor in the synthesis of norepinephrine. (17)

Double-blind—Technique of scientific investigation in which neither the investigator nor the subject knows what treatment, if any, the subject is receiving. (16)

Double bond—A type of chemical connection in which, for example, a fatty acid has two neighboring carbon atoms, each lacking one hydrogen atom. (4)

Drink—An alcoholic beverage; one drink is usually 12 ounces of beer, 4 ounces of wine, or 1.5 ounces of liquor. (20)

Dual-energy x-ray absorptiometry (DEXA)—Diagnostic test using two x-ray beams to determine body composition; used to measure bone mineral density as an indicator of osteopenia and osteoporosis. (2)

Duct—A structural tube designed to allow secretions to move from one body part to another body part. (10, 19)

Dumping syndrome—A condition in which the contents of the stomach empty too rapidly into the duodenum; mostly occurs in patients who have had gastric resections. (22)

Duodenum—The first part of the small intestine between the stomach and the jejunum. (10)

Dysphoria—A speech disorder characterized by hoarseness. (18)

Dyspnea—Difficulty breathing. (24)

Ebb phase—The first phase in the stress response; the body reduces blood pressure, cardiac output, body temperature, and oxygen consumption to meet increased demands. (24)

Eclampsia—An obstetrical emergency involving hypertension, proteinuria, and convulsions appearing after the twentieth week of pregnancy. (11)

Eczema—Skin inflammation, acute or chronic; caused by external (chemical irritation or microbial invasion) or internal (genetic or psychological) factors. (12)

Edema—The accumulation of excessive amounts of fluid in interstitial spaces. (9)

Edentulous—The state of having no teeth. (13)

Efferent—Directed away from a center; used to describe arteries, veins, lymphatic vessels, and nerves. (18)

Efferent arteriole—Small blood vessel by which blood leaves the nephron. (21)

Efficacy—Ability of a drug to achieve the desired effect. (16)

Eicosapentaenoic acid (EPA)—Omega-3 fatty acid found in fish oils. (20)

Electrocardiogram (ECG)—A graphic record produced by an electrocardiograph that shows the electrical activity of the heart. (9)

Electroencephalogram (EEG)—The record obtained from an electroencephalograph that shows the electrical activity of the brain. (9)

Electrolyte—An element or compound that when dissolved in water separates (dissociates) into ions that are capable of conducting an electrical current; acids, bases, and salts are common electrolytes. (9)

Element—A substance that cannot be separated into simpler parts by ordinary means. (3)

Elemental or "predigested" formula—Formula that contains either partially or totally predigested nutrients. (15)

Embolus—A circulating mass of undissolved matter in a blood or lymphatic vessel; may be composed of tissues, fat globules, air bubbles, clumps of bacteria, or foreign bodies, including pieces of medical devices. (20)

Embryo—A developing infant in the prenatal period between the second and eighth weeks inclusive. (11)

Empty kilocalories—Refers to a food that contains kilocalories and almost no other nutrients. (6)

Emulsification—The physical breaking up of fat into tiny droplets. (10)

Emulsifier—A molecule that attracts both water- and fat-soluble molecules. (14)

Emulsion—One liquid evenly distributed in a second liquid with which it usually does not mix. (4)

Endemic—The constant presence of a disease or infectious agent within a given geographic area; the usual prevalence of a given disease within such an area. (5, 8)

Endogenous—Produced within or caused by factors within the organism. (16)

Endoscope—A device consisting of a tube and an optical system for observing the inside of a hollow organ or cavity. (15)

End-stage renal failure—A state in which the kidneys have lost most or all of their ability to maintain internal homeostasis and produce urine. (21, 25)

Energy—The capacity to do work. (1)

Energy balance—A situation in which kilocaloric intake equals kilocaloric output. (6)

Energy expenditure—The amount of fuel the body uses for a specified period. (6)

Energy imbalance—Situation in which kilocalories eaten do not equal the number of kilocalories used for energy. (18)

Energy nutrients—The chemical substances in food that are able to supply fuel; refers collectively to carbohydrate, fat, and protein. (1)

Enrichment—The addition of nutrients previously present in a food but removed during food processing or lost during storage. (3)

Enteral tube feeding—The feeding of a formula by tube into the gastrointestinal tract. (15)

Enteric-coated—A type of drug preparation designed to dissolve in the intestine rather than in the stomach. (17)

Enteritis—Inflammation of the intestines, particularly the small intestine. (12)

Enzyme—Complex protein produced by living cells that acts as a catalyst. (5, 6)

Epidemic—Occurrence in a region of more than the expected number of cases of a communicable disease. (25)

Epinephrine—Hormone of the adrenal gland; produces the fight-or-flight response. (24)

Epithelial tissue—A type of tissue that forms the outer layer of skin and lines body surfaces opening to the outside; functions include protection, absorption, and secretion. (7)

Ergocalciferol—Vitamin D_2 formed by the action of sunlight on plants. (7)

Ergot poisoning—Poisoning resulting from excessive use of the drug ergot or from the ingestion of grain or grain products infected with the *Claviceps purpurea* fungus. (14)

Erikson, Erik—Psychologist who devised a theory of human development consisting of eight stages of life, each with a psychosocial developmental task to be mastered. (12)

Erosion—Destruction of the surface of a tissue, either on the external surface of the body or internally. (22)

Erythropoietin—Hormone released by the kidney to stimulate red blood cell production. (21)

Esophagostomy—A surgical opening in the esophagus. (15)

Esophagus—A muscular canal extending from the mouth to the stomach. (10, 22)

Essential amino acid—One of the amino acids that cannot be manufactured by the human body; must be obtained from food or artificial feeding. (5)

Essential (primary) hypertension—Elevated blood pressure that develops without apparent cause. (20)

Essential nutrient—A substance found in food that must be present in the diet because the human body lacks the ability to manufacture it in sufficient amounts for optimal health. (1)

Estimated Average Requirement—Intake that meets the estimated nutrient need of 50 percent of the individuals in a life-stage and gender group; used to set the RDA and to assess or plan the intake of groups. (2)

Ethanol—Grain alcohol; ounces of ethanol in beverages can be estimated with the conversion factors of 0.045 for beer, 0.121 for wine, and 0.409 for liquor. (20)

Ethnocentrism—Belief that one's own view of the world is superior to anyone else's. (2)

Etiology—the cause of a disease. (8)

Evaluation—The final step in the nursing process in which the actual outcome is compared to the desired outcome. (2)

Evaporative water loss—Insensible water loss through the skin. (9)

Exchange—A defined quantity of food on the American Dietetic and Diabetes associations' food exchange list or on another, similar exchange list. (2)

Exchange list—A food guide developed by the American Dietetic and Diabetes Associations; often used in clinical practice to aid in meal planning. (2)

Excretion—The elimination of waste products from the body in feces, urine, exhaled air, and perspiration. (10)

Exogenous—Outside the body. (19)

External muscle layer—Muscle layer of the alimentary canal. (6)

External water loss—Water lost to the outside of the body. (9)

Extracellular fluid—Fluid found between the cells and within the blood and lymph vessels. (9)

Extrinsic factor—Vitamin B_{12}, necessary for proper red blood cell development. (7)

Failure to thrive (FTT)—Medical diagnosis for infants who fail to gain weight appropriately or who lose weight. (12)

Fasting—The state of having had no food or fluid enterally or no parenteral nutrition. (15)

Fasting blood sugar (FBS)—Blood glucose measured in the fasting state; normal values are 70–110 mg per deciliter. (3, 19)

Fat-free mass—Lean body mass plus nonfat components of adipose tissue. (2)

Fatty acid—Part of the structure of a fat. (4)

Fatty liver—Accumulation of lipids in the liver cells; may be reversible if the cause, of which there are many, is removed. (22)

Feedback cycle—Control system of many bodily functions involving the interaction between a stimulus and an effect; in positive feedback, the effect increases the stimulus as uterine contractions increasing oxytocin secretion; in negative feedback, the effect decreases the stimulus as blood levels of thyroid hormone decrease secretion of thyroid-stimulating hormone. (8)

Ferric iron—Oxidized iron, which is less absorbable from the gastrointestinal tract than ferrous iron; abbreviated Fe^{3+}. (8)

Ferritin—An iron-phosphorus-protein complex formed in the intestinal mucosa by the union of ferric iron with apoferritin; the form in which iron is stored in the tissues, mainly in liver, spleen, and bone marrow cells. (8, 21)

Ferrous iron—The more absorbable form of iron for humans; abbreviated Fe^{2+}. (8)

Fetal alcohol syndrome (FAS)—A condition characterized by mental and physical abnormalities in an infant caused by the mother's consumption of alcohol during pregnancy. (11)

Fetus—The human child in utero from the third month until birth; also applicable to the later stages of gestation of other animals. (11)

Fiber, dietary—Material in foods, mostly from plants, that the human body cannot break down or digest. (3)

Fibrin—Insoluble protein formed from fibrinogen by the action of thrombin; forms the meshwork of a blood clot. (8)

Fibrinogen—Protein in blood essential to the clotting process; also called Factor I; see fibrin. (8)

Filtration—The process of removing particles from a solution by allowing the liquid to pass through a membrane or other partial barrier. (21)

First-degree relative—An individual's parents, siblings, or children. (11, 22)

First pass effect—Process whereby drugs are extensively metabolized by the small intestine or liver enzymes; result is that less drug reaches the systemic circulation. (17)

Flatus—Gas in the digestive tract, averaging 400 to 1200 milliliters per day. (22)

Flavonoids—Nonnutritive antioxidant compounds that occur naturally in certain foods such as onions, apples, tea, and red wine; inhibit oxidation of LDL in laboratory experiments. (20)

Flow phase—The second phase in the stress response; marked by pronounced hormonal changes. (24)

Fluorosis—Condition due to excessive prolonged intake of fluoride; tissues affected are teeth and bones. (8)

Folate conjugase—Enzyme needed to separate folic acid from the amino acids that usually bind to it in foods; found in salivary, gastric, pancreatic, and jejunal secretions. (7)

Folic acid—B-complex vitamin necessary for DNA formation and proper red blood cell formation. (7)

Food acceptance record—A checklist that indicates food items accepted or rejected by the client. (15)

Food allergy—Sensitivity to a food that does not cause a negative reaction in most people. (10, 12)

Food faddism—An unusual pattern of food behavior enthusiastically adapted by its adherents. (25)

Food frequency—A usual food intake or a description of what an individual usually eats during a typical day. (2)

Food quackery—The promotion for profit of a medical scheme or remedy that is unproven or known to be false. (25)

Food infection—Infection acquired through contact with food or water contaminated with disease-producing microorganisms. (14)

Food intoxication—An illness caused by the consumption of a food in which bacteria have produced a poisonous toxin. (14)

Food record—A diary of a person's self-reported food intake. (2)

Fortification—Process of adding nutritive substances not naturally occurring in the given food to increase its nutritional value; for example, milk fortified with vitamins A and D. (7)

Free-living—Following a way of life in which one freely indulges one's appetites and desires, as opposed to living in an institution. (7)

Free radicals—Atoms or molecules that have lost an electron and vigorously pursue its replacement; in doing so, free radicals can damage normal cell constituents. (7)

Fructose—A monosaccharide found in fruits and honey; a simple sugar. (3)

Fundus—Larger part of a hollow organ; the part of the stomach above its attachment to the esophagus. (22)

Galactose—A monosaccharide derived mainly from the breakdown of the sugar in milk, lactose; a simple sugar. (3)

Galactosemia—Lack of an enzyme needed to metabolize galactose. (12)

Gallbladder—A pear-shaped organ on the underside of the liver that concentrates and stores bile. (10, 22)

Gastric bypass—A surgical procedure that routes food around the stomach. (18)

Gastric lipase—An enzyme in the stomach that aids in the digestion of fats. (10)

Gastric stapling—A surgical procedure on the stomach to induce weight loss by reducing the size of the stomach; also known as gastroplasty. (18)

Gastrin—A hormone secreted by the gastric mucosa; stimulates the secretion of gastric juice. (10)

Gastritis—Inflammation of the stomach. (22)

Gastroesophageal reflux (acid-reflux disorder) (GERD)—Regurgitation of stomach contents into the esophagus. (22)

Gastroparesis—Partial paralysis of the stomach. (19)

Gastrostomy—A surgical opening in the stomach. (15)

Gene—Basic unit of heredity; linear segment of deoxyribonucleic acid (DNA) that occupies a specific location on a specific chromosome; provides the instructions for protein synthesis. (5, 23)

Generativity—The seventh of Erikson's developmental stages, in which the middle-aged adult guides the next generation. (13)

Generic name—The name given to a drug by its original developer; usually the same as the official name given to it by the Food and Drug Administration. (17)

Genetic susceptibility—The likelihood of an individual developing a given trait as determined by heredity. (3)

Geriatrics—The branch of medicine involved in the study and treatment of diseases of the elderly. (13)

Gestation—The time from fertilization of the ovum until birth; in humans, the length of gestation is usually 38–42 weeks. (11)

Gestational diabetes (GDM)—Hyperglycemia and altered carbohydrate, protein, and fat metabolism related to the increased physiological demands of pregnancy. (11, 19)

Globin—The simple protein portion of hemoglobin. (5)

Glomerular filtrate—The fluid that has been passed through the glomerulus. (21)

Glomerular filtration rate (GFR)—An index of kidney function; the amount of filtrate formed each minute in all the nephrons of both kidneys. (21)

Glomerulonephritis—Inflammation of the glomeruli. (21)

Glomerulus—The network of capillaries inside Bowman's capsule. (21)

Glossitis—Inflammation of the tongue. (7)

Glucagon—A hormone secreted by the alpha cells of the pancreas; increases the concentration of glucose in the blood. (5, 19)

Gluconeogenesis—The production of glucose from non-carbohydrate sources such as amino acids and glycerol. (22, 24)

Glucose—A monosaccharide (simple sugar) commonly called the blood sugar; the same as dextrose. (3)

Glucose tolerance test—A test of blood and urine after the patient receives a concentrated dose of glucose; used to diagnose abnormalities of glucose metabolism. (19)

Gluteal-femoral obesity—Excess body fat centered around an individual's buttocks, hips, and thighs. (18, 20)

Gluten—A type of protein found in wheat, rye, and barley; may contaminate oats through processing. (10, 22)

Gluten-sensitive enteropathy (celiac disease)—An intestinal disorder caused by an abnormal response following the consumption of gluten. (10, 22)

Glycemic index—A measure of how much the blood glucose level increases following consumption of a particular food that contains a given amount of carbohydrate. (19)

Glycerol—The backbone of a fat molecule; pharmaceutical preparation is glycerin. (4)

Glycogen—The form in which carbohydrate is stored in liver and muscle. (3)

Glycogenolysis—The breakdown of glycogen. (24)

Glycosuria—Glucose in the urine. (19)

Glycosylated hemoglobin—Hemoglobin to which a glucose group is attached; in diabetes mellitus, if the blood glucose level has not been controlled over the previous 120 days, the glycosylated hemoglobin level is elevated. (19)

Goiter—Enlargement of the thyroid gland characterized by pronounced swelling in the neck. (8)

Goitrogens—Substances that block the absorption of iodine, thereby causing goiter; found in cabbage, rutabaga, and turnips, but only related to goiter in cassava. (8)

Gout—A hereditary metabolic disease that is a form of acute arthritis and is marked by inflammation of the joints. (21)

GRAS List—Food additives categorized by the U.S. Food and Drug Administration to be Generally Recognized As Safe. (16)

Growth—Progressive increase in size of a living thing that entails the synthesis of new protoplasm and multiplication of cells. (12)

Gut failure—Impaired absorption due to structural damage to the small intestine; symptoms include diarrhea, malabsorption, and unsuccessful absorption of oral food. (10)

Harris-Benedict equation—A formula commonly used to estimate resting energy expenditure in a stressed client. (24, 25)

Health—The state of complete physical, mental, and social well-being, not just the absence of disease or infirmity. (1)

Healthy body weight (HBW)—Estimate of a weight suitable for an individual based on frame size and height and weight tables. (2)

Healthy Eating Index—Measure of diet quality devised by the United States Department of Agriculture Center for Nutrition Policy and Promotion. (12)

Helminthiasis—Infestation with intestinal parasites or worms. (8)

Hematocrit—Percent of total blood volume that is red blood cells; normal levels are 40–54 percent for men, 37–47 percent for women. (8)

Hematuria—Blood in the urine. (21)

Heme—The iron-containing portion of the hemoglobin molecule. (8)

Heme iron—Iron bound to hemoglobin and myoglobin in meat, fish, and poultry; 10–30 percent of the iron in these foods is absorbed. (8)

Hemochromatosis—A genetic disease of iron metabolism in which iron accumulates in the tissues. (8)

Hemodialysis—A method for cleansing the blood of wastes by circulating blood through a machine that contains tubes made of synthetic semipermeable membranes. (21)

Hemoglobin—The iron-carrying pigment of the red blood cells; carries oxygen from the lungs to the tissues. (5, 8)

Hemolysis—Rupture of red blood cells releasing hemoglobin into the plasma; causes include bacterial toxins, chemicals, inappropriate medications, vitamin E deficiency. (9)

Hemolytic anemia—An abnormal reduction in the number of red blood cells due to hemolysis. (8)

Hemosiderin—An iron oxide–protein compound derived from hemoglobin; a storage form of iron. (8)

Hemosiderosis—Condition resulting from excess deposits of hemosiderin, especially in the liver and spleen; caused by destruction of red blood cells, which occurs in diseases such as hemolytic anemia, pernicious anemia, and chronic infection. (8)

Heparin—A chemical, found naturally in many tissues, that inhibits blood clotting by preventing the conversion of prothrombin to thrombin; also given as an anticoagulant medication. (7)

Hepatic portal circulation—A subdivision of the vascular system in which blood from the digestive organs and spleen circulates through the liver before returning to the heart. (10)

Hepatitis—Inflammation of the liver, caused by viruses, drugs, alcohol, or toxic substances. (22)

Heterozygous—Having two different genes, one from each parent, governing a particular trait; the dominant gene will produce the given trait in the individual. (11)

Hiatal hernia—A protrusion of part of the stomach into the chest cavity. (22)

High-density lipoprotein (HDL)—A plasma protein that carries fat in the bloodstream to the tissues or to the liver to be excreted; elevated blood levels are associated with a decreased risk of heart disease. (20)

High-fructose corn syrup (HFCS)—A common food additive used as a sweetener; made from fructose. (3)

Hives (urticaria)—Sudden swelling and itching of skin or mucous membranes, often caused by allergies; if the respiratory tract is involved, may be life-threatening. (12)

Homeostasis—Tendency toward balance in the internal environment of the body, achieved by automatic monitoring and regulating mechanisms. (6)

Homozygous—Having two identical genes, one from each parent, governing a particular trait; necessary condition to produce a disease caused by a recessive gene, such as sickle cell anemia. (11)

Hormone—A substance produced by cells of the body that is released into the bloodstream and carried to target sites to regulate the activity of other cells and organs. (4, 5)

Human immunodeficiency virus (HIV)—The virus that causes AIDS. (25)

Humoral immunity—Development of antibodies to specific antigens by the B-lymphocytes, some of which retain the ability to recognize the antigen if it is encountered again; basis of immunizations. (23)

Humulin—Exact duplicate of human insulin manufactured by altering bacterial DNA. (19)

Hunger—The sensation resulting from a lack of food, characterized by dull or acute pain around the lower part of the chest. (18)

Hydrochloric acid (HCl)—Strong acid secreted by the stomach that aids in protein digestion. (10)

Hydrogenation—The process of adding hydrogen to a fat to make it more highly saturated. (4)

Hydrolysis—A chemical reaction that splits a substance

into simpler compounds by the addition of water; in hydrolyzed infant formulas, whole proteins are split into smaller pieces. (10, 12)

Hydrostatic pressure—The pressure created by the pumping action of the heart on the fluid in the blood vessels. (9)

Hyperalimentation—Another name for total parenteral nutrition. (15)

Hyperbilirubinemia—Excessive bilirubin in the blood; bilirubin is produced by the breakdown of red blood cells. (12)

Hypercalcemia—A serum calcium level that is too high; in adults, more than 5.5 milliequivalents per liter. (8)

Hypercholesterolemia—Excessive cholesterol in the blood. (20)

Hyperemesis gravidarum—Severe nausea and vomiting persisting after the fourteenth week of pregnancy of unknown etiology. (11)

Hyperglycemia—An elevated level of glucose in the blood; fasting value above 110 milligrams per deciliter, depending on measuring technique used. (19)

Hyperglycemic hyperosmolar nonketotic syndrome (HHNS)—Life-threatening complication of NIDDM characterized by blood glucose levels greater than 600 milligrams per deciliter, absence of or slight ketosis, profound cellular dehydration, and electrolyte imbalances. (19)

Hyperkalemia—Excessive potassium in the blood; greater than 5.0 milliequivalents per liter of serum in adults. (8)

Hyperlipoproteinemia—Increased lipoproteins and lipids in the blood. (20)

Hypermetabolism—An abnormal increase in the rate at which fuel or kilocalories are burned. (24)

Hypernatremia—An excess of sodium in the blood; greater than 145 milliequivalents per liter of serum in adults. (8)

Hyperparathyroidism—Excessive secretion of parathyroid hormone, causing changes in the bones, kidney, and gastrointestinal tract. (8)

Hyperphosphatemia—Excessive amount of phosphates in the blood; in adults, greater than 4.7 milligrams per 100 milliliters of serum. (8)

Hypertension—Condition of elevated blood pressure; diagnosed if blood pressure is greater than 140/90 on three successive occasions or if person is receiving antihypertensive medication. (20)

Hypertensive disorders of pregnancy—Blood pressure greater than 140 mmHg systolic or greater than 90 mmHg diastolic occurring in pregnancy. Subcategories are chronic hypertension, gestational hypertension, preeclampsia, and eclampsia. (11)

Hypertensive kidney disease—A condition in which vascular or glomerular lesions cause hypertension but not total renal failure. (21)

Hyperthyroidism—Oversecretion of thyroid hormones, which increases the metabolic rate above normal. (8)

Hypertonic—A solution that contains more particles and exerts more osmotic pressure than the plasma. (9)

Hypervitaminosis—Condition caused by excessive intake of vitamins. (7)

Hypocalcemia—A depressed level of calcium in the blood; less than 4.5 milliequivalents per liter of serum in adults. (8)

Hypoglycemia—A depressed level of glucose in the blood; less than 70 milligrams per deciliter. (19)

Hypokalemia—Potassium depletion in the circulating blood; less than 3.5 milliequivalents per liter of serum in adults. (8, 17, 21)

Hyponatremia—Too little sodium per volume of blood; less than 135 milliequivalents per liter of serum in adults. (8)

Hypophosphatemia—Too little phosphate per volume of blood; in adults, less than 2.4 milligrams per 100 milliliters of serum. (8)

Hypothalamus—A portion of the brain that helps to regulate water balance, thirst, body temperature, carbohydrate and fat metabolism, and sleep. (9)

Hypothyroidism—Undersecretion of thyroid hormones; reduces the metabolic rate. (8)

Hypotonic—A solution that contains fewer particles and exerts less osmotic pressure than the plasma does. (9)

Iatrogenic malnutrition—Excessive or deficit intake of one or more nutrients induced by the oversight or omissions of health-care workers. (15)

Ideal body weight—A person's weight as compared with the 1943 Height/Weight Tables. (18)

Identity—The fifth developmental task in Erikson's theory, in which the adolescent decides on an appropriate role. (12)

Idiopathic—Without a recognizable cause. (13)

Ileocecal valve—The valve between the ileum and cecum. (10)

Ileostomy—Surgical procedure in which an opening to the small intestine (ileum) is constructed on the abdomen. (22)

Ileum—The lower portion of the small intestine. (10, 22)

Immune—Produced by, involved in, or concerned with resistance or protection against a specified disease. (23)

Immune system—The organs in the body responsible for fighting off substances interpreted as foreign. (23)

Immunity—The state of being protected from a particular disease, especially an infectious disease. (5, 25)

Immunoglobulin—Blood proteins with known antibody activity; five classes of immunoglobulins have been identified: IgA, IgD, IgE, IgG, and IgM. (5)

Immunosuppressive agent—Medication that interferes with the body's ability to fight infection. (14)

Impaired glucose tolerance (IGT)—A type of classification for hyperglycemia; for persons who have a glucose intolerance but do not meet the criteria for classification as having diabetes. (19)

Implantation—Embedding of the fertilized egg in the lining of the uterus 6 or 7 days after fertilization. (11)

Incidence—The frequency of occurrence of any event or condition over a given time and in relation to the population in which it occurs. (18)

Incomplete protein—Protein lacking one or more of the essential amino acids that humans need; found primarily in plant sources such as grains and vegetables; gelatin is an animal product but is an incomplete protein. (5)

Incubation period—The time it takes to show disease symptoms after exposure to the causative organism. (14)

Indication—A circumstance that indicates when a treatment should or can be used. (15)

Indoles—Compounds found in vegetables of the cruciferous family that activate enzymes to destroy carcinogens. (23)

Industry—The fourth stage of development in Erikson's theory in which the school-age child learns to work effectively. (12)

Infection—Entry and development of parasites or entry and multiplication of microorganisms in the bodies of persons or animals; may or may not cause signs and symptoms. (25)

Initiation—The first step in the cell's becoming cancerous, when physical forces, chemicals, or biologic agents permanently alter the cell's DNA. (23)

Initiative—The third stage of development in Erikson's theory, in which the preschooler learns to set and achieve goals. (12)

Insensible water loss—Water that is lost invisibly through the lungs and skin. (9)

Insoluble—Incapable of being dissolved in a given substance. (3)

Insulin—Hormone secreted by the beta cells of the pancreas in response to an elevated blood glucose level. (5)

Insulin-dependent diabetes mellitus (IDDM)—Type 1 diabetes; persons with this disorder must take insulin to survive. (18)

Insulin resistance—A disorder characterized by elevated levels of both glucose and insulin; thought to be related to a lack of insulin receptors. (19)

Intact feeding—A feeding consisting of nutrients that have not been predigested. (15)

Intact nutrients—Nutrients that have not been predigested. (15)

Intact or "polymeric" formula—An oral or enteral feeding that contains all the essential nutrients in a specified volume. (15)

Integrity—The final stage of Erikson's theory of psychosocial development, in which the older adult learns to look back on his or her life as worthwhile. (13)

Intermittent feeding—Giving a 4- to 6-hour volume of a tube feeding over 20–30 minutes. (15)

Intermittent peritoneal dialysis—Method of dialysis treatment in which the dialysate remains in a patient's abdominal cavity for about 30 minutes and then drains from the body by gravity. (21)

International Unit (IU)—Individually scaled measure of vitamins A, D, and E agreed to by a committee of scientists; largely replaced by finer measures. (7)

Interstitial fluid—Extracellular fluid located between the cells. (9)

Intimacy—The sixth stage of development in Erikson's theory, in which the young adult builds reciprocal, caring relationships. (13)

Intracellular fluid—Fluid located within the cells. (9)

Intravascular fluid—Fluid found in the blood and lymph vessels. (9)

Intravenous—Through a vein. (3)

Intrinsic factor—Specific protein-binding factor secreted by the stomach, necessary for the absorption of vitamin B_{12}. (7)

Invisible fat—Dietary fats that cannot be seen easily; hidden fats in foods such as baked goods, peanut butter, emulsified milk, and so forth. (4)

Ion—An atom or group of atoms carrying an electrical charge; an ion with a positive charge is called a cation; an ion with a negative charge is called an anion. (9)

Ionic bond—A chemical bond formed between atoms by the loss and gain of electrons. (9)

Iron deficiency—State of inadequate iron stores measured by laboratory tests such as serum ferritin and transferrin saturation; may progress to anemia when the person's hemoglobin value drops. (8)

Irrigation—Flushing a prescribed solution through a tube or cavity. (15)

Irritable bowel syndrome—Diarrhea or alternating constipation-diarrhea with no discernible organic cause. (22)

Islet cell antibody—A protein found to be elevated in a person with insulin-dependent diabetes mellitus. (19)

Islets of Langerhans—Clusters of cells in the pancreas including alpha, beta, and delta cells; alpha cells produce glucagon, beta cells produce insulin, and delta cells produce somatostatin. (19)

Isotonic—A solution that has the same osmotic pressure as blood plasma. (9, 15)

Jaundice—Yellowing of skin, whites of eyes, and mucous membranes due to excessive bilirubin in the blood; causes may be obstructed bile duct, liver disease, or hemolysis of red blood cells. (7)

Jejunoileal bypass—A surgical procedure that removes a portion of the small intestine, bypassing about 90 percent of it. (18)

Jejunostomy—A surgical opening into the jejunum. (15)

Jejunum—The second portion of the small intestine. (8, 10)

Kaposi's sarcoma—A type of cancer often related to the immunocompromised state that accompanies AIDS; characterized by multiple areas of cell proliferation, initially in the skin and eventually in other body sites. (25)

Keshan disease—Deterioration of the heart due to selenium deficiency, but heart failure not reversible by supplementation; named for the province of Keshan, China; fatality rate as high as 80 percent; in mice, linked to a mutation of an avirulent virus to a virulent one producing myocardial disease; virulent strain then caused heart disease in mice not selenium-deficient. (8)

Keto acid—Amino acid residue left after deamination. (19)

Ketoacidosis—Acidosis due to an excess of ketone bodies. (19)

Ketone bodies—Compounds such as acetone and diacetic acid that are formed when fat is metabolized incompletely. (4)

Ketonuria—The presence of ketone bodies in the urine. (19)

Ketosis—The physical state of the human body with ketones elevated in the blood and present in the urine; one example is diabetic ketoacidosis. (3, 24)

Kilocaloric density—The kilocalories contained in a given volume of a food. (6)

Kilocalorie—A measurement unit of energy; the amount of heat required to raise 1 kilogram of water 1 degree Celsius; often referred to as calories by the general public. (6)

Kilocalorie: nitrogen ratio—A mathematical relationship expressed as the number of kilocalories per gram of nitrogen provided in a feeding. (24)

Kilojoule—A measurement unit of energy; one kilocalorie equals 4.184 kilojoules. (6)

Konzo—An irreversible paralytic disease of the lower extremities caused by consumption of inadequately processed cassava roots that contain cyanide along with a diet deficient in sulphur-based amino acids. (5)

Korsakoff's psychosis—Amnesia, often seen in chronic alcoholism, caused by degeneration of the thalamus due to thiamin deficiency; characterized by loss of short-term memory and inability to learn new skills. (7)

Krebs cycle—A complicated series of reactions that results in the release of energy from carbohydrates, fats, and proteins, also known as the TCA (tricarboxylic acid) cycle. (10)

Kussmaul respirations—Pattern of rapid and deep breathing due to the body's attempt to correct metabolic acidosis by eliminating carbon dioxide through the lungs. (19)

Kwashiorkor—Severe protein deficiency in child after weaning; symptoms include edema, pigmentation changes, impaired growth and development, and liver pathology. (5, 9)

Lactalbumin—Simple soluble protein found in greater concentration in human breast milk than in cow's milk; easily absorbed by the infant. (12)

Lactase—An intestinal enzyme that converts lactose into glucose and galactose. (10)

Lacteal—The central lymph vessel in each villus. (10)

Lactose—A disaccharide found mainly in milk and milk products. (3)

Large intestine—The part of the alimentary canal that extends from the small intestine to the anus. (10)

LCAT deficiency—A lack of LCAT, an enzyme that transports cholesterol from the tissues to the liver for removal from the body. (21)

Lean body mass—Also called fat-free mass; the weight of the body minus the fat content but including essential fats that are associated with the central nervous system, the viscera, the bone marrow, and cell membranes. (5)

Legumes—Plants that have nitrogen-fixing bacteria in their roots; a good alternative to meat as a protein source; examples are dried beans, lentils. (5)

Lesion—Area of diseased or injured tissue. (21)

Leukopenia—Abnormal decrease in the number of white blood corpuscles; usually below 5000 per cubic millimeter. (25)

Life expectancy—The probable number of years that persons of a given age may be expected to live. (13)

Limiting amino acid—Particular essential amino acid lacking or undersupplied in a food that classifies the food as an incomplete protein. (5)

Linoleic acid—An essential fatty acid. (4)

Lipectomy—Surgical removal of adipose tissue. (18)

Lipid—Any one of a group of fats or fat-like substances that are insoluble in water; includes true fats (fatty acids and glycerol), lipoids, and sterols. (4)

Lipoid—Substances resembling fats but containing groups other than glycerol and fatty acids that make up true fats; example: phospholipids. (4)

Lipolysis—The breakdown of adipose tissue for energy. (19, 24)

Lipoprotein—Combination of a protein with lipid components such as cholesterol, phospholipids, and triglycerides. (4)

Lipoprotein lipase—An enzyme that breaks down chylomicrons. (20)

Liposuction—Surgical removal of adipose tissue through a vacuum hose. (18)

Listeriosis—Bacterial infection caused by *Listeria monocytogenes* that is particularly virulent for fetuses; transmitted from the mother to the fetus in utero or through the birth canal; outbreaks associated with raw or contaminated milk, soft cheeses, contaminated vegetables, and ready-to-eat meats. (11)

Liver—A digestive organ that aids in the metabolism of all the energy nutrients, screens toxic substances from the blood, manufactures blood proteins, and performs many other important functions. (10, 22)

Loop of Henle—The segment of the renal tubule that follows the proximal convoluted tubule. (21)

Low birth weight (LBW)—Characterizing an infant that weighs less than 2500 g (5.5 lb) at birth. (11)

Low-density lipoprotein (LDL)—A plasma protein containing more cholesterol and triglycerides than protein; elevated blood levels are associated with increased risk of heart disease. (20)

Luminal effect—Drug-induced changes within the intestine that affect the absorption of nutrients and drugs without altering the intestine. (17)

Lycopene—A red pigmented carotenoid with powerful antioxidant functions but no provitamin A activity; found in tomatoes and various berries and fruits. (23)

Lymph—A body fluid collected from the interstitial fluid all over the body and returned to the bloodstream via the lymphatic vessels. (10)

Lymphatic system—All the structures involved in the transportation of lymph from the tissues to the bloodstream. (10)

Lysine—Amino acid often lacking in grains. (5)

Macrocytic anemia—Anemia in which the red blood cells are larger than normal; one characteristic of pernicious anemia also found in folic acid deficiency. (7)

Major minerals—Those present in the body in quantities greater than 5 grams (approximately 1 teaspoonful); humans need at least 100 milligrams daily (approximately 1/50 teaspoonful); also called macrominerals. (8)

Malabsorption—Inadequate movement of digested food from the small intestine into the blood or lymphatic system. (10)

Malignant—Tumor that infiltrates surrounding tissue and spreads to distant sites of the body. (23)

Malnutrition—Poor nutrition; results when the body's cells receive either an excess or a deficiency of one or more nutrients. (1)

Maltase—An intestinal enzyme that converts maltose into glucose. (10)

Maltose—A disaccharide produced when starches are broken down by the body into simpler units; two units of glucose joined together. (3)

Marasmus—Malnutrition due to a protein and kilocalorie deficit. (5)

Mastication—The process of chewing. (10)

Mechanical digestion—The digestive process that involves the physical breaking down of food into smaller pieces. (10)

Megadose—Dose providing 10 times or more of the recommended dietary allowance. (7)

Megaloblastic anemia—Anemia characterized by large immature red blood cells in the bloodstream that cannot carry oxygen properly; occurs in folic acid deficiency and pernicious anemia. (7)

Menaquinone—Vitamin K that is synthesized by intestinal bacteria; also called vitamin K_2. (7)

Meninges—Three membranes covering the brain and spinal cord; from the outside named the dura, arachnoid, and pia maters. (11)

Meningocele—Congenital protrusion of the meninges through a defect in the skull or the spinal column. (11)

Meningoencephalocele—Protrusion of the brain and its coverings through a defect in the skull. (11)

Menkes' disease—Metabolic defect blocking the absorption of copper in the gastrointestinal tract. (8)

Meta-analysis—Statistical procedure for combining data from a number of studies to analyze therapeutic effectiveness. (16)

Metabolic syndrome—Combination of atherosclerotic risk factors, including dyslipidemia, insulin resistance, obesity, and hypertension, that produces an increased risk for CAD. (20)

Metabolism—The sum of all physical and chemical changes that take place in the body; the two fundamental processes involved are anabolism and catabolism. (1, 6, 10)

Metastasis—The "seeding" of cancer cells to distant sites of the body; spread via blood or lymph vessels or by spilling into a body cavity. (23)

Methionine—Amino acid often lacking in legumes. (5)

Microalbuminuria—Small amounts of protein in the urine. Detected by a laboratory using methods more sensitive than traditional urinalysis. (19)

Microgram—One-millionth of a gram or one-thousandth of a milligram; abbreviated mcg or *u*. (7)

Micronize—To pulverize a substance into very tiny particles. (17)

Microvilli—Microscopic, hair-like rodlets (resembling bristles on a brush) covering the edge of each villus. (10)

Midarm circumference—Measure of the distance around the middle of the upper arm; used to assess body protein stores. (2)

Mildly obese—Twenty to 40 percent overweight; 120–140 percent healthy body weight. (18)

Milk-alkali syndrome—Condition characterized by high blood calcium and a more alkaline urine that predisposes to the precipitation of calcium in the kidney; caused by ingestion of excessive absorbable alkali and milk; associated with the milk and cream and antacid treatment of peptic ulcers used years ago. (8)

Milliequivalent—Unit of measure used for determining the concentration of electrolytes in solution; expressed as milliequivalents per liter; abbreviated mEq. (9)

Milling—The process of grinding grain into flour. (3)

Milliosmole—Unit of measure for osmotic activity. (9)

Mineral—An inorganic element or compound occurring in nature; in the body, some minerals help regulate bodily functions and are essential to good health. (8)

Mixed malnutrition—The result of a deficiency or excess of more than one nutrient. (15)

Moderately obese—Forty-one to 100 percent overweight; 141 to 200 percent healthy body weight. (18)

Modified diet—A term used in health-care institutions to mean the food served to a client has been altered or changed from that served to clients on regular diets, usually by physician order. (1)

Modular supplement—A nutritional supplement that contains a limited number of nutrients, usually only one. (15)

Mold—Any of a group of parasitic or other organisms living on decaying matter; fungi. (14)

Molecule—The smallest quantity into which a substance may be divided without loss of its characteristics. (3)

Monoamine oxidase inhibitor (MAO inhibitor)—A class of drugs that may have critical interactions with foods. (16, 17)

Monoglyceride—One fatty acid joined to a glycerol molecule. (4)

Monosaccharide—A simple sugar composed of one unit of $C_6H_{12}O_6$; examples include glucose, fructose, and galactose. (3)

Monounsaturated fat—A lipid in which the majority of fatty acids contain one carbon-to-carbon double bond. (4)

Morbidity—The state of being diseased; number of cases of disease in relation to population. (15)

Mortality—The death rate; number of deaths per unit of population. (13)

Motility—Power to move spontaneously. (13)

Mucosa—A mucous membrane that lines body cavities. (10)

Mucosal effect—Drug-induced changes within the intestine that affect the absorption of drugs or nutrients by damaging the tissues. (17)

Mucus—A thick fluid secreted by the mucous membranes and glands. (10)

Multiparous— Having borne more than one child. (11)

Muscular dystrophy—A disease characterized by wasting away of skeletal muscle with replacement of muscle cells by fat and connective tissue; most forms are genetic, but one form is associated with a vitamin E deficiency. (7)

Mutation—Permanent transmissible change in a gene; natural mutation produces evolutionary change in organisms; induced mutation results from exposure to environmental influences such as physical forces, chemicals, or biologic agents. (23)

Mycotoxin—A substance produced by mold growing in food that can cause illness or death when ingested by humans or animals. (14)

Myelin sheath—Fatty covering surrounding the long appendages of some nerves; serves to increase the transmission speed of impulses. (7)

Myocardial infarction (MI)—Area of dead heart muscle; usually the result of coronary occlusion. (20)

Myocardium—The heart muscle. (20)

Myoglobin—A protein located in muscle tissue that contains and stores oxygen. (8)

MyPyramid—USDA food guide balanced by healthy activity; food groups are grains, vegetables, fruits, oils, milk, meat and beans. (2)

Myxedema—A condition that occurs in older children and adults, resulting from hypofunction of the thyroid gland characterized by a drying and thickening of the skin and slowing of physical and mental activity. (8)

NANDA (originally North American Nursing Diagnosis Association)—An organization of nurses, established in 1973, that fosters the use of standard terminology in describing client problems; renamed to reflect global scope. (2)

Narcolepsy—A chronic condition consisting of recurrent attacks of drowsiness and sleep. (18)

Nasoduodenal tube (ND tube)—A tube inserted via the nose into the duodenum. (15)

Nasogastric tube (NG tube)—A tube inserted via the nose into the stomach. (15)

Nasojejunal tube (NJ tube)—A tube inserted via the nose into the jejunum. (15)

Neoplasm—A new and abnormal formation of tissue (tumor) that grows at the expense of the healthy organism. (23)

Nephritis—General term for inflammation of the kidneys. (21)

Nephron—The structural and functional unit of the kidney. (20)

Nephropathy—A kidney disease characterized by inflammation and degenerative lesions. (19)

Nephrosclerosis—A hardening of the renal arteries; may be caused by arteriosclerosis of the kidney arteries. (21)

Nephrotic syndrome—The end result of a variety of diseases that cause the abnormal passage of plasma proteins into the urine. (21)

Neuropathy—Any disease of the nerves. (19)

NHANES—National Health and Nutrition Examination Survey, a nationally representative cross-sectional survey of civilian noninstitutionalized population of the U.S.; conducted by the Centers for Disease Control's National Center for Health Statistics. (12)

Niacin—A B-vitamin that functions as a coenzyme in the production of energy from glucose; obtained from meat or produced from the amino acid tryptophan, present in milk, eggs, and meat; also called nicotinic acid. (7)

Niacin equivalent (NE)—Measure of niacin activity; equal to 1 milligram of preformed niacin or 60 milligrams of tryptophan. (7)

Night blindness—Vision that is slow to adapt to dim light; caused by vitamin A deficiency or hereditary factors or, in the elderly, by poor circulation. (7)

Nitrogen—Colorless, odorless, tasteless gas forming about 80 percent of the earth's air. (5)

Nitrogen balance—The difference between the amount of nitrogen ingested and that excreted each day; when intake is greater, a positive balance exists; when intake is less, a negative balance exists. (5)

Nitrogen-fixing bacteria—Organisms that absorb nitrogen from the air, which, upon the death of the bacteria, is released for legume plants to use in the anabolism of protein. (5)

Nomogram—A chart that shows a relationship between numerical values. (18)

Nonessential—In nutrition, refers to a chemical substance or nutrient the body normally can manufacture. (1)

Nonessential amino acid—Any amino acid that can normally be synthesized by the body in sufficient quantities. (5)

Nonheme iron—Iron that is not bound to hemoglobin or myoglobin; all the iron in plant sources. (8)

Non–insulin-dependent diabetes mellitus (NIDDM)—Type 2 diabetes; insulin resistance commonly occurs; although some persons with this disorder take insulin, it is not necessary for their long-term survival. (19, 20)

Norwalk virus—A causative organism that is responsible for more than 50 percent of the reported cases of epidemic viral gastroenteropathy. The incubation period ranges from 18 to 72 hours, and the outbreaks are usually self-limiting. Flu-like intestinal symptoms last for 24–48 hours. (14)

Nulliparous—Never having borne a child. (11)

Nursing action (intervention)—Specific care to be administered, including physical and psychological care, teaching, counseling, and referring. (2)

Nursing-bottle syndrome—A condition in which an infant has many dental caries caused by drinking milk or other sweet liquids during sleep. (3)

Nursing diagnosis—Statement of a client's nursing problem that the nurse is licensed to treat. (2)

Nursing process—Systematic and orderly method of delivering nursing care, composed of five steps: assessment, analysis, planning, implementation, and evaluation. (2)

Nutrient—Chemical substance supplied by food that the body needs for growth, maintenance, and/or repair. (1)

Nutrient density—The concentration of nutrients in a given volume of food compared with the food's kilocalorie content. (6)

Nutrition—The science of food and its relationship to living beings. (1)

Nutrition support service—A team service for clients on enteral and parenteral feedings that assesses, monitors, and counsels these clients. (15)

Nutritional assessment—The evaluation of a client's nutritional status based on a physical examination, anthropometric measurements, laboratory data, and food intake information. (2)

Nutritional status—Condition of the body as it relates to the intake and use of nutrients. (1)

Obese—Body fat content greater than 24 percent in males or 33 percent in females. (18)

Obesity—Excessive amount of fat on the body; obesity for women is a fat content greater than 33 percent; obesity for men is a fat content greater than 24 percent. (18)

Objective data—Findings verifiable by another through physical assessment or diagnostic tests, also termed signs. (2)

Obligatory excretion—Minimum amount of urine production necessary to keep waste products in solution, amounting to 400 to 600 milliliters per day. (9)

Oliguria—A decreased output of urine. (21)

Oncogene—Carcinogenic gene that stimulates excessive reproduction of the cell. (23)

Opportunistic infection—Infection caused by normally nonpathogenic organisms in a host with decreased resistance. (25)

Opsin—A protein that combines with vitamin A to form rhodopsin, a chemical in the retina necessary for vision. (7)

Optic nerve—The second cranial nerve, which transmits impulses for the sense of sight. (7)

Oral cavity—The cavity in the skull bounded by the mouth, palate, cheeks, and tongue. (10)

Organ—Somewhat independent body part having specific functions. Examples: stomach, liver. (10)

Orthostatic hypotension—A drop in blood pressure producing dizziness, fainting, or blurred vision when arising from a lying or sitting position or when standing motionless in a fixed position. (9)

Osmolality—Measure of osmotic pressure exerted by the number of dissolved particles per weight of liquid; clinically usually reported as mOsm/kg. (9)

Osmolarity—Measure of osmotic pressure exerted by the number of dissolved particles per volume of liquid; clinically usually reported as mOsm/L. (9)

Osmosis—The movement of water across a semipermeable cell membrane from an area with fewer particles to one with more particles. (9)

Osmotic pressure—The pressure that develops when a concentrated solution is separated from a less-concentrated solution by a semipermeable membrane. (9)

Osteoarthritis—Progressive deterioration of the cartilage in the joints; risk factors are aging, obesity, occupational or athletic abuse of joints, and trauma. (13)

Osteoblasts—Bone cells that build bone. (8)

Osteocalcin—Hormonally regulated calcium-binding protein made almost exclusively by the bone-building cells called osteoblasts; vitamin K facilitates synthesis of osteocalcin. (7)

Osteoclasts—Bone cells that break down bone. (8)

Osteodystrophy—Defective bone formation. (21)

Osteomalacia—Adult form of rickets. (7)

Osteopenia—Bone mineral density 1 to 2.5 standard deviations below the mean of healthy young adults. (8)

Osteoporosis—Bone mineral density more than 2.5 standard deviations below the mean of young adults. (8)

Ostomy—A surgically formed opening to permit passage of urine or bowel contents to the outside. (15)

Overnutrition—The result of an excess of one or more nutrients in the diet. (1)

Overweight—Ten to 20 percent above healthy body weight; 110–120 percent healthy body weight. (18)

Ovum—The egg cell that, after fertilization by a sperm cell, develops into a new individual. (11)

Oxalates—Salts of oxalic acid found in some plant foods; bind with the calcium in the plant, making it unavailable to the body. (8)

Oxidation—The process in which a substance is combined with oxygen. (7, 10)

Oxytocin—A hormone produced by the posterior pituitary gland in the brain; effects are uterine contractions and release of milk. (11)

Pancreas—An abdominal gland that secretes enzymes important in the digestion of carbohydrates, fats, and proteins; also secretes the hormones insulin and glucagon. (10, 22)

Pancreatic lipase—An enzyme produced by the pancreas; used in fat digestion. (10)

Pancreatitis—Inflammation of the pancreas. (22, 25)

Pantothenic acid—A B-complex vitamin found in almost all foods; deficiencies from lack of food have not been documented. (7)

Paralytic ileus—A temporary cessation of peristalsis that causes an intestinal obstruction. (24)

Paralytic shellfish poisoning—Disease caused by the consumption of poisonous clams, oysters, mussels, or scallops. (14)

Parasite—An organism that lives within, upon, or at the expense of a living host. (14)

Parathyroid hormone (PTH)—Hormone secreted by the parathyroid glands; regulates calcium and phosphorus metabolism in the body. (7, 8, 21)

Parenteral feeding—A feeding administered by any route other than the gastrointestinal tract. (15)

Parietal—Two bones that form the sides and roof of the skull; also two lobes of the cerebrum lying roughly under those bones. (16)

Parity—Condition of having carried a pregnancy to viability (20 weeks or 500-gram birth weight) regardless of whether resulted in a live birth; nulliparous—never carried a child to viability; multiparous—more than once. (13)

Parotid glands—One of the salivary glands of the mouth, located just below and in front of the ears; the mumps virus causes infectious parotitis. (10)

Pectin—Purified carbohydrate obtained from peel of citrus fruits or apple pulp; gels when cooked with sugar at correct pH to thicken jelly and jam; contained in mashed raw apple, applesauce, firm banana; recommended for diarrhea to contribute firmness to stools. (22)

Pellagra—Deficiency disease due to lack of niacin and tryptophan; characterized by the three Ds: dermatitis, diarrhea, and dementia. (7)

Pepsin—An enzyme secreted in the stomach that begins protein digestion. (10)

Pepsinogen—The antecedent of pepsin; activated by hydrochloric acid, a component of gastric juice. (10)

Peptidases—Enzymes that assist in the digestion of protein by reducing the smaller molecules to single amino acids. (10)

Peptide bond—Chemical bond that links two amino acids in a protein molecule. (5, 10)

Percutaneously—Affected through the skin. (15)

Perforated ulcer—Condition in which an ulcer penetrates completely through the stomach or intestinal wall, spilling the organ's contents into the peritoneal cavity. (22)

Periodontal disease—Disorder of the gingiva (gums) and the supporting structures of the teeth. (13)

Peripheral parenteral nutrition (PPN)—An intravenous feeding via a vein away from the center of the body. (15)

Peristalsis—A wave-like muscular movement that propels food along the alimentary canal. (10, 24)

Peritoneal dialysis—Method of removing waste products from the blood by injecting the flushing solution into a client's abdomen and using the client's peritoneum as the semipermeable membrane. (21)

Peritoneum—The membrane that covers the internal abdominal organs and lines the abdominal cavity. (21)

Peritonitis—Inflammation of the peritoneal cavity. (22)

Pernicious anemia—Inadequate red blood cell formation due to lack of intrinsic factor from the stomach, which is required for the absorption of vitamin B_{12}; leads to neural deterioration. (7)

Pesticides—A chemical used to kill insects or rodents. (14)

Petechiae—Pinpoint, flat, round, red lesions caused by intradermal or submucosal hemorrhage. (7)

pH—*Potential of Hydrogen*; a scale representing the relative acidity or alkalinity of a solution; a value of 7 is neutral, less than 7 is acidic, and greater than 7 is alkaline. (9)

Pharmacokinetics—The study of the action of drugs, emphasizing absorption time, duration of effect, distribution in the body, and method of excretion. (16)

Pharynx—The muscular passage between the oral cavity and the esophagus. (10)

Phenylalanine—Essential amino acid, which is indigestible if a person lacks a particular enzyme. Accumulation of phenylalanine in the blood can lead to mental retardation. (5)

Phenylketonuria (PKU)—Hereditary disease caused by the body's failure to convert phenylalanine to tyrosine because of a defective enzyme. (5)

Phospholipid—Diglyceride containing phosphorus; primary lipid constituent of cell membranes; examples include lecithin and myelin. (8)

Photosynthesis—Process by which plants containing chlorophyll are able to manufacture carbohydrates from carbon dioxide and water using the sun's energy. (3)

Phylloquinone—Vitamin K_1, found in foods. (7)

Phytic acid—A substance found in grains that forms an insoluble complex with calcium; phytates. (8)

Phytochemicals—Nonnutritive food components that provide medical or health benefits including the prevention or treatment of a disease. (1)

Phytonadione—Synthetic, water-soluble pharmaceutical form of vitamin K_1; can be administered orally or by injection. (7)

Pica—The craving to eat nonfood substances such as clay and starch. (11)

Pitting edema—Usually of the skin of the extremities; firm pressure by a finger produces an indentation that remains for 5 seconds. (9)

Placenta—The organ in the uterus through which the unborn child exchanges carbon dioxide for oxygen and wastes for nourishment; lay term is afterbirth. (11)

Plant sterols—Compounds, structurally similar to cholesterol, that in prescribed amounts interfere with the absorption of cholesterol and thus lower LDL-C levels; marketed as table spreads (butter substitutes) and salad dressings. (20)

Plasma—The liquid portion of the blood including the clotting elements. (9)

Plasma transferrin receptor—Measure of iron status; increases even in mild deficiency; unaffected by inflammation. (8)

Plumbism—Lead poisoning. (8)

Pneumocystis pneumonia—A type of lung infection frequently seen in AIDS patients; caused by the organism *Pneumocystis carinii.* (25)

Polycythemia—Increase in red blood cells (RBCs); may be physiologic due to demand for oxygen-carrying capacity or pathologic as in p. vera, a chronic, life-shortening disorder of unknown etiology involving hematologic stem cells. (8)

Polydipsia—Excessive thirst. (19)

Polymer—A natural or synthetic substance formed by combining two or more molecules of the same substance. (3)

Polypeptide—A chain of amino acids linked by peptide bonds that form proteins. (5, 10)

Polyphagia—Excessive appetite. (19)

Polysaccharide—Complex carbohydrates composed of many units of $C_6H_{12}O_6$ joined together; examples important in nutrition include starch, glycogen, and fiber. (3)

Polyunsaturated fat—A fat in which the majority of fatty acids contain more than one carbon-to-carbon double bond; intake is associated with a decreased risk of heart disease. (4, 20)

Polyuria—Excessive urination. (19)

Positive feedback cycle—Situation in which a condition provokes a response that worsens the condition. Example: low blood pressure due to a failing heart stimulates the kidney to save sodium and water. (20)

Postprandial—Following a meal. (22)

Potable water—Water that is safe for drinking, free of harmful substances. (11)

Potassium pump—Proteins located in cell membranes that provide an active transport mechanism to move potassium ions across a membrane to their area of greater concentration; moves potassium ions into the cells. (9)

Prebiotic—Nondigestible food ingredients that encourage the growth of favorable intestinal microorganisms. (16)

Precursor—A substance from which another substance is derived. (7)

Preeclampsia—Hypertension and proteinuria, appearing after the twentieth week of pregnancy. (11)

Preformed vitamin—A vitamin already in a complete state in ingested foods, as opposed to a provitamin, which requires conversion in the body to be in a complete state. (7)

Pressure ulcer—Tissue breakdown from external force impairing circulation. (13, 15)

Prevalence—The number of cases of a disease or condition present in a specified population at a given time. (18)

Primary malnutrition—A nutrient deficiency due to poor food choices or a lack of nutritious food to eat. (15)

Principle of complementarity—Combining incomplete-protein foods so that each supplies the amino acids lacking in the other. (5)

Prion—A proteinaceous infectious agent, extremely difficult to destroy; resistant to heat, pressure cooking, ultraviolet light, irradiation, bleach, formaldehyde, and weak acids; even autoclaving at 135 degrees for 18 minutes does not eliminate infectivity. (14)

Probiotic—Live microbial food supplements that improve the microbial balance of the intestine, mainly by reinforcing the intestinal mucosal barrier against harmful agents. (16)

Prognosis—Probable outcome of an illness based on client's condition and natural course of the disease. (25)

Promotion—The second step in a cell turning cancerous, through the action of environmental substances on the altered, initiated gene. (23)

Prostaglandins—Long-chain, unsaturated fatty acids mostly synthesized in the body from arachidonic acid; have hormone-like effects. (4)

Protein—Nutrient necessary for building body tissue; composed of carbon, hydrogen, oxygen, and nitrogen (and sometimes with sulfur, phosphorus, or iron); amino acids represent the basic structure of proteins. (5)

Protein binding sites—Various sites in the body tissues to which drugs may become attached, rendering the drug temporarily inactive. (17)

Proteinuria—Protein in the urine. (21)

Protein-calorie malnutrition (PCM)—Condition in which the person's diet lacks both protein and kilocalories. (5)

Prothrombin—A protein essential to the blood-clotting process; manufactured by the liver using vitamin K. (7)

Protocol—A description of steps to be followed when performing a procedure or providing care for a particular condition. (15)

Proto-oncogene—Gene that in the normal cell stimulates growth and maintenance; when mutated, becomes an oncogene. (23)

Provitamin—Inactive substance that the body converts to an active vitamin. (7)

Provitamin A—Carotenoids that are precursors of vitamin A, the most powerful of which is beta-carotene. (7)

Proximal convoluted tubule—The first segment of the renal tubule. (21)

Psychology—The science of mental processes and their effects on behavior. (18)

Psychosis—Severe mental disturbance with personality derangement and loss of contact with reality. (7)

Psychosocial development—The maturing of an individual in relationships with others and within himself or herself. (12)

Ptyalin—A salivary enzyme that breaks down starch and glycogen to maltose and a small amount of glucose; also known as salivary amylase. (10)

Puberty—The period of life at which the physical ability to reproduce is attained. (12)

Pulmonary—Concerning or involving the lungs. (24)

Pulmonary edema—The accumulation of fluid in the lungs. (20)

Pulse pressure—The difference between systolic and diastolic blood pressure; normally 30–40 mmHg; narrows in deficient fluid volume and widens in excess fluid volume. (9)

Purging—The intentional clearing of food out of the human body by vomiting and/or using enemas, laxatives, and/or diuretics. (18)

Purines—One of the end products of the digestion of some nitrogen-containing compounds. (21)

Pyelonephritis—An inflammation of the central portion of the kidney. (21)

Pyloric sphincter—The sphincter muscle guarding the opening between the stomach and small intestine. (10)

Pyridoxine—Pharmaceutical name for vitamin B_6. (7)

Pyruvate—An intermediate in the metabolism of energy nutrients. (10)

Quality assurance—A planned and systematic program for evaluating the quality and appropriateness of services rendered. (15)

Quetelet's Index—Body Mass Index. (2)

Radiologist—Physician with special training in diagnostic imaging and radiation treatments. (14)

Rancid—Having the rank smell and sour taste of stale fat or oil from decomposition. (1)

Rate—The speed or frequency of an event per unit of time. (18)

Rationale—Reason certain actions are likely to achieve a desired outcome; in nursing, ideally based on research indicating a nursing action was effective in similar circumstances. (2)

Rebound scurvy—Vitamin C deficiency produced in a person following cessation of megadosing due to a habitually lessened rate of absorption. (7)

Recessive trait—One that requires two recessive genes for the trait, one from each parent, for the trait to be expressed (to be manifested) in the individual. (22)

Recommended Dietary Allowance—Intake that meets the needs of 97–98 percent of the individuals in a life-stage and gender group; intended as a goal for daily intake by individuals, not for assessing adequacy of an individual's nutrient intake. (2)

Rectum—The lower part of the large intestine. (10)

Refeeding—The reintroduction of kilocalories and nutrients into a patient either orally or parenterally. (24)

Refeeding syndrome—A detrimental state that results when a previously severely malnourished person is reintroduced to food and/or nutrients and kilocalories improperly. (24)

Regurgitate—To cause to flow backward, as with an infant "spitting up." (15)

Relative risk—In epidemiological studies, the ratio of the frequency of a certain disorder in groups exposed and groups not exposed to a particular hereditary or environmental factor. (19)

Renal—Pertaining to the kidney. (9, 12, 21)

Renal corpuscle—Refers collectively to both Bowman's capsule and the glomerulus. (21)

Renal exchange lists—A specialized type of exchange list for clients with kidney disease who require restriction of one or more of the following: protein, sodium, phosphorus, and potassium. (21)

Renal osteodystrophy—Defective bone development caused by phosphorus retention, a low or normal serum calcium level, and increased parathyroid activity. (21)

Renal pelvis—A structure inside the kidney that receives urine from the collecting tubules. (21)

Renal threshold—The blood glucose level at which glucose begins to spill into the urine. (19)

Renal tubule—The second major portion of the nephron; appears rope-like. (21)

Renin—An enzyme produced by the kidney that catalyzes the conversion of angiotensinogen to angiotensin I. (9)

Rennin—An enzyme that coagulates milk. (10)

Reservoir—Place that an infectious agent normally lives and multiplies so that it can be transmitted to a susceptible host. (14)

Residue—Trace amount of any substance in a product at the time of sale; substance remaining in the bowel after absorption. (14, 22)

Respiration—The exchange of oxygen and carbon dioxide between a living organism and the environment. (24)

Respirator—A machine used to assist respiration. (24)

Respiratory acidosis—Blood pH less than 7.35 caused by pulmonary disease, characterized by a retention of carbon dioxide. (24)

Respiratory alkalosis—Blood pH greater than 7.45 caused by pulmonary disease, characterized by a loss of carbon dioxide. (24)

Resting energy expenditure (REE)—The amount of fuel the human body uses at rest for a specified period of time; often used interchangeably with basal metabolic rate (BMR). (6)

Retina—Inner lining of eyeball that contains light-sensitive nerve cells; corresponds to film in camera. (7)

Retinoic acid syndrome—Characteristic fetal deformities, including small ears or no ears, abnormal or missing ear canals, brain malformation, and heart defects caused by excessive preformed vitamin A or isotretinoin. (7, 11)

Retinol—One of the active forms of preformed vitamin A. (7)

Retinol equivalent (RE)—A measure of vitamin A activity that considers both preformed vitamin A (retinol) and its precursor (carotene); 1 RE equals 3.3 International Units from animal foods and 10 International Units from plant foods; 1 RE corresponds to 1 microgram of retinol. (7)

Retinopathy—Any disorder of the retina. (19)

Retrolental fibroplasia (RLF)—A disease of the vessels of the retina present in premature infants; often caused by exposure to high postnatal oxygen concentration. (12)

Rhodopsin—Light-sensitive protein in the retina that contains vitamin A; also called visual purple. (7)

Riboflavin—Coenzyme in the metabolism of protein; also called vitamin B_2. (7)

Ribonucleic acid (RNA)—A substance in the cell nucleus that controls protein synthesis in all living cells. (5)

Rickets—Disease caused by a deficiency of vitamin D that affects the young during the period of skeletal growth, resulting in bones that are abnormally shaped and weak. (7)

Ritter syndrome—An inflammatory skin disease seen in newborns, characterized by pustules that fill with a straw-colored fluid and become encrusted. (14)

Rooting reflex—The infant's natural response to a stroke on its cheek, which turns the head toward that side to nurse. (12)

Rotavirus—Most common cause of infectious enteritis in human infants; associated with about one-third of the cases of diarrhea requiring hospitalization in children younger than 5 years old. (12)

Roux-en-Y—A surgical connection between the distal end of the small bowel and another organ such as the stomach. (18)

Rugae—Folds of mucosa of organs such as the stomach. (10)

Salivary amylase—An enzyme that initiates the breakdown of starch in the mouth. (10)

Salivary glands—The glands that secrete saliva into the mouth. (10)

Salmonella—A genus of bacteria responsible for many cases of foodborne illness. (14)

Salmonellosis—A bacterial infection manifested by the sudden onset of headache, abdominal pain, diarrhea, nausea, and vomiting. Fever is almost always present. Contaminated food is the predominant method of transmission. (14)

Sarcoma—A malignant neoplasm that occurs in connective tissue such as muscle or bone. (23)

Satiety—The feeling after consuming food that enough has been eaten; the sensation of satisfaction. (3)

Saturated fat—A fat in which the majority of fatty acids contain no carbon-to-carbon double bonds. (4)

Scurvy—Disease due to deficiency of vitamin C marked by bleeding problems and, later, by bony skeleton changes. (7)

Seasonal variation—Refers to differences during spring, summer, fall, and winter. (1)

Sebaceous gland—Oil-secreting gland of the skin; most sebaceous glands have a hair follicle associated with them. (4)

Secondary diabetes—A World Health Organization (WHO) classification for diabetes when the hyperglycemia occurs as a result of another disorder. (19)

Secondary hypertension—High blood pressure that develops as the result of another condition. (20)

Secondary malnutrition—A nutrient deficiency due to improper absorption and distribution of nutrients. (15)

Secretin—A hormone that stimulates the production of bile by the liver and the secretion of sodium bicarbonate juice by the pancreas. (10)

Self-efficacy—One's belief in his or her ability to perform a task or behavior. (23)

Self-monitoring of blood glucose (SMBG)—A procedure that persons with diabetes follow to test their own blood glucose levels. (19)

Sensible water loss—Visible water loss through perspiration, urine, and feces. (9)

Sensitivity—Characteristic of diagnostic test; the proportion of people correctly identified as having the condition in question; a score of 100% would indicate that all the affected persons were identified by the test. (22)

Sepsis—A condition in which disease-producing organisms are present in the blood. (24)

Serosa—A serous membrane that covers internal organs and lines body cavities. (6)

Serotonin—A body chemical that assists the transmission of nerve impulses; it produces constriction of blood vessels and is thought to be related to sleep. (7, 18)

Serum—The liquid portion of the blood minus the clotting elements. (9)

Serum transferrin—Globulin in the blood that binds and transports iron; level increases in early iron deficiency, before hemoglobin and hematocrit readings drop. (8)

Severely obese—Greater than 100 percent overweight; also expressed as greater than 201 percent healthy body weight. (18)

Shelf life—The duration of time a product can remain in storage without deterioration. (4)

Shigella—Organisms causing intestinal disease; spread by fecal-oral transmission from a client or carrier via direct contact or indirectly by contaminated food. (14)

Shock—Acute peripheral circulatory failure due to loss of circulatory fluid or derangement of circulatory control producing decreased blood pressure, increased pulse rate; skin becomes cool and clammy from perspiration; urine output decreased. (9)

SIADH (Syndrome of Inappropriate Secretion of Antidiuretic Hormone)—Pathological excretion of ADH; result is dilutional hyponatremia. (9)

Signs—See Objective data. (2)

Simple carbohydrate—Composed of one or two units of $C_6H_{12}O_6$; includes the monosaccharides (glucose, fructose, and galactose) and the disaccharides (sucrose, lactose, and maltose). (3)

Simple fat—Lipids that consist of fatty acids or a simple filler such as a hydroxyl (OH) molecule joined to glycerol. (4)

Small for gestational age (SGA)—Infant weighing less at birth than considered normal for the calculated length of the pregnancy. (12)

Small intestine—The part of the alimentary canal between the stomach and the large intestine, where most absorption of nutrients occurs. (10)

Sodium pump—Proteins located in cell membranes that provide an active transport mechanism to move sodium ions across a membrane to their area of greater concentration; moves sodium ions out of the cells and water follows. (9)

Solubility—The ability of one substance to dissolve into another in solution. (3)

Soluble—Able to be dissolved. (3)

Solute—The substance that is dissolved in a solvent. (9)

Solvent—A liquid holding another substance in solution. (9)

Somatostatin—A hormone produced by the delta cells of the islets of Langerhans that inhibits both the release of insulin and the production of glucagon. (19)

Specific gravity—The weight of a substance compared to an equal volume of a standard substance; usual standard for liquids is water; its specific gravity set at 1.000. (17)

Specificity—Characteristic of diagnostic test; the proportion of people correctly identified as not having the condition in question; a score of 100 percent would indicate that all of the unaffected persons were identified by the test. (22)

Sphincter—A circular band of muscles that constricts a passage. (10)

Spina bifida—Congenital defect in spinal column whereby the vertebrae fail to close; clinical manifestations may or may not include protrusion of the meninges outside the spinal canal. (11)

Spore—A form assumed by some bacteria that is highly resistant to heat, drying, and chemicals. (12)

Sprue—Chronic form of malabsorption syndrome affecting the small intestine; subcategories: tropical and nontropical. (10, 22)

Staphylococcus aureus—One of the most common species of bacteria, which produces a poisonous toxin. The main reservoir is nose and throat discharge. Food can act as a vehicle for transmission, so proper hand washing is an essential means of control. (14)

Starches—Polysaccharides; many units of $C_6H_{12}O_6$ joined together; complex carbohydrates. (3)

Steatorrhea—The presence of greater than normal amounts of fat in the stool, producing foul-smelling, bulky excrement. (10, 22)

Sterol—Substance related to fats and belonging to the lipoids; for example, cholesterol. (4)

Stimulus control—The identification of cues that precede a behavior and rearranging daily activities to avoid such cues. (18)

Stoma—A surgically created opening in the abdominal wall. (22)

Stomach—The portion of the alimentary canal between the esophagus and small intestine. (10)

Stomatitis—An inflammation of the mouth. (17, 21)

Stress—Any threat to a person's mental or physical well-being. (24)

Stress factor—A number used to predict how much a client's kilocalorie need has increased as a result of a disease state. (24)

Subcutaneously—Beneath the skin. (19)

Subdural hematoma—Collection of blood under the outermost membrane covering the brain and spinal cord; usually resulting from head injury. (16)

Subjective data—Experiences the client reports, also termed symptoms. (2)

Submucosa—Structural layer of the alimentary canal below the mucosa; contains tissues and blood vessels. (10)

Sucrase—An enzyme in the intestinal mucosa that splits sucrose into glucose and fructose. (10)

Sucrose—A disaccharide; one unit of glucose and one unit of fructose joined together; ordinary white table sugar. (3)

Superior vena cava—One of the largest diameter veins in the human body; used to deliver total parenteral nutrition. (15)

Symptoms—See Subjective data. (2)

System—An organized grouping of related structures or parts. (10)

Systolic pressure—Pressure exerted against the arteries when the heart contracts; the upper number of the blood pressure reading. (9, 20)

T-lymphocytes (T-cells)—White blood cells that recognize and fight foreign cells such as cancer; thymic lymphocytes. (23)

Tapeworm—A parasitic intestinal worm that is acquired by humans through the ingestion of raw seafood or undercooked beef or pork. (14)

Tardive dyskinesia—Neurological syndrome involving involuntary, slow, rhythmic, movements often seen in the mouth and tongue; side effect of psychotropic drugs, especially phenothiazines. (7)

Target heart rate—Seventy percent of maximum heart rate (number of heartbeats per minute); a person's target heart rate can be objectively determined by a stress test. Individuals can estimate their target heart rate by subtracting their age from 220 and multiplying the difference by 70 percent. A person's target heart rate is the rate at which the pulse should be maintained for at least 20 minutes during aerobic exercise. (6)

Teratogenic—Capable of causing abnormal development of the embryo; results in a malformed fetus. (11)

Term infant—One born between the beginning of the 38th week through the 42nd week of gestation. (12)

Tetany—Muscle contractions, especially of the wrists and ankles, resulting from low levels of ionized calcium in the blood; causes include parathyroid deficiency, vitamin D deficiency, and alkalosis. (7)

Therapeutic index—Maximum tolerated dose of a drug divided by the minimum curative dose; a narrow index indicates greater potential for adverse side effects. (17)

Thermic effect of exercise (TEE)—The number of kilocalories used above resting energy expenditure as a result of physical activity. (6)

Thermic effect of foods (diet-induced thermogenesis, specific-dynamic action)—The energy cost to extract and utilize the kilocalories and nutrients in foods; the heat produced after eating a meal. (6)

Thiamin—Coenzyme in the metabolism of carbohydrates and fats; vitamin B_1. (7)

Thiaminase—An enzyme in raw fish that destroys thiamin. (7)

Third-space losses—Sequestering of fluid in body cavities such as the chest and abdomen; in the abdominal cavity, it produces ascites. (9)

Thoracic—Pertaining to the chest, or thorax. (10)

Thoracic duct—Major lymphatic vessel draining all except the right upper half of the body; empties into left internal jugular and left subclavian veins. (9)

Threonine—Essential amino acid often lacking in grains. (5)

Thrombus—A blood clot that obstructs a blood vessel; obstruction of a vessel of the brain or heart is among the most serious effects. (20)

Thrush—An infection caused by the organism *Candida albicans;* characterized by the formation of white patches and ulcers in the mouth and throat. (25)

Thymus—Gland in the chest, above and in front of the heart, that contributes to the immune response, including the maturation of T-lymphocytes. (23)

Thyroid-stimulating hormone (TSH)—A hormone secreted by the pituitary gland that stimulates the thyroid gland to secrete thyroxine and triiodothyronine; thyrotropin. (8)

Thyrotropin-releasing factor (TRF)—Stimulates the secretion of thyroid-stimulating hormone; produced in the hypothalamus. (8)

Thyroxine (T4)—A hormone secreted by the thyroid gland; increases the rate of metabolism and energy production. (8)

Tissue—A group or collection of similar cells and their similar intercellular substance that acts together in the performance of a particular function. (5)

Tolerable Upper Intake Level (UL)—Highest average daily intake by an individual that is unlikely to pose risks of adverse health effects in 97–98 percent of individuals in specified life-stage and gender group; ordinarily refers to intake from food, fortified food, water, and supplements. (2)

Tolerance level—The highest dose at which a residue causes no ill effects in laboratory animals. (14)

Total parenteral nutrition (TPN)—An intravenous feeding that provides all nutrients known to be required. (15)

Trace minerals—Those present in the body in amounts less than 5 grams; daily intake of less than 100 milligrams needed; also called microminerals or trace elements. (8)

Traction—The process of using weights to draw a part of the body into alignment. (15)

Transcellular fluid—Located in body cavities and spaces; constantly being secreted and absorbed; examples: cerebrospinal fluid, pericardial fluid, pleural fluid. (9)

Transferrin—Protein in the blood that binds and transports iron. (8)

Trauma—A physical injury or wound caused by an external force; an emotional or psychological shock that usually results in disordered behavior. (24)

Triceps skinfold—Measure of skin and subcutaneous tissue over the triceps muscle in the upper arm; used in body fat assessment. (2)

Trichinella spiralis—A worm-like parasite that becomes embedded in the muscle tissue of pork. (14)

Trichinosis—The infestation of *Trichinella spiralis,* a parasitic roundworm, transmitted by eating raw or insufficiently cooked pork. (14)

Triglyceride—Three fatty acids joined to a glycerol molecule. (4)

Triiodothyronine (T3)—A hormone secreted by the thyroid gland that increases the rate of metabolism and energy production. (8)

Trousseau's sign—Spasms of the forearm and hand upon inflation of the blood pressure cuff; sign of tetany or lack of ionized calcium in the blood. (8)

Trust—First stage of Erikson's theory of psychosocial development, in which the infant learns to rely on those caring for it. (12)

Trypsin—An enzyme formed in the intestine that assists in protein digestion. (10)

Tryptophan—An essential amino acid, often lacking in legumes; serves as provitamin for the production of niacin by the liver. (7)

Tubular reabsorption—The movement of fluid back into the blood from the renal tubule. (19)

Tubule—A small tube or canal. (21)

Tumor suppressor gene—Gene that inhibits growth and division of the cell. (23)

Turgor—Resilience of skin; when pinched, quickly returns to original shape in well-hydrated young person; test for deficient fluid volume that is not reliable for elderly clients. (9)

Type 1 diabetes—Persons with this disorder must take insulin to survive and are prone to ketoacidosis; also called insulin-dependent diabetes mellitus (IDDM), type II diabetes, and juvenile diabetes. (19)

Type 2 diabetes—Although some persons with this disorder take insulin, it is not necessary for their survival; also called non–insulin-dependent diabetes (NIDDM) and adult-onset diabetes mellitus. (19)

Tyramine—A monoamine present in various foods that will provoke a hypertensive crisis in persons taking monoamine oxidase (MAO) inhibitors. (17)

Ulcer—An open sore or lesion of the skin or mucous membrane. (22)

Ulcerative colitis—Inflammatory disease of the large intestine that usually begins in the rectum and spreads upward in a continuous pattern. (22)

Ultrasound bone densitometer—Machine that uses sound waves to estimate bone density as a screening test. (2)

Uncomplicated starvation—A food deprivation without an underlying stress state. (24)

Undernutrition—The state that results from a deficiency of one or more nutrients. (1)

Underwater weighing—Most accurate measure of body fatness. (2)

Universal precautions—A list of procedures developed by the Centers for Disease Control for when blood and certain other body fluids should be considered contaminated and treated as such. (25)

Unsaturated fat—A fat in which the majority of fatty acids contain one or more carbon-to-carbon double bonds. (9)

Urea—The chief nitrogenous constituent of urine; the final product, along with CO_2, of protein metabolism. (10)

Uremia—A toxic condition produced by the retention of nitrogen-containing substances normally excreted by the kidneys. (21)

Ureter—The tube that carries urine from the kidney to the bladder. (21)

Urinary calculus—A kidney stone, or deposit of mineral salts. (21)

Urinary tract infection (UTI)—The condition in which disease-producing microorganisms invade a client's bladder, ureter, or urethra. (21)

USDA Dietary Guidelines—Guidelines for health promotion issued by the U.S. Departments of Agriculture and Health and Human Services; revised in 2005. (2)

Usual food intake—A description of what a person habitually eats. (2)

Vaginitis—Inflammation of the vagina, most often caused by an infectious agent. (19)

Vasopressin—Antidiuretic hormone; abbreviated ADH. (9)

Ventilation—Process by which gases are moved into and out of the lungs; two aspects of ventilation are inhalation and exhalation. (24)

Very-low-calorie diet (VLCD)—Diet that contains less than 800 kilocalories per day. (18)

Very-low-density lipoprotein (VLDL)—A plasma protein containing mostly triglycerides with small amounts of cholesterol, phospholipid, and protein; transports triglycerides from the liver to tissues. (20)

Villi—Multiple minute projections on the surface of the folds of the small intestine that absorb fluid and nutrients; plural of villus. (10)

Virus—Very small noncellular parasite that is entirely dependent on the nutrients inside host cells for its metabolic and reproductive needs. (14)

Visible fat—Dietary fat that can be easily seen, such as the fat on meat or in oil. (4)

Vitamin—Organic substance needed by the body in very small amounts; yields no energy and does not become part of the body's structure. (7)

Waist-to-Hip Ratio (WHR)—Waist measurement divided by hip measurement; if >0.8 in women or >0.95 in men, indicates increased risk of health problems related to obesity. (2)

Warfarin—Anticoagulant that interferes with the liver's synthesis of vitamin K–dependent clotting factors II, VII, IX, and X. (7)

Water intoxication—Excess intake or abnormal retention of water. (9)

Weight cycling—The repeated gain and loss of body weight. (18)

Wernicke-Korsakoff syndrome—A disorder of the central nervous system resulting from thiamine deletion; often seen in chronic alcoholism; signs and symptoms include motor, sensory, and memory deficits. (7, 22)

Wernicke's encephalopathy—Inflammatory, hemorrhagic, degenerative lesions in several areas of the brain resulting in double vision, involuntary eye movements, lack of muscle cordination, and mental deficits; caused by thiamin deficiency, often seen in chronic alcoholism but also in gastrointestinal tract disease and hyperemesis gravidarum. (7)

Whey—Component of milk; in human milk, contains soluble proteins that are easily digested; major whey protein in breast milk is alpha-lactalbumin, with an amino acid pattern much like that of the body tissues. (12)

Wilson's disease—Rare genetic defect of copper metabolism. (8, 17)

Women, Infants, and Children (WIC)—Federal program providing nutrition education and supplemental food to low-income pregnant or breast-feeding women and children up to 5 years of age. (12)

Xerophthalmia—Drying and thickening of the epithelial tissues of the eye; can be caused by vitamin A deficiency. (7)

Xerostomia—Dry mouth caused by decreased salivary secretions. (13)

Yo-yo effect—The repeated loss and gain of body weight. (18)

Zoochemical—Physiologically active ingredient in animals. (1)

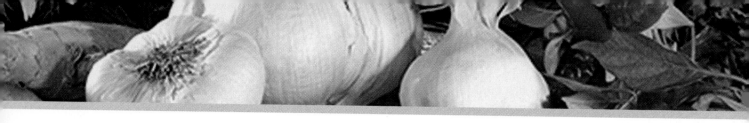

Index

Soy isoflavones, cancer risk and, 511
Soy protein, cardiovascular disease and, 436, 437
Soy protein formulas, 230
Specific gravity, 172
Specificity, 491
Sphincter(s)
  in alimentary canal, 181
  cardiac, 183
    achalasia in, 475
  pyloric, 184
Spina bifida, 203
Spores, botulism, in honey, 225
Sprue
  malabsorption in, 483, 484
  nontropical, 190–191
Stanols, plant, 64
Staphylococcus aureus food intoxication, 288
  food vehicles for, 288
  preventing, food-handling tips for, 292
  symptoms of, 288
Starch(es), 43–44
  consistency modifications of, 307
  food sources of, 47
  production of, 41
Starvation, stress of, 530–536
Stavudine, for AIDS, 550
Steatorrhea, 190
  in celiac disease, 484
Sterols, 53, 58
  plant, 64
Stevia, 43
Stimulus control, in behavior modification for weight control, 386
Stoma, 485
Stomach
  digestive functions of, 183–185
  disorders of, 477–481
  irritation of, drugs causing, 353–354
Stomatitis
  from antineoplastic drugs, 353
  in renal failure, 457
  in terminally ill, 563
Stones, kidney, 464, 466–467
Stress
  mental, nutrition and, 529–530
  nutrition during, 529–544
  of starvation, 530–536
Stress factor, in determining kilocalorie needs, 535
Stress response, 534–533
Stroke *See* Cerebrovascular accident (CVA)
  heat, 170
Structure/function claim, on food label, 292
Subcutaneous administration, of insulin, 404
Subdural hematoma, from ginkgo, 333
Subjective data, in assessment, 14, 16
Sucralose, 43
Sucrase, in digestion of carbohydrates, 185
Sucrose, 42
Sugar alcohols, 43
Sugars, food sources of, 46–47
Sulfasalazine, reduced folic acid absorption and, 355
Sulfonylureas, in diabetes management, 405
Sulfur, 135, 136
Sunlight, vitamin D from, 103
Superior vena cava, for total parenteral nutrition, 317

Supplemental feedings, 310–311
Supplements
  mineral. *See* Minerals, supplemental
  for vegetarian diets, 80
  vitamin. *See* Vitamin(s), supplemental
  vitamin D, 103
Surgery
  as hypermetabolic condition, 535
  for inflammatory bowel disease, 485–486
  for peptic ulcer, 480
  weight-loss, 387
Surgical clients, dietary considerations with, 471–475
Survival rates, for cancer, 503–504
Survival skills, in diabetes management, 407
Swallowing, difficult, nutritional interventions for, 520
Sweat, evaporation of, water loss by, 168
Sweeteners
  artificial, 43
  intense, 43
Sweets, consistency modifications of, 307
Swordfish, avoidance of, in pregnancy, 210
Symptoms, in assessment, 14
Syncope, heat, 169
Syndrome of inappropriate secretion of antidiuretic hormone (SIADH), 165
Systems, biological, 182
Systolic pressure, 163, 425

T

Tanacetum parthenium, 332, 335
Tannates, iron absorption and, 139
Tapeworms, 290
Tardive dyskinesia, pyridoxine for, 119
Taste
  alterations in
    in cancer, 518
      nutritional interventions for, 520
    in terminally ill, 561
  drugs affecting, 353
Taste receptors, in older adulthood, 264
TB (tuberculosis), in AIDS, 548
TCA (tricarboxylic acid) cycle, in catabolic reactions, 193–194, 195
Teacher, as nursing role, 5
TEF (thermic effect of food), 88–89
Temperature, of food, high, cancer risk and, 508
Teratogenic chemicals, 216
Teratogenicity, of hypoglycemia, 398
Terminal illness. *See also* Death
  case study on, 566
  dying process in, 557–559
  ethical and legal considerations in, 563–565
  nutritional assessment in, 560–563
  nutritional care in, 557–572
  nutrition screening in, 559–560
  palliative care in, 559
  symptom control in, dietary, 560–563
Tetany
  calcium deficiency and, 130–132
  vitamin D deficiency and, 102–103
Tetracycline, iron-containing foods and, 360
Therapeutic index, 363
Thermic effect
  of exercise, 89
  of food (TEF), 88–89

Thiamin (vitamin B$_1$), 106, 109–110, 116
  deficiency of, in alcoholism, 489
  dietary reference intakes for, in pregnancy and lactation, 205
  food sources of, by food groups, 117
  stability of, factors affecting, 107
  thiaminase, 110
Third-space losses, 173
Thirst, mechanism of, 164
Thoracic lymphatic duct, in absorption, 188
Threonine, 72
Throat disorders, 475
Thrombus, in coronary heart disease, 426
Thrush, in AIDS, 548
Thymus, t-lymphocytes maturing in, 519
Tilefish, avoidance of, in pregnancy, 210
Tissue(s)
  adipose, 53
  depletion of nutrients in, drugs and, 357
  fetal, protein needs for, 202
  growth and maintenance of, nutrition for, 6–7
  scar, protein in, 69
T-lymphocytes, in immune response, 519
Tobacco. *See* Smoking
  avoidance of, in pregnancy, 210
Toddlers
  diet of, quality of, 244
  inadequate fat intake in, 244
  iron-deficiency anemia in, 244
  mealtimes for, 243
  nutrition fundamentals for, 242–244
  nutrition of, 241–244
  physical growth and development of, 241–242
  psychosocial development of, 241
Tolerable upper intake level (UL), *See also specific nutrient, e.g. Iron*
  of calcium, 126
  for copper, 147
  in Dietary Reference Intakes, 28
  for iodine, 143
  for manganese, 148
  for zinc, 146
Tolerance level, for pesticide residues in foods, 297
Tongue, in older adulthood, 264
Total parenteral nutrition (TPN), 316, 317–319
  in cancer management, 521
  drug interactions with, preventing, 365
  home, 319
  indications for, 317
  monitoring of, 318, 319
  pantothenic acid and biotin deficiency in, 115
  PIC line for, 316, 317–319
  solutions for
    calculation of, 536
    energy nutrient content of, calculation of, 318
    kilocalories in, calculation of, 317
  transition and combination feedings in, 318–319
Toxic chemicals, maternal exposure to, as contraindication to breast-feeding, 216
Toxic plants, as botanical remedies, 336
Toxic seafood, 291
Toxoplasmosis, congenital, prevention of, 210
TPN. *See* Total parenteral nutrition (TPN)
Trace minerals, 137–151. *See also specific trace mineral, e.g.* Iron